Clinical Perio-dontology

Jan Lindhe

Textbook of Clinical Periodontology

2nd edition

Munksgaard

Textbook of Clinical Periodontology

2nd edition, 1st printing

Cover by Lars Thorsen
Typesetting and composition by Jens Lund Kirkegaard
Printed in Denmark 1989 by P.J. Schmidt, Vojens

ISBN 87-16-06453-4

List of Contributors

Ainamo, Jukka, LDS, O.D.,
Professor and Chairman
Department of Periodontology
School of Dentistry
University of Helsinki
Finland

Bergenholtz, Gunnar, LDS, O.D.,
Professor and Chairman
Department of Oral Diagnosis
School of Dentistry
University of Gothenburg
Sweden

Carlsson, Jan, LDS, O.D.,
Professor and Chairman
Department of Oral Microbiology
School of Dentistry
University of Umeå
Sweden

Ericsson, Ingvar, LDS, O.D.,
Associate Professor
Department of Periodontology
School of Dentistry
University of Gothenburg
Sweden

Evers, Hans, LDS,
ASTRA
Södertälje
Sweden

Frandsen, Asger, LDS, Dr.Odont.,
Professor and Chairman
Department of Periodontology
Royal Dental College
University of Copenhagen
Denmark

Glantz, Per-Olof, LDS, O.D.,
Professor and Chairman
Department of Prosthetic Dentistry
School of Dentistry
University of Lund
Sweden

Hamp, Sven-Erik, LDS, O.D.,
Associate Professor and Chairman
Specialist Dental Services
Linköping
Sweden

Heijl, Lars, LDS, O.D.,
Associate Professor
Department of Periodontology
School of Dentistry
University of Gothenburg
Sweden

Karring, Thorkild, LDS, Dr. Odont.,
Professor
Royal Dental College
University of Aarhus
Denmark

Kristoffersen, Tore, LDS, Dr. Odont.,MS,
Professor and Chairman
Department of Periodontology
School of Dentistry
University of Bergen
Norway

Lang, Niklaus P., DDS, DMD, MS, PhD,
Professor and Chairman
Department of Comprehensive Dental Care
School of Dental Medicine
University of Berne
Switzerland

Lie, Tryggve, LDS, Dr. Odont.,
Professor
Department of Periodontology
School of Dentistry
University of Bergen
Norway

Lindhe, Jan, LDS, O.D., DMD, MD(hc),
Professor and Chairman
Department of Periodontology
School of Dentistry
University of Gothenburg
Sweden

Meyer, Knut, LDS,
Assistant Professor
Department of Periodontology
School of Dentistry
University of Bergen
Norway

Nyman, Sture, LDS, O.D., MD(hc),
Associate Professor Emeritus
Department of Periodontology
School of Dentistry
University of Gothenburg
Sweden

Pindborg, Jens J., LDS, Dr. Odont.,
Professor and Chairman
Department of Oral Pathology
Royal Dental College
University of Copenhagen
Denmark

Rosling, Bengt, LDS, O.D.,
Associate Professor
Department of Periodontology
School of Dentistry
University of Gothenburg
Sweden

Rylander, Harald, LDS, O.D.,
Associate Professor
Department of Periodontology
School of Dentistry
University of Gothenburg
Sweden

Seibert, Jay, DMD,
Professor
Department of Periodontology
School of Dental Medicine
University of Pennsylvania
USA

Slots, Jörgen, LDS, Dr. Odont.,
Professor
Department of Periodontology
School of Dental Medicine
University of Pennsylvania
USA

Taichman, Norton, DMD,
Professor and Chairman
Department of Pathology
School of Dental Medicine
University of Pennsylvania
USA

Theilade, Jørgen, DDS, BScD, MS,
and Subdean Professor
Department of Periodontology and
Public Health
Faculty of Dentistry
University of Hong Kong
Hong Kong

Thilander, Birgit, LDS, O.D.,
Professor and Chairman
Department of Ortodontics
School of Dentistry
University of Gothenburg
Sweden

Wennström, Jan, LDS, O.D.,
Associate Professor
Department of Periodontology
School of Dentistry
University of Gothenburg
Sweden

Illustrations:
Berglundh, Tord, LDS
Research Associate
Department of Periodontology
School of Dentistry
University of Gothenburg
Sweden

Acknowledgement

In the preparation of this edition of **Textbook of Clinical Periodontology** illustration material has kindly been placed at our disposal by a number of distinguished research workers and clinicians. In some chapters reference to the original contribution has been made in the legends. It is a pleasure for me to acknowledge these contributors as well as the contributions of the following scientists:

B. Bergman, Anna-Lisa Björn, J. Egelberg, P.A. Knudsen, M. Listgarten, D. Lundgren, S.W. Meitner, P. Milleding, B. Moskow, R. Page, A.M. Polson, H.E. Schroeder, K.A. Selvig, E. Strandman, R.E. Walton, Jytte Westergaard, Jens Waerhaug, H.A. Zander.

Foreword 1st Edition

Upon reading this book - and as I sit down pen in hand, to introduce the reader to this text on Periodontology - I become literally overwhelmed by the memory of Dr. Jens Waerhaug, the father of modern periodontology, my tutor and friend. Thus, this could easily become an emotional outlet for personal affection and devotion on the part of his first student; feelings which in thereserved climate of Scandinavian collegiality were never adequately expres while he was alive. Byt it will not. The man, the friend, had passed on, but the scientist, the revolutionary, the genius is very much alive in every chapter of this treatise on periodontal diseases and their treatment and prevention.

It all began with the publishing og Jens Waerhaug's dissertation "*The Gingival Pocket*" in 1952, through which he laid the intellectual foundation for an entirely new era in periodontology. This was followed by a rapid succession of experiments, designed to answer questions one by one, reflecting a delightfully imaginative mind and profound clinical perception. In this way, step by step, he unveiled the mysteries surrounding periodontal diseases.

The reaction was - reactionary, especially among authoritarians. To other of us, the novelty of the dynamic approach to the experiments and the clarity of the clinical trials opened a lage window on to a realm never heretofore seen. The Scandinavian school of periodontal research was born.

Some 30 years have elapsed, but as this text bears forceful witness to, the torch has been passed on.

The reader will find that this book is somewhat traditional in its infrastructure and layout. Its uniqueness lies in the consistency of the basic paradigm from one chapter to the next and in the weight of scientific evidence brought to bear. This book affords both an intelligent synthesis and an excellent overview of the progress in the science and practicalities of modern periodontology and brings together a large amount of current experimental data compiled by the editor and the authors themselves in the context of their own clinical experience.

The problem of periodontal diseases and their clinical management are not solved. However, the authors are all committed to the idea that at the present stage of development, there is enough knowledge to formulate clinical concepts for the practical man agement of these diseases. The strong message that emerges is that, although the technology may not be ideal, periodontal diseases can today be prevented and treated.

At a time of an information explosion in dental literature, this text is a most refreshing example of how scientific advances can be communicated for the clinician's comprehension and use.

The style is bold without being reckless; it is provocative without being presumptuous. The word "proper" is used profusely throughout the chapters. They still make proper reading, and I propose to recommend this book for general practitioners and specialists, students and teachers, clinicians and scientists, and for anyone else interested in the transfer of basic and clinical science to patient management in periodontal diseases.

Harald Löe, D.D.S., Dr. Odont., Director, National institute of Dental Research, National Institutes of Health, Bethesda, Maryland 20205, U.S.A

March 1983

Preface 1st Edition

This **Textbook of Clinical Periodontology** was prepared with the needs of undergraduated and gratuate students of dentistry in mind. It is our hope, however, that the text may be of interrest and use also to general practitioners and dentists with a special interrest in periodontology.

This book is devided into tow parts. The first part deals with the biology of the periodontal tissues and the epidemiology, etiology and pathogenesis of periodontal disease. Special emphasis has been given to bacterial plaque as the main etiologicval factor in periodontal disease and to the pathogenesis of various forms of plaque associated periodontal disorders. In two separate chapters material is presented illustrating how systemic disorders may influence periodontal disease and how the periodontal tissues may become the seat of tumors of both benign and malignant character.

The second part of the book deals with the clinical management of periodontal disease; examination procedures, diagnosis, treatment planning, treatment and maintenance therapy. It was our intention to create en analytical and critical text describing the present state of clinical periodontology. Particular efforts have been made to distinguish between facts obtained from pertinent research and unsubstantiated assumptions regarding the effect of different treatment procedures often utilized in periodontal therapy.

Textbook of Clinical Periodontology is the result of the inspiring collaboration, loyalty and never failing efferts of many past and present members and close friends of the staff of the Department of Periodontology, School of Dentistry, University of Gothenburg, Sweden. During various periods of time we have had the privilege of the cooperation of research workers and clinicians from all over the world. I would not like to complete this preface without expressing our sincere appreciation to Drs. Hilding Björn (University of Lund), Harald Löe (NIDR, Bethesda), Helmut Zander (Eastman Dental Center, Rochester), Hubert Schroeder (University of Zurich), Sigmund Socransky (Forsyth Dental Center, Boston), Max Listgarten (University of Pennsylvania) and Roy Page (University of Washington) for introdicing us to and guiding our work in different fields of periodontal research.

We should also like to express our sincere gratitude to Dr. Tord Berglundh who was responsible not only for editing the photographical material but also for producing most of the drawings and schematic illustrations included in the various chapters of this book.

Last but not least it is a privilege to thank the publisher and the editional and technical staff of Munksgaard International Publishers for their generosity and their skill in handling the printing and reproduction of our material.

The text was completed in the early Fall of 1982. Research findings published in the literature since then have added to our knowledge and understanding of periodontal disease but have not, in any significant way, altered or invalidated the conclusions made in the various chapters of this book.

Gothenburg, March 1983

Jan Lindhe

Preface 2nd Edition

It is with great pleasure and pride we present the second and revised edition of **Textbook of Clinical Periodontology**. In the five years that have elapsed since the publishing of the first edition of this text many advances have occurred in *Periodontology*. Both basic science and clinical research have provided information that have enabled the clinician to better understand the function of the normal periodontium, the etiology of various diseases in the periodontium, pathogenic mechanisms through which the periodontal tissues may be destroyed and through which the function of the periodontium may be jeopardized. New therapeutic procedures have been introduced and their efficacy tested in clinican trials.

Much of this new material has been incorporated in this revised edition of **Textbook of Clinical Periodontology**. Several chapters have been added and several new authors have made important contributions. No doubt the efforts of this team of authors have improved the quality of **Textbook of Clinical Periodontology**.

This textbook is intended for undergraduate and graduate students of dentistry as well as for practicing dentists.

The text was completed in the spring of 1988. Findings published since then have added to our knowledge of periodontal disease, but not altered or invalidated the conclusions made in the various chapters of this book.

Gothenburg, February 1989

Jan Lindhe

Contents

CHAPTER 1

The Anatomy of the Periodontium

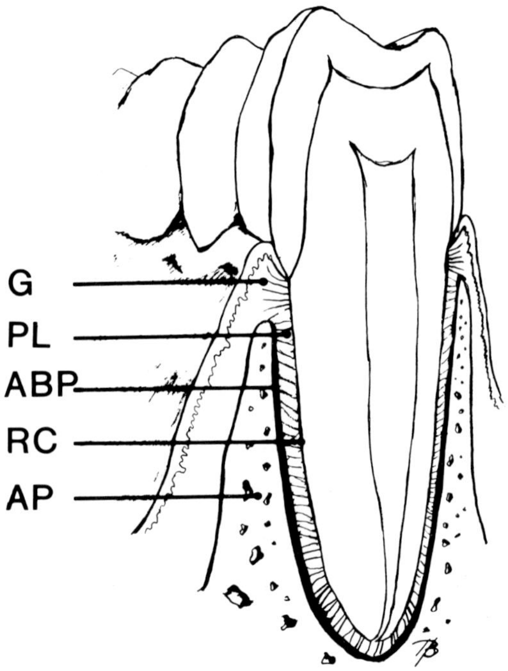

Fig. 1-1 is a schematic drawing of the tooth with its periodontium: the gingiva (G), the periodontal ligament (PL), the root cementum (RC) and the alveolar bone (i.e. the alveolar bone proper (ABP) and the alveolar process (AP)).

This chapter includes a brief description of the characteristics of the normal periodontium. It is assumed that the reader has prior knowledge of oral embryology and histology.

The periodontium (peri = around, odontos = tooth) comprises the following tissues: the *gingiva*, the *periodontal ligament*, the *root cementum* and the *alveolar bone*. The alveolar bone consists of two components, the *alveolar bone proper* and the *alveolar process*. The alveolar bone proper is continuous with the alveolar process and forms the thin bone plate that is located immediately lateral to the periodontal ligament. Three of the periodontal tissues, i.e. the cementum, the periodontal ligament and the alveolar bone proper, are formed by cells which are contained in the dental follicle of the developing tooth. The fourth tissue component of the periodontum, i.e. the gingiva, is not derived from the dental follicle. The gingiva is, however, a tooth-related structure which grows in height with the erupting tooth.

The main function of the periodontum is to attach the tooth to the bone tissue of the jaws and to maintain the integrity of the surface of the masticatory mucosa of the oral cavity. The periodontum, also called "the attachment apparatus" or "the supporting tissues of the teeth" establishes a developmental, biological and functional unit which undergoes certain changes with age and is, in addition, subjected to morphological and functional alterations as well as to changes related to alterations in the oral environment.

The gingiva

Macroscopic anatomy

The oral mucosa (mucous membrane) is continuous with the skin of the lips and the mucosa of the soft palate and pharynx. The oral mucous membrane consists of (1) the *masticatory mucosa* which includes the gingiva and the covering of the hard palate, (2) the *specialized mucosa* which covers the dorsum of the tongue and (3) the remaining part, called the *lining mucosa*.

Fig. 1-2. *The gingiva* is that part of the *masticatory* mucosa which covers the alveolar process and surrounds the cervical portion of the teeth. The gingiva obtains its final shape and texture in conjunction with eruption of the teeth.

In coronal direction the coral pink gingiva terminates in the *free gingival margin* which has a scalloped outline. In apical direction the gingiva is continuous with the loose, darker red *alveolar mucosa* (lining mucosa) from which the gingiva is separated by a, usually, easily recognizable borderline called either the *mucogingival junction* (arrows) or the *mucogingival line*.

Fig. 1-3. There is no mucogingival line present in the palate since the hard palate and the maxillary alveolar process are covered by the same type of masticatory mucosa.

Fig. 1-4. Two parts of the gingiva can be differentiated:

1) the *free gingiva* (FG)
2) the *attached gingiva* (AG)

The *free gingiva* is coral pink, has a dull surface and firm consistency, and comprises the gingival tissue at the vestibular and lingual/palatal aspects of the teeth, and the *interdental gingiva* or the *interdental papillae*. On the vestibular and lingual side of the teeth, the free gingiva extends from the gingival margin in apical direction to the *free gingival groove* which is positioned at a level corresponding to the level of the *cemento-enamel junction* (CEJ). In clinical examinations it has been observed that a free gingival groove is only present in about 30-40% of adults. The free gingival groove is often most pronounced on the vestibular aspect of the teeth, occurring most frequently in the incisor and premolar regions of the mandible, and least frequently in the mandibular molar and maxillary premolar regions *(mucogingival junction*: MGJ).

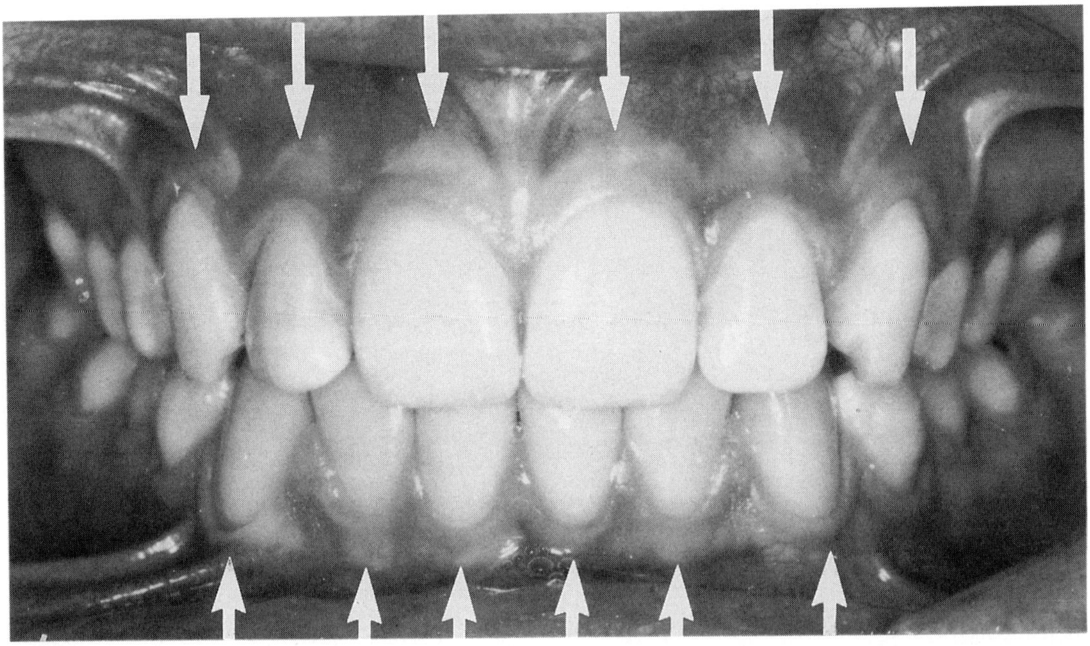

Fig. 1-2.

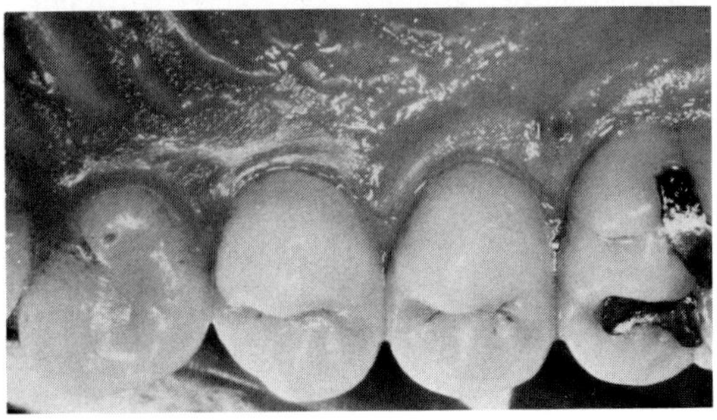

Fig. 1-3.

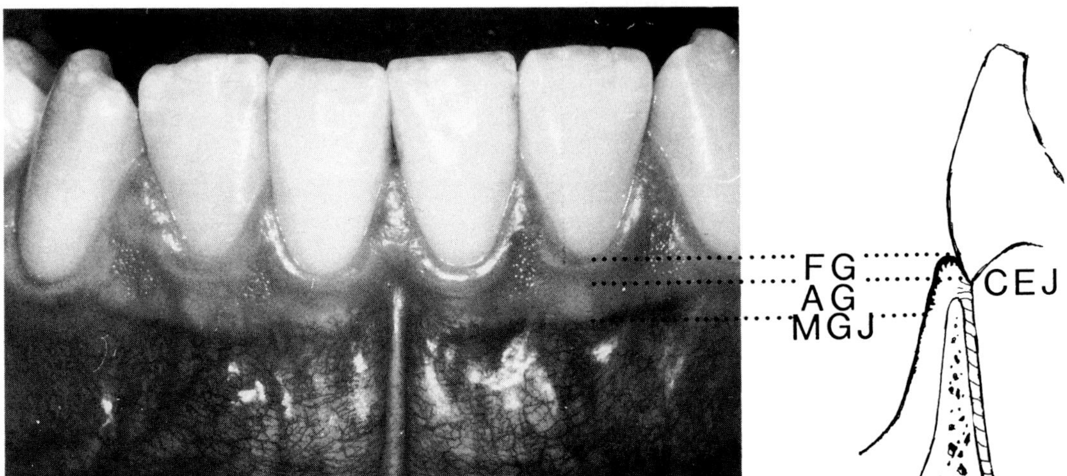

Fig. 1-4.

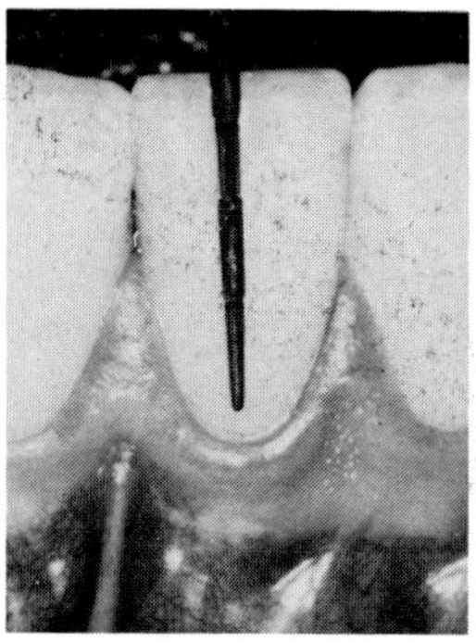
Fig. 1-5a.

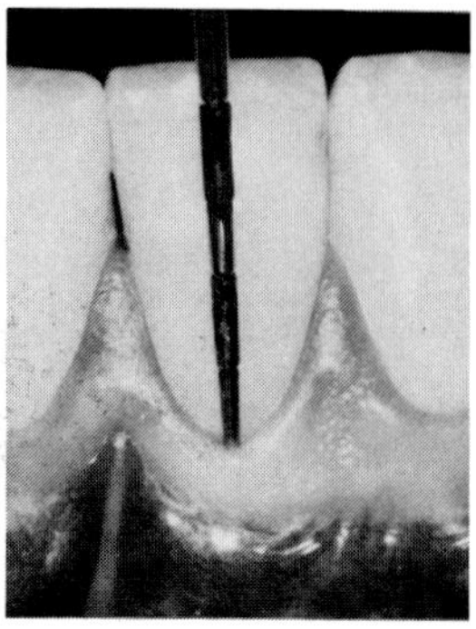
Fig. 1-5b.

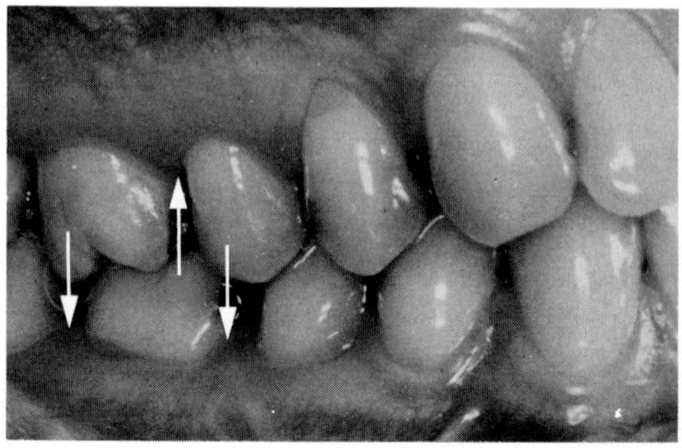
Fig. 1-6.

Fig. 1-5. The *free gingival margin* is often rounded in such a way that a small invagination or sulcus is formed between the tooth and the gingiva (Fig. 1-5a).

When a periodontal probe is inserted into this invagination and, further, apically towards the cemento-enamel junction, the gingival tissue is separated from the tooth and a "*gingival pocket*" or "*gingival crevice*" is artificially opened. Thus, in normal or *clinically healthy gingiva* there is in fact no "gingival pocket" or "gingival crevice" present but the gingiva is in close contact with the enamel surface. In the illustration to the right (Fig. 1-5b) a periodontal probe has been inserted in the tooth/gingiva interface and artificially opened a "gingival crevice" approximately to the level of the cemento-enamel junction.

After completed tooth eruption, the free gingival margin is located on the enamel surface approximately 0.5-2 mm coronal to the cemento-enamel junction.

Fig. 1-6. The shape of the *interdental gingiva* (the *interdental papilla*) is determined by the contact relationships between the teeth, the width of the approximal tooth surfaces and the course of the cemento-enamel junction. In anterior regions of the dentition, the interdental papilla is of pyramidal form while in the molar regions, the papillae are more flattened in bucco-lingual direction (arrows). Due to the presence of interdental papillae, the free gingival margin follows a more or less accentuated, scalloped course through the dentition (see also Fig. 1-2).

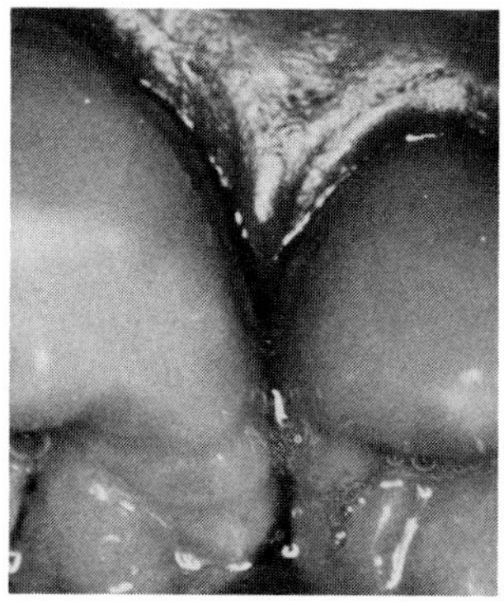
Fig. 1-7a.

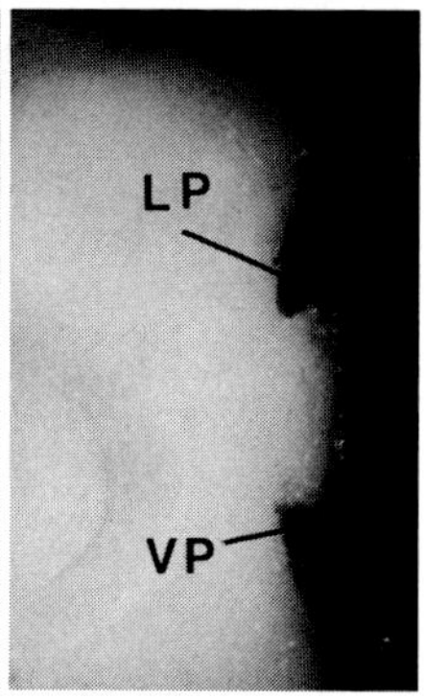

Fig. 1-7b.

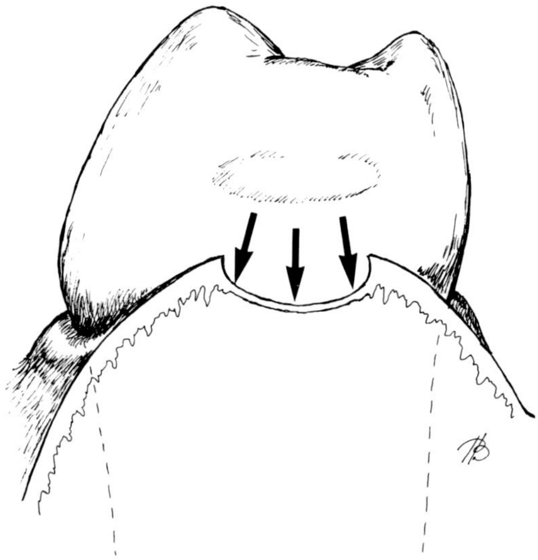
Fig. 1-7c.

Fig. 1-7. In the premolar/molar regions of the dentition, the teeth have approximal contact

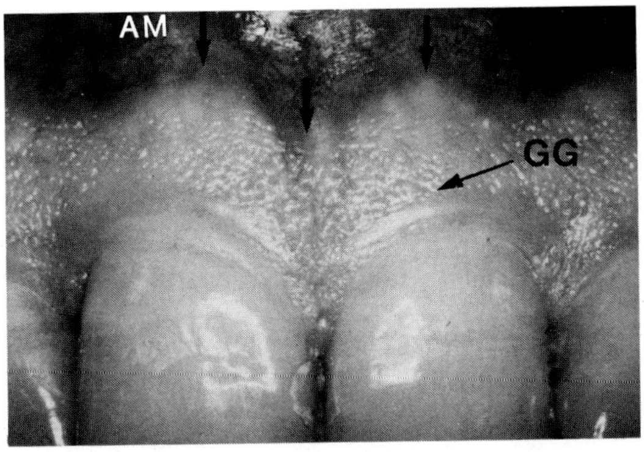

Fig. 1-8.

surfaces (Fig. 1-7a) rather than contact points. Since the interdental papilla has a shape in conformity with the outline of the interdental contact surfaces, a concavity - *a col* - is established in the premolar and molar regions, as demonstrated in Fig. 1-7b where the distal tooth has been removed. Thus, the interdental papillae in these areas often have one vestibular (VP) and one lingual/palatal portion (LP) separated by the col region.

The col region, as demonstrated in the schematic drawing (Fig. 1-7c), is covered by a thin non-keratinized epithelium (arrows).

Fig. 1-8. The *attached gingiva* is, in coronal direction, demarcated by the *free gingival groove* (GG) or, when such a groove is not present, by a horizontal plane placed at the level of the cemento-enamel junction. The attached gingiva extends in apical direction to the mucogingival junction (arrows), where it becomes continuous with the alveolar (lining) mucosa (AM).

The attached gingiva is of firm texture, coral pink in color, and often shows a fine, surface stippling giving it the appearance of orange peel. The stippling, however, is only present in about 40% of adults.

This type of mucosa is firmly attached to the underlying alveolar bone and cementum by connective tissue fibers and is, therefore, comparatively immobile in relation to the underlying tissue.

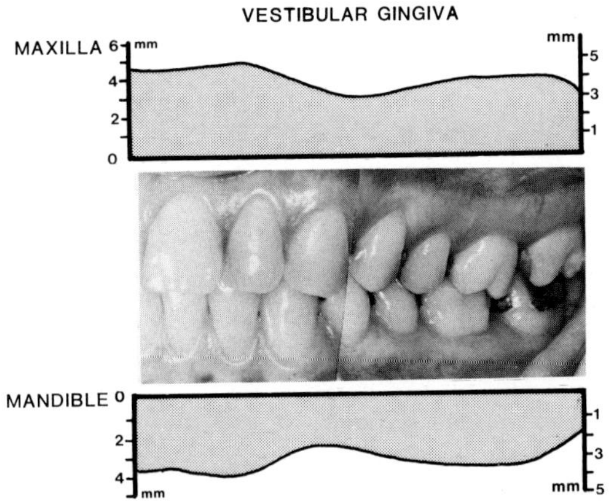

Fig. 1-9a.

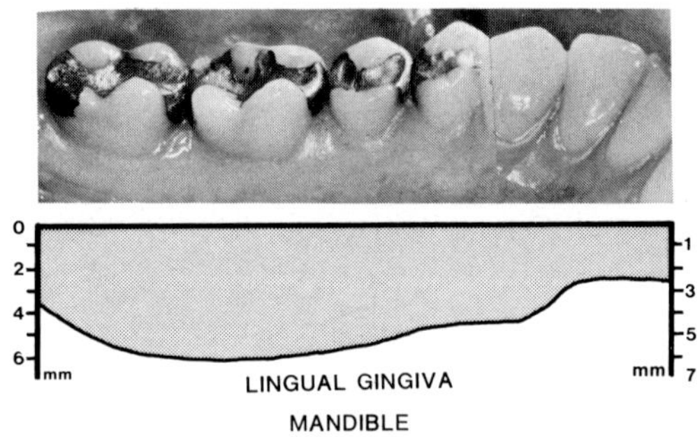

Fig. 1-9b.

The darker red, alveolar mucosa (AM) located apical to the mucogingival junction, on the other hand, is loosely bound to the underlying bone. Therefore, in contrast to the attached gingiva, the alveolar mucosa is mobile in relation to the underlying tissue.

Fig. 1-9 describes how the width of the gingiva varies in different parts of the mouth. In the maxilla (1-9a), the vestibular gingiva is generally widest in the area of the incisors and most narrow adjacent to the premolars. In the mandible (1-9b), the gingiva on the lingual aspect is particularly narrow in the area of the incisors and wide in the molar region. The range of variation is 1-9 mm.

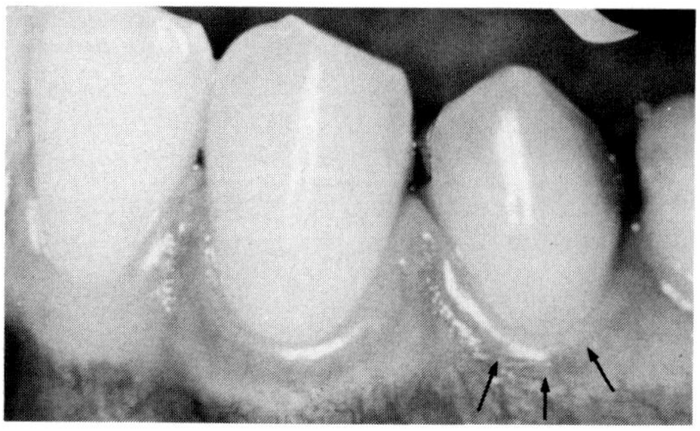

Fig. 1-10.

Fig. 1-10 illustrates an area in the mandibular premolar region where the gingiva is extremely narrow. The arrows indicate the location of the mucogingival junction.

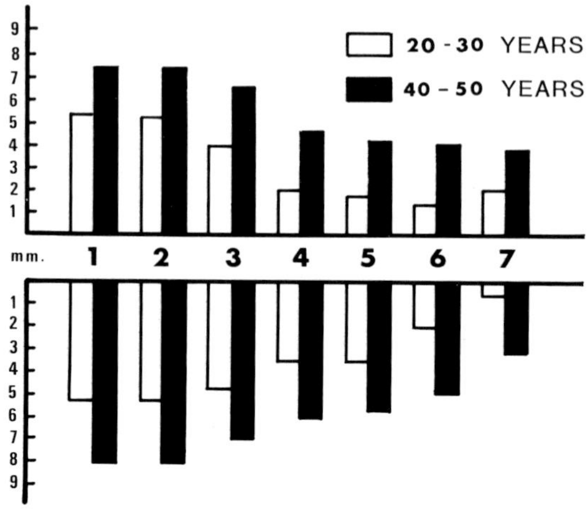

Fig. 1-11.

Fig. 1-11 depicts the result of a study in which the width of the attached gingiva was assessed and related to the age of the patients examined. It was found that the gingiva in 40-50 year olds was significantly wider than that in 20-30 year olds. This observation indicates that the width of the gingiva tends to increase with increasing age. Since the mucogingival junction remains stable throughout life in relation to the lower border of the mandible, the increasing width of the gingiva may suggest that the teeth, as a result of occlusal wear, slowly erupt throughout life.

Microscopic anatomy

The oral epithelium

Fig. 1-12a. A schematic drawing of the histological section, presented in *Fig. 1-12b*, describing the composition of the gingiva and the contact area between the gingiva and the enamel (E). The free gingiva comprises all tissue structures located coronal to a horizontal line placed at the level of the cemento-enamel junction (CEJ). The epithelium covering the free gingiva may be differentiated as follows:

oral epithelium (OE) which faces the oral cavity

oral sulcular epithelium (OSE) which faces the tooth without being in contact with the tooth surface

junctional epithelium (JE) which participates in the contact between the gingiva and the tooth.

The boundary between the oral epithelium (OE) and the underlying connective tissue (CT) has a wavy course. The connective tissue portions which project into the epithelium are called *connective tissue papillae* and are separated from each other by *epithelial ridges* - so-called rete pegs. In normal, non-inflamed gingiva, rete pegs and connective tissue papillae are lacking at the boundary between the junctional epithelium and its underlying connective tissue. Thus, a characteristic morphological feature of the oral epithelium and the oral sulcular epithelium is the presence of rete pegs while these structures are lacking in the junctional epithelium.

Fig. 1-13. A model of the *oral epithelium* of the gingiva after the connective tissue has been removed is presented in Fig. 1-13. The *subsurface* (i.e. the surface of the epithelium facing the connective tissue) of the oral epithelium exhibits several depressions corresponding to the

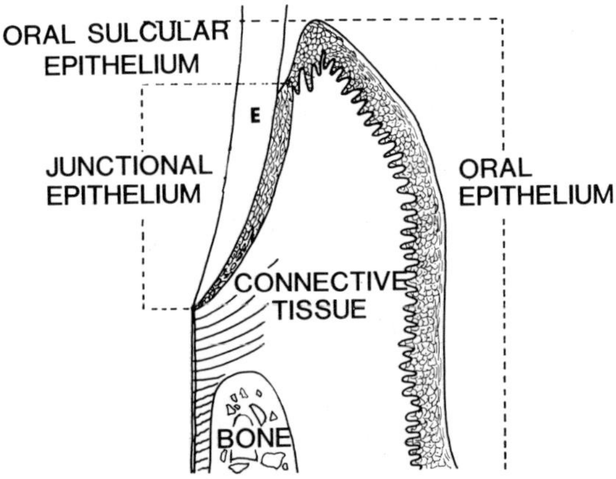

Fig. 1-12a.

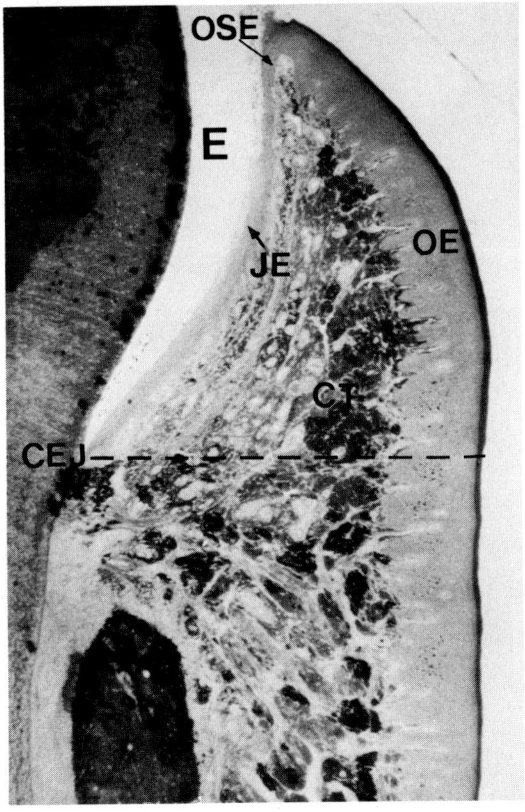

Fig. 1-12b.

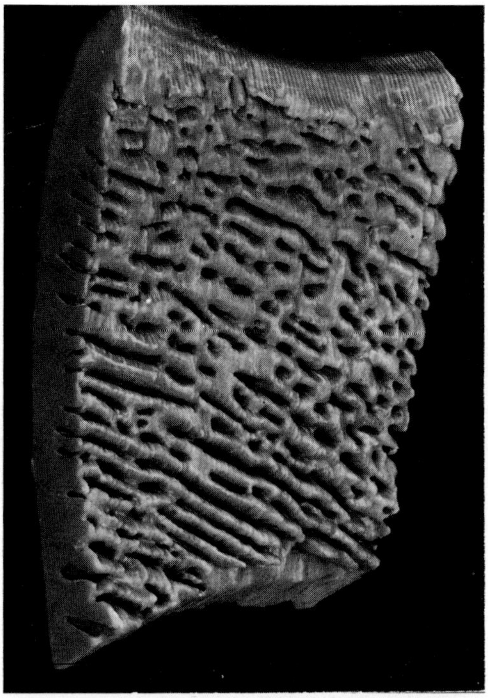

Fig. 1-13.

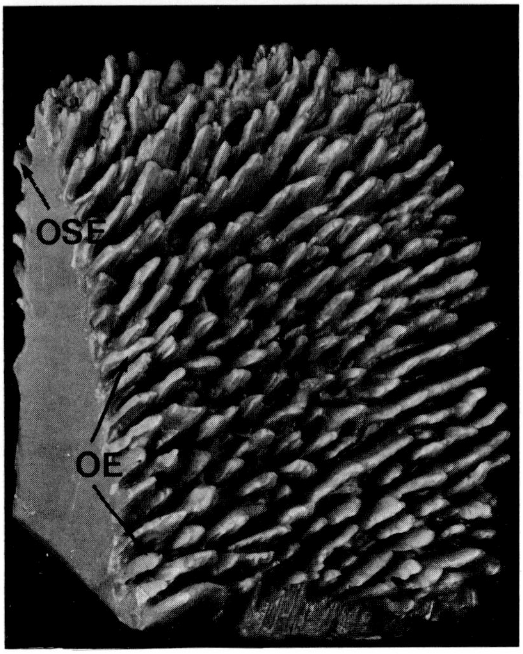

Fig. 1-14.

connective tissue papillae which project into the epithelium. It can be seen that the epithelial projections, which in histological sections separate the connective tissue papillae, constitute a more continuous system of epithelial ridges.

Fig. 1-14 presents a model of the *connective tissue*, corresponding to the model of the epithelium shown in Fig. 1-13. The tooth surface is located at the left-hand side of the illustra-

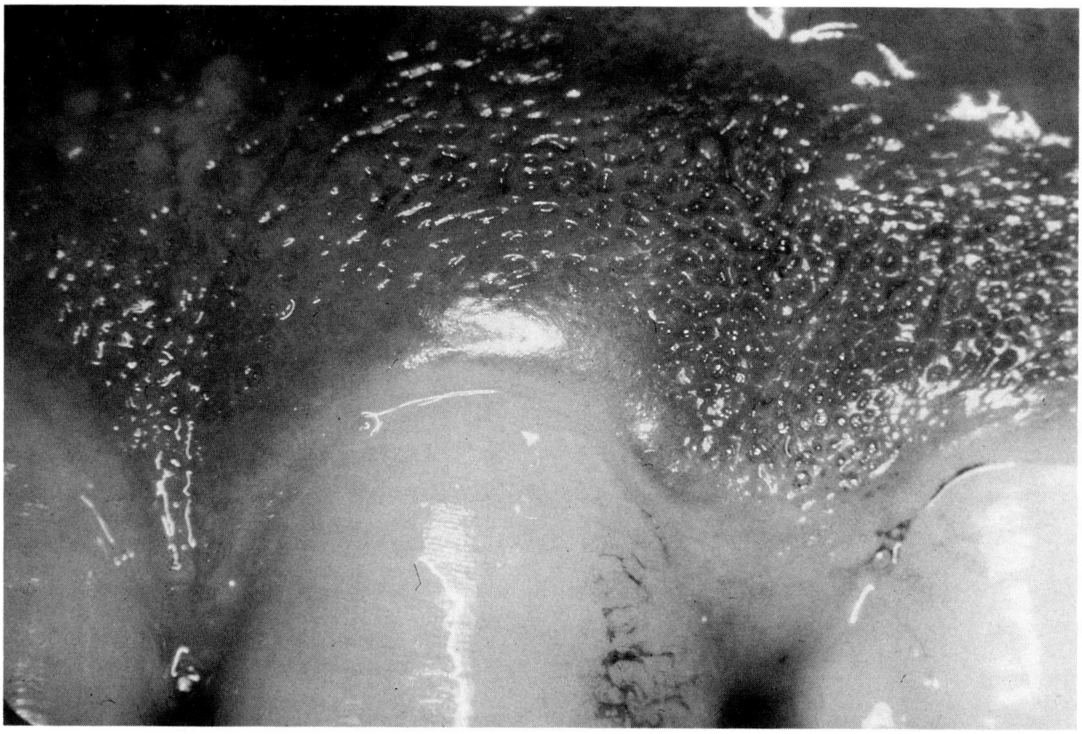

Fig. 1-15a.

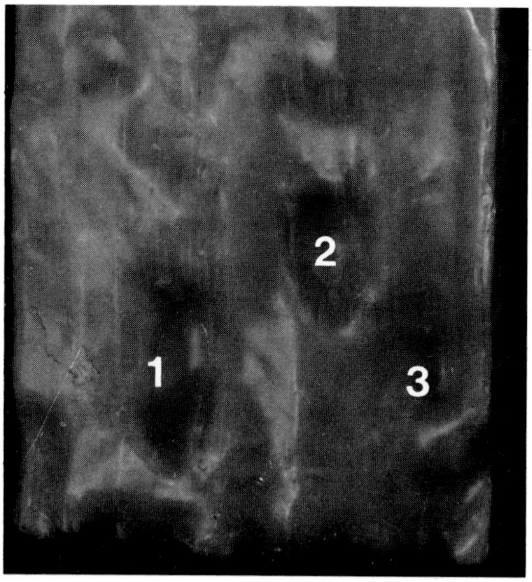

Fig. 1-15b.

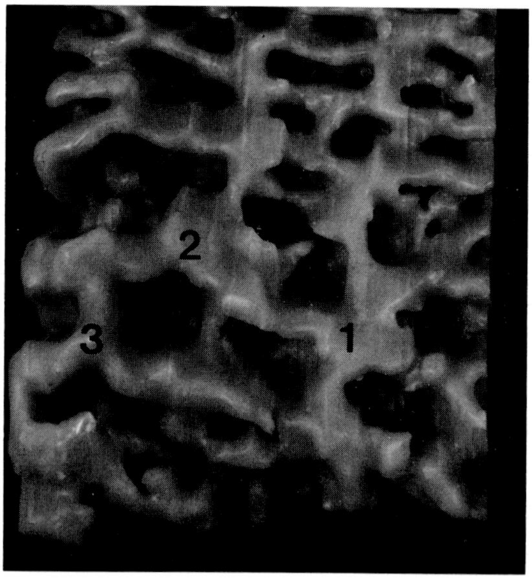

Fig. 1-15c.

tion. The epithelium is removed. Notice the connective tissue papillae which project into the space occupied by the oral epithelium (OE) and the oral sulcular epithelium (OSE).

Fig. 1-15a. In 40% of adults the attached gingiva shows a stippling on the surface. The photograph shows a case where this stippling is very conspicuous. *Fig. 1-15b* presents a model of the outer surface of the *oral epithelium* of the attached gingiva. The surface exhibits the minute depressions (1,2,3) which, when present, give the gingiva its characteristic stippled appearance.

Fig. 1-15c. A photograph of the *subsurface* (i.e. the surface of the epithelium facing the connective tissue) of the same model as described in Fig. 1-15b. The subsurface of the epithelium is characterized by the presence of epithelial ridges which merge at various locations (1,2,3). The depressions (1-3) seen on the outer surface of the epithelium (shown in Fig. 1-15b) correspond with the fusion sites (1-3) between epithelial ridges (shown in Fig. 1-15c) at the subsurface of the epithelium. Thus, the depressions on the surface of the gingiva are established at the areas of fusion between various epithelial ridges.

Fig. 1-16a. A portion of the oral epithelium which covers the free gingiva is illustrated in this photomicrograph. The oral epithelium is a keratinized, stratified, squamous epithelium which on the basis of the degree to which the *keratin producing* cells are differentiated can be divided into the following cell layers:

1) *basal layer* (stratum basale or stratum germinativum)
2) *spinous cell layer* (stratum spinosum)
3) *granular cell layer* (stratum granulosum)
4) *keratinized cell layer* (stratum corneum)

It should be observed that in this section cell nuclei are lacking in the outer cell layers. Such an epithelium is denoted *orthokeratinized.*

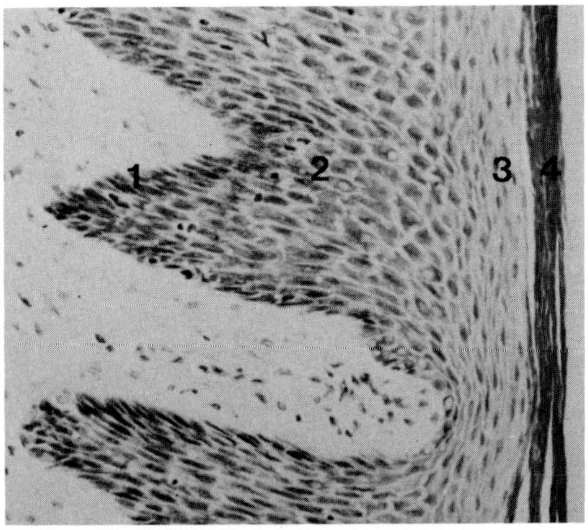

Fig. 1-16a.

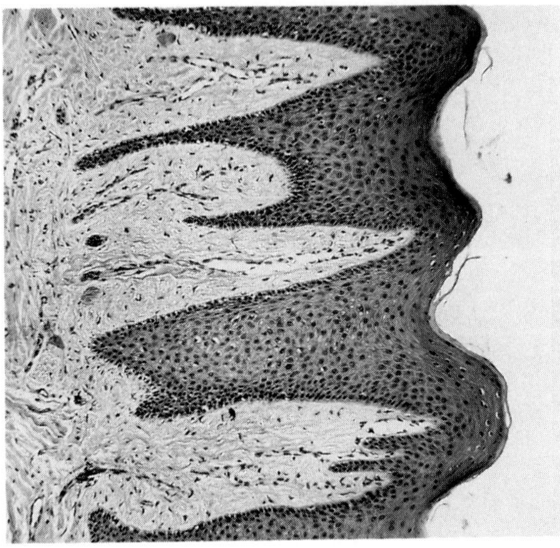
Fig. 1-16b.

Often, however, the cells of the stratum corneum of the epithelium of human, masticatory mucosa contain remnants of the nuclei. In such case the epithelium is denoted *parakeratinized.* (Fig. 1-16b).

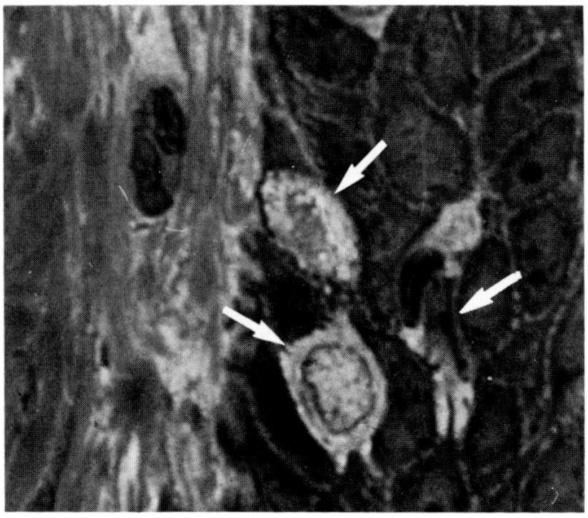

Fig. 1-17.

Fig. 1-17. In addition to the keratin producing cells, which comprise about 90% of the total cell population, the oral epithelium contains the following 3 types of cell:

1) melanocytes
2) Langerhans cells
3) non-specific cells (i.e. cells which do not exhibit the same ultrastructural characteristics as the other 2 cell types).

All 3 cell types are stellate and have cytoplasmic extensions of various size and appearance. These cells are also called "clear cells" (arrows) since in the histological section they appear lighter than the surrounding keratin producing cells.

The photomicrograph shows 3 "clear cells" (arrows) located in the region of the stratum basale and stratum spinosum of the oral epithelium. Thus, these "clear cells" which are not producing keratin can be either melanocytes, Langerhans cells or nonspecific cells. The melanocytes are pigment-containing cells while the Langerhans cells are believed to play a role in the defense mechanism of the oral mucosa. It has been suggested that the Langerhans cells react with antigens which are in the process of penetrating the epithelium. An early immunological response is initiated, inhibiting or preventing further antigen penetration of the tissue.

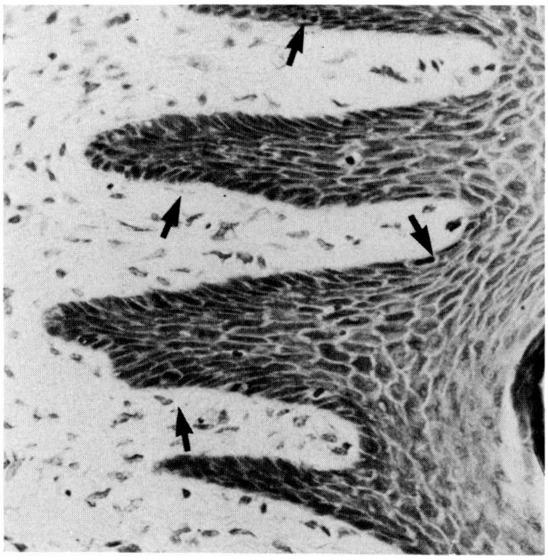

Fig. 1-18.

Fig. 1-18. The cells in the *basal layer* are either cylindrical or cuboid, and are in contact with the *basement membrane*. The basal cells possess the ability to divide, i.e. undergo mitotic cell division. The cells marked with arrows in the photomicrograph are in the process of dividing. It is in the basal layer that the epithelium is renewed and therefore this layer is also termed *stratum germinativum*.

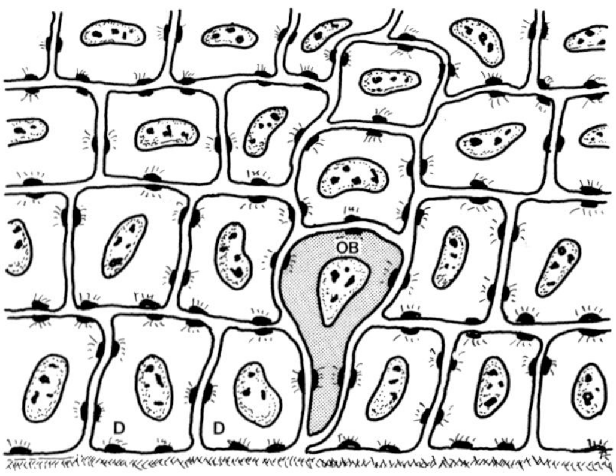

Fig. 1-19.

Fig. 1-19. When 2 daughter cells (D) have been formed by cell division, an adjacent "older" basal cell (OB) is pushed into the *spinous cell layer* and starts, as a keratinocyte, to traverse the epithelium. It takes approximately 1 month for a keratinocyte to reach the outer epithelial surface where it becomes desquamated from the stratum corneum. In a given time, the number of cells which divide in the basal layer equals the number of cells which become desquamated from the surface. Under normal conditions there is complete equilibrium between cell renewal and desquamation. As the basal cell migrates through the epithelium it becomes flattened and has its long axis parallel to the tissue surface.

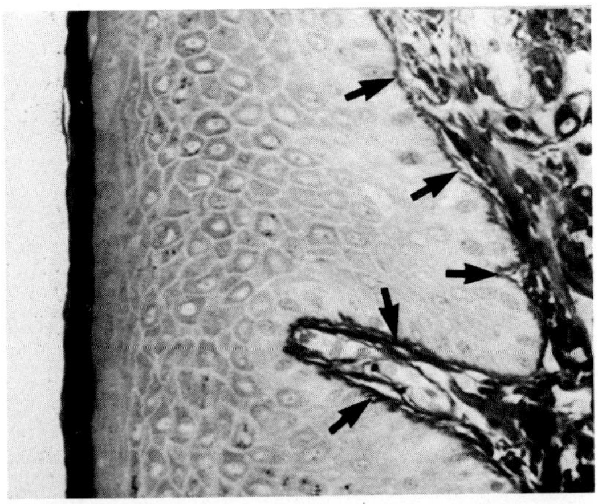

Fig. 1-20.

Fig. 1-20. The basal cells are found immediately adjacent to the connective tissue and are separated from this tissue by a *basement membrane*, probably produced by the basal cells. Under the light microscope this membrane appears as a zone approximately 1 μm wide (arrows), which reacts positively to a PAS stain (periodic acid Schiff stain). This positive reaction demonstrates that the basement membrane (arrows) contains carbohydrate (glycoproteins). The epithelial cells are surrounded by an extracellular substance which also contains protein-polysaccharide complexes.

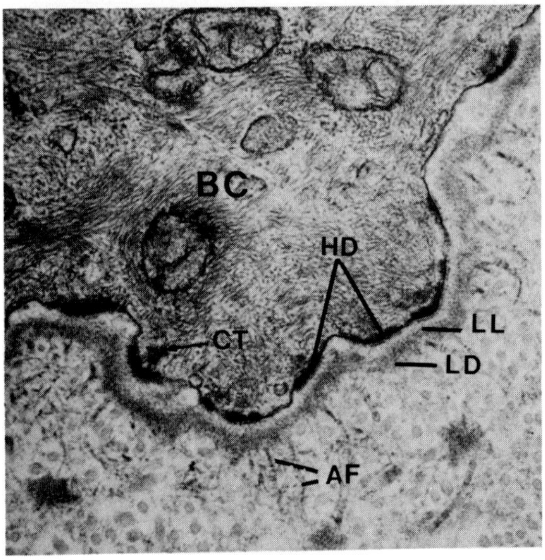

Fig. 1-21.

Fig. 1-21 is an electronmicrograph (magnification x 70,000) of an area including part of a basal cell, the basement membrane and part of the adjacent connective tissue. The basal cell (BC) occupies the upper portion of the picture. Immediately beneath the basal cell an approximately 400 Å wide electron lucent zone can be seen which is called *lamina lucida* (LL). Beneath the lamina lucida an electron dense zone of approximately the same thickness can be observed. This zone is called *lamina densa* (LD). From the lamina densa so-called *anchoring fibers* (AF) project in fan-shaped fashion into the connective tissue. The anchoring fibers are approximately 1 μm in length and terminate freely in the connective tissue.

The basement membrane, that appeared as an entity under the light microscope, thus, in the electronmicrograph, appears to comprise one lamina lucida and one lamina densa with adjacent connective tissue fibers (anchoring fibers). The cell membrane of the epithelial cells facing the lamina lucida harbors a number of electron dense, thicker zones appearing at various intervals along the cell membrane. These structures are called *hemidesmosomes* (HD). The cytoplasmic *tonofilaments* (CT) in the cell converge towards such hemidesmosomes. The hemidesmosomes are involved in the attachment of the epithelium to the underlying basement membrane.

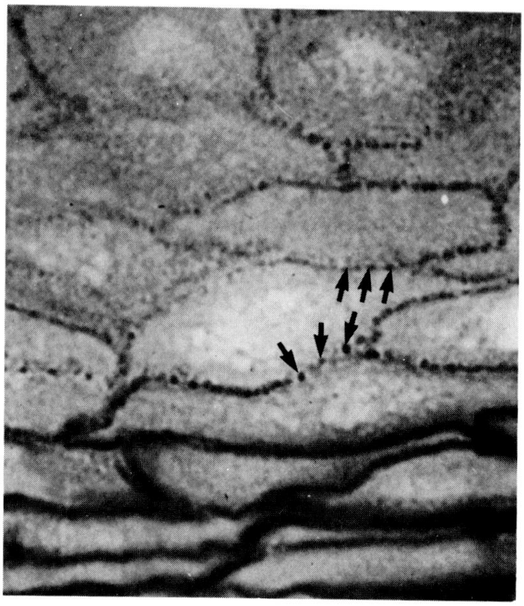

Fig. 1-22.

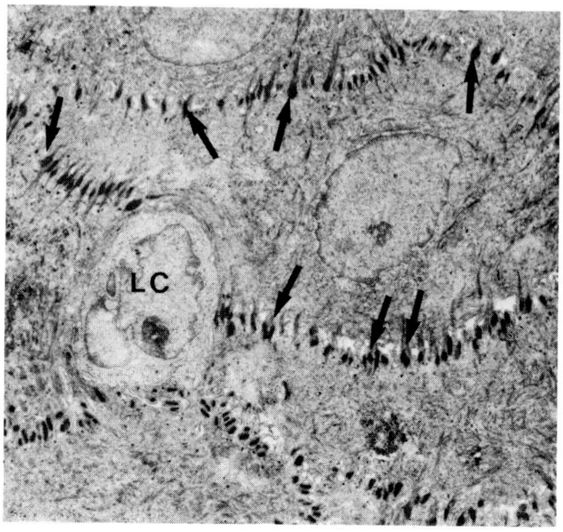

Fig. 1-23.

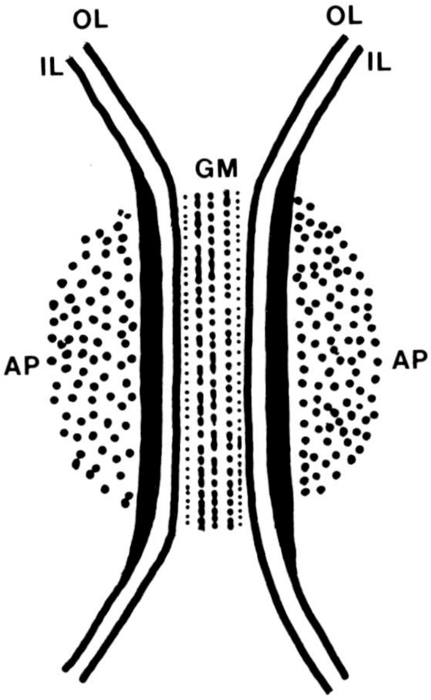

Fig. 1-24.

Fig. 1-22 illustrates an area of stratum spinosum in the gingival oral epithelium. Stratum spinosum consists of 10-20 layers of relatively large, polyhedral cells, equipped with short cytoplasmic processes resembling spines. The cytoplasmic processes (arrows) occur at regular intervals and give the cells a prickled appearance. The cells are attached to one another by numerous "desmosomes" (pairs of hemidesmosomes) which are located between the cytoplasmic processes of adjacent cells.

Fig. 1-23 shows an area of stratum spinosum in an electron micrograph. The dark-stained structures between the individual epithelial cells represent the desmosomes (arrows). As stated above, a desmosome may be considered as 2 hemidesmosomes facing one another. The presence of a large number of desmosomes indicates that the attachment between the epithelial cells is solid. The light cell (LC) in the center of the illustration harbors no hemidesmosomes and is, therefore, not a keratinocyte but rather a "clear" cell (see also Fig. 1-17).

Fig. 1-24 is a schematic drawing describing the composition of a desmosome. A desmosome consists of 2 adjoining hemidesmosomes separated by a zone containing electron dense granulated material (GM). In addition, a hemidesmosome comprises the following structural components: 1) the outer leaflets (OL) of the cell membrane of 2 adjoining cells, 2) the thick

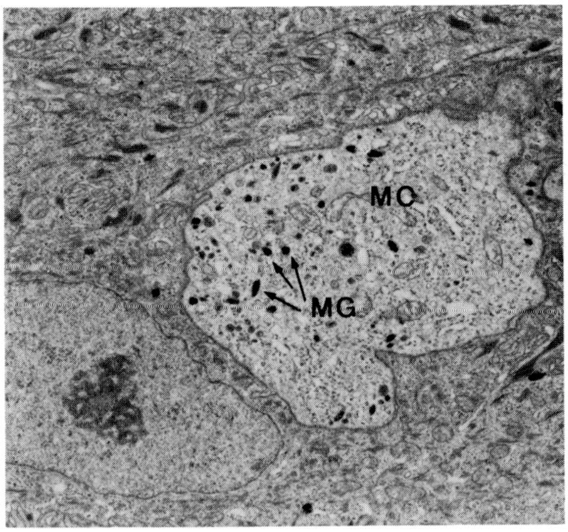

Fig. 1-25.

inner leaflets (IL) of the cell membranes and 3) the attachment plaques (AP) which represent granular and fibrillar material in the cytoplasm.

Fig. 1-25. As mentioned previously, the oral epithelium also contains *melanocytes* which are responsible for the production of the pigment melanin. Melanocytes are present in individuals with marked pigmentation of the oral mucosa (Indians and Negroes) as well as in individuals where no clinical signs of pigmentation can be seen. In this electron micrograph a melanocyte (MC) is present in the lower portion of the stratum spinosum. In contrast to the keratinocytes, this cell contains melanin granulae (MG) and has no tonofilaments or hemidesmosomes. Note the large amount of tonofilaments in the cytoplasm of the adjacent keratinocytes.

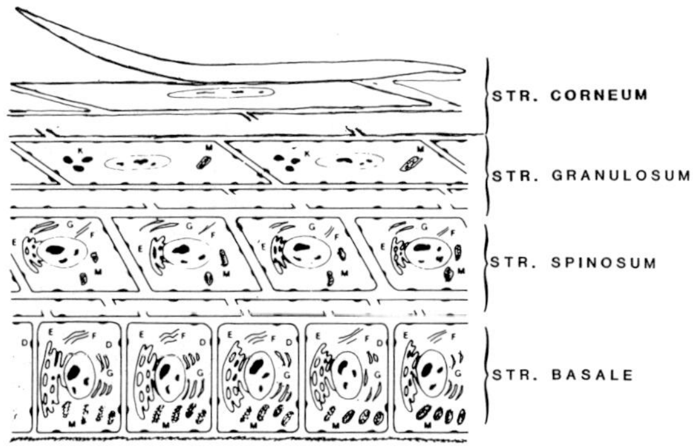

Fig. 1-26.

Fig. 1-26. When traversing the epithelium from the basal layer to the epithelial surface, the keratinocytes undergo continuous differentiation and specialization. The many changes which occur during this process are indicated in this diagram of a keratinized, stratified, squamous epithelium. From the basal layer (Str. basale) to the granular layer (Str. granulosum) both the number of tonofilaments (F) in the cytoplasm and the number of desmosomes (D) increase. In contrast, the number of organelles such as mitochondria (M), lamellae of rough endoplasmic reticulum (E) and Golgi complexes (G) decreases in the keratinocytes on their way from the basal layer towards the surface. In the stratum granulosum, electron dense keratohyalin bodies and clusters of glycogen containing granula start to occur. Such granula are believed to be related to the synthesis of keratin.

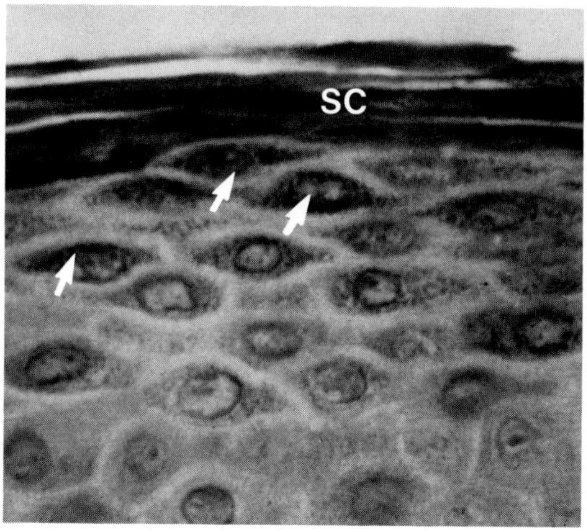

Fig. 1-27.

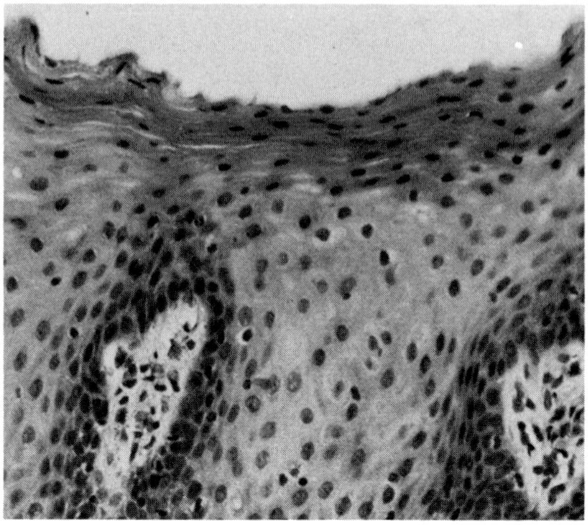

Fig. 1-28.

Fig. 1-27 is a photomicrograph of the stratum granulosum and stratum corneum. Keratohyalin granula (arrows) are seen in the stratum granulosum. There is often an abrupt transition of the cells from the stratum granulosum to the stratum corneum. This is indicative of the keratinization of the cytoplasm of the keratinocyte and its conversion into an "acellular" structure bordered by a cell membrane. The cytoplasm of the cells in the stratum corneum (SC) is filled with keratin and the entire apparatus for protein synthesis and energy production, i.e. the nucleus, the mitochondria, the endoplasmic reticulum and the Golgi complex is lost. In parakeratinized epithelia, however, the cells of the stratum corneum contain remnants of nuclei. Keratinization is considered as a process of differentiation rather than degeneration. It is a process of protein synthesis which requires energy and is dependent on functional cells, i.e. cells containing a nucleus and a normal set of organelles.

In summary:
The keratinocyte undergoes continuous differentiation on its way from the basal layer to the surface of the epithelium. Thus, once the keratinocyte has left the basement membrane it can no longer divide but maintains a capacity for production of protein (tonofilaments and keratohyalin granules). In the granular layer, the keratinocyte is deprived of its energy and protein producing apparatus (probably by enzymatic breakdown) and is abruptly converted into a keratin filled cell which from the stratum corneum is shed from the tissue surface.

Fig. 1-28 illustrates a portion of the epithelium covering the alveolar (lining) mucosa. In contrast to the epithelium of the masticatory mucosa, the lining mucosa has no stratum corneum. Notice that cells containing nuclei can be identified in all layers, from the basal layer to the surface of the epithelium.

The dento-gingival epithelium
The tissue components of the dento-gingival region achieve their final structural characteristics in conjunction with the eruption of the teeth. This is illustrated in Fig. 1-29.

a) When the enamel of the tooth is fully developed, the enamel-producing cells (ameloblasts) become reduced in height, produce a basal lamina and form, together with cells from the outer enamel epithelium, the so-called *reduced enamel epithelium* (RE). The basal lamina (*epithelial attachment lamina:* EAL) lies in direct contact with the enamel; the contact between this lamina and the epithelial cells is

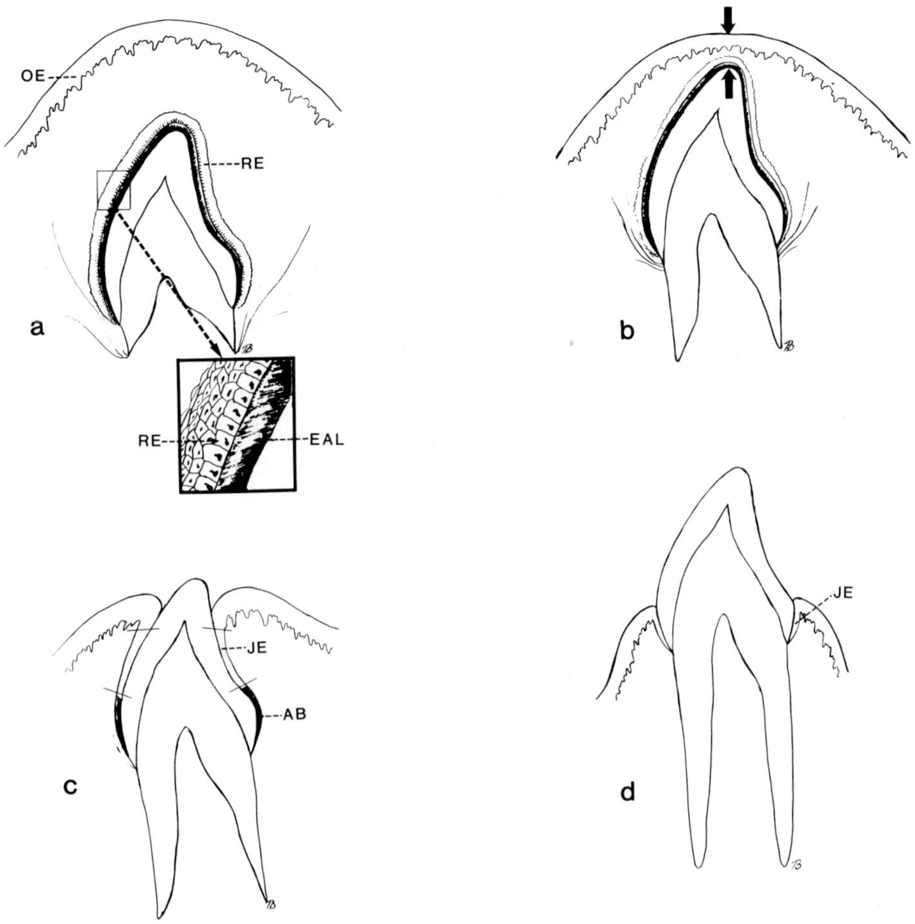

Fig. 1-29.

maintained by hemidesmosomes. The reduced enamel epithelium surrounds the crown of the tooth from the moment the enamel is properly mineralized until the tooth starts to erupt.

b) As the erupting tooth approaches the oral epithelium, the cells of the outer layer of the reduced enamel epithelium, as well as the cells of the basal layer of the oral epithelium (OE), show increased mitotic activity (arrows); the former ameloblasts do not divide. The reduced enamel epithelium is gradually transformed during tooth eruption into a *junctional epithelium*.

c) When the tooth has penetrated into the oral cavity, the reduced enamel epithelium and the oral epithelium fuse at the incisal edge of the tooth. Large portions immediately apical to the incisal area of the enamel are then covered by a junctional epithelium (JE) containing only few layers of cells. The cervical region of the enamel, however, is still covered by ameloblasts (AB) and outer cells of the reduced enamel epithelium.

d) During the later phases of tooth eruption, all cells of the reduced enamel epithelium are transformed into a junctional epithelium. This transformed epithelium is continuous with the oral epithelium and participates in the attachment between the tooth and the gingiva. The

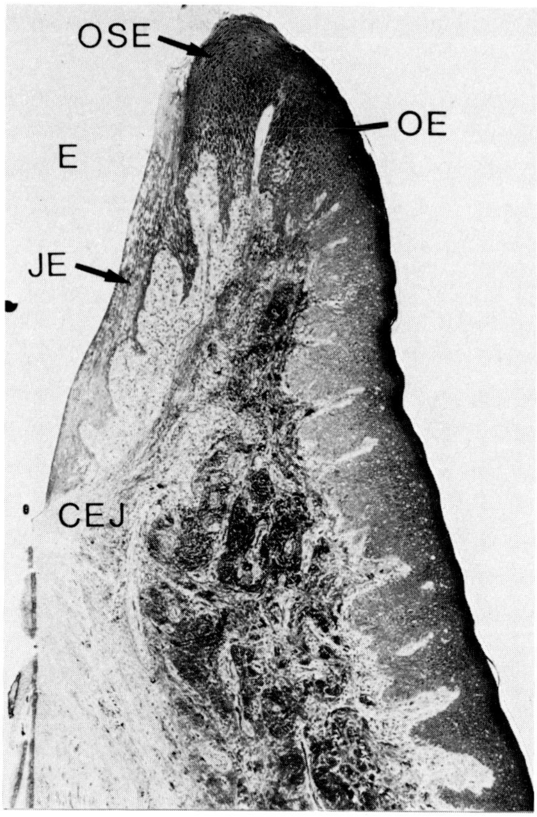

Fig. 1-30

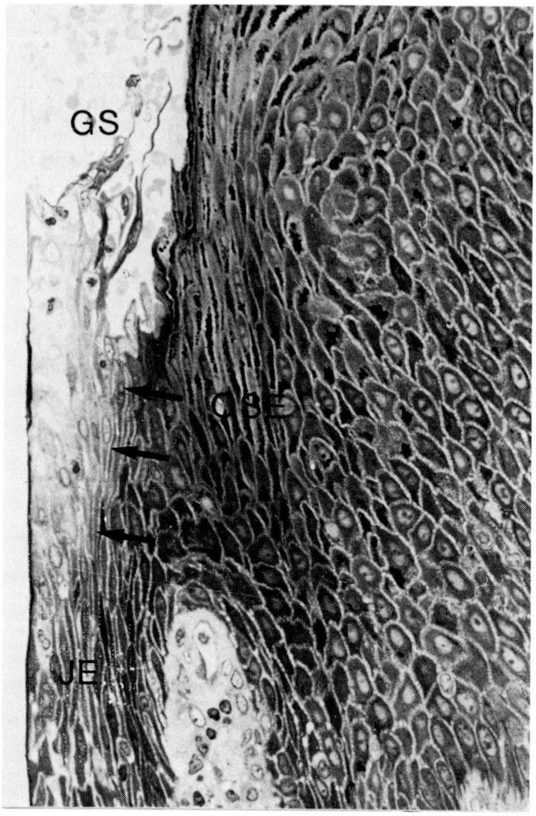

Fig. 1-31.

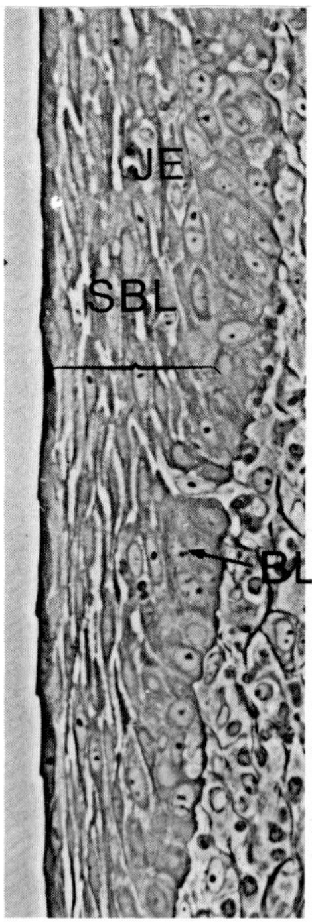

Fig. 1-32a.

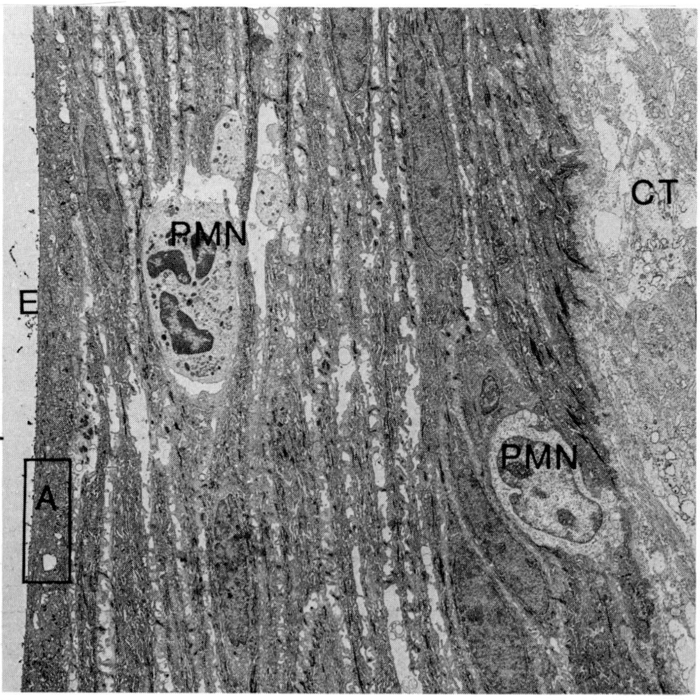

Fig. 1-32b

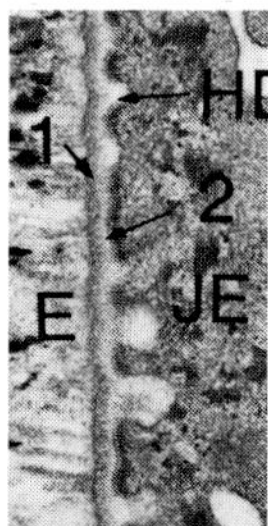

Fig

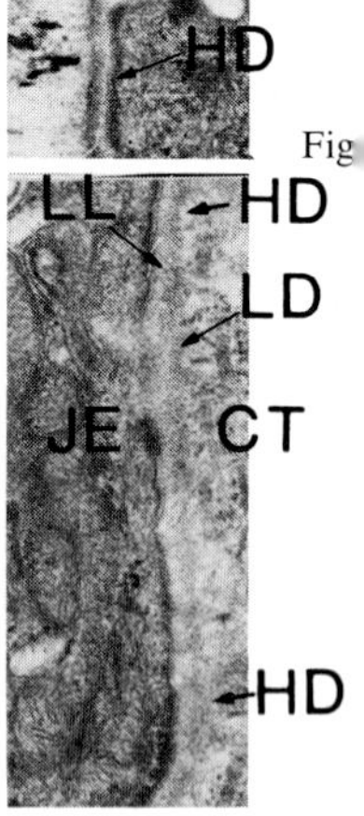

Fig.1-32d.

secondary epithelial attachment, produced by the basal cells of the junctional epithelium, is composed of the former *epithelial attachment lamina* and the hemidesmosomes of the basal cells of this junctional epithelium.

If the free gingiva is excised after the tooth has fully erupted, a new junctional epithelium and new attachment lamina, indistinguishable from the ones found following tooth eruption, will develop during healing. The fact that this new junctional epithelium and new attachment lamina have developed from the oral epithelium indicates that the cells of the oral epithelium possess the ability to differentiate into cells of junctional epithelium, and to synthesize and secrete basal lamina material.

Fig. 1-30 is a histological section cut through the border area between the tooth and the gingiva, i.e. the dento-gingival region. The enamel (E) is to the left. Towards the right follow the junctional epithelium (JE), the oral sulcular epithelium (OSE) and the oral epithelium (OE). The junctional epithelium differs morphologically from the oral sulcular epithelium and oral epithelium, while the two latter are structurally very similar. The junctional epithelium is widest in its coronal portion (about 15-20 cell layers), but becomes thinner towards the cemento-enamel junction (CEJ).

Fig. 1-31. The junctional epithelium has a free surface at the bottom of the *gingival sulcus* (GS). It is from this surface that the epithelial cells of the junctional epithelium are desquamated. Like the oral sulcular epithelium and the oral epithelium, the junctional epithelium is continuously renewed through cell division in the basal layer. The cells migrate to the base of the gingival sulcus from where they are shed. The border between the junctional epithelium (JE) and the oral sulcular epithelium (OSE) is indicated by arrows. The cells of the oral sulcular epithelium are cuboid and the surface of this epithelium is keratinized.

Fig. 1-32 illustrates different characteristics of the junctional epithelium.

Fig. 1-32a shows that the cells of the junctional epithelium (JE) are arranged into one basal layer (BL) and several suprabasal layers (SBL).

Fig. 1-32b. The basal cells as well as the suprabasal cells are flattened with their long axis parallel to the tooth surface. (CT = connective tissue, E = enamel space).

There are distinct differences between the oral sulcular epithelium, the oral epithelium and the junctional epithelium:

1) the size of the cells in the junctional epithelium is, relative to the tissue volume, larger than in the oral epithelium
2) the intercellular space in the junctional epithelium is, relative to the tissue volume, comparatively wider than in the oral epithelium
3) the number of desmosomes is smaller in the junctional epithelium than in the oral epithelium.

Note the comparatively wide intercellular spaces between the oblong cells of the junctional epithelium, and the presence of 2 neutrophilic granulocytes (PMN) which are traversing the epithelium.

The framed area (A) is shown in a higher magnification in Fig. 1-32c, from which it can be seen that the basal cells of the junctional epithelium are not in direct contact with the enamel (E). Between the enamel and the epithelium (JE) one electron lucent zone (1) and one electron dense zone (2) can be seen. The electron lucent zone is in contact with the cells of the junctional epithelium (JE). These 2 zones have a structure very similar to that of the lamina densa (LD) and lamina lucida (LL) in the basement membrane area (i.e. the epithelium (JE) - connective tissue (CT) interface) de-

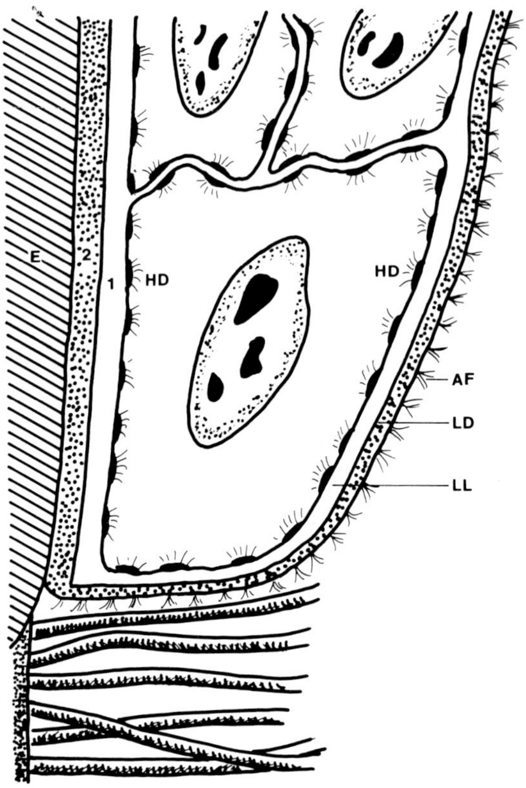

Fig. 1-33.

scribed in Fig. 1-21. Furthermore, as seen in Fig. 1-32d the cell membrane of the junctional epithelial cells harbors hemidesmosomes (HD) towards the enamel as it does towards the connective tissue. Thus, the interface between the enamel and the junctional epithelium is similar to the interface between the epithelium and the connective tissue.

Fig. 1-33 is a schematic drawing of the most apically positioned cell in the junctional epithelium. The enamel (E) is depicted to the left in the drawing. It can be seen that the electron dense zone (2) between the junctional epithelium and the enamel can be considered as a continuation of the lamina densa (LD) in the basement membrane of the connective tissue side. Similarly, the electron lucent zone (1) can be considered as a continuation of the lamina lucida (LL). It should be noticed, however, that

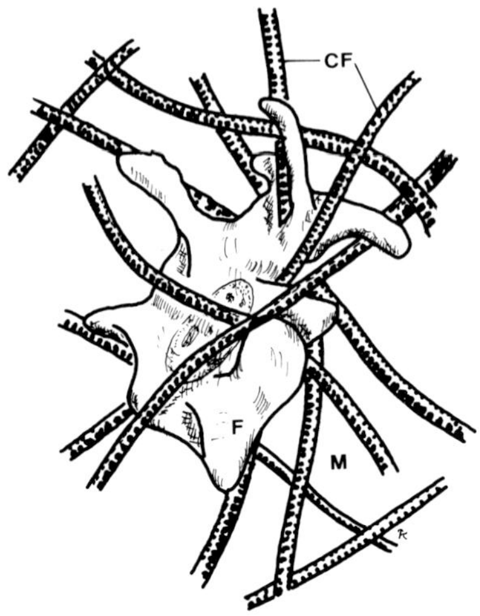

Fig. 1-34.

in variance with the epithelium-connective tissue interface, there are no anchoring fibers (AF) attached to the lamina densa-like structure. However, like the basal cells adjacent to the basement membrane (at the connective tissue interface), the cells of the junctional epithelium facing the lamina lucida-like structure (1) harbor hemidesmosomes. Thus, the interface between the junctional epithelium and enamel is structurally very similar to the epithelium-connective tissue interface, which means that the junctional epithelium is not only in contact with the enamel but is actually physically attached to the tooth via hemidesmosomes.

The connective tissue

The predominant tissue component of the gingiva and periodontal ligament is the connective tissue. The major components of the connective tissue are *collagen fibers* (around 60% of connective tissue volume), *fibroblasts* (around 5%), *vessels*, *nerves* and *matrix* (around 35%).

Fig. 1-34. The drawing illustrates a fibroblast (F) residing in a network of connective tissue fibers (CF). The intervening space is filled with matrix (M) which constitutes the "environment" for the cell.

Cells

The different types of cell present in the connective tissue are a) fibroblasts, b) mast cells, c) macrophages, d) neutrophilic granulocytes, e) lymphocytes and f) plasma cells.

Fig. 1-35. The fibroblast is the most predominant connective tissue cell (65% of the total cell population). The fibroblast is engaged in the production of various types of fibers found in the connective tissue, but is also instrumental in the synthesis of the connective tissue matrix. The fibroblast is a spindle shaped or stellate cell. Fig. 1-35 shows part of a fibroblast in electron microscopic magnification. The cytoplasm contains a well developed granular endoplasmic reticulum (E) with ribosomes.

The Golgi complex (G) is usually of considerable size and the mitochondria (M) are large and numerous. Furthermore, the cytoplasm contains many fine tonofilaments (F). Adjacent to the cell membrane, all along the periphery of the cell, a large number of vesicles (V) can be found.

Fig. 1-36. The *mast cell* is responsible for the production of certain components of the matrix. This cell also produces vasoactive substances, which can affect the function of the microvascular system and control the flow of blood through the tissue. Fig. 1-36 presents a mast cell in electron microscopic magnification. The cytoplasm is characterized by the presence of a large number of vesicles (V) of varying size. These vesicles contain biologically active substances such as proteolytic enzymes, histamin and heparin. The Golgi complex (G) is well developed, while rough surface endoplasmic reticulum structures are scarce. A large number of small cytoplasmic projections, i.e. microvilli (MV), can be seen along the periphery of the cell.

Fig. 1-37. The *macrophage* has a number of different phagocytic and synthetic functions in

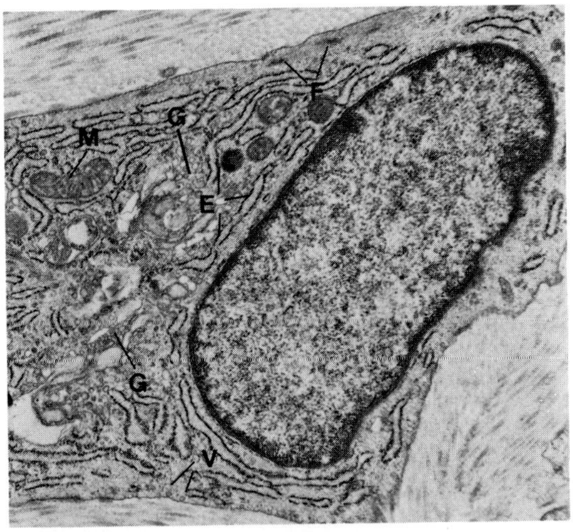

Fig. 1-35.

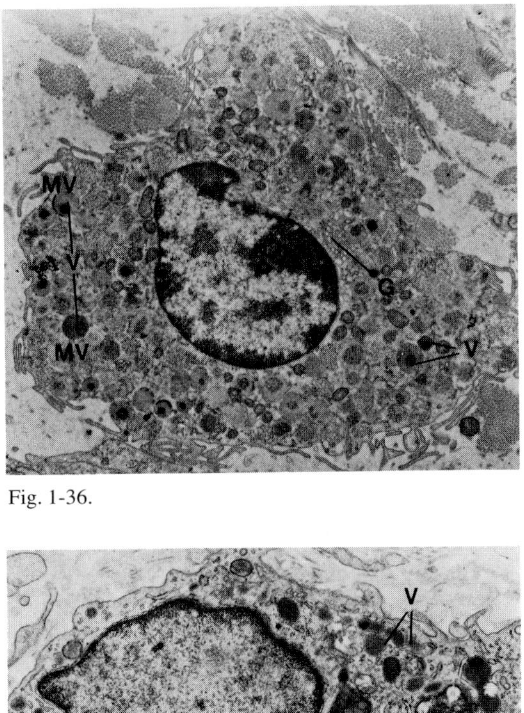

Fig. 1-36.

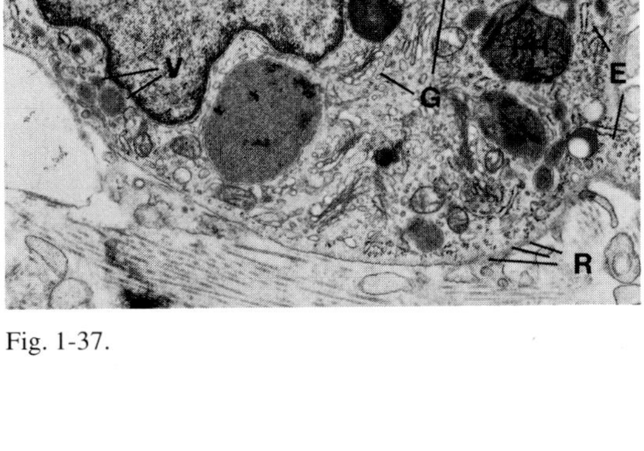

Fig. 1-37.

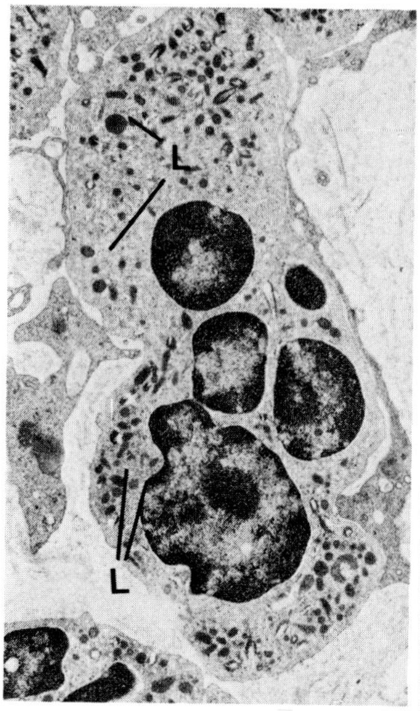

Fig. 1-38a.

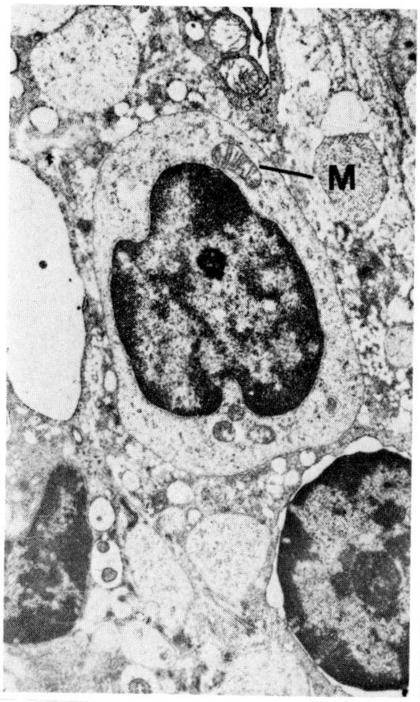

Fig. 1-38b.

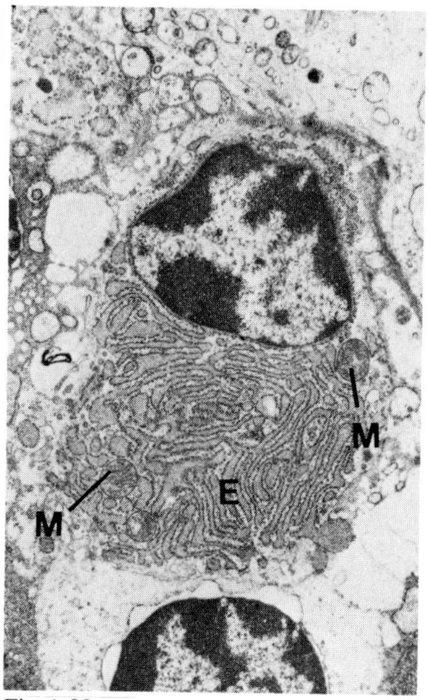

Fig. 1-38c.

the tissue. Fig. 1-37 shows a macrophage in electron microscopic magnification. The nucleus is characterized by numerous invaginations of varying size. A zone of electron dense chromatin condensations can be seen along the periphery of the nucleus. The Golgi complex (G) is well developed and numerous vesicles (V) of varying size are present in the cytoplasm. Rough surface endoplasmic reticulum (E) is scarce, but a certain number of free ribosomes (R) are evenly distributed in the cytoplasm. Remnants of phagocytosed material are often found in lysosomal vesicles: phagosomes (PH). In the periphery of the cell a large number of microvilli of varying size can be seen.

The macrophage as well as the mast cell is actively involved in the defense of the tissue against foreign and/or irritating substances.

Besides fibroblasts, mast cells and macrophages, the connective tissue also contains undifferentiated mesenchymal cells, the function of which is not properly understood.

The connective tissue also harbors *inflammatory cells* of various types, for example neutrophilic granulocytes, lymphocytes and plasma cells.

Fig. 1-38. The *neutrophilic granulocytes*, also called *polymorphonuclear leukocytes* (Fig. 1-38a), have a characteristic appearance. The nucleus is lobulate and numerous lysosomes (L), containing lysosomal enzymes, are found in the cytoplasm.

The *lymphocytes* (Fig. 1-38b) are characterized by an oval to spherical nucleus containing localized areas of electron dense chromatin. The narrow border of cytoplasm surrounding the nucleus contains numerous free ribosomes, a few mitochondria (M) and in localized areas endoplasmic reticulum with fixed ribosomes. Lysosomes are also present in the cytoplasm.

The *plasma cells* (Fig. 1-38c) contain an eccentrically located spherical nucleus with radially deployed electron dense chromatin. Endoplasmic reticulum (E) with numerous ribosomes is found randomly distributed in the cytoplasm. In addition, the cytoplasm contains numerous mitochondria (M) and a well developed Golgi complex.

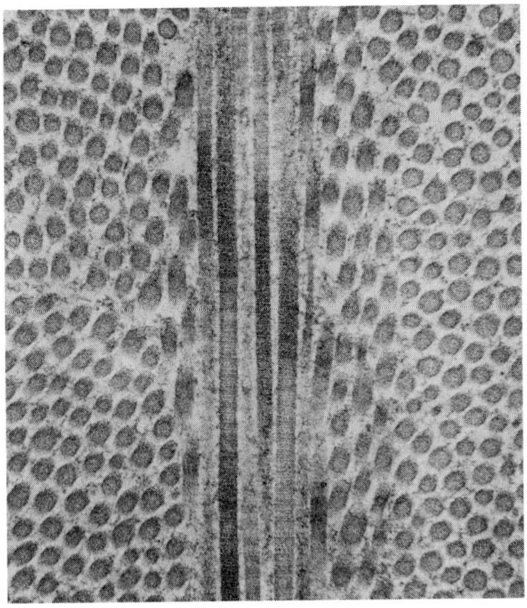

Fig. 1-39.

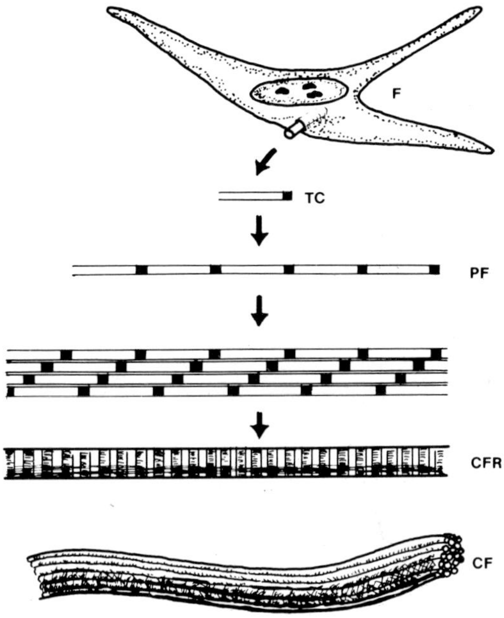

Fig. 1-40.

Fibers

The connective tissue fibers are produced by the fibroblasts and can be divided into: a) *collagen fibers* , b) *reticulin fibers*, c) *oxytalan fibers*, and d) *elastic fibers*.

Fig. 1-39. The *collagen fibers* predominate in the gingival connective tissue and they comprise the most essential components of the periodontium. The electron micrograph shows cross- and longitudinal sections of collagen fibers. The collagen fibers have a characteristic cross-banding with a periodicity of 700 Å between the individual dark bands.

Fig. 1-40 illustrates some important features of the production and the composition of collagen fibers; (F = fibroblast). The smallest unit, the collagen molecule, is often referred to as *tropocollagen.* A tropocollagen molecule (TC) which is seen in the upper portion of the drawing is approximately 3,000 Å long and has a diameter of 15 Å. It consists of 3 polypeptide chains intertwined to form a helix. Each chain contains about 1,000 amino acids. One third of these are glycine and about 20% proline and hydroxyproline, the latter being practically only found in collagen. Tropocollagen synthesis takes place inside the fibroblast from which the tropocollagen molecule is secreted into the extracellular space. Thus, the polymerization of tropocollagen molecules to collagen fibers takes place in the extracellular compartment. First, tropocollagen molecules are aggregated longitudinally to *protofibrils* (PF), which are subsequently laterally aggregated in parallel to *collagen fibrils* (CFR), with an overlapping of the tropocollagen molecules by about 25% of their length. Due to the fact that special refraction conditions develop after staining at the sites where the tropocollagen molecules adjoin, a cross-banding with a periodicity of approximately 700 Å occurs under light microscopy. The *collagen fibers* (CF) are bundles of collagen fibrils, aligned in such a way that the fibers also exhibit a cross-banding with a periodicity of 700 Å. In the tissue, the fibers are usually arranged in bundles. As the *collagen fibers* mature, covalent cross-links are formed

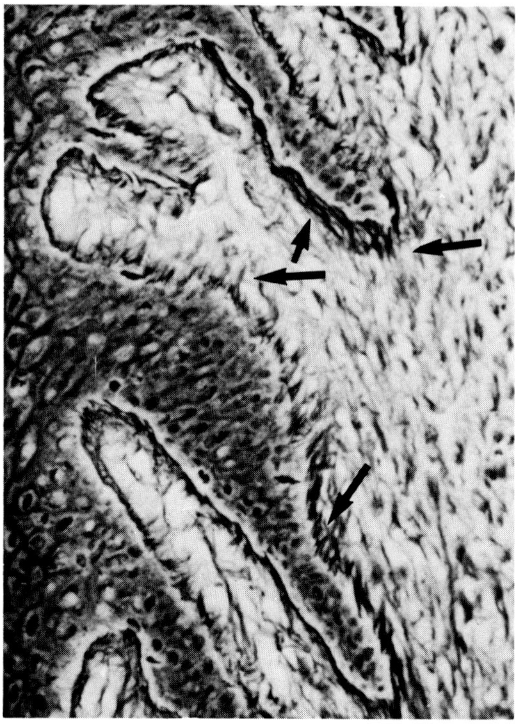

Fig. 1-41.

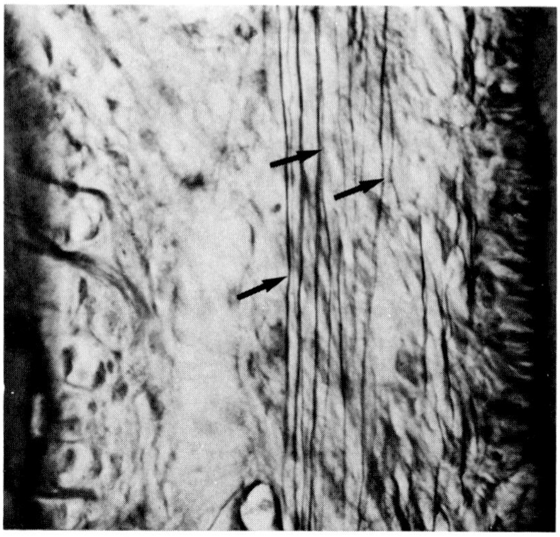

Fig. 1-42.

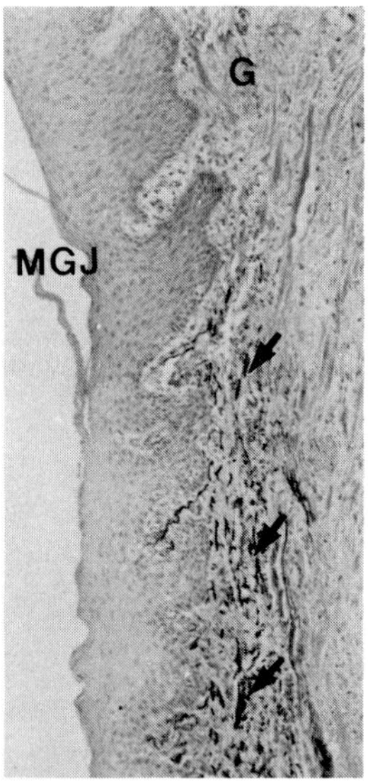

Fig. 1-43.

between the tropocollagen molecules resulting in an age-related reduction in collagen solubility.

Cementoblasts and *osteoblasts* are cells which also possess the ability to produce collagen.

Fig. 1-41. Reticulin fibers - as seen in this photomicrograph - exhibit argyrophilic staining properties and are numerous in the tissue adjacent to the basement membrane (arrows). However, reticulin fibers also occur in large numbers in the loose connective tissue surrounding the blood vessels. Thus, reticulin fibers are present at the epithelium-connective tissue- and the endothelium-connective tissue interfaces.

Fig 1-42. Oxytalan fibers are present in all connective tissue structures of the periodontium and seem to be composed of long thin fibrils with a diameter of approximately 150 Å. The photomicrograph illustrates oxytalan fibers (arrows) in the periodontal ligament, where they have a course mainly parallel to the long axis of the tooth. The function of these fibers is as yet unknown.

Fig. 1-43. Elastic fibers are in the connective tissue of the gingiva and periodontal ligament only present in association with blood vessels. However, in the connective tissue of the alveolar (lining) mucosa, elastic fibers are numerous. In this photomicrograph they can be seen in the loose alveolar mucosa (arrows). The gingiva (G) seen coronal to the mucogingival junction (MGJ) contains no elastic fibers.

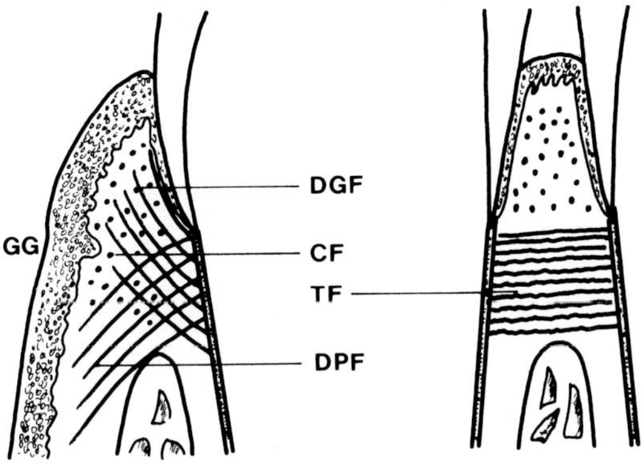

Fig. 1-44.

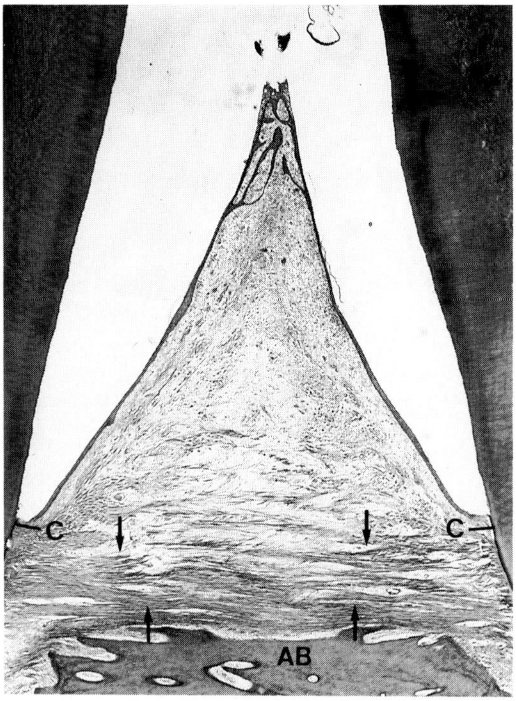

Fig. 1-45.

Fig. 1-44. Although many of the collagen fibers in the gingiva and the periodontal ligament are irregularly or randomly distributed, most tend to be arranged in groups of bundles with a distinct orientation. According to their insertion and course in the tissue, the oriented bundles in the gingiva can be divided into the following groups:

a) *Circular fibers* (CF) are fiber bundles which run their course in the free gingiva and encircle the tooth in a cuff- or ring-like fashion.
b) *Dentogingival fibers* (DGF) are embedded in the cementum of the supraalveolar portion of the root and project from the cementum in a fan-like configuration out into the free gingival tissue of the facial, lingual and interproximal surfaces.
c) *Dentoperiosteal fibers* (DPF) are embedded in the same portion of the cementum as the dentogingival fibers, but run their course apically over the vestibular and lingual bone crest and terminate in the tissue of the attached gingiva. In the border area between the free and attached gingiva, the epithelium often lacks support by underlying oriented collagen fiber bundles. In this area the free gingival groove (GG) is often present.
d) *Transseptal fibers* (TF), seen on the drawing to the right, extend between the supraalveolar cementum of approximating teeth. The transseptal fibers run straight across the interdental septum and are embedded in the cementum of adjacent teeth.

Fig. 1-45 illustrates in a histological section the orientation of the transseptal fiber bundles (arrows) in the supraalveolar portion of the interdental area. It should be observed that the transseptal fibers also connect the supraalveolar cementum (C) with the crest of the alveolar bone (AB). The 4 groups of collagen fiber bundles reinforce the interdental papilla and provide the resilience and tone which is necessary for maintaining its architectural form.

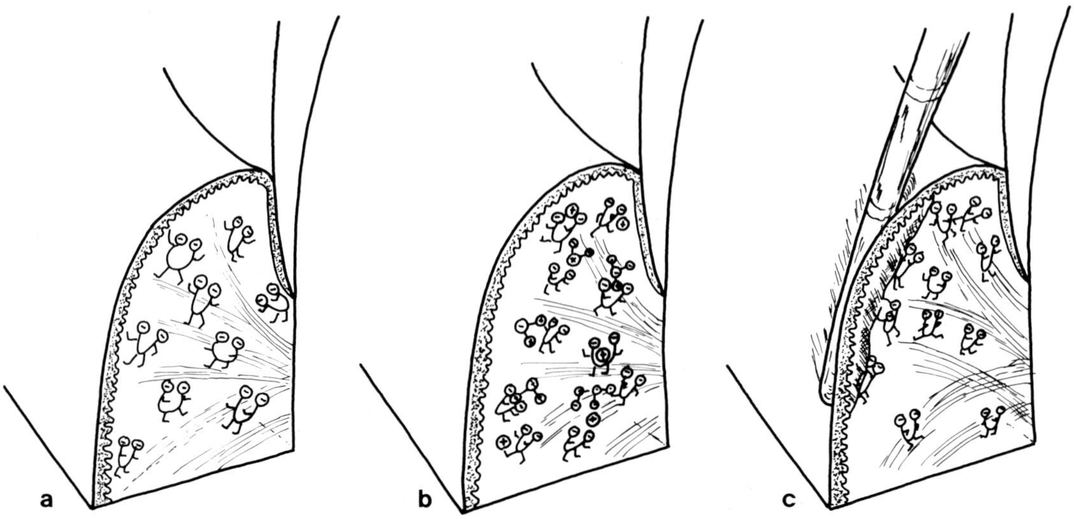

Fig. 1-46.

Matrix

The matrix of the connective tissue is first produced by the fibroblasts, although some constituents are produced by mast cells, and other components are derived from the blood. The matrix is the medium in which the connective tissue cells are embedded and it is essential for the maintenance of the normal function of the connective tissue. Thus, the transportation of water, electrolytes, nutrients, metabolites, etc., to and from the individual connective tissue cells occurs within the matrix. The main constituents of the connective tissue matrix are proteinpolysaccharide macromolecules. These complexes are normally differentiated into *proteoglycans* and *glycoproteins*. The *proteoglycans* contain glycosaminoglycans as the polysaccharide units (chondroitin sulfate etc.) which, via covalent bonds, are attached to one or more protein chains. The polysaccharide component is always predominant in the proteoglycans. The glycosaminoglycan called "hyaluronic acid" is probably not bound to protein. The *glycoproteins* also contain polysaccharides, but these macromolecules are different from glycosaminoglycans. The protein component is predominating in glycoproteins. In the macromolecules, mono- or oligosaccharides are, via covalent bonds, connected with one or more protein chains.

Fig. 1-46a. Normal function of the connective tissue depends on the presence of proteoglycans and glycosaminoglycans. The polysaccharide moiety of the proteoglycan, the glycosaminoglycans ( ), are large, flexible, chain formed, negatively charged molecules, each of which occupies a rather large space.

Fig. 1-46b. In such a space, smaller molecules, e.g. water and electrolytes, can be incorporated while larger molecules are prevented from entering. The proteoglycans thereby regulate diffusion and fluid flow through the matrix and are important determinants for the fluid content of the tissue and the maintenance of the osmotic pressure. In other words the proteoglycans act as a molecule filter and, in addition, play an important role in the regulation of cell migration (movements) in the tissue.

Fig. 1-46c. Due to their structure and hydration, the macromolecules exert resistance towards deformation, thereby serving as regulators of the consistency of the connective tissue. If the gingiva is suppressed, the macromolecules become deformed. When the pressure is eliminated the macromolecules regain their original form. Thus, the macromolecules are of importance for the resilience of the gingiva.

Epithelial differentiation

There are many examples of the fact that during the embryonic development of various organs, a mutual inductive influence occurs between the epithelium and the connective tissue. The development of the teeth is a characteristic example of such phenomena. The connective tissue is on the one hand a determining factor for a normal development of the tooth bud while, on the other, the enamel epithelia exert a definite influence on the development of the mesenchymal components of the teeth. It has been suggested that tissue differentiation in the adult organism can be influenced by environmental factors. The skin and mucous membranes for instance often display increased keratinization and hyperplasia of the epithelium in areas which are exposed to mechanical stimulation. Thus, the tissues seem to adapt to environmental stimuli. The presence of keratinized epithelium on the masticatory mucosa has been considered to represent an adaptation to mechanical irritation released by mastication. However, research has demonstrated that the characteristic features of the epithelium in such areas are genetically determined. Some pertinent observations are reported in the following:

Fig. 1-47 shows an area in a monkey where the gingiva (G) and the alveolar mucosa (AM) have been transposed by a surgical procedure. The alveolar mucosa is placed in close contact with the teeth while the gingiva is positioned in the area of the alveolar mucosa.

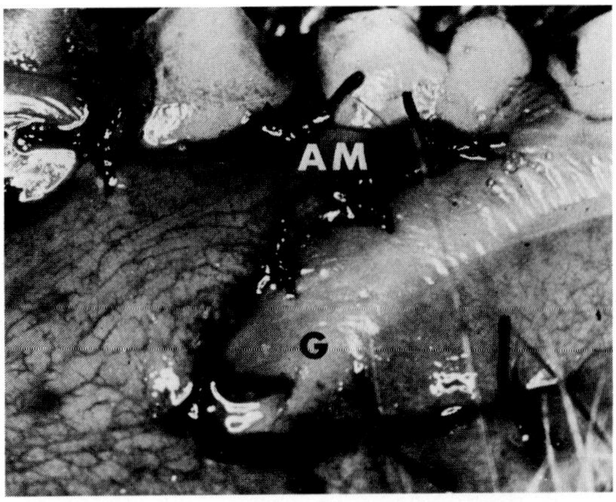

Fig. 1-47.

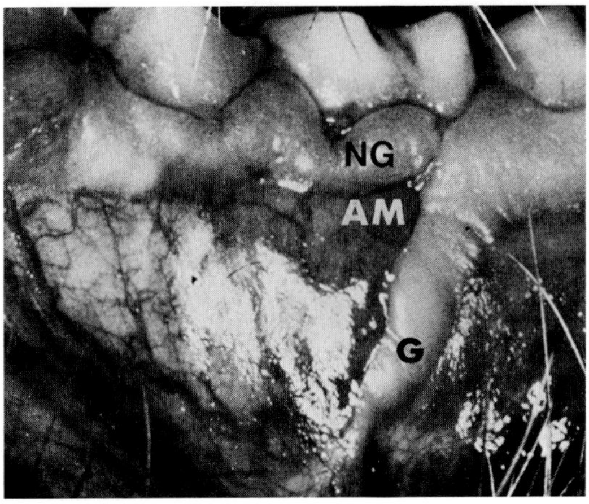

Fig. 1-48.

Fig. 1-48 shows the same area 4 months later. Despite the fact that the transplanted gingiva (G) is movable in relation to the underlying bone, like an alveolar mucosa, it has retained its characteristic, morphological features of a masticatory mucosa. However, a narrow zone of new keratinized gingiva (NG) has regenerated between the alveolar mucosa (AM) and the teeth. The alveolar mucosa (AM) is interposed between the transplanted gingiva (G) and the newly formed gingiva (NG).

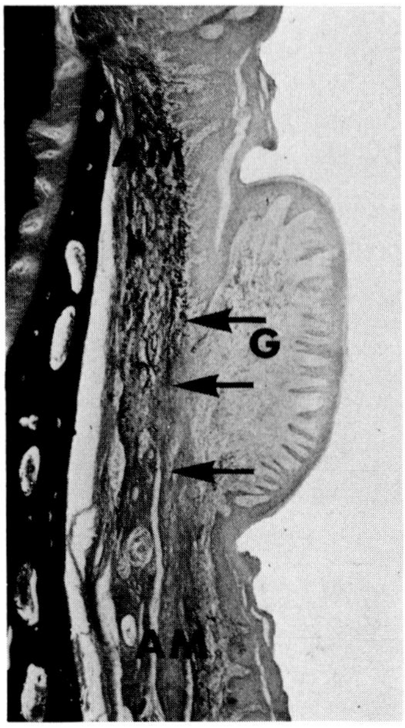

Fig. 1-49.

Fig. 1-49 presents a histological section cut through the transplanted gingiva seen in Fig. 1-48. Since elastic fibers are lacking in the gingival connective tissue (G), but are numerous in the connective tissue of the alveolar mucosa (AM), the transplanted tissue can readily be identified. The epithelium covering the transplanted gingival tissue exhibits a distinct keratin layer on the surface and also the configuration of the epithelium-connective tissue interface (i.e. rete pegs and connective tissue papillae) is similar to that of normal nontransplanted gingiva. Thus, the heterotopically located gingival tissue has maintained its original specificity. *This observation demonstrates that the characteristics of the gingiva are genetically determined rather than being the result of functional adaptation to environmental stimuli.*

Fig. 1-50 shows a histological section cut through the coronal portion of the area of transplantation. The transplanted gingival tissue (G) shown in Fig. 1-49 can be seen in the lower portion of the photomicrograph. The alveolar mucosa transplant (AM) is seen between the arrows in the middle of the illustration. After surgery, the alveolar mucosa was positioned in close contact with the teeth as seen in Fig. 1-47. After healing, a narrow zone of keratinized gingiva (NG) developed coronally to the alveolar mucosa transplant (see Fig. 1-48). This new zone of gingiva (NG), seen in the upper portion of the histological section, is covered by keratinized epithelium and the connective tissue contains no dark-stained elastic fibers. In addition, it is important to notice that the junction between keratinized and nonkeratinized epithelium corresponds exactly to the junction between "elastic" and "nonelastic" connective tissue. The connective tissue of the new gingiva has regenerated from the connective tissue of the supraalveolar and periodontal ligament compartments and has separated the alveolar mucosal transplant from the tooth. It is likely that the epithelium which covers the new gingiva has migrated from the adjacent epithelium of the alveolar mucosa.

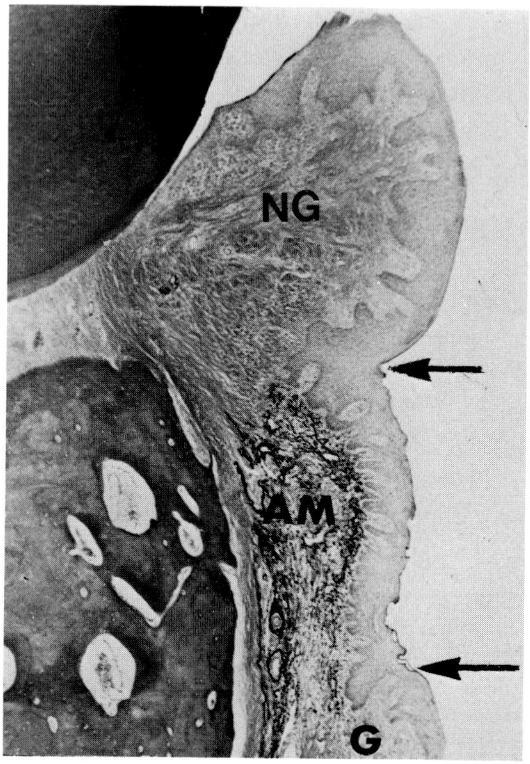

Fig. 1-50.

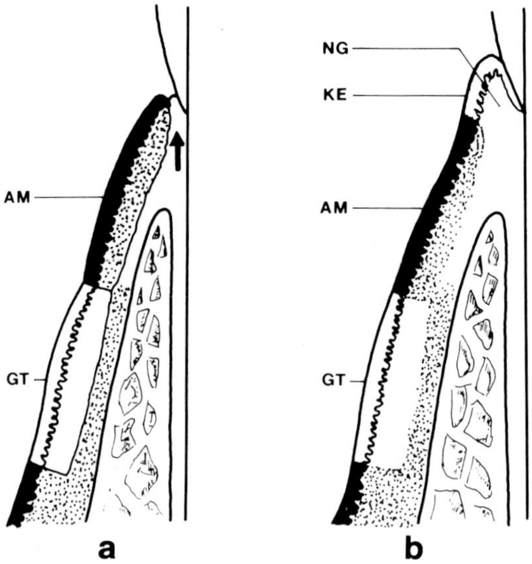

Fig. 1-51.

Fig. 1-51 presents a schematic drawing of the development of the new, narrow zone of keratinized gingiva (NG) seen in Figs. 1-48 and 1-50.

a) Granulation tissue has proliferated coronally along the root surface (arrow) and has separated the alveolar mucosa transplant (AM) from its contact with the tooth surface.
b) Epithelial cells have migrated from the alveolar mucosal transplant (AM) onto the newly formed gingival connective tissue. Thus, the newly formed gingiva has become covered with a keratinized epithelium (KE) which has originated from the nonkeratinized epithelium of the alveolar mucosa (AM). This implies that the newly formed gingival connective tissue (NG) possesses the ability to induce changes in the differentiation of the epithelium originating from the alveolar mucosa. This epithelium which is normally nonkeratinized, apparently, differentiates to keratinized epithelium because of stimuli arising from the newly formed gingival connective tissue; (*Gingival transplant:* GT).

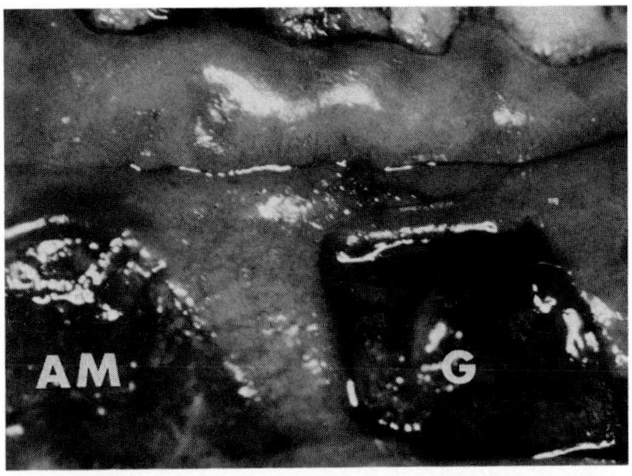

Fig. 1-52.

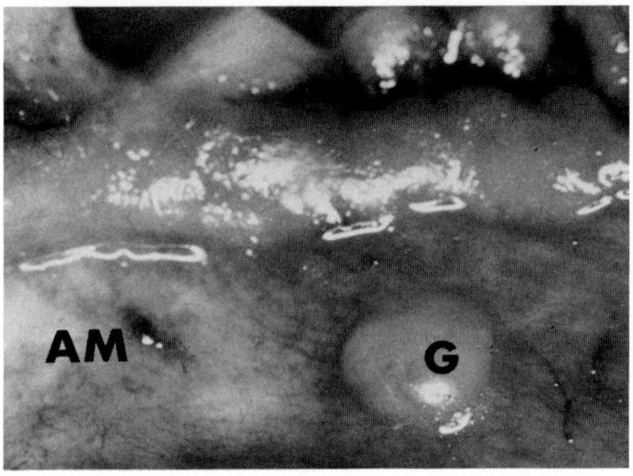

Fig. 1-53.

Fig. 1-52 illustrates a portion of gingival connective tissue (G) and alveolar mucosal connective tissue (AM) which, after a particular transplantation, has healed into wound areas in the alveolar mucosa. Epithelialization of these transplants can only occur through migration of epithelial cells from the surrounding alveolar mucosa.

Fig. 1-53 shows the transplanted gingival connective tissue (G) after reepithelialization. This tissue portion has attained an appearance similar to that of the normal gingiva, indicating that this connective tissue is now covered by keratinized epithelium. The transplanted connective tissue from the alveolar mucosa (AM) is covered by nonkeratinized epithelium and has the same appearance as the surrounding alveolar mucosa.

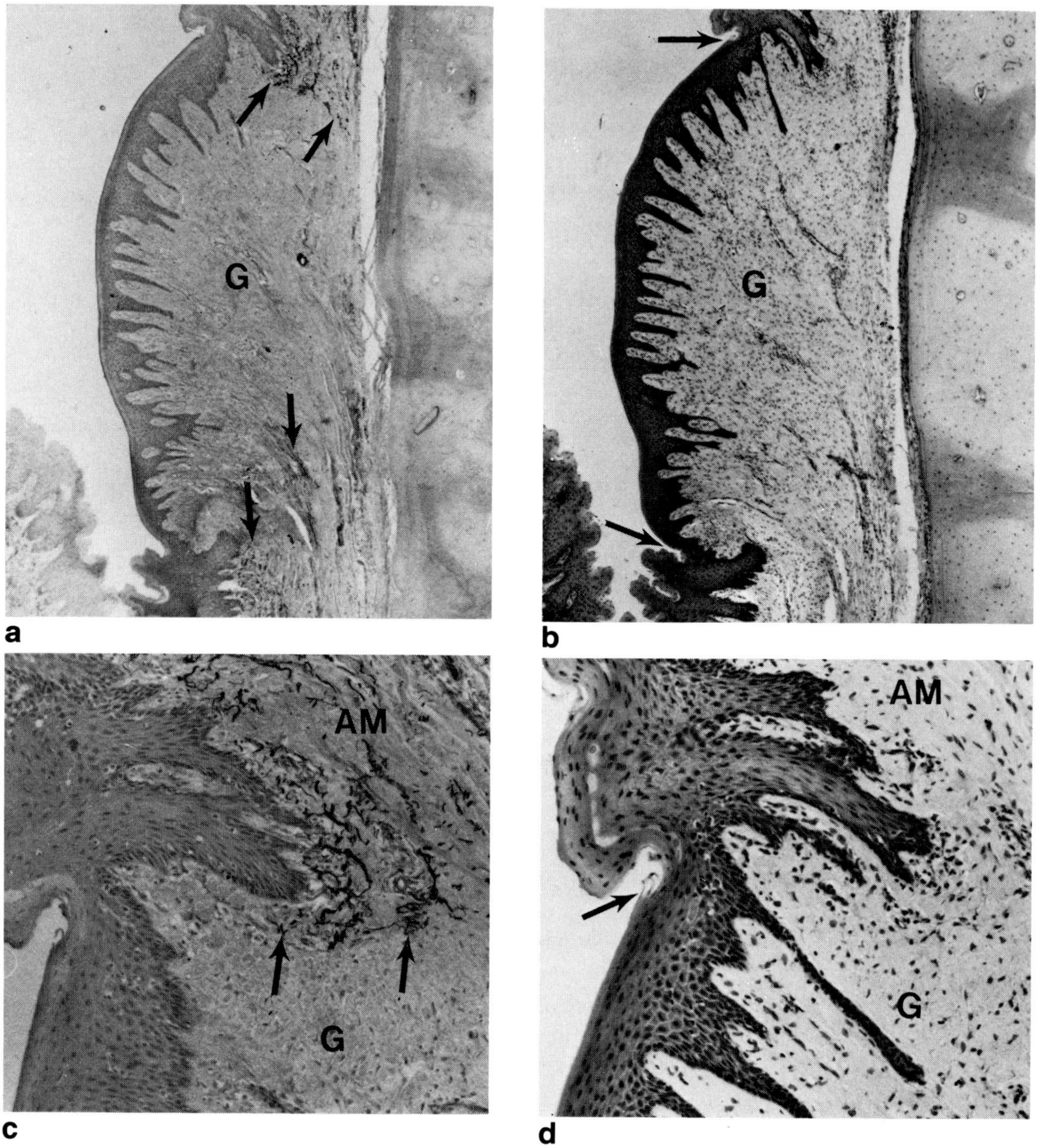

Fig. 1-54.

Fig. 1-54 presents 2 histological sections through the area of the transplanted gingival connective tissue. The section shown in Fig. 1-54a is stained for elastic fibers (arrows). The tissue in the middle is the transplanted gingival connective tissue (G). Fig. 1-54b shows an adjacent section stained with hematoxylin and eosin. By comparing Figs. 1-54 a and b it can be seen that:

1) the transplanted gingival connective tissue is covered by keratinized epithelium (between arrows)
2) the epithelium-connective tissue interface

has the same wavy course (i.e. rete pegs and connective tissue papillae) as seen in normal gingiva.

The photomicrographs seen in Figs. 1-54c and 1-54d illustrate, at a higher magnification, the border area between the alveolar mucosa (AM) and the transplanted gingival connective tissue (G). Note the distinct relationship between keratinized epithelium and "inelastic" connective tissue, and between nonkeratinized epithelium and "elastic" connective tissue (arrows). This relationship implies that the transplanted gingival connective tissue possesses the ability to alter the differentiation of epithelial cells as previously suggested (Fig. 1-51). From being nonkeratinizing cells, the cells of the epithelium of the alveolar mucosa have evidently become keratinizing cells. *This means that the specificity of the gingival epithelium is determined by genetical factors inherent in the connective tissue.*

The periodontal ligament

The periodontal ligament is the soft, richly vascular and cellular connective tissue which surrounds the roots of the teeth and joins the root cementum with the alveolar bone proper. In the coronal direction, the periodontal ligament is continuous with the lamina propria of the gingiva and is separated from the gingiva by the collagen fiber bundles which connect the alveolar bone crest with the root (the alveolar crest fibers).

Fig. 1-55 is a radiograph of a mandibular premolar-molar region. The periodontal ligament is included in the space between the roots (R) of the teeth and the alveolar bone proper

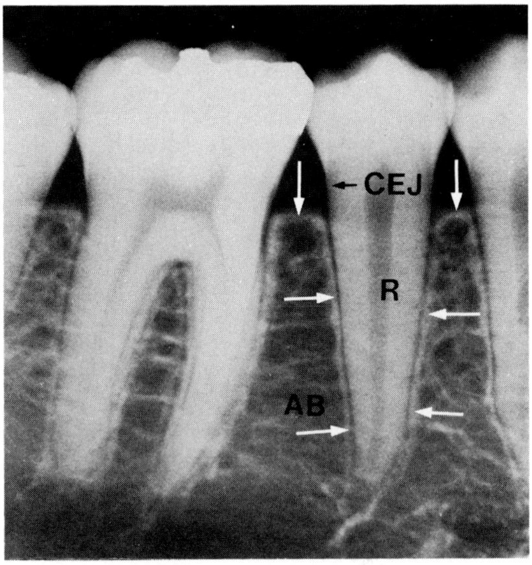

Fig. 1-55.

(ABP; lamina dura). The alveolar bone surrounds the tooth to a level approximately 1 mm apical to the cementoenamel junction (CEJ). In radiographs, two types of alveolar bone can be distinguished: (1) The part of the alveolar bone which covers the alveolus, also called the cortical bone, and sometimes referred to as "lamina dura" (arrows); (2) The portion of the alveolar process which, in the radiograph, has the appearance of a meshwork. This is also called the spongy bone; the periodontal ligament communicates via the alveolar bone proper with the marrow spaces of the alveolar bone. The periodontal ligament space has the shape of an hourglass and is narrowest at the mid-root level. The width of the periodontal ligament is approximately 0.25 mm ± 50%. The presence of a periodontal ligament makes it possible to distribute and resorb forces, elicited during function, into the alveolar process via the alveolar bone proper. The periodontal ligament is also essential for the mobility of the teeth. Tooth mobility is to a large extent (see Chapter 12) determined by the width, height and quality of the periodontal ligament.

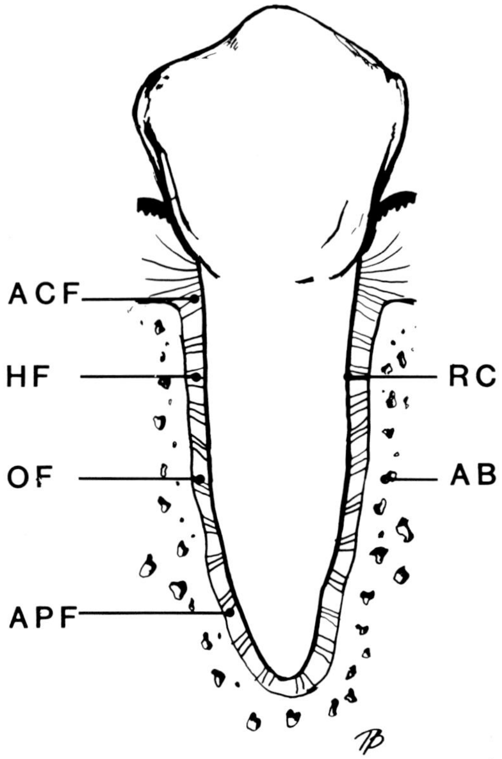

Fig. 1-56.

Fig. 1-56 illustrates in a schematic drawing how the periodontal ligament is positioned between the alveolar bone proper (ABP) and the root cementum (RC). The tooth is joined to the bone by bundles of collagen fibers which can be divided into the following main groups:

1) Alveolar crest fibers (ACF)
2) Horizontal fibers (HF)
3) Oblique fibers (OF)
4) Apical fibers (APF)

Fig. 1-57. The periodontal ligament and the root cementum develop from the loose connective tissue (the follicle) which surrounds the tooth bud. The schematic drawing depicts the various stages in the organization of the periodontal ligament which forms concomitantly with the development of the root and the eruption of the tooth.

a) The tooth bud is formed in a crypt of the bone. The collagen fibers produced by the fibroblasts in the loose connective tissue of the tooth bud are, during the process of their maturation, embedded into the newly formed cementum immediately apical to the cemento-enamel junction (CEJ). The fibers fasciculate, oriented towards the coronal portion of the bone crypt. These fiber bundles will later form the *dentogingival fiber group,* the *dentoperiosteal fiber group* and the *transseptal fiber group* which belong to the oriented fibers of the gingiva (see Fig. 1-44).
b) The true periodontal ligament fibers, the *principal fibers* develop in conjunction with the eruption of the tooth. First fibers can be identified which are entering the most marginal portion of the alveolar bone.
c) Later, more apically positioned bundles of oriented collagen fibers are seen.
d) The orientation of the collagen fiber bundles alters continuously during the phase of the tooth eruption. First, when the tooth has reached contact in occlusion and is in proper function, the fibers of the periodontal ligament associate into groups of well oriented *dentoalveolar collagen fibers:*

   1) Alveolar crest fibers (ACF)
   2) Horizontal fibers (HF)
   3) Oblique fibers (OF)
   4) Apical fibers (APF) (see Fig. 1-56).

Fig. 1-58. This schematic drawing illustrates the development of the principal fibers of the periodontal ligament. The alveolar bone proper (ABP) is seen to the left, the periodontal ligament (PL) is depicted in the center and the root cementum (RC) is seen to the right.

a) First small, fine, brush-like fibrils are detected arising from the root cementum and projecting into the PL space. The surface of the bone is, at this stage, covered by osteoblasts. From the surface of the bone only a

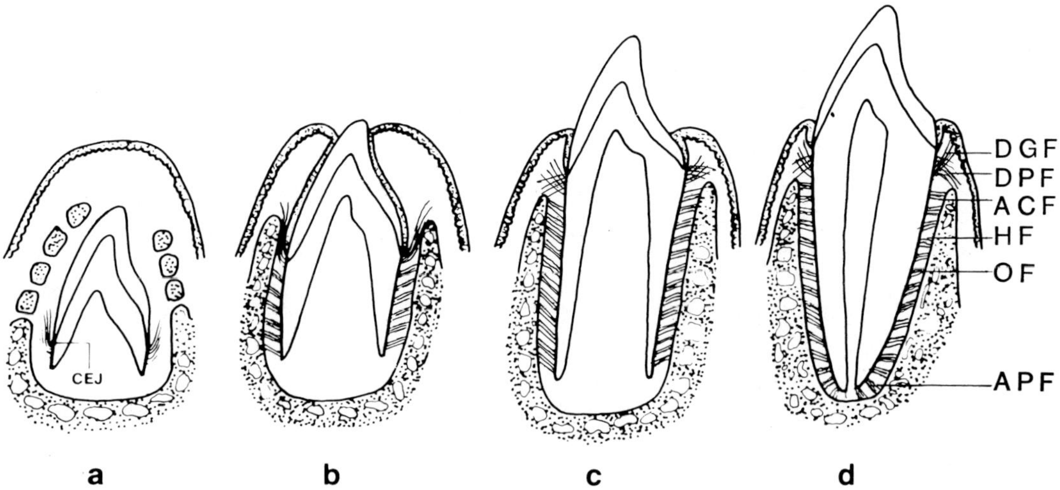

Fig. 1-57.

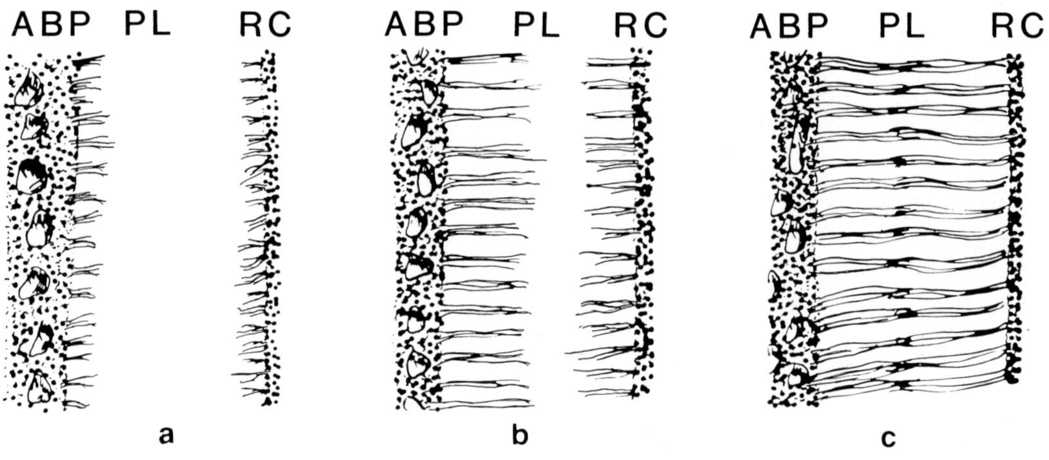

Fig. 1-58.

small number of radiating, thin, collagen fibrils can be seen.

b) Later on, the number and thickness of fibers entering the bone increase. These fibers radiate towards the loose connective tissue in the mid-portion of the periodontal ligament area (PL), which contains more or less randomly oriented collagen fibrils. The fibers originating from the cementum are still short while those entering the bone gradually become longer. The terminal portions of these fibers carry finger-like projections.

c) The fibers originating from the cementum subsequently increase in length and thickness and fuse in the periodontal membrane space with the fibers originating from the alveolar bone. When the tooth, following eruption, reaches contact in occlusion and starts to function, the principal fibers become organized in bundles and run continuously from the bone to the cementum.

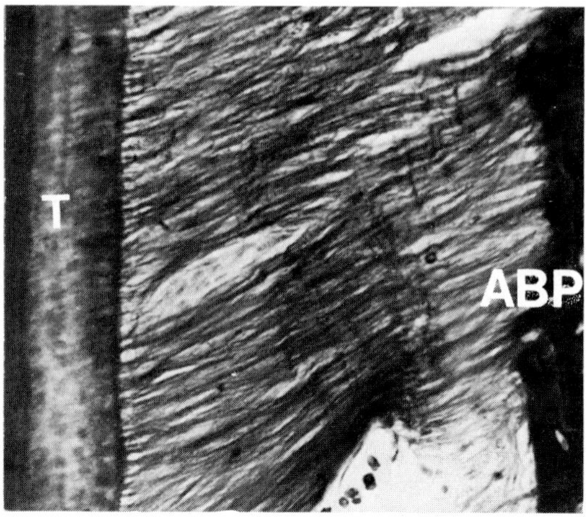

Fig. 1-59.

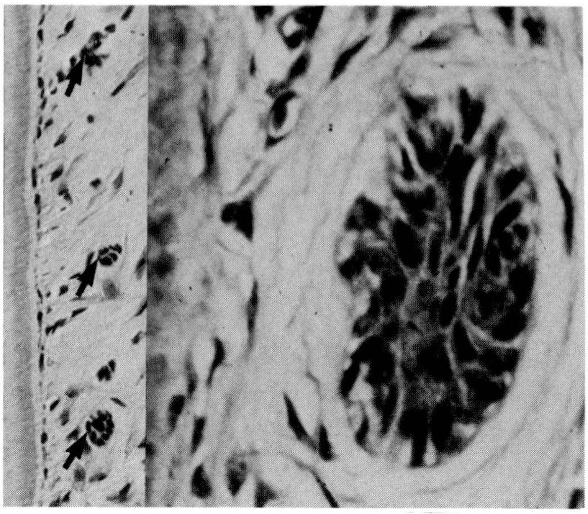

Fig. 1-60a. Fig. 1-60b.

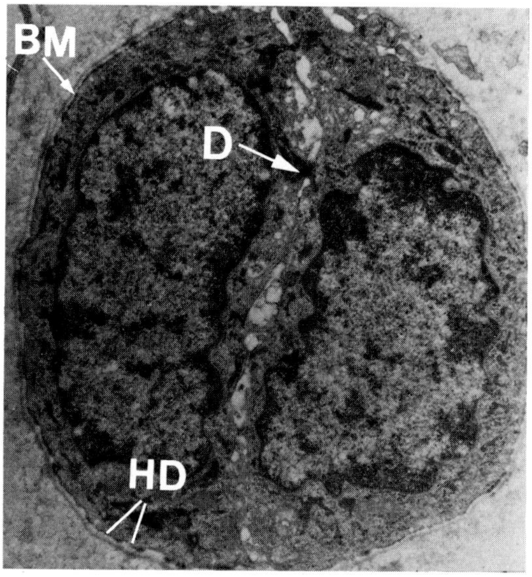

Fig. 1-61.

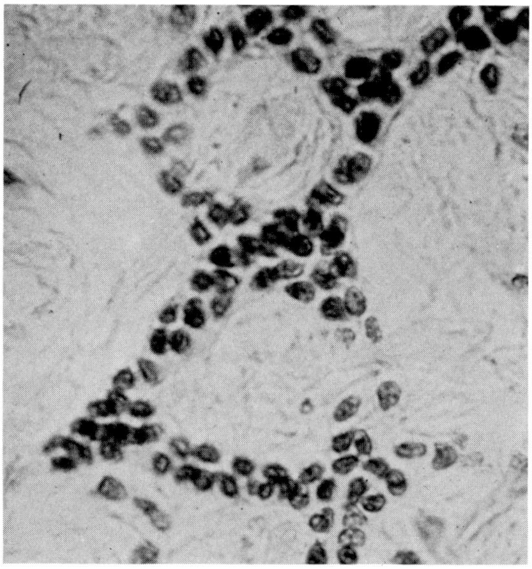

Fig. 1-62.

Fig. 1-59 illustrates how the principal fibers of the periodontal ligament run continuously from the tooth (T) to the alveolar bone proper (ABP). The individual bundles have a slightly wavy course which allows the tooth to move within its socket - physiological mobility. The principal fibers, embedded in the cementum, have a smaller diameter but are more numerous than those embedded in the alveolar bone. The cells of the periodontal ligament are: fibroblasts, osteoblasts, cementoblasts, osteoclasts, as well as epithelial cells and nerve cells.

Fig. 1-60a shows the presence of small clusters of epithelial cells (arrows) in the periodontal ligament. These cells, called the epithelial cell "*rests of Mallassez*", represent remnants of the *epithelial sheath of Hertwig*. The "rests of Mallassez" are situated in the periodontal ligament at a distance of 15-75 μm from the root surface. A group of such cells is seen in a higher magnification in *Fig. 1-60b*.

Fig. 1-61. Electron microscopically it can be seen that the "rests of Mallassez" are surrounded by a basement membrane (BM) and that the cell membranes of the epithelial cells exhibit the presence of desmosomes (D) as well as hemidesmosomes (HD). The epithelial cells contain only few mitochondria and have a poorly developed endoplasmic reticulum. This means that they are vital, but resting, cells with minute metabolism.

Fig. 1-62 is a photomicrograph of a periodontal ligament removed from an extracted tooth. The "rests of Mallassez", which in ordinary histological sections appear as isolated groups of epithelial cells, form, in this specimen, a continuous network of epithelial cells surrounding the root; their function is presently unknown.

The root cementum

The cementum is a specialized calcified tissue covering the root surfaces and, occasionally, small portions of the crown of the teeth. It has many features in common with bone tissue; however, the cementum (1) contains no blood or lymph vessels, (2) has no innervation, (3) does not undergo physiological resorption and remodelling, but *is* characterized by continuing deposition throughout life. Cementum serves different functions. It attaches the periodontal ligament fibers to the root and contributes to the process of repair after damage to the root surface. Two different types of cementum are recognized:

1) *primary cementum* or *acellular cementum* which forms in conjunction with root formation and tooth eruption
2) *secondary cementum* or *cellular cementum* which forms after tooth eruption and in response to functional demands.

Fig. 1-63 shows a portion of the periodontal ligament. The root cementum (RC) which is in contact with the root dentin to the left is called the *primary cementum.* This primary cementum contains no cells and is thus also denoted *acellular cementum.* This primary or acellular

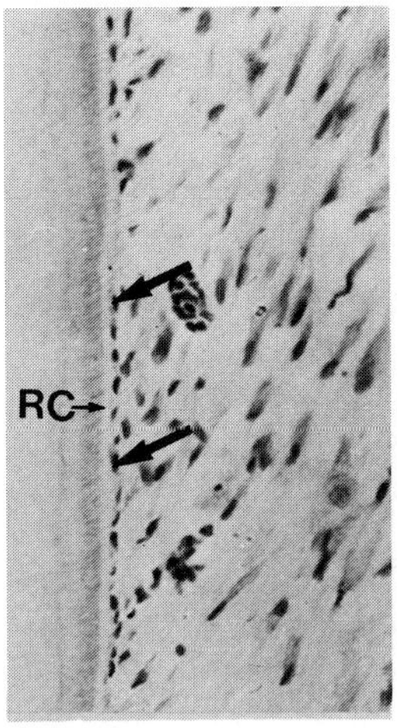

Fig. 1-63.

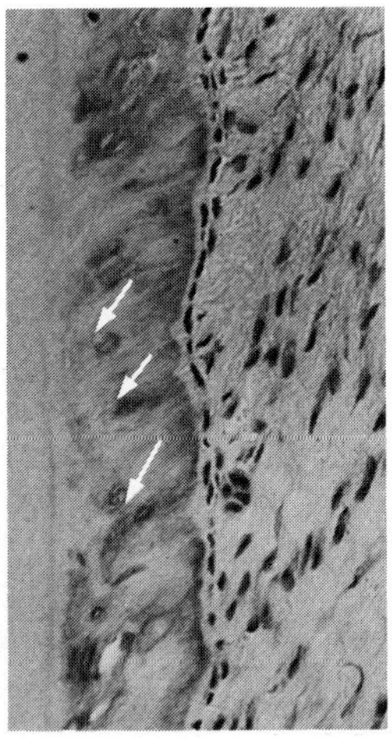

Fig. 1-64.

cementum is formed concomitantly with the formation of the root dentin and in the presence of the epithelial sheath of Hertwig. At a certain stage during tooth formation the epithelial sheath of Hertwig, which lines the newly formed predentin, is broken. The epithelial cells migrate into the loose connective tissue lateral of the tooth bud. Fibroblasts from this loose connective tissue occupy the area next to the predentin and produce a layer of randomly oriented collagen fibrils which make contact with, but do not enter, the newly formed dentin. The fibroblasts differentiate into cementoblasts and remain on the lateral surface of the cementoid.

Fig. 1-64 describes the structure of the *secondary cementum* which, in contrast to the primary cementum, contains cells. This structure is also called *cellular cementum.* Secondary or cellular cementum is laid down on top of the primary cementum throughout the functional period of the tooth. It is often only found on the intra-alveolar part of the root. Both cellular and acellular cementum are produced by cementoblasts. Some of these cells (arrows) become incorporated into the cementoid which subsequently calcifies to form cementum. The cells which are incorporated in the cementum are called *cementocytes.*

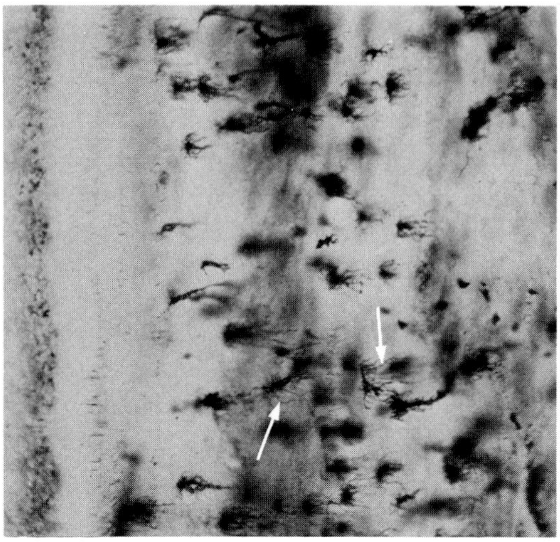

Fig. 1-65.

Fig. 1-65 illustrates how cementocytes (black cells) reside in lacunae in cellular cementum. They are linked together by cytoplasmic processes (arrows) running in canaliculi in the cementum. The cementocytes are also, via cytoplasmic processes, linked with the cementoblasts on the surface. The presence of cementocytes allows transportation of nutrients through the cementum, and contributes to the maintenance of the vitality of this mineralized tissue.

Fig. 1-66a is a photomicrograph of a horizontal section through the periodontal ligament (PL) in an area where the root is covered with acellular cementum (AC). The portions of the principal fibers which are embedded in the root cementum and in the alveolar bone (AB) are called *Sharpey's fibers*. A major portion of the acellular cementum consists of Sharpey's fiber bundles which have become mineralized. In the photomicrograph it can be seen that these often start close to the cemento-dentin junction (arrows). In the acellular cementum they have a smaller diameter and are more densely packed than those in the alveolar bone. During the continuous formation of acellular cementum portions of the periodontal ligament fibers (principal fibers) adjacent to the root become embedded with mineral crystals, i.e. mineralized.

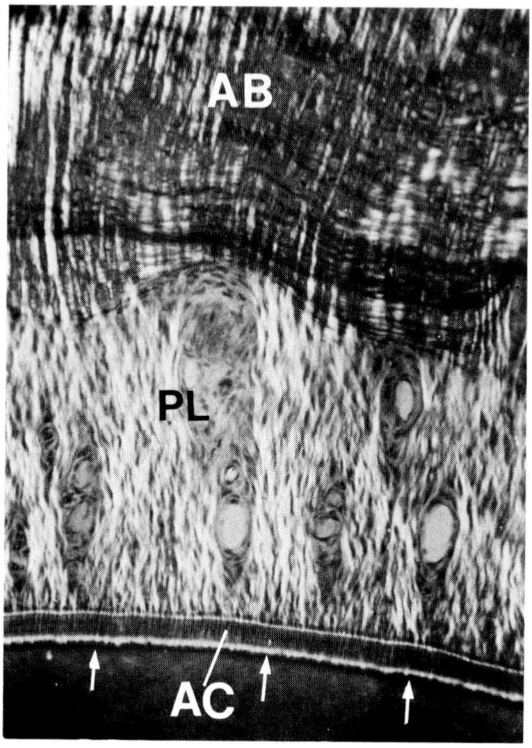

Fig. 1-66a.

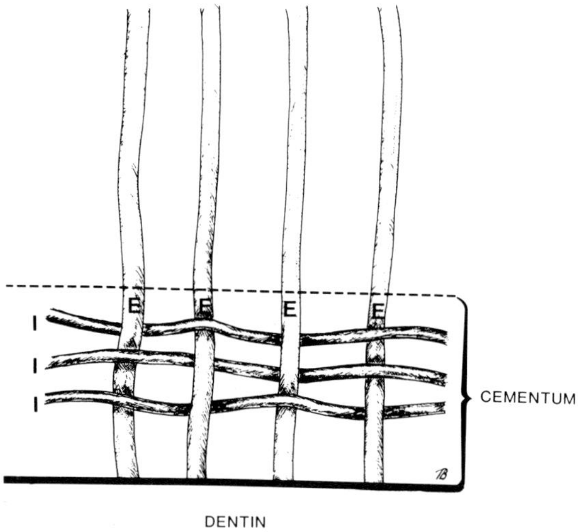

Fig. 1-66b.

Thus, the Sharpey's fibers in the cementum should be regarded as a direct continuation of the collagen fibers in the supraalveolar connective tissue and the periodontal ligament (Fig. 1-66b). The Sharpey's fibers form the so-called

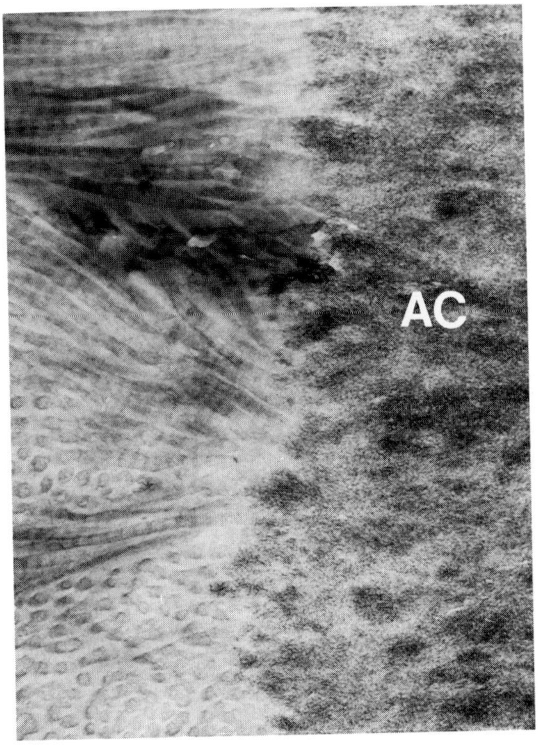

Fig. 1-67.

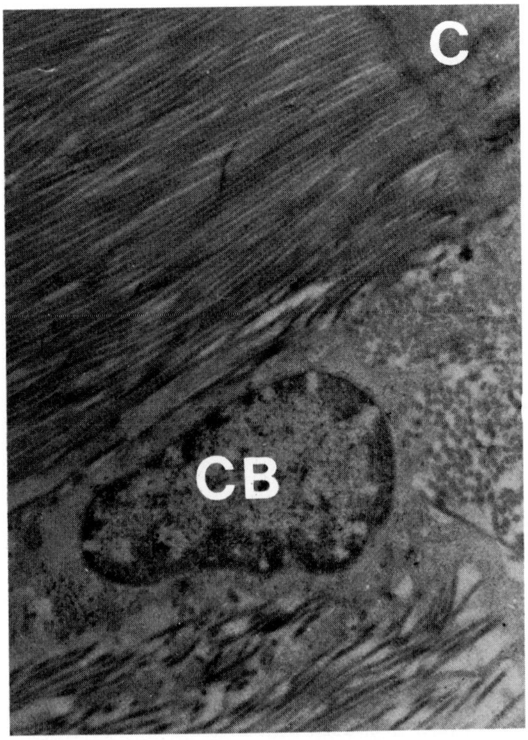

Fig. 1-68.

extrinsic fiber system (E) of the cementum and are produced by fibroblasts in the periodontal ligament. The *intrinsic fiber system* (I) is produced by cementoblasts and is composed of fibers oriented more or less parallel to the long axis of the root.

Fig. 1-67 shows principal fibers entering acellular cementum (AC). The characteristic cross-banding of the collagen fibers is masked in the cementum because apatite crystals have become deposited in the fiber bundles during the process of mineralization.

Fig. 1-68. In contrast to the bone, the cementum (C) contains no nerves and no blood or lymph vessels. The cementum does not exhibit alternating periods of resorption and apposition, but increases in thickness throughout life by deposition of successive new layers of tissue. During this process of gradual apposition, the particular portion of the principal fibers which resides immediately adjacent to the root surface becomes calcified. Mineralization occurs by the deposition of hydroxyapatite crystals, first within the collagen fibers, later upon the fiber surface and finally in the interfibrillar matrix. Fig. 1-68 shows a cementoblast (CB) located near the surface of the cementum and between 2 inserting principal fiber bundles. Generally the acellular cementum is more mineralized than the cellular cementum. Sometimes only the periphery of the Sharpey's fibers of the *cellular cementum* is calcified, leaving an uncalcified core within the fiber.

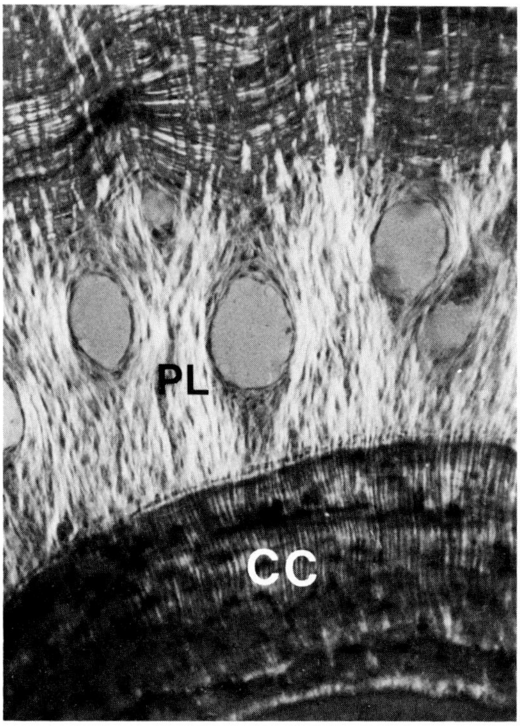

Fig. 1-69.

Fig. 1-69 is a photomicrograph showing a horizontal section through the periodontal ligament (PL) in an area where the root surface is covered with cellular cementum (CC). This cementum, which is formed after the termination of tooth eruption and often in response to functional demands, is densely packed with coarse collagen fibrils oriented parallel to the root surface (intrinsic fiber system) and Sharpey's fibers (extrinsic fiber system) which run more or less perpendicularly to the cementodentin junction. These Sharpey's fibers, which are thicker and more dispersed than those in the acellular cementum, continue as principal fibers, undisrupted from the cementum into the periodontal ligament. The cementoid on the surface increases in thickness by gradual apposition throughout life and is considerably more pronounced in the apical portion of the root than in the cervical portion where the thickness is only 20-50 μm. In the apical root portion the cementoid is often 150-250 μm thick.

The alveolar bone

The alveolar process is defined as the parts of the maxilla and the mandible that form and support the sockets of the teeth. The alveolar process develops in conjunction with the development and eruption of the teeth and is gradually resorbed if the teeth are lost. The alveolar process consists of bone which is formed both by cells from the dental follicle (alveolar bone proper) and cells which are independent of tooth development. Together with the root cementum and the periodontal membrane, the alveolar bone constitutes the attachment apparatus for the teeth, the main function of which is to distribute and resorb forces generated by e.g. mastication and other tooth contacts.

Fig. 1-70 illustrates a cross-section through the alveolar process of the maxilla at the mid-root level of the teeth. Note that the bone which covers the root surfaces is considerably thicker at the palatal than at the buccal aspect of the jaw. The walls of the sockets are lined by *compact* bone (arrows) which interproximally is connected with mainly *cancellous* bone. The cancellous bone contains bone trabeculae, the architecture and size of which are partly genetically determined and partly the result of the forces to which the teeth are exposed during function.

Fig. 1-71 shows cross-sections through the mandibular alveolar process (pars alveolaris) at levels corresponding to the coronal (1) and apical (2) thirds of the roots. The bone lining the wall of the sockets (alveolar bone proper) is often continuous with the compact or cortical bone at the lingual (L) and buccal (B) aspects of the alveolar process (arrows).

Note how the bone on the buccal and lingual aspects of the alveolar process varies in thickness from one region to another. In the incisor and premolar regions, the cortical bone plate at

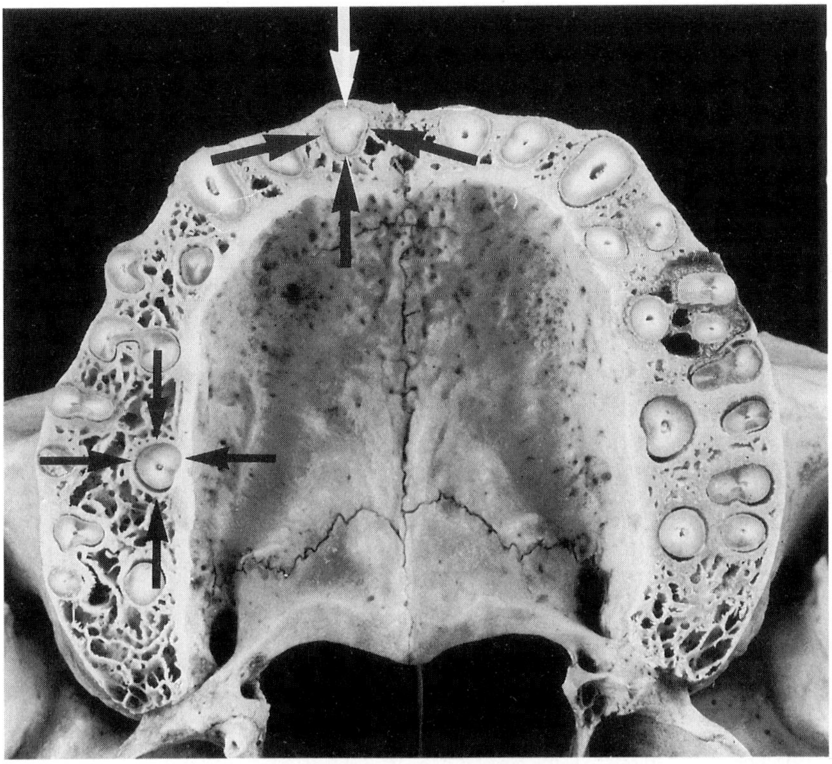

Fig. 1-70.

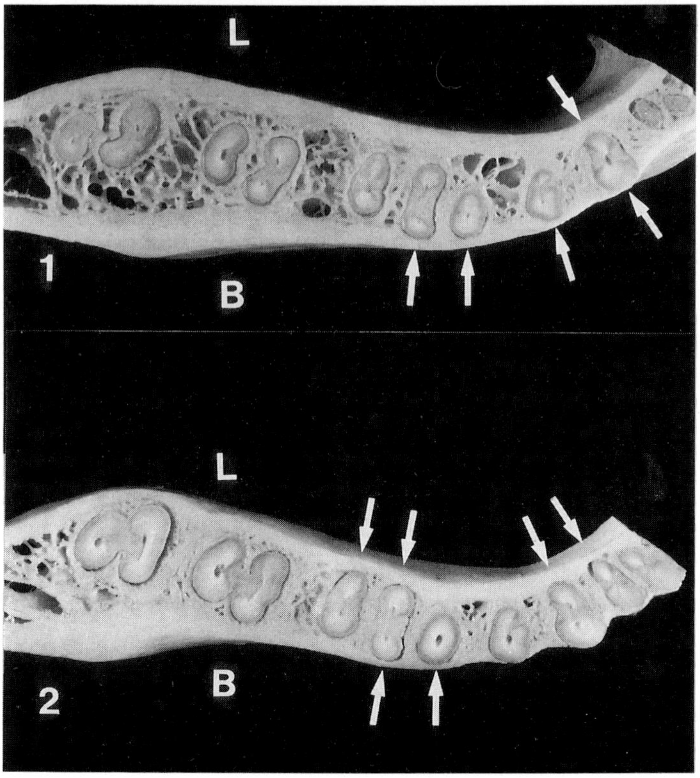

Fig. 1-71.

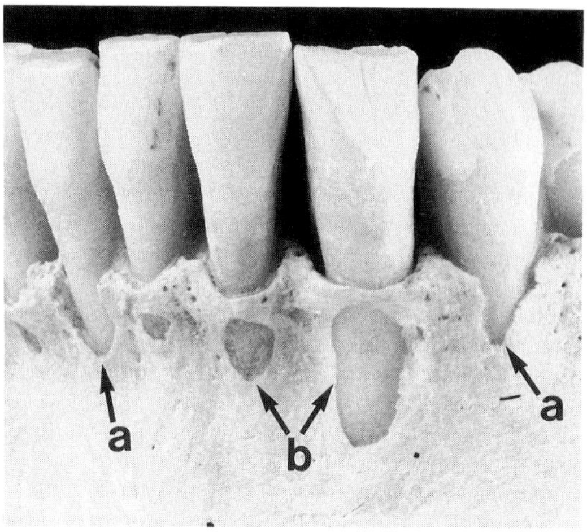

Fig. 1-72.

the buccal aspects of the teeth is considerably thinner than at the lingual aspect. In the molar region, the bone is thicker at the buccal than at the lingual surfaces.

Fig. 1-72. At the buccal aspect of the jaws the bone coverage is sometimes missing at the coronal portion of the roots, forming a so-called dehiscense. If some bone is present in the most coronal portion of such an area the defect is called a fenestration.

Fig. 1-73 presents vertical sections through various regions of the mandibular dentition. The bone wall at the buccal (B) and lingual (L) aspects of the teeth varies considerably in thickness, e.g. from the premolar to the molar region. Note, for instance; how the presence of the oblique line (*linea obliqua*) results in a shelf-like bone process (arrows) at the buccal aspect of the second and third molars.

Fig. 1-74 shows a section through the periodontal ligament (PL), tooth (T), and the alveolar bone (AB). The compact bone, that in a radiograph (Fig. 1-55) appears as "lamina dura" (LD), lines the tooth socket and is perforated by numerous *Volkmann's canals* (arrows) through which blood vessels and nerves pass from the alveolar bone (AB) to the periodontal ligament (PL). The layer of bone into which the Sharpey's fiber bundles are inserted is called "*bundle bone*" (alveolar bone proper) and lies at the inner surface of the bony wall of the socket. Thus, from a functional point of view this "bundle bone" has many features in common with the cementum layer on the root surfaces.

Fig. 1-75. The alveolar process starts to form early in fetal life, with mineral deposition at small foci in the mesenchymal matrix surrounding the tooth buds. These small calcified areas increase in size, fuse, become resorbed and remodelled until a continuous mass of

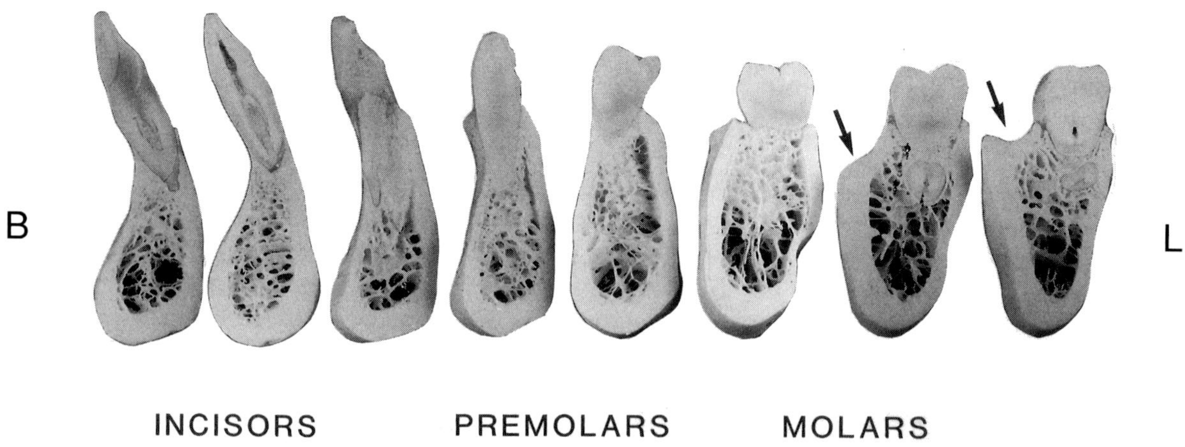

Fig. 1-73.

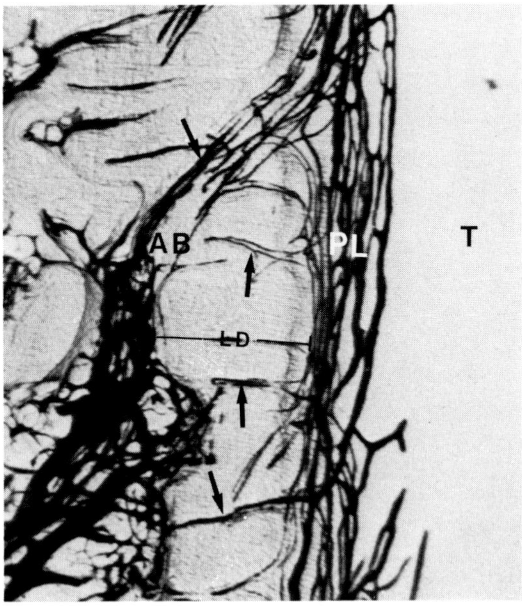

Fig. 1-74.

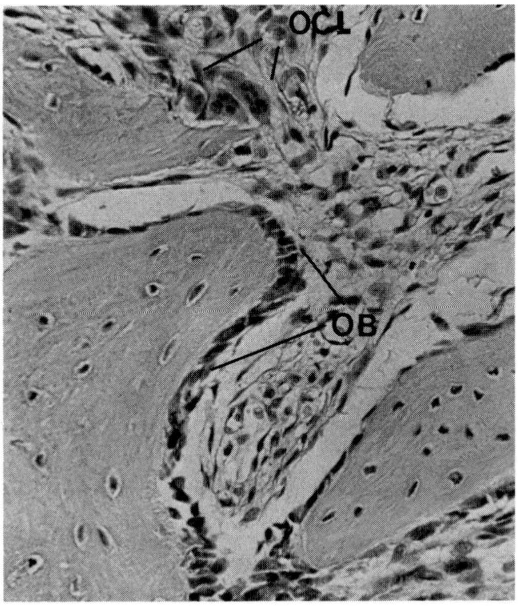

Fig. 1-75.

bone has formed around the fully erupted teeth. The outer surface of the bone is always lined with a nonmineralized zone of tissue, an *osteoid* which in turn is covered by the *periosteum*. The periosteum contains *collagen fibers*, *osteoblasts* and *osteoclasts*. The marrow spaces inside the bone are lined with *endosteum* which has many features in common with the periosteum at the outer surface of the bone. The photomicrograph in Fig. 1-75 illustrates the presence of bone forming osteoblasts (OB) and bone resorbing osteoclasts (OCL) in the endosteum.

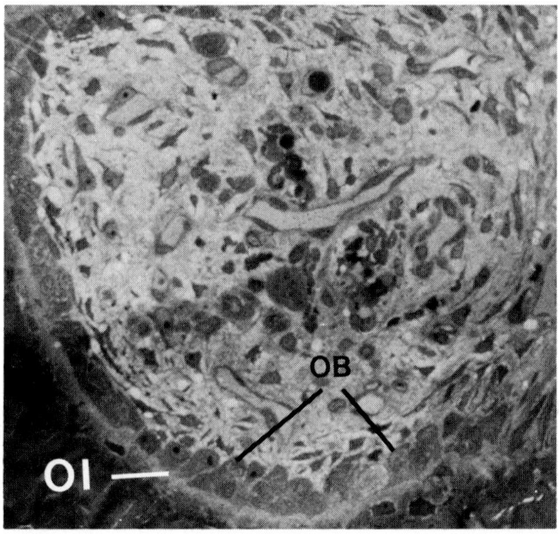

Fig. 1-76.

Fig. 1-76. Osteoblasts and osteoclasts are present in the following areas:

1) On the surface of the bone trabeculae in cancellous bone
2) On the outer surface of cortical bone which delineates the jaws
3) In the sockets towards the periodontal membrane
4) On the inside of the cortical bone towards the marrow spaces.

In the photomicrograph of Fig. 1-76 osteoblasts (OB) reside on the surface of a bone trabecula. The osteoblasts produce osteoid (OI) consisting of collagen fibers and a matrix which contains mainly glycoproteins and proteoglycans. This bone matrix or osteoid (OI) undergoes calcification by the deposition of minerals which are subsequently transformed to hydroxyapatite.

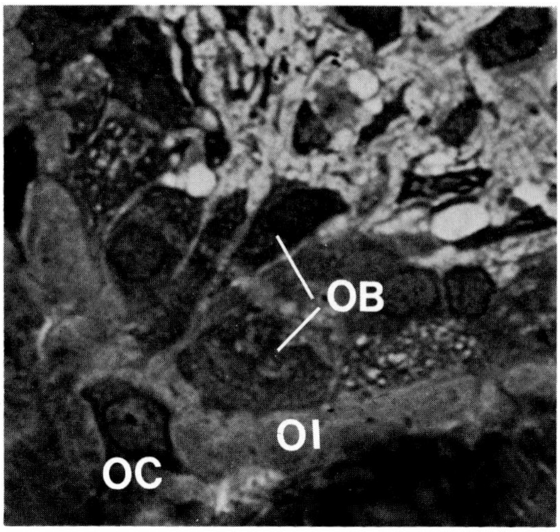

Fig. 1-77.

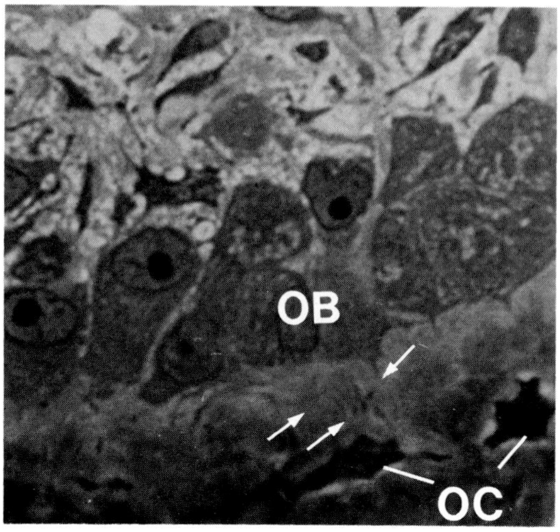

Fig. 1-78.

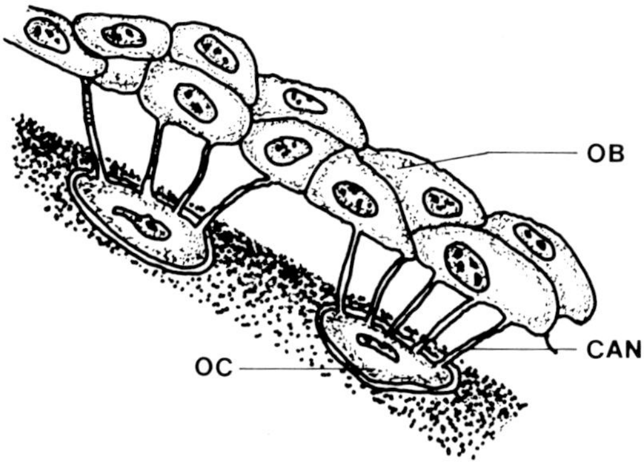

Fig. 1-79.

Fig. 1-77. During the process of maturation and calcification of the osteoid some of the osteoblasts (OB) are trapped in the osteoid (OI) as seen in this photomicrograph. Cells which are present in the osteoid, and later on in the calcified bone tissue, are termed *osteocytes* (OC).

Fig. 1-78. Osteocytes (OC) resident in lacunae in calcified bone are linked to each other and to osteoblasts on the bone surface through cyto-

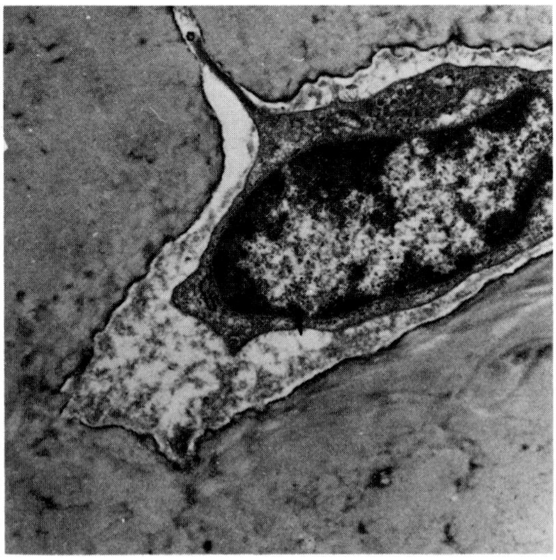

Fig. 1-80.

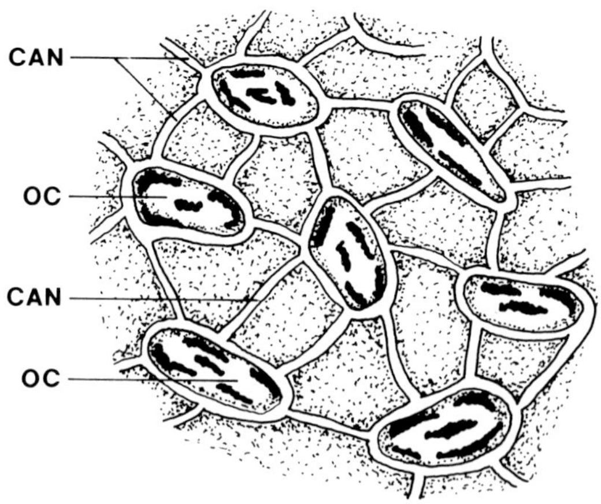

Fig. 1-81.

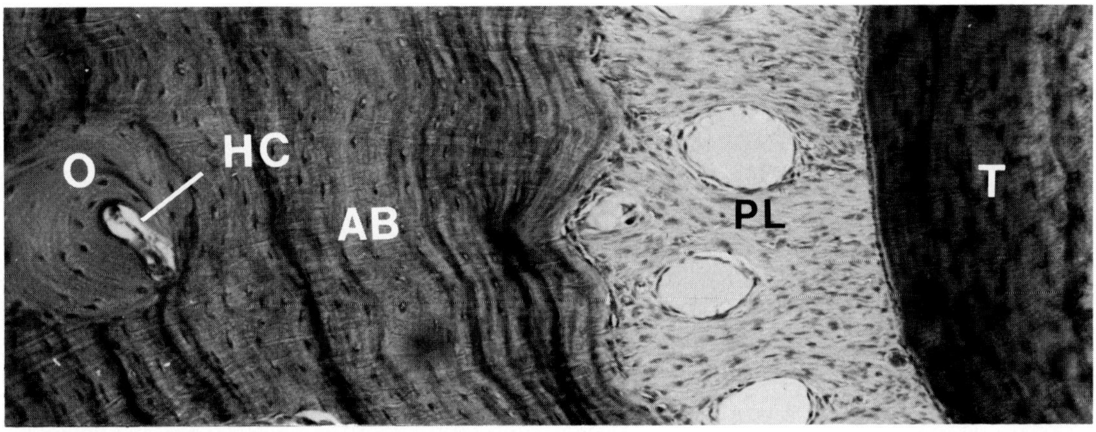

Fig. 1-82.

plasmic processes running in canaliculi (arrows). The drawing in *Fig. 1-79* illustrates how osteoblasts (OB) and osteocytes (OC) are linked to each other by cytoplasmic processes running in canaliculi (CAN).

Fig. 1-80 illustrates an osteocyte residing in a lacuna in the bone. The cytoplasmic processes radiate in different directions.

Fig. 1-81 illustrates how the osteocytes (OC) make contact with each other via cytoplasmic processes running in canaliculi (CAN) in the bone. The surface between the osteocytes with their cytoplasmic processes on the one side, and the calcified matrix on the other, is very large. It has been calculated that the interface between cells and matrix in a cube of bone, 10×10×10 cm, amounts to approximately 250 m^2. This enormous surface of exchange serves as a regulator, e.g. for the serum calcium and the serum phosphate levels via hormonal control mechanisms.

Fig. 1-82 shows a horizontal section through the alveolar bone (AB), periodontal ligament (PL) and tooth (T). The nutrition of the bone is secured by the incorporation of blood vessels in the bone tissue. These blood vessels surrounded by bone lamellae, eventually constitute the center of an *osteon* (O). The central canal (which mainly contains the blood vessel) in an osteon is called the *Haversian canal* (HC). The osteon is also called a *Haversian system*. The blood vessels in the *Haversian canals* are connected with each other by anastomoses running in the *Volkmann's canals*. The alveolar bone is continually renewed in response to functional demands. The teeth erupt and migrate in mesial direction throughout life to compensate for attrition. Such movement of the teeth implies remodelling of the alveolar bone. During the process of remodelling, the bone trabeculae are continuously resorbed and reformed and the cortical bone mass is dissolved and replaced by new bone. During breakdown of the cortical bone, resorption canals are formed by proliferating blood vessels. Such canals, which in their center contain a blood vessel, are subsequently refilled with new bone by the formation of lamellae arranged in concentric layers around the blood vessel. Thus, a new *Haversian system* (O), as seen in the photomicrograph, is established.

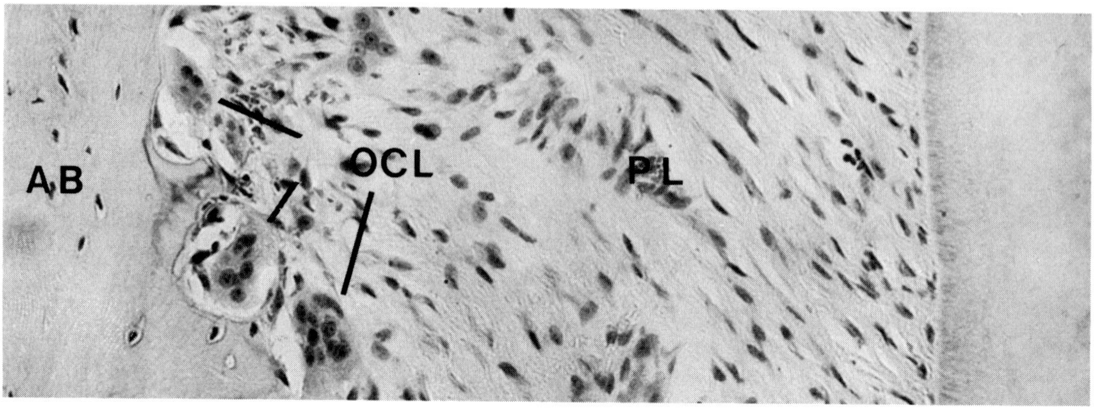

Fig. 1-83.

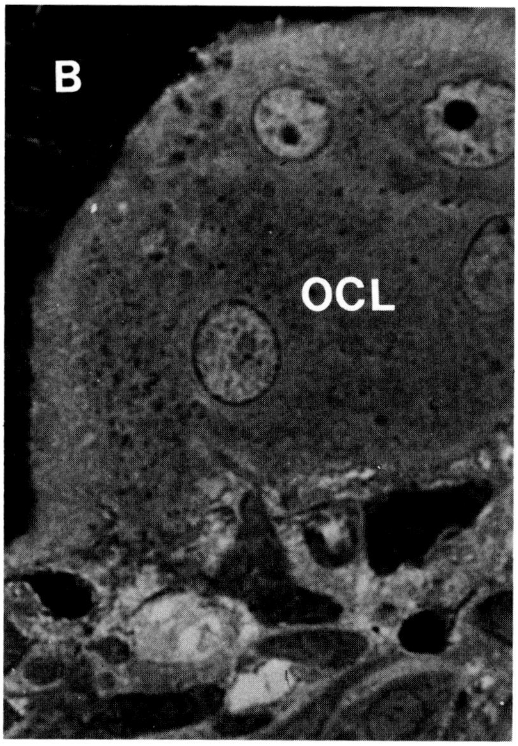

Fig. 1-84.

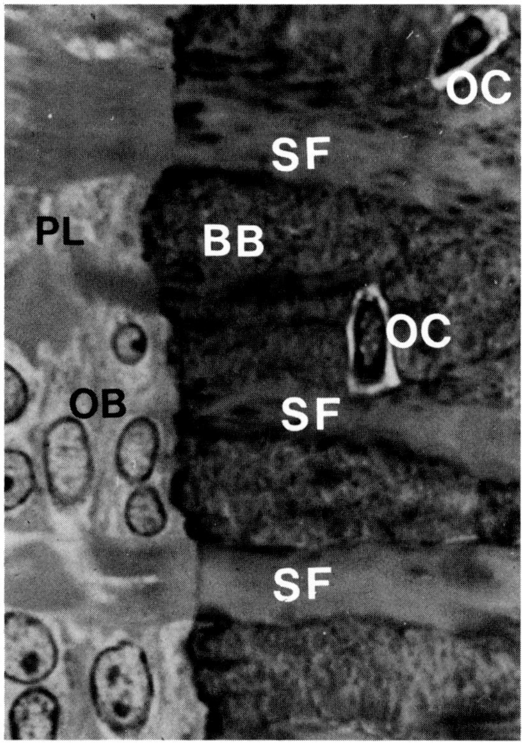

Fig. 1-85.

Fig. 1-83. The apposition of new bone is always associated with osteoblasts. These cells produce an osteoid which subsequently undergoes calcification. Osteolysis (i.e. breakdown of bone) is an active cellular process associated with osteoclasts, probably developed from blood monocytes. The photomicrograph demonstrates osteoclastic activity at the surface of the bone (AB) facing the periodontal ligament (PL). The osteoclasts (OCL) are multinucleated cells which frequently reside in so-called *Howship's lacunae* on the bone surface.

Fig. 1-84 shows an osteoclast (OCL) residing in a *Howship's lacuna* on the surface of the bone (B). The osteoclast resorbs organic as well as inorganic substances. The resorption occurs by the release of acid substances (lactic acid, etc.) which form an acidic environment in which the mineral salts of the bone tissue become dissolved. Remaining organic substances are eliminated by osteoclastic phagocytosis.

Fig. 1-85. Collagen fibers of the periodontal ligament (PL) are inserting in the mineralized bone which lines the wall of the tooth socket. This bone, which as previously described is called *bundle bone* (BB), has a high turnover rate. The portions of the collagen fibers which are inserted inside the bundle bone are called Sharpey's fibers (SF). These fibers are mineralized at their periphery, but often have a nonmineralized central core. The collagen fiber bundles inserting in the bundle bone generally have a larger diameter and are less numerous than the corresponding fiber bundles in the cementum on the opposite side of the periodontal ligament. Individual bundles of fibers can be followed all the way from the alveolar bone to the cementum. However, despite being in the same bundle of fibers, the collagen adjacent to the bone is always less mature than that adjacent to the cementum. The collagen on the tooth side has a low turn-over rate. Thus, while the collagen adjacent to the bone is renewed relatively rapidly, the collagen adjacent to the root surface is renewed slowly or not at all.

Note the occurrence of osteoblasts (OB) and osteocytes (OC).

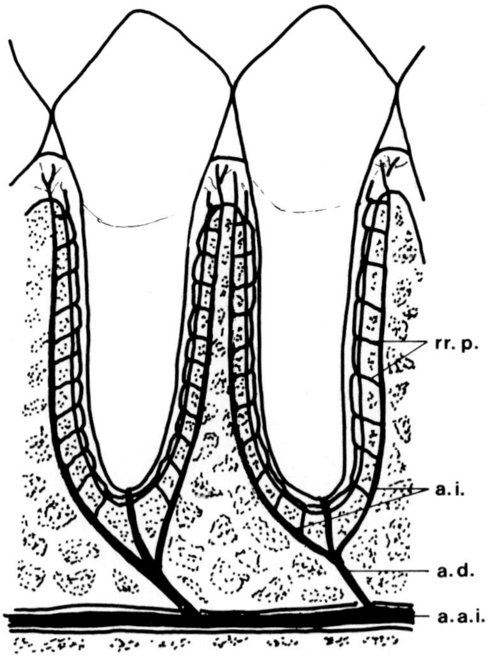

Fig. 1-86.

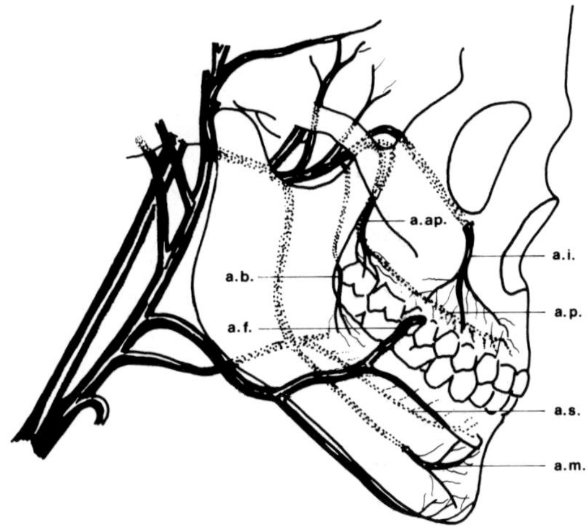

Fig. 1-87.

The blood supply of the periodontium

Fig. 1-86. The schematic drawing depicts the blood supply to the teeth and the periodontal tissues. The *dental artery* (a.d.) which is a branch of the *superior* or *inferior alveolar (dental) artery* (a.a.i.) dismisses the *intraseptal artery* (a.i.) before it enters the tooth socket. The terminal branches of the intraseptal artery (*rami perforantes,* rr.p.) penetrate the lamina dura in canals at all levels of the socket. They anastomose in the periodontal ligament space, together with blood vessels originating from the apical portion of the periodontal ligament and with other terminal branches, from the intraseptal artery (a.i.). Before the dental artery (a.d.) enters the root canal it puts out branches which supply the apical portion of the periodontal ligament.

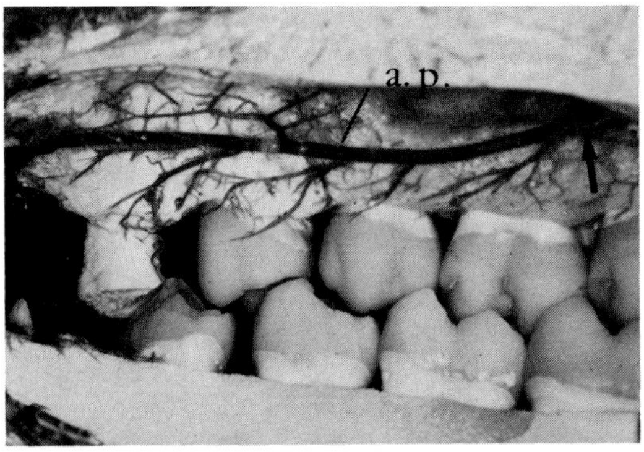

Fig. 1-88.

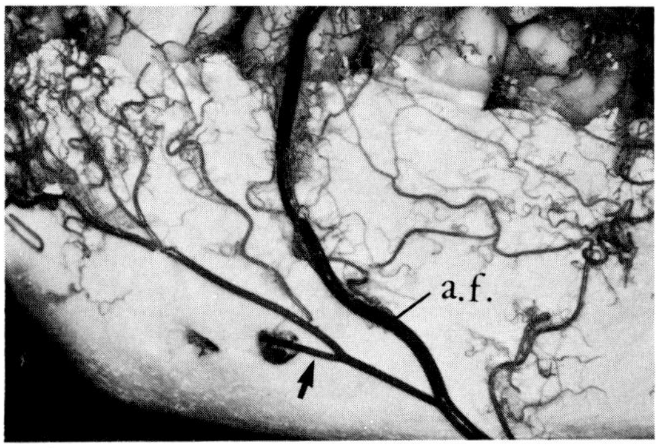

Fig. 1-89.

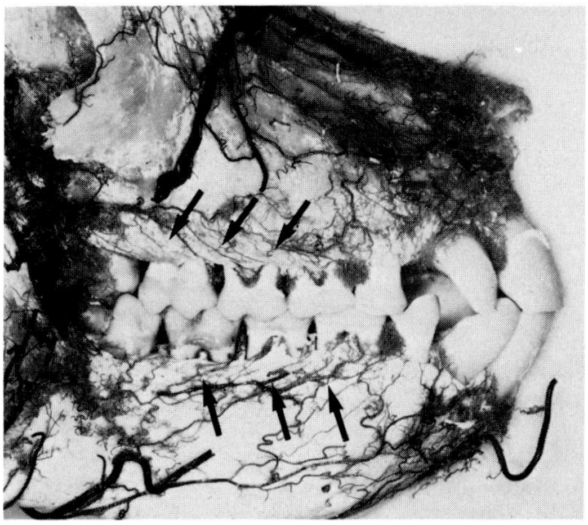

Fig. 1-90.

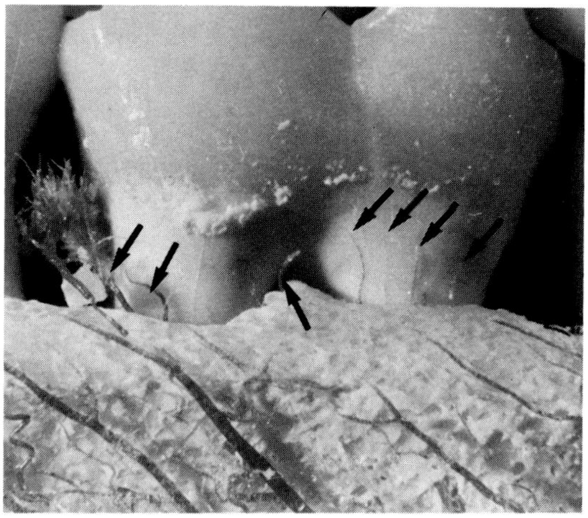

Fig. 1-91.

Fig. 1-87. The gingiva receives its blood supply mainly through *supraperiosteal* blood vessels which are terminal branches of the *sublingual artery* (a.s.), the *mental artery* (a.m.), the *buccal artery* (a.b.), the *facial artery* (a.f.), the *greater palatine artery* (a.p.), the *infra orbital artery* (a.i.) and the *posterior superior dental artery* (a.ap.).

Fig. 1-88 depicts the course of the greater palatine artery (a.p.) in a specimen of a monkey which at sacrifice was perfused with plastic. Subsequently, the soft tissue was dissolved. The greater palatine artery (a.p.) which is a terminal branch of the ascending *palatine artery* (from the *maxillary,* "internal maxillary", artery) runs through the *greater palatine canal* (arrow) to the palate. As this artery runs in frontal direction it puts out branches which supply the masticatory mucosa of the palate.

Fig. 1-89. The various arteries are often considered to supply certain well defined regions of the dentition. In reality, however, there are numerous anastomoses present between the different arteries. Thus, the *entire system of blood vessels,* rather than individual groups of vessels, should be regarded as the unit supplying the soft and hard tissue of the maxilla and the mandible, e.g. in this figure there is an anastomosis (arrow) between the *facial artery* (a.f.) and the blood vessels of the mandible.

Fig. 1-90 illustrates a vestibular segment of the maxilla and mandible from a monkey which at sacrifice was perfused with plastic. Notice that

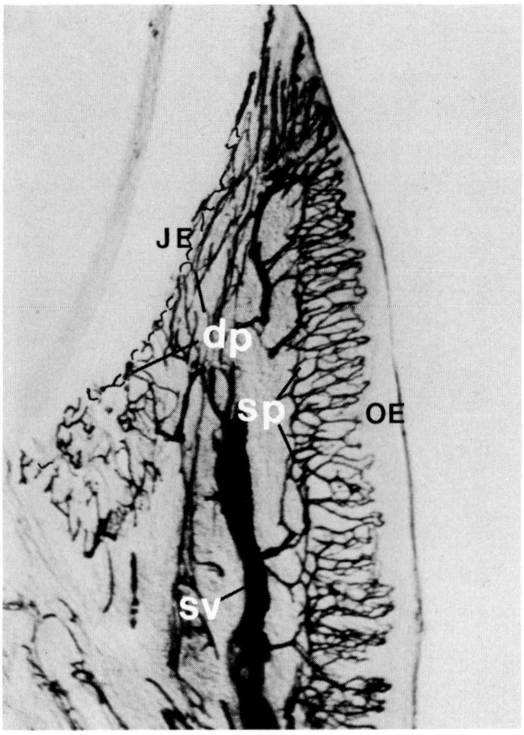

Fig. 1-92.

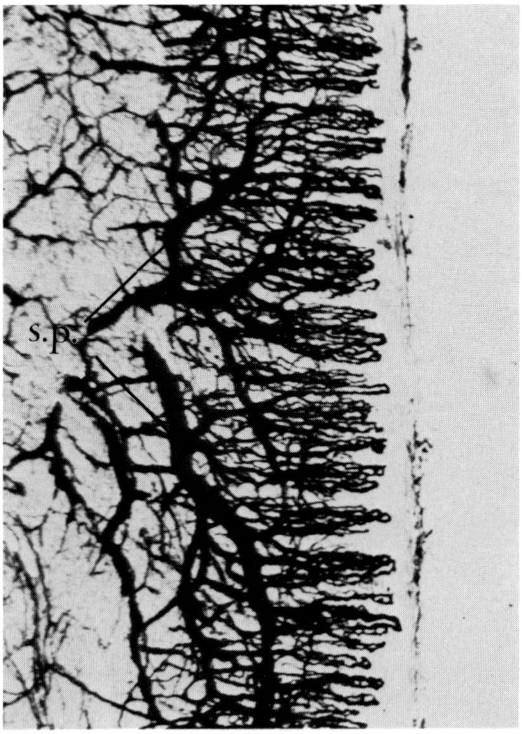

Fig. 1-93.

the vestibular gingiva is supplied with blood mainly through supraperiosteal blood vessels (arrows).

Fig. 1-91. As can be seen, blood vessels (arrows) terminate at the alveolar bone crest. They originate from vessels in the periodontal ligament and contribute to the blood supply of the free gingiva.

Fig. 1-92 shows a specimen from a monkey which at the time of sacrifice was perfused with ink. Subsequently, the specimen was treated to make the tissue transparent (cleared specimen). To the right, the supraperiosteal blood vessels (sv) can be seen, which during their course towards the free gingiva put forth numerous branches to a subepithelial plexus (sp) located immediately beneath the oral epithelium of the free and attached gingiva. This subepithelial plexus in turn yields thin capillary loops to each of the connective tissue papillae projecting into the oral epithelium (OE). The number of such capillary loops is constant over a very long time and is not altered by application of epinephrine or histamine to the gingival margin. This implies that the blood vessels of the lateral portions of the gingiva, even under normal circumstances, are fully utilized and that the blood flow to the free gingiva is regulated entirely by velocity alterations. In the free gingiva, the supraperiosteal blood vessels (sv) anastomose with blood vessels from the periodontal ligament and the bone. To the left (in Fig. 1-92), beneath the junctional epithelium (JE), is a plexus of blood vessels termed the *dentogingival plexus* (dp). The blood vessels in this plexus have a thickness of approximately 40 µm which means that they are mainly venules. In healthy gingiva, no *capillary loops* occur in the dentogingival plexus.

Fig. 1-93. This figure illustrates how the subepithelial plexus (sp), beneath the oral epithelium of the free and attached gingiva, yields

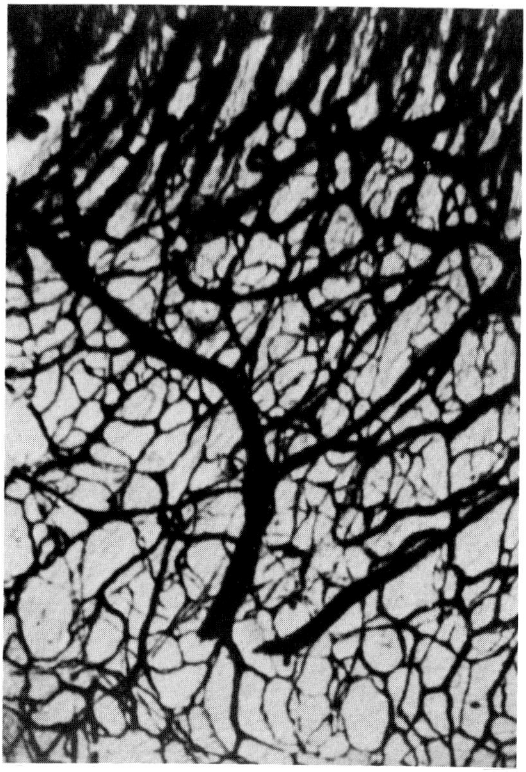

Fig. 1-94.

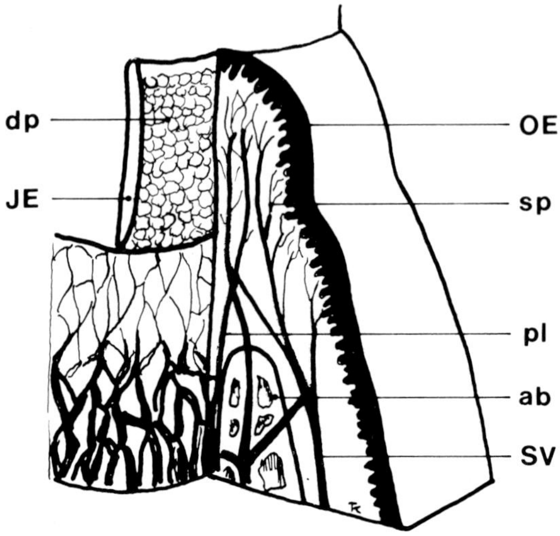

Fig. 1-95.

thin capillary loops to each connective tissue papilla. These capillary loops have a diameter of approximately 7 μm which means they have the size of true capillaries.

Fig. 1-94 illustrates the *dentogingival plexus* in a section cut parallel to the subsurface of the junctional epithelium. As can be seen, the dentogingival plexus consists of a finemeshed network of blood vessels. In the upper portion of the picture, capillary loops can be detected belonging to the subepithelial plexus beneath the oral sulcular epithelium.

Fig. 1-95 is a schematic drawing of the blood supply to the free gingiva. As stated above, the main blood supply of the free gingiva is derived from the *supraperiosteal blood vessels* (sv) which, in the gingiva, anastomose with blood vessels from the alveolar bone (ab) and periodontal ligament (pl). To the right in the drawing, the oral epithelium (OE) is depicted with its underlying subepithelial plexus of vessels (sp). To the left beneath the junctional epithelium (JE) the *dentogingival plexus* (dp) can be seen which, under normal conditions, is comprised of a fine-meshed network without capillary loops.

Fig. 1-96 illustrates a section prepared through a tooth (T) with its periodontium. Blood vessels (perforating rami; arrows) arising from the intraseptal artery in the alveolar bone run through canals (Volkmann's canals) in the socket wall (VC) into the periodontal ligament (PL) where they anastomose.

Fig. 1-97 shows blood vessels in the periodontal ligament in a section cut parallel to the root surface. After entering the periodontal ligament, the blood vessels (perforating rami; ar-

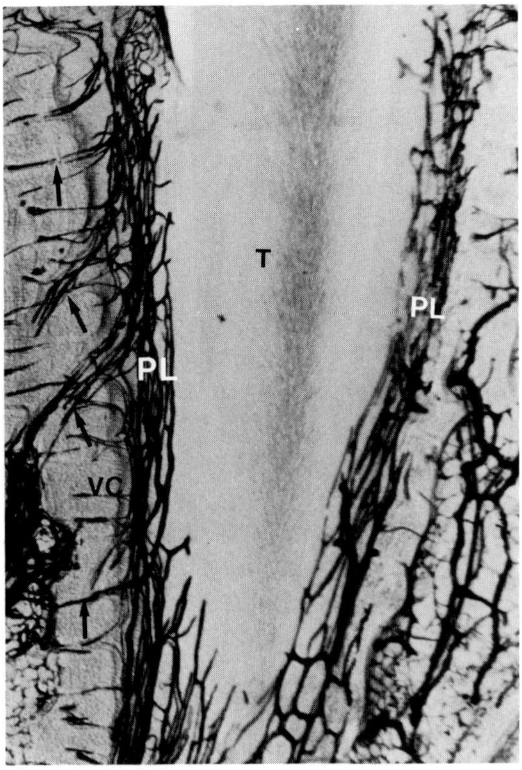

Fig. 1-96.

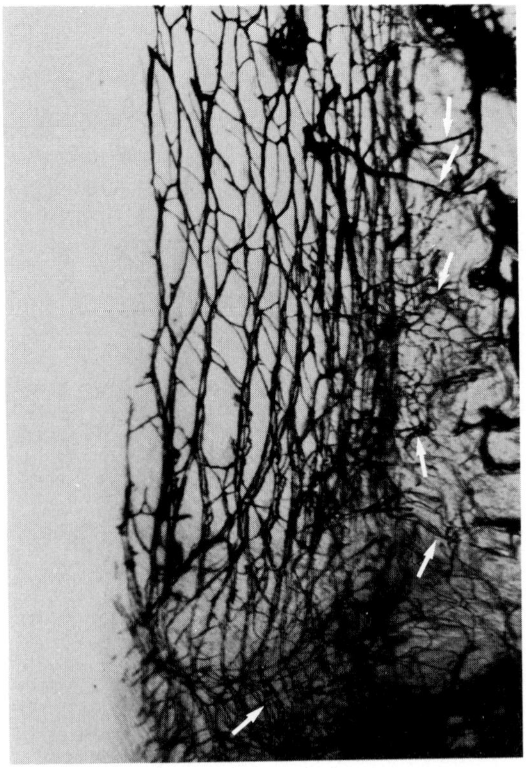

Fig. 1-97.

rows) anastomose and form a polyhedral network which surrounds the root like a stocking. The majority of the blood vessels in the periodontal ligament are found close to the alveolar bone. In the coronal portion of the periodontal ligament blood vessels run in coronal direction, passing the alveolar bone crest, into the free gingiva (see Fig. 1-91).

Fig. 1-98 is a schematic drawing of the blood supply of the periodontium. The blood vessels in the periodontal ligament form a polyhedral network surrounding the root. Note that the free gingiva receives its blood supply from 1) supraperiosteal blood vessels, 2) the blood vessels of the periodontal ligament and 3) the blood vessels of the alveolar bone.

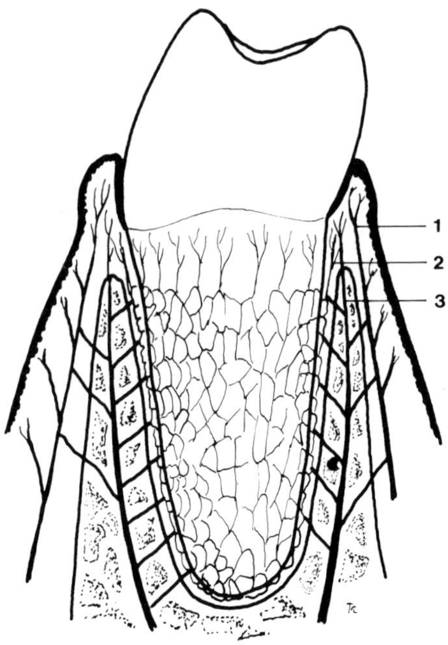

Fig. 1-98.

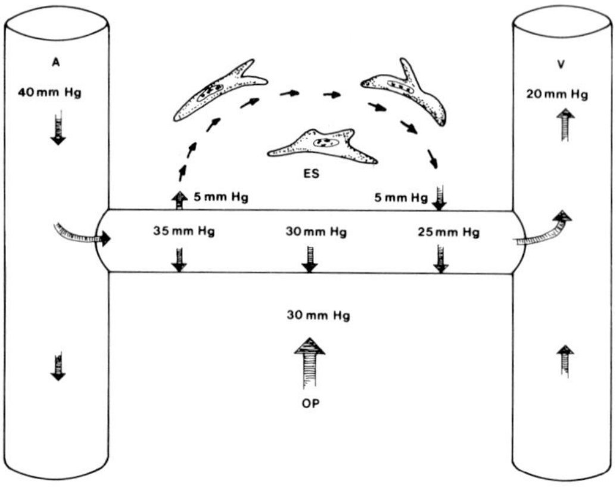

Fig. 1-99.

Fig. 1-99 illustrates schematically, the so-called "extravascular" circulation through which nutrients and other substances are carried to the individual cells and metabolic products are removed from the tissue. In the arterial (A) end of the capillary, to the left in the drawing, a hydraulic pressure of approximately 35 mm Hg is maintained as a result of the pumping function of the heart. Since the hydraulic pressure is higher than the osmotic pressure (OP) in the tissue (which is approximately 30 mm Hg), a transportation of substances will occur from the blood vessels to the extravascular space (ES). In the venous (V) end of the capillary system, to the right in the drawing, the hydraulic pressure has decreased to approximately 25 mm Hg (i.e. 5 mm lower than the osmotic pressure in the tissue). This allows a transportation of substances from the extravascular space to the blood vessels. Thus, the difference between the hydraulic pressure and the osmotic pressure results in a transportation of substances from the blood vessels to the extravascular space in the arterial part of the capillary while, in the venous part, a transportation of substances occurs from the extravascular space to the blood vessels. Hereby an extravascular circulation is established (arrows).

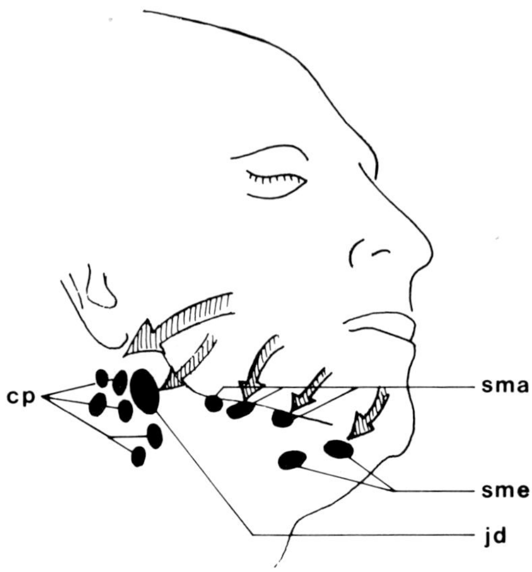

Fig. 1-100.

The lymphatic system of the periodontium

Fig. 1-100. The smallest lymph vessels, the *lymph capillaries*, form an extensive network in the connective tissue. The wall of the lymph capillary consists of a single layer of endothelial cells. For this reason such capillaries are difficult to identify in an ordinary histological section. The lymph is absorbed from the tissue fluid through the thin walls into the lymph capillaries. From the capillaries, the lymph passes into larger *lymph vessels* which are often in the vicinity of corresponding blood vessels. Before the lymph enters the blood stream it passes through one or more *lymph nodes* in which the lymph becomes filtered and supplied with lymphocytes. The lymph vessels are like veins provided with valves. The lymph from the periodontal tissues is drained to the lymph nodes of the head and the neck. The labial and lingual gingiva of the mandibular incisor region is drained to the *submental lymph nodes* (sme). The palatal gingiva of the maxilla is drained to the *deep cervical lymph nodes* (cp). The buccal gingiva of the maxilla and the buccal and lingual gingiva in the mandibular premolar-molar region are drained to *submandibular lymph nodes* (sma). Except for the third molars and mandibular incisors, all teeth with their adjacent periodontal tissues are drained to the *submandibular lymph nodes* (sma). The third molars are drained to the *jugulodigastric lymph node* (jd) and the mandibular incisors to the *submental lymph nodes* (sme).

The nerves of the periodontium

Like other tissues in the body, the periodontium contains receptors which record pain, touch and pressure. The periodontal ligament, but not the gingiva, cementum and alveolar bone, also contains proprioceptors, giving information concerning movements and positions (i.e. deep sensibility). In addition to the different types of sensory receptors which belong to the somatic nervous system, nerve components are found innervating the blood vessels of the periodontium. Such nerve components belong to the autonomic nervous system. Nerves recording pain, touch, and pressure have their trophic center in the *semilunar ganglion*, while the proprioceptive nerves have the trophic center in the more centrally positioned *mesencephalic nucleus*. Both types of nerves are brought to the periodontium via the *trigeminal nerve* and its end branches. Due to the presence of receptors in the periodontal membrane, small forces applied on the teeth may be identified. For example, the presence of a very thin (10-30 μm) metal foil (strip) placed between the teeth during occlusion can readily be identified. It is also well known that a movement which brings the teeth of the mandible in contact with the occlusal surfaces of the maxillary teeth is arrested reflexively and altered into an opening movement if an inert particle is detected in the chew. Thus, the receptors in the periodontal ligament together with the proprioceptors in muscles and tendons, play an essential part in the regulation of chewing movements and chewing forces.

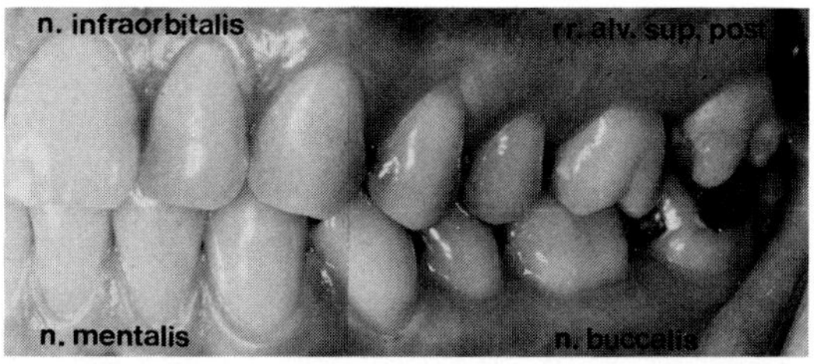

Fig. 1-101a.

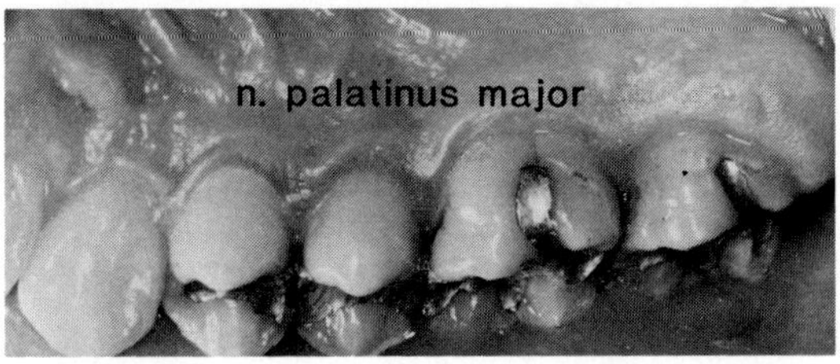

Fig. 1-101b.

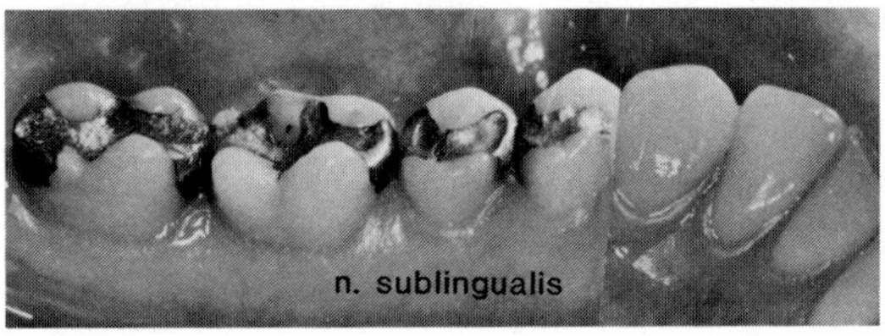

Fig. 1-101c.

Fig. 1-101 shows the various regions of the gingiva which are innervated by end branches of the trigeminal nerve. The gingiva on the labial aspect of maxillary incisors, canines and premolars is innervated by *superior labial branches* from the *infraorbital nerve,* n. infraorbitalis (Fig. 1-101a). The buccal gingiva in the maxillary molar region is innervated by branches from the *posterior superior dental nerve,* rr. alv. sup. post. (Fig. 1-101a). The palatal gingiva is innervated by the *greater palatal nerve,* n. palatinus major (Fig. 1-101b), except for the area of the incisors which is innervated by the *long sphenopalatine nerve,* n. pterygopalatini. The lingual gingiva in the mandible

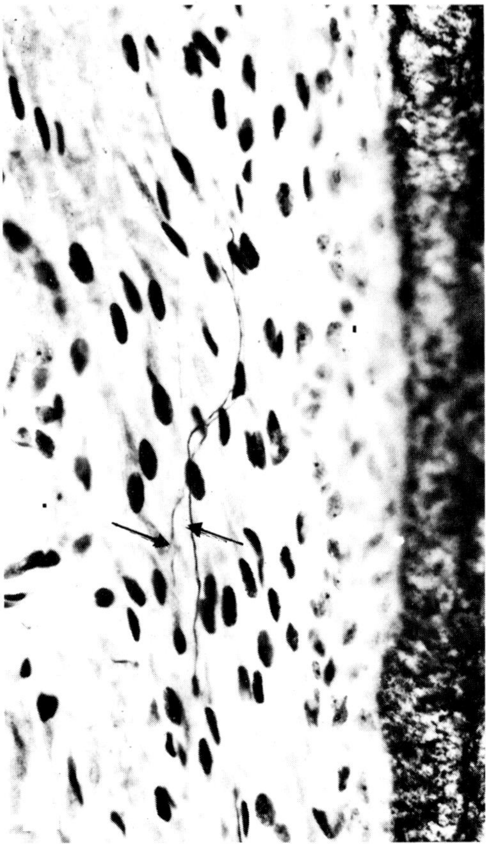

Fig. 1-102.

is innervated by the *sublingual nerve,* n. sublingualis (Fig. 1-101c), which is an end branch of the *lingual nerve.* The gingiva at the labial aspect of mandibular incisors and canines is innervated by the *mental nerve,* n. mentalis, and the gingiva at the buccal aspect of the molars by the *buccal nerve,* n. buccalis (Fig. 1-101a). The innervation areas of these 2 nerves frequently overlap in the premolar region. The teeth in the mandible including their periodontal ligament are innervated by the *inferior alveolar nerve,* n. alveolaris inf., while the teeth in the maxilla are innervated by the *superior alveolar plexus,* n. alveolares sup.

Fig. 1-102. The small nerves of the periodontium follow almost the same course as the blood vessels. The nerves to the gingiva run in the tissue superficial to the periosteum and put out several branches to the oral epithelium on their way towards the free gingiva. The nerves enter the periodontal membrane through the perforations (Volkmann's canals) in the socket wall. In the periodontal membrane, the nerves join larger bundles which take a course parallel to the long axis of the tooth. The photomicrograph illustrates small nerves (arrows) which have emerged from the larger bundles in order to supply certain parts of the periodontal ligament tissue.

References:

Ainamo, J. & Talari, A. (1976) The increase with age of the width of attached gingiva. *Journal of Periodontal Research* **11**, 182-188.

Anderson, D.T., Hannam, A.G. & Matthews, G. (1970) Sensory mechanisms in mammalian teeth and their supporting structures. *Physiological Review* **50**, 171-195.

Carranza, F.A., Itoiz, M.E., Cabrini, R.L. & Dotto, C.A. (1966) A study of periodontal vascularization in different laboratory animals. *Journal of Periodontal Research* **1**, 120-128.

Egelberg, J. (1966) The blood vessels of the dento-gingival junction. *Journal of Periodontal Research* **1**, 163-179.

Fullmer, H.M., Sheetz, J.H. & Narkates, A.J. (1974) Oxytalan connective tissue fibers. A review. *Journal of Oral Pathology* **3**, 291-316.

Karring, T. (1973) Mitotic activity in the oral epithelium. *Journal of Periodontal Research, Suppl.* **13**, 1-47.

Karring, T., Lang, N.P. & Löe, H. (1974) The role of gingival connective tissue in determining epithelial differentiation. *Journal of Periodontal Research* **10**, 1-11.

Karring, T. & Löe, H. (1970) The three-dimensional concept of the epithelium-connective tissue boundary of gingiva. *Acta Odontologica Scandinavia* **28**, 917-933.

Karring,T., Ostergaard, E. & Löe, H. (1971) Conservation of tissue specificity after heterotopic transplantation of gingiva and alveolar mucosa. *Journal of Periodontal Research* **6**, 282-293.

Kvam, E. (1973) Topography of principal fibers. *Scandinavian Journal of Dental Research* **81**, 553-557.

Listgarten, M.A. (1966) Electron microscopic study of the gingivo-dental junction of man. *American Journal of Anatomy* **119**, 147-178.

Listgarten, M.A. (1972) Normal development, structure, physiology and repair of gingival epithelium. *Oral Science Review* **1**, 3-67.

Lozdan, J. & Squier, C.A. (1969) The histology of the mucogingival junction. *Journal of Periodontal Research* **4**, 83-93.

Melcher, A.H. (1976) Biological processes in resorption, deposition and regeneration of bone. In *Periodontal Surgery, Biologic Basis and Technique,* ed. S.S. Stahl, pp. 99-120. Springfield: C.C. Thomas.

Page, R.C., Ammons, W.F., Schectman, L.R. & Dillingham, L.A. (1974) Collagen fiber bundles of the normal marginal gingiva in the marmoset. *Archives of Oral Biology* **19**, 1039-1043.

Schroeder, H.E. & Listgarten, M.A. (1971) *Fine Structure of the Developing Epithelial Attachment of Human Teeth.* 2nd ed., p. 146. Basel:Karger.

Schroeder, H.E. & Münzel-Pedrazzoli, S. (1973) Correlated morphometric and biochemical analysis of gingival tissue. Morphometric model, tissue sampling and test of stereologic procedure. *Journal of Microscopy* **99**, 301-329.

Schroeder, H.E. & Theilade, J. (1966) Electron microscopy of normal human gingival epithelium. *Journal of Periodontal Research* **1**, 95-119.

Schultz-Haudt, S.P. & Aas, E. (1962) Dynamics of the periodontal tissues. II. The connective tissue. *Odontologisk Tidsskrift* **70**, 397-428.

Selvig, K.A. (1965) The fine structure of human cementum. *Acta Odontologica Scandinavica* **23**, 423-441.

Selvig, K.A. (1968) Differences between cementum and bone tissue. *Norske Tannlaegeforenings Tidsskrift*78, 71-86.

Stallard, R.E. (1963) The utilization of H^3-proline by the connective tissue elements of the periodontium. *Periodontica* **1**, 185-188.

Valderhaug, J.P. & Nylen, M.U. (1966) Function of epithelial rests as suggested by their ultrastructure. *Journal of Periodontal Research* **1**, 67-78.

CHAPTER 2

Epidemiology of Periodontal Disease

General principles in epidemiological research

The word epidemiology is defined as the science of epidemics. In medicine, epidemiological methods are utilized for determining what proportion of the population, at a given time, is affected by a disease. In such studies the basic unit is the individual member of the community to be studied. With modern possibilities for automatic data processing, the results from epidemiological research have become of increasing importance in the planning and administration of health care.

Epidemiological methodology

Epidemiological research may have various objectives. One objective is to assess the treatment needs of a disease of known etiology. Especially when repeated at given time intervals, such studies can provide health care planners with valuable information about the need of manpower and other resources. Another objective may be to clarify the factors contributing to, or directly causing, the disease under study. In such cases, a simple clarification of disease prevalence is seldom sufficient. Instead, the full range of systematic epidemiological research may have to be utilized. The strategy of such an approach has been summarized by MacMahon et al. (1960) as follows:

1) *Descriptive epidemiology* - description of the distribution of disease, with comparison of its frequency in different populations and different segments of the same population.
2) *Formulation of hypotheses* - tentative theories designed to explain the observed distribution of the disease in terms of the most direct causal associations.
3) *Analytic epidemiology* - observational studies designed specifically to examine the hypotheses resulting from the descriptive studies.

4) *Experimental epidemiology* - experimental studies on human populations to stringently test those hypotheses which stand the test of observational and analytic studies.

A classic example of the utilization of the full range of epidemiological strategy in dentistry is represented by the progressive research leading to the clarification of the role of fluorides in the frequency and prevention of dental caries. During the last few decades, the use of the same 4 stages of systematic epidemiological research has also given us our present knowledge of the directly causative and contributory factors of periodontal disease. A description of the various steps taken and achievements made in this progressive development may enhance the understanding of the need for the large variety of periodontal indices which are available in current dental literature.

Specific problems in dental epidemiology

In studies on the frequency and distribution of medical conditions such as tuberculosis, cardiac disease, etc., the number of subjects affected is given in per cent of the number of subjects examined. The problem in dentistry has been that, in many populations, practically all subjects have experienced either dental caries or periodontal disease, or both. Consequently, comparison of proportions of the population affected by these 2 oral diseases has proved to be of little value. Instead, researchers interested in the epidemiology of dental diseases have utilized individual teeth or tooth surfaces as the basic unit of examination and have analyzed their data accordingly.

The simple and straightforward DMF Index for assessment of past caries experience has been successfully used since the 1930's. As a result, epidemiological data from different parts of the world is now available for those researchers and health administrators who are interested in oral health promotion, both locally and on a global basis. Already in the late 1940's Massler was concerned with the fact that there was no index system for periodontal disease, the simplicity and applicability of which could be compared with the DMF Index for past caries experience (Massler et al. 1950). To date, although some progress has been made, this concern still partly exists.

Epidemiology of periodontal disease

Before any periodontal indices had been developed, periodontal health was commonly classified as being good, medium or poor. This way of classifying the periodontal condition was used as late as the 1950's. Such subjective criteria did not permit results from different studies to be compared because the good ones in one group and with one examiner could well be worse than the poor ones in another group with another examiner. The use of the criteria was strongly dependent on the interest and training of the examiner, as shown by prevalence rates for gingivitis which ranged from 8-98% in similar populations (see reviews by Schour & Massler 1947, Ramfjord 1959).

A review of currently available indices for the evaluation of periodontal health or disease reveals a confusing abundance of classification systems. Because it is difficult to choose an appropriate index from among the many which aim to measure periodontal disease and related factors, the individual investigator usually finds it laborious to perform a meaningful comparison of his own results with those of another investigator. The following review is an attempt to clarify the origin of some periodontal indices by presenting their purpose in the perspective of time. The intention is to demonstrate why so many different index systems have been considered necessary and how their use has as-

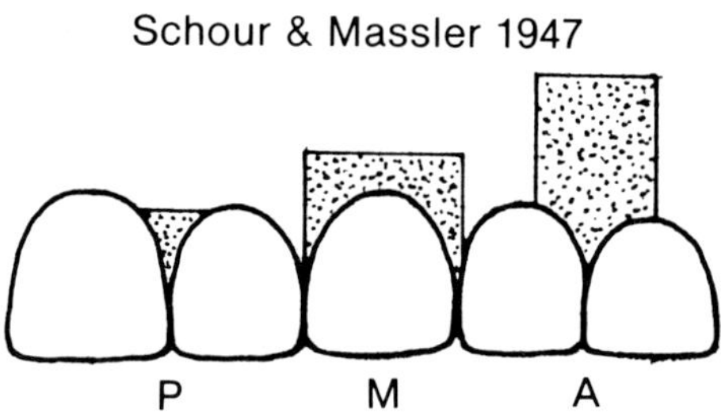

Fig. 2-1. Schour & Massler's PMA-index (1947) is based on recording of inflamed papillae (P), gingival margins (M) and areas of attached gingiva (A) on the facial aspects of anterior teeth.

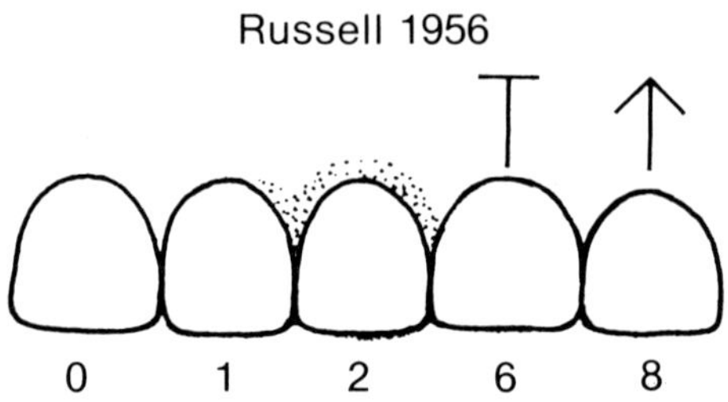

Fig. 2-2. Russell's Periodontal Index (PI) (1956) has been widely used for assessment of average severity of periodontal disease in large population groups. Scores 1 and 2 indicate gingivitis along part of or the total circumference of the tooth, score 6 indicates pathological pocketing and score 8 stands for loss of function due to excessive mobility.

sisted us in reaching the degree of knowledge of periodontology which we have today.

Descriptive and analytic studies

The first well defined classification system for gingivitis was published by Schour & Massler (1947). These investigators examined the gingival conditions of children in post-war Italy. The essence of the PMA Index is to determine the number of (1) inflamed papillae (P), (2) gingival margins (M) and (3) areas of attached gingiva (A) at the labial surface of each anterior tooth (Fig. 2-1). The PMA Index was later modified by Parfitt (1957) and has been used extensively, particularly in the United States and Britain. Although limited to describe only gingivitis around anterior teeth, the PMA Index offered, for the first time, a possibility to compare prevalence and severity scores recorded from different populations.

In the 1950's WHO became interested in the assessment of periodontal disease in the Far East where caries at that time was not a major health problem. The PMA Index was inadequate for this purpose because it lacked criteria describing actual periodontal breakdown. A suitable instrument for the purpose was developed by Russell who published the Periodontal Index (PI) in 1956 (Fig. 2-2). In the epidemiological determination of periodontal health or disease the PI was, until the 1980's, the most widely used index. Its criteria are applied to each tooth in the mouth and scoring is performed as follows: a tooth with a healthy periodontium (0), gingivitis around only part of the tooth (1), gingivitis encircling the tooth (2), pocket formation (6) and loss of function due to excessive mobility (8). Mean PI scores for individuals and population groups have usually been used for describing the average severity of disease. It should be noted that due to the nature of its criteria the PI is a reversible scoring system, i.e. the individual can, following proper treatment, have his score lowered or reduced to 0.

In contrast to the PI, the Periodontal Disease Index (PDI) of Ramfjord (1959), when used to assess destructive disease, measures loss of tooth attachment instead of pocket depth. This particular part of the PDI includes an irreversible change which cannot be influenced by treatment. The main difference between the PI and the PDI is thus that the former records the need for treatment (periodontal disease status) while the latter scores the accumulated consequences of the disease (periodontal status). For example, with horizontal loss of alveolar bone support, the periodontal status of a given tooth would be the same before and after proper treatment.

Mainly by the use of the PI (Russell 1956),

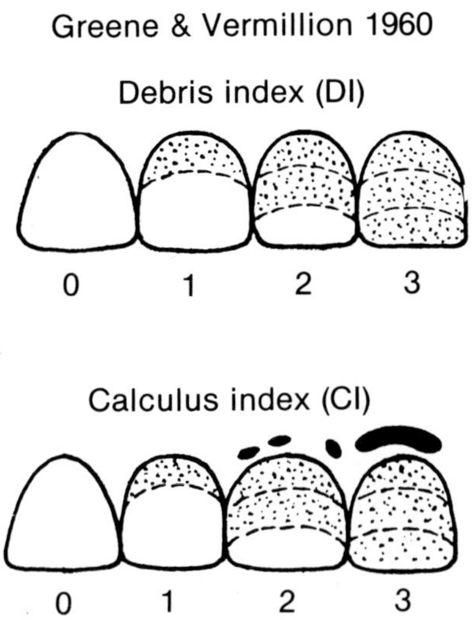

Fig. 2-3. The Oral Hygiene Index (OHI) consists of 2 separate components. The Debris Index (DI) measures coronal extension of soft deposits up to the first, second, or last third of the facial or lingual tooth surface. The Calculus Index (CI) measures the corresponding coronal extension of supragingival calculus and/or the presence of separate flecks or a continuous band of subgingival calculus. The OHI score is the sum of the DI and CI scores.

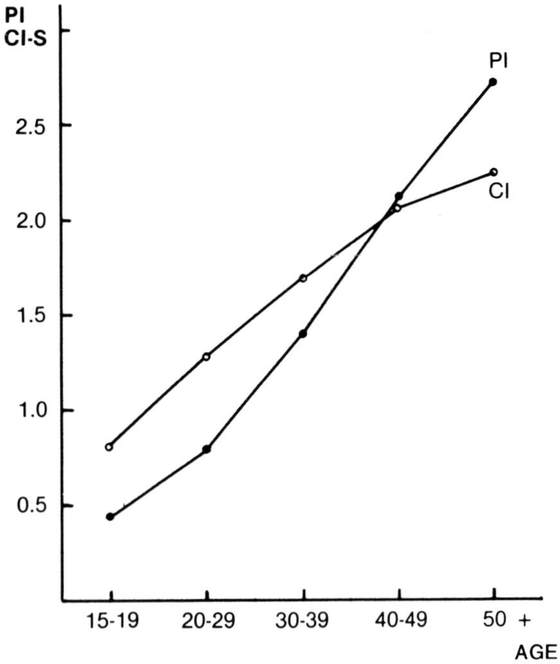

Fig. 2-4. On the population level the increase of Periodontal Index scores with age is found to correlate closely to a corresponding increase in the amount of dental calculus (Greene 1963).

extensive data has been collected from populations all around the world. Analyses of the findings have revealed that differences in prevalence and severity of periodontal disease are associated with race, geographic area, sex, socioeconomic status, educational level, etc.

For proper understanding of the rapid development which has taken place within research on the epidemiological aspects of periodontal disease, one should realize that the first classification systems for assessment of oral hygiene were developed only some 20 years ago. An oral hygiene classification was included in the PDI system (Ramfjord 1959). With the use of the better known Oral Hygiene Index (OHI) of Greene & Vermillion (1960) it has been shown that all the apparent racial, geographic and other demographic differences in the severity of periodontal disease disappear when disease levels are related directly to levels of oral hygiene (see reviews by Löe 1963, Scherp 1964, Waerhaug 1966). Russell himself suggested that the amount of plaque and calculus, together with the age of the group of subjects, may explain as much as 90% of their periodontal disease experience (Russell 1963).

The crude criteria of the OHI were based on 2 components: the coronal extension of plaque (Debris Index) and, likewise, the coronal extension of supragingival calculus and/or concurrent occurrence of subgingival calculus on the tooth surface (Calculus Index). A schematic description of the Oral Hygiene Index is presented in Fig. 2-3.

By means of descriptive and analytic studies it was possible to demonstrate that a strong positive correlation exists between increasing age and pocket formation and progressive periodontal breakdown (Fig. 2-4). In diagrams representing disease levels of populations, the lines illustrating Russell's PI scores and the CI scores of the OHI increase in an almost parallel

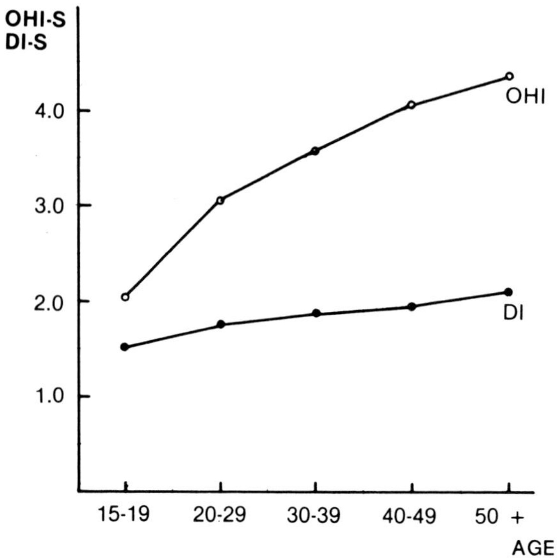

Fig. 2-5. That Oral Hygiene Index scores tend to increase with advancing age is mainly due to increasing Calculus Index scores (cf. Fig. 2-4). The Debris Index scores remain more or less constant through life (Greene 1963).

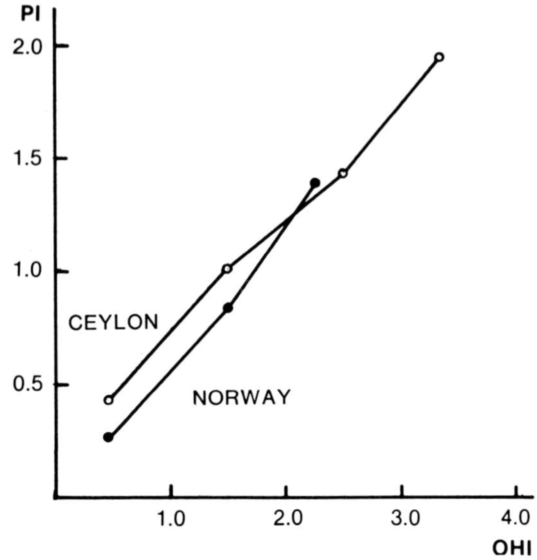

Fig. 2-6. A close association between PI and OHI scores was demonstrated by Waerhaug (1967) in both Norwegian recruits ($\bar{x}$ PI = 0.80) and students of corresponding age in Ceylon ($\bar{x}$ PI = 1.14). The difference in disease level was thus due to different oral hygiene levels.

manner with advancing age. Up to about 40 years of age the CI score is slightly higher than the PI score. After 40 the calculus score starts to approach its maximum level whereas the periodontal disease score continues to progress (Fig. 2-4).

There are many difficulties in interpreting the results from cross-sectional epidemiological studies. One source of confusion has been the lack of correlation between plaque scores and the amount of attachment loss. The simple explanation is that all plaque indices, the debris component of the OHI included, measure only the amount of supragingival plaque. Comparisons between age groups indicate that the amount of supragingival plaque does not vary to any obvious extent with age (Fig. 2-5). A large amount of plaque on the teeth thus seems to reflect a permanent characteristic of the oral hygiene behavior of a particular individual rather than the end result of a life-long accumulation of microbial deposits. Indeed, plaque scores, as the concept is understood today, can not be expected to correlate to pocket formation and loss of alveolar bone. The steep ascent of the OHI scores with age (Fig. 2-5) is thus mainly due to the rapidly increasing scores for the calculus component (CI) of the OHI (Fig. 2-4).

During the past 2 decades ample evidence has accumulated of the existence of an inferior periodontal health situation in developing countries as compared with that observed in countries of the affluent western world. For example, the mean PI score of 206 Norwegian Army recruits was found to be 0.80 whereas a group of 281 University students of the same age in Ceylon scored as high as 1.14 (Waerhaug 1967). However, when the groups were reorganized according to their individual OHI and PI scores, no difference was found which could have been indicative of racial variations in tissue response to the suggested etiological agent (Fig. 2-6). Further comparisons between these 2 countries seem to confirm strongly the view that on a population level the amount of plaque and calculus found in the dentition is the discriminating factor for differences between levels of periodontal disease (Löe et al. 1978, Ånerud et al. 1979).

The most recent purely descriptive epidemiological methodology was described by Carlos et al. (1986). Their Extent and Severity Index (ESI) is based on scoring of gingival bleeding, pocket depth and loss of attachment on buccomesial and buccal aspects of all teeth in either the left or right half of the maxilla and in the contralateral half of the mandibular jaw of the same individual. The choice of examination sites is based on good reproducibility of the measurements, ensuring reliable comparison of results from consecutive cross-sectional studies.

Experimental epidemiology

Both the OHI and its later modification OHI-S (Greene & Vermillion 1964) are rather crude indices, best suited for rapid screening of large population groups. Once the association between periodontal disease and oral hygiene had been demonstrated epidemiologically, an increasing interest in experimental research and clinical trials developed. In most cases the objective of such trials was to evaluate the relative effectiveness of various therapeutic measures. For this purpose more sensitive index systems were required.

In attempts to measure the inhibition of calculus formation, the Calculus Surface Index (CSI) (Ennever et al. 1961) and the V-M Index (Volpe & Manhold 1962, Volpe et al. 1965) were developed. These indices were designed for use in clinical trials of short duration. The CSI measures the prevalence of calculus on the 4 surfaces of the 4 mandibular incisors (Fig. 2-7) and is recommended for studies of less than 8 weeks' duration, whereas the V-M Index measures the coronal extension of supragingival calculus on the lingual surfaces of the 6 mandibular anterior teeth (Fig. 2-8) and is suitable also for longer study periods (Mühlemann 1968). Both indices have been used for clinical evaluation of the effect of potential anticalculus agents (for review see Mühlemann 1968, Schroeder 1969).

In an attempt to quantify plaque removal with electric as compared to manual tooth-

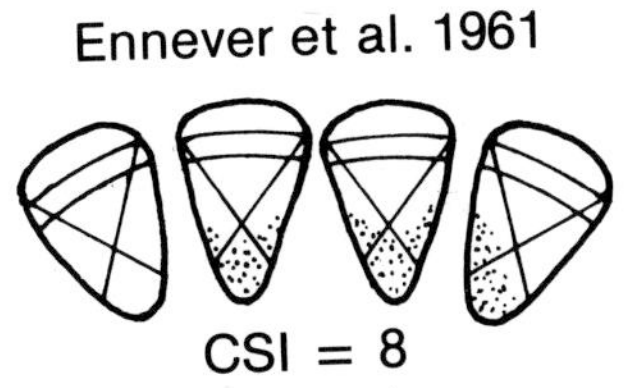

Fig. 2-7. The Calculus Surface Index (CSI) was designed for assessment of supragingival calculus formation during short-term experimental studies. Presence or absence of mineralized deposits is determined for the 4 surfaces of the mandibular incisors. The score per subject ranges from 0 to 16.

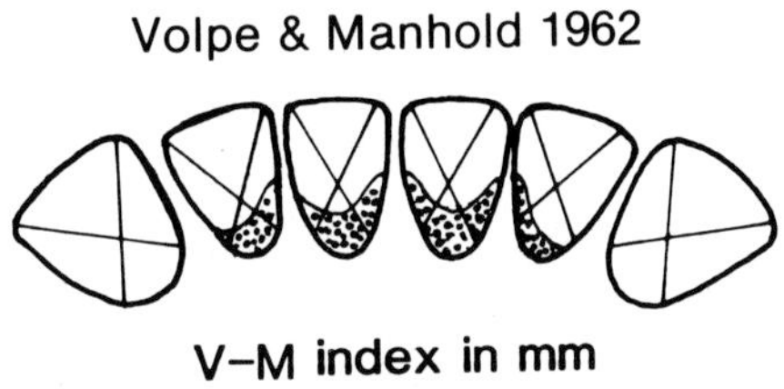

Fig. 2-8. The V-M index was designed for assessment of the formation of supragingival calculus in long-term experiments. The amount of calculus is measured in mm along the 2 diagonal lines drawn over the lingual surface of each one of the lower anteriors. The score is expressed in mm of calculus.

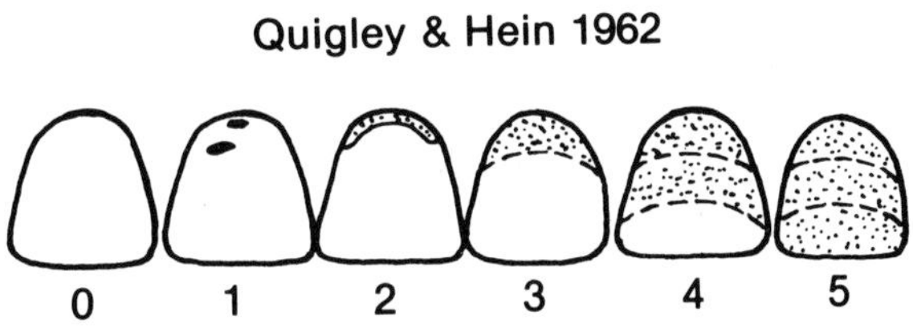

Fig. 2-9. For use in experimental studies Quigley & Hein (1962) augmented the OHI with 2 low scores between Greene & Vermillion's (1960) recordings 0 and 1.

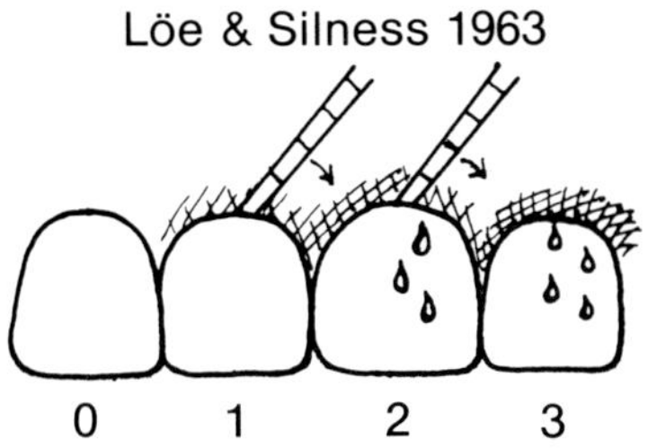

Fig. 2-10a. According to the Gingival Index, severity of gingivitis is assessed separately at the 4 smooth surfaces of the tooth. Whenever the gingival margin looks inflamed, it is massaged with the side of the periodontal probe. If this massage does not result in bleeding, the unit scores 1; if bleeding occurs, score 2 is given. Ulceration and "spontaneous" bleeding scores 3.

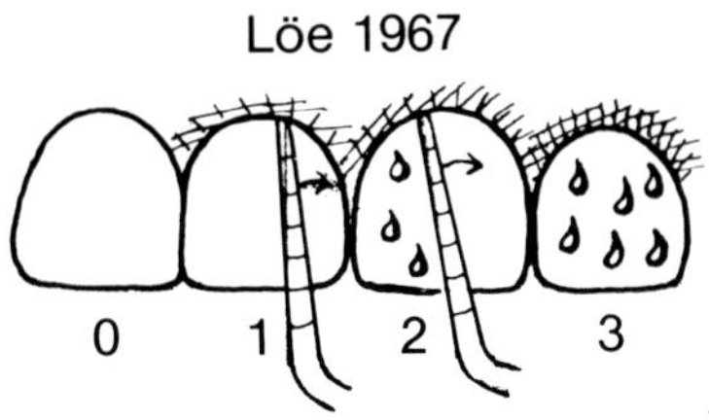

Fig. 2-10b. Subsequently "bleeding after pressure" (Löe & Silness 1963, Fig. 2-10a) was replaced with "bleeding after probing" (Löe 1967). Currently presence or absence of bleeding (score 2) is determined after running a blunt probe along the soft tissue wall of the entrance of the gingival crevice.

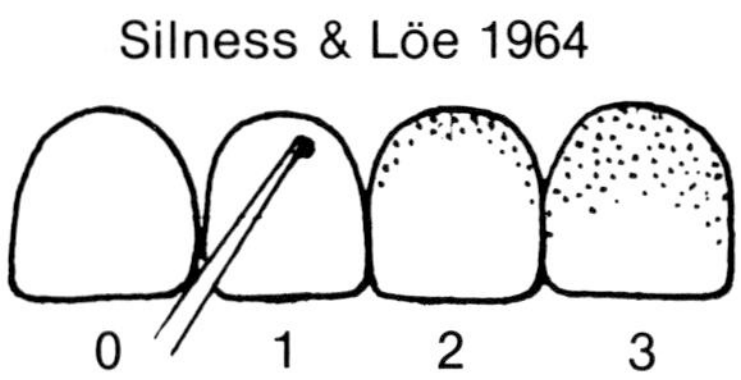

Fig. 2-11. According to the Plaque Index, a tooth surface scores 0 when it is clean and 1 when it looks clean but material can be removed from its gingival third with a sharp explorer. Visible plaque scores 2 and a tooth surface covered with abundant plaque scores 3.

brushes, Quigley & Hein (1962) found the criteria of the OHI too crude to differentiate between small changes in the amount of plaque. These investigators, therefore, added 2 criteria between scores 0 and 1 in the OHI system (Fig. 2-9).

At about the same time in Norway, Löe & Silness attempted to compare the health of gingival tissues in various stages of pregnancy. For such a study, an index system was needed by which also the most subtle differences could be detected. The development and presentation of the Gingival Index (GI) system by Löe & Silness (1963) and the Plaque Index system (PlI) by Silness & Löe (1964) opened up a new era in experimental periodontology (Figs. 2-10a,b and 2-11).

In the PlI and GI system, separate recordings are made for the 4 smooth surfaces of each tooth. The maximum number of recordings made per subject thus increases from 28 tooth scores to $4 \times 28 = 112$ tooth surface scores. In the PlI system, the previous method of scoring the coronal extension of plaque was replaced by the assessment of plaque thickness at the gingival margin. In the GI system, the extension of signs of inflammation around a part or the total circumference of the tooth (the basis of the gingivitis component of the PI) was replaced by 4 degrees of severity at each tooth surface. The scoring of signs of reversible gingival inflammation was no longer combined with an assessment of irreversible loss of tooth attachment as was the case in earlier periodontal indices. Also, the very name of the PlI system reflected the improved understanding at that time of the primarily bacterial character of the soft deposits, which earlier had commonly been denoted debris or materia alba.

By the use of the PlI and GI system it was possible to perform the well known and now classical study on "Experimental gingivitis in man" which definitely proved the direct cause and effect relationship between plaque and gingivitis (Löe et al. 1965).

The Gingival Index has since been modified with regard to the manner in which testing for

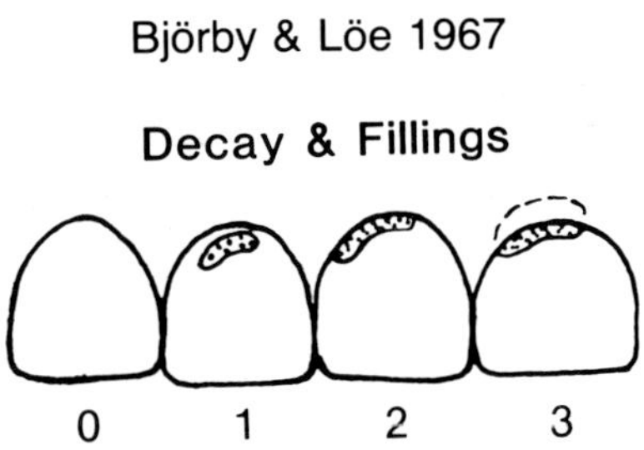

Fig. 2-12. The Retention Index has 3 components which can be used separately or combined. An open caries lesion or a defective margin of a filling or crown within the gingival third of the tooth surface is given score 1 when it does make contact with the gingiva, score 2 when it contacts the gingival margin, and score 3 when it extends 1 mm or more beneath the gingiva.

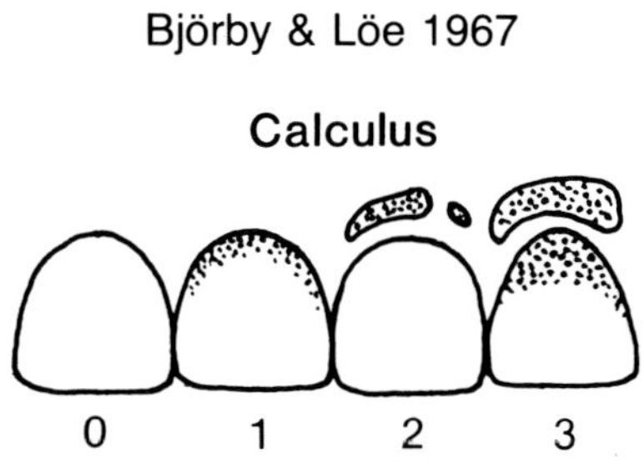

Fig. 2-13. The third component of the Retention Index measures calculus, also at the gingival margin only. A strand of mineralized material at the orifice of the pocket is given the same score as supragingival calculus (1). Subgingival calculus is given score 2 and presence of abundant calculus results in score 3 for the tooth surface.

bleeding tendency is performed. Originally, score 2 was given to a gingival unit if bleeding occurred after "pressure" (Löe & Silness 1963), as illustrated in Fig. 2-10a. This criterion was changed to bleeding after "probing" (Fig. 2-10b) by Löe in 1967. With both methods the probe is used for the detection of bleeding only when visible signs of inflammation are present in the marginal gingiva.

That gingivitis does not, in all cases, lead to progressive destruction of tooth attachment is a common finding in the clinic and has also been demonstrated in experimental studies (Lindhe et al. 1975). It is generally accepted, however, that dental calculus, in spite of epidemiological "evidence", is not the etiologic agent in progressive periodontal disease. The causative factor is the layer of viable microorganisms which always covers subgingival calculus deposits. The strong positive correlation that exists between the PI and CI scores in Fig. 2-4 thus results from the fact that the dental calculus is the retention factor for the subgingival plaque.

For scoring of factors which contribute to gingival inflammation through plaque retention, yet another index was developed by Björby & Löe (1967). By the use of the Retention Index it became possible, on the 4 surfaces of each tooth, to evaluate the degree of plaque retention caused by untreated carious lesions and fillings or crowns with defective gingival margins (Fig. 2-12), or by supra- or subgingivally located calculus deposits (Fig. 2-13).

In order to make the recording of the periodontal disease status complete, the Plaque Index, the Gingival Index, and the Retention Index should, according to Löe and collaborators, be augmented with measurements of pocket depth to the nearest mm (Glavind & Löe 1967).

By the end of the 1960's any previous doubts about the etiology of gingivitis and the causes of periodontal tissue breakdown had been dispelled. In the 1970's, therefore, experimental periodontal research was directed mainly towards the clarification of the relative effects that could be obtained by different modalities for plaque control. By the use of the already available index systems it became possible to confirm more accurately the positive effect of oral hygiene measures on periodontal health, already reported by Lövdal et al. in 1961. In addition to the documentation of the preventive effect of periodontal treatment (Lightner et al. 1971, Suomi et al. 1971), the decisive role of personal oral hygiene combined with proper maintenance care in the form of regular professional cleaning of the patients' teeth was also clearly demonstrated by means of controlled longitudinal studies (Suomi et al. 1973, Ram-

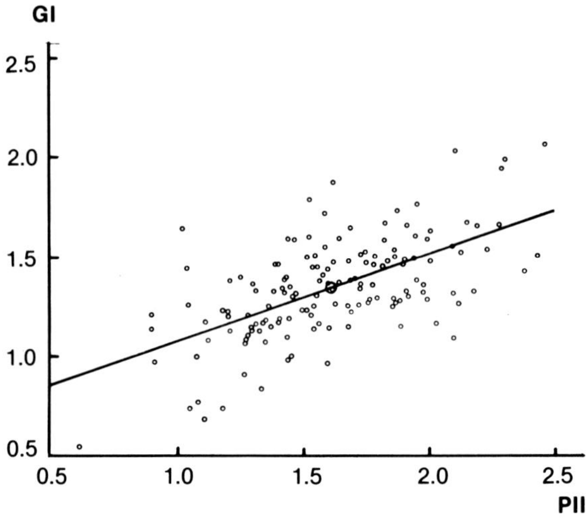

Fig. 2-14. The scatter diagram is based on the individual PlI and GI scores of 154 young adult males. Within the group the positive correlation between PlI and GI is quite high (r = 0.62). However, there are individuals with high GI and low PlI scores and vice versa (Ainamo 1970).

fjord et al. 1975, Rosling et al. 1976, Axelsson & Lindhe 1981a,b).

Individual variation

Epidemiological, clinical and laboratory research have shown, beyond doubt, that plaque and calculus are associated with gingivitis and periodontal tissue breakdown. Yet, in discussion with practising dentists, one is repeatedly told about the individual patient who has had abundant plaque, calculus and ill-fitting restorations for a lifetime, without evidence of destructive changes in the attachment apparatus. Another typical exception is the young patient with relatively good oral hygiene and advanced breakdown of the attachment of incisors and first molars. The very fact that such cases do not conform to generally accepted rules makes them easy to remember. No doubt, both extremes exist. It should be realized, however, that they are in no way in conflict with epidemiological findings.

Epidemiological studies are expected to fulfil certain requirements. One of these is that the study group is representative of the population whose periodontal disease status is to be assessed. The requirement of representativeness means that each individual in the population should have an equal possibility to become included in the sample. Another requirement is that the sample is sufficient in size so that the effect of the exceptional case is eliminated. A simple example would be a study for determining whether men are taller than woman. It is possible that the first woman measured is found to be taller than all the men and the other women in the sample. Only measurement of a large group of people will eventually eliminate the effect of this one giant lady, and thus give the expected result, i.e. that men *on average* seem to be slightly taller than women.

In the individual patient, the degree of periodontal disease is not determined by the microbial plaque alone. The "individual host (or tissue) response", which contains a number of immunological and other systemic components, is also of marked importance. According to the Plaque Principle the following equations can be used to simplify the relation between plaque and periodontal disease:

$$\text{Gingivitis} = \frac{\text{Plaque}}{\text{Host response}}$$

$$\text{Periodontitis} = \text{Age} \times \frac{\text{Plaque}}{\text{Host response}}$$

These equations indicate that a difference in quantity or quality of plaque results in different amounts of disease only when the host response is constant. On the other hand, similar amounts and compositions of bacterial deposits can develop more or less dramatic signs of gingivitis depending on individual differences in the tissue reaction of the host. For example, it has been shown in clinical trials that the deciduous dentition in general is extremely resistant to plaque (Mackler & Crawford 1973, Matsson 1978).

In the case of destructive periodontal disease, the duration of plaque irritation is an additional factor to be considered. Each individual seems to have a characteristic equilibrium between plaque irritation and host response. If this equilibrium is negative, sooner or later periodontal disease will develop. In order to assess the host response of an individual it is, therefore, not sufficient to determine the amount or quality of the plaque or various plaque retentive elements. The additional explaining factor is the age of the patient. Loss of one third of the tooth attachment may indicate a fair host response if the patient is 50 years or older, whereas the same situation would be alarming in an individual aged 15-20 years.

The presence of a varying host response to plaque accumulation was already noted by Löe et al. (1965) in their experimental gingivitis study. All test subjects started the experiment with clean teeth and healthy gingivae. However, when all oral hygiene measures were discarded, some subjects reached Gingival Index score 1.0 in 10 days and others in 21 days.

Indeed, it should be understood that correlations calculated from epidemiological studies can only indicate that *on average* there seems to be a strong positive or negative association between a potential etiologic factor and the disease under study. Russell's argument, for instance, that 90% of all periodontal disease can be explained by oral hygiene and age, is valid only on a population level or in population groups which are large enough to eliminate the effect of variation between individuals (Fig. 2-14).

During recent years research in microbiology has indicated that the composition of supra- and subgingival plaque may be of decisive importance in the development of periodontal disease. Such a claim can neither be confirmed nor rejected by means of epidemiological research. The problem is similar to that of isolating the causative factor when a window is broken by throwing a stone: it is difficult to judge whether it was the weight of the stone or the weakness of the glass which caused the end result. In the field of dermatology it is well known that it is the susceptibility of the individual patient, rather than the presence of pathogenic fungi *per se*, which determines whether or not a dermatitis develops. The possibility thus remains that the presence of a certain type of bacterial flora in periodontal disease is the result, rather than the cause, of disease.

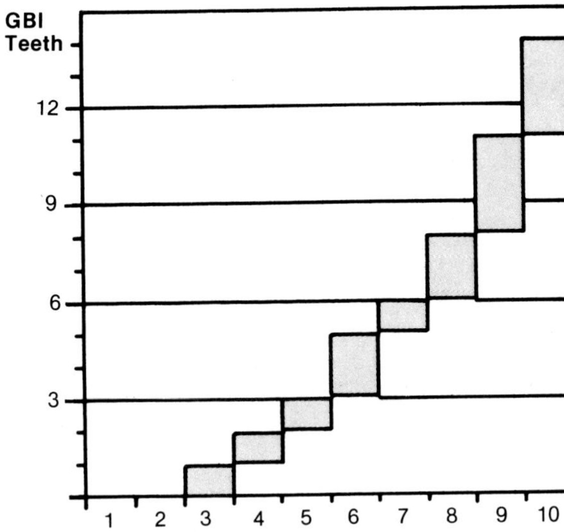

Fig. 2-15. A group of 3500 Finnish recruits was organized according to increasing gingival bleeding tendency in the right sides of the jaws. The group was then divided into 10 subgroups of equal size (deciles). The first 3 deciles were practically free of bleeding whereas in the worst 20% (deciles 9 and 10) bleeding occurred after gentle probing around 8-14 of the 14 teeth examined (Ainamo et al. 1980).

Identification of risk groups

Considering the fact that there are individuals who show minor or no signs of irreversible periodontal breakdown after life-long exposure to irritation from dental plaque, it seems important to try to utilize epidemiological methods to identify individuals with an unfavorable host response, i.e. individuals who are susceptible to periodontal disease.

In a survey of 3500 Finnish young adult males, pockets with a depth of 4 mm or more were found in 11%, whereas a total of 73% of the recruits demonstrated gingival bleeding around one or more of the 14 teeth probed in the right half of the jaw (Ainamo et al. 1980). In a more detailed analysis, the group was organized into 10 subgroups of equal size according to increasing numbers of teeth involved in the disease process (Fig. 2-15). It then became evident that the number of teeth with bleeding gingivae in the 700 subjects with "worst periodontal disease status" was larger than the corresponding figure for all the remaining 2800 subjects. The presentation of the data in this way certainly gives better information for use in treatment planning than do either average severity scores or simple prevalence rates.

In the identification of high susceptibility groups several different approaches can be utilized. Traditionally, on the basis of early epidemiological studies on large populations, the main interest has been to determine oral hygiene levels, i.e. quantification of the etiologic factor. Especially in preventive programs, plaque has thus been considered equal to early gingivitis. According to the study on young Finnish males (Fig. 2-15) a more realistic approach may be to assess susceptibility on the basis of already existing signs of pathology, such as bleeding tendency, subgingival calculus and early loss of alveolar bone. Assessment of disease rather than of a potentially pathogenic microbiota is common practice also among medical professionals.

As bacterial plaque seems to explain only part of the periodontal disease status, one can only hope that future research will result in possibilities to determine also those indirect systemic factors which influence the individual's host response. By means of biochemical, cytological and immunological tests it may one day be possible to reliably identify those individuals who are most likely to become affected

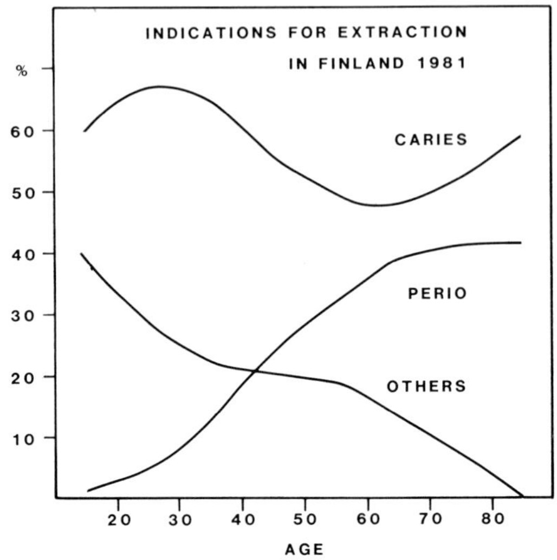

Fig. 2-16. Reasons for extraction of 3883 teeth from 2542 patients as assessed, according to detailed instructions, by 222 randomly selected Finnish dentists in 1981. In the category "Others", impacted teeth and orthodontic extractions dominated at ages 16-20 years and prosthetic extractions from age 31-40 onwards (Ainamo et al. 1984b).

by periodontal disease and give priority to such individuals in programs aimed at prevention.

Tooth mortality due to periodontitis

After 40 years of age, periodontal disease has been traditionally assumed to be the main cause of tooth loss (Carranza 1984). In this respect, recent epidemiological data are contradictory (Fig. 2-16). Although in some studies it has been found that after the age of 40 years, periodontal extractions slightly outnumber the extractions performed due to dental caries (Curilovic 1979, Cahen et al. 1985), there are other studies suggesting that even in the oldest age groups of the population the number of periodontal extractions is lower than the number of teeth extracted because of caries (Ainamo et al. 1984b, Ekanayaka 1984, Bailit et al. 1987).

Assessment of treatment needs

In epidemiological surveys of earlier years periodontal data were usually given as mean scores for the population studied (Greene 1963, Scherp 1964, Ramfjord et al. 1968, Carranza 1984). Such data were suitable for comparison of one population with another but gave little information about the distribution of disease within the population. In the 1970's, an increasing interest in health services research could be observed also in the area of periodontology. In order to improve periodontal health on a global level, it became necessary to clarify the magnitude of the periodontal problem by establishing to what extent each age group of various populations was affected with what level of periodontal disease (WHO 1978).

The Periodontal Treatment Need System (PTNS)

During the very productive years of periodontal research in the 1960's, the general trend was to develop increasingly sensitive index systems for the clarification of the etiology and pathogenesis of periodontal disease. In the 1970's efforts were made to create simplified methods for scoring periodontal treatment needs in a given population (Bellini & Gjermo 1973, Johansen et al. 1973, Oliver 1977). The Periodontal Treatment Need System (PTNS), introduced by Johansen et al. (1973), represented an entirely new approach to the assessment of treatment needs. The system allows fairly accurate determination of the amount and type of periodontal treatment required by individual patients. The assessment can be made in just 1-3 min.

According to the PTNS, the dentition is divided into 4 quadrants. For each quadrant assessments are made to determine whether the worst affected tooth would require periodontal surgery, scaling, or improved personal oral hygiene. Only the worst condition is recorded since, for example, a quadrant requiring surgical therapy would also need scaling, and a patient having either one of these two treatment needs would also need instructions for improved oral hygiene.

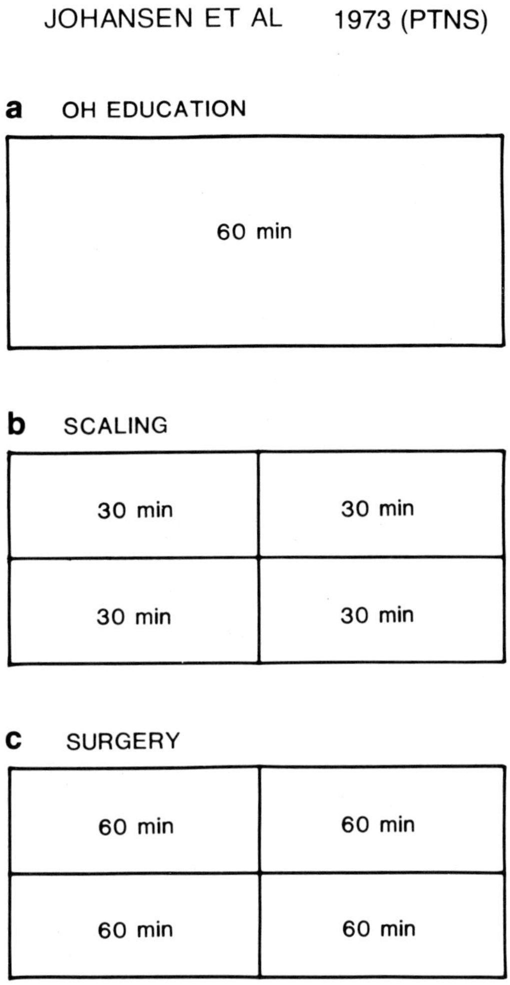

Fig. 2-17. According to assessments using the Periodontal Treatment Need System (PTNS: Johansen et al. 1973), the average time required for treatment of adult patients is 60 min for oral hygiene instruction, including follow-ups and reinstruction, and 30 min for scaling and 60 min for surgery per quadrant of the dentition.

The next step in the development of the PTNS was to assess the time required for delivering the 3 different types of treatment

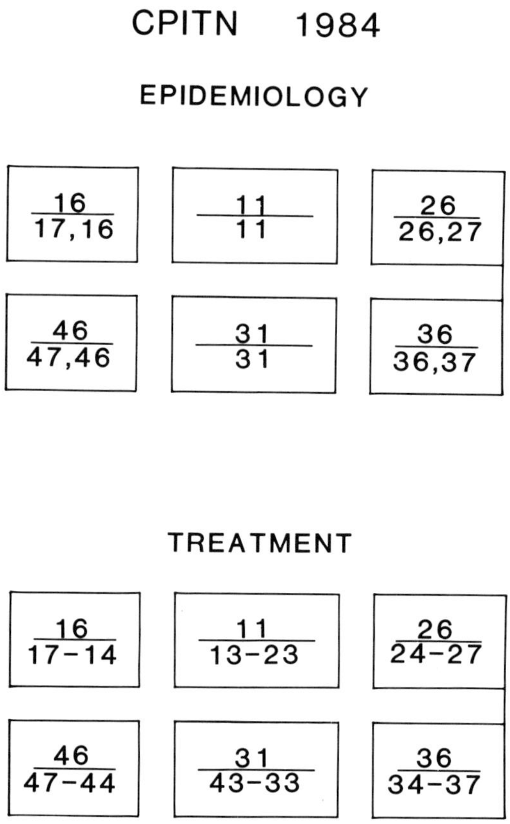

Fig. 2-18. For scoring according to the Community Periodontal Index of Treatment Needs (CPITN) the dentition is divided into 6 segments (sextants). Each sextant is given one code number, regardless of number of teeth examined. In epidemiological surveys of adults, the code number is scored for the highest treatment need observed after examination of 10 index teeth (Epidemiology, below horizontal line) or of all teeth in each sextant (Treatment, below horizontal line). In subjects under 20 years of age, the code number is given after examination of 6 index teeth only (Epidemiology and Treatment, above horizontal line) (Ainamo 1984).

(Johansen et al. 1973). Treatment time is thus used as a common denominator for all 3 categories of treatment. In a group of 42 periodontal patients the average time required was 60 min per quadrant for surgery, 30 min per quadrant for scaling, and 60 min per person for improving personal oral hygiene to an acceptable level (Fig. 2-17).

Although the PTNS is both rapid and easy to use, it does not seem to have gained much attention. The method is more informative in the screening of adult patients (Bellini & Gjermo 1973) than in the assessment of early treatment needs in children and adolescents.

Dichotomous scoring

During the 1970's emphasis was also laid on improving opportunities for general dental practitioners to implement the knowledge acquired from periodontal research. To practising dentists the assessment of different severities of disease on 4 surfaces of each tooth did not seem to be the most attractive way of clinical charting. Instead of scoring severity per tooth surface, recording of the presence or absence of plaque and gingival bleeding per tooth was suggested by Ainamo & Bay (1975). The resulting indices, the Visible Plaque Index (VPI) and the Gingival Bleeding Index (GBI) are reported as the number of teeth affected in per cent of the number of teeth examined. Subsequently, the same principle was applied to other periodontal disease indicators as well (Ainamo & Ainamo 1978). Such efforts were particularly welcomed by practising dentists and public dental health administrators. Dichotomous scoring was adopted for epidemiological purposes by the WHO (1978) and found suitable for use also in clinical trials (Ainamo et al. 1977).

The Periodontal Screening Examination (PSE)

The Periodontal Screening Examination represents another type of approach for determining treatment needs. The method was introduced by Oliver in 1977 and has gained a relatively wide use, e.g. by practising dentists, particularly in the United States. The PSE involves assessment of probing depth at the mesiobuccal and distobuccal line angle of each remaining tooth. Bleeding after probing and probing depths of 0-3 mm, 4-5 mm, and 6 mm or more,

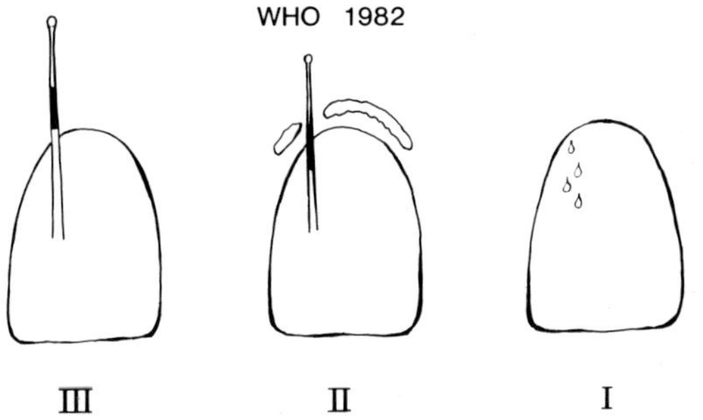

Fig. 2-19. Classification of treatment needs according to the CPITN. Complex treatment (III) is required when the color coded area (3.5-5.5 mm) of the WHO probe disappears underneath the gingival margin. The finding of a 6 mm or deeper pocket is recorded by giving code 4 to the sextant. Scaling (II) is indicated if the deepest pocket is 4 or 5 mm (code 3) or if supra- or subgingival calculus or defective margins of fillings or crowns (code 2) are found. If no pockets or plaque retentions are observed but bleeding occurs after probing, code 1 is given to the sextant. The corresponding treatment need is oral hygiene instruction (I).

are the indicators of the actual treatment need.

The PTNS and the PSE both give direct indications as to whether the patient can be taken care of by the dental hygienist, whether treatment should be delivered by the examining general practitioner or whether the services of a specialist periodontist are required. For such purposes the PTNS would seem more reliable than the PSE. Through the examination of all surfaces of all teeth *all* patients with at least one 6 mm or deeper pocket will be identified even when only 1 score per quadrant is recorded (PTNS). The PSE, though it records 2 surfaces of each tooth, still harbors the inherent shortcoming of partial examination systems; in this case a single deep pocket on the lingual aspect of a tooth is inevitably overlooked. It has recently been demonstrated that partial examination offers a fair estimate of average periodontal disease severity levels in population groups but fails to identify a considerable proportion of individuals with localized periodontal disease of the more advanced type (Ainamo & Ainamo 1981).

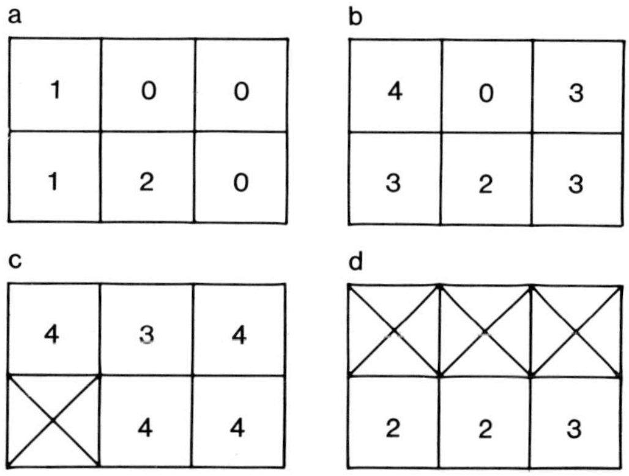

Fig. 2-20. Examples of CPITN recordings. Case a needs scaling in the mandibular anterior sextant and oral hygiene instructions for elimination of the bleeding also in the right side posterior sextants. In case b complex treatment is needed in 1 and scaling in all but 1 sextant. If this is a young patient the possibility of juvenile periodontitis should be considered. Case c needs complex treatment in 4 sextants and scaling in all but the edentulous mandibular right sextant. In case d the maxilla is edentulous (or only 1 tooth remains). The lower jaw requires scaling in all 3 sextants. In addition, cases b, c and d all require oral hygiene instruction as well.

The Community Periodontal Index of Treatment Needs (CPITN)

A new era in periodontal health services research was started when, at the initiative of the World Health Organization (WHO 1978), the Community Periodontal Index of Treatment Needs (CPITN) was developed (Ainamo et al. 1982), and after years of collaborative research, testing and refining, subsequently adopted by the International Dental Federation (FDI 1985) for use both in epidemiological studies and for screening of patients in general dental practice (Figs. 2-18, 2-19 and 2-20). The CPITN has been widely used in all parts of the world. The many studies from varying geographic and socio-economic areas already included in the WHO Global Data Bank (Pilot et al. 1986, 1987a) have substantially increased the knowledge and understanding of the prevalence and distribution of periodontal disease and have made it possible to start the planning of preventive periodontal services on a population level as well as for individuals. Knowledge of the current situation has also made it possible to plan periodontal health goals for the year 2000 (Frandsen 1984).

The CPITN is a combination of the dichotomous scoring principle, the treatment need assessment used in the PTNS, and the division of the full dentition into 6 segments as suggested by O'Leary (1967). Instead of quadrants, sextants are thus used as basic units of examination for and recording of treatment needs (Fig. 2-18). For a sextant to qualify for recording, it must contain at least 2 functioning teeth. The observations made from only 1 remaining tooth are included in the recording for the adjoining sextant (Ainamo et al. 1982, Cutress et al. 1987, WHO 1987).

Only 1 recording is given to each sextant. In developing countries with little experience of dental caries and reparative treatment, loss of tooth attachment may proceed rather evenly in all areas of the dentition. In such cases, the sextant recording may be determined after examination of the first and second molars in the posterior, and 1 central incisor in the anterior, sextants. This selection of 10 index teeth is recommended for epidemiological surveys of adults (Fig. 2-18, Epidemiology, below horizontal line). The results thus obtained overestimate periodontal treatment needs in young individuals and may, as with the use of the PSE, fail to identify an occasional adult subject with localized advanced breakdown of the periodontium.

In adult inhabitants of affluent industrialized countries advanced periodontal breakdown is often observed at only one or a limited number of sites. To ensure that in such populations all subjects in need of treatment for advanced periodontitis are identified, the examination of all teeth in the sextant is recommended (Fig. 2-18, Treatment, below the horizontal line).

In subjects under the age of 20 it is uncommon to find deep pockets with loss of attachment around other teeth if the first molars and/or incisors are not affected. In determining the periodontal treatment needs in children and adolescents it is therefore recommended to restrict the examination to 6 index teeth (Fig. 2-18, Epidemiology and Treatment, above horizontal line). The second molars included in the screening of adults are deleted because of their tendency to give false positives with regard to deep pockets during the eruptive stage of these teeth (Ainamo 1984). False pockets may also occur in adults, e.g. between the distal surface of the second molar and a hyperplastic retromolar pad.

For further simplification of the examination, a special WHO periodontal probe was developed. The probe has a "ball point", 0.5 mm in diameter, for easy detection of subgingival calculus and to decrease the risk of overmeasurement of pocket depth (Fig. 2-19). The force used at probing should correspond to 20 g or less. The color coded area extends from 3.5 to 5.5 mm:

Code 4 is given to the sextant if at one or more teeth the color coded area of the WHO probe disappears into the inflamed pocket indicating pocket depth of 6mm or more. Such a sextant requires "complex treatment", i.e. either deep scaling, curettage or surgical intervention. In most cases the patient would be referred to a specialist periodontist for treatment.

Code 3 is given to the sextant if the color coded area of the probe remains partially visible when inserted into the deepest pocket. Pocket depth is now 4 or 5 mm and treatment of the sextant can usually be managed with thorough scaling and proper personal oral hygiene measures.

Code 2 is assigned to the sextant if there are no pocket depths exceeding 3 mm (colored area remains totally visible) but dental calculus or other plaque retentions are seen at, or recognized underneath, the gingival margin. The treatment need for code 2 is the same as for code 3, scaling and improved oral hygiene.

Code 1 is given to a sextant when there are no pockets and no calculus or overhangs of fillings but bleeding occurs after gentle probing of one or more pockets. A maximum score of 1 indicates a need only for instructions in improved oral hygiene.

As shown in Fig. 2-20, only the highest code number per sextant is recorded. The need for complex treatment (code 4) thus includes also the needs for scaling and oral hygiene instruction, and codes 3 and 2, correspondingly, always require improved oral hygiene in addition to scaling.

As with the PTNS, recording of the CPITN codes can be performed in just 1-3 min. Like the PTNS, the method is thus practical for preliminary assessment of the need for periodontal treatment during initial screening of the oral health status of a new patient. The advantage of the CPITN over the PTNS is that the CPITN allows scoring of, for example, calculus occurring in the lower anterior sextant alone. Using the PTNS, calculus on the two central incisors would be scored as a need for scaling of both mandibular quadrants. This difference has special bearing in the assessment of periodontal treatment needs at young age. The CPITN is already in use for initial screening of patients in the Departments of Oral Diagnosis and Treatment Planning of a number of Dental Schools. On the basis of the 6 code numbers, the patient can be referred to a hygienist for a prophylaxis or to a specialist periodontist for detailed recording of disease status. After treatment, the CPITN can be used for monitoring of the maintenance phase following periodontal treatment.

Treatment needs in populations

Instead of using average scores for a given population, the CPITN is designed to directly indicate what percentage of a given age group requires complex treatment, scaling, or oral hygiene instructions. For treatment planning in clinical practice it is also essential to know whether 4 deep pockets in a dentition are located all in one (Fig. 2-20b) or in 4 different sextants (Fig. 2-20c).

With the CPITN, it is not meaningful to use the various code numbers for calculating average scores for individuals or population groups. As with the PTNS (Johansen et al. 1973), the possibility exists with the CPITN to use the separately calculated treatment time per sextant and per type of treatment as a common de-

Table 2-1

Age	No. examined	No. dentate	Highest treatment need recorded per person (in %)				
			TN 0 Health	TN 1 Bleeding	TN 2 Calc + OF Pockets ≤ 5 mm	TN 3 Pockets ≥ 6 mm	Missing sextants
25	313	312	2 (0.8)	7 (1.7)	91 (3.3)	1 (0.0)	(0.2)
35	318	299	2 (0.5)	7 (0.7)	85 (3.3)	6 (0.1)	(1.5)
50	317	192	1 (0.2)	1 (0.3)	82 (2.7)	18 (0.4)	(2.4)
65	306	92	2 (0.1)	2 (0.2)	69 (2.2)	27 (0.6)	(3.0)

Table 2-1. Number of Finnish rural subjects examined and distribution of dentate subjects according to their highest treatment need. TN 0 = no treatment, TN 1 = oral hygiene education, TN 2 = scaling and removal of overhangs in pockets ≤ 5 mm, TN 3 = complex treatment of pockets ≥ 6 mm. The mean number of sextants involved per dentate person is given in brackets (Ainamo et al. 1986).

nominator for assessment of the total amount of treatment required.

Prevalence of advanced disease in adults

According to CPITN data from Europe, about 25-50% of dentate 64-year-olds have advanced periodontal disease, indicated by the presence of one or more 6 mm or deeper pathological pockets. In a Finnish rural population, the prevalence figure started at values close to zero at age 25 and increased steadily with advancing age (Table 2-1, Ainamo et al. 1986). A comparable prevalence (23%) was recorded by Vogel and Strohmenger in Italy (1985) whereas Neissen and Lange found as many as 42% of 55-year-olds in Münster, Germany, to be affected with advanced periodontal disease (unpublished data).

One of the most important recent findings in periodontal epidemiological research is that, of all those subjects with one or more teeth or sextants affected, more than 50% seem to have the advanced disease limited to one or two teeth or one sextant only (Schaub 1984, Hunt 1986, Ismail et al. 1986, Ainamo et al. 1987) (Table 2-2). Thus, the extent of treatment required seems to be much smaller than previously assumed. This epidemiological finding strongly supports the concept originating from clinical research that periodontal disease is "site specific" (Socransky et al. 1983). It also

Table 2-2

Age (N)	No. of sextants scoring TN 3 (in %)						
	0	1	2	3	4	5	6
25 (312)	99	1	0	0	0	0	0
35 (299)	94	5	0	1	0	0	0
50 (192)	83	9	3	1	3	1	1
65 (92)	73	13	7	3	2	0	2

Table 2-2. Distribution of Finnish rural adults with one or more sextants scoring TN 3, according to number of sextants affected. Each horizontal lines equals 100% (Ainamo et al. 1987).

SUBJECTS AND QUADRANTS AFFECTED
ADVANCED DISEASE

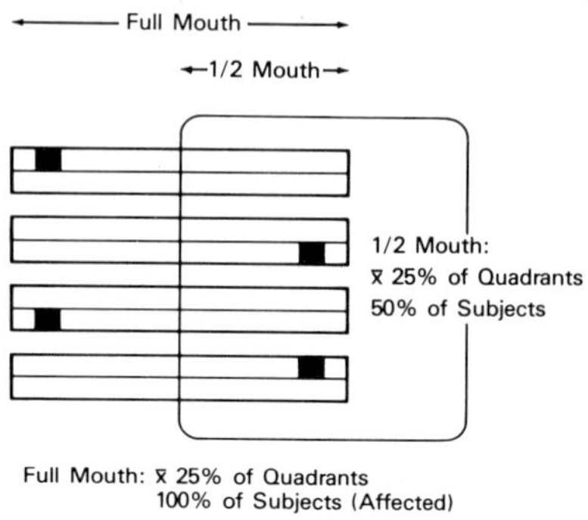

Fig. 2-21. Of subjects with advanced periodontal disease over 50% have only one site, sextant or quadrant affected. Half-mouth examination, for example, thus gives a correct evaluation of extent (x number of quadrants) but results in a 50% or higher underestimate of prevalence (% of subjects affected) of 6 mm or deeper pockets. N.B., on the average, the distribution of advanced disease in the 4 subjects is symmetrical.

supports the suggestion that the balance between the bacterial challenge and the tissue response of an individual may vary from one tooth and even from one tooth surface to another (Haffajee et al. 1983), and indirectly confirms the assumption that the single affected site may undergo only infrequent bursts of destructive activity between lengthy time periods of quiescence (Goodson et al. 1982).

The site specificity of advanced periodontal disease also importantly influences the choice of methods to be applied in epidemiological research. Thus, full mouth examination can be expected to result in a higher prevalence of advanced periodontal disease than any partial examination suggested so far (Ainamo & Ainamo 1985). The Extent and Severity Index (Carlos et al. 1986), limited to half-mouth examination, would fail to identify more than 50% of those individuals who have advanced disease in one site or segment only (Table 2-2), in addition to missing all those subjects whose deep pocket(s) occur on the lingual aspects of the teeth (Fig. 2-21).

Table 2-3

Age	No. examined	Highest treatment need (TN) recorded per person (in %) TN 0 Healthy	TN 1 Bleeding	TN 2 Calc+OF Pockets ≤ 5 mm	TN 3 Pockets ≥ 6 mm	Missing index teeth
7	101	5 (2.7)	89 (3.2)	6 (0.1)	0 (0)	(0)
12	100	2 (0.9)	74 (4.8)	24 (0.3)	0 (0)	(0)
17	98	2 (1.9)	59 (3.5)	39 (0.6)	0 (0)	(0)

Table 2-3. Distribution of the three groups of Finnish schoolchildren aged 7, 12 and 17 years according to highest treatment need (TN) recorded per subject. The mean number of sextants (index teeth) involved per subject is given in brackets (Nordblad et al. 1986).

Both the PTNS and the treatment version of the CPITN are based on full mouth examination but partial recording, as only the highest treatment need in a group of teeth is scored. Although subsequent actual treatment of subjects with advanced disease requires also full mouth or full sextant recordings, the identification of each patient with 6 mm or deeper pockets can be achieved with only the 4 (PTNS) or 6 (CPITN) segment recordings.

Data from subjects under 20 years of age

The constant period of inflammation around erupting and exfoliating teeth in the mixed dentition has discouraged many researchers from assessing periodontal disease in young age groups. With the CPITN this problem has been solved by scoring only those 6 permanent teeth (Fig. 2-18) which are the first ones to erupt into the mouth. From age 7 to 11, the index teeth are scored for bleeding and calculus only while from 12 (Ainamo et al. 1984a) or 15 (WHO 1987) to 19 years of age, also probing for pocket depth is performed. Results from such studies are illustrated with the example in Table 2-3. The increasing prevalence and number of sextants affected with calculus (TN2) are in agreement with other, unpublished reports from Europe but are considerably lower than those recorded in developing countries (Nordblad et al. 1986, Pilot et al. 1987a,b).

From a public health point of view, there is an urgent need to develop improved methods for the prevention of periodontal disease. A look at Table 2-1 reveals that already among young adults there are considerable needs for clinical treatment. At a recent EEC sponsored symposium, tentative goals for periodontal health in the year 2000 were formulated (Frandsen 1984). Total periodontal health being rare, the concept of "acceptable" health, indicated by the presence of 3 or more healthy (CPITN code 0) sextants, was introduced. This criterion seems particularly useful for those under 20 years of age when the presence of one or more healthy posterior sextants can be interpreted to reflect an "acceptable" level of self care. In a group of Finnish schoolchildren, the proportion of subjects with "acceptable" health

Table 2-4

Age (N)	No. of sextants scoring TN 0 (in %) 0	1	2	3	4	5	6
7 (101)	4	19	20	25	22	5	5
12 (100)	36	33	14	10	4	1	2
17 (98)	13	22	18	12	25	7	3

Table 2-4. Distribution of three groups of Finnish schoolchildren aged 7, 12 and 17 years according to number of healthy sextants (TN 0). Each horizontal line equals 100% (Nordblad et al. 1986).

decreased from 57% at age 7 to 17% at age 12 years (Table 2-4). However, most probably due to an increased concern about self care at that specific age, the proportion of subjects with "acceptable" health was again up at 47% in 17-year-olds, in spite of the concurrent linear increase in prevalence and extent of dental calculus shown in Table 2-3.

Of the 3 European periodontal health goals (Frandsen 1984), the one requiring that 90% of 18-year-olds should present "acceptable" periodontal health, seems to be the most meaningful one. The 2 goals for adults are more difficult to implement because of the limited effect of self care measures in adults who already have developed both calculus and pathological pockets. In order to effectively decrease periodontal disease in future adults and to reach the periodontal health goal for 18-year-olds, it would seem necessary to start preventive measures from the time when the first permanent teeth erupt. At the same time, however, the associated risk of using an excessive brushing force, resulting in loss of attachment due to recession of the gums (Paloheimo et al. 1987), should be given careful consideration.

Current and future trends

The epidemiology of periodontal disease is a relatively young science. Research conducted during the last few decades indicates that periodontal disease is one of the most common plagues of mankind. The direct causal association between bacterial colonization on the tooth surface and the inflammatory destruction of tooth attachment has been clearly demonstrated. The rate of destruction has further been found to vary considerably from one subject to another, and even from one site to the next in the same mouth, depending mainly on individual differences in tissue response to the bacterial irritation.

Although, from a practical point of view the etiology of periodontal disease has been clarified, this does not mean that research in the area of periodontal epidemiology has become redundant. For the interested researcher, epidemiological methodology offers fascinating possibilities for solving periodontal problems also in the future.

Further development is needed in the area of simple charting of periodontal disease status in dental practice so that treatment needs can be identified. The main challenge for the immediate future is to find ways to identify potential risk groups before irreversible breakdown of periodontal tissue has taken place. In this respect, further research on both microbiological aspects and tissue response factors should be given continued attention.

Also, epidemiological methods will continue to be required for the monitoring of periodontal health, and for the evaluation of the effect of various preventive and therapeutic programs and procedures.

References

Ainamo, J. (1970) Concomitant periodontal disease and dental caries in young adult males. *Proceedings of the Finnish Dental Society* **66**, 303-366.

Ainamo, J. (1984) Assessment of periodontal treatment needs. Adaptation of the WHO Community Periodontal Index of Treatment Needs (CPITN) to European conditions. In *Public Health Aspects of Periodontal Disease in Europe*, ed. Frandsen, A. Berlin: Quintessenz Verlag.

Ainamo, J. & Ainamo, A. (1978) Development of oral health during dental studies in India and Finland. *International Dental Journal* **28**, 427-433.

Ainamo, J. & Ainamo, A. (1985) Partial indices as indicators of the severity and prevalence of periodontal disease. *International Dental Journal* **35**, 322-326.

Ainamo, J., Ankkuriniemi, O. & Parviainen. K. (1980) The prevalence of caries and periodontal disease in the same subjects. In *The Borderland between Caries and Periodontal Disease. II*, ed. Lehner, T. & Cimasoni, G., pp. 9-29. Academic Press, London-Toronto-Sydney, Grune & Stratton, New York-San Fransisco.

Ainamo, J., Barmes, D., Beagrie, G., Cutress, T., Martin, J. & Sardo-Infirri, J. (1982) Development of the World Health Organization (WHO) Community Periodontal Index of Treatment Needs (CPITN). *International Dental Journal* **32**, 281-291.

Ainamo, J. & Bay, I. (1975) Problems and proposals for recording gingivitis and plaque. *International Dental Journal* **25**, 229-235.

Ainamo, J., Nordblad, A. & Kallio, P. (1984a) Use of the CPITN in populations under 20 years of age. *International Dental Journal* **34**, 285-291.

Ainamo, J., Sarkki, L., Kuhalampi, M.L., Palolampi, L. & Piirto, O. (1984b). The frequency of periodontal extractions in Finland. *Community Dental Health* **1**, 165-172.

Ainamo, J., Sjöblom, M., Ainamo, A. & Tiainen, L. (1977) Growth of plaque while chewing sucrose and sorbitol flavoured gum. *Journal of Clinical Periodontology* **4**, 151-160.

Ainamo, J., Tervonen, T., & Ainamo, A. (1986) CPITN-assessment of periodontal treatment needs among adults in Ostrobothnia, Finland. *Community Dental Health* **3**, 153-161.

Ainamo, J., Tervonen, T., Nordblad, A. & Kallio, P. (1987) Use of CPITN cross-tabulations - A research perspective. *International Dental Journal* **37**, 173-178.

Ånerud, Å., Löe, H., Boysen, H. & Smith, H. (1979) The natural history of periodontal disease in man. Changes in gingival health and oral hygiene before 40 years of age. *Journal of Periodontal Research* **14**, 526-540.

Axelsson, P. & Lindhe, J. (1981a) Effect of controlled oral hygiene procedures on caries and periodontal disease in adults. Results after 6 years. *Journal of Clinical Periodontology* **8**, 239-248.

Axelsson, P. & Lindhe, J. (1981b) The significance of maintenance care in the treatment of periodontal disease. *Journal of Clinical Periodontology* **8**, 281-294.

Bailit, H.L., Braun, R., Maryniuk, G.A. & Camp, P. (1987) Is periodontal disease the primary cause of tooth extraction in adults? *Journal of American Dental Association* **114**, 40-45.

Bellini, H.T. & Gjermo, P. (1973) Application of the Periodontal Treatment Need System (PTNS) in a group of Norwegian industrial employees. *Community Dentistry and Oral Epidemiology* **1**, 22-29.

Björby, A. & Löe, H. (1967) The relative significance of different local factors in the initiation and development of periodontal inflammation. *Journal of Periodontal Research* **2**. Abstr., 76-77.

Cahen, P.M., Frank, R.M. & Turlot, J.C. (1985) A survey of the reasons for dental extractions in France. *Journal of Dental Research* **64**, 1087-1093.

Carlos, J.P., Wolfe, M.D. & Kingman, A. (1986) The extent and severity index: a simple method for use in epidemiologic studies on periodontal disease. *Journal of Clinical Periodontology* **13**, 500-505.

Carranza, F.A. (ed.) (1984). *Glickman's Clinical Periodontology*. 6th ed., pp. 309-341, Philadelphia, W.B. Saunders.

Curilovic, Z. (1979) Die Ursachen des Zahnverlustes in der Schweiz. Resultate einer Umfrage bei Privatzahnärzten. *Schweizerische Monatsschrift für Zahnheilkunde* **89**, 727-737.

Cutress, T., Ainamo, J. & Sardo-Infirri, J. (1987) The community periodontal index of treatment needs (CPITN) procedure for population groups and individuals. *International Dental Journal* **37**, 223-233.

Ekanayaka, A. (1984) Tooth mortality in plantation workers and residents in Sri Lanka. *Community Dentistry and Oral Epidemiology* **12**, 128-135.

Ennever, J., Sturzenberger, O.P. & Radike. A.W. (1961) The Calculus Surface Index method for scoring clinical calculus studies. *Journal of Periodontology* **32**, 54-57.

FDI (1985) A simplified periodontal examination for dental practices. *FDI Newsletter* No. 142.

Frandsen, A. (ed.) (1984) *Public Health Aspects of Periodontal Disease*, p. 250, Berlin, Quintessence.

Glavind, L. & Löe, H. (1967) Errors in the clinical assessment of periodontal destruction. *Journal of Periodontal Research* **2**, 180-184.

Goodson, J.M., Tanner, A.C.R., Haffajee, A.D., Somberger, G.C. & Socransky, S.S. (1982) Patterns of progression and regression of advanced destructive periodontal disease. *Journal of Clinical Periodontology* **9**, 472-481.

Greene, J.C. (1963) Oral hygiene and periodontal disease. *American Journal of Public Health* **53**, 913-922.

Greene, J.C. & Vermillion, J.R. (1960) The Oral Hygiene Index: A method for classifying oral hygiene status. *Journal of American Dental Association* **61**, 172-179.

Greene, J.C. & Vermillion, J.R. (1964) The simplified oral hygiene index. *Journal of American Dental Association* **68**, 7-13.

Haffajee, A.D., Socransky, S.S. & Goodson, J.M. (1983) Comparison of different data analyses for detecting changes in attachment level. *Journal of Clinical Periodontology* **10**, 298-310.

Hunt, R.J. (1986) Periodontal treatment needs in an elderly population in Iowa. *Gerodontics* **2**, 24-27.

Ismail, A.I., Eklund, S.A., Burt, B.A. & Calderone, J.J. (1986) Prevalence of deep periodontal pockets in New Mexico adults aged 27 to 74 years. *Journal of Public Health Dentistry* **46**, 199-206.

Johansen, J.R., Gjermo, P. & Bellini, H.T. (1973) A system to classify the need for periodontal treatment. *Acta Odontologica Scandinavica* **31**, 297-305.

Lightner, L.M., O'Leary, T.J., Drake, R.B., Crump, P.P. & Allen, M.F. (1971) Preventive periodontic treatment procedures: results after 46 months. *Journal of Periodontology* **42**, 555-561.

Lindhe, J., Hamp, S.E. & Löe, H. (1975) Plaque-induced periodontal disease in beagle dogs. *Journal of Periodontal Research* **10**, 243-255.

Löe, H. (1963) Epidemiology of periodontal disease. *Odontologisk Tidsskrift* **71**, 479-503.

Löe, H. (1967) The Gingival Index, the Plaque Index and the Retention Index system. *Journal of Periodontology* **38**, 610-616.

Löe, H., Ånerud, Å., Boysen, H. & Smith, M. (1978) The natural history of periodontal disease in man. Study design and baseline data. *Journal of Periodontal Research* **13**, 550-562.

Löe. H. & Silness, J. (1963) Periodontal disease in pregnancy. I. Prevalence and severity. *Acta Odontologica Scandinavica* **21**, 533-551.

Löe, H., Theilade. E. & Jensen, S.B. (1965) Experimental gingivitis in man. *Journal of Periodontology* **36**, 177-187.

Lövdal, A., Arno, A., Schei, O. & Waerhaug, J. (1961) Combined effect of subgingival scaling and controlled oral hygiene on the incidence of gingivitis. *Acta Odontologica Scandinavica* **19**, 537-555.

Mackler, S.B. & Crawford, J.J. (1973) Plaque development and gingivitis in the primary dentition. *Journal of Periodontology* **44**, 18-24.

MacMahon, B., Pugh, T.F. & Ipsen, J. (1960) *Epidemiologic Methods*. Boston: Little and Brown.

Massler, M., Schour, I. & Chopra, B. (1950) Occurrence of gingivitis in suburban Chicago school children. *Journal of Periodontology* **21**, 146-164.

Matsson, L. (1978) Development of gingivitis in pre-school children and young adults. *Journal of Clinical Periodontology* **5**, 24-34.

Mühlemann, H.R. (1968) *In vivo* measurements of dental calculus. *Annals of the New York Academy of Sciences* **153**, 164-196.

Nordblad, A, Kallio, P., Ainamo, J. & Dusadeepan, A. (1986) Periodontal treatment needs in populations under 20 years of age in Espoo, Finland and Chiangmai, Thailand. *Community Dentistry and Oral Epidemiology* **14**, 129-131.

O'Leary, T.J. (1967) The periodontal screening examination. *Journal of Periodontology* **38**, 617-624.

Oliver,R.C. (1977) Patient evaluation. *International Dental Journal* **27**, 103-106.

Paloheimo, L., Ainamo, J., Niemi, M-L. & Viikinkoski, M. (1987) Prevalence of and factors related to gingival recession in Finnish 15- to 20-year olds. *Community Dental Health* **4**, 425-436.

Parfitt, G.J. (1957) A five year longitudinal study of the gingival condition of a group of children in England. *Journal of Periodontology* **26**, 26-32.

Pilot, T., Barmes, D.E., Leclercq, M.H., McCombie, B.J. & Sardo Infirri, J. (1986) Periodontal conditions in adults, 35-44 years of age: An overview of CPITN data in the WHO Global Oral Data Bank. *Community Dentistry and Oral Epidemiology* **14**, 310-312.

Pilot, T., Barmes, D.E., Leclercq, M.H., McCombie, B.J. & Sardo Infirri, J. (1987a) Periodontal conditions in adolescents, measured by CPITN. *Community Dentistry and Oral Epidemiology* **15**, 336-338.

Pilot, T., Effendi, I., Sunu, N.P. & Wibowo, D. (1987b) Periodontal conditions in different regions in Indonesia. *Community Dental Health* **4**, 239-243.

Quigley, G.A. & Hein, J.W. (1962) Comparative cleansing efficiency of manual and power brushing. *Journal of American Dental Association* **65**, 26-29.

Ramfjord, S.P. (1959) Indices for prevalence and incidence of periodontal disease. *Journal of Periodontology* **30**, 51-59.

Ramfjord, S.P., Emslie, R.D., Greene, J.C., Held, A.J. & Waerhaug, J. (1968) Epidemiological studies of periodontal disease. *American Journal of Public Health* **58**, 1713-1722.

Ramfjord, S.P., Knowles, J.W., Nissle, R.R., Burgett, F.G. & Shick, R.A. (1975) Results following three modalities of periodontal therapy. *Journal of Periodontology* **46**, 522-526.

Rosling, B., Nyman, S., Lindhe, J. & Jern, B. (1976) The healing potential of the periodontal tissues following different techniques of periodontal surgery in plaque-free dentitions. A 2 year clinical study. *Journal of Clinical Periodontology* **3**, 233-250.

Russell, A.L. (1956) A system of classification and scoring for prevalence surveys of periodontal disease. *Journal of Dental Research* **35**, 350-359.

Russell, A.L. (1963) International nutrition surveys: A summary of preliminary dental findings. *Journal of Dental Research* **42**, 232-244.

Schaub, R.M.H. (1984) *Barriers to Effective Periodontal Care*. Thesis, University of Groningen, The Netherlands.

Schour, I. & Massler, M. (1947) Gingival disease in postwar Italy (1945) I. Prevalence of gingivitis in various age groups. *Journal of the American Dental Association* **35**, 475-482.

Schroeder, H.E. (1969) *Formation and Inhibition of Dental Calculus*. Berne and Stuttgart: Hans Huber Publishers.

Scherp, H.W. (1964) Current concepts in periodontal disease research: epidemiological contributions. *Journal of the American Dental Association* **68**, 667-675.

Silness, J. & Löe, H. (1964) Periodontal disease in pregnancy. II. Correlation between oral hygiene and periodontal condition. *Acta Odontologica Scandinavica* **24**, 747-759.

Socransky, S.S., Haffajee, A.D., Goodson, J.M. & Lindhe, J. (1983) New concepts of destructive periodontal disease. *Journal of Clinical Periodontology* **11**, 21-32.

Suomi, J.D., Greene, J.C., Vermillion, J.R., Doyle, J., Chang, J.J. & Leatherwood, E.C. (1971) The effect of controlled oral hygiene procedures on the progression of periodontal disease in adults: results after third and final year. *Journal of Periodontology* **42**, 152-160.

Suomi, J.D., Smith, L.W., Chang, J.J. & Barbano, J.P. (1973) Study on the effect of different prophylaxis frequencies on the periodontium of young adults. *Journal of Periodontology* **44**, 406-410.

Volpe, A.R. & Manhold, J.H. (1962) A method of evaluating the effectiveness of potential calculus inhibiting agents. *New York State Dental Journal* **28**, 289-290.

Volpe, A.R., Manhold, J.H. & Hazen, S.P. (1965) *In vivo* calculus assessment. I. A method and its examiner reproducibility. *Journal of Periodontology* **36**, 292-298.

Waerhaug, J. (1966) Epidemiology of periodontal disease. In *Workshop in Periodontics*. ed. Ramfjord, S.P., Kerr, D.A., Ash, M.M., pp. 179-211, Michigan: Ann Arbor.

Waerhaug, J. (1967) Prevalence of periodontal disease in Ceylon. Association with age, sex, oral hygiene, socioeconomic factors, vitamin deficiencies, malnutrition, betel and tobacco consumption and ethnic group. *Acta Odontologica Scandinavica* **25**, 205-231.

WHO (1978) *Epidemiology, Etiology and Prevention of Periodontal Diseases*. Geneva: Technical Report Series 621.

WHO (1987) *Oral Health Surveys, Basic Methods*. 3rd ed., pp. 31-33. Geneva: WHO, Oral Health Unit.

Vogel, G. & Strohmenger, L. (1985) Periodontal Treatment Needs (CPITN) of 54961 Subjects Aged 15-64. Faculty of Medicine, University of Milano.

CHAPTER 3

Dental Plaque and Dental Calculus

Proper oral hygiene has for centuries been recommended in dental textbooks as a preventive measure against dental diseases. However, the significance of dental deposits for the development of periodontal disease lacked a scientific basis until the middle of this century, when well designed epidemiological studies were performed. From such surveys it is now established that the presence of dental deposits, whether mineralized or not, is undoubtedly the most important factor in the development of periodontal disease.

Final evidence for this statement was presented as a result of clinical studies in which gingivitis was experimentally initiated by the abolition of oral hygiene procedures (Löe et al. 1965, Theilade et al. 1966). When a correct regime of oral hygiene was reinstituted, gingival inflammation resolved within a week, restoring gingival health.

The transition from gingivitis to destructive periodontal disease has not been demonstrated experimentally in man. However, in dogs gingivitis develops as the result of plaque accumulation (Egelberg 1965a) and, if it is allowed to continue for a sufficiently long period, permanent destruction of the supporting tissues of the teeth may occur typical of human periodontal disease (Saxe et al. 1967, Lindhe et al. 1973). These results indicate that destructive periodontal disease may develop from longstanding gingivitis, and thus support the conclusions drawn from epidemiologic studies.

Additional evidence for the role of dental deposits in the development of periodontal disease in man has been derived from studies in which the progression of periodontal desease has been markedly retarded by the introduction of improved oral hygiene measures (e.g. Lövdal et al. 1961, Suomi et al. 1971, Ramfjord et al. 1973, Knowles et al. 1979). In highly motivated individuals optimal plaque control may practically arrest the progression of periodontal desease (Lindhe & Axelsson 1973, Axelsson & Lindhe 1974, 1981 Söderholm 1979, Pihlstrom et al. 1983, Lindhe & Nyman 1984, Saxen et al. 1986, Wennström et al. 1986). Thus, there is excellent reason for the interest, developed over the last 25 years, in the subject of dental deposits.

Unfortunately, the successful plaque preventive measures available today are time consuming for the individual as well as for the dental profession. It is therefore unlikely that a significant proportion of the population of the world will benefit from the available knowledge of plaque control in this century. Less demanding plaque control methods are sought and a better understanding of the nature of dental deposits is essential for the development of safe alternative inhibitors of plaque and calculus formation.

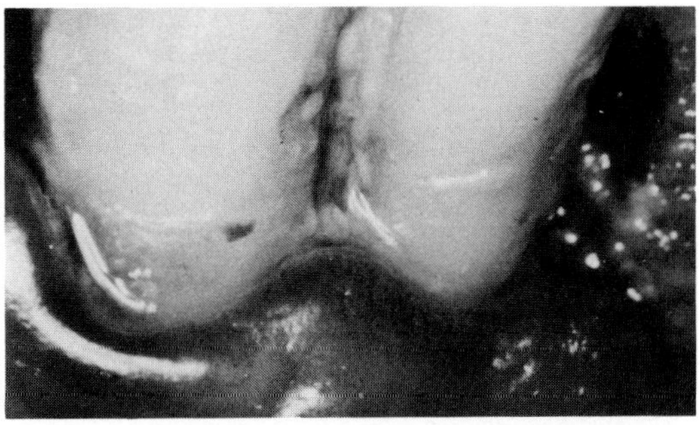

Fig. 3-1 Supragingival plaque of a thickness which makes it clinically visible. The interproximal space between the two teeth is completely occupied by plaque.

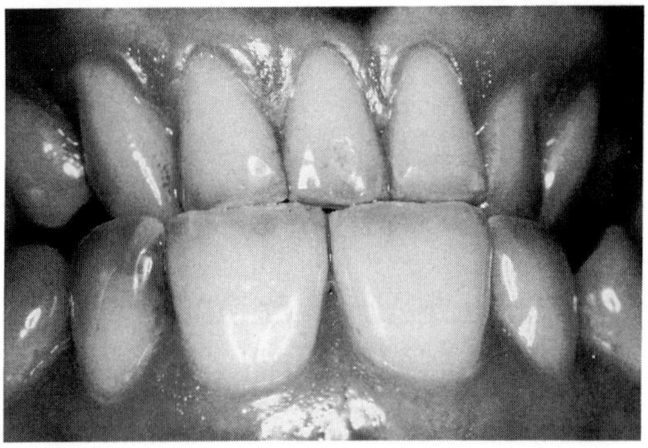

Fig. 3-2. No visible plaque is apparent.

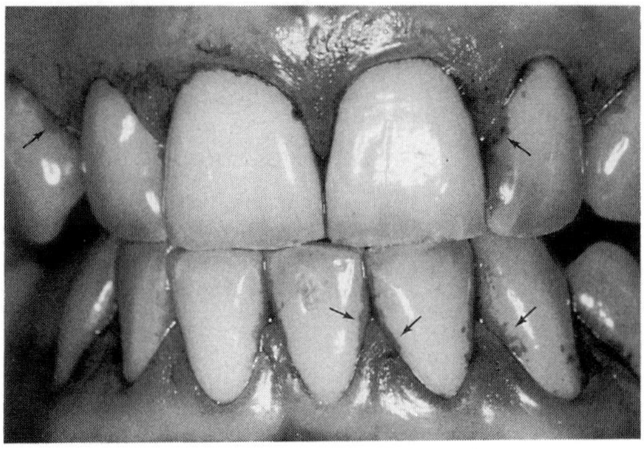

Fig. 3-3. The same teeth as seen in Fig. 3-2 are now stained with a disclosing solution, revealing plaque interproximally along the gingival margin of the teeth (arrows).

Dental Plaque

Definition and classification of dental plaque

Dental plaque may be defined as bacterial aggregations on the teeth or other solid oral structures (Dawes et al. 1963, Egelberg 1970, Kelstrup & Theilade 1974).

However, this definition is not employed universally although, for clinical purposes, it seems adequate and simple. Another definition distinguishes dental plaque from materia alba, the latter comprising the soft white material consisting of bacterial aggregations, leukocytes and desquamated oral epithelial cells accumulating in an unclean mouth at the surface of plaque or teeth (Mühlemann & Schroeder 1964). According to this definition the differentiation between dental plaque and materia alba is determined by the strength of adherence of the deposit. If it is removed by the mechanical action of a strong water spray, the material is termed materia alba; if it withstands the water spray, it is called dental plaque. The distinction between these two types of bacterial accumulation is of questionable value and is often impractical to use clinically. Hence, the term dental plaque will be used in this chapter to designate both types of bacterial aggregations on the solid surfaces in the mouth.

Plaque in the dentogingival region is of primary concern to the therapist dealing with periodontal disease. Dentogingival plaque may arbitrarily be classified as surpragingival plaque deposited on clinical crowns of teeth, and subgingival plaque located in the gingival sulcus or the periodontal pocket. Of course, this classification of dentoginival plaque is only precise at a given moment, as the separating border between the two types of plaque, i.e. the gingival margin, may shift coronally due to swelling of the gingival tissues, or it may migrate apically as a result of gingival recession. If this shift in the position of the gingival margin occurs, the classification of the plaque located between the previous and the new location of the gingival margin is automatically changed. However, in spite of the theoretical inaccuracies of the classification, its value in practice is well documented.

Clinical appearance and distribution of plaque

Supragingival plaque is clinically detectable once it has reached a certain thickness and then it appears as a whitish, yellowish layer primarily along the gingival margins of the teeth (Fig. 3-1). Plaque may be difficult to identify if it is present in small quantities (Fig. 3-2). In this case its presence may be ascertained by scraping the tooth surface along the gingival margin with the end of a probe or by using a disclosing solution (Fig. 3-3). This may be a conventional dye staining the plaque, or a fluorescent dye which can be demonstrated by illumination with ultraviolet light (Hefferren et al. 1971, Lang et al. 1972).

Subgingivally situated plaque cannot be diagnosed directly *in situ*. And since subgingival plaque is normally present in thin layers, it is not possible to diagnose such deposits by clinical inspection unless it is revealed by removal from the gingival sulcus or pocket, or by displacing the soft tissues. Plaque may form anywhere on solid structures in the mouth, if the site is protected from the normal mechanical cleaning action of the food, the tongue, the cheeks and the lips. Plaque deposits are, thus, regularly present in the fissures of the occlusal surfaces, in pits and irregularities, even on the smooth tooth surfaces, on fillings and artificial crowns and especially along ill-fitting restorations, on orthodontic bands and on removable orthodontic appliances and dentures.

Composition of dental plaque

The easiest way to get information on the composition of dental plaque is to remove a small sample from the tooth surface, transfer it to a microscope slide and stain it with a bacterial stain (Fig. 3-4). Examination of the preparation in a microscope with transillumination will reveal a multitude of bacteria of different morphological forms. Some host cells will also be present, either epithelial cells from the desquamated oral epithelia or blood cells, primarily polymorphonuclear leukocytes.

Well established plaque may contain microorganisms other than bacteria. Mycoplasms have been demonstrated, and small numbers of yeasts and protozoa may also be present (Lange et al. 1983). In spite of the fact that plaque has often previously been considered as food debris, at least by the lay public, recognizable dietary remains are infrequently encountered in dental plaque.

Microbiology of dental plaque

In 1 mm^3 of dental plaque weighing about 1 mg, more than 10^8 bacteria may be counted. A multitude of different species of microorganisms is present and it is not currently possible to identify them all. Studies of the microbial composition of gingival plaque have been performed ever since it was discovered that specific organisms were the cause of many diseases affecting mankind. Such studies will continue for the foreseeable future as improved methods become available for culturing and

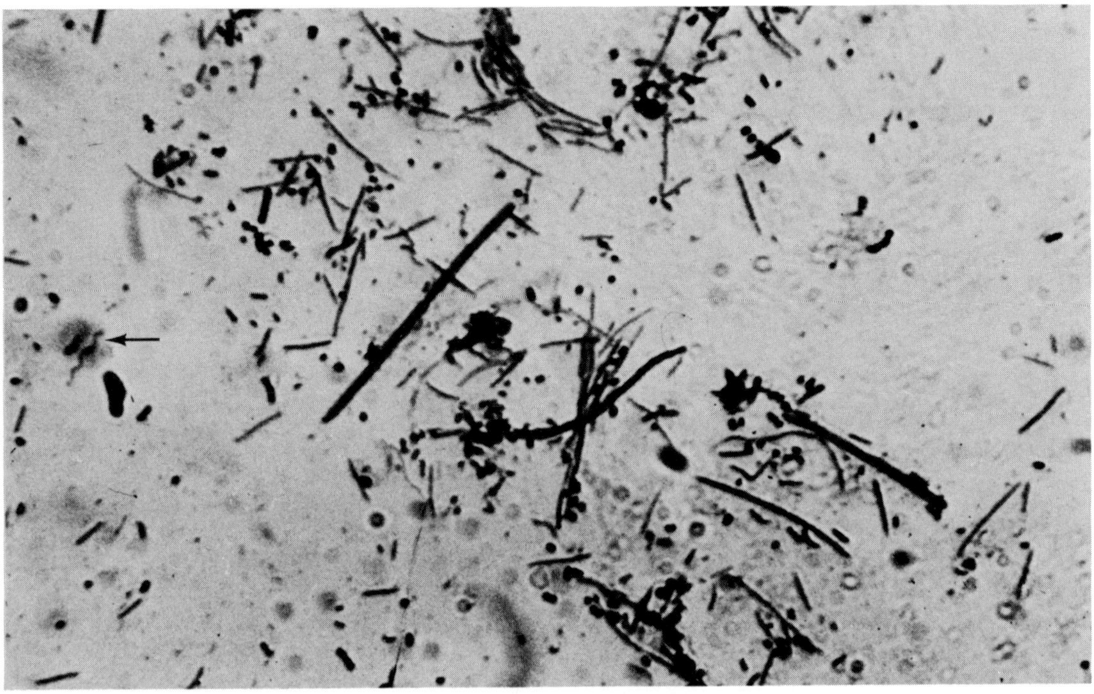

Fig. 3-4. Gram-stained smear of old human supragingival plaque. Cocci constitute a relatively small porportion of the bacterial flora. Filamentous organisms predominate, and a spirochete is present in the field (arrow).

identifying the individual species present. There are still microorganisms in the mouth (such as spirochetes) for which the available culturing techniques are insufficient. This means that such microorganisms cannot be adequately studied. Other types, though culturable, cannot be correctly determined because of the lack of taxonomic data and reference strains essential for the final identification of a bacterial species. However, certain patterns of microbial composition of plaque at different sites in the mouth have become evident. Apparently, the characteristic environment of each location favors development of a certain microbial community (Theilade & Theilade 1985).

Supragingival plaque

In an investigation called "Experimental gingivitis in man" (Löe et al. 1965, Theilade et al. 1966), the oral hygiene of a group of dental students was improved during several weeks of intensive instruction in the use of toothbrush and toothpicks. This resulted in a very low occurrence of plaque and excellent gingival conditions. Then, all oral hygiene measures were withdrawn allowing plaque to reaccumulate along the gingival margin. After 2-3 weeks, all subjects had developed gingivitis. During the experimental period plaque samples were obtained at regular intervals and subjected to a bacteriological examination of Gram-stained smears. The bacteria present in the samples were classified according to their Gram reaction and morphology. The results of this analysis were tabulated as the percentage distribution of the various types of microorganisms.

At commencement, with healthy gingivae, very few bacteria were present on the cervical surfaces of the teeth. The removable deposit was dominated by desquamated epithelial cells on, or between which, few bacteria could be seen. Of these, about 90% were Gram positive cocci and rods, the remainder primarily Gram negative. When all oral hygiene measures were

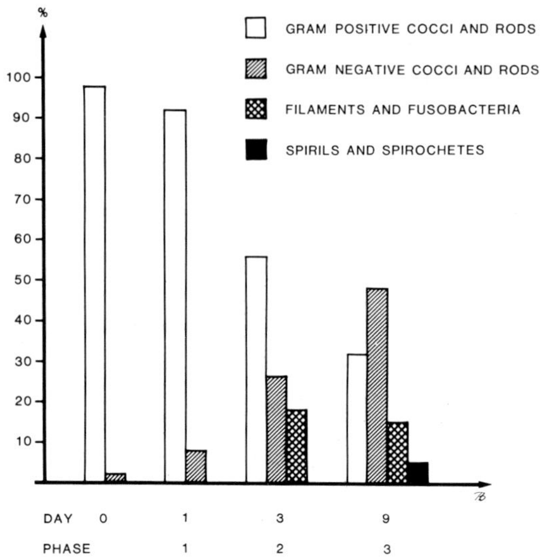

Fig. 3-5. Percentage distribution of different types of organisms on the mesial surface of the lower left premolar in a particular human subject at days 0, 1, 3, and 9 of experimental gingivitis. In the first phase of the plaque development, represented by day 1, the relative number of Gram negative cocci and rods increases. In the second phase, represented by day 3, the percentage of Gram negative cocci and rods further increases and fusobacteria and filamentous bacteria appear. In the third phase, represented by day 9, the Gram negative cocci and rods have augmented again in relative number, and in addition spirils and spirochetes are present. In contrast Gram positive cocci and rods constitute a continuously decreasing proportion of the plaque during development. Based on results presented by Theilade et al. (1966).

withdrawn, the simple bacterial plaque composition changed drastically. During the first phase of plaque development comprising the initial 2 days of the experiment, not only the number of all types of bacteria increased, but their proportional distribution changed as well. Gram negative cocci and rods now comprised a greater proportion of the flora. The second phase of plaque development, days 3 and 4, was characterized by a proliferation of fusobacteria and filamentous bacteria. During the third phase, days 5-9, spirilla and spirochetes appeared, so that the complex flora seen in old plaque had become established. After about 7 days, the various groups of bacteria had proliferated to the extent that the Gram positive cocci and rods, which initially predominated, now constituted only 50% of the complex flora. During the remaining period up to 3 weeks, no further major changes in the bacterial distribution occurred (Fig. 3-5).

A more detailed classification of the bacteria present in early stages of supragingival plaque development has become available from cultural studies (Rönstrom et al. 1977, Socransky et al. 1977, Theilade et al. 1982a, Moore et al. 1982, Liljemark et al. 1986). It is now apparent that the very early flora, 3-8 h after proper tooth cleaning, is dominated by streptococci. Most of these have been identified as *Streptococcus mitior*, while *Streptococcu sanguis* and *Streptococcus milleri* are present in smaller numbers. *Streptococcus mutans* is either absent or present only in very low numbers. Gram positive rods constitute a small proportion of this early flora, primarily *Actinomyces viscosus, Actinomyces naeslundii* and *Actinomyces odontolyticus*. Furthermore, during this initial formative stage, the microorganisms adhere very loosely to the tooth surface, so that a spray of water will remove most of them (Theilade & Mikkelsen 1972, Brecx et al. 1981). As previously mentioned, some authors do not consider such loose deposits as plaque and recommend that material that may be removed by a water-spray be termed materia alba. However, as even loosely adhering bacteria may eventually become irreversibly attached to the tooth and are therefore potential determinants of the composition of the plaque established at a later stage, the interest in the early bacterial populations is justified, regardless of the term ascribed to this deposit.

It is not until after 24 h without cleaning that a clinically demonstrable layer of plaque has formed. The number of microorganisms adhering to the tooth at this time represents the net balance between (1) previously attached bacteria which have subsequently been detached and rinsed away by the salivary flow, (2) those which have become irreversibly adherent and started to multiply, and finally (3) bacteria arriving later from the saliva to the site where they are trapped and aggregated to those already there. Recent studies indicate that multiplication of initially adhering microorganisms accounts for a major portion of the increased number of bacteria collected on the tooth after 24 h (Ørstavik & Ruangsri 1979, Brecx et al. 1983). It has been estimated that during this first day of plaque formation the mean generation time, that is the time it takes for the bacteria to double their number, is about 3 h (Socransky et al. 1977, Brecx et al. 1983). This means that 1 microorganism during the first 24-h period may multiply to a total of 256 microorganisms. A large number of these are detached and lost in saliva, which is constantly swallowed. Saliva thus has an important rinsing effect but is unfortunately insufficient to prevent plaque formation.

After the first day of plaque growth the flora becomes increasingly more complex. The proportion of streptococci decreases to 45% at 24 h while Gram negative anaerobic cocci (*Veillonella*) rapidly increase to about 20%. Facultative and obligate anaerobic species of *Actinomyces* also become more prominent, constituting about 25% after 3 days. Gram negative anaerobic rods make up about 5% of the cultivable flora after 3 days (Theilade et al. 1982 a). Facultative Gram negative rods, mainly *Haemophilus* species, also constitute a significant proportion (Liljemark et al. 1986).

During the following 3 weeks of undisturbed plaque formation the relative proportions of the various types of bacteria in the cultivable flora continue to change (Syed & Loesche 1978). The Gram positive cocci decrease in relative numbers particularly because the Gram positive rods increase, especially due to the appearance of a high proportion of *Actinomyces israelii*. Among the Gram negative bacteria, *Veillonella* is the most prominent organism while rods such as *Bacteroides* and *Fusobacterium* still constitute small proportions. Although the details of the complex bacterial composition of older plaque are far from complete, the general trend is clear. As the dentogingival plaque layer increases in thickness, the milieu changes to favor anaerobic microorganisms and an increasing number of Gram negative rods may now grow, especially in the deeper layers next to the tooth (Ritz 1969). The changed growth condition may be influenced by the concomitantly developing inflammation in the gingiva, resulting in a marked increase in the flow of gingival exudate which contains a number of growth factors not readily available in saliva. Additional nutrition is also provided by microbial symbiosis and through the death and disruption (lysis) of microorganisms in the plaque. After 3 weeks of plaque growth significant numbers of plaque bacteria are no longer viable (Theilade & Theilade 1970).

Subgingival plaque

Colonization of the gingival sulcus and the subsequently developing periodontal pocket initially starts from an already occurring deposit of supragingival plaque. Thus, the bacterial composition of subgingival plaque is partly influenced by that existing in the adjacent portion of the supragingival bacterial deposit.

However, the subgingival environment will influence the growth conditions of this area. The access to the oral cavity is limited, which favors anaerobic development. Nutrients are readily available from the gingival exudate, the volume of which is increased as a result of inflammation in the gingiva. Detachment of already established microorganisms is limited due to the protecting gingival tissues, making it possible for organisms without special adhesion mechanisms to survive. On the other hand, the chance of the arrival of additional salivary bacteria is limited or impossible. These factors may explain why the bacterial composition of

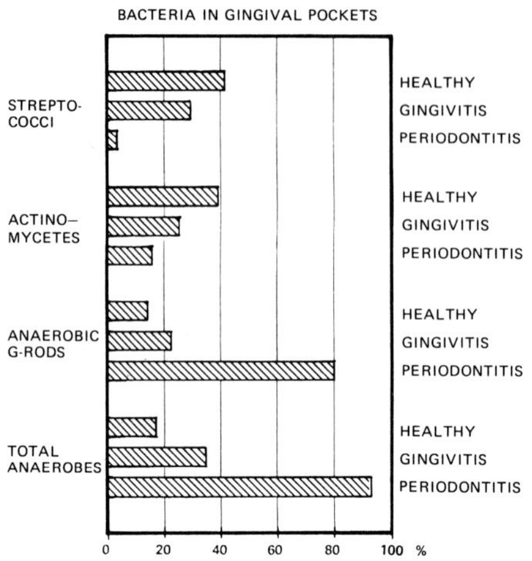

Fig. 3-6. Percentage predominantly cultivable bacteria in gingival sulci of patients with healthy gingiva and moderate gingivitis, and in periodontal pockets from patients with advanced marginal periodontitis. As periodontal disease progresses the relative numbers of Gram positive organisms such as streptococci and *Actinomyces* decrease at the expense of anaerobic bacteria, particularly Gram negative rods. Based on results from Slots (1976,1977) and from Slots et al. (1978).

subgingival plaque is different from that of the adjacent supragingival plaque.

In patients who have suffered from mild to moderate gingivitis for at least 2-3 months, streptococci only account for around 25% of the microbial flora of subgingival plaque. *Streptococcus mitis* and *S. sanguis* are predominant species. Approximately another 25% of the subgingival bacteria is comprised of various *Actinomyces* species. Gram negative anaerobic rods contribute a further 25% of the subgingival flora with *Fusobacterium, Bacteroides, Wolinella* and *Campylobacter* prominent (Slots et al. 1978, Moore et al. 1987).

Since spirochetes are not readily cultured, they are not represented in this account of the predominantly cultivable flora. However, their presence may be ascertained by darkfield microscopy, and may constitute up to 2% in gingival sulci at sites characterized as relatively healthy (Listgarten & Helldén 1978).

In advanced periodontal disease with pathologically deepened pockets along the root surface, the flora of subgingival deposits is somewhat different. The cultivable microbiota is dominated by up to 90% of anaerobic microorganisms. The Gram negative bacteria, almost exclusively rods, constitute 75% *Bacteroides* species and *Fusobacterium nucleatum* are prominent (Slots 1977, Tanner et al. 1984, Moore et al. 1985). Again, the spirochetes have not been included in this account, but darkfield microscopy reveals that in the deep pockets of advanced periodontal disease they comprise up to 50% of the flora (MacPhee & Muir 1986).

In a special form of periodontal disease in young patients, termed juvenile periodontitis, the subgingival flora is somewhat different from that described above. The cultivable flora has the same overall characteristics as other deep pockets, such as the predominance of anaerobic Gram negative rods which constitute up to 60% (Slots 1976). Among the facultative Gram negative rods, much attention has been paid to *Actinobacillus actinomycetemcomitans*, which is almost always present in juvenile periodontitis and less prevalent in adult periodontitis. It has consequently been implied that it may be a specific pathogen (Genco et al. 1986). However, this suggestion is far from universally accepted (Moore et al. 1985, Theilade 1986). Also total counts by darkfield microscopy have revealed that in juvenile periodontitis sites, spirochetes only accounted for about 7% of the flora (Liljenberg & Lindhe 1980). Thus, in juvenile periodontitis, the proportion of spirochetes is intermediate between that found in mild gingivitis and that of advanced periodontal disease.

From this review of the subgingival microbial flora of the gingival crevice in health and disease certain general trends become apparent. As disease progresses the proportion of streptococci and *Actinomyces* decreases, while the Gram negative rods increase drastically, as compared to the anaerobic bacteria (Fig. 3-6).

Structure of dental plaque

Supragingival plaque

Supragingival plaque has been examined in a multitude of studies by light and electron microscopy to gain information on its internal structure (Mühlemann & Schneider 1959, Turesky et al. 1961, Theilade 1964, Frank & Brendel 1966, Leach & Saxton 1966, Frank & Houver 1970, Schroeder & De Boever 1970, Theilade & Theilade 1970, Eastcott & Stallard 1973, Saxton 1973, Rönström et al. 1975, Tinanoff & Gross 1976, Lie 1978).

The introduction of the electron microscope in dental research was a significant development for studies of dental plaque, both because the size of many bacteria approaches the ultimate resolving power of the light microscope, and because the resins used for embedding allowed for sections thinner than the smallest bacterial dimension. Hereby the substructure of plaque could be identified. Simultaneously, advances in biochemistry made it possible to interpret the structural details revealed by electron microscopy.

In studies of the internal details of plaque, samples are required in which the deposits are kept in their original relation to the surface on which they have formed. This may be accomplished by removing the deposits with the tooth. If plaque of known age is the object of study, the tooth surfaces are cleaned at a predetermined time before removal (McDougall 1963, Frank & Houver 1970, Schroeder & De Boever 1970). If the removal of the tooth on which the plaque is located becomes impractical, pieces of natural teeth or artificial surfaces may be attached to solid structures in the mouth and removed after a given interval. This method of plaque collection was used at the beginning of the century by Black (1911), who used a glass slide attached to his upper denture as a substrate for the developing plaque. The systematic use of artificial surfaces for collection of plaque was reintroduced during the 1950's. Thin plastic foils of Mylar® were attached to lower incisor teeth for known periods, after which they were removed for histologic, histochemical and electron microscopic examination of the deposited material (Mandel et al. 1957, Mühlemann & Schneider 1959, Zander et al. 1960, Schroeder 1963, Theilade 1964). Later, other types of plastic materials such as Westopal®, Epon®, Araldite®, and spray plast have been employed for this purpose (Berthold et al. 1971, Kandarkar 1973, Lie 1975, Listgarten et al. 1975, Rönström et al. 1975). Results from several such studies indicate that plaque formed on natural or artificial surfaces does not differ significantly in structure or microbiology (Hazen 1960, Berthold et al. 1971, Nyvad et al. 1982, Theilade et al. 1982 a & b), indicating that at least some of the principal mechanisms involved in plaque formation are unrelated to the nature of the solid surface colonized. However, there are small but important differences in the chemical composition of the first layer of organic material formed on these artificial surfaces compared with that formed on natural tooth surfaces (Sönju & Rölla 1973, Sönju & Glantz 1975, Öste et al. 1980). Tooth surfaces, enamel as well as exposed cementum, are normally covered by a thin acquired pellicle of glycoproteins (Fig. 3-7, 3-9, 3-10). If removed, e.g. by mechanical instrumentation, it reforms within minutes. The pellicle is believed to play an active part in the selective adherence of bacteria to the tooth surface. For details of the proposed mechanisms, see Chapter 4.

The first cellular material adhering to the pellicle on the tooth surface or other solid surfaces consists of coccal bacteria with small numbers of epithelial cells and polymorphonuclear leukocytes (Fig. 3-8). The bacteria are either encountered on or within the pellicle as single organisms or as aggregates of microorganisms (Figs. 3-11, 3-14). Larger numbers of microorganisms may be carried to the tooth surface by epithelial cells (Figs. 3-12, 3-13).

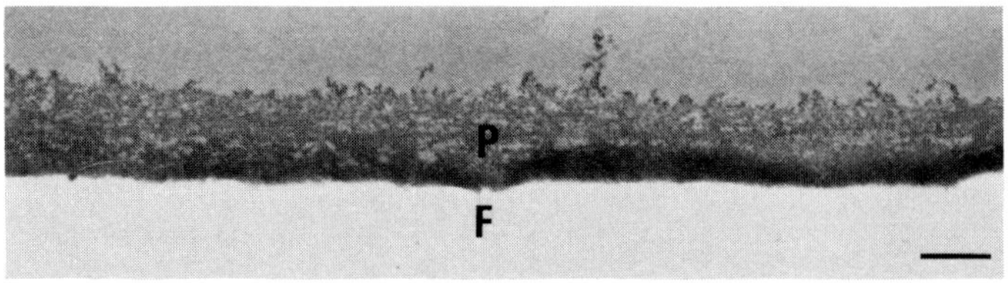

Fig. 3-7. Thin section of pellicle (P) deposited within minutes on a Mylar film (F) attached to the buccal surface of a premolar. Magnification 6 000. Bar: 1 μm.

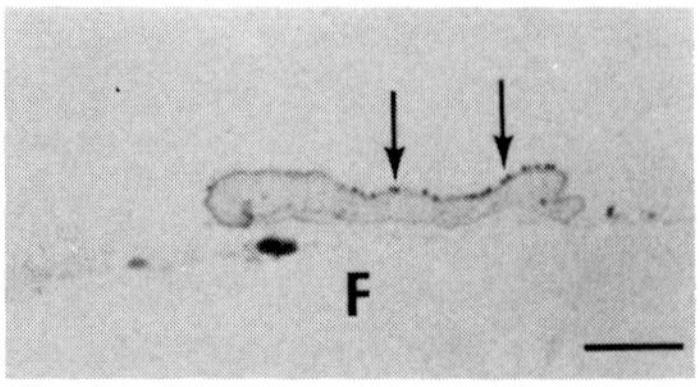

Fig. 3-8. Semithin section of deposit collected on plastic film (F) applied to the buccal surface of a premolar during a 4 h period. A thin layer of pellicle material covers the plastic film and an adhering epithelial cell is covered by coccal bacteria (arrows). Magnification X 615. Bar: 10 μm.

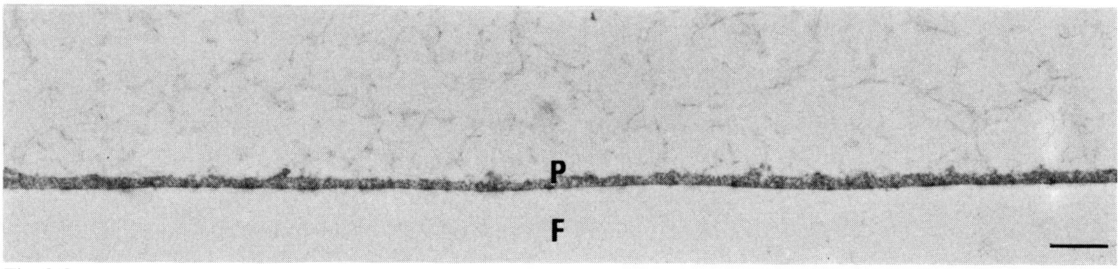

Fig. 3-9.

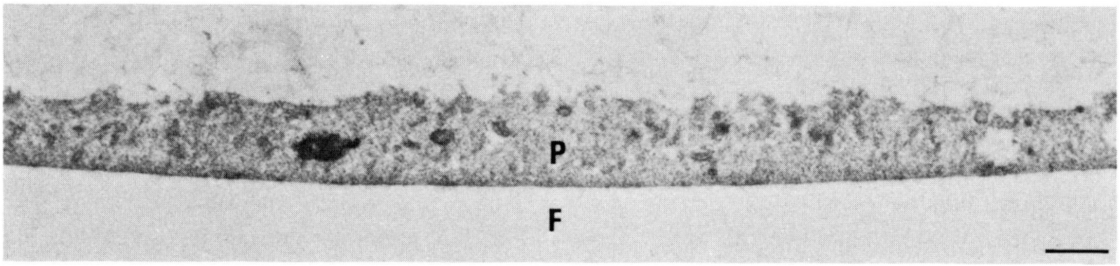

Figs. 3-9 & 3-10. Thin section of pellicle (P) deposited on plastic film (F) applied to the buccal surface of a premolar during a 4 h period. Magnification X 14 000. Bar: 0.5 μm.

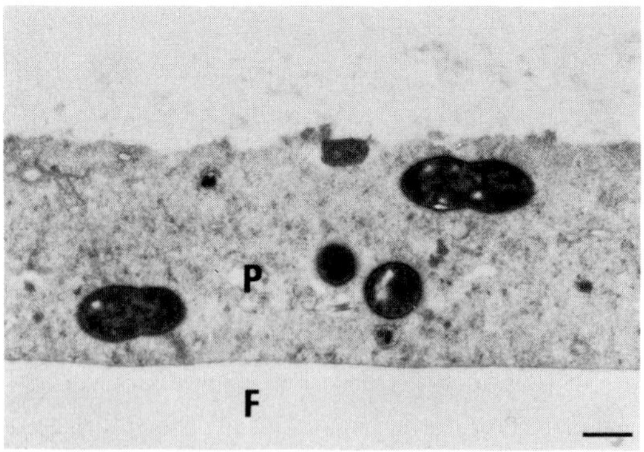

Fig. 3-11. Thin section of pellicle (P) collected within 4 h on a plastic film (F) applied to the buccal surface of a premolar. Within the pellicle material 4 microorganisms are deposited. Magnification X 10 000. Bar: 0.5 μm.

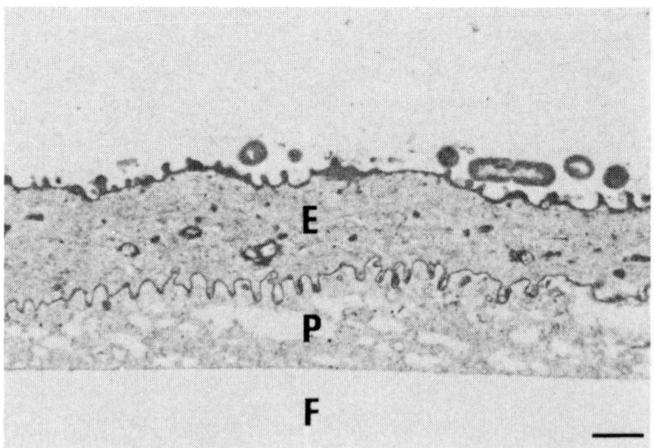

Fig. 3-12. Thin section of pellicle (p) formed on plastic film (F) applied to the buccal surface of a premolar during a 4 h period. An epithelial cell (E) carrying a few bacteria on its surface is adhering to the pellicle material. Magnification X 5 000. Bar: 1 μm.

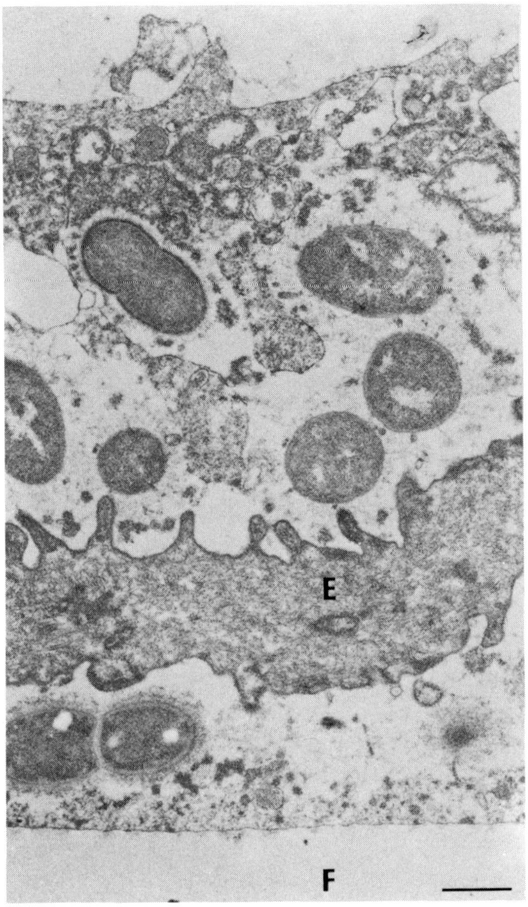

Fig. 3-13. Thin section of 4-h-old plaque formed on plastic film (F) containing bacteria and an epithelial cell (E). Magnification X 17 000. Bar: 0.5 µm.

The number of bacteria found on the surface a few hours after cleaning depends on the procedures applied to the sample before examination, the reason being that adherence to the solid surface is initially very weak. If no special precautions are taken during the preparatory processing, the early deposits are easily lost (Brecx et al. 1981). Apparently the adherence of microorganisms to solid surfaces takes place in 2 steps:

1) a reversible phase in which the bacteria adhere loosely, and later
2) an irreversible phase during which their adherence becomes consolidated (Gibbons & van Houte 1975, 1980).

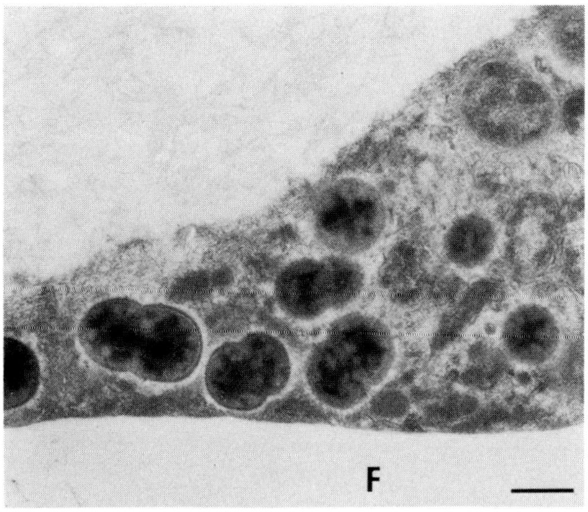

Fig. 3-14. Thin section of 8 h plaque formed on plastic film (F) containing an aggregate of bacteria. Magnification X 16 500. Bar: 0.5 µm.

Another factor which may modify the number of bacteria in early plaque deposits is the presence of gingivitis, which increases the plaque formation rate so that the more complex bacterial composition is attained earlier (Saxton 1973, Hillam & Hull 1977, Brecx et al. 1980). Plaque growth may also be initiated by microorganisms harbored in minute irregularities in which they are protected from the natural cleaning of the tooth surface.

During the first few hours, bacteria that resist detachment from the pellicle may start to proliferate and form small colonies of morphologically similar organisms (Fig. 3-15). However, since other types of organisms may also proliferate in an adjacent region, the pellicle becomes easily populated by a mixture of different microorganisms (Fig. 3-16). In addition, some organisms seem able to grow between already established colonies (Fig. 3-17) and, finally, it is likely that clumps of organism of different species will become attached to the tooth surface or to the already attached microorganism. Such clumps will also produce mixed colonies when they proliferate. Therefore, the overall impression of plaque composition after a few days is characterized by complexity. At this time it also becomes evident

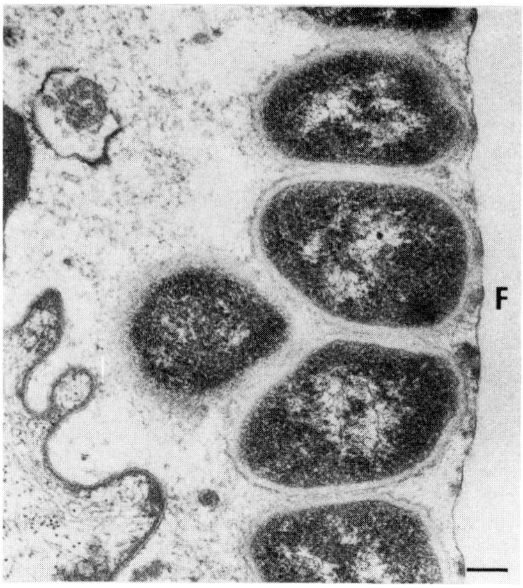

Fig. 3-15. Thin section of plaque colony consisting of morphologically similar bacteria deposited on plastic film (F) applied to the buccal surface of a premolar during an 8 h period. Magnification X 33 000. Bar: 0.2 μm.

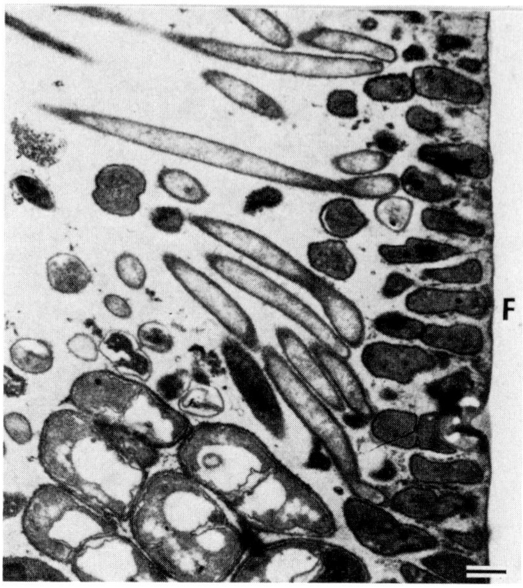

Fig. 3-16. Thin section of plaque colony containing different types of bacteria formed on Mylar film (F) during a 3 day period. Magnification X 9 100. Bar: 0.5 μm.

that different types of organisms may benefit from each other. One example is the corncob configurations resulting from the growth of cocci on the surface of a filamentous microorganism (Listgarten et al. 1973). Another feature of older plaque is the presence of dead and lysed bacteria (Fig. 3-18) which may provide additional nutrients to the still viable bacteria in the neighborhood (Theilade & Theilade 1970).

The material present between the bacteria in dental plaque is called the intermicrobial matrix and accounts for approx. 25% of the plaque volume. Three sources may contribute to the intermicrobial matrix: the plaque microorganisms, the saliva, and the gingival exudate.

The bacterial metabolism may release various end products. Some bacteria may produce various extracellular carbohydrate polymers, serving as energy storage or as anchoring material to secure their retention in plaque (Fig. 3-19). Degenerating or dead bacteria may also contribute to the intermicrobial matrix. Different bacterial species often have distinctly different metabolic pathways and capacity to synthesize extracellular material. The intermicrobial matrix in plaque, therefore, varies considerably from region to region. A fibrillar component is often seen in the matrix between Gram positive cocci (Fig. 3-20), and is in accordance with the fact that several oral streptococci synthesize levans and glucans from dietary sucrose. In other regions, the matrix appears granular or homogeneous (Fig. 3-21). In parts of the plaque with the presence of Gram negative organisms, the intermicrobial matrix is regularly characterized by the presence of small vesicles surrounded by a trilaminar membrane, which is similar in structure to that of the outer envelope of the cell wall of the Gram negative microorganisms (Fig. 3-22). Such vesicles probably contain endotoxins and proteolytic enzymes, and may also be involved in adherence between bacteria (Hofstad et al. 1972, Grenier & Mayrand 1987).

It must be remembered, however, that the transmission electron microscope does not reveal all organic components of the intermicro-

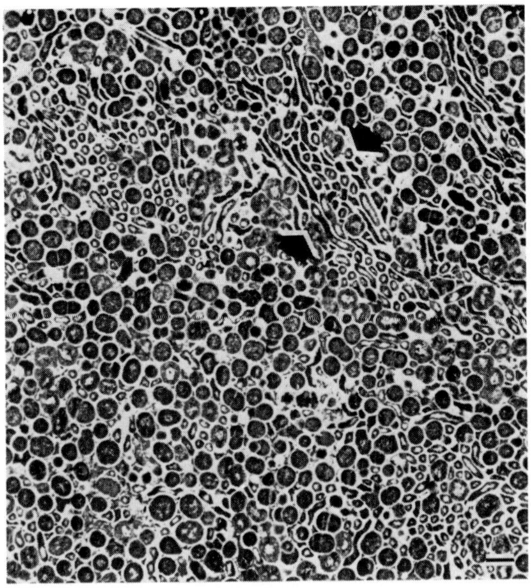

Fig. 3-17. Thin section of 3-day-old plaque. The predominant organisms appear to be cocci and rods into which strands of filamentous organisms grow (arrows). Magnification X 2 800. Bar: 1 µm.

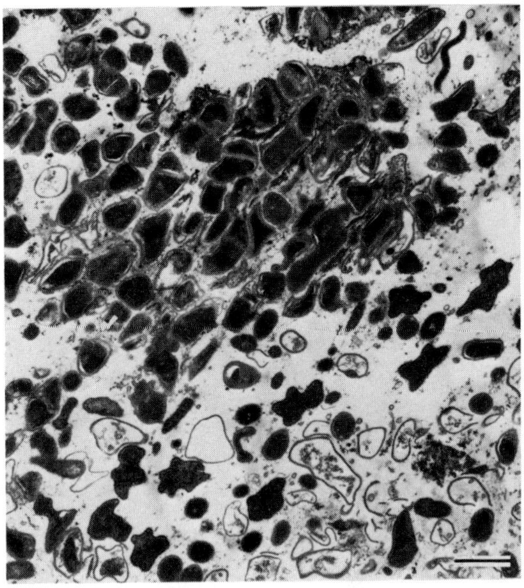

Fig. 3-18. Thin section of 23-day-old plaque, which contains a considerable number of dead or lysed bacteria as evidenced by partly or completely empty bacterial cell walls termed ghosts. A spirochete is seen in the upper right corner of the illustration. Magnification X 58 000. Bar: 1 µm.

bial matrix and the more soluble constituents may be lost during the procedures required prior to sectioning and examination of the plaque sample. Biochemical techniques may be used to identify such compounds (Silvermann & Kleinberg 1967, Krembel et al. 1969, Kleinberg 1970, Hotz et al. 1972, Rölla et al. 1975, Bowen 1976). Such studies indicate that proteins and carbohydrates constitute the bulk of the organic material while lipids appear in much lower amounts. However, studies are few in which bacteria and intermicrobial matrix have been analyzed separately, and thus the total compositional nature of the matrix is still far from being finally established. Some of the proteins in the matrix are altered salivary glycoproteins, probably partly degraded by the microorganisms utilizing the sugar moiety, others have been identified as salivary or bacterial enzymes and as immunoglobulins.

The carbohydrates of the matrix have received a great deal more attention, and at least some of the polysaccharides in the plaque ma-

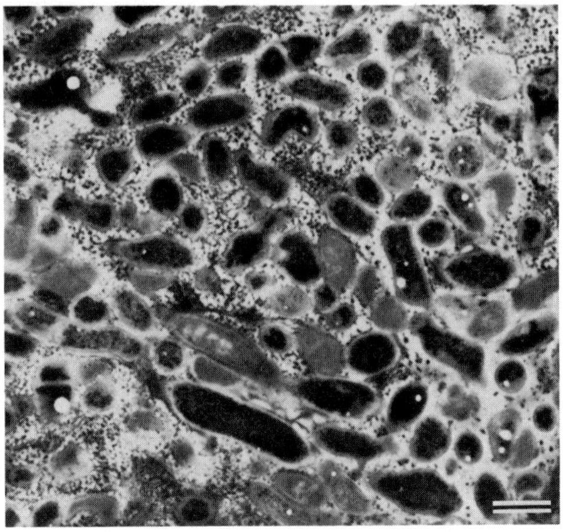

Fig. 3-19. Thin section of old plaque stained for the demonstration of polysaccharides by reacting them with electron-dense material appearing dark in the illustration. Many bacteria contain large amounts of intracellular polysaccharide, and the intermicrobial matrix contains extracellular polysaccharides. Magnification X 6 600. Bar: 1 µm.

trix are well characterized. These are fructans (levans) and glucans. Fructans are synthesized in plaque from dietary sucrose and provide a

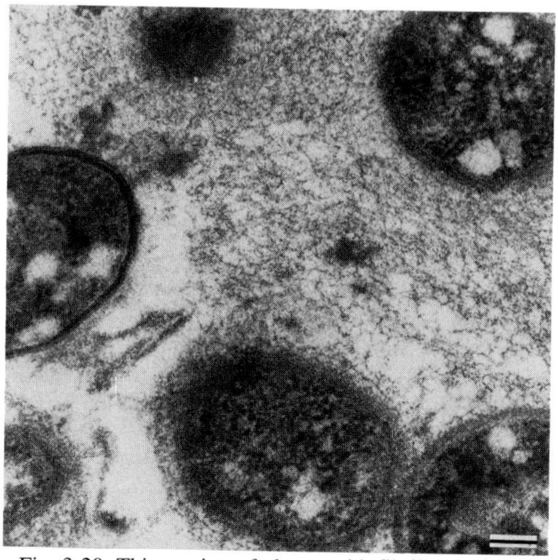

Fig. 3-20. Thin section of plaque with fibrillar intermicrobial matrix. Magnification X 47 500. Bar: 0.1 µm.

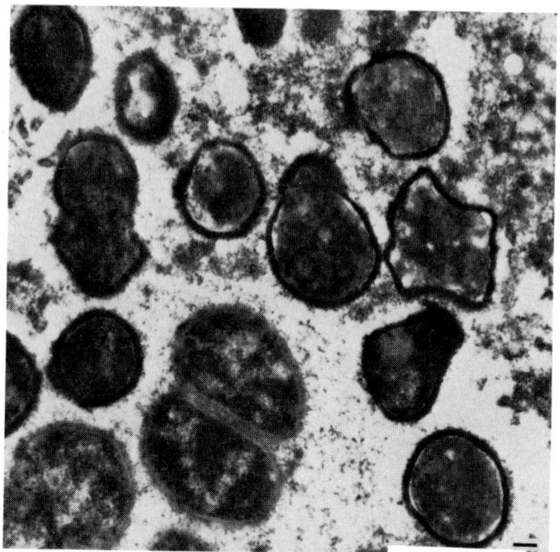

Fig. 3-21. Thin section of plaque with a granular or homogeneous intermicrobial matrix. Magnification X 19 000. Bar: 0.1 µm.

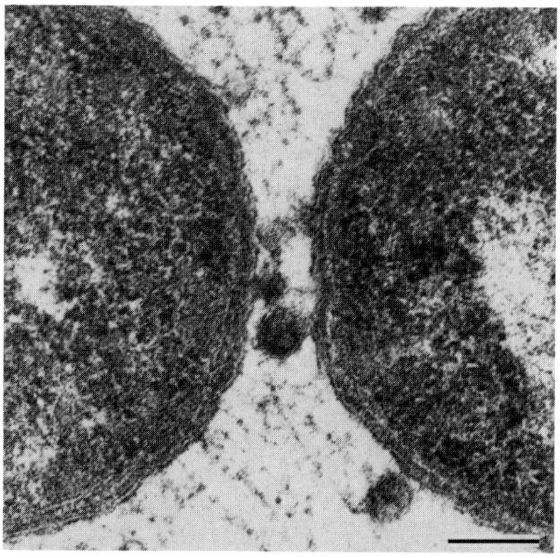

Fig. 3-22. Thin section of plaque with a region predominated by Gram negative bacteria. Between them vesicles surrounded by a trilaminar membrane (two thin electron-dense layers with an electron-lucent layer interposed between them). This substructure is also seen in the outermost endotoxin containing cell wall layer of the adjacent Gram negative bacteria. Magnification X 100 000. Bar: 0.1 µm.

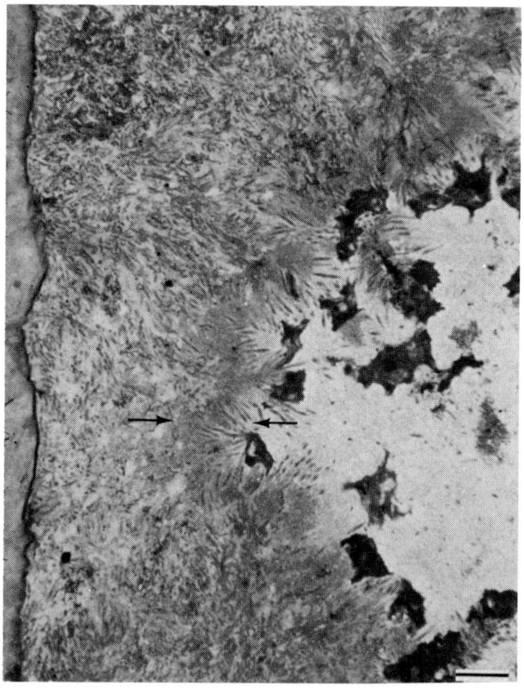

Fig. 3-23. Semithin section of subgingival plaque. To the left an electron-dense cuticle bordering the enamel space. Filamentous bacteria are less predominating than in supragingival plaque. The surface toward the gingival tissue contains many spirochetes (between arrows). To the right in the illustration various host tissue cells. Magnification X 724. Bar: 10 µm. From Listgarten (1976).

storage of energy, which may be utilized by microorganisms in time of low sugar supply. The glucans are also synthesized from sucrose. One type of glucan is dextran, which may also serve as energy storage. Another glucan is mutan which is not readily degraded. It acts primarily, therefore, as a skeleton in the matrix

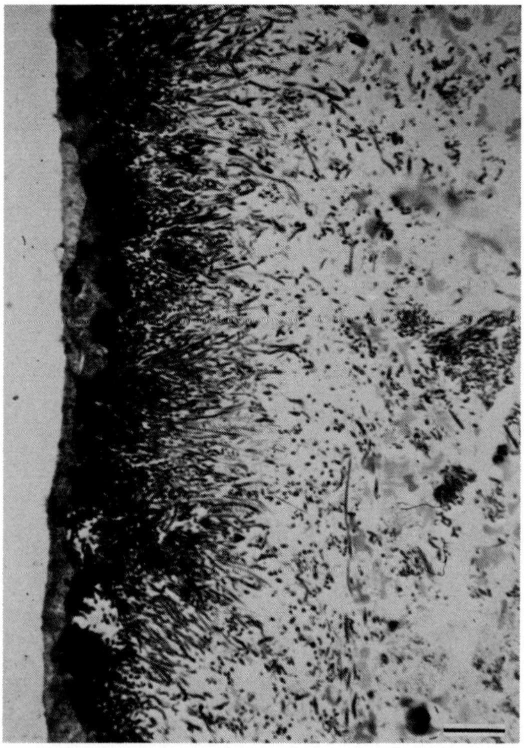

Fig. 3-24. Semithin section of supragingival plaque with a predominantly filamentous bacterial layer adherent to the enamel (to the left).Calcification of part of the plaque close to the tooth is evidenced by lighter staining. Magnification X 700. Bar: 10 μm. From Listgarten (1976).

in much the same way as collagen stabilizes the intercellular substance of connective tissue. It has been suggested that such carbohydrate polymers may be responsible for the change from a reversible to an irreversible adherence of plaque bacteria.

The small amount of lipids in the plaque matrix is as yet largely uncharacterized. Part of the lipid content is found in the small extracellular vesicles which may contain lipopolysaccharide endotoxins of Gram negative bacteria.

Subgingival plaque

The mechanisms involved in the formation of subgingival plaque are only partly elucidated. One reason is the difficulty in obtaining samples with subgingival plaque preserved in its original position between the soft tissues of the

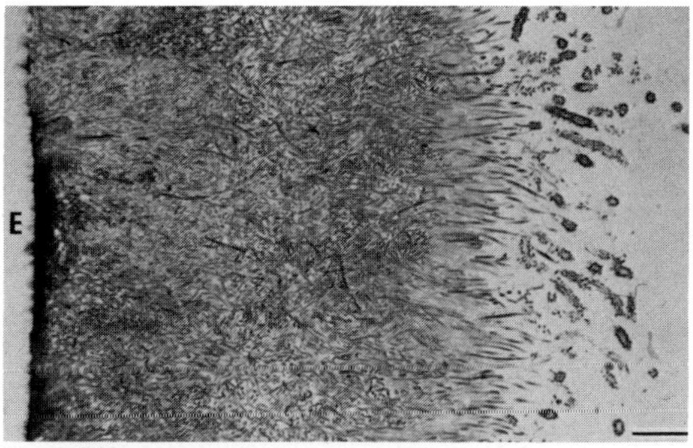

Fig. 3-25.

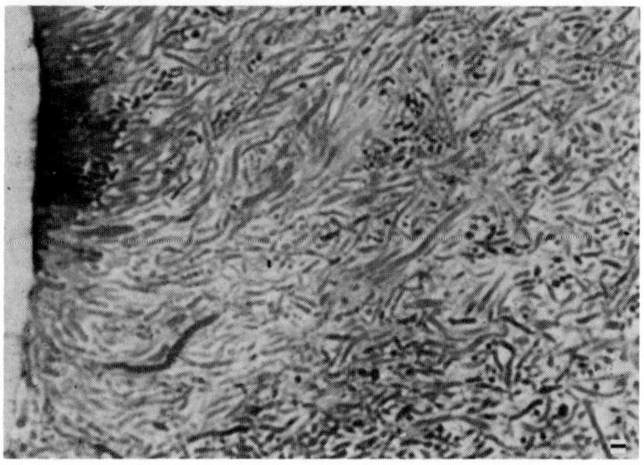

Figs. 3-25 & 3-26. Semithin section of supragingival plaque on enamel (E), which has been dissolved prior to sectioning. Filamentous organisms predominate, and at the surface some of these are surrounded by cocci giving rise to corncob-like aggregations. Magnification X 708 and 1 300 X. Bars: 10 μm and 1 μm. From Listgarten (1976).

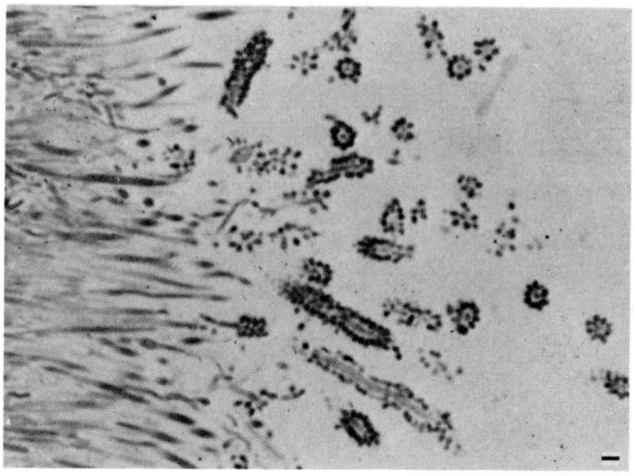

Fig. 3-27. The corncob formations seen at the plaque surface in Fig. 3-25. Magnification X 1 200. Bar: 1 μm. From Listgarten (1976).

gingiva and the hard tissues of the tooth. Thus, there are only a limited number of studies on the detailed internal structure of human subgin-

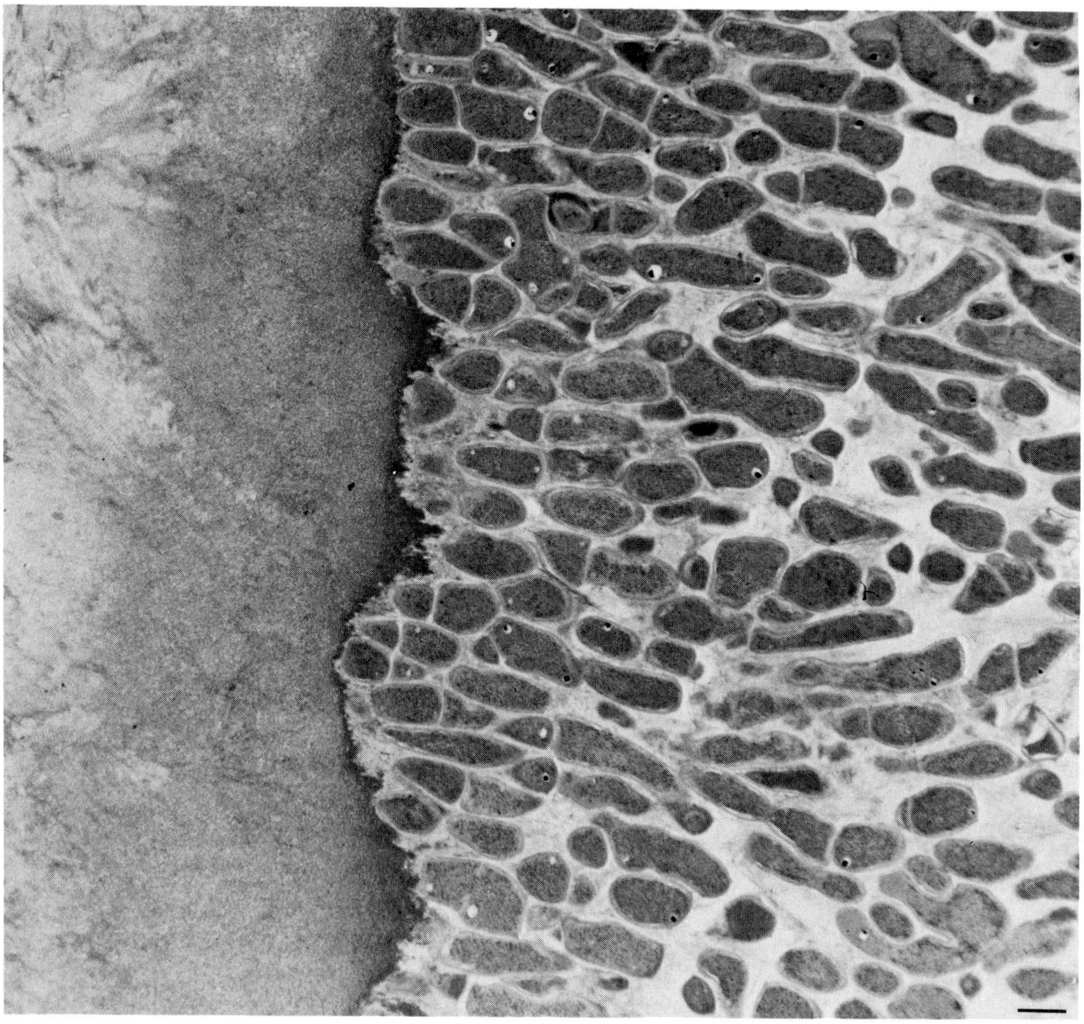

Fig. 3-28. Thin section of supragingival plaque on a root surface (to the left). The Gram positive bacteria are oriented in a palisading arrangement. Magnification X 6 000. Bar: 1 µm. From Listgarten (1976).

gival plaque (Schroeder 1970, Listgarten et al. 1975, Listgarten 1976, Westergaard et al. 1978). From these it is evident that in many respects subgingival plaque resembles the supragingival variety, although the predominant types of microorganisms found vary considerably from those present coronally to the gingival margin.

Between subgingival plaque and the tooth an electron-dense organic material is interposed, termed a cuticle (Fig. 3-23). This cuticle probably contains the remains of the epithelial attachment lamina originally connecting the junctional epithelium to the tooth with the addition of material deposited from the gingival exudate (Frank & Cimasoni 1970, Lie & Selvig 1975, Eide et al. 1983). It has also been suggested that the cuticle represents a secretory product of the adjacent epithelial cells (Schroeder & Listgarten 1977). Information is lacking concerning its chemical composition, but its location in the subgingival area makes it unlikely that salivary constituents contribute to its formation.

The structure of subgingival plaque has some similarity to the supragingival variety,

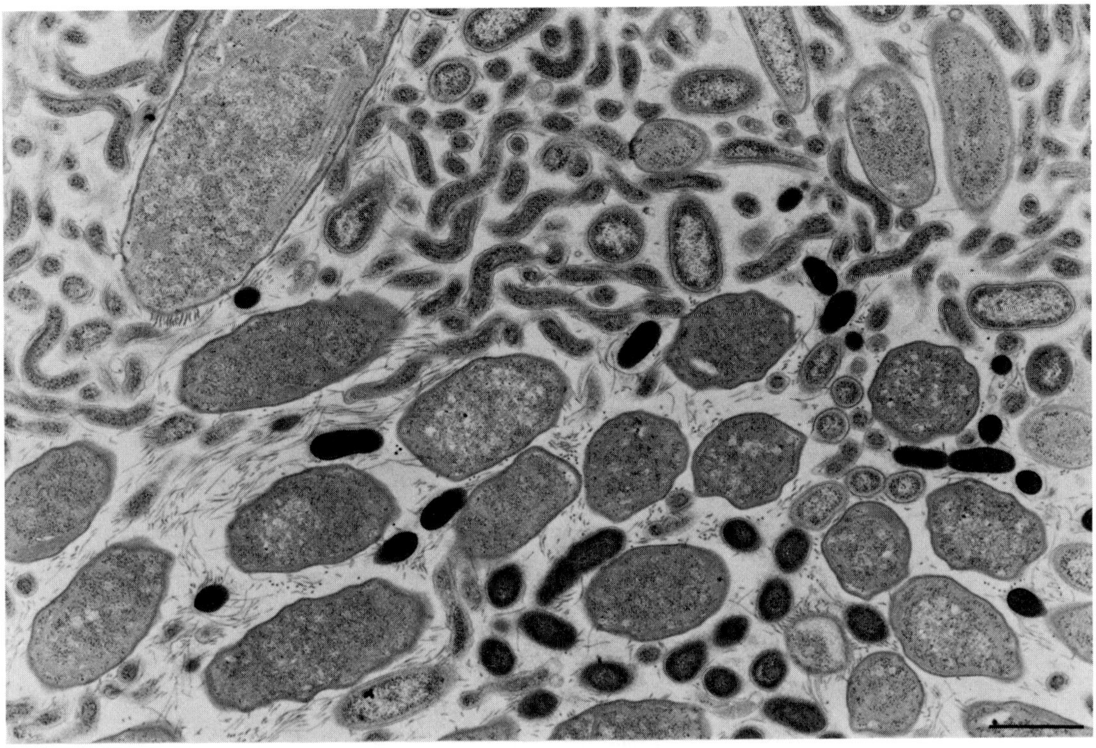

Fig. 3-29. Thin section of subgingival plaque from a deep periodontal pocket. Small microorganisms predominate, many of which are spirochetes. Magnification X 12 000. Bar: 1 μm. From Listgarten (1976).

particularly when it concerns plaque associated with gingivitis without the formation of deep pockets. A densely packed accumulation of microorganisms is seen adjacent to the cuticular material covering the tooth surface (Fig. 3-24). The bacteria comprise Gram positive and Gram negative cocci, rods, and filamentous organisms. Spirochetes and various flagellated bacteria may also be encountered, especially at the apical extension of the plaque. The surface layer is often less densely packed and leukocytes are regularly interposed between the plaque and the epithelial lining of the gingival sulcus.

When periodontal disease has resulted in a periodontal pocket, the appearance of the subgingival bacterial deposit becomes much more varied. The tooth surface may in this case either represent enamel or cementum from which the periodontal connective tissue is detached. Plaque accumulation on the portion of the tooth previously covered by periodontal tissues does not differ markedly from that observed in gingivitis (Fig. 3-25). In this layer filamentous microorganisms dominate (Figs. 3-26, 3-27, 3-28), but cocci and rods also occur. However, in the deeper parts of the periodontal pocket, the filamentous organisms become fewer in number, and in the apical portion they seem to be virtually absent. Instead, the dense, tooth-facing part of the bacterial deposit is dominated by smaller organisms without particular orientation (Fig. 3-29).

The surface layers of microorganisms in the periodontal pocket facing the soft tissue are distinctly different from the adherent layer along the tooth surface, and no definite intermicrobial matrix is apparent (Figs. 3-29, 3-30). The microorganisms comprise a large number spirochetes and flagellated bacteria. Gram negative cocci and rods are also present. The multitude of spirochetes and flagellated organ-

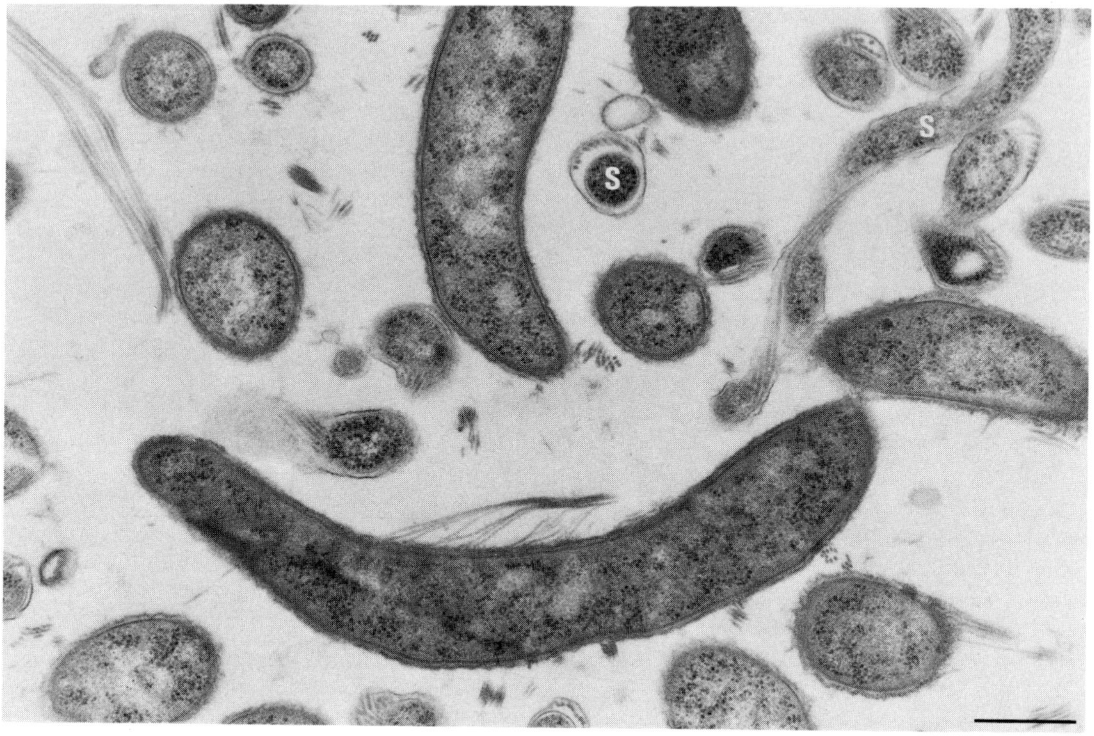

Fig. 3-30. Thin section of subgingival plaque from a deep periodontal pocket with many spirochetes (S) which are recognised by their axial filaments. In the lower part of the figure a curved organism with flagella at its concave surface. Magnification X 24 000. Bar: 0.5 μm. From Listgarten (1976).

isms are motile bacteria, and since there is no intermicrobial matrix between them, this outer part of the microbial accumulation in the periodontal pocket no doubt adheres very loosely, the soft-tissue pocket wall no doubt being responsible for their retention. As plaque is, by definition, bacteria that aggregate to the tooth, it has been suggested that subgingival microorganisms should be redesignated subgingival flora rather than subgingival plaque, as the latter term may exclude the significant motile portion of the bacterial population (Listgarten 1976).

Subgingival plaque has also been studied in cases of juvenile periodontitis (Listgarten 1976, Westergaard et al. 1978). It appears that the bacterial deposit in deep pockets from such patients is much thinner than found in adult forms of periodontal disease and that areas of the tooth surface in the periodontal pocket may be devoid of adherent microbial deposits. The cuticular material is characterized by an uneven thickness (Figs. 3-31, 3-32). The adherent layer of microorganisms, which also varies considerably in thickness, shows, equally, considerable variation in arrangement and may exhibit a palisaded organization of the bacteria (Fig. 3-33). The microorganisms in this layer are mainly cocci, rods or filamentous bacteria, primarily of the Gram negative type (Fig. 3-34). A surface layer with some Gram positive cocci frequently associated with filamentous organisms in the typical corncob formation may also be found with spirochetes in between.

The sequential events taking place during the development of subgingival plaque have not been studied in man. However, in dogs subgingival plaque may develop in the gingival sulcus within a few days, if oral hygiene is discontinued (Matsson & Attström 1979, Ten

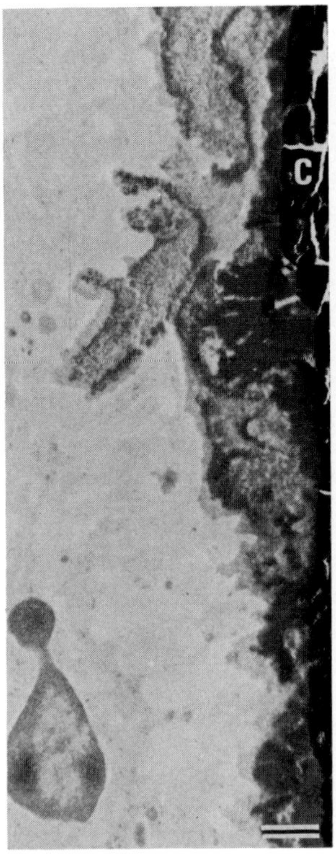

Fig. 3-31.

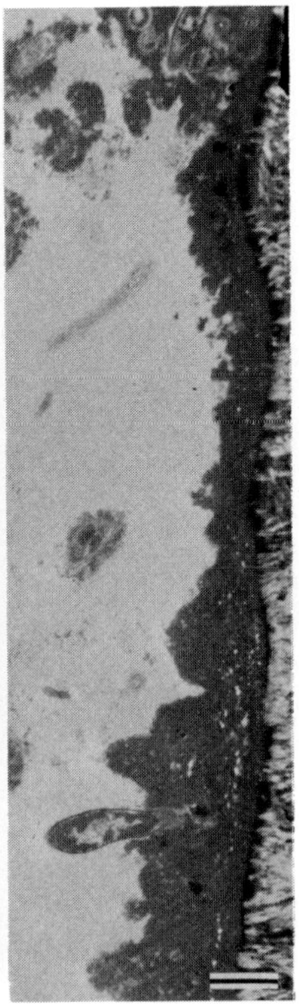

Fig. 3-32.

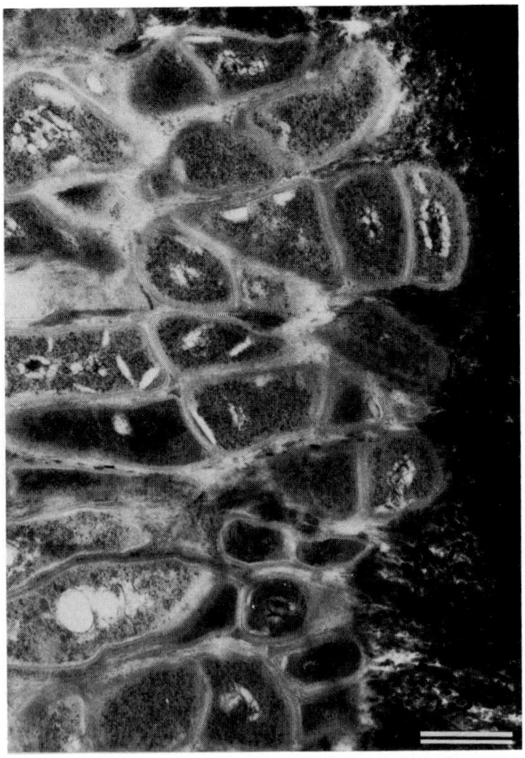

Fig. 3-33. Thin section of plaque in deep pocket of patient with juvenile periodontitis. Densely packed Gram positive rods grow perpendicular to the cementum to the right in the illustration. Magnification X 21 500. Bar: 0.5 μm. From Westergaard et al. (1978).

Fig. 3-31. Thin section of deposit in deep pocket of patient with juvenile periodontitis. The cementum (C) is covered with cuticular material and cellular remnants. Magnification X 5 200. Bar: 1 μm. From Westergaard et al. (1978).

Fig. 3-32. Thin section of deposit in deep pocket of patient with juvenile periodontitis. A cuticle of uneven thickness is seen to the right on the cementum. A small colony of degenerating bacteria adheres to the cuticle in the upper part of the illustration, and below a single rod-shaped microorganism is partly embedded in the cuticle. Magnification X 5 400. Bar: 1 μm. From Westergaard et al. (1978).

Napel et al. 1985). From these studies it has been established that early dental plaque in the dog has many structural similarities with that occurring in man. This applies to the supragingival plaque (Fig. 3-35) as well as to the subgingival accumulations (Figs. 3-36, 3-37, 3-38, 3-39). These deposits may either appear as an apical continuation of the supragingival plaque, or as discrete aggregates at some distance from the supragingival deposit (Fig. 3-37). Old established subgingival plaque shows considerable variation of the bacterial composition between dogs: in some, a subgingival flora dominated by spirochetes is seen, in others colonies of Gram negative cocci and rods are found in the gingival crevice, whereas spirochetes are virtually absent (Soames & Davies 1975, Theilade & Attström 1985). A characteristic feature of the subgingival plaque is the presence of a number of leukocytes interposed between the surfaces of the bacterial deposit and the gingival sulcular epithelium (Fig. 3-40). Some bacteria may be found between the epithelial cells, and evidence of phagocytosis (by polymorphonuclear leukocytes) is frequently encountered (Fig. 3-41).

Although subgingival plaque formation in the dog may not develop identically to that in

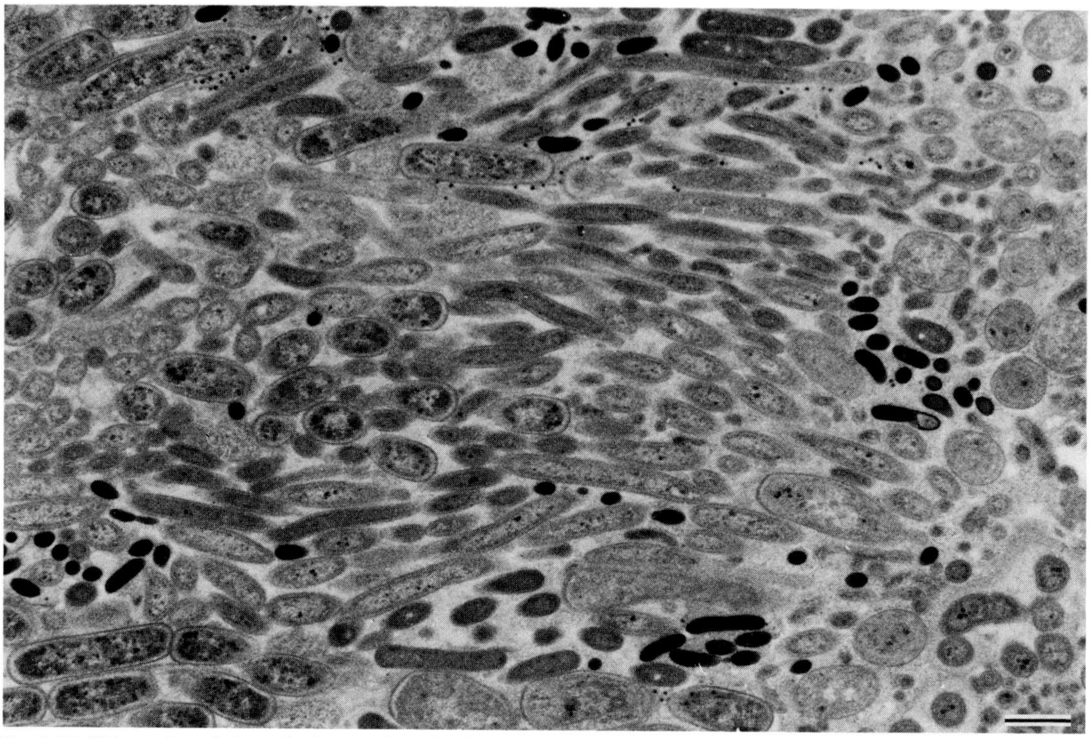

Fig. 3-34. Thin section of plaque in deep pocket of patient with juvenile periodontitis. The bacterial flora is characterized by cocci, rods or filamentous organisms, primarily of the Gram negative type. Magnification X 8 600. Bar: 1 µm. From Westergaard et al. (1978).

man, the dog may still serve as a convenient model for investigating the basic phenomena governing the formation of subgingival plaque (Schroeder & Attström 1979).

Diet and plaque formation

Diet has frequently been considered to play a significant part in the development of dental plaque, yet for more than 50 years it has been known that dental plaque may form on human teeth in the absence of oral food intake (Howitt et al. 1928). Similar results have been obtained from studies in dogs (Egelberg 1965b) and monkeys (Bowen 1974).

On the other hand, it is similarly well established that diet may modify both the amount of plaque formed and its composition. Two different plaque-forming modes of action may be operating. The diet may be such as to require vigorous chewing, thus activating the cleansing action of saliva, lips, cheeks and tongue, or it may be such as to favor plaque formation.

Consistency of diet

The plaque-reducing effect of a hard, fibrous diet has been shown in dogs receiving raw bovine trachea (Egelberg 1965a). However, a similar marked effect of diets requiring vigorous chewing has not been demonstrated in man. The most likely explanation for this lack of effect is that there are major differences in tooth anatomy. The tapered form of dog teeth and the diastemata between them probably make the surfaces more accessible for cleansing action, while in man the dental plaque, located along the gingival margin of the teeth and interproximally, is not subject to friction from food during mastication (Wilcox & Everett 1963). It is, therefore, not surprising that

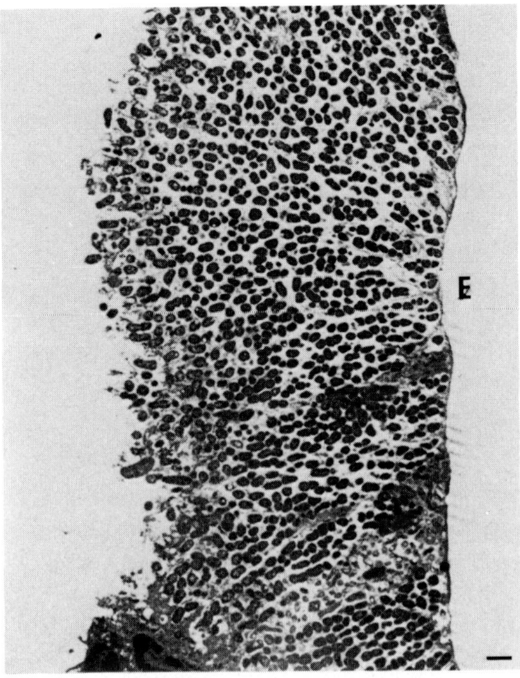

Fig. 3-35. Thin section of 14-day-old supragingival plaque in the Beagle dog. Cocci or rods are present in a palisading arrangement perpendicular to the enamel (E). Magnification X 2 260. Bar: 1 µm.

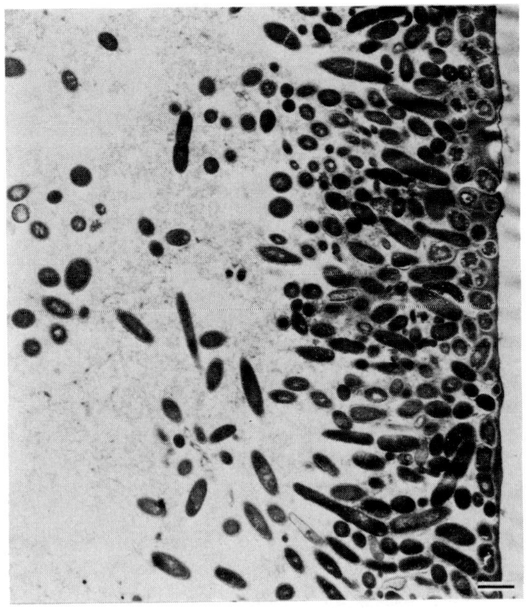

Fig. 3-36. Thin section of 4-day-old subgingival plaque near the orifice of the gingival sulcus in the Beagle dog. Magnification X 5 000. Bar: 1 µm.

several investigators have failed to demonstrate any effect on human plaque accumulation, even after excessive chewing of raw carrot, apple, etc. (Bergenholtz et al. 1967, Lindhe & Wicen 1969, Wade 1971).

Composition of diet

The composition of diet has been considered to have a marked influence on plaque formation, because diet together with saliva provides nutrients for plaque microorganisms. Most studies of dietary effect on plaque pertain to the carbohydrates. Fermentable sugars might be expected to increase plaque formation because of their action as additional energy supply for the plaque microbiota; they may also act as substrate for the production of extracellular polysaccharides (Guggenheim 1970). However, the results from a number of studies regarding the effect of carbohydrates on plaque formation are contradictory, probably because of varying trial

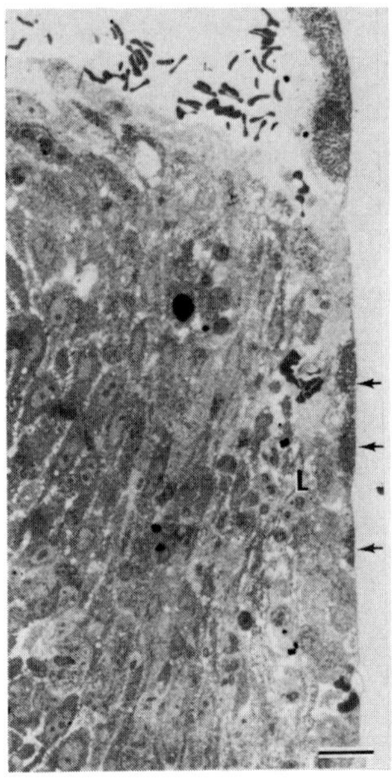

Fig. 3-37. Thin section of the gingival sulcus area in the Beagle dog. Plaque is seen at the orifice of the gingival sulcus in the upper part of the illustration. Subgingival plaque is deposited as discrete separate colonies on the tooth (arrows). Many leukocytes (L) migrate through the junctional epithelium to the subgingival portion of the tooth. Magnification X 700. Bar: 10 µm.

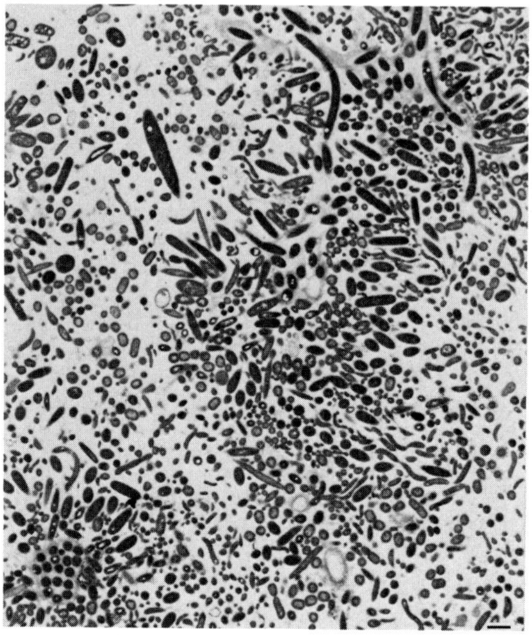

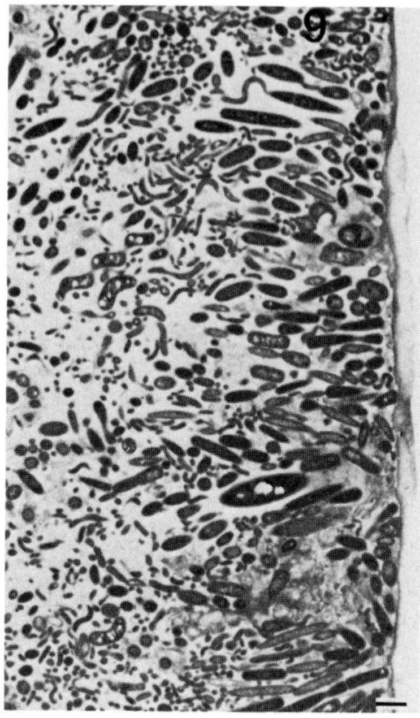

Figs. 3-38 & 3-39. Thin sections of 14-day-old plaque in dog. The subgingival flora is characterized by a variety of different types of microorganisms including spirochetes with no apparent order of arrangement. Magnification X 2 750. Bar: 1 μm.

design and limited subject availability as well as large individual variations in plaque formation (Carlsson & Egelberg 1965, Sheinin & Makinen 1971, Folke et al. 1972, Brecx et al. 1981, Rateitschak-Pluss & Guggenheim 1982, Lim et al. 1986). However, these studies may indicate that the effect of dietary sugars on the amount of plaque forming in man is, generally, far less than theoretical expectation. Some studies show no effect and others show statistically significant increases which, however, may be too small to have clinical significance, e.g. an increased extension of plaque coronally on the clinical crowns of the teeth may be inconsequential to the marginal periodontium.

Several studies have been performed to investigate whether dietary carbohydrates, and especially sucrose, have an influence on the bacterial composition of dental plaque. It has been known for many years that large numbers of lactobacilli in saliva are related to a high consumption of fermentable carbohydrates, and that following restrictions of dietary sugar the lactobacillus counts are reduced. However, lactobacilli constitute a very small proportion of the plaque flora (van Houte et al. 1972). Streptococci also might be expected to be influenced by dietary sugars. *S. mutans* and *S. sanguis* produce extracellular polysaccharides from sucrose but not from other sugars. Sucrose seems to favor *S. mutans* but not *S. sanguis* in plaque (de Stoppelaar et al. 1970). It is evident that the quantitative proportions of some bacterial species may to some extent be modified by diet. Plaque flora is dependent to a much greater extent on the oral environment than on the transient presence of food (Bibby 1976).

The assessment of the effect of diet on the chemical composition of plaque has dealt mainly with the carbohydrate metabolism. Plaque carbohydrates are primarily present as structural components of the microorganisms, as storage granules in the bacteria termed intracellular polysaccharides, and as extracellular polysaccharides in the matrix between the microorganisms (Wood 1969); carbohydrate constitutes about 20% of plaque dry weight (Hotz et al. 1972).

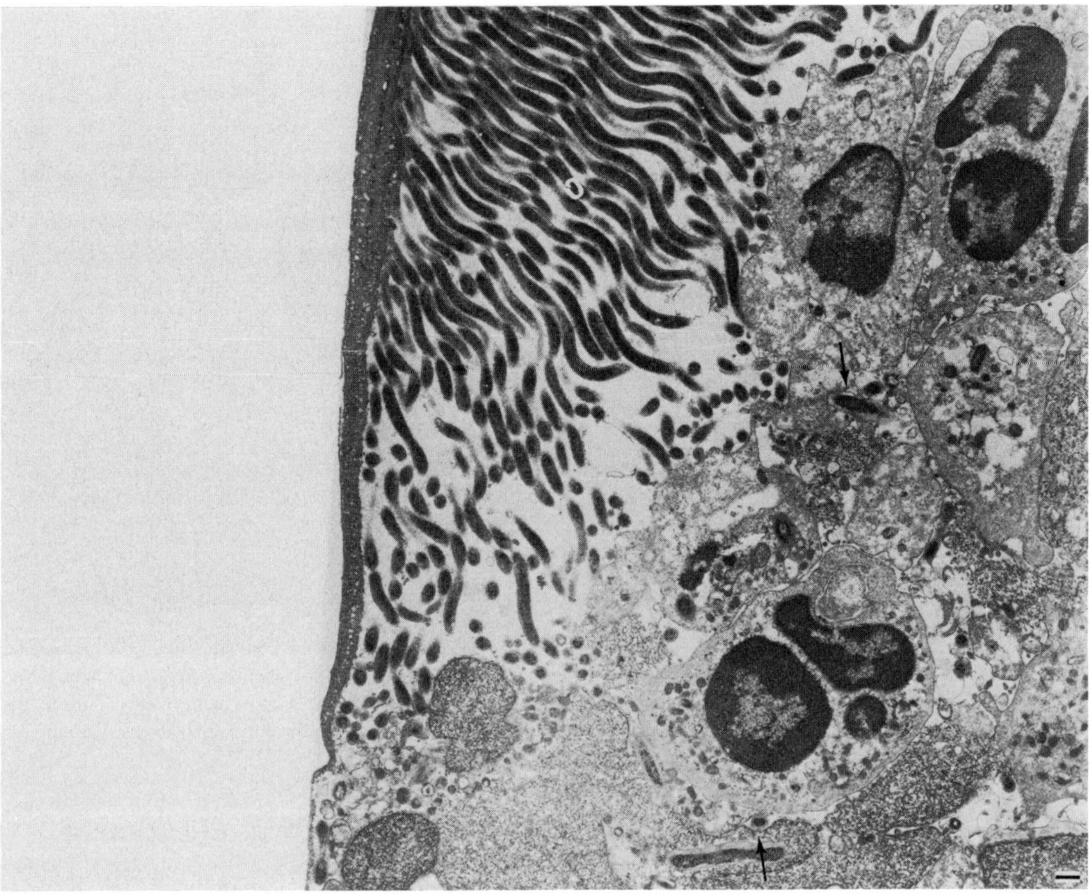

Fig. 3-40. Thin section of old subgingival plaque in a dog with long-standing gingivitis. The most apical colony consists primarily of spirochetes attached to a dense cuticle and surrounded by migrated leukocytes. Single microorganisms are seen between them (arrows). Magnification X 2 650. Bar: 1 μm.

Intracellular polysaccharides of the glycogenamylopectin type are synthesized by plaque bacteria from dietary sugars, such as sucrose, glucose and others, and in the absence of a sugar supply they are catabolized (Gibbons & Socransky 1962, Saxton 1969, Wood 1969). Thus, dietary restriction of carbohydrate seems to cause a marked reduction in the number of polysaccharide storing bacteria in plaque (van Houte 1964).

Extracellular polysaccharides in plaque comprise a variety of sugar polymers. Of these, fructans (levans) and glucans have received much attention in recent years. Fructans are synthesized in plaque from dietary sucrose, and, as with intracellular polysaccharides, they provide a storage component which is broken down when the sugar supply is insufficient. Thus, fructans constitute a variable, but always minor proportion of the extracellular polysaccharides in plaque (Critchley et al. 1967, Wood 1967, Higuchi et al. 1970, Leach et al. 1972, Gold et al. 1974). Glucans, which are also synthesized from sucrose, seem to be more important both quantitatively and functionally and comprise a variety of different types of polymers. One of these is dextran, which has predominance of α-1.6 linkages, and as some plaque bacteria possess the enzyme dextranase, the dextrans may also act as a storage carbohydrate. Another type of glucan characterized mainly by α-1.3 linkages is called mutan and does not seem to be broken down in plaque, so that its function is primarily that of structural

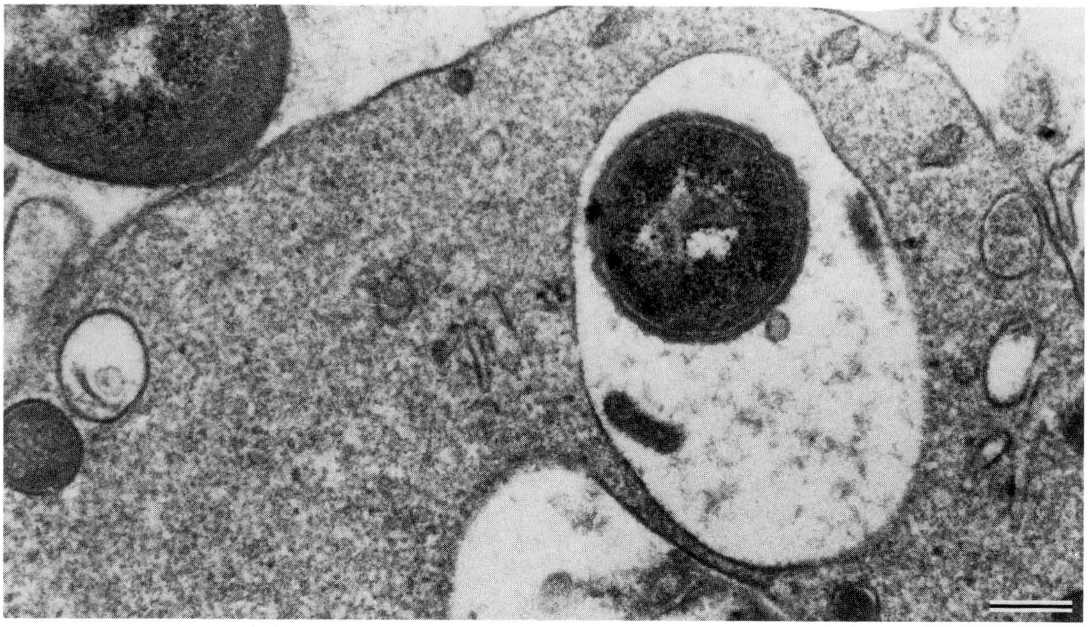

Fig. 3-41. Thin section of part of a leukocyte situated between subgingival plaque and the junctional epithelium in dog. The large membrane bound compartment of the leukocyte cytoplasm contains a phagocytized Gram negative microorganism. Another bacteria is in close apposition to the cytoplasmic membrane of the leukocyte. Magnification X 20 000. Bar: 0.5 μm.

stabilizer of the intermicrobial matrix (Guggenheim 1970, Hotz et al. 1972, Dewar & Walker 1975).

The carbohydrates, thus, play an important part in plaque development and maintenance. However, with the diversity of possible metabolic pathways that dietary sugars can take in plaque, the lack of exact knowledge concerning the details of the clinical impact of variations in sugar consumption is not surprising.

Dental Calculus

The calcified deposits termed tartar or dental calculus have been recognized for centuries together with their detrimental effect on gingival tissue. In the middle of this century, renewed interest in dental calculus developed as a result of improved research methods, primarily the introduction of modern epidemiology applied to periodontal disease, and by the application of biochemical and biophysical techniques in the investigation of dental calculus.

Definition and classification of dental calculus

Dental calculus may be defined as calcified or calcifying deposits on the teeth and other solid structures in the oral cavity. It is classified as supragingival calculus when present on the visible clinical crowns of the teeth above the gingival margin. Calculus located apically to the gingival margin in the gingival sulcus or the periodontal pocket is termed subgingival calculus.

Clinical appearance and distribution of calculus

Supragingival calculus comprises yellow, white accretions usually located along the gingival margins of the teeth. However, the color may change to brown as a result of secondary staining from the use of tobacco or from food pigments. The distribution of supragingival calculus does not entirely follow that of supragingival plaque, as the tendency for the latter to

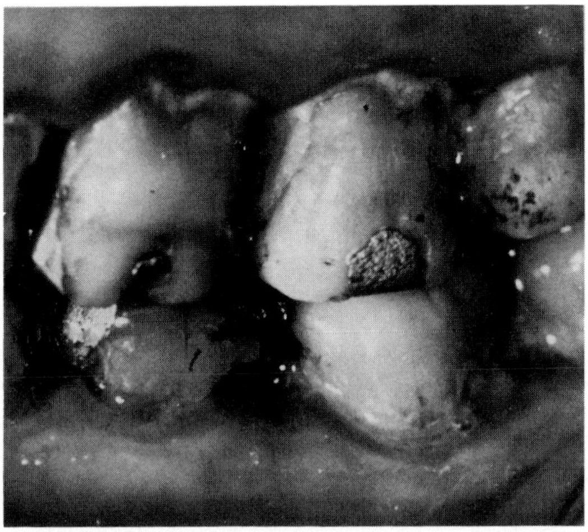

Fig. 3-42. Supragingival calculus along the gingival margin on the buccal surfaces of maxillary molars.

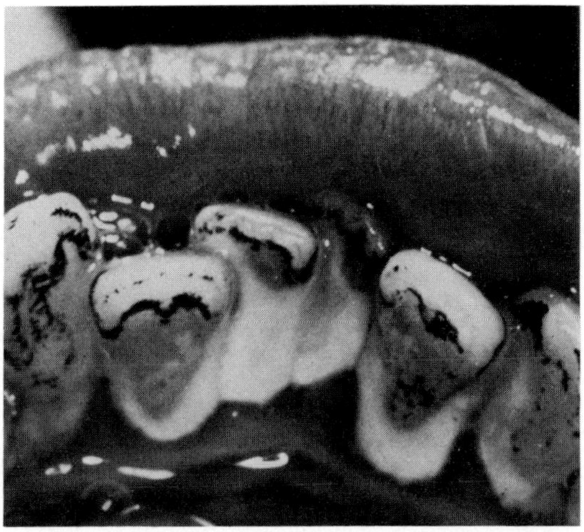

Fig. 3-43. Supragingival calculus along the gingival margin on the lingual surfaces of the mandibular cuspids and incisors.

calcify into calculus varies within the oral cavity. The largest amounts of supragingival calculus are found opposite the openings of the major salivary ducts. Thus, copious amounts of supragingival calculus are often seen on the buccal aspects of the maxillary molars in the vicinity of the opening of the Stensen's duct of the parotid salivary gland, and on the lingual and even buccal surfaces of the mandibular incisors opposite the orifice of the Warton's duct of the submandibular and the Bartholin's duct of the sublingual, salivary glands (Figs. 3-42, 3-43).

Subgingival calculus is brown to black in color and harder and often more tenaciously adherent to the tooth surface (Fig. 3-44). It is more evenly distributed on the various teeth, but on the individual tooth subgingival calculus is more prevalent on the approximal and lingual than on the buccal tooth surfaces.

Diagnosis of dental calculus

Supragingival calculus may be recognized by clinical inspection when present in sufficient amounts. Thin layers may, however, be overlooked if the tooth surface is moistened by saliva, which penetrates the porous surface of calculus. If the tooth surface is dried, a thin layer of calculus may have an appearance similar to that of a hypoplastic tooth surface, and its detection therefore requires probing or scraping with an instrument. Subgingival calculus is often difficult to detect by clinical inspection, though its presence below the gingival margin may be indirectly diagnosed if its dark color shines through the thin gingival margin in the same way as a dark restoration or a dark endodontically treated root. Subgingival calculus

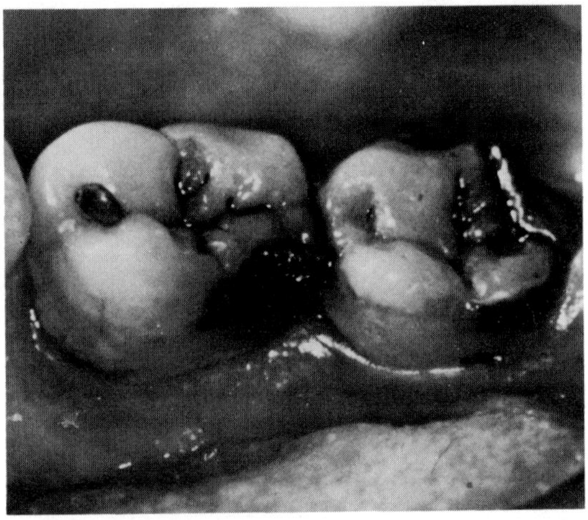

Fig. 3-44. Subgingival calculus partly visible as a dark concrement in the orifice of the gingival sulcus of the mandibular molars.

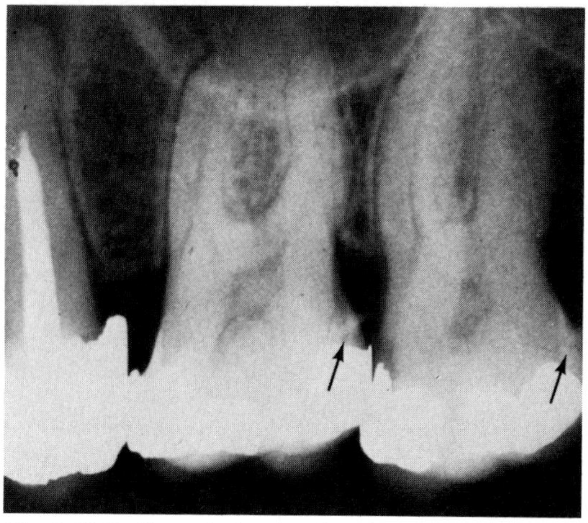

Fig. 3-45. Radiograph showing dental calculus (arrows) on the distal surfaces of two maxillary molars.

may be seen by the detachment of the gingival margin from the tooth by air blast or by appropriate instrument. Calculus in deeper periodontal pockets may be disclosed by probing, but this method of calculus detection is highly inefficient (Waerhaug 1978). Under certain circumstances calculus on the approximal surfaces of the teeth may be visible on radiographs (Fig. 3-45). This method of detection is also very uncertain, because the image of the calculus is dependent both on its density and on the radiographic technique. The correct diagnosis of subgingival calculus in deeper periodontal pockets, therefore, sometimes necessitates the reflection of the covering periodontal tissues during periodontal surgery.

Composition of dental calculus

Calculus consists of 70-80% inorganic salts, of which two-thirds are in crystalline form (Leung & Jensen 1958). Calcium and phosphorus constitute the major elements with a Ca/P ratio ranging from 1.66 to more than 2 (Leung & Jensen 1958, Little et al. 1963, Schroeder 1963, Little & Hazen 1964). Calcium usually accounts for up to 40% of the inorganic weight, while the proportion of phosphorus approaches 20%. Small amounts of magnesium, sodium, carbonate and fluoride may be present as well, together with traces of other elements (for review see Theilade & Schroeder 1966, Schroeder 1969, Leach 1973, Mandel & Gaffar 1986).

The crystal forms in which inorganic constituents are present have been determined by various physical techniques of analysis, primarily X-ray and electron diffraction. The 4 principal crystal forms are hydroxyapatite, $Ca_{10}(OH)_2(PO_4)_6$, magnesium whitlockite, $Ca_3(PO_4)_2$ in which the magnesium ion substitutes a small number of the calcium ions; octacalcium phosphate, $Ca_4H(PO_4)_3$, $2H_2O$; and brushite $CaHPO_4$, $2H_2O$ (Rowles 1964). Of these crystal types, the first 3 are variants of the hydroxyapatite lattice, which dominates many biological mineralized tissues such as bone, cementum, dentin and enamel. Brushite is the simple secondary calcium phosphate. The 4 crystal forms do not occur with the same frequency in all calculus samples; generally 2 or more are present in a sample. Their incidence varies with the age of the calculus sample (Schroeder & Baumbauer 1966) as well as with its location. Thus brushite is more common in supragingival calculus, while magnesium whitlockite is present particularly in the subgingival variety.

The organic portion of calculus has been analyzed biochemically and histochemically in a number of studies (Mandel 1963, Little et al. 1964, 1966, Stanford 1966), from which it is evident that the bulk of the organic portion of calculus consists of proteins and carbohydrates, while lipids account for only a minor fraction; this composition is comparable to that of dental plaque (Silverman & Kleinberg 1967).

Structure of dental calculus

Study of the internal structure of dental calculus has been hampered by the high amount of inorganic constituents, which restricts sufficiently thin sectioning for subsequent examin-

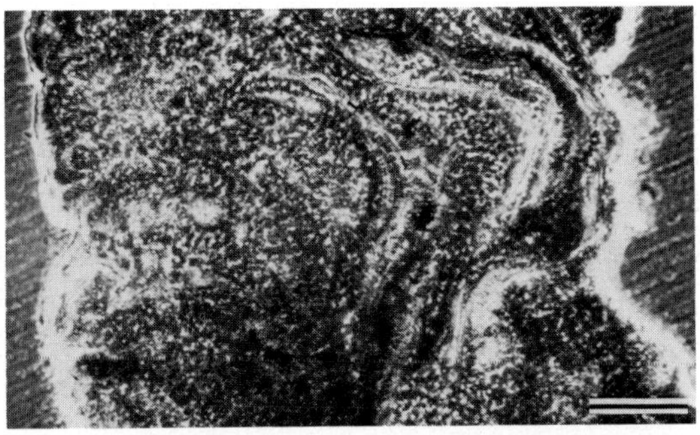

Fig. 3-46. Ground section of subgingival calculus. The tooth surface is represented to the left. A definite layering of the deposit is evident. Magnification X 90. Bar: 100 μm.

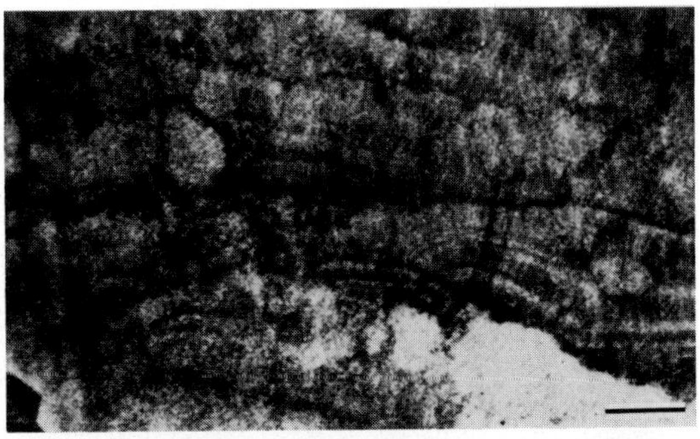

Fig. 3-47. Microradiograph of ground section of calculus. The tooth surface is at the bottom of the illustration. The degree of calcification varies from region to region. Unmineralized resting or incremental lines appear as radiolucent dark lines. Magnification X 77. Bar: 100 μm.

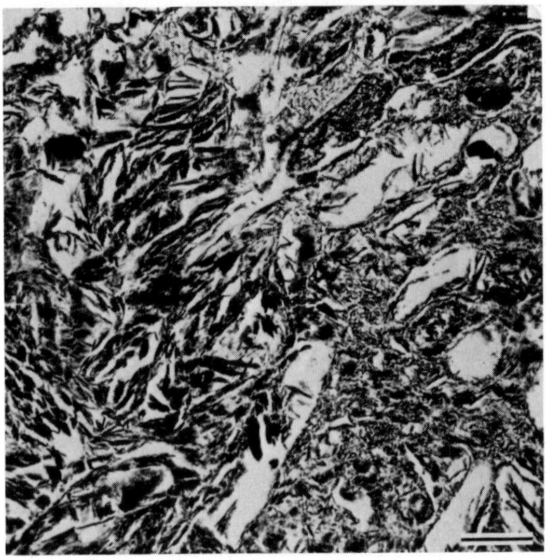

Fig. 3-48. Thin section of old calculus. Crystals of varying size are deposited in random orientation. The outlines of microorganisms are discernible; in the upper right corner a fully mineralized filamentous organism can be seen. Magnification X 17 000. Bar: 0.5 μm.

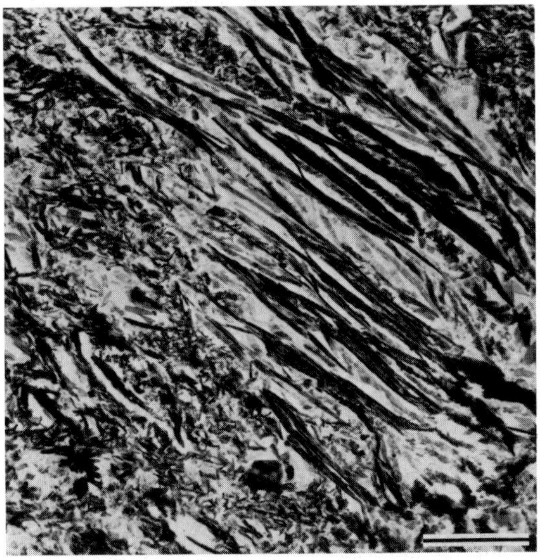

Fig. 3-49. Thin section of old calculus with a region of long ribbon-shaped crystal with a preferred orientation. Magnification X 25 000. Bar: 0.5 μm.

ation. Calculus has been studied in a variety of ways including ground sections of undemineralized samples as well as regular sections of decalcified specimens with or without the presence of the adjacent tooth structure, and soft tissues. With the introduction of electron microscopy and the concomitant possibility of ultrathin sections, a clearer understanding of the nature of dental calculus emerged (Gonzales & Sognnaes 1960, Theilade 1960, Zander et al. 1960).

The examination of ground sections reveals that calculus is often a layered structure (Fig. 3-46) in which the degree of calcification varies in the different layers (Fig. 3-47) between which resting lines are frequently evident. In thin undecalcified sections, calculus is dominated by small needle-shaped, inorganic crystals revealed by electron diffraction to consist of apatite. Other crystals appear as platelets or long rods. Generally, the crystals are randomly orientated (Fig. 3-48), although in certain re-

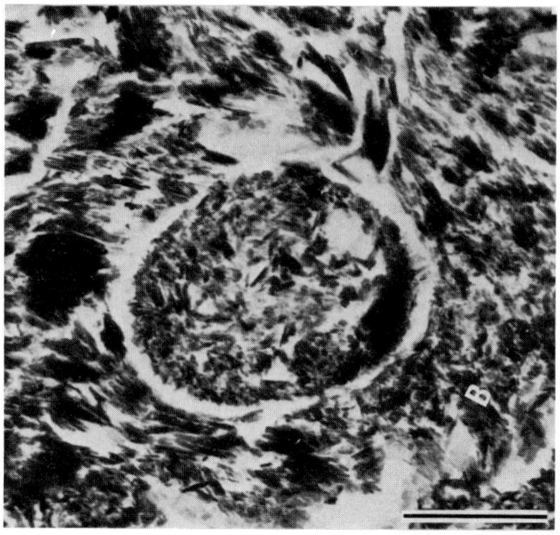

Fig. 3-50. Thin section of old calculus. The intermicrobial matrix and the microorganism are calcified to the same extent. Only the outline distinguishes the bacterium. Magnification X 31 000. Bar: 0.5 μm.

gions a particular orientation may prevail (Fig. 3-49). Within the mineralized material, it is possible to discern the outlines of calcified microorganisms (Fig. 3-50). A very significant feature of calculus (Fig. 3-51) is that its surface is covered by a layer of unmineralized plaque (Gonzales & Sognnaes 1960, Theilade 1960, Zander et al. 1960, Schroeder 1969).

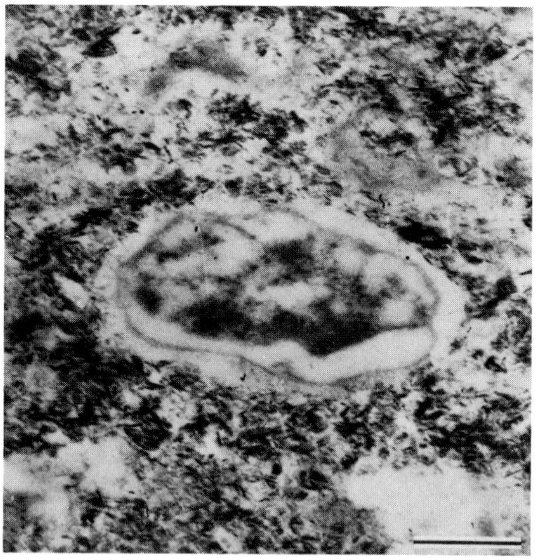

Fig. 3-52. Thin section of old plaque. A degenerating organism is surrounded by intermicrobial matrix in which initial mineralization has started by the deposition of small needle-shaped electron-dense apatite crystals. Magnification X 25 000. Bar: 0.5 μm. From Zander et al. (1960).

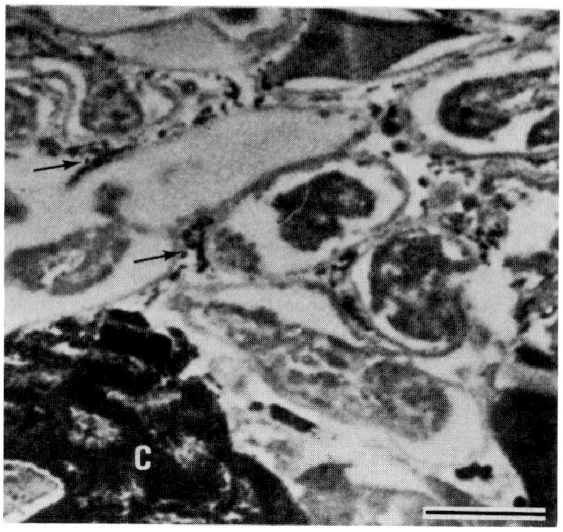

Fig. 3-51. Thin section of calculus (C). At its surface a layer of plaque with only small amounts of mineral precipitates (arrows) between the bacteria. Magnification X 28 000. Bar: 0.5 μm.

Formation of calculus

Information on how calculus develops has to a large extent been obtained from studies in which Mylar® films were attached, for set periods, to tooth surfaces known to form calculus. After removal the films were processed for either light or electron microscopy (Mandel et al.

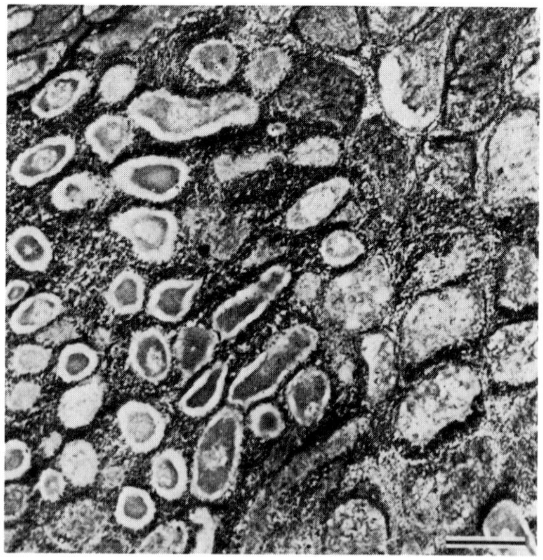

Fig. 3-53. Thin section of old mineralizing plaque. The intermicrobial matrix is totally calcified, and many microorganisms show intracellular crystal deposition. Magnification X 9 000. Bar: 1 μm.

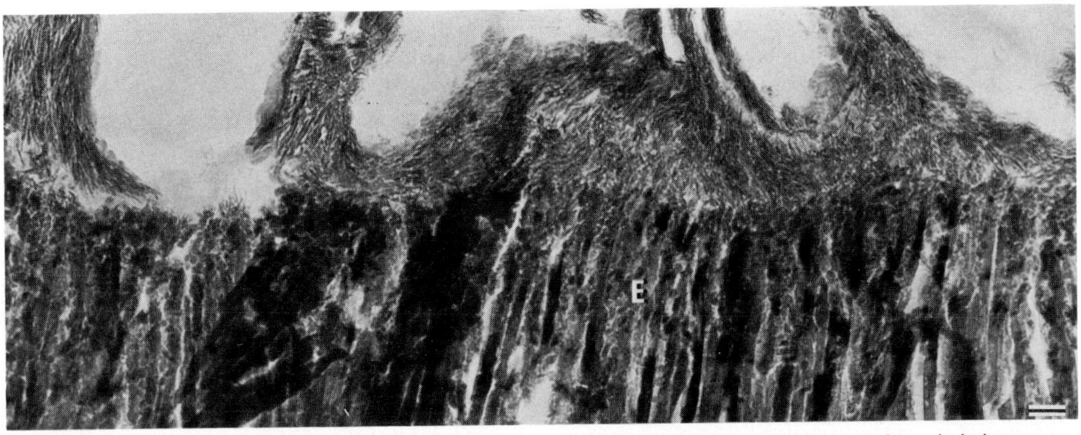

Fig. 3-54. Thin section of enamel surface (E) with overlying calculus. The enamel and calculus crystals are in intimate contact, and the latter extends into the minute irregularities of the enamel. Magnification X 35 000. Bar: 0.1 µm. From Selvig (1970).

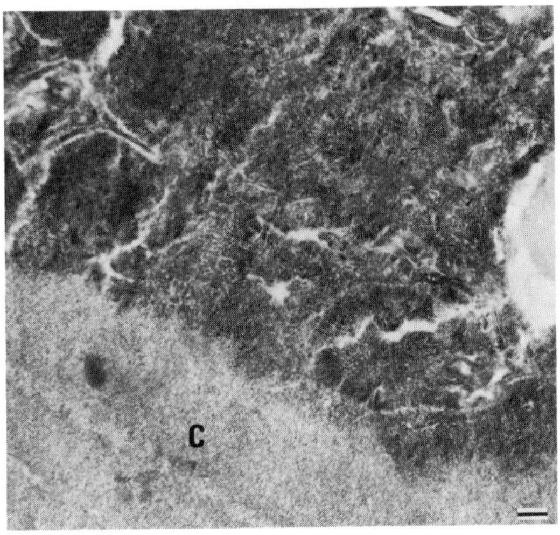

Fig. 3-55. Thin section of cementum surface (C) with overlying calculus. The calculus is closely adapted to the irregular cementum and is more electron-dense and therefore harder than the adjacent cementum. To the right in the illustration part of an uncalcified microorganism. Magnification X 30 000. Bar: 0.1 µm. From Selvig (1970).

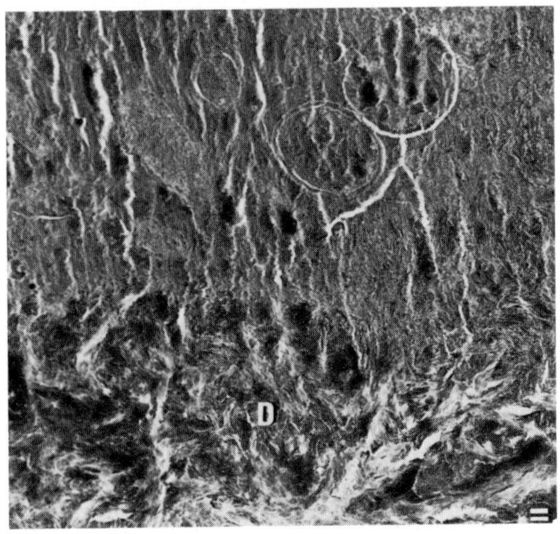

Fig. 3-56. Thin section of dentin (D) surface with overlying calculus. The interface between the calculus and dentin cannot be precisely determined as the calculus crystals fill in the irregularities of the dentin surface, which is devoid of cementum as a result of a previous scaling of the root surface. The circular profiles in the calculus surround completely calcified bacteria. Magnification X 18 000. Bar: 1 µm. From Selvig (1970).

1957, Voreadis & Zander, 1958, Mühleman & Schneider 1959, Hazen 1960, Turesky et al. 1961, Schroeder et al. 1964, Theilade 1964, Schroeder 1965). From these studies it is evident that calculus formation is always preceded by plaque formation. The plaque accumulations serve as an organic matrix for the subsequent mineralization of the deposit.

Initially, small crystals are seen in the intermicrobial matrix (Fig. 3-52) frequently in close apposition to the external aspect of the bacteria. Gradually, the matrix between the microorganisms becomes entirely calcified, and eventually the bacteria also become mineralized (Fig. 3-53).

While the deposition of crystals within preformed plaque is the usual mode of calculus formation, minerals may also be deposited at the surface of supragingival plaque accumulations. In such foci the crystals are rod-shaped. X-ray diffraction indicates that these crystals are calcium phosphate precipitated as brushite, $CaHPO_4$, $2H_2O$ (Schroeder 1964, Schroeder & Baumbauer 1966).

The time required for the formation of supragingival calculus is, in some persons, less than 2 weeks, at which time the deposit may already contain about 80% of the inorganic material found in mature calculus (Mühlemann & Schroeder 1964).

The first evidence of calcification may already occur after a few days (Theilade 1964). However, the development of a deposit with a crystal composition characteristic of old calculus requires months or years (Schroeder & Baumbauer 1966).

Attachment of calculus to the teeth

Calculus often adheres tenaciously to the teeth, and hard subgingival calculus may be especially difficult to remove. One reason for its firm attachment to the tooth surface may be that the pellicle beneath the plaque also calcifies, and thereby the calculus crystals come into intimate contact with the enamel, cementum or dentin crystals (Figs. 3-54, 3-55, 3-56) (Kopczyk & Conroy 1968, Selvig 1970, Canis et al. 1979). In addition, the surface irregularities are also penetrated by calculus crystals, so that the calculus is virtually locked to the tooth. This is particularly the case on exposed cementum where small pits occur at sites where the Sharpey's fibers were previously inserted (Bercy & Frank 1980). Uneven root surfaces may be the result of carious lesions, small pieces of cementum may have been lost as a result of wear when the periodontal ligament was still attached (Moskow 1969) and, under such conditions, it becomes impossible to remove all calculus without the loss of some of the hard tissue of the teeth.

Mineralization theories

The question of why calcium phosphates precipitate as calculus has puzzled scientists for many years. Two aspects must be explained, first the nucleation of the crystalites, and secondly their growth. Saliva is a metastable solution for some calcium phosphates, namely apatite, octocalcium phosphate and whitlockite, and under certain conditions also with respect to brushite. This means that saliva is supersaturated with respect to the salts and thus able to support crystal growth, but that spontaneous precipitation does not occur unless the solution is seeded, e.g. by the presence of crystals on which new crystals can form. Crystals for this nucleation process are present in the tooth surface, but since they are covered by a pellicle, they are not readily available for this function. Several explanatory hypotheses have been offered for the initiation of the mineralization process, but the question remains unresolved; discussion of some hypotheses follows: the carbon dioxide theory propounds that freshly secreted saliva leaving the openings of the salivary ducts has a CO_2 tension of about 60 mm Hg, while that prevailing in the oral cavity is considerably lower, somewhere between the CO_2 tension of the expired air (29 mm Hg) and that of the atmosphere (0.3 mm). This discrepancy will result in the escape of CO_2 from saliva, the pH of which will rise. When the pH of saliva increases, less calcium and phosphates can be accomodated in the ionized form, and consequently spontaneous precipitation may occur. Once crystallites are present, the physiological supersaturation accounts for this growth. This theory offers a plausible explanation for the occurrence of copious amounts of supragingival calculus near the orifice of the major salivary ducts. It cannot explain, however, the formation of subgingival calculus, which probably derives from the salts in the gingival exudate. Other mechanisms, however, might raise the pH in saliva or plaque, such as ammonia production (Driessens et al. 1985). It has been observed that rapid calculus formers have an increased urea concentration of saliva (Mandel & Thompson 1967). Ammonia is a breakdown product from urea and might result in a local pH increase in plaque. The pH of plaque is actually frequently above that of saliva. This is attributed to proteolytic activity which may result in the formation of amines, urea and ammonia. Proteolytic enzymes are present in plaque, and a positive correlation has been found between their proteolytic activity and calculus formation (Watanabe et al. 1982).

When it was established that calculus forms by the calcification of plaque, and that certain changes could be demonstrated in plaque when the process of mineralization begins, it was proposed that the organic matrix could be acting as a seeding agent. When crystallization is nucleated by a compound of different chemical composition, the phenomenon is termed epitaxis. Although epitaxis has been claimed for the last 25 years to occur in biological mineralization including calculus (Glimcher 1960), the compound(s) responsible has still not been identified. However, recently some progress has been made in characterizing fractions of the organic matrix that might be initiators. Thus, *in vitro* experiments with decalcified calculus have shown that extraction of the lipid component prevented remineralization of the calculus matrix, and later a proteolipid with nucleating property was partly characterized (Ennever et al. 1973, 1979). This does not preclude other organic compounds as nucleating factors. Furthermore, specific nucleators of apatite may not be essential, as it is possible for apatite crystals to transform from brushite and octocalcium phosphate (Barone et al. 1976).

The synthesis of the nucleating organic compounds is largely unknown, but it has been established that degenerating oral bacteria may calcify *in vitro* by deposition of calcium phosphate crystals of the same type as those found in calculus (Ennever 1960, Bowen & Gilmour 1961, Lie & Selvig 1974, Sidaway 1979). Recently a protease has been isolated from cultures of *Bacteroides loeschii*, an oral microorganism regularly present in plaque. This enzyme breaks down the specific salivary peptides that are responsible for maintaining the supersaturated state of saliva with respect to calcium and phosphate ions, and may thus promote calculus formation (Morishita et al. 1986).

Pyrophosphate present in saliva and plaque also assists in maintaining calcium and phosphate ions in the supersaturated solution (Edgar & Jenkins 1972). Pyrophosphate in plaque may be hydrolysed by phosphatase, and a significant positive relation has been found between calculus formation and pyroshosphatase activity in plaque (Bercy & Vreven 1979). The inhibitory effect of pyrophosphates on mineralization has been used in the formulation of toothpastes to reduce supragingival calculus formation (Zacherl et al. 1985, Lobene 1986, Schiff 1986). However, since plaque formation is not reduced concurrently, improvement in gingival inflammation cannot be expected as a result of the addition of pyrophosphates.

It is reasonable to assign bacteria a key role in a possible mechanism for the mineralization process. This does not mean that they alone are responsible for producing nucleating compounds, since calculus formation, to a small extent, does occur in germ-free rats by calcification of an organic matrix probably originating from saliva (Baer & Newton 1959, Fitzgerald & McDaniel 1960, Theilade et al. 1964)

Effect of calculus on periodontal tissues

The presence of calculus is invariably associated with periodontal disease (Waerhaug 1952,

1955, Lövdal et al. 1958). However, as calculus is always covered by an unmineralized plaque layer, it may be difficult to assess whether calculus *per se* has a detrimental effect on the periodontal tissue. From epidemiologic data, however, it is evident that the correlation between plaque and gingivitis is much stronger than that between calculus and gingivitis (Silness & Löe 1964, Buckley 1980). It has been proposed that calculus may exert a detrimental effect on the soft tissues of the periodontium because of its rough surface. However, it has been clearly demonstrated that the roughness of a surface does not initiate gingivitis (Waerhaug 1956), and under certain circumstances a normal attachment may even be seen between the junctional epithelium and calculus (Listgarten & Ellegaard 1973). It has also been shown that autoclaved calculus may be encapsulated in connective tissue without causing marked inflammation (Allen & Kerr 1965).

The primary effect of calculus in periodontal disease, therefore, seems to be its retention site role for plaque. Large amounts of calculus may hamper the efficacy of daily oral hygiene and thereby accelerate plaque formation. In addition the calcified deposit may contain products toxic to soft tissue. Such products may either persist in the calculus from the period prior to its calcification, or they may enter its porous surface from the overlying plaque layer. Thus calculus may be considered to be slowly delivering pathogenic products to the adjacent soft tissues (Friskopp & Hammerström 1980, Patters et al. 1982, Mandel & Gaffar 1986).

In conclusion, calculus is not the most significant etiological factor in periodontal disease. However, its presence makes adequate plaque removal impossible for the therapist, and prevents patients from performing an efficient plaque control.

References

Allen, D.L. & Kerr, D.A. (1965) Tissue response in the guinea pig to sterile and non-sterile calculus. *Journal of Periodontology* **36**, 121-126.

Axelsson, P. & Lindhe, J. (1974) The effect of a preventive programme on dental plaque, gingivitis and caries in schoolchildren. Results after one and two years. *Journal of Clinical Periodontology* **1**, 126-138.

Axelsson, P. & Lindhe, J. (1981) Effect of controlled oral hygiene procedures on caries and periodontal disease in adults. Results after 6 years. *Journal of Clinical Periodontolology* **8**, 239-248.

Baer, P.N. & Newton, W.L. (1959) The occurrence of periodontal disease in germ-free mice. *Journal of Dental Research* **38**, 1238.

Barone, J.P., Nancollas, G.H. & Tomson, M. (1976) The seeded growth of calcium phosphates. The kinetics of growth of calcium phosphates. The kinetics of growth of dicalcium dihydrate on hydroxyapatite. *Calcified Tissue Research* **21**, 171-182.

Bercy, P. & Frank, R.M. (1980) Microscopie électronique à balayage de la surface du cément humain normal et carié. *Journal Biologie Buccale* **8**, 331-352.

Bercy, P. & Vreven, J. (1979) Correlation between calculus index and acid and alcaline pyrophosphatases activities of dental plaque and saliva *Journal de Biologie Buccale* **7**, 31-36.

Bergenholtz, A., Hugoson, A. & Sohlberg, F. (1967) Den plaqueavlägsnande förmaga hos nogre mundhygieniske hjälpmedel. *Svensk Tandläkare Tidsskrift* **60**, 447-454.

Berthold, C.-H., Berthold, P. & Söder, P.-O. (1971) The growth of dental plaque on different materials. *Svensk Tandläkare Tidsskrift* **64**, 863-877.

Bibby, B.G. (1976) Influence of diet on the bacterial composition of plaques. In *Microbial Aspects of Dental Caries*, ed. Stiles, H.M., Loesche, W.J. O'Brien, T.C., Special Supplement, *Microbiology Abstracts*, Vol. II, pp. 477-490. Washington D.C.: Information Retrieval Inc.

Black, G.V. (1911) Beginnings of pyorrhea alveolaris - treatment for prevention. *Dental Items of Interest* **33**, 420-455.

Bowen, W.H. (1974) Effect of restricting oral intake to invert sugar or casein on the microbiology of plaque in *Macaca fascicularis (irus)*. *Archives of Oral Biology* **19**, 231-239.

Bowen, W.H. (1976) Nature of plaque. *Oral Sciences Reviews* **9**, 3-21.

Bowen, W.H. & Gilmour, M.N. (1961) The formation of calculus-like deposits by pure cultures of bacteria. *Archives of Oral Biology* **5**, 145-148.

Brecx, M., Rönström A., Theilade, J. & Attström R. (1981) Early formation of dental plaque on plastic films. II. Electron microscopic observations. *Journal of Periodontal Research* **16**, 213-227.

Brecx, M., Theilade, J. & Attström, R. (1980) Influence of optimal and excluded oral hygiene on early formation of dental plaque on plastic films. A quantitative and descriptive light and electron microscopic study. *Journal of Clinical Periodontology* **7**, 361-373.

Brecx, M., Theilade, J. & Attström, R. (1981) Ultrastructural estimation of the effect os sucrose and glucose rinses on dental plaque formed on plastic films. *Scandinavian Journal of Dental Research* **89**, 157-164.

Brecx, M., Theilade, J. & Attström, R (1983) An ultrastructural quantitative study of the significance of microbial multiplication during early dental plaque growth. *Journal of Periodontal Research* **18**, 177-186.

Burckley, L.A. (1980) The relationships between irregular teeth, plaque, calculus and gingival disease. *British Dental Journal* **149**, 67-69.

Canis, M.F., Kramer, G.M. & Pameijer, C.M. (1979) Calculus attachment. Review of the literature and new findings. *Journal of Periodontology* **50**, 406-415.

Carlsson, J. & Egelberg, J. (1965) Effect of diet on early plaque formation in man. *Odontologisk Revy* **16**, 112-125.

Critchley, P., Wood, J.M., Saxton, C.A. & Leach, S.A. (1967) The polymerisation of dietary sugars by dental plaque. *Caries Research* **1**, 112-129.

Dawes, C., Jenkins, G.N. & Tonge, C.H. (1963) The nomenclature of the integuments of the enamel surface of teeth. *British Dental Journal* **16**, 65-68.

De Stoppelaar, J.D., van Houte, J. & Dirks, D.B. (1970) The effect of carbohydrate restriction on the presence of *Streptococcus mutans*, *Streptococcus sanguis* and iodophilic polysaccharide-producing bacteria in human dental plaque. *Caries Research* **4**, 114-123.

Dewar, M.D. & Walker, G.J. (1975) Metabolism of the polysaccharides of human dental plaque. I. Dextranase activity of streptococci, and the extracellular polysaccharides synthesized from sucrose. *Caries Research* **9**, 21-35.

Driessens, F.C.M., Borggreven, J.M.P.M., Verbeeck, J.W.E. van Dijk & Feagin, F.F. (1985) On the physicochemistry of plaque calcification and the phase composition of dental calculus. *Journal of Periodontal Research* **20**, 329-336.

Eastcott, A.D. & Stallard, R.E. (1973) Sequential changes in developing human dental plaque as visualized by scanning electron microscopy. *Journal of Periodontology* **44**, 218-244.

Edgar, W.M. & Jenkins, G.N. (1972) Inorganic pyrophosphate in human parotid saliva and dental plaque. *Archives of Oral Biology* **17**, 219-223.

Egelberg, J. (1965a) Local effect of diet on plaque formation and development of gingivitis in dogs. I. Effect of hard and soft diets. *Odontologisk Revy* **16**, 31-41.

Egelberg, J. (1965b) Local effect of diet on plaque formation and development of gingivitis in dogs. III. Effect or frequency of meals and tube feeding. *Odontologisk Revy* **16**, 50-60.

Egelberg, J. (1970) A review of the development of dental plaque. In *Dental Plaque*, ed. McHugh, W.D., pp. 9-16. Edinburgh: Livingstone.

Eide, B., Lie, T. & Selvig, K.A. (1983) Surface coatings on dental cementum incident to periodontal disease. I. A scanning electron microscopic study. *Journal of Clinical Periodontology* **10**, 157-171.

Ennever, J. (1960) Intracellular calcification by oral filamentous organisms. *Journal of Periodontology* **3**, 304-307.

Ennever, J., Streckfuss, J.L. & Takazoe, I. (1973) Calcification of bacillary and streptococcal variants of *Bacterionema matruchotii*. *Journal of Dental Research* **52,** 305-308.

Ennever, J., Vogel, J.J., Boyan-Salyers, B. & Riggan, L.J. (1979) Characterization of calculus matrix calcification nucleator. *Journal of Dental Research* **58**, 619-623.

Fitzgerald, R.J. & McDaniel, E.G. (1960) Dental calculus in the germ-free rat. *Archives of Oral Biology* **2**, 239-240.

Folke, L.E.A., Gawronski, T.H., Staat, R.H. & Harris, R.S. (1972) Effect of dietary sucrose on quantity and quality of plaque. *Scandinavian Journal of Dental Research* **80**, 529-533.

Frank, R.M. & Brendel, A. (1966) Ultrastructure of the approximal dental plaque and the underlying normal and carious enamel. *Archives of Oral Biology* **11**, 883-912.

Frank, R.M. & Cimasoni, G. (1970) Ultrastructure de l'epithelium cliniquement normal du sillon et de jonction gingivo-dentaires. *Zeitschrift für Zellforschung und Mikroskopische Anatomie* **109**, 356-379.

Frank, R.M. & Houver, G. (1970) An ultrastructural study of human supragingival dental plaque formation. In *Dental Plaque*, ed. McHugh, W.D., pp. 85-108. Edinburgh: Livingstone.

Friskopp, J. & Hammerström, L. (1980) A comparative scanning electron microscopic study of supragingival and subgingival calculus. *Journal of Periodontology* **51**, 553-562.

Genco, R.J., Christerson, L.A. & Zambon, J.J. (1986) Juvenile periodontitis. *International Dental Journal* **36**, 168-176.

Gibbons, R.J. & Socransky, S.S. (1962) Intracellular polysaccharide storage by organisms in dental plaques. *Archives of Oral Biology* **7**, 73-80.

Gibbons, R.J. & van Houte, J. (1975) Bacterial adherence in oral microbial ecology. *Annual Review of Microbiology* **29**, 19-44.

Gibbons, R.J. & van Houte, J. (1980) Bacterial adherence and the formation of dental plaques. In *Bacterial Adherence* (Receptors and Recognition, series B, vol. 6), ed. Beachey, E.H. pp. 60-104. London: Chapman and Hall.

Glimcher, M.J. (1960) Specificity of the molecular structure of organic matrices in mineralization. In *Calcification in Biological Systems*, ed. Sognnaes, R.F., pp. 421-487. Washington, D.C.: AAAS Publication No. 64.

Gold, W., Preston, F.B., Lache, M.G. & Blechman, H. (1974) Production of levan and dextran in plaque in vivo. *Journal of Dental Research* **53**, 442-446.

Gonzales, F. & Sognnaes, R.F. (1960) Electron microscopy of dental calculus. *Science* **131**, 156-157.

Grenier, D. & Mayrand, D. (1987) Functional characterization of vesicular vesicles produced by *Bacteroides gingivales. Infection and Immunity* **55**, 111-117.

Guggenheim, B. (1970) Extracellular polysaccharides and microbial plaque. *International Dental Journal* **20**, 657-678.

Hazen, S.P. (1960) *A Study of Four Week Old in Vivo Calculus Formation.* Thesis. Rochester, N.Y.: University of Rochester.

Hefferren, J.J., Cooley. R.O., Hall, J.B., Olsen, N.H. & Lyon, H.W. (1971) Use of ultraviolet illumination in oral diagnosis.*Journal of the American Dental Association* **82**, 1353-1360.

Higuchi M., Iwami, Y., Ymada, T. & Araya, S. (1970) Levan synthesis and accumulation by human dental plaque. *Archives of Oral Biology* **15**, 563-567.

Hillam, D.G. & Hull, P.S. (1977) The influence of experimental gingivitis on plaque formation. *Journal of Clinical Periodontology* **4**, 56-61.

Hofstad, T., Kristoffersen, T. & Selvig, K.A. (1972) Electron microscopy of endotoxic lipopolysaccharide form *Bacteroides, Fusobacterium* and *Sphaerophorus. Acta Pathologica et Microbiologica Scandinavica*, Section B **80**, 413-419.

Hotz, P., Guggenheim, B. & Schmid, R. (1972) Carbohydrates in pooled dental plaque. *Caries Research* **6**, 103-121.

Howitt, B.F., Fleming, W.C. & Simonton, F.V. (1928) A study on the effects upon the hygiene and microbiology for the mouth of various diets without and with the use of the toothbrush. *Dental Cosmos* **70** , 575-588.

Kandarkar, S.V. (1973) Ultrastructure of dental plaque and acquired pellicle formed on the artificial tooth surface (araldite plate). *Journal of the Indian Dental Association* **45**, 122-129.

Kelstrup, J. & Theilade E. (1974) Microbes in periodontal disease. *Journal of Clinical Periodontology* **1**, 15-35.

Kleinberg, I. (1970) Biochemistry of the dental plaque. *Advances in Oral Biology* **4**, 43-90.

Knowles, J.W., Burgett, F.G., Nissle, R.R., Schick, R.A., Morrison, E.C. & Ramfjord, S.P. (1979) Results of periodontal treatment related to pocket depth and attachment level. Eight years. *Journal of Periodontology* **50**, 225-233.

Kopczyk, R.A. & Conroy, C.W. (1968) The attachment of calculus to root-planed surfaces. *Periodontics* **6**, 78-83.

Krembel, J., Frank, R.M. & Deluzarche, A. (1969) Fractionation of human dental plaque. *Archives of Oral Biology* **14**, 563-565.

Lang, N.P., Østergaard, E. & Löe, H (1972) A fluorescent plaque disclosing agent. *Journal of Periodontal Research* **7**, 59-67.

Lange, D.E., Stockman, H. & Höcker, K. (1983) Vorkommen und Identifizierung von Protozoen in der menschlichen Mundhöle. *Deutsche Zahnärztliche Zeitschrift* **38**, 906-910.

Leach, S.A. (1973) Dental calculus. In *Biological Mineralization*, ed. Zipkin, I., pp. 587-606. New York: John Wiley & Sons.

Leach, S.A., Appleton, J., Dada, O.A. & Hayes, M.L. (1972) Some factors affecting the metabolism of fructan by human oral flora. *Archives of Oral Biology* **17**, 137-145.

Leach, S.A. & Saxton, C.A. (1966) An electron microscopic study of the acquired pellicle and plaque formed on the enamel of human incisors. *Archives of Oral Biology* **11**, 1081-1094.

Leung, S.W. & Jensen, A.T. (1958) Factors controlling the deposition of calculus. *International Dental Journal* **8**, 613-626.

Lie, T. (1975) Growth of dental plaque on hydroxyapatite splints. A method of studying early plaque morphology. *Journal of Periodontal Research* **9**, 137-145.

Lie, T. (1978) Ultrastructural study of early dental plaque formation. *Journal of Periodontal Research* **13**, 391-409.

Lie, T. & Selvig, K. (1974) Calcification of oral bacteria - an ultrastructural study of two stains of *Bacterionema matruchotii. Scandinavian Journal of Dental Research* **82**, 8-18.

Lie, T. & Selvig, K.A. (1975) Formation of an experimental dental cuticle. *Scandinavian Journal of Dental Research* **83**, 145-152.

Liljemark, W.F., Fenner, L.J. & Bloomquist, C.G. (1986) In vivo colonization of salivary pellicle by *Haemophilus, Actinomyces* and *Streptococcus* species. *Caries Research* **20**, 481-497.

Liljenberg, B. & Lindhe, J. (1980) Juvenile periodontitis. Some microbiological, histopathological and clinical characteristics. *Journal of Periodontology* **7**, 48-61.

Lim, L.P., Tay, F.B.K., Waite, I.M. & Cornick, D.E.R. (1986) A comparison of 4 techniques for clinical detection of early plaque formed during different dietary regimens. *Journal of Clinical Periodontology* **13**, 658-665.

Lindhe, J. & Axelsson, P. (1973) The effect of controlled oral hygiene and topical fluoride application on caries and gingivitis in Swedish schoolchildren. *Community Dentistry and Oral Epidemiology* **1**, 9-16.

Lindhe, J., Hamp, S.-E. & Löe, H. (1973) Experimental periodontitis in the Beagle dog. *Journal of Periodontal Research* **8**, 1-10.

Lindhe, J. & Nyman, S. (1984) Long-term maintenance of patients treated for advanced periodontal disease. *Journal of Clinical Periodontology* **11**, 504-514.

Lindhe, J. & Wicen P.-O. (1969) The effects on the gingivae of chewing fibrous foods. *Journal of Periodontal Research* **4**, 193-201.

Listgarten, M.A. (1976) Structure of the microbial flora associated with periodontal health and disease in man. A light and electron microscopic study. *Journal of Periodontology* **47**, 1-18.

Listgarten, M.A. & Ellegaard, B. (1973) Electron microscopic evidence of a cellular attachment between junctional epithelium and dental calculus. *Journal of Periodontal Research* **8**, 143-150.

Listgarten, M.A. & Helldén, L. (1978) Relative distribution of bacteria at clinically healthy and periodontally diseased sites in humans. *Journal of Clinical Periodontology* **5**, 115-132.

Listgarten, M.A., Mayo, H. & Amsterdam, M. (1973) Ultrastructure of the attachment device between coccal and filamentous microorganisms in "corn cob" formations in dental plaque. *Archives of Oral Biology* **8**, 651-656.

Listgarten, M.A., Mayo, H. & Tremblay, R. (1975) Development of dental plaque on epoxy resin crowns in man. A light and electron microscopic study. *Journal of Periodontology* **46**, 10-26.

Little, M.F., Bowman, L., Casciani, C.A. & Rowley, J. (1966) The composition af dental calculus. III. Supragingival calculus - the amino acid and saccharide component. *Archives of Oral Biology* **11**, 385-396.

Little, M.F., Bowman, L.M. & Dirksen, T.R. (1964) The lipids of supragingival calculus. *Journal of Dental Research* **43**, 836.

Little, M.F., Casciani, C.A. & Rowley, J. (1963) Dental calculus composition. I. Supragingival calculus. ash, calcium, phosphorus, sodium, and density. *Journal of Dental Research* **42**, 78-86.

Little, M.F. & Hazen, S.P. (1964) Dental calculus composition. II. Subgingival calculus: ash, calcium, phosphorus and sodium. *Journal of Dental Research* **43**, 645-651.

Lobene, R.R. (1986) A clinical study of the anticalculus effect of a dentifrice containing soluble pyrophosphate and sodium fluoride. *Clinical Preventive Dentistry* **8**, 5-7.

Löe, H., Theilade E. & Jensen, S.B. (1965) Experimental gingivitis in man. *Journal of Periodontology* **36**, 177-187.

Lövdal, A., Arnö, A., Schei, O. & Waerhaug, J. (1961) Combined effect of subgingival scaling and controlled oral hygiene on the incidence of gingivitis. *Acta Odontologica Scandinavica* **19**, 537-555.

Lövdal, A., Arnö, A., & Waerhaug, J. (1958) Incidence of clinical manifestations of periodontal disease in light of oral hygiene and calculus formation. *Journal of the American Dental Association* **56**, 21-33.

MacPhee, I.T. & Muir, K.F. (1986) Dark ground microscopy in relation to 3 clinical parameters of chronic inflammatory periodontal disease. *Journal of Clinical Periodontology* **13**, 900-904.

Mandel, I.D. (1963) Histochemical and biochemical aspects of calculus formation. *Periodontics* **1**, 43-52.

Mandel, I.D. & Gaffar, A. (1986) Calculus revisited: A review. *Journal of Clinical Periodontology* **31**, 249-257.

Mandel, I.D., Levy, B.M. & Wasserman, B.H. (1957) Histochemistry of calculus formation. *Journal of Periodontology* **28**, 132-137.

Mandel, I.D. & Thompson, R.H. (1967) The chemistry of parotid and submaxillary saliva in heavy calculus formers and non-formers. *Journal of Periodontology* **38**, 310-315.

Matsson, L. & Attström, R. (1979) Histologic characteristics of experimental gingivitis in the juvenile and adult beagle dog. *Journal of Clinical Periodontology* **6**, 334-350.

McDougall, W.A. (1963) Studies on dental plaque. II. The histology of the developing interproximal plaque. *Australian Dental Journal* **8**, 398-407.

Moore, L.V.H., Moore, W.E.C., Cato, E.P., Smibert, R.M., Burmeister, J.A., Best, A.M. & Ranney, R.R. (1987) Bacteriology of human gingivitis. *Journal of Dental Research* **66**, 989-995.

Moore, W.E.C., Holdeman, L.V., Cato, E.P., Smibert, R.M., Burmeister, J.A., Palcanis, K.G. & Ranney, R.R. (1985) Comparative bacteriology of juvenile periodontitis. *Infection and Immunity* **48**, 507-519.

Moore, W.E.C., Holdeman, L.V., Smibert, R.M., Good, I.J., Burmeister, J.A., Palcanis, K.G. & Ranney, R.R. (1982) Bacteriology of experimental gingivitis in young adult humans. *Infection and Immunity* **38**, 651-667.

Morishita, M., Tokumoto, K., Watanabe, T. & Iwamoto Y. (1986) Effect of a protease derived from the oral bacterium *Bacteroides loescheii* on the inhibition of calcium-phosphate precipitation by human parotic saliva. *Archives of Oral Biology* **31**, 555-557.

Moskow, B.S. (1969) Calculus attachment in cemental separations. *Journal of Periodontology* **40**,

125-130.

Mühlemann, H.R. & Schneider, U.K. (1959) Early calculus formation. *Helvetica Odontologica Acta* **3**, 22-26.

Mühlemann, H.R. & Schroeder, H.E. (1964) Dynamics of supragingival calculus. I *Advances in Oral Biology*, ed. Staple, P.H., pp. 175-203. New York: Academic Press.

Nyvad, B., Fejerskov, O., Theilade J., Melsen, B., Rölla, G. & Karring, T. (1982) The effect of sucrose or casein on early microbial colonization on Mylar and tooth surfaces in monkeys. *Journal of Dental Research* **61**, 570.

Ørstavik, D. & Ruangsri, P. (1979) Effects of bactericidal treatments on bacterial adherence and dental plaque formation.*Scandinavian Journal of Dental Research* **87**, 296-301.

Öste, R., Rönström, A., Birkhed, D., Edwardsson, S. & Stenberg, M. (1981) Gas-liquid chromatographic analysis of amino acids in pellicle formed on tooth surface and plastic film in vitro. *Archives of Oral Biology* **26**, 635-641.

Patters, M.R., Landesberg, R.L., Johansson, L.A., Trummel, C.L. & Robertson, P.B. (1982) *Bacteroides gingivalis* antigens and bone resorping activity in root surface fractions of periodontally involved teeth. *Journal of Periodontal Research* **17**, 122-130.

Pihlstrom, B.L., McHugh, B., Oliphant, T.H. & Campos, C.O. (1983) Comparison of surgical and nonsurgical treatment of periodontal disease - a review of current studies and additional results after 6.5 years. *Journal of Clinical Periodontology* **10**, 524-541.

Ramfjord, S.P., Knowles, J.W., Nissle, R.R., Schick, R.A. & Burgett, F.G. (1973) Longitudinal study of periodontal therapy. *Journal of Periodontology* **46**, 66-77.

Rateitschak-Plüss, E.M. & Guggenheim, B. (1982) Effects of a carbohydrate-free diet and sugar substitutes on dental plaque accumulation. *Journal of Clinical Periodontology* **9**, 239-251.

Ritz, H.L. (1967) Microbial population shifts in developing human dental plaque. *Archives of Oral Biology* **12**, 1561-1568.

Ritz, H.L. (1969) Fluorescent antibody staining of Neisseria, Streptococcus and Veillonella in frozen sections of dental plaque. *Archives of Oral Biology* **14**, 1073-1084.

Rölla, G., Melsen, B. & Sönju, T. (1975) Sulphated macromolecules in dental plaque in the monkeys *Macaca irus*. *Archives of Oral Biology* **20**, 341-343.

Rönström, A., Attström, R. & Egelberg, J. (1975) Early formation af dental plaque on plastic films. 1. Light microscopic observations. *Journal of Periodontal Research* **10**, 28-35.

Rönström, A., Edwardsson, S. & Attström, R. (1977) *Streptococcus sanguis* and *Streptococcus salivarius* in early plaque formation on plastic films. *Journal of Periodontal Research* **12**, 331-339.

Rowles, S.L. (1964) The inorganic composition of dental calculus. In *Bone and Tooth*, ed. Blackwood, H.J.J., pp. 175-183. Oxford: Pergamon Press.

Saxe, S.R., Greene, J.C., Bohannan, H.M. & Vermillion, J.R. (1967) Oral debris, calculus and periodontal disease in the Beagle dog. *Periodontics* **5**, 217-225.

Saxén, L., Asikainen, S., Sandblom, L. & Kari, K. (1986) Treatment of juvenile periodontitis without antibiotics. A follow-up study. *Journal of Clinical Periodontology* **13**, 714-719.

Saxton, C.A. (1969) An electron microscope investigation of bacterial polysaccharide synthesis in human dental plaque. *Archives of Oral Biology* **4**, 1275-1284.

Saxton, C.A. (1973) Scanning electron microscope study of the formation of dental plaque. *Caries Research* **7**, 102-119.

Schiff, T.G. (1986) The effect on calculus deposits of a dentifrice containing soluble pyrophosphate and sodium fluoride. A 3-month clinical study. *Clinical Preventive Dentistry* **8**, 8-10.

Schroeder, H.E. (1963) Inorganic content and histology of early calculus in man. *Helvetica Odontologica Acta* **7**, 17-30.

Schroeder, H.E. (1964) Two different types of mineralization in early dental calculus. *Helvetica Odontologica Acta* 7, 117-127.

Schroeder, H.E. (1965) Crystal morphology and gross structures of mineralizing plaque and calculus. *Helvetica Odontologica Acta* **9**, 73-86.

Schroeder, H.E. (1969) *Formation and Inhibition of Dental Calculus*. Berne: Hans Huber Publishers.

Schroeder, H.E. (1970) The stucture and relationship of plaque to the hard and soft tissues: electron microscopic interpretation. *International Dental Jounal* **20**, 353-381.

Schroeder, H.E. & Attström, R. (1979) Effects of mechanical plaque control on development of subgingival plaque and initial gingivitis in neutropenic dogs. *Scandinavian Journal of Dental Research* **87**, 279-287.

Schroeder, H.E. & Baumbauer, H.U. (1966) Stages of calcium phosphate crystallization during calculus formation. *Archives of Oral Biology* **11**, 1-14.

Schroeder, H.E. & De Boever, J. (1970) The structure of microbial dental plaque. In *Dental Plaque*, ed. McHugh, W.D., pp. 49-74, Edinburgh: Livingstone.

Schroeder, H.E., Lenz, H. & Mühlemann, H.R. (1964) Microstructures and mineralization of early dental calculus. *Helvetica Odontologica Acta* **8**, 1-16.

Schroeder, H. E. & Listgarten, M.A. (1977) *Fine Structure of the Developing Epithelial Attachment of Human Teeth*. Basel: S. Karger.

Selvig, K.A. (1970) Attachment of plaque and calculus to tooth surfaces. *Journal of Periodontal Research* **5**, 8-18.

Sheinin, A. & Mäkinen, K.K. (1971) The effect of various sugars on the formation and chemical composition of dental plaque. *International Dental Journal* **21**, 302-321.

Sidaway, D.A. (1979) A microbiological study of dental calculus. III. A comparison of the in vitro calcification of viable and non-viable microorganisms. *Journal of Periodontal Research* **14**, 167-172.

Silness, J. & Löe, H. (1964) Periodontal disease in pregnancy. II. Correlation between oral hygiene and periodontal condition. *Acta Odontologica Scandinavica* **22**, 121-135.

Silverman, G. & Kleinberg, I. (1967) Fractionation of human dental plaque and the characterization of its cellular and acellular components. *Archives of Oral Biology* **12**, 1387-1405.

Slots, J. (1976) The predominant cultivable flora in juvenile periodontitis. *Scandinavian Journal of Dental Research* **84**, 1-10.

Slots, J. (1977) The predominant cultivable microflora of advanced periodontitis. *Scandinavian Journal of Dental Research* **85**, 114-121.

Slots, J., Möenbo, D., Langebaek, J. & Frandsen, A. (1978) Microbiota of gingivitis in man. *Scandinavian Journal of Dental Research* **86**, 174-181.

Soames, J.V. & Davies, R.M. (1975) The structure of subgingival plaque in a beagle dog. *Journal of Periodontal Research* **9**, 333-341.

Socransky, S.S., Manganiello, A.D., Propoas, D., Oram, V. & van Houte, J. (1977) Bacteriological studies of developing supragingival dental plaque. *Journal of Periodontal Research* **12**, 90-106.

Söderholm, G. (1979) *Effect of a Dental Care Program on Dental Health Conditions. A Study of Employees of a Swedish Shipyard.* Malmö: Department of Periodontology, Faculty of Odontology, University of Lund, Sweden.

Sönju, T. & Glantz, P.-O. (1975) Chemical composition of salivary integuments formed in vivo on solids with some established surface characteristics. *Archives of Oral Biology* **20**, 687-691.

Sönju, T. & Rölla, G. (1973) Chemical analysis of the acquired pellicle formed in two hours on cleaned human teeth. *Caries Research* **7**, 30-38.

Stanford, J.W. (1966) Analysis of the organic portion of dental calculus. *Journal of Dental Research* **45**, 128-135.

Suomi, J.D., Greene, J.C., Vermillion, J.R., Doyle, J., Chang, J.J. & Leatherwood, E.C. (1971) The effect of controlled hygiene procedures on the progression of periodontal disease in adults: results after third and finial year. *Journal of Periodontology* **42**, 152-160.

Syed, S.A. & Loesche, W.J. (1978) Bacteriology of human experimental gingivitis: effect of plaque age. *Infection and Immunity* **21**, 821-829.

Tanner, A.C.R., Socransky, S.S. & Goodson, J.M. (1984) Microbiota of periodontal pockets losing crestal alveolar bone. *Journal of Periodontal Research* **9**, 279-291.

Ten Napel, J., Theilade, J., Matsson, L. & Attström, R. (1983) Ultrastructure of developing subgingival plaque in beagle dogs. *Journal of Clinical Periodontology* **12**, 507-524

Theilade, E. (1986) The non-specific theory in microbial etiology of inflammatory periodontal diseases. *Journal of Clinical Periodontology* **13**, 905-911.

Theilade, E. & Theilade, J. (1970) Bacteriological and ultrastructural studies of developing dental plaque. In *Dental Plaque*, ed., McHugh, W.D., pp. 27-40. Edinburgh: Livingstone.

Theilade, E. & Theilade, J. (1985) Formation and ecology of plaque at different locations in the mouth. *Scandinavian Journal of Dental Research* **93**, 90-95.

Theilade, E., Theilade, J. & Mikkelsen, L. (1982a) Microbiological studies on early dentogingival plaque on teeth and Mylar strips in humans. *Journal of Periodontal Research* **17**, 12-25.

Theilade, E., Wright, W.H., Jensen, S.B. & Löe, H. (1966) Experimental gingivitis in man. II. A longitudinal clinical and bacteriological investigation. *Journal of Periodontal Research* **1**, 1-13.

Theilade, J. (1960) *The Microscopic Structure of Dental Calculus.* Thesis. Rochester, NY: University of Rochester.

Theilade, J. (1964) Electron microscopic study of calculus attachment to smooth surfaces. *Acta Odontologica Scandinavica* **22**, 379-387.

Theilade, J. & Attström, R. (1985) Distribution and ultrastructure of subgingival plaque in beagle dogs with gingival inflammation. *Journal of Periodontal Research* **20**, 131-145.

Theilade, J., Fejerskov, O., Karring, T., Rölla, G. & Melsen, B. (1982b) TEM of the effect of sucrose on plaque formation on Mylar and tooth surfaces in monkeys. *Journal of Dental Research* **61**, 570.

Theilade, J., Fitzgerald, R.J., Scott, D.B. & Nylén, M.U. (1964) Electron microscopic observations of dental calculus in germ-free and conventional rats. *Archives of Oral Biology* **9**, 97-100.

Theilade, J. & Mikkelsen, L. (1972) Ultrastructural study of dental plaque formation during the first 3-hour period. *Caries Research* **6**, 79.

Theilade, J. & Schroeder, H.E. (1966) Recent results in dental calculus research. *International Dental Journal* **16**, 205-221.

Tinanoff, N. & Gross, A. (1976) Epithelial cells associated with the development of dental plaque. *Journal of Dental Research* **55**, 580-583.

Turesky, S., Renstrup, G. & Glickman, I. (1961) Histologic and histochemical observations regarding early calculus formation in children and adults.

Journal of Periodontology **32**, 7-14.

Van Houte, J. (1964) Relationship between carbohydrate intake and polysaccharide-storing organisms in dental plaque. *Archives of Oral Biology* **9**, 91-93.

Van Houte, J., Gibbons, R.J. & Pulkkinen, A.J. (1972) Ecology of human oral lactobacilli. *Infection and Immunity* **6**, 723-729.

Voreadis, E.G. & Zander, H.A. (1958) Cuticular calculus attachment. *Oral Surgery, Oral Medicine and Oral Pathology* **11**, 1120-1125.

Wade, A.B. (1971) Effect on dental plaque of chewing apples. *Dental Practitioner* **21**, 194-196.

Watanabe, T., Toda, K., Morishita, M. & Iwamoto Y. (1982) Correlations between salivary protease and supragingival and subgingival calculus. *Journal of Dental Research* **61**, 1048-1051.

Waerhaug, J. (1952) The gingival pocket. *Odontologisk Tidskrift* **60**, Supplement 1.

Waerhaug, J. (1955) Microscopic demonstration of tissue reaction incident to removal of dental calculus. *Journal of Periodontology* **26**, 26-29.

Waerhaug, J. (1956) Effect of rough surfaces upon gingival tissues. *Journal of Dental Research* **35**, 323-325.

Waerhaug, J. (1978) Healing of dento-epithelial junction following subgingival plaque control. II. As observed on extracted teeth, *Journal of Periodontology* **49**, 119-134.

Wennström, A., Wennström, J. & Lindhe, J. (1986) Healing following surgical and non-surgical treatment of juvenile periodontitis. A 5-year longitudinal study. *Journal of Clinical Periodontology* **13**, 869-882.

Westergaard, J., Frandsen, A. & Slots, J. (1978) Ultrastructure of the subgingival flora in juvenile periodontitis. *Scandinavian Journal of Dental Research* **86**, 421-429.

Wilcox, C.E. & Everett, F.G (1963) Friction on the teeth and the gingiva during mastication. *Journal of the American Dental Association* **66**, 513-520.

Wood, J.M. (1967) The amount, distribution and metabolism of soluble polysaccharides in human dental plaque. *Archives of Oral Biology* **12**, 849-858.

Wood, J.M. (1969) The state of hexose sugar in human dental plaque and its metabolism by the plaque bacteria. *Archives of Oral Biology* **14**, 161-168.

Zacherl, W.A., Pheiffer, H.J. & Swancar, J.R. (1985) The effect of soluble pyrophosphates on dental calculus in adults. *Journal of the Americal dental Association* **110**, 737-738.

Zander, H.A., Hazen, S.P. & Scott, D.B. (1960) Mineralization of dental calculus. *Proceedings of the Society for Experimental Biology and Medicine*, New York **103**, 257-260.

CHAPTER 4

Microbiology of Plaque-associated Periodontal Disease

A retrospective survey

The first described bacteria

In one of his letters to the Royal Society of London, Anton van Leeuwenhoek (1632-1723) wrote on September 17, 1683:

> "Tis my wont of a morning to rub my teeth with salt, and then swill my mouth out with water: and often, after eating, to clean my back teeth with a toothpick, as well as rubbing them hard with a cloth: wherefore my teeth, back and front, remain as clean and white as falleth to the lot of few men of my years, and my gums (no matter how hard the salt be that I rub them with) never start bleeding. Yet notwithstanding, my teeth are not so clean thereby, but what there sticketh or groweth between some of my front ones and my grinders (whenever I inspected them with a magnifying

> mirror), a little white matter, which is as thick as if 'twere batter. On examining this, I judged (albeit I could discern nought a-moving in it) that there yet were living animalcules therein" (Dobell 1960).

Then follows the first description of bacteria from the human oral cavity. Anton van Leeuwenhoek further remarks:

> "That all the people living in our United Netherlands are not as many as the living animals that I carry in my own mouth this very day."

He was obviously not far from the conclusion that bleeding of the gums was caused by the living animalcules he was studying. But it took over 200 years to realize that microorganisms cause disease.

The specificity of microbial action

The concept of the specific action of microbes was introduced by Louis Pasteur (1822-1895) in his studies on fermentation (Collard 1976). To prove his hypothesis that each type of fermentation was caused by specific microorganisms, Pasteur had to develop methods for the cultivation of each organism uncontaminated by any other species. He also had to develop methods for the sterilization of his media and glassware, as well as aseptic techniques for handling bacterial samples. The use of the naked flame, the hot-air oven and the autoclave all originated in his laboratory. By applying the concept of specificity of microbial action Pasteur was able to solve many of the problems arising in the production of wine and beer. Using the microscope, he was also able to show (1865) that a disease in silkworms was caused by a protozoan parasite.

Robert Koch (1843-1910) developed methods for staining bacteria in smears and he showed by the use of the microscope that a specific microorganism caused anthrax in cattle (1876). He was also the first to publish photomicrographs of bacteria (1877). The identity of microorganisms, however, can not usually be disclosed by microscopy. So when Koch in 1881 introduced the solid-media technique, he initiated a veritable revolution in bacteriology. To obtain pure cultures of bacteria Pasteur had to use tedious liquid dilution methods, but with the solid-media technique, mixed cultures could be isolated and pure single species cultures easily obtained. In the last two decades of the 19th century, the "Golden Era" of medical bacteriology, the causal organisms of the majority of the bacterial infections were isolated and characterized. Then studies on the mechanisms of pathogenicity, host response, and methods of prevention and treatment followed.

Koch's postulates

The criteria for distinguishing a pathogenic microorganism from an adventitious one are known as Koch's postulates:

1. The pathogenic organism is regularly found in the lesions of disease.
2. It can be isolated in pure culture on artificial media.
3. Inoculation of this culture produces a similar disease in experimental animals.
4. The organism can be recovered from the lesions in the animals.

Specific bacteria in periodontal disease

In Koch's laboratory worked a dentist, Willoughby Dayton Miller (1853-1907), who applied all the current bacteriological techniques to studies of the oral microbiota (Miller 1890). He was interested in many aspects of oral diseases and also in finding out whether any specific bacterium caused periodontal disease. From his studies in 1888-89 he drew the following conclusion:

> "Pyorrhaea alveolaris is not caused by any specific bacterium, which occurs in every case (like the tubercle bacillus in tuberculosis), but various bacteria may participitate in it, just as in suppurative processes not only one but generally various species have been found. Besides, as far as we know, there is no bacterium which, inoculated under the gums is able to provoke the disease in healthy persons."

but he also made the important remark:

> "if there is a specific bacterium of pyorrhaea alveolaris it does not readily grow on gelatine... At the same time the thought suggests itself that possibly the bacterium of pyorrhaea alveolaris, like so many mouth bacteria, is cultivable on none of the artificial nutrient media, which would of course render all experimenting useless."

It was not until quite recently that bacteriological techniques were developed which permit cultivation of the majority of the microorganisms of the oral cavity. The breakthrough came when careful dispersion of samples was combined with strict anaerobic techniques in which bacteria were protected from exposure to oxygen during various phases of the work in the laboratory. Now we have reached the point where the concept of specific bacteria in periodontal disease can again be tested.

The unique microbiota of the oral cavity

The oral cavity - an ecological system

The oral cavity with its microbiota is an ecological system of bewildering complexity (Bowden et al. 1979). It has been characterized as a river system (Appleton 1944), where sterile saliva arises from the salivary glands, washes all surfaces in the mouth, and passes many sites of prospering microbial life becoming, thus, strongly polluted before leaving the mouth. In running-water systems, life is proverbially rich and varied on solid surfaces, where the organisms achieve firm anchorage and a favorable nutritional environment. The mouth is the only site in the human body where such hard solid surfaces are found, i.e. the surfaces of the teeth.

From an ecological point of view the oral cavity is an open growth system. This means that nutrients and microbes are repeatedly introduced into and removed from the system (Lynch & Poole 1979). The flow rate of saliva is so high that the only organisms that are successful are those which can adhere to the surfaces of the oral cavity, or are, in some other way, retained. Not only the flow of saliva, but also the flow of the gingival fluid, chewing, oral hygiene procedures and desquamation of epithelial cells from the mucous membranes serve to remove bacteria from the oral surfaces. Some bacteria may be retained simply by obtaining a refuge in pits and fissures, or in the protected areas in between the teeth. Other microorganisms have to rely on specific mechanisms of adherence in order to overcome the strong removal forces on the oral surfaces. The characteristics of the oral surfaces are unique and only specific bacteria have the ability to adhere. This means that the oral cavity harbors a unique microbiota and most of its members are not able to colonize any other site of the human body. The oral cavity consists of several distinct sites, each of which will support the growth of a characteristic microbial community. Enormous differences, thus, exist in the composition of the microbiota on the mucous membranes, the tongue, the teeth and in the gingival sulcus area. It has even been demonstrated that the composition of the microbiota may vary from site to site on a single tooth surface.

Factors involved in the adherence of the microbes to the surfaces of the oral cavity are of primary ecological importance. An import-

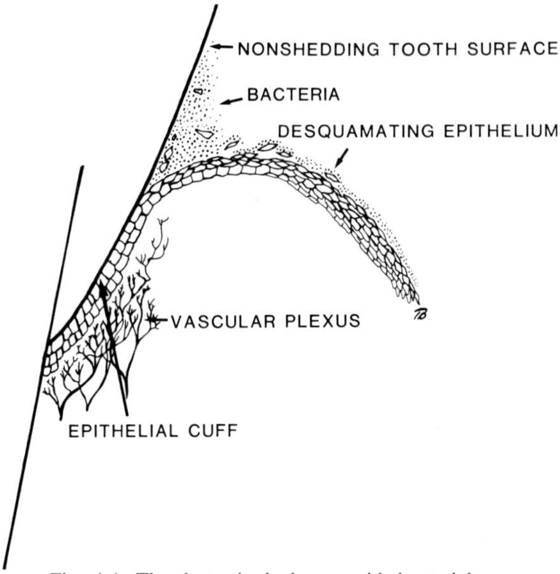

Fig. 4-1. The dentogingival area with bacterial aggregations on the solid tooth surface and bacteria colonizing the surface of the desquamating epithelium. In the gingival crevice area the epithelial cuff and the dense vascular plexus play an important part in the host defense against microbial invasion.

ant ecological determinant of the oral cavity is also the nutritional interrelation between the host and the microbes. The composition of the microbiota is to a significant degree determined by the efficiency of various organisms to utilize the available nutrients.

For those organisms which become established the oral cavity will be like the "Garden of Eden". The humidity is high. The temperature, pH and carbon dioxide tension are optimal for growth. The oxygen tension varies in various sites and permits growth of aerobic as well as strictly anaerobic organisms. Saliva not only provides nutrients to the microbiota but also buffers acidic fermentation products of the microbiota and removes inhibitory waste products.

In addition to the primary ecological determinants, bacterial adherence and nutrition, many other factors also influence the establishment of the organisms in the oral cavity, but before these factors are discussed, the primary determinants should be further considered.

Bacterial adherence

Bacterial adherence involves specific physicochemical mechanisms and is influenced not only by the interaction between surface structures of bacteria and colonizable surfaces, but also by the activity of saliva as a suspending fluid.

Characteristics of oral surfaces

The surfaces of lips, cheeks, palate, tongue, gums and teeth all provide different characteristics for bacterial colonization. All these surfaces are covered, however, by a highly hydrophilic confluent film of salivary mucins. These mucins have the form of a complex hydrated gel composed of a variety of high molecular weight glycoproteins. This surface film may be of importance in lubrication of the mucosa, in waterproofing and in protection against sudden changes in osmotic pressure, but it will also interfere with the bacterial adherence (McNabb & Tomasi 1981).

The most important difference among the oral surfaces is the one between the mucosa, with its desquamating epithelium, and the solid tooth surface (Gibbons & van Houte 1975). On the tooth surface the salivary mucins are denatured (Pruitt 1977) and form a highly structured organic film called pellicle which serves as solid ground for long-lasting microbial life. On the desquamating epithelial surface, the bacteria must continually colonize 'virgin soil' (Fig. 4-1). The shedding surface of the oral mucosa is an important part of the host defence against bacterial invasion. Although the epithelial turnover is higher in the dentogingival area than anywhere else in the mouth, this defence mechanism does not work very efficiently at this particular site. The reason is that the bacteria in contact with the epithelium are in addition firmly anchored to the solid non-shedding tooth surface. This is one of the reasons why this area presents so many unique features of host parasite interactions.

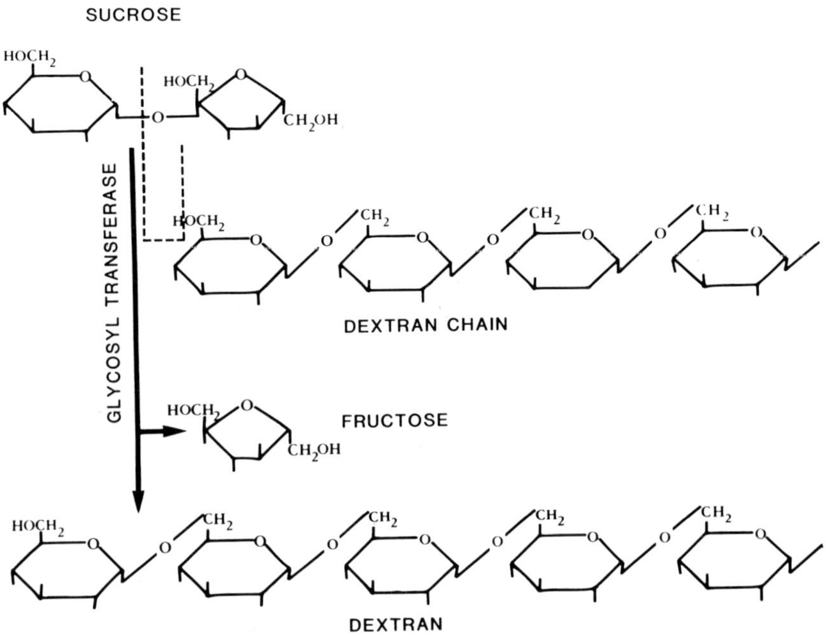

Fig. 4-2. Synthesis of dextran (1,6-α-glucan) from sucrose catalyzed by a glycosyl transferase.

Characteristics of bacterial surfaces

Most bacteria in nature are surrounded by highly hydrated matrices called glycocalyces (Costerton et al. 1981). These structures had for a long time been overlooked. The reason was that bacteria rapidly lose these structures when cultured in the laboratory and the glycocalyces are not visualized by conventional light or electron microscopy. In some bacteria the glycocalyx consists of a regular array of rod-like glycoprotein appendages, but more often bacteria are surrounded by a glycocalyx composed of a matrix of polysaccharide fibers. The glycocalyx may be a coherent capsule or a more loosely, cell-associated, extracellular polysaccharide. Many bacteria bear long nonflagellar appendages at their surfaces, which extend beyond the surface of the glycocalyx. These appendages can vary in length between 0.2 and 20 μm and the width of these structures ranges between 30 and 140 Å. They have many names but are usually called pili or fimbriae.

The glycocalyces are often made up of heteropolysaccharides, which bacteria can produce from any carbohydrate source. Some bacteria have in addition the capacity to form extracellular homopolysaccharides from sucrose (Guggenheim 1970, Walker & Jacques 1987). These polysaccharides are synthesized from sucrose by enzymes, glycosyl transferases, excreted by *Streptococcus sanguis, S. mitis, S. salivarius* and *S. mutans*. There are different types of glycosyl transferases. Some cleave sucrose, release fructose and obtain energy for the extracellular conversion of the glucose moieties of sucrose into highly branched glucans (Fig. 4-2). These glucans can be both 1.3-α- and 1.6-α-polymers. Those glucans which have a high percentage of 1.3-α-linkages are highly insoluble and are called mutan, while those with predominantly 1.6-α-linkages are soluble and are called dextran. The insoluble glucans are considered to play an important role as a matrix in the microbial aggregations on the teeth. Other glycosyl transferases cleave sucrose, release glucose and convert the fruc-

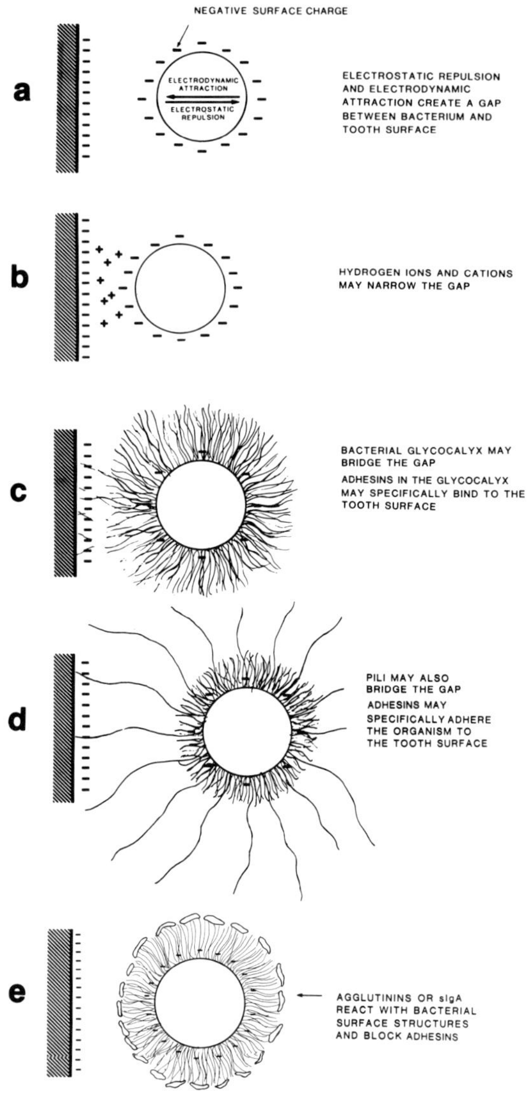

Fig. 4-3. Some factors which influence the adherence of a bacterial cell to a tooth surface.

tose moieties of sucrose into fructan. This fructan is usually highly soluble and can be used as a source of carbohydrate by some of the bacteria of the oral microbiota (McGhee & Michalek 1981).

Physicochemical characteristics of bacterial adherence

An important characteristic of living cells is that they carry a net negative electric charge and thus tend to repel each other electrostatically. The tooth surface is also negatively charged and repels the cells (Gristina 1987). The cells are further influenced, however, by electrodynamic or van der Waal's force. These forces are attractive and of longer range than the repulsive electrostatic force. The attractive and repulsive forces will favor a separation of the bacteria at specific distances from the tooth surface (Fig. 4-3a). This separation gap is influenced by the presence of ions. An acid pH or an increased concentration of cations will decrease the gap (Fig. 4-3b). The importance of the glycocalyx for bacterial adherence is that the glycocalyx constitutes a hydrophilic extension beyond the highly charged surface of the bacterial cell and can thus bridge the separation gap between the bacteria and the tooth surface (Fig. 4-3c). When the glycocalyx comes into contact with the tooth surface other attractive forces such as hydrogen bonding, ion pair formation and dipole-dipole interaction can be established. The bacterial pili or fimbriae are usually long enough to protrude beyond the glycocalyx and may therefore assist in bridging the separation gap and establishing the contact between the bacteria and the tooth surface (Fig. 4-3d).

The adhesion of bacteria to the tooth surface is probably in most cases determined by highly specific mechanisms (Mergenhagen et al. 1987). Molecules called adhesins on the bacteria recognize specific receptor molecules on the tooth surface (Figs. 4-3c, d). These adhesins are often located on the pili or fimbriae. Adhesins which are proteins and recognize carbohydrate structures are called lectins. The carbohydrate groups of the glycoproteins of the pellicle may serve as receptors for such bacterial adhesins (Sharon 1987). While the mucinous denatured film covering the solid tooth surface, pellicle, seems to facilitate the bacterial adherence, the mucinous film covering the oral mucosa may prevent bacteria from reaching receptor sites on the epithelial surfaces. Some of

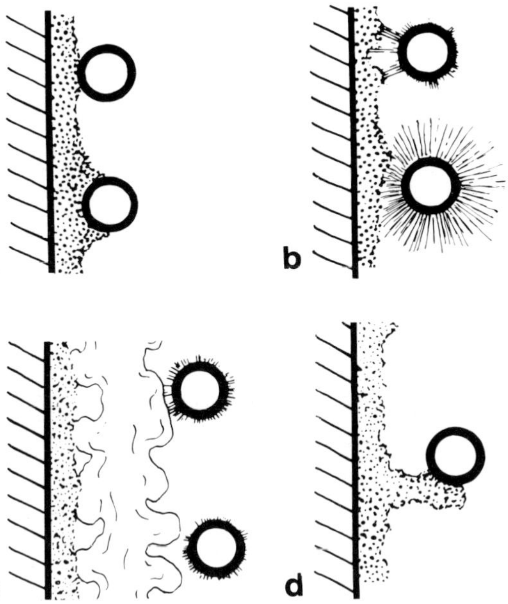

Fig. 4-4. Different modes of bacterial adherence to the tooth surface (Lie 1979).

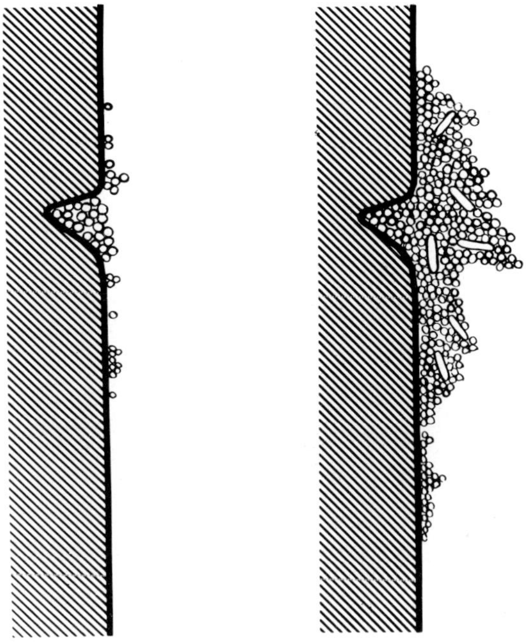

Fig. 4-5. Early bacterial aggregations in pits and grooves of the tooth surface (a). These bacteria increase rapidly in number and spread over the tooth surface (b) (Lie 1979).

the salivary mucins (agglutinins) as well as secretory immunoglobulin A (sIgA) may react with bacterial surface structures (Fig. 4-3e) and in that way prevent the bacteria from adhering to the oral surfaces (Gibbons & van Houte 1975).

Structure of the pellicle

The appearance of the pellicle may vary considerably. The mean thickness of 2 h pellicle is about 100 nm and increases to about 400 nm in 24-48 h. The structure of the pellicle is heterogeneous. Initially, there are small globules or aggregations of amorphous material adsorbed to the tooth surface. Later globules of varying size and 3 and 7 nm wide fiber can be distinguished in the internal structure of the pellicle. In other areas of the pellicle there are laminated granular patterns (Lie 1979).

Structure of the microbial community on the tooth surface

In microscopic studies on the initial colonization of the tooth surface, single bacteria are usually seen to adhere to small irregularities in the surface of the pellicle (Figs. 4-4a, d). Some bacteria are attached to the pellicle by pili or fimbriae (Fig. 4-4b). Sometimes epithelial cells colonized by bacteria are seen on the tooth surface (Fig. 4-4c). The attached bacteria start to grow and multiply, and microorganisms in pits and grooves especially increase rapidly in number (Fig. 4-5a). From these initial areas of colonization, single layers of cells spread over the surface (Fig. 4-5b) and coalesce with neighboring areas of bacterial accumulation (Lie 1979). At this stage of bacterial accumulation, the mean bacterial generation time has been estimated to be 3-4 h (Socransky et al. 1977). When germ-free rats were infected with *Actinomyces viscosus*, the generation time on the tooth surface was 2.9 h. The generation time of *Streptococcus mutans* was 1.1 h (Beckers & van der Hoeven 1982).

The replicating bacteria will be unable to accumulate on the tooth surface unless there are

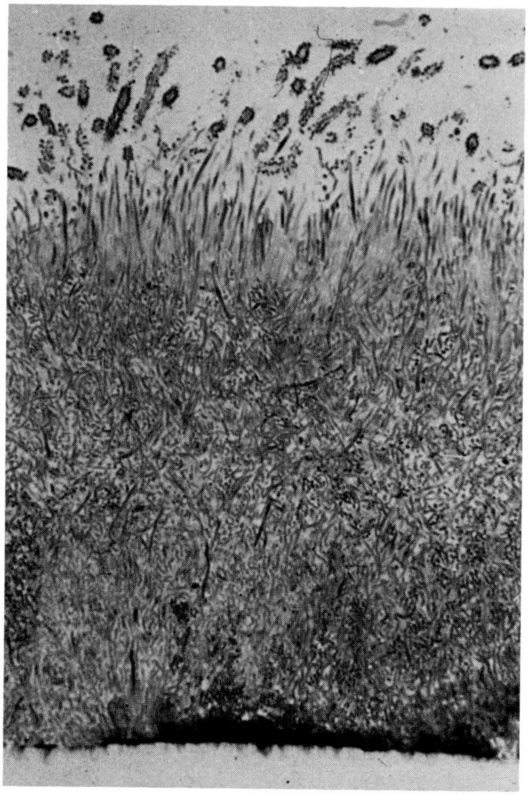

Fig. 4-6. Supra-gingival microbial mass adhering to a tooth with advanced periodontal disease. There are dense masses of filamentous organisms and "corncob" formations are seen on the surface of the microbial mass (Listgarten 1976). The tooth surface is located at the bottom of the illustration.

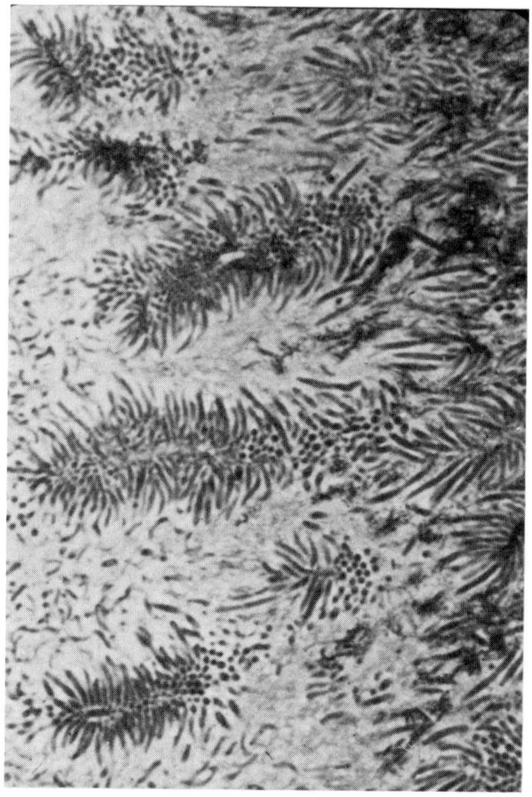

Fig. 4-7. "Test-tube brush" formations among the microbial masses in a gingival pocket. These structures are composed of filamentous bacteria to which the "bristles" (Gram negative rods) of the "brush" attach (Listgarten 1976).

retention mechanisms in operation. Mechanisms involved in bacterial adhesion to the tooth surface are also in effect when bacteria adhere to each other. Bacterial glycocalyces and salivary glycoproteins constitute a matrix which retains the microbial mass to the tooth surface. The cohesion of the mass is dependent on both unspecific and specific binding mechanisms. The "corncob" formations (Fig. 4-6) in which streptococci adhere to filaments of *Bacterionema matruchotii* (Mouton et al. 1980) or of Actinomyces (Cisar 1982), are very spectacular. Another example of intermicrobial cohesion is the "bristle brush" or "test-tube brush" formation commonly observed in the superficial layers of microbial masses in gingival pockets (Fig. 4-7). A characteristic of the microbial aggregations on the tooth is that the organisms are organized in a pattern perpendicular to the tooth surface (Figs. 4-8, 4-9). Filamentous organisms could thus play an important role in keeping the microbial mass together (Fig. 4-6; Listgarten 1976).

When gingival pockets develop, surfaces with new characteristics for bacterial colonization become exposed. The cemental root surface will be covered by an organic film composed of gingival fluid proteins instead of the salivary proteins which cover those parts of the teeth exposed to saliva. Although there is a flow of cells and fluid out of the gingival pocket, this is a rather stagnant environment compared to most other areas of the mouth. This means that the adherence capacity of the

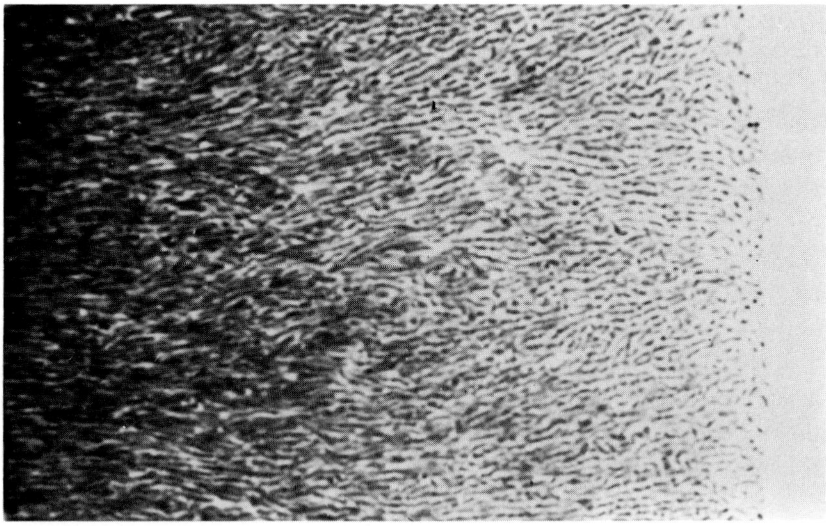

Fig. 4-8. A dense microbial mass adhering to the enamel of a tooth with healthy gingiva (Listgarten 1976). The tooth surface is located on the lefthand side of the illustration.

bacteria is not as decisive for their colonization in this area as in most other parts of the oral cavity. Along the gingival sulcus and in the gingival pocket there are usually many motile bacteria. It is likely that these bacteria have become established in the periodontal pocket because of their motility, although they may not be able to adhere either to the sulcular epithelial cells or to the root surface (Gibbons & van Houte 1975).

Microbial aggregations on the teeth often become mineralized by calcium phosphates. Dental calculus is formed. This calcified structure provides excellent sites for microbial retention on the teeth and in the deepened gingival pockets.

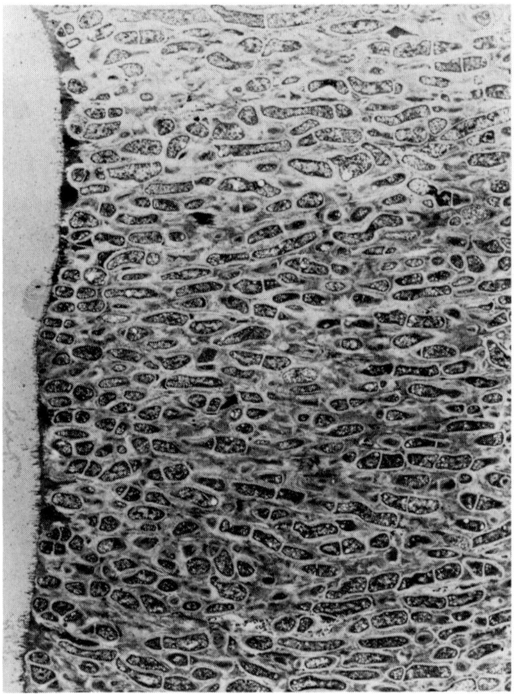

Fig. 4-9. Electron micrograph of the microbial mass (Fig. 4-8) close to the enamel surface. The bacteria are arranged perpendicular to the tooth surface and are embedded in an amorphous matrix (Listgarten 1976). The tooth surface is on the left-hand side of the illustration.

Nutritional interrelations between bacteria and the host

Bacterial nutritional requirements

In order to grow, the bacterial cell must be supplied with sources of carbon and of energy in addition to nitrogen and essential inorganic ions. Of the bacteria that adhere to specific sites of the oral cavity, only those will become established which are able to utilize efficiently the nutrients normally available. They must also have the capacity to respond rapidly to environmental change. Bacteria with simple nutritional requirements are able to grow and multiply if the environment supplies sugar, ammonium and other essential inorganic ions.

From these molecules the bacterial cell synthesizes its own cell constituents. In order to accomplish this, the bacterial cell has to have a complete set of enzymes to catalyze all the required chemical reactions. If some of these enzymes are lacking, essential molecules will not be formed and the organism will not be able to grow or multiply unless these molecules are provided by the environment. Many oral bacteria have incomplete cellular machineries and, therefore, require a number of amino acids, vitamins, purines and pyrimidines from the environment in order to grow and multiply (Mandelstam et al. 1982).

Nutrients provided by the host

The nutritional environment on the tooth surface is completely different from that in the periodontal pocket. On the tooth surface, the nutrients are provided by the saliva. The concentration of nutrients in saliva is, however, very low and our knowledge about the nutritional value of saliva is far from complete. In order to grow and multiply on the tooth surface, where saliva is the main source of nutrients, the bacteria must obviously have a high capacity to utilize nutrients available at low concentrations (de Jong & van der Hoeven 1987).

In the gingival pocket all the nutrients of the tissue fluid are available and the growth of very fastidious organisms will be supported. When epithelial and connective tissue cells disintegrate, valuable nutrients may also be available. The value of the diet as a source of nutrients for the oral microbiota is very limited (Carlsson 1980). One reason is that the dietary components remain in the mouth for only a short time. Another reason is that in order to grow, an organism has to be supplied with all the essential nutrients more or less simultaneously and the diet may lack some specific nutrients.

Bacteria, like mammalian cells, cannot utilize macromolecules, but only simple molecules such as sugars, amino acids, peptides and vitamins. In the digestive tract, proteins, lipids and polysaccharides are hydrolyzed by various enzymes into such simple molecules. The only digestive enzyme present in salivary secretions is amylase and it is relatively inefficient in converting starch. However, many bacteria which colonize the gingival pocke produce very potent hydrolytic enzymes which can break down macromolecules. But such hydrolytic enzymes break down not only macromolecules of saliva and gingival fluid, but also attack the host tissue with deleterious results.

Food webs

The bacterial cellular machinery is subject to an elaborate system of control mechanisms in order to modulate all the different enzymatic processes (Mandelstam et al. 1982). It may happen, however, that in a given bacterial cell some amino acids, vitamins, purines or pyrimidines are produced in higher quantities than can be assimilated. These products may then leak from the cell and be used as nutrients by neighbor cells in the microbial community. In the microbial communities established on the teeth and in the gingival pockets it is likely that such exchange of nutrients will play an important nutritional role. In Fig. 4-10 some possible nutritional interrelations are illustrated. The majority of the bacteria colonizing the mucous membranes and the teeth, such as streptococci and Actinomyces, utilize saliva as the main nutrient source and sugars as the main energy source, while microorganisms colonizing the gingival pockets often utilize amino acids and simple peptides as energy sources (Loesche 1968). When amino acids are used as an energy source, carboxylic acid, ammonia and hydrogen sulfide are produced. The concentration of these substances may reach toxic levels in the gingival pockets. Butyrate and propionate formed by many of the bacteria colonizing the gingival pockets have recently been shown to be highly cytotoxic even in moderate concentration (Singer & Bruckner 1981). Although

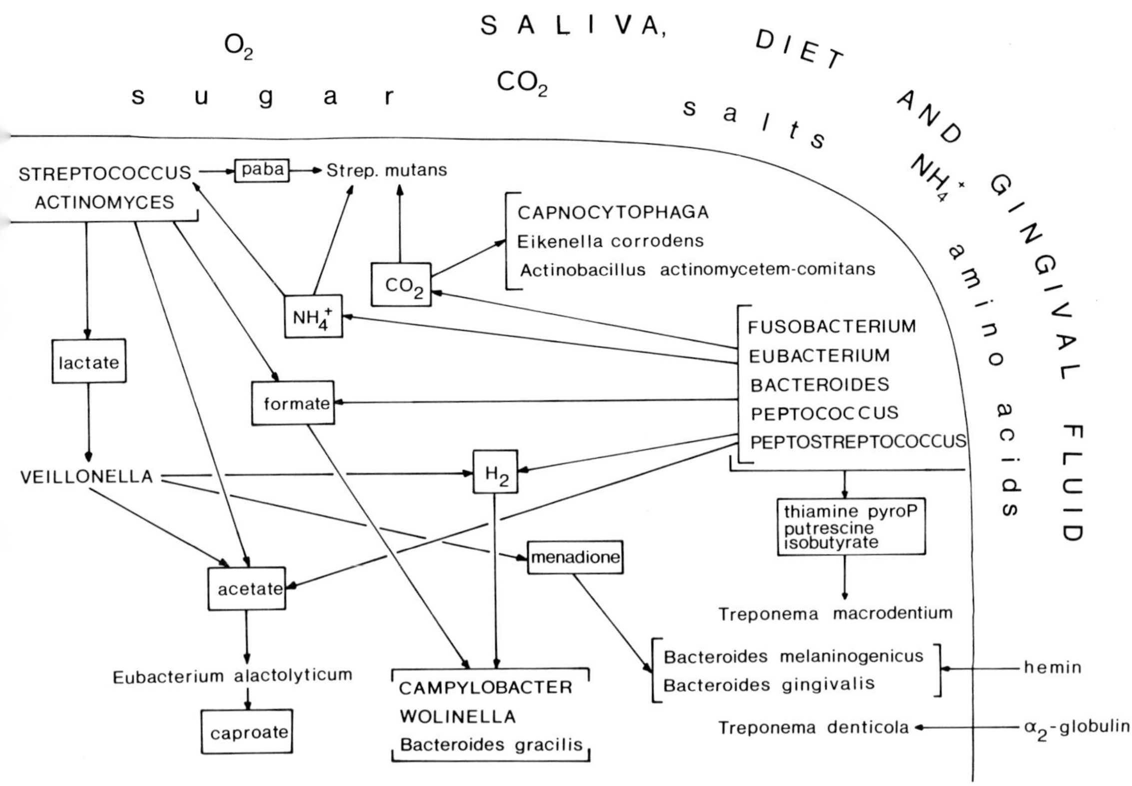

Fig. 4-10. Some possible nutritional interrelations in the dentogingival area.

some of these substances may be toxic to the host, they may also be significant as nutrients for other bacteria. Ammonia is toxic at high concentration but is also a very important source of nitrogen for many bacteria, even for streptococci. Ammonia is available in saliva as a result of bacterial hydrolysis of salivary urea and bacterial catabolism of amino acids. Carbon dioxide is an essential nutrient for many bacteria especially those colonizing gingival pockets. Some so-called "capnophilic" bacteria will not grow unless carbon dioxide is available.

Lactate, formate and hydrogen are excreted by many bacteria as a result of their energy metabolism. These products are subsequently used by other bacteria as an energy source. Fig. 4-10 shows that streptococci and Actinomyces produce lactate from sugars and that lactate is used by Veillonella as an energy source. In the catabolism of lactate by Veillonella hydrogen gas is formed which can be used by a number of organisms in the gingival pockets such as Campylobacter, Wolinella and *Bacteroides gracilis* (Tanner et al. 1981). Another organism colonizing the gingival pockets, *Eubacterium alactolyticum*, has the interesting ability to form caproic acid from acetic and butyric acids (Moore et al. 1982), and in this way the acidity of the environment is lowered. Some bacteria have very specific nutritional requirements (Fig. 4-10). *Streptococcus mutans* requires p-amino benzoate and this compound is produced by *S. sanguis* (Carlsson 1971). Black pigmented Bacteroides species may require vitamin K and hemin (Gibbons & MacDonald 1960). Vitamin K can be produced by many bacteria (Gibbons & Engle 1964) and hemin is made available when hemoglobin is broken down in the gingival pockets. Some bacteria also produce hemins. The requirement of vitamin K by *Bacteroides intermedius* and *B. melaninogenicus*

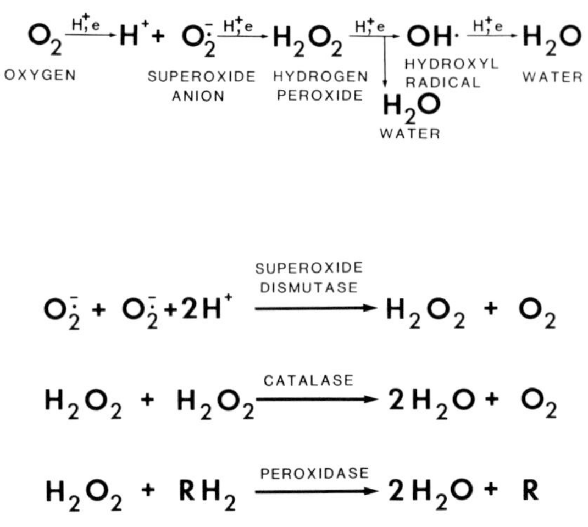

Fig. 4-11. Reduction of oxygen into water in 4 one-electron steps and detoxification of the oxygen intermediates by the concerted action of superoxide dismutase, catalase and peroxidase.

could be substituted with the steroids, estradiol or progesterone (Kornman & Loesche 1982). *Treponema denticola* has a specific requirement for α_2-globulin and this globulin is only available in the gingival pockets (Socransky & Hubersak 1967). The requirement of *T. macrodentium* for thiamine pyrophosphate, putrescine and isobutyrate is satisfied by the concerted action of a number of organisms living in the gingival pockets (Socransky et al. 1964).

Oxygen and oxygen products as ecological determinants

Oxygen and oxygen products are very important ecological determinants because there are great variations in the ability of bacteria to grow and multiply at various levels of oxygen. Some bacteria are killed at extremely low oxygen levels, while others will grow only in the presence of oxygen. In relation to this spectrum of oxygen tolerance, the separation of bacteria into anaerobic and aerobic organisms is quite arbitrary. Microorganisms are identified as being anaerobic if they do not grow on the surface of blood agar in the presence of air, while bacteria that only grow in presence of air are called aerobic. Facultatively anaerobic are microorganisms which grow under anaerobic as well as aerobic conditions.

Most bacteria, even oral streptococci, consume large quantities of oxygen and develop a low redox potential in their environment. This low redox potential may favor the growth of some anaerobic bacteria, but the actual redox potential is usually of less importance for the survival and growth of the bacteria than the level of oxygen (Walden & Hentges 1975).

Intracellular, or in any site characterized by low redox potential, oxygen is converted into highly reactive, potentially destructive products. Oxygen is reduced in one-electron stages, and superoxide anions ($O_2^{\bullet -}$), hydrogen peroxide (H_2O_2), and hydroxyl radicals ($OH^{\bullet}$) are formed (Fig. 4-11). Of these products hydrogen peroxide and superoxide anions are not very toxic *per se*, but they can generate the more devastating hydroxyl radicals (Vuillaume 1987). Hydroxyl radicals are so very reactive that they fail to diffuse away from their site of formation. Hydrogen peroxide and superoxide anions become dangerous because they can reach the lethal target sites of the cell and generate *in situ* the highly reactive hydroxyl radicals. The oxygen products may damage cell membranes and inactivate enzymes, but one of the primary sites of damage in bacteria, as well as in mammalian cells exposed to hydrogen peroxide, is chromosomal DNA. The DNA molecule may be randomly split into pieces.

In order to survive in an aerobic environment, bacterial as well as mammalian cells have to be equipped with an elaborate system of enzymes which disarms the harmful oxygen products. The concerted action of superoxide dismutase, catalase and peroxidases converts superoxide anions and hydrogen peroxide into water and thereby prevents the formation of hydroxyl radicals (Fig. 4-11). The cells are also equipped with enzyme systems which repair DNA and other cellular sites damaged by oxygen products. Organisms lacking some of these enzymes may not be able to survive in an aerobic environment and are, *de facto*, anaerobic.

Bacterial growth within the mouth creates sites with various oxygen levels. The oxygen level and the redox potential are especially low in sites characterized by heavy accumulations of bacteria, *e.g.* in the gingival pockets where growth of even the extremely oxygen - sensitive obligate anaerobes is supported (Globerman & Kleinberg 1979). In sites with high oxygen levels such as the mucous membranes, the bacterial oxygen uptake, especially by the oral streptococci, may result in excretion of high amounts of hydrogen peroxide. This hydrogen peroxide is potentially dangerous for the epithelial cells of the mucous membrane, but saliva contains a peroxidase which converts hydrogen peroxide in the presence of salivary thiocyanate into water and hypothiocyanite (Hoogendoorn et al. 1977).

Hypothiocyanite is much less toxic to the cells than hydrogen peroxide and is, in addition, a potent inhibitor of glycolysis and hydrogen peroxide production by oral streptococci. So peroxidase-thiocyanate of saliva has a dual function. It detoxifies hydrogen peroxide and the product of this reaction, hypothiocyanite, serves as feed-back inhibitor of hydrogen peroxide production by the oral streptococci (Carlsson 1987).

Other factors of ecological importance

Lactoferrin

Lactoferrin is an iron-binding protein in saliva, milk and other exocrine secretions such as bile, pancreatic juice, and small intestinal secretions. Lactoferrin is also found in polymorphonuclear leukocytes. Several biological functions have been proposed for lactoferrin. Iron-saturated lactoferrin may be involved in the transport of iron across the intestinal brush border, and it may play a part in the regulation of myelopoiesis (Pelus et al. 1981). It has also been shown to potentiate the hydroxyl-radical formation from polymorphonuclear leukocytes (Ambruso et al. 1981). The unsaturated form of lactoferrin is bacteriostatic because it may deplete the environment of iron to a concentration which fails to support bacterial growth.

Lysozyme

Lysozyme like lactoferrin is found in polymorphonuclear leukocytes and in secretions like saliva and tears. It is an enzyme which splits the bond between N-acetyl glucosamine and N-acetyl muramic acid in the murein of the bacterial cell wall.

Lysozyme may have bacteriostatic or bactericidal effects *in vitro*, but the efficiency of the enzyme is strongly dependent on pH, ionic strength and various cell surface structures, and it is not clear what role this enzyme has in the microbial ecology of the oral cavity (Iacono et al. 1982).

Bacteriocins

A bacteriocin is a protein, produced by a microorganism, which has the capacity to inhibit the growth of a limited number of the other strains. The formation of a given bacteriocin is dependent on the presence of a corresponding plasmid. Bacteriocins are much more potent than antibiotics and have a more narrow antimicrobial spectrum. One molecule only may kill a microorganism. Some bacteriocins are nucleases and attack DNA. Others act on the cytoplasmic membrane, increasing its permeability to ions or inhibiting active transport. Although bacteriocins produced by oral bacteria have not yet been fully characterized, it is possible that bacteriocins may influence the microbial ecology of the oral cavity.

Composition of the microbiota in the dentogingival area

Oral bacteria

Classification

More than 300 morphologically and biochemically distinct bacterial groups or species of bacteria are today recognized as normal inhabitants of the human oral cavity (Moore 1987). Many bacterial strains isolated from the human oral cavity still remain to be classified.

The object of classification is to group together bacteria with similar properties and to separate those with dissimilar properties. It is important to remember, however, that this is an arbitrary process, and the form it takes is decided by the interest and knowledge of the persons making the classification. This means that new species will usually be created when the interest in a particular group of organisms increases. In recent years many new species from the human oral cavity have been described, and it is important that this work on classification is continued as the association of specific bacteria with particular diseases cannot be disclosed unless the bacteria have been identified. It will take many years before the oral microbiota has been properly described and classified. Until then our descriptions of the microbiota colonizing the dentogingival area will be incomplete. Demonstrated differences in composition of the microbiota at various pathological conditions of gingiva and periodontium will not necessarily be of pathogenic significance (Socransky et al. 1987).

Cultivation

By using current bacteriological techniques about 70% of the bacteria disclosed by microscopy in a sample from the gingival margin may be cultivated in the laboratory. There are several reasons why not all bacteria are detected (Moore 1987). Some of the bacteria do not find the conditions in the laboratory suitable for growth. Others may be killed by the methods we use in dispersing the bacterial masses we have sampled. On the other hand, if the bacterial sample is not properly dispersed the number and types of bacteria in the sample will be underestimated.

Gingivally accumulating bacteria

Clinically healthy gingiva

If the teeth are kept clean with proper oral hygiene measures, the gingiva remains healthy and few bacteria are found along the gingival margin. If a person with such a healthy gingiva abstains from oral hygiene measures, bacteria accumulate on the teeth. After the first 4 h of abstention there are 10^3-10^4 bacteria per mm^2 tooth surface (Nyvad & Kilian 1987). Streptococcus and Actinomyces predominate, but also Gram negative, facultatively anaerobic rods such as Haemophilus, Eikenella and *Actinobacillus actinomycetemcomitans* are found (Kilian et al. 1979). Within a day the number of bacteria increase 100- to 1000-fold. This rapid increase is above all dependent on the growth of streptococci.

In Fig. 4-12 the relative proportion of various bacterial groups in clinically healthy gingiva is presented. Most of the bacteria are facultatively anaerobic and the anaerobic bacteria only make up a minor portion of the flora (Slots 1977a). Among the facultatively anaerobic cocci streptococci are of particular interest since they adhere to the pellicle of the tooth surface and produce extracellular homopolysaccharides from sucrose. These polysaccharides play an important part in the accumulation of bacteria on the teeth. Among the facultatively anaerobic rods, *Actinomyces viscosus* seems to have specific affinity for the root surface (Ellen 1982). When hamsters or rats are infected with *Actinomyces viscosus* these bac-

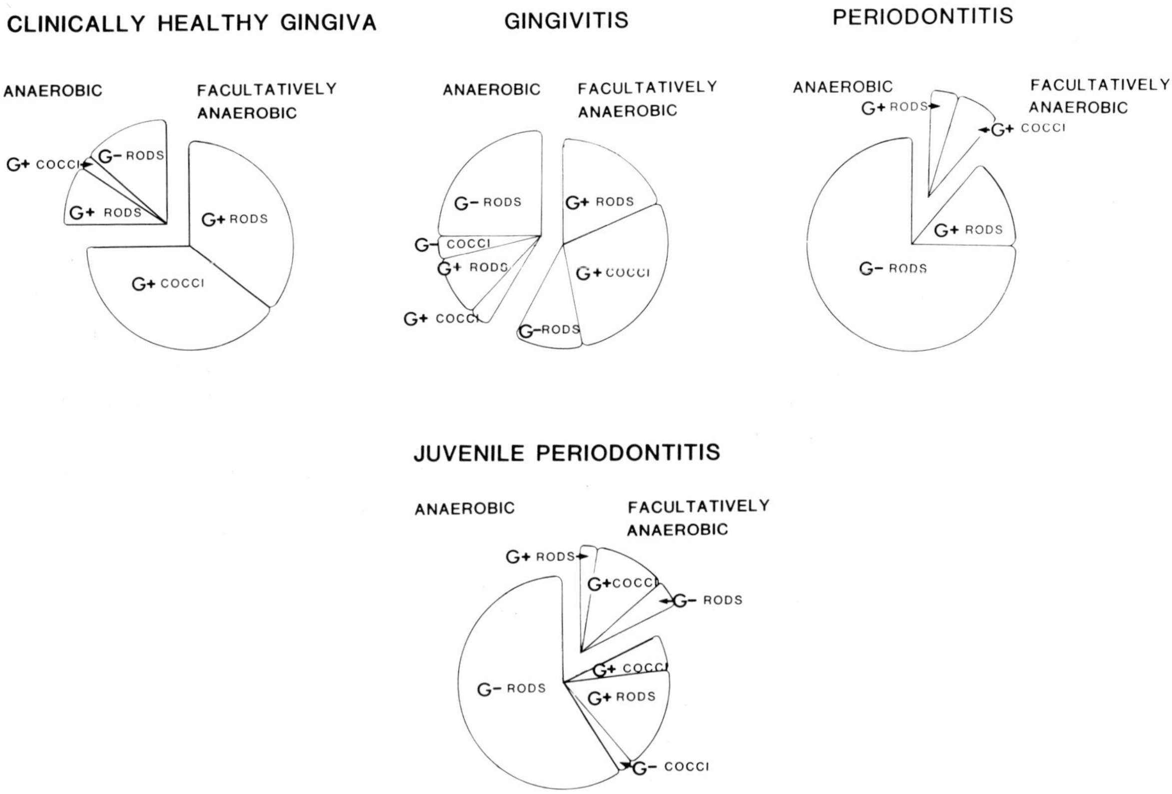

Fig. 4-12. Relative proportions of various bacterial groups in clinically healthy gingiva and in microbial masses associated with gingivitis, periodontitis and juvenile periodontitis. (Adapted from Slots et al. 1976-1978).

teria adhere to the root surfaces and there is a rapid breakdown of the alveolar bone (Keyes & Jordan 1964).

Gingivitis

Accumulation of bacteria along the gingival margin for 3-4 days results in gingivitis. This inflammatory condition creates new opportunities for the growth of bacteria and a continuous change in the composition of the microbial community is initiated. Microscopic studies uncover 3 phases in the changes of the microbiota in a 2-week period (Theilade et al. 1966). During the first phase, the microbiota is dominated by Gram positive cocci, Gram positive rods and Gram negative cocci. During the second phase filamentous organisms appear and during the third phase spirilla and spirochetes (Theilade et al. 1966). When gingivitis has become established, cultivation of the bacteria from the infected sites discloses an increase in a number of anaerobic bacteria in relation to the facultatively anaerobic ones (Fig. 4-12; Slots et al. 1978).

Advanced periodontal disease

In the early stages of periodontitis, the bacterial flora of the gingival pocket is similar to that of gingivitis (Moore et al. 1987). Cultivation of samples from advanced cases of periodontal disease demonstrates a predominance of Gram negative anaerobic rods (Fig. 4-12; Slots 1977b). In the microscope it can also be observed that samples from advanced cases of periodontal disease usually contain high numbers of spirochetes (Listgarten & Helldén 1979). In juvenile periodontitis special attention has been paid to the presence of *Actinoba-*

cillus actinomycetemcomitans (Zambon 1985; Moore 1987). It should be remembered, however, that the composition of the microbiota varies not only between various stages of periodontal disease, but also between individuals with similar symptoms. In addition the microbiota of the pockets may be different in various parts of the mouth and in various parts of a particular gingival pocket.

The criteria used by Koch for distinguishing a pathogenic microorganism from an adventitious one are not easily applicable to the pathogens in periodontal disease. Many potentially pathogenic organisms are, thus, regularly found both in healthy and in diseased sites. Some of them cannot be implanted in the oral cavity of experimental animals, and from those organisms which can be implanted, it is not always clear whether the disease induced is the same disease as in humans.

In evaluating the etiologic role of a given microorganism in periodontal disease a number of characteristics of the organism have to be considered (Socransky 1979). A potential pathogen should be present in higher numbers at sites of pathology than in healthy sites or sites with different forms of disease. Elimination of this organism from the diseased sites should stop the progress of the active lesion. An increased or decreased cellular or humoral immune response to that organism in the presence of a consistent response to other organisms might also be suggestive of a special role of that organism in the disease process. Animal pathogenicity testing could also give important information if the specific organism can actually be implanted in animals. The most important criterion, however, which could contribute to the understanding of its role as an oral pathogen is the possession of unique characteristics which could contribute to the pathogenesis of the disease. Some such characteristics of oral microorganisms will be discussed in the following parts of this chapter.

Host defense in the dentogingival area

Host-parasite interrelations

The microorganisms colonizing the oral cavity constitute a constant threat to the host tissues. In the healthy mouth, the host defense mechanisms match the attacks of the microorganisms, but as soon as the microorganisms at any site overcome this defense, an infection with tissue damage will develop.

The host defense works at various levels. An efficient defense against the microorganisms is provided by the intact surface of the mucous membranes, the desquamation of the epithelial cells, the salivary flow and various components of the salivary secretions. When the intact mucosal surface is broken, further protection is offered by various components of the body fluids and by the phagocytic cells.

In the dentogingival area the epithelial layer of the gingiva is penetrated by a solid body, the tooth. This creates a unique morphological situation, which the host defense mechanisms have to deal with. The contact area between the tooth and the soft tissues (i.e. the junctional epithelium) is a very weak structure in the host defense even if the capacity for defense in this region is reinforced by the epithelial cuff and the vascular plexus surrounding the tooth (Fig. 4-1) (Egelberg 1967). The unique feature to be handled by the host defense is that the bacteria may obtain a firm anchorage on the nonshedding tooth surface and will thereby remain in close contact, for a long time, with the soft tissues surrounding the tooth. This contact relationship triggers the defense mechanisms of tissues. The high efficiency of this gingival host defense is convincingly demonstrated, however, by the fact that periodontal disease in most situations progresses at a slow pace.

Defense by saliva

An important part of the defense is constituted by factors which interfere with bacterial adherence and prevent microorganisms from colonizing the dentogingival area. The salivary flow, the flow of gingival fluid, chewing, and oral hygiene procedures have previously been considered as important ecological determinants, but may equally be conceived as an important part of the host defense. Most of the bacteria entering the oral cavity are rapidly washed away by the salivary flow and swallowed. Only organisms which have capacity to adhere to the surfaces of the oral cavity have a potential to remain in the oral cavity. But the salivary secretions also contain substances that can interfere with the bacterial adherence: agglutinins and secretory immunoglobulin A (sIgA). In addition, the salivary component lysozyme may kill bacteria by lysing their cell wall, and the salivary lactoferrin may deprive the bacteria of essential iron.

Microbial perturbation of the salivary defense

The actual pathogens in periodontal disease have to be sought among those organisms which, having survived defense by saliva, have found an adequate environment for their growth and multiplication in the dentogingival area. Of ultimate importance for these bacteria are the surface characteristics which contribute to their capacity for adherence or retention. They may also release products which interact with the humoral defense factors of saliva. Many strains of *Streptococcus sanguis* and *Streptococcus mitis* produce an IgA protease which breaks down the sIgA, thus removing this obstacle to their colonization of the oral surfaces (Kilian & Reinholdt 1986). Another way oral bacteria perturb the salivary immune defense is by "antigenic shift and drift". The bacteria change their surface characteristics so they escape being recognized by the salivary immune systems (Gibbons & Qureshi 1980). Little is known about the significance of the salivary lactoferrin and lysozyme in the host defense and how bacteria may evade these defense factors.

Humoral factors in the local defense

One of the first signs that the defense mechanisms against the bacteria colonizing the teeth are put into action is a swelling of the vessels of the gingival margin (Egelberg 1967). This is followed by an increased vascular permeability, exudation of gingival fluid and migration of polymorphonuclear leukocytes into the gingival sulcus. This means that already, in this early phase, the gingival tissues have mobilized very potent parts of their defense forces. The tissues become inflamed.

The gingival fluid contains both complement factors and specific antibodies. Many members of the gingival microbiota induce an immune response in the host (Seymour 1987). The classical pathway of complement activation will be initiated when specific antibodies of IgG or IgM classes react with the bacteria. The alternative pathway of complement activation will be initiated by various bacterial cell constituents such as lipopolysaccharides, lipoteichoic acids and polysaccharides. The tissue consequences of this activation will be described elsewhere, and we will here consider only what the activation of the complement cascade means as far as protection of the tissues against bacterial invasion is concerned.

Among the fragments formed in the activation of the complement cascade, C3a and C5a play an important part in releasing histamine in the tissue. This leads to increased vascular permeability and to extensive transudation of serum components including complement and antibodies. C5a also has a strong chemotactic effect on polymorphonuclear leukocytes and will, thus, help in mobilizing these important defense forces. C3b is fixed to the bacterial cell surfaces and facilitates phagocytosis of the bacteria by the polymorphonuclear leukocytes and macrophages. An activation of the entire complement system leads to membrane damage and can cause lysis of Gram negative bacteria in the presence of lysozyme.

In addition to the part played by specific IgG and IgM antibodies in the activation of the complement system, IgG antibodies facilitate phagocytosis by binding to the bacterial cell surface. Antibodies of IgA, IgG and IgM classes prevent tissue damage by neutralizing exotoxins released by the bacteria.

Microbial perturbation of the local humoral defense

Some of the bacteria colonizing the gingival pockets produce proteases which may degrade not only IgA but also other immunoglobulins and complement factors (Kilian 1981; Carlsson et al. 1986). This means that the humoral immune defense mechanisms can actually be paralyzed in infected gingival pockets. The degradation of IgA may facilitate the penetration and spread of potentially toxic substances, lytic enzymes and antigens released by the entire subgingival microbiota. Due to the importance of IgG antibodies and complement in the defense mediated by phagocytes, the efficiency of this cellular defense may be impaired. The significance of the immune defense against chronic infections has been demonstrated in experimental root canal infections in monkeys (Dahlen et al. 1982). In animals immunized against bacteria in the root canals, the periapical lesions were encapsulated and not so diffusely spread in the tissue as in non-immunized animals. An important point here is that, although the immune defense mechanisms may lead to inflammation and tissue damage, as described in Chapter 5, they are in most cases beneficial for the host by preventing the spread of an infection into the tissue.

Microorganisms can also contrive sophisticated mechanisms capable of interfering with the productions of humoral antibodies and cell-mediated immune responses (Seymour 1987). There may be inhibition of lymphoid tissue maturation as well as quantitative and qualitative modulations of the immune response. The immunocompetence of the host is maintained by a delicate balance between stimulatory and suppressor cells, and bacterial constituents such as peptidoglycans, lipopolysaccharides, and lipoteichoic acids can interfere with the function of these cells.

Defense by phagocytes

Both polymorphonuclear and mononuclear leukocytes take part in the phagocytic defense of the dentogingival area and this defense is dependent on the presence of complement and often specific antibodies. In order to be effective, the phagocytes have to recognize the site of the microbial invasion. They have to leave the blood vessels and migrate through the tissue to the site of invasion, where they have to ingest and kill the microorganisms (Van Dyke et al. 1985). An activation of the complement cascade has an important function in this process. The binding of the complement fragment C5a to the surface of polymorphonuclear leukocytes determines the adherence of the leukocytes to the vascular endothelium close to the site of the microbial invasion. The migration of the leukocytes through the tissue to the site of infection (chemotaxis) may be determined by C5a and by substances released by metabolizing bacteria. Chemotactic substances are also produced by lymphocytes stimulated by specific antigens or mitogens, and by mast cells and basophils interacting with the complement fragments C3a or C5a. Metabolites of the lipoxygenation of arachidonic acid are also chemotactic (Samuelsson et al. 1987).

During chemotaxis the leukocytes release some of the contents of their lysosomal enzymes. The next step in the process of phagocytosis is the attachment of the organism to the surface of the leukocyte. To achieve this attachment, C3b and/or specific antibodies must often attach to the surface of the microorganism. After the attachment the organism is ingested and enclosed into a phagosome. This process causes the leukocyte to release oxygen products and lysosomal granule contents into the phagosome and the extracellular milieu. The oxygen products include both singlet oxygen and superoxide anions as well as hydrogen peroxide and hydroxyl radicals. These oxygen products are in themselves microbicidal, but the most potent microbicidal mechanism of the leukocyte is a reaction catalyzed by the lysosomal enzyme, myeloperoxidase, in the presence of hydrogen peroxide and chloride ions (Forman & Thomas 1986). The leukocytes also have microbicidal systems that work under anaerobic conditions (Spitznagel & Shafer 1985, Rice et al. 1987). The products released by the leukocytes not only kill invading microorganisms, but the oxygen products and the lysosomal proteases may cause extensive tissue injuries (Fantone & Ward 1982).

Microbial perturbation of the phagocytic defense

Microorganisms can elude the phagocytic defense in many ways (Densen & Mandell 1980). They can fail to induce chemotaxis and will, thus, not be detected by the phagocytes. The reason may be that their metabolism does not result in the production of a chemotactic substance, or that the microorganisms are not able to activate the chemotactic complement fragment C5a. Bacteria may also influence chemotaxis by producing substances which inhibit the motility of the leukocytes. Capnocytophaga, a member of the subgingival microbiota, has this capacity and it has been demonstrated that patients with their gingival pockets infected with this organism have a systemic defect in leukocyte function (Shurin et al. 1979). The normal functions of the leukocytes may also be impaired by subtoxic levels of some leukotoxins (Arbuthnott 1981).

Bacteria may also perturb the phagocytic defense by avoiding attachment to the leukocytes. Bacterial surface structures may prevent the attachment. Often such structures are capsules composed of polysaccharides but may also be proteins. Such bacteria can normally not be phagocytosed until the host has produced specific antibodies against the surface structures. These antibodies have to react with the surface, initiate the complement cascade, and thereby fragment C3b is fixed to the bacterial surface. As the leukocytes have receptors for C3b as well as for the Fc portion of IgG, the attachment to the bacteria can now be accomplished. The organisms may avoid this by the aforementioned "antigenic shift and drift" (Gibbons & Qureshi 1980) or by degrading antibodies and complement factors (Carlsson et al. 1986).

After the microorganism has become attached to the leukocyte, it is usually ingested and killed. Some pathogenic bacteria such as gonococci may, however, prevent ingestion after the attachment by increasing, in an unknown way, the rigidity of the leukocyte membrane (Densen & Mandell 1980). It is presently unknown whether members of the subgingival microbiota can exert such effects on the leukocytes.

The attachment and ingestion of an organism induce a burst of metabolic oxidative activity in the leukocyte. This is essential for the normal bactericidal activity of this particular phagocyte. Some pathogenic bacteria can inhibit this metabolic oxygen burst, but it is not known if any of the members of the subgingival microbiota have this ability.

After the microorganism has been enclosed in a phagosome, it becomes exposed to toxic oxygen products, the myeloperoxidase system, lytic lysosomal enzymes and cationic proteins (Root & Cohen 1981). Usually, few of the pathogens can resist these very potent microbicidal activities for any significant length of time. Such pathogens, the intracellular parasites, have not yet been described from gingival pockets or the oral cavity.

An efficient way for the organism to elude all the phagocytic defenses is to kill the phagocytes. Many pathogens possess leukotoxins and these toxins often play a key role in the pathogenicity of such organisms (Arbuthnott 1981). One predominant member of the subgingival microbiota, *Actinobacillus actinomycetemcomitans*, possesses such a leukotoxin (Baehni et al. 1979). The presence of this toxin in the gingival pocket will paralyze the phagocytic defense against all the subgingival microbiota. Even subtoxic levels of the toxin may impair normal function of the leukocytes such as motility and phagocytic activity. The host defense in the form of specific antibodies may, however, have the capacity of neutralizing these effects of the leukotoxins (Tsai & Taichman 1986).

The important part played by polymorphonuclear leukocytes in the defense of the periodontal tissues was nicely demonstrated in dogs with low numbers of polymorphonuclear leukocytes after treatment with antileukocyte serum (Attström & Schroeder 1979). In the serum-treated dogs bacteria advanced much more rapidly along the epithelial junction of the gingival crevice than in controls.

Microbial invasion of the periodontal tissue

The combined humoral and phagocytic defense of the dentogingival area efficiently protects the periodontal tissues from bacterial invasion. This protection is actually so efficient that it has been claimed that the members of the subgingival microbiota should be unable to invade tissues. A bacterial invasion of the junctional epithelium of the gingival pocket has been demonstrated, however, in acute ulcerative gingivitis (Fig. 4-13, Listgarten 1965) and in advanced cases of periodontal disease (Frank, 1980; Saglie et al. 1982; Liakoni et al. 1987).

Bacteria growing in the tissue may damage the tissue by releasing toxins, enzymes and metabolic waste products. No exotoxins other than the leukotoxin produced by *Actinobacillus actinomycetemcomitans* have been shown to be produced by members of the subgingival microbiota. Various enzymes are produced, however, which may degrade intercellular tissue components. Phosphatases, aminopeptidases, proteases, phosphoamidases and glycosidases have been demonstrated (Slots 1981) as well as hyaluronidase, chondroitin sulfatase and fibrinolysin (Nitzan et al. 1978, Steffen & Hentges 1981). Black pigmented Bacteroides may produce proteases which degrade a number of proteins. Some of these proteins may play important roles in the host defense against bacterial infections. Not only the immunoglobulins IgG, IgA and IgM may be degraded, but also many other plasma proteins (Carlsson et al. 1986). Also phospholipase A is formed by members of the subgingival microbiota (Bulkacz et al. 1979), an enzyme which may contribute to the formation of prostanoids in the tissue (Needleman et al. 1986). Bacteria in the gingival pockets may also release waste products from their metabolism at cytotoxic levels. These may be ammonia, hydrogen sulfide, indol or carboxylic acids such as butyrate and propionate. To what extent these products may contribute to the periodontal tissue destruction remains unknown.

Much has been learned in the past few years about the microbiology of plaque-associated periodontal disease. This growth in our understanding has given us a solid basis for formulating new questions concerning the microbiology and pathophysiology of this disease. The answers to these questions will not only increase our knowledge but also influence our way of treating the various phases of periodontal disease.

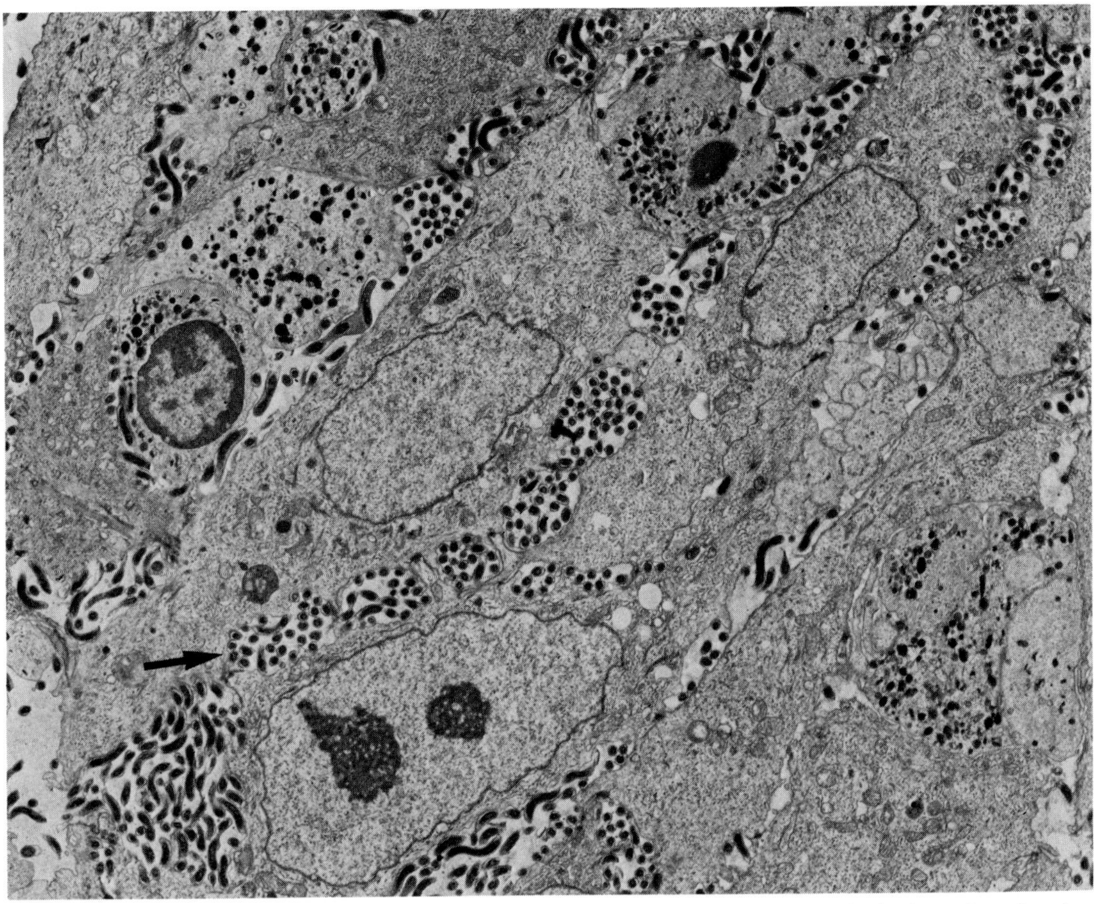

Fig. 4-13. Junctional epithelium in acute necrotizing ulcerative gingivitis with dense masses of spirochetes distending the space between the epithelial cells. (Listgarten 1965).

References

Ambruso, D.R., & Johnston Jr., R.B. (1981) Lactoferrin enhances hydroxyl radical production by human neutrophils, neutrophil particulate fractions, and an enzymatic generating system. *Journal of Clinical Investigation* **67**, 352-360.

Appleton, J.L.T. (1944) In: *Bacterial Infection with Special Reference to Dental Practice*. 3rd ed., pp.301-316. Philadelphia: Lea & Febiger.

Arbuthnott, J.P. (1981) Membrane-damaging toxins in relation to interference with host defense mechanisms. In *Microbial Perturbation of Host Defenses*, ed. Grady, F.O. & Smith, H., pp. 97-120. London: Academic Press.

Attström, R. & Schroeder, H.E. (1979) Effect of experimental neutropenia on initial gingivis in dogs. *Scandinavian Journal of Dental Research* **87**, 7-23.

Baehni, P., Tsai, C.-C., McArthur, W.P., Hammond, B.F. & Taichman, N.S. (1979) Interaction of inflammatory cells and oral microorganisms. VIII. Detection of leukotoxic activity of a plaque-derived gram-negative microorganism. *Infection and Immunity* **24**, 233-243.

Beckers, H.J.A. & van der Hoeven, J.S. (1982) Growth rates of *Actinomyces viscosus* and *Streptococcus mutans* during early colonization of tooth surfaces in gnotobiotic rats. *Infection and Immunity* **35**, 583-587.

Bowden, G.H.W., Ellwood, D.C. & Hamilton, I.R. (1979) Microbial ecology of the oral cavity. *Advances in Microbial Ecology* **3**, 135-217.

Bulkacz, J., Newmann, M.G., Sokransky, S.S., Newbrun, E. & Scott, D.F. (1979) Phospholipase A activity of microorganisms from dental plaque.

Microbios Letters **10**, 79-88.

Carlsson, J. (1971) Growth of *Streptococcus mutans* and *Streptococcus sanguis* in mixed culture. *Archives of Oral Biology* **16**, 963-965.

Carlsson, J. (1980) Symbiosis between host and microorganisms in the oral cavity. *Scandinavian Journal of Infectious Diseases,* Supplement 24, 74-78.

Carlsson, J. (1987) Salivary peroxidase - An important part of our defense against oxygen toxicity. *Journal of Oral Pathology* **8**, 412-416.

Carlsson, J., Nilsson, T., & Sundqvist, G. (1986) Effect of proteinases from black-pigmented Bacteroides on human plasma proteins. In *The Borderland Between Caries and Periodontal disease III,* ed. Lehner, T. & Cimasoni, G., pp. 155-163. Genève, Editions Médecine et Hygiène.

Cisar, J.O. (1982) Coaggregation reactions between oral bacteria: Studies of specific cell-to-cell adherence mediated by microbial lectins. In *Host-Parasite Interactions in Periodontal Diseases,* ed. Genco, R.J. & Mergenhagen, S.E., pp. 121-131. Washington, D.C.: American Society for Microbiology.

Collard, P. (1976) *The Development of Microbiology.* Cambridge: Cambridge University Press.

Costerton, J.W., Irvin, R.T. & Cheng, K.-J. (1981) The bacterial glycocalyx in nature and disease. *Annual Review of Microbiology* **35**, 299-324.

Dahlen, G., Fabricius, L., Heyden, G., Holm, S.E. & Möller,Å.J.R. (1982) Apical periodontitis induced by selected bacterial strains in root canals of immunized and non-immunized monkeys. *Scandinavian Journal of Dental Research* **90**, 207-216.

De Jong, M.H. & Van Der Hoeven, J.S. (1987) The growth of bacteria on saliva. *Journal of Dental Research* **66**, 498-505.

Densen, P. & Mandell.G.L. (1980) Phagocyte strategy vs. microbial tactics. *Reviews of Infectious Diseases* **2**, 817-838.

Dobell, C. (1960) *Antony van Leeuwenhoek and His "Little Animals". New York: Dover Publications.*

Egelberg, J. (1967) The topography and permeability of the vessels at the dento-gingival junction in dogs. *Journal of Periodontal Research,* Supplement Nr. 1.

Ellen, R. (1982) Oral colonization by Gram-positive bacteria significant to periodontal disease. In *Host-Parasite Interactions in Periodontal Diseases* ed. Genco, R.J. & Mergenhagen, S.E., pp. 98-111. Washington, D.C.: American Society for Microbiology.

Fantone, J.C. & Ward, P.A. (1982) Role of oxygen-derived free radicals and metabolites in leukocyte-dependent inflammatory reactions. *American Journal of Pathology* **107**, 397-418.

Forman, H.J. & Thomas, M.J. (1986) Oxidant production and bactericidal activity of phagocytes. *Annual review of Physiology* **48**, 669-680.

Frank, R.M. (1980) Bacterial penetration in the apical pocket wall of advanced human periodontitis. *Journal of Periodontal Research* **15**, 563-573.

Gibbons, R.J. & Engle, L.P. (1964) Vitamin K compounds in bacteria that are obligate anaerobes. *Science* 146, 1307-1309.

Gibbons, R.J. & MacDonald, J.B. (1960) Hemin and vitamin K compounds as required factors for the cultivation of certain strains of *Bacteroides melaninogenicus. Journal of Bacteriology* **80**, 164-170.

Gibbons, R.J. & Qureshi, J.V. (1980) Virulence-related physiological changes and antigenic variation in populations of *Streptococcus mutans* colonizing gnotobiotic rats. *Infection and Immunity* **29**, 19-44.

Gibbons, R.J. & van Houte, J. (1975) Bacterial adherence in oral microbial ecology. *Annual review of Microbiology* **29**, 19-44.

Globerman, D.Y. & Kleinberg, I. (1979) Intraoral PO_2 and its relation to bacterial accumulation on the oral tissues. In *Saliva and Dental Caries,* ed. Kleinberg, I., Ellison, S.A. & Mandel, I.D., pp. 275-291. Washington, D.C.: Information Retrieval.

Gristina, A.G. (1987) Biomaterial-centered infection: Microbial adhesion versus tissue integration. *Science* **237**, 1588-1595.

Guggenheim, B. (1970) Extracellular polysaccharides and microbial plaque. *International Dental Journal* **20**, 657-678.

Hoogendoorn, H., Piessens, J.P., Scholtes, W & Stoddard,L.A. (1977) Hypothiocyanite ion; the inhibitor formed by the system lactoperoxidase-thiocyanate-hydrogen peroxide. I. Identification of the inhibiting compound. *Caries Research* **11**, 77-84.

Iacono., V.J., MacKay, B.J., Pollock, J.J., Boldt, P.R., Ladenheim, S., Grossbard, B.L. & Rochon,M.L. (1982) Roles of lysozyme in the host response to periodontopathic microorganisms. In *Host-Parasite Interactions in Periodontal Diseases,* ed. Genco, R.J. & Mergenhagen, S.E., pp. 318-342. Washington, D.C.: American Society for Microbiology.

Keyes, P.H. & Jordan, H.V. (1964) Periodontal lesions in the Syrian hamster. III: Findings related to an infectious and transmissible component. *Archives of Oral Biology* **9**, 377-400.

Kilian, M. (1981) Degradation of immunoglobalins A1, A2, and G by suspected principal periodontal pathogens. *Infection and Immunity* **34**, 757-765.

Kilian, M. & Reinholdt, J. (1986) Interference with IgA defense mechanisms by extracellular bacterial enzymes. *Medical Microbiology* **5**, 173-208.

Kilian, M., Larsen, J., Fejerskov, O. & Thylstrup, A. (1979) Effects of fluoride on the initial colonization of teeth in vivo. *Caries Research* **13**, 319-329.

Kornman, K.S. & Loesche, W.J. (1982) Effects of estradiol and progesterone on *Bacteroides melaninogenicus* and *Bacteroides gingivalis*. *Infection and Immunity* **35**, 256-263.

Liakoni, H., Barber, P. & Newman, H.N. (1987) Bacterial penetration of pocket soft tissues in chronic adult and juvenile periodontitis cases. *Journal of Clinical Periodontology* **14**, 22-28.

Lie, T. (1979) Morphologic studies on dental plaque formation. *Acta Odontologica Scandinavica* **37**, 73-85.

Listgarten, M.A. (1965) Electron microscopic observations on the bacterial flora of acute necrotizing ulcerative gingivitis. *Journal of Periodontology* **36**, 328-339.

Listgarten, M.A. (1976) Structure of the microbial flora associated with periodontal health and disease in man. *Journal of Periodontology* **47**, 1-18.

Listgarten, M.A. & Helldén, L. (1979) Relative distribution of bacteria at clinically healthy and periodontally diseased sites in humans. *Journal of Clinical Periodontology* **5**, 115-132.

Loesche, W.J. (1968) Importance of nutrition in gingival crevice microbial ecology. *Periodontics* **6**, 245-249.

Lynch, J.M. & Poole, N.J. (ed.) (1979) *Microbial Ecology: A Conceptual Approach*. Oxford: Blackwell Scientific Publications.

Mandelstam, J., McQuillen, K., & Dawes, I. (ed.) (1982) *Biochemistry of Bacterial Growth*. Oxford: Blackwell Scientific Publications.

McGhee, J.R. & Michalek, S.M. (1981) Immunobiology of dental caries: Microbial aspects and local immunity. *Annual Review of Microbiology* **35**, 595-638.

McNabb, P.C. & Tomasi, T.B. (1981) Host defense mechanisms at mucosal surfaces. *Annual Review of Microbiology* **35**, 477-496.

Mergenhagen, S.E., Sandberg, A.L., Chassy, B.M., Brennan, M.J., Yeung, M.K., Dondersloot & Cisar, J.O. (1987) Molecular basis of bacterial adhesion in the oral cavity. *Reviews of Infectious Diseases*, Supplement 5, **9**, 467-474.

Miller, W.D. (1890) *The Micro-Organisms of the Human Mouth*. Reprint 1973. Basel: S.Karger.

Moore, L.V.H., Moore, W.E.C., Cato, E.P., Smibert, R.M., Burmeister, J.A. & Best, A.M. (1987) Bacteriology of human gingivitis. *Journal of Dental Research* **66**, 989-995.

Moore, W.E.C. (1987) Microbiology of periodontal disease. *Journal of Periodontal Research* **22**, 335-341.

Moore, W.E.C., Ranney, R.R. & Holdeman, L.V. (1982) Subgingival microflora in periodontal disease: Cultural studies. In *Host-Parasite Interactions in Periodontal Disease,* ed. Genco, R.J. & Mergenhagen, S.E., pp. 13-26. Washington, D.C.: American Society for Microbiology.

Mouton, C., Reynolds, H.S. & Genco, R.J. (1980) Characterization of tufted streptococci isolated from the "corn cob" configuration of human dental plaque. *Infection and Immunity* **25**, 235-245.

Needleman, P., Turk, J., Jakschik, B.A., Morrison, A.R. & Lefkowith, J.B. (1986) Arachidonic acid metabolism. *Annual Review of Biochemistry* **55**, 69-102.

Nitzan, D., Sperry, J.F. & Wilkins, T.D. (1978) Fibrinolytic activity of oral anaerobic bacteria. *Archives of Oral Biology* **23**, 465-470.

Nyvad, B. & Kilian, M. (1987) Microbiology of the early colonization of human enamel and root surfaces in vivo. *Scandinavian Journal of Dental Research* **95**, 369-380.

Pelus, L.M., Broxmeyer, H.E. & Moore,M.A.S. (1981) Regulation of human myelopoiesis by prostaglandin E and lactoferrin. *Cell and Tissue Kinetics* **14**, 514-526.

Pruitt, K.M. (1977) Macromolecular components of oral fluids at tooth surfaces. *Swedish Dental Journal* **1**, 225-240.

Rice, W.G., Ganz, T., Kinkade, J.M., Jr, Selsted, M.E., Lehrer, R.I. & Parmley, R.T. (1987) Defensin-rich dense granules of human neutrophils. *Blood* **70**, 757-765.

Root, R.K. & Cohen, M.S. (1981) The microbicidal mechanisms of human neutrophils and eosinophils. *Reviews of Infectious Diseases* **3**, 565-598.

Saglie, R., Newman, M.G., Carranza Jr., F.A. & Pattison, G.L. (1982) Bacterial invasion of gingiva in advanced periodontitis in humans. *Journal of Periodontology* **53**, 217-222.

Samuelsson, B., Dahlén, S.-E., Lindgren, J.Å., Rouzer, C.A. & Serhan, C.N. (1987) Leukotrienes and lipoxins: Structures, biosynthesis, and biological effects. *Science* **237**, 1171-1176.

Seymour, G.J. (1987) Possible mechanisms involved in the immunoregulation of chronic inflammatory periodontal disease. *Journal of Dental Research* **66**, 2-9.

Sharon, N. (1987) Bacterial lectins, cell-cell recognition and infectious disease. *FEBS Letters* **217**, 145-157.

Shurin, S.B., Socransky, S.S., Sweeney, E. & Stossel, T.P. (1979) A neutrophil disorder induced by Capnocytophaga, a dental microorganism. *New England Journal of Medicine* **301**, 849-854.

Singer, R.E. & Buckner, B.A. (1981) Butyrate and propionate: Important components of toxic dental plaque extracts. *Infection and Immunity* **32**,458-463.

Slots,J. (1976) The predominant cultivable organisms in juvenile periodontitis. *Scandinavian Journal of Dental Research* **84**, 1-10.

Slots, J. (1977a) Microflora in the healthy gingival sulcus in man. *Scandinavian Journal of Dental Research* **85**, 247-254.

Slots, J. (1977b) The predominant cultivable microflora of advanced periodontitis. *Scandinavian Journal of Dental Research* **85**, 114-121.

Slots, J. (1981) Enzymatic characterization of some oral and nonoral Gram-negative bacteria with the API ZYM system. *Journal of Clinical Microbiology* **14**, 288-294.

Slots, J., Möenbo, D., Langebaek, J. & Frandsen, A. (1978) Microbiota of gingivitis in man. *Scandinavian Journal of Dental Research* **86**, 174-181.

Socransky, S.S. (1979) Criteria for the infectious agents in dental caries and periodontal disease. *Näringsforskning* **23**, Supplement 17, 16-21.

Socransky, S.S. & Hubersak, C. (1967) Replacement of ascitic fluid or rabbit serum requirement of *Treponema dentium* by α-globulin. *Journal of Bacteriology* **94**, 1795-1796.

Socransky, S.S., Haffajee, A.D., Smith, G.L.F. & Dzink, J.L. (1987) Difficulties encountered in the search for the etiologic agents of destructive periodontal diseases. *Journal of Clinical Periodontology* **14**, 588-593.

Socransky, S.S., Loesche, W.J., Hubersak, C. & MacDonald, J.B. (1964) Dependency of *Treponema microdentium* on other oral organisms for isobutyrate, polyamines, and a controlled oxidation-reduction potential. *Journal of Bacteriology* **88**, 200-209.

Socransky, S.S., Manganiella, A.D., Propas, D., Oram, V. & van Houte, J. (1977) Bacteriological studies of developing supra-gingival dental plaque. *Journal of Periodontal Research* **12**, 90-106.

Spitznagel, J.K. & Shafer, W.M. (1985) Neutrophil killing of bacteria by oxygen-independent mechanisms: A historical summary. *Reviews of Infectious Diseases* **7**, 398-403.

Steffen, E.K. & Hentges, D.J. (1981) Hydrolytic enzymes of anaerobic bacteria isolated from human infections. *Journal of Clinical Microbiology* **14**, 153-156.

Tanner, A.C.R., Badger, S., Lai, C.-H., Listgarten, M.A., Visconti, R.A. & Socransky, S.S. (1981) Wolinella gen. nov., *Wolinella succinogenes (Vibrio succinogenes* Wolin et al.) comb. nov., and description of *Bacteroides gracilis* sp. nov., *Wolinella recta* sp. nov., *Campylobacter concisus* sp. nov., and *Eikenella corrodens* from humans with periodontal disease. *International Journal of Systematic Bacteriology* **31**, 432-445.

Theilade, E., Wright, W.H., Jensen, S.B. & Löe, H. (1966) Experimental gingivitis in man. II. A longitudinal clinical and bacteriological investigation. *Journal of Periodontal Research* **1**, 1-13.

Tsai, C.-C. & Taichman, S. (1986) Dynamics of infection by leukotoxic strains of *Actinobacillus actinomycetemcomitans* in juvenile periodontitis. *Journal of Clinical Periodontology* **11**, 330-331.

Van Dyke, T.E., Levine, M.J. & Genco, R.J. (1985) Neutrophil function and oral disease. *Journal of Oral Pathology* **141**, 95-120.

Vuillaume, M. (1987) Reduced oxygen species, mutation, induction and cancer initiation. *Mutation Research* **186**, 43-72.

Walden, W.C. & Hentges, D.C. (1975) Differential effects of oxygen and oxidation-reduction potential on the multiplication of three species of anaerobic intestinal bacteria. *Applied Microbiology* **30**, 781-785.

Walker, G.J. & Jacques, N.A. (1987) Polysaccharides of oral streptococci. In *Sugar transport and metabolism in Gram-positive bacteria*, ed. Reizer, J. & Peterkofsky, A., pp. 39-68. Chichester: Ellis Horeword Ltd.

Zambon, J.J. (1985) *Actinobacillus actinomycetemcomitans* in human periodontal disease. *Journal of Clinical Periodontology* **12**, 1-20.

CHAPTER 5

Pathogenesis of Plaque-Associated Periodontal Disease

Pathogenesis of periodontal disease

Infection and inflammation are the hallmarks of periodontal disease. The inflammatory reaction is visible microscopically and clinically in the affected periodontium and represents the host's response to the plaque microbiota and its products. As in other infections, inflammation in the gingival tissues protects us against local microbial attack and prevents microorganisms from spreading beyond the immediate target area. However, the inflammatory reaction may not be altogether beneficial because it can also damage surrounding cells and connective tissue structures, including alveolar bone. This probably accounts for much of the tissue injury observed in gingivitis and destructive periodontal disease.

While inflammation in periodontal tissues may be similar in many respects to that seen in other parts of the body, there are significant differences. In part, this is a consequence of the anatomy of the periodontium. More importantly, it is essential to understand that inflammatory processes in periodontal tissues are not simply stereotyped events caused by one microorganism or a single microbial product acting over a relatively short period of time. As discussed in Chapter 4, the bacteria which provoke inflammatory reactions in the gingiva and periodontium vary from one form of periodontal disease to another. Further, periodontal pockets are teeming with numerous species of microorganisms, each of which has different biological potentials. Periodontal disease has sometimes been referred to as a "mixed bacterial infection" to denote that more than one microbial species contributes to the development of disease (Mayrand 1985). Synergisms probably exist amongst many species. In fact, some microorganisms may not be overt pathogens but still play a role in the disease process by providing factors or conditions that promote the virulence potential of other microbes. The microbiota in periodontal pockets is in a state of continual flux; species which are relevant at one stage of disease may not be important at another. In other words, periodontal disease, or rather periodontal diseases, represent dynamic infections caused by combinations of bacterial vectors which vary over time. This stands in contrast with most other classical infectious diseases (e.g., tuberculosis, syphilis, gonorrhea) where the host contends with one rather than a multitude of organisms. As a result, the molecular events which trigger and sustain the inflammatory reaction in periodontal diseases constantly change.

It is also important to note that in some instances disease progression may be an episodic phenomenon as opposed to a continuous process. We used to believe that the periodontium was destroyed as a consequence of a slowly progressive inflammatory process of the tooth-supporting tissues. Recent data indicate that tissue destruction in some lesions occurs during relatively "acute" bursts of "disease activity" followed by "quiescent" periods (Haffagee et al. 1983, Lindhe et al. 1983, Socransky et al. 1984). The burst is characterized by rapid deepening of the periodontal pocket, detachment of periodontal fibers from root cementum and loss of alveolar bone. By contrast, the quiescent phase is not associated with clinical or radiographic evidence of disease progression, and this phase may last for extended periods of time. Unfortunately, complete healing of the area is not likely to be realized during the quiescent period because infection (subgingival plaque) remains on the root surface and inflammation persists in the connective tissues. At present, we cannot explain the pathogenic basis for these active and inactive phases of periodontal tissue destruction. Theoretically, the burst may represent a transient impairment of the inflammatory response to defend the host, thereby permitting organisms in the area to gain an advantage. Lowered host resistance may also allow "new", opportunistic pathogens to infect the pocket. By contrast, it is possible that during the burst the inflammatory reaction is activated in such a way that it hurts more than protects the affected site. In this context, the host's response to the organisms rather than microbial virulence *per se* actually damages tissues and causes loss of fiber attachment and alveolar bone. Some of these possibilities will be discussed below.

It is also relevant to point out that, even within the same individual, the severity of periodontal tissue injury often varies from tooth to tooth and from one tooth surface to another. Thus, while many teeth may suffer from advanced loss of connective tissue attachment and alveolar bone, other teeth or tooth surfaces (sites) may be almost unaffected and surrounded by a normal periodontium. In addition, the inflammatory lesion may be contained within the gingiva (gingivitis) for prolonged periods of time without any apparent progression of the disease into deeper tissues. Hence, a patient with periodontal disease is not afflicted with a "homogeneous" condition. Each affected site in his/her mouth represents an "individualized" or "specific" microenvironment.

Current concepts regarding the etiology and pathogenesis of periodontal disease are mainly derived from the results of *epidemiological studies, analyses of autopsy and biopsy material, clinical trials and animal experimentation.*

Findings from *epidemiological studies* have consistently revealed that the frequency and severity of periodontal disease increase with age and with inadequate oral hygiene (see Chapter 2). *Histologic studies* of human tissues (e.g. Waerhaug 1952, 1979) indicate that a close topographical relationship exists between the location of the plaque deposit on the tooth surface and the extension of the inflammatory lesion in the adjacent soft tissue. As long as the microbial deposit remains on the crown of the tooth, the lesion is limited to the supraalveolar gingival connective tissue. However, as microbial plaque growth extends onto the root cementum, the adjacent tissue compartments (which were occupied by periodontal ligament and alveolar bone) become replaced by inflammatory cell infiltrates.

Subjects maintaining a high standard of oral hygiene are not likely to develop gingival or periodontal disease. However, *experimental, short-term clinical studies* have shown that microorganisms quickly start to colonize clean tooth surfaces once an individual abstains from mechanical tooth cleaning; within a few days microscopical and clinical signs of gingivitis are then apparent. These inflammatory alterations are resolved or reversed when proper tooth-cleaning measures are resumed (Löe et al. 1965). Further, inflammation can be prevented by daily use of chlorhexidine digluconate (an antimicrobial compound which prevents the colonization of bacteria on the tooth surface) as a substitute for mechanical tooth cleaning (Löe & Rindom Schiott 1970). These findings demonstrate that microorganisms which form plaques on the teeth contain or release components which induce gingivitis. In agreement with this conclusion is the finding that topical applications of soluble plaque extracts produce inflammatory alterations in gingival tissues (Hellden & Lindhe 1973).

Long-term clinical trials provide additional information regarding the relationship between plaque and periodontal disease in humans. In general, further progression of existing or established periodontal lesions can be arrested by judicious measures to remove bacterial plaque from subgingival areas (Ramfjord et al. 1968, Axelsson & Lindhe 1978, 1981, Lindhe & Nyman 1975, 1984). Such measures include scaling and root planing in conjunction with pocket elimination and subsequent adoption of an effective oral hygiene program. In subjects with untreated periodontal disease, on the other hand, further loss of attachment and alveolar bone can be anticipated (Axelsson & Lindhe 1978, 1981). Thus, the progressive and destructive character of periodontal disease is maintained in areas which continue to harbor subgingival plaque.

Finally, *experiments in animals* (especially dogs and non-human primates) have confirmed the infectious etiology of gingival/periodontal lesions. Long-term observations in beagles, for example, indicate that gingivitis develops only in animals that accumulate bacterial plaque deposits. The inflammatory changes remain confined to the gingival area for several years, but at some sites gingivitis eventually shifts to destructive periodontal disease resulting in loss of connective tissue attachment and alveolar bone (Saxe et al 1967, Lindhe et al. 1975).

Taken together, the research data strongly imply that most forms of periodontal disease are plaque-associated disorders which start as an overt inflammation in the gingiva. If left untreated, inflammation may spread in an apical direction. It is not presently understood why some lesions remain localized to the marginal portion of the gingival tissues while others progress to involve the loss of connective tissue attachment and supporting alveolar bone.

Progression of periodontal disease: the burst hypothesis of disease activity

Results from epidemiologic studies and long-term clinical trails in human populations prior

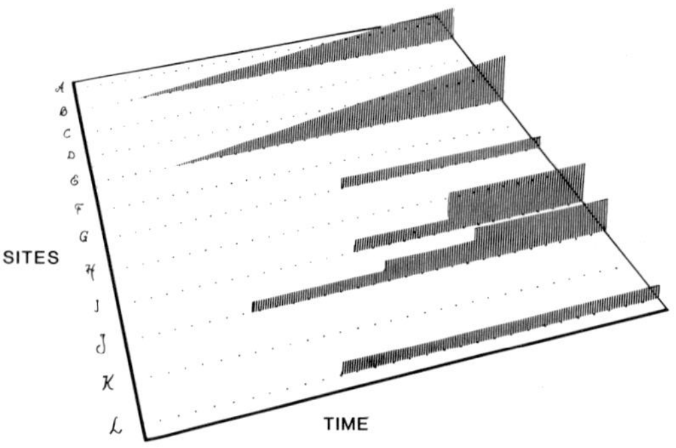

Fig. 5-1.

to the 1980's allowed one to conclude that, in the presence of plaque and calculus, periodontal disease increased in severity with age (see Chapter 2). The data also seemed to suggest that once initiated, the disease continued to relentlessly destroy the periodontium more or less continuously throughout the life of the individual. Thus, time and "improper oral hygiene" appeared to be the primary variables in determing the extent of disease. Based on such findings and interpretations, it was estimated that the disease progressed in small increments and that adult patients experienced an *overall* loss of attachment of around 0.1-0.2 mm per tooth surface per year (or 1-5 μm per day; Waerhaug 1977). The word *overall* is underlined to emphasize that the analytical methods employed in these early investigations tended to "homogenize" or "spread" the disease activity, more or less uniformly throughout the entire dentition. This approach obscured or ignored the fact that within the same dentition individual teeth and individual sites exhibit different degrees of pathology: some areas are healthy while others may be severely affected. If this is taken into consideration and the rate of disease progression is monitored at individual sites over time, an entirely different picture of progressive periodontal disease emerges.

It is apparent that periodontal disease develops and progresses at different rates at different surfaces of the dentition. For example, some advanced diseased sites fail to continue to lose attachment or alveolar bone for extended periods of time. This was shown by Lindhe et al. (1983) who studied the progression of periodontal disease (attachment level changes) over a period of 6 years in a group of 65 untreated adult periodontal patients. While the annual *overall* loss of attachment per individual was found to be 0.18 mm (a figure similar to that reported from earlier epidemiological studies), only 12% of all the surfaces examined actually suffered additional attachment loss during the period of observation. Moreover, only 40% of the tooth surfaces which exhibited attachment loss within the first 3 years showed further tissue breakdown in the next 3 years of the study. In another study, Haffajee and her collaborators (1983) monitored attachment levels in 22 patients with untreated periodontal disease: 3,414 tooth surfaces were examined every 2 months for 1 year. Only about 3% of these surfaces lost additional attachment and when this occurred the amount of attachment loss experienced within a 2-month interval ranged between 2-5 mm (a figure that is considerably higher than the 0.1-0.2 mm/year calculated in earlier studies). Thus, the rate and extent of destruction at individual sites appear to be much greater than previously appreciated; if tissue loss actually continued at this pace affected teeth would be lost in a few years. It is evident, therefore, that periodontal disease may not simply be an unrelenting, slowly progressive process. In some instances, tissue destruction occurs within a very short period of time. This may be followed by a long quiescent interval when some sort of equilibrium is established which minimizes or prevents continued loss of tissue.

Fig. 5-1 depicts the concept of the continuous as well as the episodic model of periodontal destruction. Certain sites (A, C, D, F, H, K) are free from disease throughout the individual's life. Other sites (G, I, J and L) demonstrate one or more active "bursts" of destructive disease resulting in a minor (G and L) or pronounced (I and J) attachment loss but may never progress beyond this point. By contrast, other sites (B and E) are exposed to several minor destructive "bursts" of short duration which give a pattern of continuous attachment loss with a cumulative effect on the functional integrity of the periodontium. Some of the possible pathogenic mechanisms which may explain the burst of disease will be discussed later in this chapter.

Histopathology of periodontal disease

Normal gingiva

In order to fully understand and evaluate different symptoms of gingival inflammatory disease, a detailed knowledge of the structural composition and function of the healthy periodontium is a fundamental prerequisite. The biology of the gingiva and the attachment apparatus were described in Chapter 1; summarized below are some important features:

Clinically, *normal gingiva* is characterized by its pink color, firm consistency and by the scalloped outline of the gingival margin. The interdental papillae are firm, do not bleed on gentle probing and occupy the entire space available below the contact area of neighboring teeth. *Normal gingivae* are free from inflammation at both the clinical and microscopical level. This "ideal" condition can be established under experimental conditions in humans who under supervision daily exercise meticulous plaque control for several weeks. Such fastidious measures are, however, seldom practiced by the average subject. *Normal gingivae* need to be distinguished, therefore, from *clinically healthy gingivae*; the latter may be attained by patients who practice more "routine" measures to prevent plaque accumulation.

As stated, *normal gingivae* are free from

a

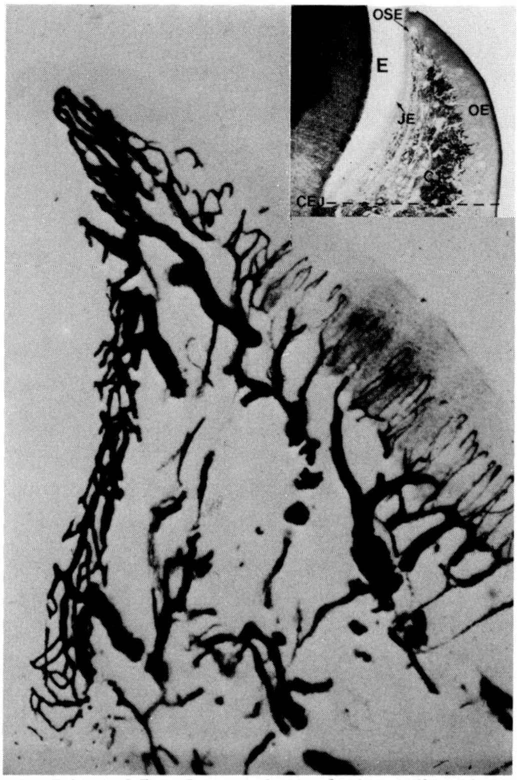

b

Fig. 5-2a, b. Microphotograph (a) of a bucco-lingual section of a normal beagle dog gingiva. The gingival vessels (b) were filled with a carbon suspension (prior to biopsy). A thin vascular network is present beneath the junctional epithelium.

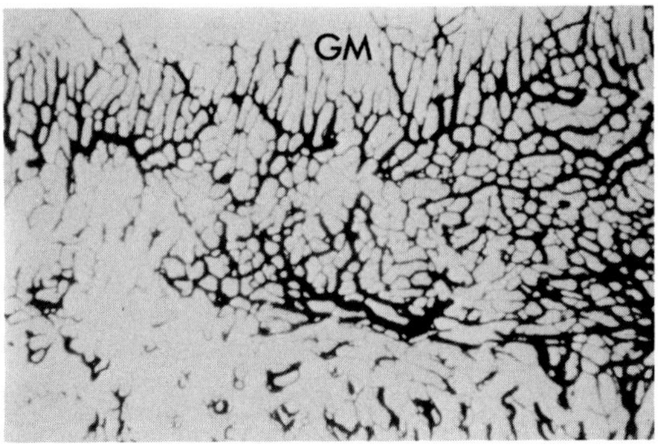

Fig. 5-2c. The thin vascular network (plexus) is shown in a mesio-distal section

"significant" accumulations of inflammatory cells and a gingival sulcus is rarely evident at the microscopic level in these tissues. The oral surface of normal gingiva is covered by a keratinized oral epithelium which fuses with the

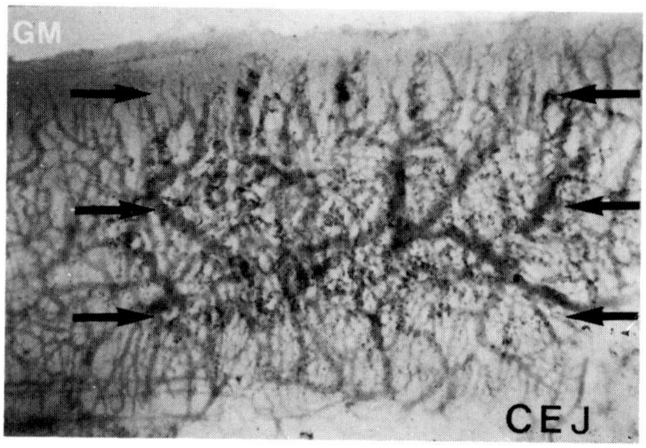

Fig. 5-3. Mesiodistal section of a gingiva showing the vascular network below the junctional epithelium. In the area between the arrows a filter paper-strip has been introduced into the junctional epithelium whereby an increased permeability of the gingival vessels has been induced. The increased vascular permeability is in this case identified by the presence of carbon particles which prior to biopsy were injected intravenously. The carbon particles have become trapped in the open endothelial junctions, and so-called vascular labelling has occurred. GM: gingival margin. (From Egelberg 1967). See also Fig. 5-8b.

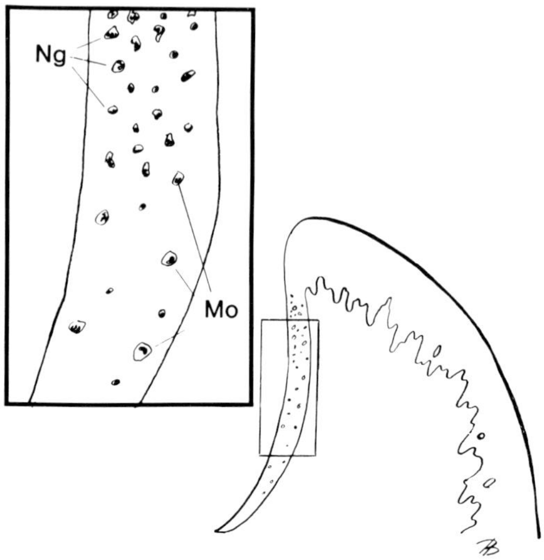

Fig. 5-4. Leokocytes in the junctional epithelium. Observe that the volume of leukocytes decreases in apical direction and approaches 0 in the most apical portion. Within the junctional epithelium, the mononuclear leukocytes are located in more basal layers, while the neutrophilic granulocytes are present primarily in the superficial portions of the junctional epithelium.

junctional epithelium (Fig. 5-2a). The latter is firmly attached to the tooth surface via hemidesmosomes and the marginal portion of the junctional epithelium harbors a few neutrophilic granulocytes and mononuclear cells. The space between the oral and junctional epithelia is occupied by collagenous structures, most of which are organized in densely packed, distinctly outlined fiber bundles. Immediately below the junctional epithelium there is a microvascular plexus, containing numerous venules (Egelberg 1967) (Fig. 5-2). Isolated inflammatory cells may be present in this area and/or around some vessels in more distant locations (Attstrom et al. 1975, Lindhe & Rylander 1975). An analysis of the composition of *normal gingiva* reveals that about 40% of its volume is occupied by epithelial structures (oral epithelium 30%, junctional epithelium 10%) and 60% by connective tissue components such as collagen fibers, matrix, cells, vessels and nerves.

In *clinically healthy gingiva* a small but definite infiltrate of inflammatory cells can be detected in the coronal portion of the connective tissue (Page & Schroeder 1976). This infiltrate (consisting of lymphocytes, neutrophils and monocytes/macrophages) occupies around 3-5% of the connective tissue volume and is in contact with the junctional epithelium. Collagen has been depleted in this infiltrated area but the tissue compartment is rich in vascular structures. Fluid and plasma proteins leak from the microvasculature, percolating through the connective tissue and the junctional epithelium into the gingival sulcus to give rise to the *gingival fluid* (Egelberg 1967, Cimasoni 1983) (Figs. 5-2 and 5-3). A *gingival sulcus*, 0.1-0.5 mm deep, is found between the coronal portion of the junctional epithelium and the tooth surface and probably develops as a result of microbial irritation. The sulcus may disappear after bacterial debridement and institution of meticulous plaque control measures to reestablish a normal gingival condition. As discussed below, the gingival sulcus should be distinguished from the so-called gingival pocket

(Schroeder 1973, 1977, Page & Schroeder 1982).

Neutrophils (PMNs) and mononuclear leukocytes are present in the junctional epithelium of *clinically healthy gingivae* (Fig. 5-4). These cells more or less continuously migrate from the dentogingival microvessels via the junctional epithelium into the gingival sulcus. Presumably, their movement through the tissues is largely mediated by chemotactic factors derived from plaque bacteria. The number of leukocytes recruited to the area increases markedly with further growth of plaque on the tooth surface and the development of overt gingivitis (Attstrom 1971).

It seems reasonable to believe that *normal* and *healthy* gingiva are continually confronted by potential pathogenic organisms and up to a certain point effectively deal with these assaults. This is probably accomplished by a combination of mechanisms including: 1) outward gingival fluid flow, 2) killing of microorganisms by neutrophils and monocytes/macrophages in the gingival sulcus, 3) shedding of organisms attached to the surface of desquamating oral junctional epithelial cells, 4) destruction of certain microorganisms by antibodies and/or activation of the complement system, 5) restriction of massive microbial growth by the normal or indigenous microflora. Theoretically, something may transpire to compromise one or more of these mechanisms and permit indigenous organisms and/or exogenous bacteria to proliferate on the gingival portion of the tooth surface. It is relatively easy to understand how this can occur in an individual who has an underlying or pre-existing defect in a primary, frontline defense system (e.g., someone who has an abnormality in neutrophil function; see below). But it is more difficult to explain why this develops in apparently healthy individuals. Are local defense systems simply overwhelmed by the sheer mass of plaque bacteria that can accumulate on the teeth as a consequence of ineffective oral hygiene? Or is the area jeopardized by an infection by a specific organism(s) which is especially adept at attacking or evading the gingival defense system? It is likely that both pathways operate to perturb the normal or healthy gingival environment. In any event, under these circumstances the host has no recourse but to intensify or augment its efforts to reestablish the normal "balance". This is reflected by the development of a conspicuous inflammatory response in the underlying tissues.

Gingival inflammation

Inflammatory changes in the gingiva develop within a couple of days of undisturbed bacterial growth on the cervical portion of the tooth surface. Clinically, inflammation is initially seen as discrete color and texture changes of the marginal tissues. After 10-20 days of plaque accumulation overt gingivitis is established in most individuals, characterized by gingival redness and swelling and increased tendency of the soft tissue to bleed on gentle probing (Fig. 5-5). As stated above, if the microbial plaque is removed at this stage and effective plaque control measures instituted, the inflammatory alterations soon disappear (Löe et al. 1965, Lindhe & Rylander 1975).

The underlying microscopic events which account for these clinical changes are apparent even before gross alterations in the appearance of the gingiva become visible. These events are associated with profound alterations in the integrity of the microcirculatory bed and by the influx and proliferation of inflammatory cells in the connective tissue beneath the dentogingival epithelium. The inflammatory cell infiltrate includes plasma cells, lymphocytes, blast cells, macrophages and neutrophils. The accumulation of these cells in the tissue compartment is associated with a significant reduction in the number of fibroblasts and the density of collagen and matrix components. The dynamics and dimensions of these changes were do-

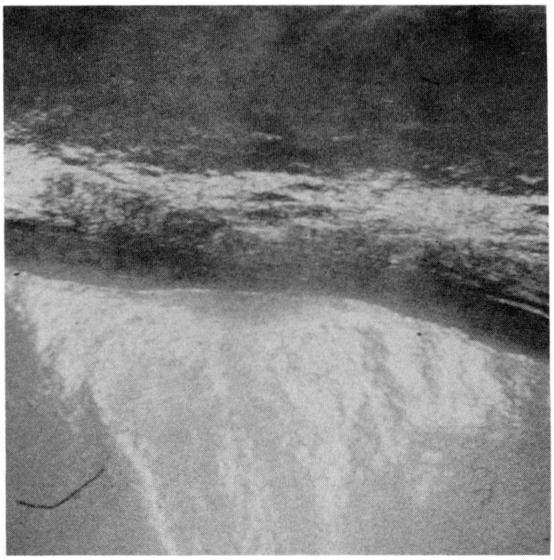

Fig. 5-5a

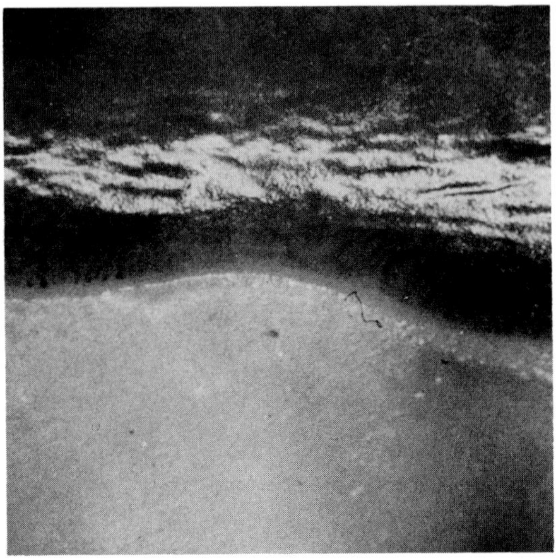

Fig. 5-5b

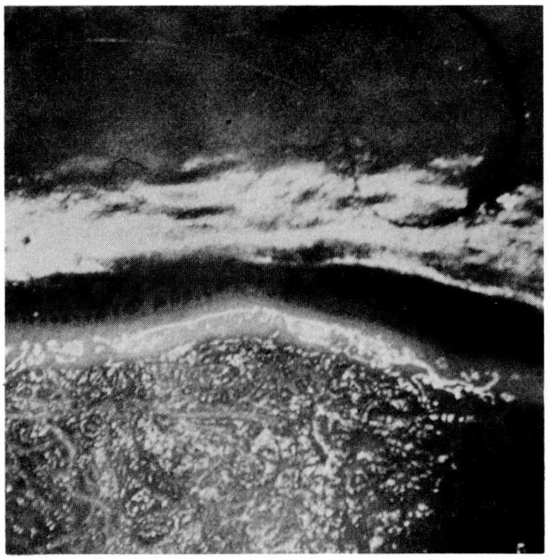

Fig. 5-5c

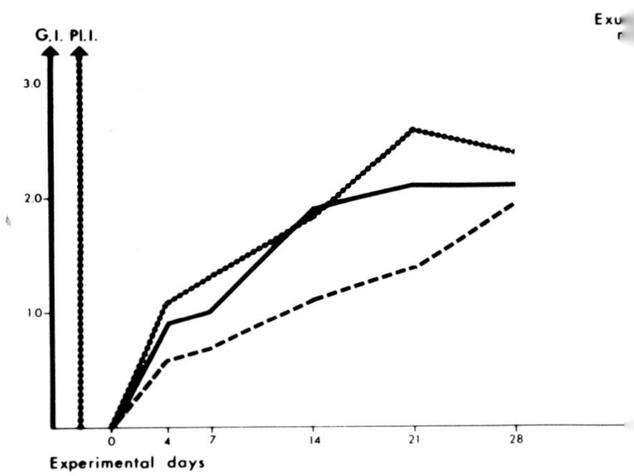

Fig. 5-5d

Fig. 5-5a-d. Gingival alterations which have occurred during a period of gingivitis development in beagles. a: day 0, b: day 4, c: day 14. Note the gradually developing plaque on the tooth surface and inflammatory changes in the gingiva. Note the vascular reaction which is illustrated by a gradually increased number of vessels in the gingival margin. Gingival Index (GI), Plaque Index (PlI) and Gingival exudate alterations during experimental gingivitis are illustrated in d (Lindhe & Rylander 1975).

cumented in an experiment comparing the cellular and structural composition of the affected area before and during the development of gingivitis over a period of 28 days (Lindhe & Rylander 1975). In this study plaque was allowed to accumulate on the teeth of dogs with initially *normal gingiva*; biopsy samples were taken at Day 0 and at Days 4, 14 and 28. The normal tissue (Day 0) is referred to below as *Noninfiltrated Connective Tissue* (NCT) and the altered area as the *Infiltrated Connective Tissue* (ICT) (Table 5-1).

Table 5-1

Parameter	Normal Connective Tissue (NCT) (Day 0)	Infiltrated Connective Tissue (ICT) Day 4	Day 14	Day 28
Size of infiltrate	0%	5%	15%	37%
Collagen fibers	60%	20%	24%	30%
Fibroblasts	13%	8%	7%	7%
Vessels	7%	22%	14%	16%
Residual tissue	20%	40%	45%	36%
Neutrophils	0.5%	8%	4%	1%
Plasma cells, lymphocytes, macrophages	0.1%	3%	7%	10%

Table 5-1. Size (%volume) of various components of the normal connective tissue (NCT) and the infiltrated connective tissue (ICT) at various days (4,14 and 28) after onset of plaque formation (from Lindhe & Rylander 1975).

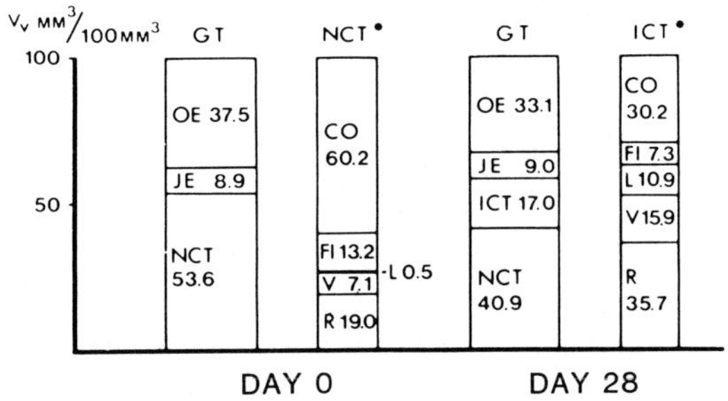

Fig. 5-6. Composition of the gingiva (GT), noninfiltrated (NCT) and infiltrated (ICT) gingival connective tissue on day 0 (normal gingiva) and on day 28 of gingivitis in beagles. Note that the infiltrated connective tissue portion amounts to 17% of the free gingival margin on day 28 and that the collagen content is reduced from approximately 60% on day 0 to 30% on day 28 in the area where the inflammatory infiltrate has become established. Note also that in this area (on day 28) a reduction in fibroblast proportion has occurred, as well as an increase of vessels and residual tissue. OE: oral epithelium, JE: junctional epithelium, NCT: noninfiltrated connective tissue, ICT: infiltrated connective tissue, CO: collagen fibers, FI: fibroblasts, V: vascular structures, L: leukocytes, R: residual tissue. (From Lindhe & Rylander 1975).

At Day 0 the *normal* gingival unit is essentially free of inflammatory cells (Fig. 5-6) and is comprised of approximately 40-45% epithelium and 55-60% connective tissue. The NCT zone consists of collagen (60%), fibroblasts (13%), vessels (7%) and other tissue constituents, such as intercellular matrix and nerves (20%). After the onset of plaque accumulation neutrophils and mononuclear leukocytes quickly move into the area. An ICT is starting to form and increases in volume over the 28-day period, becoming populated by lymphocytes, plasma cells and macrophages (Fig. 5-6). The influx of neutrophils is also sustained throughout this interval, but most of them leave the ICT, emigrating into the gingival sulcus. As inflammatory cells populate the ICT there is a marked reduction in the amount of collagen and the number of fibroblasts in the lesion, with a concomitant increase in the volume of residual tissue (intercellular matrix, degraded collagen, exudate material, degenerated or dead cells) and small blood vessels.

In order to gain additional perspectives on the development of gingival and periodontal inflammation, Page & Schroeder (1976) have suggested that it would be useful to describe or divide lesion progression into four phases: *initial, early, established* and *advanced* stages. The initial and early lesions represent relatively "acute" stages of gingivitis and the established lesion designates more "chronic" gingivitis. The advanced lesion actually refers to the progression of gingivitis into periodontitis. It should be understood that there is no clear dividing line between these stages. Most general pathology textbooks describe the inflammatory reaction as being separated into "acute" and "chronic" phases. While this classification is helpful for descriptive purposes, it is of limited use when one considers the pathogenesis of gingival/periodontal inflammation. During the initial and early stages of gingivitis the classical histological features of the acute inflammatory reaction tend to dominate in the affected

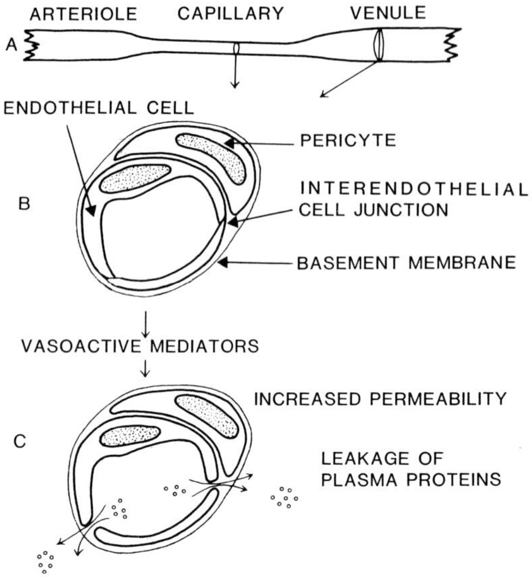

Fig. 5-7. Schematic illustrations depicting the terminal vascular bed and the mechanisms of increased vascular permeability. Under normal conditions the terminal vessels are freely permeable to small molecules, salt and water. The intercellular junctions between the endothelial cells are closed. Via the influence of vasoactive mediators the endothelial cells become separated and increased vascular permeability occurs. Large molecules and plasma proteins leak into surrounding tissue. A number of inflammatory mediators present in plasma are activated when they enter the perivascular tissue.

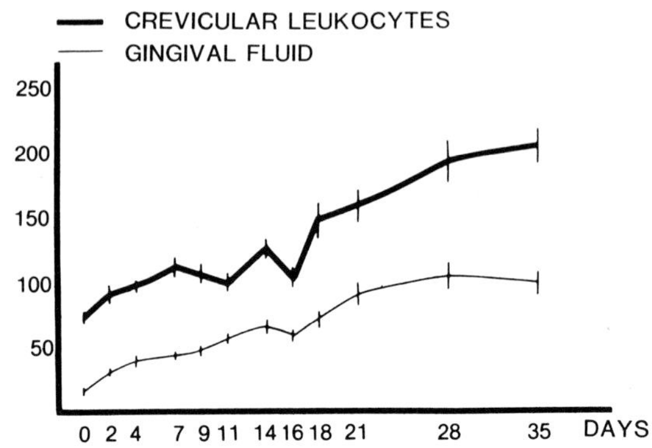

Fig. 5-8. Alterations in number of crevicular leukocytes and in gingival fluid during a period of developing gingivitis in beagles. Note the gradual increase of leukocytes and fluid flow during the experimental period. (From Attström & Egelberg 1971).

area. Subsequently, chronic inflammatory changes become superimposed so that both acute and chronic elements co-exist in early, established and advanced lesions. The explanation for this may be due to the simultaneous and sustained operation of numerous etiologic, pro-inflammatory pathways within the lesions.

The initial gingival lesion

As previously stated inflammation quickly develops as plaque starts to be deposited on the tooth. Within 24 hours marked changes are evident in the microvascular plexus beneath the junctional epithelium. More blood is brought to the area as manifested by dilation of the arterioles, capillaries and venules of the dentogingival plexus. At the same time, the hydrostatic pressure within the microcirculation is elevated coupled with the formation of intercellular gaps between adjacent capillary or venular endothelial cells. This results in a profound increase in the permeability of the microvascular bed to fluids and proteins which leak into the tissues (Fig. 5-7).These changes represent an important defense reaction. For example, the outward flow of edema fluid from the blood into the tissues and gingival sulcus may dilute irritants (such as microbial toxins) and flush bacteria and their products from the sulcus into the oral cavity. Plasma proteins escaping from the microcirculation include fibrinogen, immunoglubulins, specific antibodies, complement peptides and albumin as well as other macromolecules which have numerous functions, many of which will be detailed below. One can readily detect this fluid by placing filter strips at the gingival margin and allowing the exudate to absorb onto the filter. In the non-inflamed gingival unit very little fluid is available to absorb onto the filter strip, but during all phases of gingivitis the amount of exudate can be used as one index of inflammatory injury (Fig. 5-5). Also, the concentration of specific plasma proteins (e.g., albumin, fibrinogen) and products released from leukocytes in the gingival sulcus can be estimated as another parameter of the

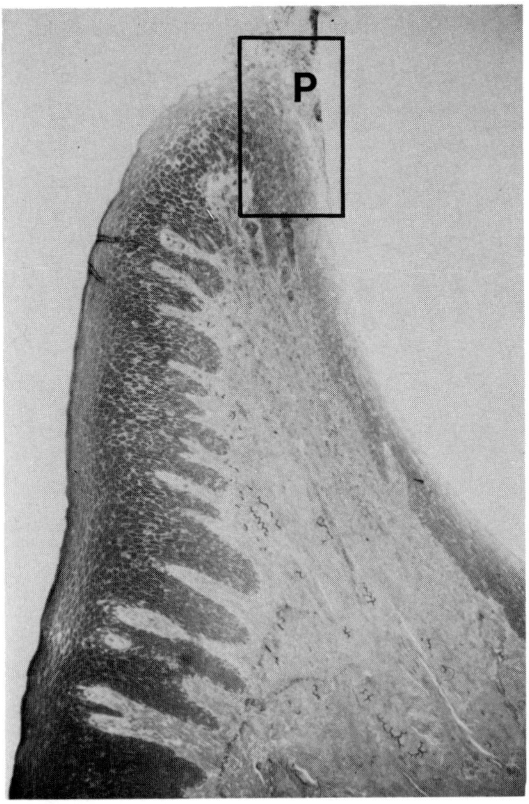

Fig. 5-9a.

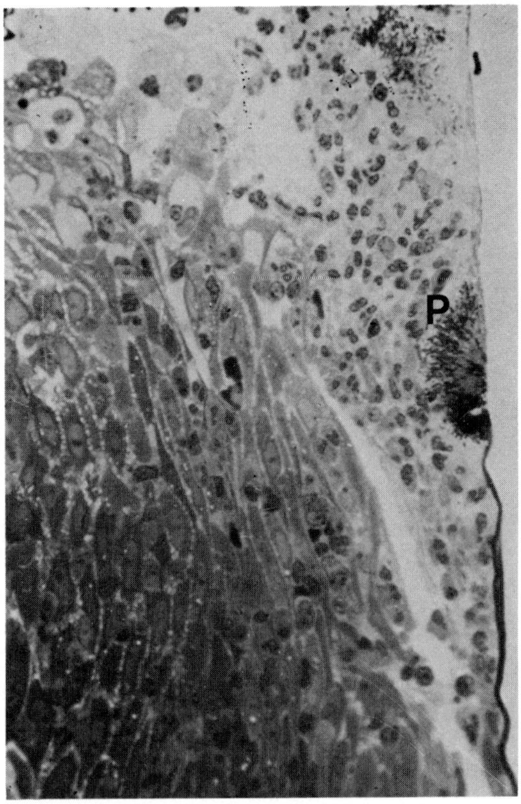

Fig. 5-9b.

Fig. 5-9a,b. Buccolingual section of the gingiva on day 4 of developing gingivitis in a beagle. Note plaque (P) in the sulcus region and increased cellularity in the coronal part of the connective tissue below the junctional epithelium. Note the presence of leukocytes in the coronal part of the junctional epithelium and at the surfaces of the subgingival plaque.

inflammatory process (review: Fine & Mandel 1986).

Co-incidentally with these vascular alterations, numerous neutrophils and monocytes/macrophages (as well as some lymphoid cells) begin to migrate from the dentogingival microvascular plexus. The cellular response is well established by 2-4 days from the onset of plaque accumulation and is mediated by chemotactic substances originating from the plaque microbiota as well as from host cells and secretions. Leukocytes move through the connective tissue and the majority seem to accumulate in the junctional epithelium and gingival sulcus region. Neutrophils appear to preferentially enter into the gingival sulcus and are often referred to as *crevicular leukocytes* (Fig. 5-8). Crevicular leukocytes can be collected by various techniques for quantitation and *in vitro* observation.

Although neutrophils and macrophages are recruited to the area to defend the host against bacterial attack, their accumulation in the coronal part of the connective tissue and junctional epithelium probably accounts for much of the damage that can be seen in this portion of the gingiva. These cells may, for example, cause focal destruction of the epithelium and deplete collagen in the infiltrated connective tissues. The mechanisms whereby inflammatory cells

a

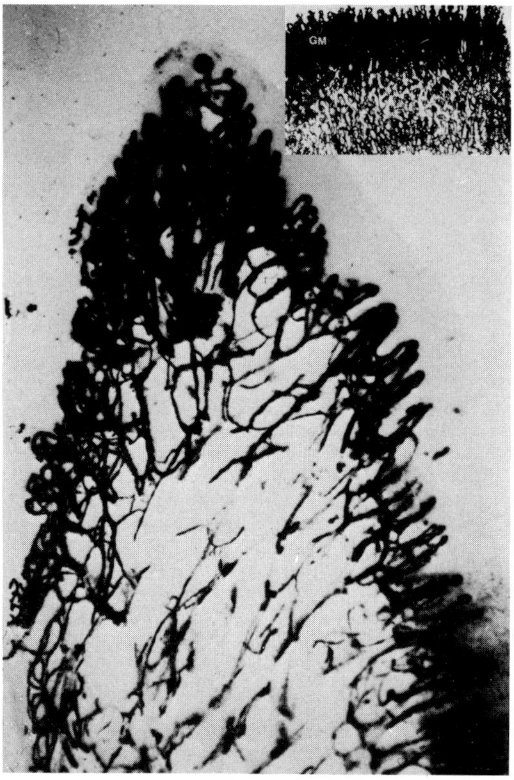

b

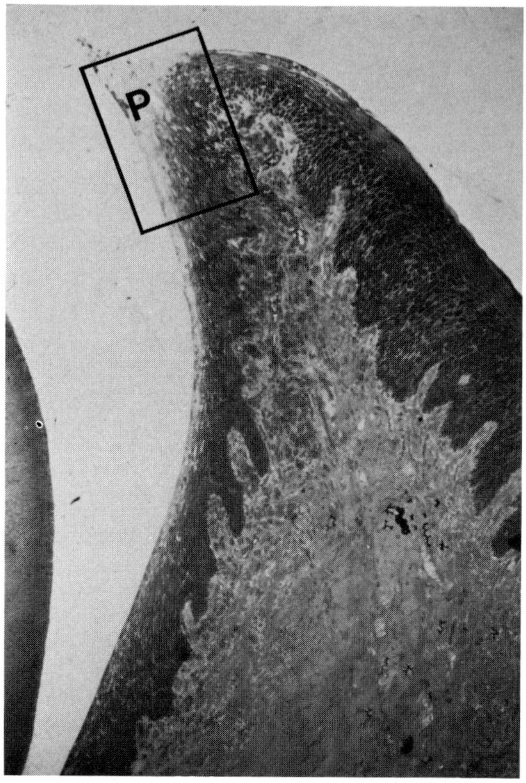

Fig. 5-10a. Buccolingual section of chronically inflamed gingiva in a dog. The vessels have been filled with a contrasting carbon suspension. Note the wide and tortuous vessels below the junctional epithelium to the left in the illustration. Compare with the vasculature in healthy gingiva in Fig. 5-8. The pronounced vascular reaction in this area is a result of plaque accumulation.

Fig. 5-10b. Mesiodistal section of a gingiva illustrating the vessels below the junctional epithelium of chronically inflamed gingiva. Note vascular dilation and proliferation at the level of the gingival margin (GM). Note also that vascular proliferation has occurred in the apical part of the vascular plexus. (From Egelberg 1967).

Fig. 5-11. Buccolingual section of the gingiva on day 7 of developing gingivitis in a beagle. Note the subgingival extension of plaque (P), as well as the increased number of inflammatory cells in the connective tissue below the dentogingival epithelium.

produce these alterations will be considered below.

The early gingival lesion

During the 4-7 day interval after microbial colonization (Fig. 5-9), the vessels of the coronal portion of the dentogingival plexus remain dilated. Moreover, the numbers of functioning vessels increase as a result of vascular proliferation and opening of previously inactive vascular units (compare Fig. 5-2 and 5-10). It is possible to visualize the course, size and number of microvasculature units by the clinical appearance of the gingival margin at this time (Fig. 5-5: Egelberg 1967, Lindhe & Rylander 1975).

With additional plaque accumulation, there is a more pronounced infiltration of neutrophils and monocytes (macrophages) in the dentogingival epithelium when compared to the initial lesion. The inflammatory cell infiltrate in the connective tissue at this stage contains small and medium-sized lymphocytes. Many of these are T cells responsible for cell-mediated immune reactions, while others represent B cells

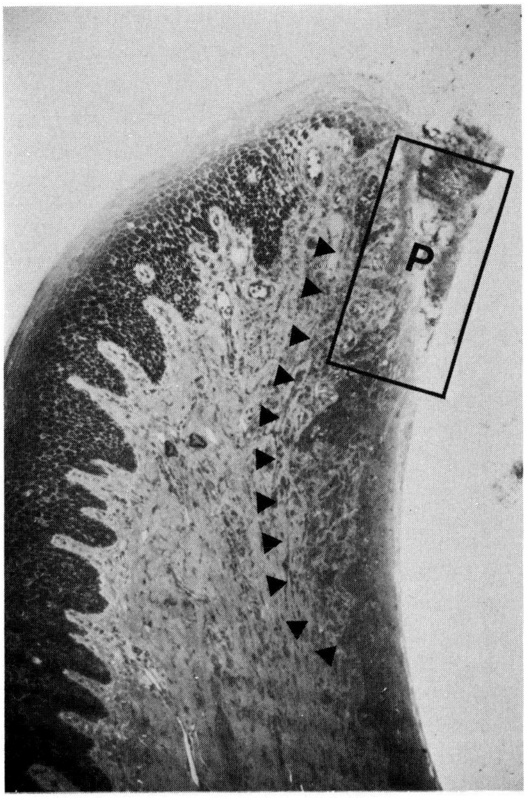

Fig. 5-12. Buccolingual section of the gingiva on day 21 of developing gingivitis in a beagle. Compare with Fig. 5-11. Note the extension of the subgingival plaque (P) as well as the apical extension of the infiltrate (the lesion) in the connective tissue.

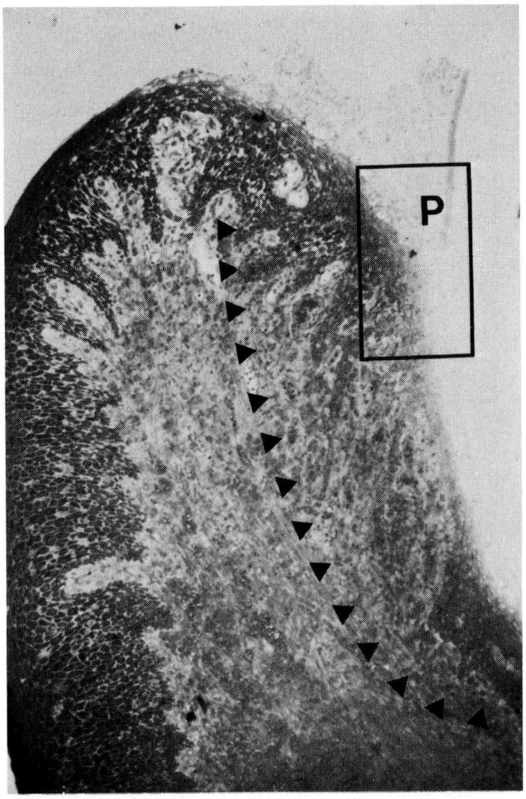

Fig. 5-13. Buccolingual section of the gingiva on day 28 of gingivitis development in a beagle. Note the extension of the subgingival plaque (P) and the increased number of leukocytes in the connective tissue below the junctional epithelium. Note rete pegs in the dentogingival epithelium.

which will probably develop into antibody-producing plasma cells. Some fibroblasts within the inflammatory cell infiltrate exhibit signs of degeneration (cellular vacuolization); presumably some of these cells have been injured by cytotoxic products originating primarily from lymphoid cells (Schroeder & Page 1972).

Towards the end of the 2nd week of abstinence from tooth cleaning, microbial plaque can frequently be found in a subgingival position. The size of the inflammatory cell infiltrate in the connective tissue has increased to occupy approximately 10-15% of the connective-tissue volume of the free gingiva. Furthermore, the basal cells of the junctional/sulcus epithelium have proliferated and rete pegs can be seen piercing and entering the coronal part of the infiltrate (Fig. 5-11).

The established gingival lesion

This phase of lesion development is commonly referred to as "chronic gingivitis". With continued exposure to plaque, the amount of fluid exuding from the vasculature and the number of leukocytes migrating into the tissues and the gingival crevice increase further. At approximately one month after the onset of plaque accumulation, the cellular as well as the permeability response appear to plateau. It would seem a "steady state" or balance has been achieved and this may last for extended periods of time without the established lesion progress-

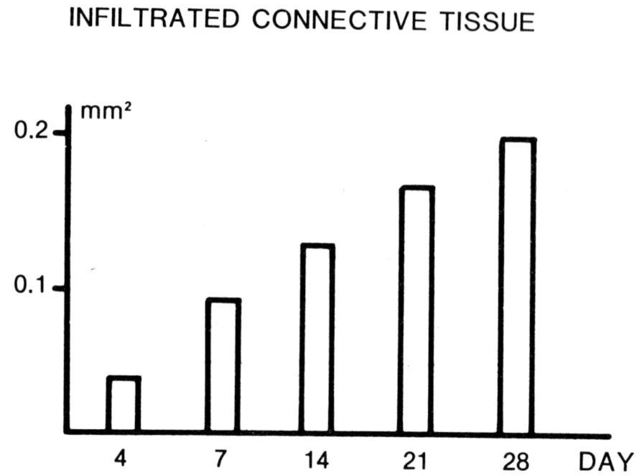

Fig. 5-14. Diagram showing the increase in size of the infiltrated connective tissue during the development of gingivitis in beagles. (From Mattsson & Attström 1979).

ing into the advanced lesion. It has not been possible to actually define the nature of this equilibrium in functional terms. The apparent balance may reflect an equilibrium that is sufficient to counteract irritation produced by the dental plaque and/or impede unrestricted growth of microorganisms down the root surface or their invasion into the connective tissues. While this may theoretically prevent rapid extension of the infection, the host response does not seem to be capable of totally eliminating microorganisms from the sulcus /pocket. Thus, plaque continues to persist and sustain the inflammatory reaction in the coronal gingiva.

Large numbers of mature plasma cells are seen in the established lesion and are situated primarily in the coronal connective tissues as well as around vessels in more distant parts of the gingival connective tissue. Collagen continues to be lost in both lateral and apical directions as the inflammatory cell infiltrate expands, resulting in collagen-depleted (ICT)

Table 5-2

Summary of some important histopathological alterations during the gradual development of gingivitis

	Day 4	Day 7	Day 14	Day 21	Day 28	
Neutrophils and mononuclear leukocytes in the junctional epithelium	———	———	———	———	———	→
Increased vascular permeability	———	———	———	———	———	→
Vascular proliferation		———	———	———	———	→
Neutrophils and monocytes/macrophages in the connective tissue	———	———	———	———	———	→
Lymphocytes	———	———	———	———	———	→
Plasma cells			———	———	———	→
Infiltrate size	———	———	———	———	———	→
Collagen destruction	———	———	———	———	———	→

Table 5-2. Solid line indicates when the change can be noted and the gradual increase to day 28. From day 28 the changes take place more slowly, probably as a result of the fact that a "balance" has been established between the bacteria in the gingival sulcus and the defense response in the tissue.

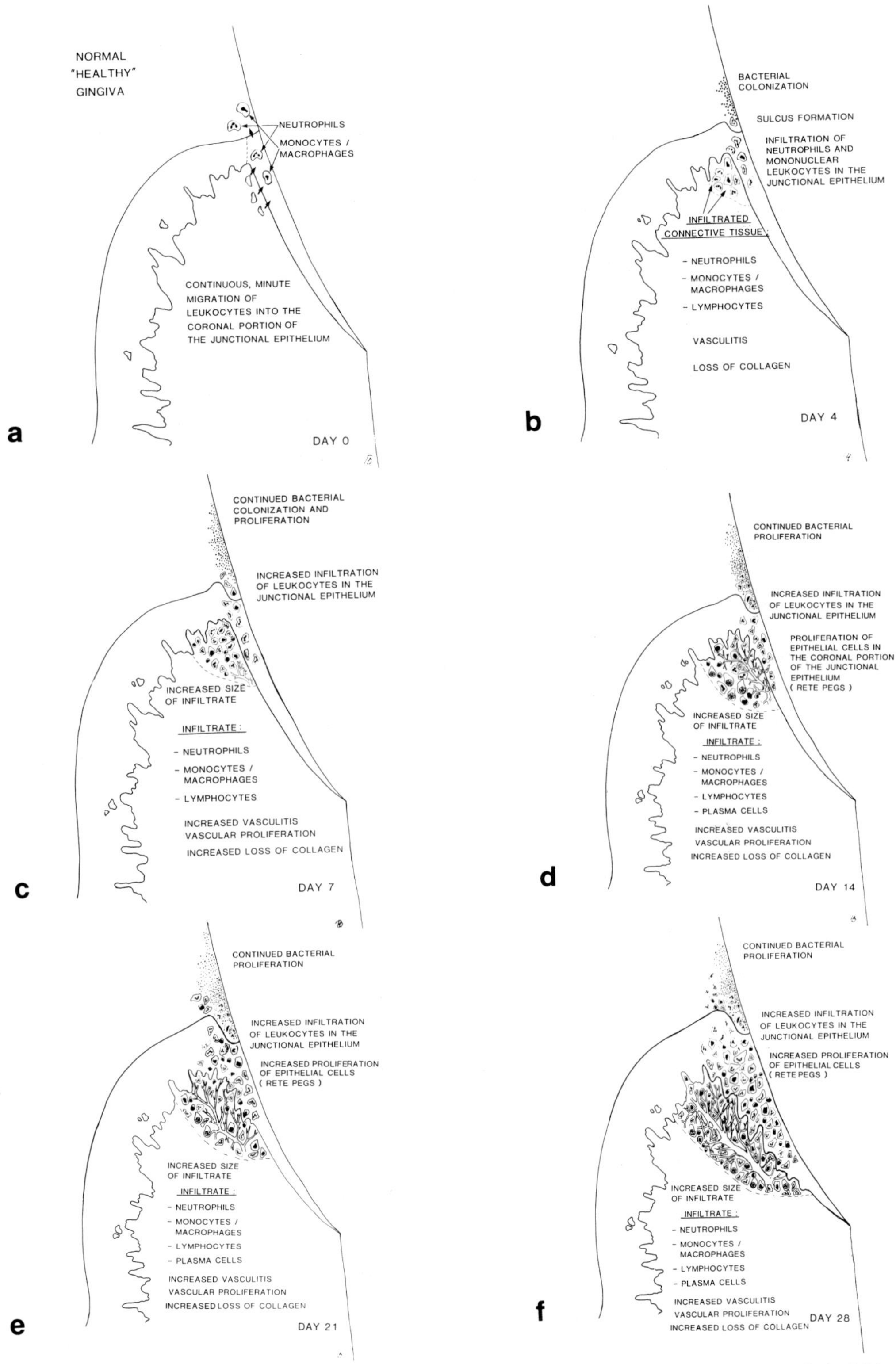

Fig. 5-15a-f. Schematic illustration depicting some alterations of the gingival tissues during the development of gingivitis. Note the continuous increase in the size of the infiltrated area in the connective tissue. Also observe the gradual development of an infiltration of leukocytes in the junctional epithelium.

areas radiating deeper into the tissue (Figs. 5-12, 5-13, 5-14). Proliferation of the dentogingival epithelium is maintained and rete pegs extend into the connective tissue infiltrate. The dentogingival epithelium adjacent to the ICT is now commonly referred to as *pocket epithelium* and forms the external boundary of the inflammatory cell infiltrate. The pocket epithelium is not attached to the tooth surface and is heavily infiltrated with neutrophils and macrophages, as well as lymphocytes and plasma cells. Most of the neutrophils eventually migrate across the epithelium into the gingival pocket. The pocket epithelium may be extremely thin and may actually be ulcerated in some areas. When compared to the junctional epithelium, the pocket epithelium is more fragile and permeable to the passage of substances into and out of the underlying tissues.

Alterations which occur in the epithelium and the connective tissue during development of gingivitis are schematically illustrated in Fig. 5-15 and Table 5-2.

The advanced gingival/periodontal lesion

As plaque continues its apical downgrowth along the crown and the cementum of the root surface, there is a concomitant deepening of the periodontal pocket. This is accompanied by the proliferation of the dentogingival epithelium over the "detached" root surface. The inflammatory cell infiltrate extends laterally and further apically into the connective tissues. Plasma cells (most of which produce IgG antibodies) dominate in the lesions, but lymphocytes, macrophages and neutrophils are also present. At this time the first indication of alveolar bone destruction can be observed histologically and appears to be primarily the consequence of osteoclastic activity. The mechanisms which account for osteoclast stimulation are not completely understood, but plaque as well as host-derived mediators are probably involved.

Pathogenic mechanisms in gingival inflammation

Most, if not all, forms of human periodontal disease are initiated and sustained by factors produced/released by the subgingival microbiota (Kahnberg, Lindhe & Hellden 1976). Some of these substances can directly damage host cells and tissues. Other microbial constituents may not actually injure the host; instead, they activate endogenous cellular and humoral inflammatory systems which secondarily affect the integrity of the periodontium. It is the combination of both the direct and indirect pathways that accounts for periodontal injury.

Direct injury by plaque microorganisms

In Chapter 4 detailed consideration was given to the way plaque organisms may overtly damage cellular and structural components of the periodontium. In this context, we are concerned with microbial invasion of soft tissues as well as the formation of noxious substances by the microbiota of the gingival pocket. Proliferation of bacteria within the gingival tissues would probably have disastrous effects on normal functions. Invasion of the dentogingival epithelium by spirochetes has been conclusively documented in acute necrotizing ulcerative gingivitis (Listgarten 1965). Recently, numerous reports suggest that microorganisms may also be found within the gingiva of subjects with advanced juvenile periodontitis or adult periodontitis (see Chapters 4 and 6). However, the significance of these observations remains to be resolved. For one thing, some researchers have failed to confirm these findings. Even if bacteria are within the tissues it is not known whether this represents true invasion (i.e. microbial colonization and proliferation within the tissues) as opposed to "simple" displacement or translocation of the bacteria into the soft tissues during late stages of disease. More research is needed to resolve this issue and to determine whether microbial invasion is significant in periodontitis, especially during acute bursts of disease activity.

The release of soluble, irritative substances is another way bacteria produce disease (see Chapter 4). For instance, bacterial hydrolytic enzymes can attack critical substrates, including collagen, elastin, fibronectin, fibrin and various other components of the intercellular matrix of epithelial and connective tissues. In addition, plaque bacteria generate numerous metabolic products, such as ammonia, indole, hydrogen sulphide and butyric acid, which may "non-specifically" perturb cellular functions. Recent studies indicate that some microorganisms elaborate more specific factors that may have profound biological potentials. For illustration, *Actinobacillus actinomycetemcomitans* synthesizes a "leukotoxin" which destroys neutrophils and monocytes (review: Taichman et al. 1984) and a substance which activates T suppressor cells (Shenker, McArthur & Tsai 1982). Both factors could impair gingival antibacterial defense. In addition, *A. actinomycetemcomitans* as well as other organisms produce factors which depress fibroblast, endothelial and epithelial cell proliferation *in vitro*. If these agents function *in vivo* they could adversely affect the capacity of the periodontium to respond to irritation.

Table 5-3

Major classes of endogenous mediators of inflammation

Vasoactive amines
histamine and serotonin

Plasma proteases
kinin system
complement system
plasmin system

Arachidonic acid metabolities
prostaglandins and leukotrienes

Lysosomal acid hydrolases

Neutral proteases
elastase, collagenase and cathepsin G

Oxygen-derived metabolities
superoxide anion, hydrogen peroxide and hydroxyl radical

Lymphokines and monokines
see Tables 5-9 and 5-11

Others

Indirect injury by plaque microorganisms via inflammation

Many microbial products have little or no direct toxic effect on the host; instead, they possess the potential to activate non-immune and/or immune inflammatory reactions which in turn actually cause the damage. A few examples will be cited here and more will be considered below. Lipopolysaccharides (*endotoxins*) of Gram negative microorganisms may be responsible for a spectrum of inflammatory events because they interact with and modulate the behavior of leukocytes. For example, endotoxin acts as a mitogen, stimulating B cell proliferation and antibody secretion; it causes macrophages to produce and secrete neutral proteinases and acid hydrolases; it promotes osteoclastic bone resorption; it has profound effects on the blood coagulation system. Further, endotoxin triggers the complement system resulting in the formation of numerous pro-inflammatory peptides. These are only a few of the properties that account for the biological expression of endotoxic activity, and lipoteichoic acids from Gram positive bacteria share many of these properties. Likewise, specific proteins or polysaccharides produced and released from several subgingival bacteria activate endogenous mediators of vascular permeability, encourage inflammatory cells to move into the tissues and cause them to dis-

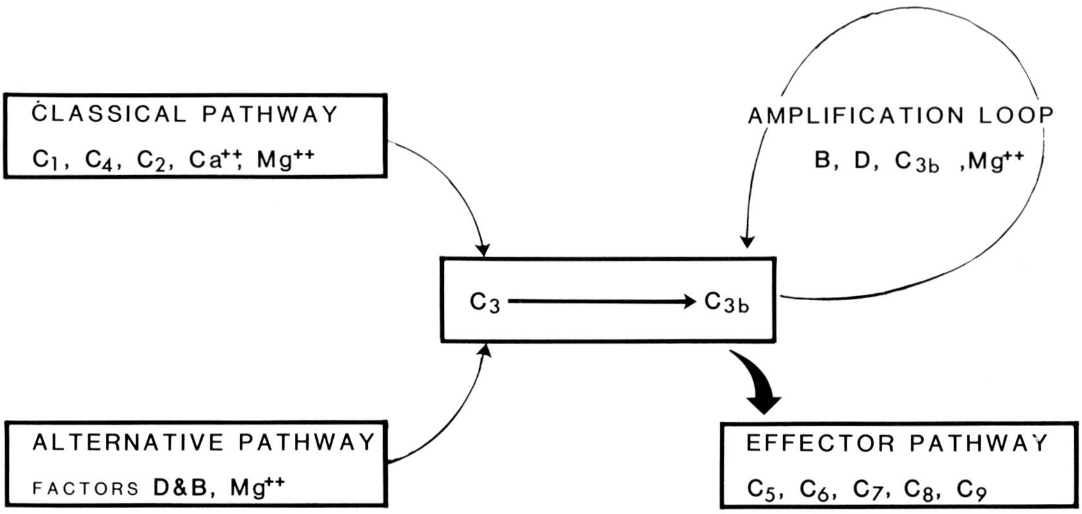

Fig. 5-16. *Simplified mechanisms of activation of the complement cascade:* The classical pathway components include C1, C4 and C2 while factor B and factor D are components of the alternative pathway. Activation of C3 to C3b is the critical step in both pathways because this triggers activation of the terminal or effector proteins (C5-C9). C3b also amplifies the formation of more C3b by a positive feedback of the alternative pathway components. The terminal or effector pathway gives rise to the "membrane attack complex" and various other peptide fragments with biological activities. Activated complement components and fragments are very labile, and several inhibitor and inactivator proteins (not shown) normally regulate or limit the extent of complement activation.

charge pro-inflammatory agents. Finally, immune reactions to antigens derived from the subgingival microbiota can be harmful to the host.

Endogenous mediators of inflammation

The major groups of endogenous mediators are listed in Table 5-3; in many instances specific factors belonging to each of these categories have been identified in gingival exudates. Sometimes, it is tempting to try to assign a more important role to one class of mediator when compared to others. This may be possible in experimental models of inflammation where one has "control" over the extent, time course and dynamics of the reaction. Thus, for example, it is known that the amines may be responsible for immediate but transitory changes in vascular permeability while other substances, such as the prostaglandins and the kinin peptides, produce a delayed but more sustained phase of plasma protein leakage. Similarly, it has been possible to dissect the evolution of various other events in the progression of the inflammatory response. But in human gingivitis and periodontitis it is not that simple because many different mediators are probably always available in the lesion and all may contribute simultaneously to the vascular, cellular and reparative phases of the disease process. Moreover, several mediators are linked to one another via positive feedback systems which amplify their biological potentials. Indeed, most mediators have more than one inflammatory function and many may have physiological effects unrelated to their pro-inflammatory activities. After being released or activated, mediators are usually rapidly inactivated in the local area. This is an important step in the control of the inflammatory process. It is conceivable that an abnormality in one or more of these control mechanisms contributes to the development of gingival exudates. A brief review of the pharmacology and biological potentials of representative endogenous mediators of inflammation is presented below.

Histamine is found primarily in mast cells and basophils. Mast cells are widely distributed in connective tissues, especially adjacent to small blood vessels. Some studies suggest that their numbers increase in long standing gingival lesions and that the concentration of histamine is higher in inflamed gingiva than in normal gingiva. Besides histamine, mast cells secrete other inflammatory mediators (e.g. heparin, lysosomal enzymes and metabolites of arachidonic acid) into surrounding tissues in response to a variety of stimuli (Siraganian 1983). Histamine causes dilation of blood vessels, increases the permeability of venules and may also have regulator activities, altering the responses of various cells to other mediators and stimuli. Mast cell activation can be induced by numerous factors including complement peptides (C3a and C5a) and binding of antigen to IgE-senitized cells. The latter refers to mast cells with IgE antibodies "fixed" or bound to homologous Fc receptors on the cell membrane. Once antigen interacts with bound antibody a series of biochemical events ensues, leading to the release of histamine and other mediators. IgE-sensitized mast cells have been identified in inflamed gingiva, and it is possible that some are coated with IgE directed against plaque-derived antigens (Nisengard 1974). Thus, local anaphylaxis-type reactions may represent a mechanism to induce mast cell degranulation in gingival tissues.

Kinins are peptides produced as a consequence of the proteolytic action of *kallikreins*, which are trypsin-like serine proteinases present in plasma and inflammatory exudates. These enzymes are normally inactive but become functional when acted upon by clotting factor XII (Hageman factor). Factor XII in turn is activated following contact with various surfaces (e.g., collagen, vascular basement membrane) which are exposed or become "available" during inflammation. Kallikreins interact with their protein substrates (*kininogens*), resulting in cleavage and liberation of vasoactive kinins. Probably the most significant of these is *bradykinin* (a nonapeptide). Pharmacological effects of bradykinin include: vascular smooth muscle relaxation and contraction, increased vascular permeability, leukocyte emigration and pain. Bradykinin probably acts on blood vessels, at least partially, by triggering the formation of arachidonic acid metabolites. It is relevant to point out that bacterial as well as neutrophil proteases can activate the kinin system.

Table 5-4

Potential biological functions of complement in inflammation

Function	Component
Mobilization of leukocytes from bone marrow	C3e
Adherence of leukocytes to endothelial surfaces	C5a
Chemotaxis of leukocytes	C5a, C567
Opsonization of microorganisms for phagocytosis	C3b
Stimulation of leukocyte oxidative metabolism	C3b, C5a
Activation of neutrophil degranulation	C5a
Induction of macrophage secretion	C3b
Lymphokine production	C3b
Mast cell degranulation (anaphylatoxin activity) resulting in an increase in vascular permeability	C3a, C5a
Bone resorption (prostaglandin E_2-mediated)	??
Lysis of certain Gram negative bacteria	C5b, C6, C7, C8, C9
Destruction of host cells	C5b, C6, C7, C8, C9

The *complement system* has numerous critical functions in inflammation (see Table 5-4) and consists of at least 20 individual proteins which can interact with each other in a specific series of cascading reactions (Fig. 5-16). These proteins are normally present in an inactive precursor state in plasma or serum. They are activated and deposited in the tissues and gingival exudates during the development gingivitis and periodonitis (review: Schenkein 1982). Presumably, this translates into some protection for the host against microbial attack, but it may also result in local tissue damage as a consequence of the formation of pro-inflammatory mediators.

It is beyond the scope of this chapter to detail the mechanisms of complement activation; suffice it to say that this occurs via 2 major routes, the "classical" and the "alternative" pathways (Fig 5-16). Both proceed in an orderly, sequential fashion giving rise to proteolytic enzymes which cleave various complement components to form biologically-active peptide fragments. The *classical pathway* is typically initiated by the union of antigen with specific antibody (IgM and IgG_1, IgG_2 or IgG_3). The antigen may be represented by a constituent found on the surface of a target cell (e.g., microorganisms or host cells) or it may be a soluble or an extracellular factor (e.g., released microbial antigen, host basement membrane, collagen, etc). The *alternative (or "properdin") pathway* is activated by a wide variety of substances, including complex polysaccharides, endotoxin and other surface components of all intact Gram negative and some Gram positive bacteria, and by proteases discharged from neutrophils and macrophages. It is a more primitive line of defense when compared to the classical pathway by providing a mechanism of "recognizing" bacteria in the absence of an immune response.

The biological properties of the classical and alternative pathways are identical because both yield the same effector or terminal molecules as a consequence of C3,5,6,7,8,9 activation (Fig. 5-16; Table 5-4).

Activation of complement can directly damage bacteria or host cells because of the formation of the so-called "membrane attack complex", which consists of C5b, C6, C7, C8 and C9. The complex binds or fuses with phospholipids in the cell membrane of target cells to form ion channels causing profound alterations in membrane permeability, and osmotic lysis ensues. However, many microorganisms are resistant to complement-mediated lysis. This could be due, for example, to steric hindrance of C5b-9 binding to complement-susceptible sites on the outer membrane, to non-covalent associations of C5b-9 with other membrane components (thereby preventing insertion of C5b-9) or to the thick peptidoglycan layer in Gram positive organisms (which protects the inner membrane from complement attack). The non-cytolytic effects of complement are due to the formation of peptides derived primarily from limited proteolytic cleavage of C3 and C5. These peptides are released into the environment to interact with receptors on the surfaces of neighboring cells, including mast cells, neutrophils, macrophages and lymphocytes. This results in a wide variety of responses depending on the type of cell affected and accounts for most of the pro-inflammatory functions of the complement system (Table 5-4).

Arachidonic acid metabolites: prostaglandins and leukotrienes

Prostaglandins and leukotrienes are synthesized by leukocytes and other cells from arachidonic acid and have biological properties that are relevant to the inflammatory process (Fig. 5-17). Most arachidonic acid is esterified within membrane phospholipids and must first be released or hydrolysed from phospholipids in order to form prostaglandins and leukotrienes. In PMNs and macrophages this occurs primarily due to activation of phospholipase A_2 (which is largely localized within lysosomes), while in mast cells and platelets arachadonic acid is hydrolysed by phospholipase C. Corticosteroids inhibit phospholipase activation and thereby reduce the formation of prostaglandins and leukotrienes.

Upon release, arachidonic acid can be metabolized via at least 3 pathways:

1) the enzyme cyclooxygenase catalyses arachidonic acid, yielding various prostaglandins and thromboxanes;
2) arachidonic acid may be attacked by lipoxygenase, giving rise to leukotrienes;
3) arachadonic acid may be non-enzymatically converted by oxygen-derived radicals into chemotactic lipids (this will be mentioned again when the formation of active oxygen metabolites by leukocytes is discussed below).

Prostaglandins

Prostaglandins (PG) are 20-carbon unsaturated, hydroxylated fatty acids, identified by a letter of the alphabet (e.g., PGA, PGB, PGD, PGE, etc.) to designate the presence of various hydroxyl and ketone groups and unsaturated carbon atoms on the cyclopane portion of the molecule. Prostaglandins are subdivided further on the number of double bonds in the aliphatic side chains (e.g., PGE_1, PGE_2, etc). The prostaglandins appear to mediate numerous events in the inflammatory process (Weissmann 1980) (Table 5-5). In recent investigations elevated levels of PGE_2 were detected in inflamed gingival tissues and crevice fluids, especially from periodontal sites exhibiting recent attachment loss (Offenbacher, Odle & Van Dyke 1986). Thus, PGE_2 levels may be an indicator of disease activity. It is of interest that the formation of prostaglandins is suppressed by aspirin and other non-steroidal anti-inflammatory drugs (e.g., indomethacin) which inhibit cyclooxygenase activity. Evidence in humans and animals suggests that such drugs may reduce alveolar bone resorption in periodontal disease (see below).

Table 5-5

Potential roles of prostaglandins and leukotrienes in inflammation

Prostaglandins as modulators of inflammation
Mediate vasodilation
Act synergistically with histamine and bradykinin to increase vascular permeability
Produce hyperalgesia by sensitizing nerve endings to other agents
Play role in platelet adherence and release reactions (thrombosis)
Modulate T lymphocyte functions including inhibition of lymphokine production
Stimulate osteoclastic bone resorption
Pharmacological actions of leukotriene B_4
Vascular permeability (effect may be due to modulating PMN activity)
Promotes aggregation of PMNs
Increases adhesion of PMNs to vascular endothelial surface
Stimulates PMN chemotaxis and random migration (chemokinesis)
Enhances expression of C3b receptors on PMNs
Induces PMN lysosomal degranulation
Stimulates eosinophil chemotaxis
Enhances T-lymphocyte chemokinesis
Suppresses T-lymphocyte lymphocyte proliferation and lymphokine production

Leukotrienes

Lipoxygenases oxidize arachidonic acid to hydroperoxy products which may subsequently undergo metabolic reduction to form a series of monohydroxy-eicosatetraenoic acids (HETEs) and leukotrienes (LTs) (Fig. 5-17). Lipoxygenases from different cells vary in their substrate specificity and can insert a hydroperoxy group at the 5-, 12- or 15- carbon position on arachidonic acid. 5-Lipoxygenase activity appears to predominate in neutrophils, monocytes, eosinophils, lymphocytes and mast cells; thus, 5-lipoxygenase products may be especially relevant in inflammatory and immune reactions (Parker 1984). The initial step in the 5-lipoxygenase pathway is the formation of 5-hydroperoxy-eicosatetraenoic acid (5-HPETE): this

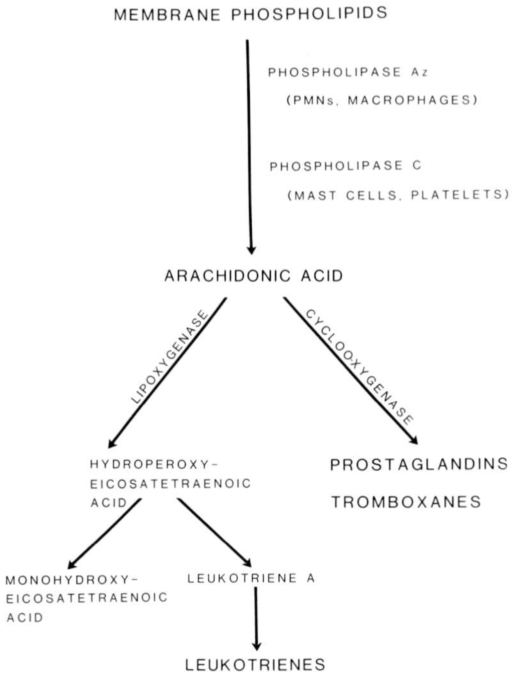

Fig. 5-17. *Simplified outline of prostaglandin and leukotriene production from arachidonic acid:* Following stimulation, arachidonic acid is released from cell membrane phospholipids by enzymatic hydrolysis mediated by phospholipases. Phospholipases are derived primarily from lysosomes and their activation can be impeded by corticosteroids. Arachiadonic acid is then converted to prostaglandins by cyclooxygenase (which is inhibited by nonsteroidal anti-inflammatory drugs), to leukotrienes by lipoxygenase and to chemotactic lipids by oxidative radicals.

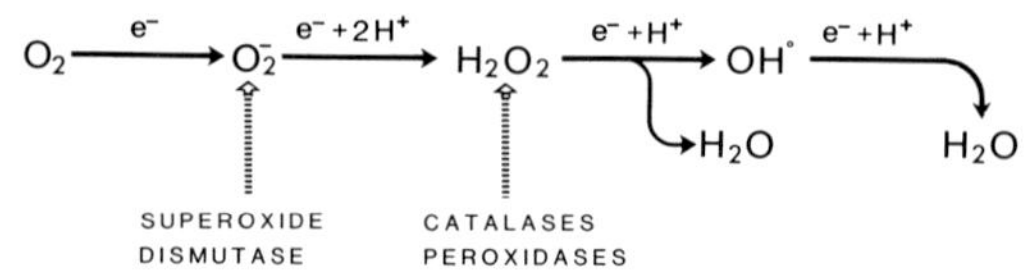

Fig. 5-18. *Simplified pathway of oxygen reduction by PMNs:* PMNs manufacture cytotoxic oxidants upon challenge by bacteria, immune complexes, complement C5a or other stimuli. This can occur even under surprisingly low oxygen tensions. For example, PMNs in 1% oxygen produce 70% and in 0.35% oxygen generate approximately 50% of superoxide radical when compared to PMNs in room air (Babior 1982). Thus, PMNs probably produce oxygen reactants even in the gingival crevice where reduced oxygen tensions are encountered. Oxidative reactants are catalytically scavenged by superoxide dismutases ($^-O_2$), catalases and peroxidases (H_2O_2). The efficient removal of $^-0_2$ and H_2O_2 by these enzymes would minimize $OH^•$ formation. In some microorganisms there may be a correlation between their ability to synthesize superoxide dismutase, catalase or peroxidase and their resistance to oxygen toxicity. However, most bacteria are killed by PMNs irrespective of whether they produce these enzymes: only a relatively few microbial species seem to be entirely unaffected by PMN oxidants.

molecule is unstable and is reduced by glutathione peroxidase to form 5-HETE and/or is converted into a family of leukotrienes containing a conjugated triene structure (LTA4, LTB4, LTC4, LTD4, LTE4). Of the lipoxygenase products discovered thus far, LTB4 seems to be the most potent in causing a variety of inflammatory alterations (Bhattacherjee & Eakins 1984). In general, there are fewer reports on lipoxygenase products in inflammatory exudates when compared to prostaglandins. In the past this was primarily due to the lack of sensitive and reliable assays for these agents, but new techniques have been developed and LTB4 activity will probably be detected in gingival crevice fluids during periodontal disease.

Oxygen radicals

Upon contact with bacteria (including several plaque organisms), microbial cell walls, immune complexes, complement peptides and a variety of other stimulants, neutrophils (and macrophages to a lesser extent) exhibit a sharp increase in oxygen consumption (Beaman & Beaman 1984). This is not related to respiratory or mitochondrial metabolism but in large measure reflects activation of NADPH oxidase, an enzyme present on the cell membrane. NADPH oxidase traps oxygen, which is then reduced in a series of steps to yield various radicals including: superoxide anion ($^-O_2$), hydroxyl radical ($OH^•$) and hydrogen peroxide (H_2O_2) (Fig 5-18). These substances are critical to the microbicidal activity of neutrophils (Table 5-6). Current evidence suggests that H_2O_2 is especially important. By itself, H_2O_2 has bacte-

Table 5-6

Antibacterial factors produced by neutrophils (PMNs)

Oxygen-dependent pathways

Reactive oxygen metabolities (H_2O_2, $^-O_2$, $OH^\bullet$)

When tested alone these reactants have limited microbicidal activities. Their mechanisms of action have not been completely resolved but may involve lipid peroxidation of the bacterial cell wall which could lead to inactivation of critical enzyme systems and/or to cross-linking of membrane proteins.

Myeloperoxidase system (myeloperoxidase + H_2O_2 + halide ions)

Myeloperoxidase is released from lysosomes into the phagosome and combines with H_2O_2 and chloride ions resulting in the formation of hypochlorous acid (HOCl). This acid is a powerful bactericidal agent.

Oxygen-independent pathways

Acid pH

The pH within the phagosome may be lowered to 4.0-6.0 due to lactate formation during glycolysis and the movement of protons and anions across the phagosome membrane. Many bacteria are intolerant to low pH.

Cationic proteins and peptides (e.g., "Bacterial permeability-increasing proteins")

Cationic proteins (rich in basic and hydrophobic amino acids) bind to microorganisms perturbing membrane permeability and transport mechanisms.

Lactoferrin

Lactoferrin binds and removes iron from the environment thereby interfering with iron uptake by bacteria.

Lysozyme

Lysozyme cleaves B-(1,4) linkages between repeating units of N-acetylmuramic acid and N-acetylglucosamine in bacterial cell wall peptidoglycans. Lysozyme alone does not appear to lyse most disease-causing bacteria. Its action may be facilitated by the disruption of the outer membrane of Gram negative organisms by antibody and complement and perhaps other factors, such as cationic proteins and cathepsin G.

Neutral proteases (elastase, collagenase, cathepsin G) and other lysosomal hydrolases

PMN and macrophage proteases may have microbicidal activity by virtue of their cationic nature. These enzymes also degrade bacterial cell walls and other components. Certain types of microbial cell walls are resistant to leukocyte proteases and are not readily broken down and removed following killing of phagocytosed organisms. Undigested bacterial "debris" may persist and trigger chronic inflammatory lesions and may conceivably represent a pathway for sustaining the inflammatory response in periodontal disease.

ricidal properties, but these are amplified in the presence of myeloperoxidase (derived from PMN granules) and halides (particularly Cl^-). It is likely that myeloperoxidase reacts with H_2O_2, producing a complex which oxidizes Cl^- to yield hypochlorous acid (HOCl). HOCl halogenates and/or oxidizes the surface of bacteria, which then undergo lysis. The significance of the production of oxidative reactants to antimicrobial defense is readily verified because patients with specific abnormalities in PMN oxygen metabolism appear to be more susceptible to certain bacterial (e.g., staphylococcal) and fungal (e.g., *Candida*) infections. These include, for example, individuals with an inherited deficiency in NADPH oxidase activity (chronic granulomatous disease). It is likely that PMN oxidative responses will be relevant to defense in the gingival pocket because these patients often present with very aggressive

Table 5-7

Potential functions of PMN oxygen radicals in inflammation
Killing of invading microorganisms
Damage to surrounding normal cells (e.g., fibroblasts, endothelial cells, erythrocytes)
Autodestruction of PMNs
Destruction of tumor cells
Depolymerization of structural matrix of tissues (e.g., proteoglycans, glycosaminoglycans and collagen)
Oxidation of arachidonic acid to produce chemotactic factor(s)
Inactivation of chemotactic factors
Suppression of protease inhibitor systems
Cytogenetic damage to eukaryotic cells

forms of periodontitis or stomatitis (Van Dyke, Levine & Genco 1985).

In addition to killing bacteria, oxygen radicals may have deleterious effects on the host because they can destroy eukaryotic cells (review: Fantone & Ward 1982). *In vitro* and *in vivo* studies suggest that these reactants injure erythrocytes, fibroblasts, vascular and pulmonary endothelial cells, as well as other cells. Moreover, there are reasons to suspect that they have other biological properties, such as the production of chemotactic lipids from arachidonic acid, inactivation of serum inhibitors of PMN proteases, and depolymerization of glycosaminoglycans, proteoglycans and collagen. Table 5-7 provides a summary of the possible pro-inflammatory potentials of oxygen-derived free radicals.

Neutral proteinases released by neutrophils and macrophages

Gingival inflammatory exudates are enriched with endogenous proteolytic enzymes derived from plasma and from cells within the lesion (Cimasoni 1983). The role of these enzymes in the pathogenesis of inflammatory injury has been the focus of countless studies for over 100 years. Metchnikoff and his contemporaries were the first to realize that neutrophils and macrophages were enriched with these "ferments" and appreciated that they contribute to the breakdown of numerous tissue substrates. Within the past 25 years our knowledge of the varied roles of leukocyte proteinases in inflammation has expanded dramatically, especially in regard to the "neutral proteases" (Havermann & Janoff 1978). These include elastase, collagenase and cathepsin G (a cationic, chymotrypsin-like enzyme). A representative list of their biological properties is given in Table 5-8. Obviously, the capacity of these proteases to degrade collagen and elastin may represent a primary pathway for initiating connective tissue breakdown. However, they also are able to digest microbial cell walls, attack immunoglobulins and proteoglycans, interact with the complement, kinin and clotting system and stimulate B lymphocytes (polyclonal activa-

Table 5-8

Potential importance of neutral proteases in inflammation (e.g., elastase, collagenase, cathepsin G)
Destruction of connective tissue components (e.g., collagen, elastin, basement membrane, proteoglycans, fibronectin)
Digestion of Gram positive and Gram negative bacteria
Production of vascular lesions (e.g, increase permeability and induce hemorrhage)
Alteration of host proteins (e.g., digestion of immunoglubulins)
Activation of alternative complement pathway
Generation of kinin-like peptides from kininogen
Procoagulant as well as anticoagulant activities
Stimulation of B lymphocyte proliferation and antibody production

tion). On the basis of these potentials it seems reasonable to suspect that they probably contribute to several pathways in gingival/periodontal inflammation. We still know relatively little about the control or inhibition of these proteases in gingival tissues. However, it has been suggested that a deficiency or dysfunction in one or more of the anti-protease systems may impede protease inactivation and elimination and thereby contribute to periodontal tissue destruction (Sandholm 1986).

Cytokines

Mediators produced by lymphocytes (lymphokines), monocytes and macrophages (monokines) and other cell types are collectively known as cytokines. Lymphoid cells dominate within the infiltrated connective tissues of established and advanced gingival lesions and this suggests that immunologic reactions may contribute to the pathogenesis of the inflammatory reaction. This will be considered in greater detail below; suffice it to mention that upon contact with antigen, sensitized T lymphocytes produce a variety of lymphokines which play a pivotal role in the progression of cell-mediated types of immune and hypersensitivity reactions (Table 5-9). It is also appropriate to note that T lymphocytes can be activated by mitogens and some lectins; thus, non-immunologic mechanisms can trigger lymphokine production. It is conceivable that surface-active factors derived from plaque may operate in an analogous fashion to stimulate these cells.

Table 5-9

Functional properties of lymphokines

Lymphokines affecting lymphocytes
- modulate antibody production by B cells
- stimulate proliferation of non-sensitized T-lymphocyte cells
- transfers specific delayed hypersensitivity reactions

Lymphokines affecting macrophages
- stimulate macrophage chemotaxis
- inhibit macrophage migration out of inflammatory lesion
- mediate macrophage activation
- induce and maintain monocyte growth *in vitro*

Lymphokines affecting PMNs
- promote chemotaxis and adhesivity
- restrict migration from inflammatory focus

Lymphokines affecting fibroblasts
- stimulate as well as inhibit chemotaxis
- modulate fibroblast proliferation and collagen synthesis

Lymphokines affecting other cells
- kill a variety of target cells including tumor cells
- modulate growth and differentiation of certain cells
- inhibit viral proliferation and augment activity of NK (natural killer) cells
- promote osteoclastic bone resorption
- procoagulant effect, decreasing clotting time

Neutrophils as mediators of gingival host defense

As outlined earlier, there is a constant traffic of neutrophils (PMNs) into the gingival tissues during all phases in the development of gingivitis. The bulk of PMNs move into the gingival sulcus/pocket in response to chemotactic factors. These include bacterial peptides as well as host-derived substances (e.g., complement peptides, leukotrienes, lymphokines, fibrin peptides). PMNs constitute over 90% of the leukocytes that emigrate into the gingival sulcus/pocket, where they come into direct contact with the subgingival microbiota. In fact, it is common to find PMNs palisading on the outer surface of plaque, seeming to form a barrier against bacterial penetration of underlying tissues. Considerable evidence indicates that PMNs are needed to defend the gingival region because patients with PMN dysfunctions often present with exaggerated forms of stomatitis and periodontitis (Van Dyke, Levine & Genco 1985). This includes individuals with qualitative (defects in the capacity of PMNs to re-

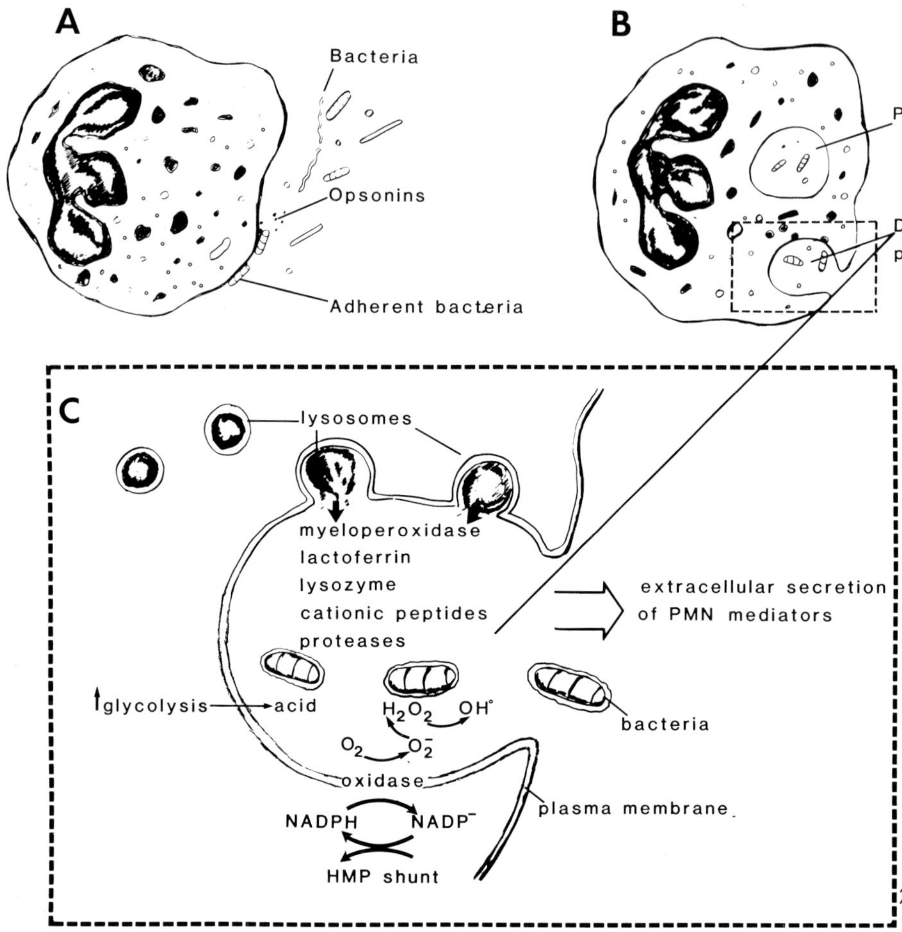

Fig. 5-19. *Major events in the encounter between PMNs and invading microorganisms:*

A. Once PMNs emigrate from the microcirculation, they migrate toward bacteria under the influence of chemotactic factors. Upon contact PMNs adhere to the organisms (many types of bacteria must be opsonized to facilitate PMN adherence and phagocytosis).

B. Coincident with adhesion, PMNs begin to phagocytose these organisms. This is accomplished as the plasma membrane flows around and then invaginates to internalize attached organisms which are now contained within phagosomes. Several bacteria can be phagocytosed simultaneously by the PMN.

C. As these events occur PMNs demonstrate dramatic metabolic alterations including: an elevation in glycolysis, a marked rise in oxygen consumption and increased glucose utilization by the hexose monophosphate shunt. Glycolytic metabolism of glucose provides the energy required by phagocytosis and also results in a drop in intracellular pH due to the formation of lactate. The oxidative burst is largely the result of NADPH oxidase activity (an enzyme associated with the cell membrane), which oxidizes NADPH to NADP and results in the reduction of oxygen to various free radicals. These oxidants ($^-O_2$, H_2O_2, $OH^\bullet$) are released into the phagosome to kill bacteria. The hexose monophosphate shunt provides for the regeneration of NADPH.

At the same time, lysosomes are mobilized toward the developing phagosome and fuse with the phagosome membrane, giving rise to a phagolysosome. Lysosomal antimicrobial compounds (myeloperoxidase, lysozyme, lactoferrin, cationic proteins, etc) are discharged into the vacuole. The combination of oxidative and non-oxidative (acid pH, lysosomal agents) pathways explains how PMNs kill ingesed organisms. Lysozyme and neutral proteases (particularly elastase) derived from lysosomes digest and dispose of the dead organisms.

Before invagination is completed, biologically-active products can be released from the phagosome into the external environment. These agents play a role in extracellular killing of microorganisms but also adversely affect surrounding host cells and tissue structures.

Table 5-10

Potential strategies of the subgingival microbiota against neutrophils (PMNs)

Destruction of PMNs
(e.g., *A. actinomycetemcomitans* leukotoxin)

Inhibition of PMN chemotaxis
(e.g., *Capnocytophaga*)

Impairment of PMN adherence and phagocytosis
(e.g., polysaccharide capsule of black pigmented *Bacteroides*)

Degeneration of opsonizing antibodies and complement peptides
(e.g., *Bacteroides* and *Capnocytophaga* spp.)

Inhibition of oxygen radical activity
(e.g., superoxide dismutase and catalase of *B. gingivalis* and *A. actinomycetemcomitans*)

Inhibition of lysosomal degranulation
(e.g., *Treponema denticola*)

Degradation of lactoferrin
(e.g., *B. gingivalis*)

Escape from phagolysosome
(no examples of plaque organisms presently availble)

Resistance to PMN digestion
(no examples of plaque organisms presently availble)

spond to infection) or with quantitative (low numbers of PMNs) neutrophil abnormalities. As described in Chapter 6, a subtle abnormality in PMN chemotaxis may help to explain why some children and young adults are at risk to develop rapidly progressive periodontitis. The mechanisms of PMN antimicrobial defense of the dentogingival region in otherwise healthy individuals, however, are not entirely understood.

PMNs generate and release a series of compounds that explain how these cells kill microorganisms (Table 5-6). These agents become available as a consequence of the oxidative burst (see above) and lysosomal degranulation during phagocytosis of most Gram positive or Gram negative bacteria (Fig. 5-19). In addition, these substances are liberated into the external environment to interact with non-phagocytosed bacteria. Thus, microbial kill in the gingival pocket may occur inside as well as outside the PMN; however, the relative importance of either mechanism in gingival defense has yet to be determined. In addition to killing bacteria, crevicular PMNs may also impede colonization of bacteria by interfering with the ability of certain microorganisms to adhere onto host tissues or other organisms (Wilton & Jarvis 1981).

It is conceivable that potential periodontal pathogens have developed strategies against PMNs, some of which are listed in Table 5-10. Of these, *A. actinomycetemcomitans* has devised one of the most effective ways to evade PMNs: these organisms produce a potent leukotoxin which destroys PMNs and macrophages (review: Taichman et al. 1984). It is possible that local depletion of PMNs during early phases of infection may represent one mechanism to allow *A. actinomycetemcomitans* to establish a firm foothold in the dentogingival region.

The gingival sulcus/pocket must represent an exceedingly formidable environment for PMNs because they are confronted by and presumably respond to pathogens as well as organisms with little or no virulence potential. PMNs probably furnish an umbrella type of protection directed against all or most bacteria which colonize the pocket. This may be an effective strategy under "normal" circumstances, but it may be "wasteful" or inefficient if the pocket is colonized by an especially aggressive organism. Under these conditions, it may theoretically be preferable for the PMN to direct its action specifically against the invader as opposed to "irrelevant" organisms. This can be realized in other types of infections where PMNs contend with only one organism. Even the availability of specific opsonizing antibodies may not augment the PMN's ability to select these pathogens in the pocket because non-aggressive organisms are

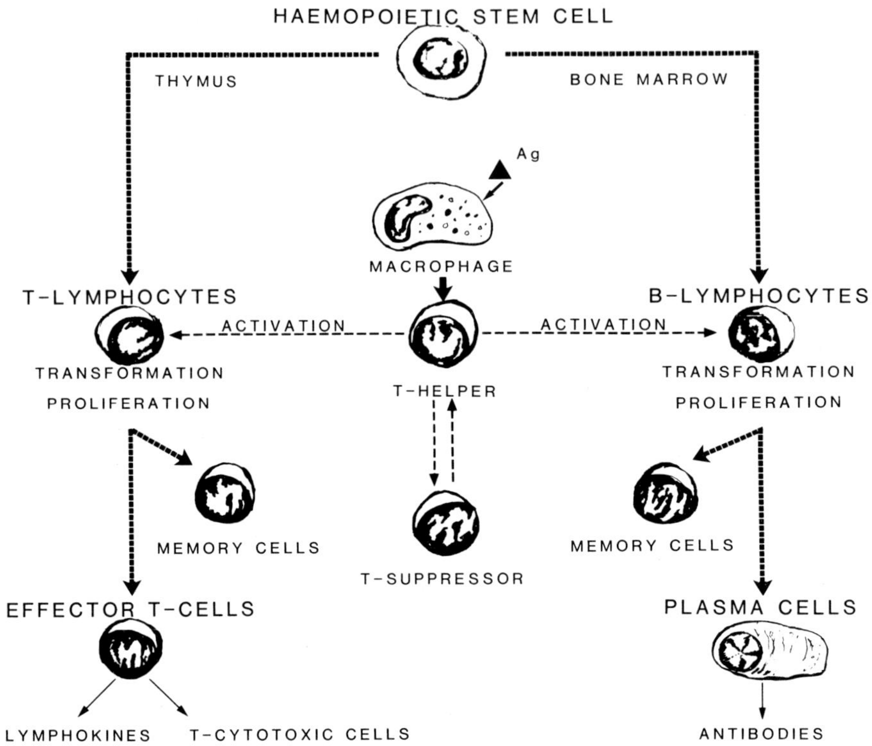

Fig. 5-20. Schematic illustration of immune reactions.

probably also opsonized for phagocytosis. Thus, when speculating about the mechanisms of PMN defense in response to plaque, one must necessarily bear in mind that this occurs in a very unique, poorly understood environment.

Neutrophils as mediators of tissue injury in periodontal inflammation

The possible contribution of PMNs to gingival inflammatory injury has been the subject of several investigations (review: Taichman et al. 1984). As PMNs emigrate out of the microcirculation and move through the tissues, they are probably constantly secreting pro-inflammatory agents into the environment (Freedman et al. 1968). These substances include lysosomal hydrolases, prostaglandins, leukotrienes, and oxygen radicals. The stimuli which provoke PMN release reactions include: intact bacteria, bacterial cell walls, bacterial toxins, immune complexes, complement (C5a) and other chemotactic peptides. Under experimental conditions one can show that PMN reactions contribute to gingival injury. To illustrate, topical application of PMN lysosomal extracts onto the gingival margin promotes an increase in vascular permeability and leukocyte migration in experimental animals (Kahnberg & Hellden 1977). Further, short-term reduction of circulating neutrophils (by cytotoxic drugs or anti-neutrophil antiserum) is accompanied by a decrease in the clinical signs of gingivitis in dogs (Attstrom et al. 1971, Attstrom & Schroeder 1979, Rylander et al. 1975). Finally, intradermal injections of plaque produce more local tissue damage in normal as compared to neutropenic rabbits (Taichman, Freedman & Uriuhara 1966). Normal rabbits exhibit abscess formation at the injection sites; by contrast, neutropenic animals seem to have less injury in the skin *but succumb to overwhelming sepsis.* These observations underscore that the host pays a price at the local level in order to prevent plaque organisms from disseminating throughout the body.

Page & Schroeder (1982) have proposed that there are two functional PMN compartments in the gingival environment: one within the tissues and the other in the pocket. They suggest that crevicular PMNs serve principally as defensive elements because pro-inflammatory products released from leukocytes in this location may largely be washed from the pocket into the oral cavity. On the other hand, PMN activation and discharge within the connective tissues or in the junctional epithelium would have the potential to harm the host. This might occur if PMN movement into the pocket was impeded and the cells accumulated in the tissues, eventually overloading local inhibitory systems which normally protect the tissues against PMN assault. If this hypothesis is correct, it may provide a reasonable explanation of one of the mechanisms through which an "acute burst" of disease activity may occur.

Immune reactions in the pathogenesis of gingival inflammation

Protection of the host by the immune response to plaque bacteria

Most of the substances produced and released by plaque microorganisms are antigenic, eliciting both cell-mediated and antibody-mediated immune reactions (Fig. 5-20). It is common to find that patients with existing diseases have antibodies and/or sensitized lymphocytes against different plaque bacteria in serum (systemic immune response) and within gingival lesions (local immune response). The immune response to many of these organisms is probably instrumental in defending the host against the plaque microbiota. It is beyond the scope of this chapter to detail the potential mechanisms of immunological defense in the dentogingival region. Both systemic and local antibody synthesis are activated in response to plaque antigens; local antibody synthesis by lymphoid cells may conceivably be more relevant in gingival defense than the systemic immune response. The reason for this speculation stems from the finding that gingival exudates usually contain higher concentrations of antibodies against specific plaque organisms when compared to serum. Thus, local antibody production may provide a more enriched or "customized" antibody cocktail in the immediate vicinity of the infection.

It is important, however, to acknowledge that there is very little precise information to explain if and how the immune response in humans actually defends against specific periodontopathic bacteria. As mentioned, most periodontal patients respond immunologically to plaque antigens, but this does not actually prove that the response is relevant to host defense or that it is successful in minimizing infection. For one thing, the dynamics of the immune response have not been defined, nor whether the response is directed against critical microbial virulence factors or mechanisms. Until this information is acquired it will not be possible to determine whether an aberration(s) in immunity contributes to the onset or continuation of infection. Thus, while the centrality of the immune system in gingival defense is acknowledged, the unequivocal proof that is required to support this theory is lacking.

Let us assume that the immune response provides protection against the development of periodontal disease and that as a consequence periodontal patients suffer from an inadequate or inappropriate immune response to gingival infection. This could be expressed in several ways; only a few possibilities will be considered below (a more extensive review has recently been published by Shenker(1987)).

a) *The host must recognize the organism as being foreign in order to mount an immune response against the invader*: It is conceivable that specific determinants of microbial pathogenicity are not identified by the immune system because their antigenic structure is similar to or closely mimics that of the host. Thus, certain plaque antigens may escape detection because the host is "tolerant" to them. It is also conceivable that some plaque organisms fail to provoke an immune response because they become coated by "irrelevant" host constituents in the gingival pocket. Under these circumstances the bacteria may be "disguised" and fail to be recognized as foreign.

b) *Some microorganisms may suppress the immune response*: The immune response against specific microorganisms or microbial products may be modulated by immunosuppressive factors elaborated by plaque bacteria. For example, the *A. actinomycetemcomitans* leukotoxin destroys monocytes which are essential in the regulation of the immune response. This microorganism also produces a non-cytotoxic factor which activates T suppressor lymphocytes (CD8 positive cells) which then depress antibody production. Spirochetes suppress immune reactivity *in vitro* by activating macrophages to secrete prostaglandins which in turn down-regulate lymphoid cells. These as well as other bacterial immunosuppressive factors may not only depress lymphoid function to homologous microorganisms but also modulate immune reactivity to other opportunistic bacteria. The effect may be long-lasting or short-lived, but even a temporary retardation in the response may be sufficient to allow large numbers of bacteria to populate the dentogingival region. In general, the immune response is more likely to provide effective protection during earlier as opposed to later phases of infection. Thus, even if the immune response is eventually restored, it may not be able to contend with "antigen overload". This could explain why plaque and disease persist in the face of a vigorous immune response; in fact, an especially aggressive immune reaction may be the cause of tissue damage (see below).

c) *Some bacteria may neutralize or degrade antibodies*: Once secreted, antibodies may be functionally unavailable to protect the host because some microorganisms, such as *B. gingivalis* and certain other black-pigmented *Bacteroides*, produce proteolytic enzymes which cleave and inactivate antibodies (as well as complement components). In addition, some organisms may constantly shed antigen into the extracellular environment. The free antigen may bind antibody and block its interaction with antigen on the microbial surface. This might, for example, minimize the chance of these organisms being destroyed by the complement system or being opsonized for phagocytosis.

d) *Some plaque bacteria may exhibit antigenic variation:* Certain infections endure because the microorganisms are able to elude the immune response by varying their antigenic structure. This phenomenon has been extensively studied in chronic protozoan (such as the African trypanosomes) and malarial infections. It also appears to be operating in relapsing fever due to spirochetes, *Borrelia recurrentis* (Turner 1980). Antigenic variation is an attractive concept because it may help to explain how some organisms persist in the gingival pocket. Here, the host responds immunologically to microbial challenge but the response is not effective because the bacteria mutate, constantly expressing new virulence-associated antigens. As a consequence, the immune response may be one step behind the microbe's ability to generate new antigenic determinants and infection continues in spite of a vigorous immune response.

e) *The host is continually infected with different periodontopathic bacteria:* As postulated earlier, periodontal lesions are not likely to be caused by one microorganism or one virulence mechanism but probably reflect successive contributions by different etiologic vectors. One set of bacteria may initiate disease and cause "significant" injury before being contained by the immune response. The lesion may remain quiescent until another group of pathogens colonizes the area, setting off a new round of disease activity until they are neutralized by the immune response. This cycle may be repeated over and over again and with time result in extensive, cumulative tissue damage at the affected site. In other words, periodontal lesions might be due to successive waves of infections, and the immune response primarily reflects protection against microorganisms and antigens that are no longer pertinent to the continued progression of the lesion.

Tissue injury by the immune response to plaque microorganisms

As in other aspects of the inflammatory reaction, the immune response against plaque organisms may cause damage to the gingiva and the periodontium. In fact, an especially vigorous or exaggerated immune response may do more harm than good. In this context, immune responses injure the host by one or more mechanisms:

1) immune complex,
2) immune cytotoxic,
3) antibody- dependent cellular cytotoxicity,
4) anaphylactic and
5) cell-mediated (delayed) hypersensitivity.

Immune complex-mediated inflammatory injury

Antibodies to various microbial constituents are probably available to interact with their respective antigens in the gingival environment. These interactions could, theoretically, trigger immune complex (Arthus type) inflammatory reactions in the connective tissues and the junctional epithelium. Immune complexes consisting of IgG or IgM antibodies activate the complement system leading to the formation of peptides which alter vascular permeability and attract PMNs. As PMNs accumulate in these areas, they phagocytose antigen-antibody complexes and in the process release oxygen radicals, prostaglandins and lysosomal products, thereby damaging neighboring cells and structures. A comparable series of events has been shown to result in periodontal injury (in experimental animals). For example, Ranney & Zander (1970) demonstrated that topical application of an antigen to the gingival sulcus in monkeys resulted in the development of an immune reaction in the gingival tissue. If antigen applications were continued for prolonged periods of time, an intense Arthus-type inflammatory reaction ensued. The reaction was associated with loss of connective tissue attachment, apical proliferation of junctional and dentogingival epithelium and loss of alveolar bone. This experiment demonstrates that immune complex-type reactions may conceivably be related to the destruction of the periodontium in human periodontal disease.

Immune cytotoxic inflammatory tissue injury

Immune cytotoxic reactions result in the destruction of host (target) cells as a consequence of complement activation. In this case, IgG or IgM antibodies are produced which interact with antigens on the surface of target cells. As described earlier, this interaction triggers the complement cascade with subsequent formation of the "membrane attack complex" and the host "accidentally" destroys his own cells. On a theoretical basis this could occur in gingival lesions under the following circumstances: a) Bacterial antigens adsorb onto the membrane

Table 5-11

Representative products secreted by activated macrophages

Product	Function
Collagenase, elastase	Inflammatory tissue degradation
Lysosomal acid hydrolases	Inflammatory tissue degradation
Cytolytic proteinase	Tumoricidal
Complement components	Antimicrobial, inflammatory
Lysozyme	Antimicrobial
Fibronectin	Opsonic, adhesive protein
Procoagulant factor	Coagulation, tissue repair
Interferon	Antiviral defense
Interleukin 1	Activation of lymphocytes, inflammatory
Fibroblast and endothelial cell mitogens	Tissue repair
Oxidative metabolities	Microbicidal, tumoricidal
Prostaglandin E1	Inflammatory, immunoregulatory
Prostaglandin E2	Inflammatory, bone resorption
Leukotriene C	Inflammatory, immunoregulatory
12-Hydroxyeicosatetranoic acid	Inflammatory, immunoregulatory

of host cells, allowing antibodies to interact with these antigens on the cell surface; b) Bacterial antigens may closely mimic the structure of host membrane antigens giving rise to antibodies which cross-react with the surface of target cells; c) An immune aberration produced during the course of long-standing infection may lead to the production of antibodies directed against the host's own membrane components (i.e., an "autoimmune" type of cellular injury). It is theoretically possible (but yet to be substantiated) that any of these processes operates during the course of periodontal disease.

Antibody-dependent cellular cytotoxicity

Antibody-dependent cellular cytotoxicity (AD CC) results in target-cell destruction by macrophages, neutrophils or by subpopulations of lymphocytes (sometimes referred to as K(killer) cells). As in immune cytotoxic reactions, IgG or IgM antibodies interact with antigens on host cell membranes. These antigens may be integral components of the membrane or adsorbed microbial antigens. Subsequently, leukocytes with receptors for the Fc region of IgG or IgM bind to these antibodies on the cell surface, resulting in activation of the effector leukocyte, which then damages the target cell. Here again, there is no evidence that such events occur in periodontal disease, but the possibility is certainly interesting and worth keeping in mind.

Anaphylactic type of inflammatory injury

As mentioned previously, IgE antibodies specifically directed against oral microorganisms have been found in patients with periodontal disease (Nisengard 1974). These antibodies may sensitize mast cells for anaphylactic-type hypersensitivity reactions, which result in the release of vascoactive compounds. Although anaphylactic reactions are usually considered to be harmful to the host, they sometimes appear to have beneficial consequences. For example, in certain types of parasitic infections the expulsion of worms from the gastrointestinal tract is associated with an IgE-dependent reaction leading to diarrhea. It is conceivable that an IgE-mediated increase in vascular permeability in the gingiva represents part of the host's attempt to remove bacteria or their products from the gingival environment.

Cell-mediated (delayed hypersensitivity) immune reactions in inflammatory tissue injury

Periodontal lesions exhibit many of the classical microscopic features of so-called cell-mediated inflammatory diseases. These features include: a) infiltration of the lesion by mononuclear leukocytes (macrophages, lymphocytes and plasma cells); b) destruction of normal connective tissues; c) replacement of destroyed cells and tissues by proliferating fibroblasts and small blood vessels (fibrosis). Tissue destruction and fibrosis in delayed hypersensitivity appear to be largely mediated by T lymphocytes and macrophages which elaborate a variety of effector molecules (Tables 5-4 & 5-11). These mediators have pro-inflammatory functions and also modulate connective tissue metabolism, resulting in destruction as well as formation of excessive amounts of connective tissue matrices (review: Wahl 1986). The interplay of lymphocytes and macrophages represents a very important area for research in explaining the pathogenesis of established and advanced stages of periodontal disease, but at present there is only a very limited understanding of the molecular mechanisms to explain how these cells function to protect as well as damage the periodontium.

Numerous studies demonstrate that periodontal patients have circulating lymphocytes which are sensitized to substances originating from subgingival plaque organisms (Ivanyi & Lehner 1970, Lang & Smith 1977, Reed et al. 1976). Some experiments seem to suggest that a correlation exists between the severity of periodontal disease and the number of sensitized lymphocytes; however, this association has not been confirmed in other studies. In any event, it is likely that periodontal lesions contain subpopulations of T cells which have been sensitized and are responding to different plaque antigens (O'Neill, Woodson & Mackler 1982, O'Neill & Woodson 1986). Sensitized T lymphocytes are produced following initial exposure of the lymphoid system to antigens, and upon reexposure to these antigens they respond by proliferating and synthesizing lymphokines. It is clear that lymphokines serve as signals which stimulate, inhibit or even kill numerous types of cells (Table 5-9). The biochemical properties of lymphokines have not been fully defined and some of their different functions are probably mediated by the same protein molecule. In addition to sensitized lymphocytes, delayed hypersensitivity lesions contain non-sensitized lymphocytes which probably form part of the inflammatory cell infiltrate in periodontal disease. They may also produce lymphokines when stimulated by mitogenic substances released either by the subgingival microbiota or by other cells in the inflammatory reaction.

The participation of macrophages is crucial to the development of cell-mediated hypersensitivity reactions. Upon being recruited into inflammatory lesions, macrophages become activated under the influence of lymphokines and other substances, such as endotoxin and bacterial cell walls. When compared to resting cells, activated macrophages adhere more avidly to various substrates, phagocytose and kill bacteria more efficiently and also acquire cytotoxic properties enabling them to destroy tumor as well as other eukaryotic target cells. As shown in Table 5-11, activated macrophages synthesize and secrete numerous products which have wide-ranging biological potentials. These include hydrolytic enzymes, complement components, binding components (fibronectin), oxygen metabolites, arachidonic acid

Table 5-12

Factors present in diseased gingiva which stimulate *in vitro* bone resorption

Soluble extracts of inflamed tissues (factors unidentified)
Lipopolysaccharides (endotoxins) of Gram negative organisms
Lipoteichoic acids and muramyl dipeptides of Gram positive organisms
Non-endotoxin substance of *Actinobacillus actinomycetemcomitans*
"Amphipathic factor" from *Actinomyces viscosus*
Prostaglandin E_2
IL1 ("osteoclast activating factor")
Activated complement components (??)

metabolites and monokines (e.g., interleukin 1). Lysosomal enzymes, collagenase and elastase probably facilitate extracellular breakdown of the connective tissue matrix while prostaglandins and monokines have a multiplicity of effects on the growth and activity of other cells, including T and B lymphocytes, fibroblasts, angioblasts, osteoblasts and osteoclasts.

Polyclonal activation of the immune response as a mechanism of periodontal injury: It has been mentioned that mitogenic factors may play a role in the pathogenesis of periodontal disease by triggering lymphocyte proliferation and production of lymphokines (T cells) or antibodies (B cells). Endotoxin and non-endotoxic bacterial components, as well as proteases released by PMNs or macrophages, have mitogenic properties. Mitogens do not operate as antigenic signals; instead they act as non-specific stimuli to provoke polyclonal reactions in which diverse as opposed to specific clones of lymphocytes are responding. If mitogens operate *in situ* they could theoretically cause an overproduction of antibodies and/or lymphokines in gingival tissues. This might provide some enhanced resistance to infection but more probably it is liable to have undesirable consequences (Clagett & Engel 1978). For instance, hypersecretion of lymphokines could adversely affect tissue homeostasis. Likewise, excessive production of antibodies could result in extensive formation of immune complexes and inappropriate activation of the complement system and PMNs to generate pro-inflammatory mediators. It is also conceivable that persistent polyclonal activation could lead to exhaustion of local immune reactivity so that the host is impaired from quickly responding to specific antigenic challenge from infecting pathogens. Here, the immune system may be depleted of its antigen-reactive B cells and considerable time may be required to repopulate the tissues with stem cells. Finally, although the evidence is very tenuous, it may also be possible for polyclonal activation to result in the induction of "self-reactive" lymphocytes giving rise to autoimmune phenomena. It is apparent, but still to be proven, that mitogenic substances could represent vectors in explaining some of the pathological features of periodontal disease.

Alveolar bone resorption in periodontal disease

Loss of alveolar bone is a critical feature of destructive periodontal disease. Most likely, bone is lost primarily as a consequence of osteoclast activity but may also result from reduced or impaired osteogenic activity. Table 5-12 presents a list of substances which have been extracted from or identified in periodontal lesions and which promote *in vitro* bone resorption. Osteoclast function may be modulated by factors derived from the plaque microbiota and/or from inflammatory or resident tissue cells (reviews: Haussmann, Nair & Dziak 1982, Goldhaber & Rabadjija 1982, Sandberg 1982). Based on current information prostaglandin E probably plays an important role in alveolar bone resorption by regulating osteoclast activity and/or by affecting the synthesis of IL1 ("osteoclast activating factor") by lymphocytes. For example, dogs treated with indomethacin (which inhibits cylooxygenase activity) suffer less bone loss in experimental periodontal lesions (Nyman, Schroeder & Lindhe 1979). In addition, Feldman et al. (1983) have reported that humans on long-term, non-steroidal anti-inflammatory drugs have reduced interproximal bone loss when compared to matched controls. These, as well as other studies, indicate that alveolar bone loss associated with periodontal disease may be retarded by anti-inflammatory agents. This does not mean that such drugs should be employed in treating the vast majority of periodontal patients. In most instances, one should strive to eliminate and control the cause of periodontal disease (i.e., microbial plaque) as opposed to treating one of the symptoms of the disease process.

Pathogenesis of the "acute burst" of disease activity

In previous sections of this chapter various ways were considered whereby microorganisms and the inflammatory response could adversely affect the status of the periodontium. Currently, there is a great deal of interest in explaining the pathogenesis of the acute burst of tissue damage that seems to be a feature of some periodontal lesions. For example, periods of active destruction may represent a time when the host is confronted by organisms which are capable of evading or interfering with gingival defense systems. At the other end of the continuum, active destruction may be precipitated by an overly aggressive or inappropriate host response to microbial stimulation. In truth, a great deal of research will be required before it will be possible to adequately explain the basis for active periodontal destruction.

From a hypothetical point of view, specific microorganisms may promote bacterial as well as host-mediated injury. To illustrate this view, *A. actinomycetemcomitans* will be discussed as a prototype model of gingival infection. When *A. actinomycetemcomitans* colonizes the sulcus it may destroy PMNs and monocytes/macrophages, thereby impairing a frontline defense mechanism. Moreover, the disintegration of PMNs in the gingival sulcus and within the tissues also results in wholesale discharge of lysosomal products into the environment, and this may produce considerable damage to surrounding structures. The destruction of monocytes/macrophages may also have an effect on the local immune response because these cells are necessary for antibody production against certain microbial antigens. In addition, *A. actinomycetemcomitans* produces an immunosuppressive factor which activates T suppressor cells. The net effect may allow *A. actinomycetemcomitans*, as well as other potential parasites, to proliferate within the crevice and may even permit microbial invasion into the underlying connective tissues. This period of unbridled microbial aggression would represent

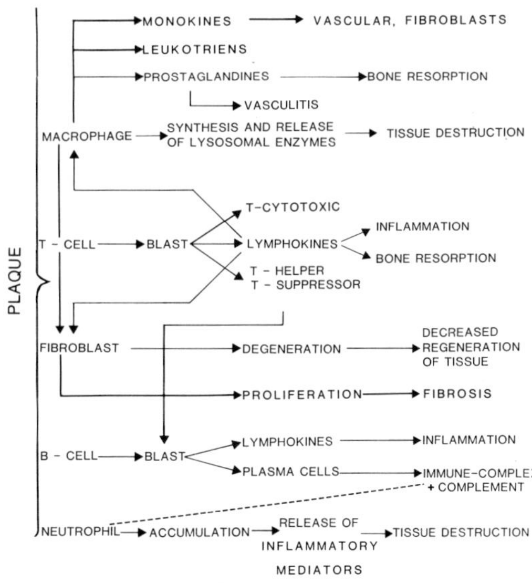

Fig. 5-21. Schematic illustration depicting the interaction between dental plaque and the immune system and the effects of this interaction on cells and tissues.

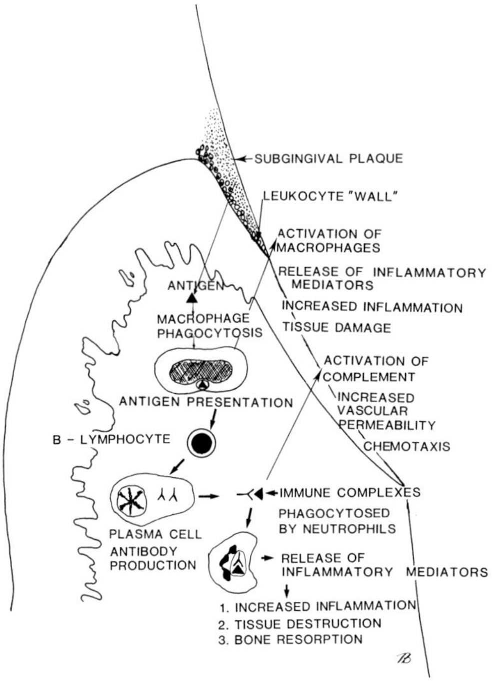

Fig. 5-22. Schematic illustration of possible effects of antigen/antibody reactions on gingival tissue. Antigens from dentogingival plaque enter the connective tissue through the junctional epithelium. In the connective tissue, the antigen is phagocytosed by macrophages, which alter the antigens into a form recognizable by the B-lymphocytes *(Recognition)*. The B-lymphocytes are stimulated to proliferate and develop into plasma cells which produce antibodies directed against the penetrating antigen. Antigen/antibody complexes are formed and activate complement which in turn induces increased vascular permeability and chemotaxis of leukocytes. Neutrophils phagocytose the immune complexes *(Elimination)* and during this process release various mediators into the surrounding tissue. Increased inflammation, tissue destruction and bone resorption can result. Activated B-lymphocytes and macrophages also release different mediators which may promote inflammation and tissue damage.

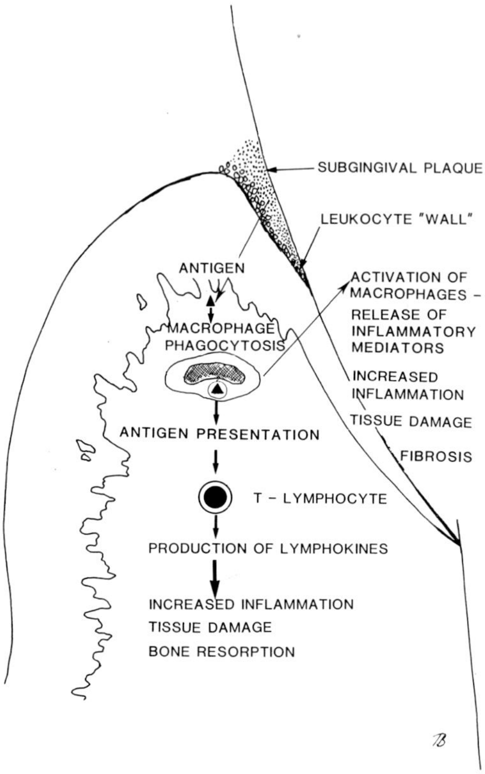

Fig. 5-23. Schematic illustration of possible effects of cell mediated immunity on the gingival tissue. Antigens from subgingival plaque penetrate into the connective tissue through the junctional epithelium. Macrophages phagocytose the antigen and alter it to a form recognizable by the immune system (Recognition). The T-lymphocytes are stimulated to proliferate and release lymphokines. Such lymphokines may cause increased inflammation, tissue damage and bone resorption. Activation of the macrophages also leads to release of mediators which cause increased inflammation, tissue damage, bone loss and fibrosis (compare Fig. 5-22).

the active phase of tissue destruction where injury is mediated by virulence factors originating from the infecting organisms as well as pro-inflammatory products released by the host. Eventually, the host's immune response is restored so that the leukotoxin is neutralized and an equilibrium is established, where PMNs, antibodies as well as other defensive functions prevent or minimize further assault by *A. actinomycetemcomitans*. At this juncture, the lesion enters into the quiescent phase where tissue damage and repair are balanced so as to prevent further progression of the disease process. The balance may be upset and another burst of tissue destruction may be triggered by a combination of one or more of these circumstances: a) *A. actinomycetemcomitans* mutates to acquire new virulence potentials; b) new pathogens gain access to the gingival sulcus; c) the intensity of the host's immune and/or non-immune inflammatory response is out of proportion to the insult originating from the subgingival microflora. The initiation of periodontal disease by other types of periodontal pathogens besides *A. actinomycetemcomitans* may involve similar or totally different pathogenic steps.

Concluding remarks

It is still not possible to entirely account for the pathogenesis of periodontal disease. The key development up to now has been the recognition that most, if not all, forms of periodontal disease are the consequence of microbial infections of the gingival sulcus/pocket (Fig. 5-21, 5-22, 5-23 and 5-24). This provides a starting point for investigating the pathogenesis of these disorders, but at this time one can only speculate on how these organisms actually hurt the host.

The purpose of this chapter was to provide concepts that may help to explain how plaque organisms contribute to the disease process. Various possibilities were considered: these as well as other ideas need to be confirmed, extended, modified or rejected by future research. Periodontal disease is a very complex, multifactorial infection in which the microbiota as well as the inflammatory reactions of the host contribute to the destruction of the periodontium. Individual lesions undergo continuous change in terms of the nature and outcome of local host-parasite confrontations. It would be unrealistic to believe that it will be possible to completely unravel or understand the complexities of these infections in the immediate future.

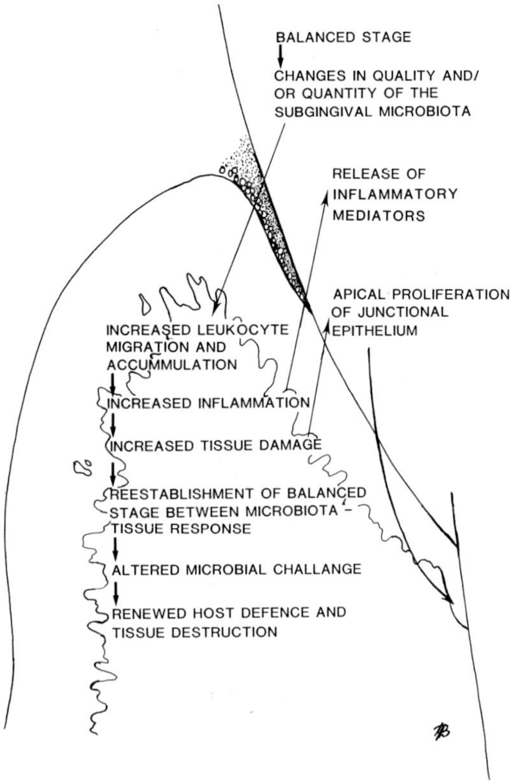

Fig. 5-24. Schematic illustration of a burst of progression in periodontal disease. The gingival tissue is in a balanced state with the microbiota in the plaque. A change in quantity and/or quality occurs in the sub-gingival microbiota. This results in an enhanced (acute) inflammatory response. The reaction counteracts the bacterial activity but also results in tissue damage. Destruction of the collagen fibers apical to the junctional epithelium enables it to further proliferate apically on the root surface.

However, sophisticated biochemical, immunological, and genetic approaches are now beginnning to be applied to the study of periodontal disease and will provide molecular insights into the microbial and host determinants of pathogenicity. This promises to open up new and exciting avenues to more effectively prevent, diagnose and treat these diseases.

References

Attstrom, R. (1971). Studies on neutrophil polymorphonuclear leukocytes at the dento-gingival junction in gingival health and disease. *Journal of Periodontial Research*, Supplement 8.

Attstrom, R., Graf-de Beer, M & Schroeder, H.E. (1975). Clinical and histological characterization of normal gingiva in dogs. *Journal of Periodontal Research* **10**, 115-127.

Attstrom, R. & Schroeder, H.E. (1979). Effect of experimental neutropenia on initial gingivitis in dogs. *Scandinavian Journal of Dental Research* **87**, 7-23.

Attstrom, R., Tynelius-Bratthall, G. & Egelberg, J. (1971). Effects of experimental leukopenia on gingival inflammation in dogs. II. Induction of leukopenia by heterologous anti-neutrophil serum. *Journal of Periodontal Research* **7**, 200-210.

Axelsson, P. & Lindhe, J. (1978). Effect of controlled oral hygiene procedures on caries and periodontal disease in adults. *Journal of Clinical Periodontology* **5**, 133-151.

Axelsson, P. & Lindhe, J. (1981). The significance of maintenance care in the treatment of periodontal disease. *Journal of Clinical Periodontology* **8**, 281-295.

Babior, B.M. (1982). The role of oxygen in microbial killing by phagocytes. In: *Pathology of Oxygen*, ed. Autor, A.P., pp 45-53. Academic Press, New York.

Beaman, L. & Beaman, B.L. (1984). The role of oxygen and its derivatives in microbial pathogenesis and host defense. *Annual Reviews of Microbiology* **38**, 27-48.

Bhattacherjee, P. & Eakins, K.E. (1984). Lipoxygenase products: mediation of inflammatory responses and inhibition of their formation. In: *The Leukotrienes*, ed. Charkin, L.W. & Bailey, D.M., pp. 195-213. Orlando: Academic Press.

Cimasoni, G. (1983). *Crevicular Fluid Updated.* Basel: Karger.

Clagett, J.A. & Engel, D. (1978). Polyclonal activation: A form of primitive immunity and its possible role in pathogenesis of inflammatory diseases. *Development and Comparative Immunology* **2**, 235-242.

Egelberg, J. (1967). The topography and permeability of vessels at the dentogingival junction in dogs. *Journal of Periodontal Research* 2O, Supplement 1.

Fantone, J.C. & Ward, P.A. (1982). Role of oxygen-derived free radicals and metabolites in leukocyte-dependent inflammatory reactions. *American Journal of Pathology* **107**, 397-418.

Feldman, R.S., Szeto, B., Chauncey, H. & Goldhaber, P. (1983). Non-steroidal anti-inflammatory drugs in the reduction of human alveolar bone loss. *Journal of Clinical Periodontology* **10**, 131-136.

Fine, D.H. & Mandel, I.D. (1986). Indicators of periodontal disease activity: an evaluation. *Journal of Clinical Periodontology* **13**, 533-546.

Freedman, H.L., Listgarten, M.A. & Taichman, N.S. (1968). Electron microscopic features of chronically inflamed human gingiva. *Journal of Periodontal Research* **3**, 313-327.

Goldhaber, P. & Rabadjija, L. (1982). Influence of pharmacological agents on bone resorption. In: *Host-Parasite Interactions in Periodontal Diseases*, ed. Genco, R.J. and Mergenhagen, S.E. pp. 363-375. Washington: American Society for Microbiology.

Haffajee, A.D., Socransky, S.S. & Goodson, I.M. (1983). Comparison of different data analyses for detecting changes in attachment level. *Journal of Clinical Periodontology* **10**, 298-310.

Havemann, K. & Janoff, A. (1978). *Neutral Proteases of Human Polymorphonuclear Leukocytes.* Baltimore: Urban and Schwarzenberg, Inc.

Hausmann, E., Nair, B.C. & Dziak, R. (1982). Bacterial components which result in bone loss. In: *Host-Parasite Interactions in Periodontal Diseases*, ed. Genco, R.J. and Mergenhagen, S.E. pp. 151-159. Washington: American Society for Microbiology.

Hellden, L. & Lindhe, J. (1973). Enhanced emigration of crevicular leukocytes mediated by factors in human dental plaque. *Scandinavian Journal of Dental Research* **8**, 123-129.

Ivanyi, L. & Lehner, T. (1970). Stimulation of lymphocyte transformation by bacterial antigens in patients with periodontal disease. *Archives of Oral Biology* **15**, 1089-1096.

Kahnberg, K.-E. & Hellden, L. (1977). Effect of topically applied neutrophil leukocyte extract on normal gingiva of dogs. *Scandinavian Journal of Dental Research* **85**, 155-163.

Kahnberg, K.-E., Lindhe, J. & Hellden, L. (1976). Initial gingivitis induced by topical application of plaque extract. A histometric study in dogs with normal gingiva. *Journal of Periodontal Research* **11**, 218-225.

Lang, N.P. & Smith, F.N. (1977). Lymphocyte blastogenesis to plaque antigens in human periodontal disease. I. Populations of varying sensitivity of disease. *Journal of Periodontal Research* **12**, 298-309.

Lindhe, J., Haffajee, A.D. & Socransky, S.S. (1983). Progression of periodontal disease in adult subjects in the absence of periodontal therapy. *Journal of Clinical Periodontology* **10**, 433-442.

Lindhe, J., Hamp, S.-E. & Löe, H. (1975). Plaque-induced periodontal disease in beagle dogs. A 4-year clinical, roentgenographical and histometric study. *Journal of Periodontal Research* **10**, 243-255.

Lindhe, J. & Nyman, S. (1975). The effect of plaque control and surgical pocket elimination on the establishment and maintenance of periodontal health. A longitudinal study of periodontal therapy in cases of advanced disease. *Journal of Clinical Periodontology* **2**, 67-79.

Lindhe, J. & Nyman, S. (1984). Long-term maintenance of patients treated for advanced periodontal disease. *Journal of Clinical Periodontology* **11**, 504-514.

Lindhe, J. & Rylander, H. (1975). Experimental gingivitis in young dogs. *Scandinavian Journal of Dental Research* **83**, 314-326.

Listgarten, M.A. (1965). Electron microscopic observations on the bacterial flora of acute necrotizing ulcerative gingivitis. *Journal of Periodontology* **36**, 328-339.

Löe, H. & Rindom Schiott, C.R. (1970). The effect of mouth rinses and topical application of clorhexidine on the development of dental plaque and gingivitis in man. *Journal of Periodontal Research* **5**, 79-83.

Löe, H., Theilade, E. & Jensen, S.B. (1965). Experimental gingivitis in man. *Journal of Periodontology* **36**, 177-187.

Mayrand, D. (1985). Virulence promotion by mixed bacterial infections. In: *The Pathogenesis of Bacterial Infections*, ed. Jackson, G.G. and Thomas H. pp. 282-291. Berlin: Springer-Verlag.

Nisengard, R.J. (1974). Immediate hypersensitivity and periodontal disease. *Journal of Periodontology* **45**, 344-350.

Nyman, S., Schroeder, H.E. & Lindhe, J. (1979). Suppression of inflammation and bone resorption by indomethacin during experimental periodontitis in dogs. *Journal of Periodontology* **50**, 450-461.

Offenbacher, S., Odle, B.M. & Van Dyke, T.E. (1986). The use of crevicular fluid prostaglandin E_2 levels as a predictor of periodontal attachment loss. *Journal of Periodontal Research* **21**, 101-112.

O'Neill, P.A. & Woodson, D.L. (1986). Lymphokine production by human gingival lymphocytes. *Journal of Periodontal Research* **21**, 338-350.

O'Neill, P.A. & Woodson, D.L. & Mackler, B.F. (1982). Functional characterization of human gingival lymphocytes. *Journal of Periodontal Research* **17**, 50-59.

Page, R.C. & Schroeder, H.E. (1976). Pathogenesis of inflammatory periodontal disease. A summary of current work. *Laboratory Investigation* **33**, 235-249.

Page, R.C. & Schroeder H.E. (1982). *Periodontitis in Man and Animals. A comparative review.* Basel: Karger.

Parker, C.W. (1984). The lipoxygenases in leukocytes and other mammalian cells. In: *The Leukotrienes*, ed. Chakrin, L.W. and Bailey, D.M. pp. 125-137. Orlando: Academic Press.

Ramfjord, S.P., Nissle, R.R., Shick, R.A. & Cooper, Jr., H. (1968). Subgingival curettage versus surgical elimination of periodontal pockets. *Journal of Periodontology* **39**, 167-175.

Ranney, R.R. & Zander, H.A. (1979). Allergic periodontal disease in sensitized squirrel monkeys. *Journal of Periodontology* **41**, 12-21.

Reed, M.J., Patters, M.R., Mashimo, P.A., Genco, R.J. & Levine, M.J. (1976). Blastogenic response of human lymphocytes to oral bacterial antigens: characterization of bacterial sonicates. *Infection and Immunity* **14**, 1202-1212.

Rylander, H., Attstrom, R. & Lindhe, J. (1975). Influence of experimental neutropenia in dogs with chronic gingivitis. *Journal of Periodontal Research* **10**, 315-323.

Sandberg, A.L. (1982). Humoral and cellular mechanisms of bone resorption. In: *Host-Parasite Interactions in Periodontal diseases*, ed. Genco, R.J. & Mergenhagen, S.E. pp. 309-317. Washington: American Society for Microbiology.

Sandholm, L. (1986). Proteases and their inhibitors in chronic inflammatory periodontal disease. *Journal of Clinical Periodontology* **13**, 19-26.

Saxe, S.R., Greene, J.C., Bohannan, H.M. & Vermillion, J.R. (1967). Oral debris, calculus and periodontal disease in the beagle dog. *Periodontics* **5**, 217-224.

Schenkein, H.A. (1982). The complement system in periodontal diseases. In: *Host-Parasite Interactions in Periodontal Diseases*, ed. Genco, R.J. & Mergenhagen, S.E. pp. 299-308. Washington: American Society for Microbiology.

Schroeder, H.E. (1973). Transmigration and infiltration of leukocytes in human junctional epithelium. *Helvetica Odontologica Acta* **17**, 6-15.

Schroeder, H.E. (1977). Histopathology of the gingival sulcus. In: *Borderland between Caries and Periodontal Disease*, ed. Lehner, T., pp. 43-78. New York: Academic Press.

Schroeder, H.E. & Page, R.C. (1972). Lymphocyte-fibroblast interactions in the pathogenesis of inflammatory gingival disease. *Experienta* **28**, 1228-1230.

Shenker, B.J., McArthur, W.P. & Tsai, C.C. (1982). Immune suppression induced by *Actinobacillus actinomycetemcomitans*. I. Effects on human peripheral blood lymphocyte response to mitogens and antigens. *Journal of Immunology* **128**, 148-154.

Shenker, B.J. (1987). Immunologic dysfunction in the pathogenesis of periodontal disease. *Journal of Clinical Periodontology* **14**, 489-498.

Siraganian, R.P. (1983). Histamine secretion from mast cells and basophils. *Trends in Pharmacological Sciences* **4**, 432-437.

Socransky, S.S., Haffajee, A.D., Goodson, J.M. & Lindhe, J. (1984). New concepts of destructive periodontal disease. *Journal of Clinical Periodontology* **11**, 21-32.

Taichman, N.S., Tsai C.C., Shenker, B.J. & Boehringer, H. (1984). Neutrophil interactions with oral bacteria as a pathogenic mechanism in periodontal disease. *Advances in Inflammation Research* **8**, 113-142.

Taichman, N.S., Freedman, H.L. & Uriuhara, T. (1966). Inflammation and tissue injury. I. The response to intradermal injections of human dentogingival plaque in normal and leukopenic rabbits. *Archives of Oral Biology* **11**, 1385-1392.

Turner, M.J. (1980). Antigenic variation. In: *The Molecular Basis of Microbnial Pathogenicity*, ed. Smith H., Skehel, J.J. & Turner, M.J. pp. 133-158.

Van Dyke, T.E., Levine, M.J. & Genco, R.J. (1985). Neutrophil function and oral disease. *Journal of Oral Pathology* **14**, 95-120.

Waerhaug, J. (1952). The gingival pocket. Anatomy pathology deepening and elimination. *Odontologisk Tidsskrift* **60**, Supplement.

Waerhaug, J. (1977). Subgingival plaque and loss of attachment of periodontosis as evaluated on extracted teeth. *Journal of Periodontology* **48**, 125-130.

Waerhaug, J. (1979). The angular bony defect and its relationship to trauma from occlusion and down growth of subgingival plaque. *Journal of Clinical Periodontology* **6**, 61-82.

Wahl, S.M. (1986). Inflammatory cell regulation of connective tissue metabolism. *Rheumatology* **10**, 404-429.

Weissmann, G. (1980). Prostaglandins in Acute Inflammation. Current Concepts, The Upjohn Company.

Wilton, J.M.A. & Jarvis, J. (1981). Detachment and killing of glass adherent bacteria by human polymorphonuclear leukocytes: a model system for the modulation of plaque formation by inflammatory cells. *Revue de l'Institut Pasteur de Lyon* **14**, 57-66.

CHAPTER 6

Periodontal Disease in Children and Young Adults

Prepubertal periodontitis and *juvenile periodontitis* are two forms of periodontal disease that can be found in children and young adults. Both diseases occur in a localized as well as in a generalized variety. *Prepubertal periodontitis* affects the primary dentition but the inflammatory disease may subsequently spread into the periodontium of the permanent teeth. *Juvenile periodontitis*, on the other hand, is a periodontal disorder that involves the permanent dentition only.

Prepubertal periodontitis

Clinical characteristics

According to Page et al. (1983) the prepubertal forms of periodontal disease may have their

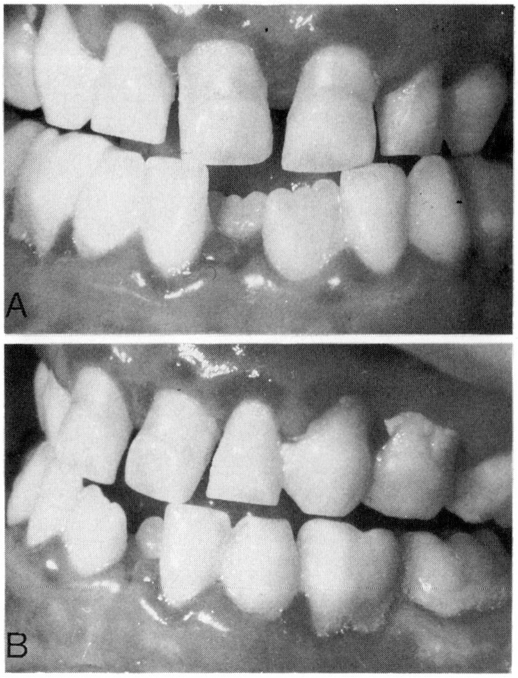

Fig. 6-1. Clinical features of generalized prepubertal periodontitis seen in a 6 1/2-year-old boy. Acute inflammation of gingival tissues is apparent with accompanying advanced recession of the gingival margin (a). Note the inflamed gingiva at the erupting mandibular permanent incisor (b) and the plaque accumulations in both the maxillary and mandibular dentition. (From Page et al. 1983).

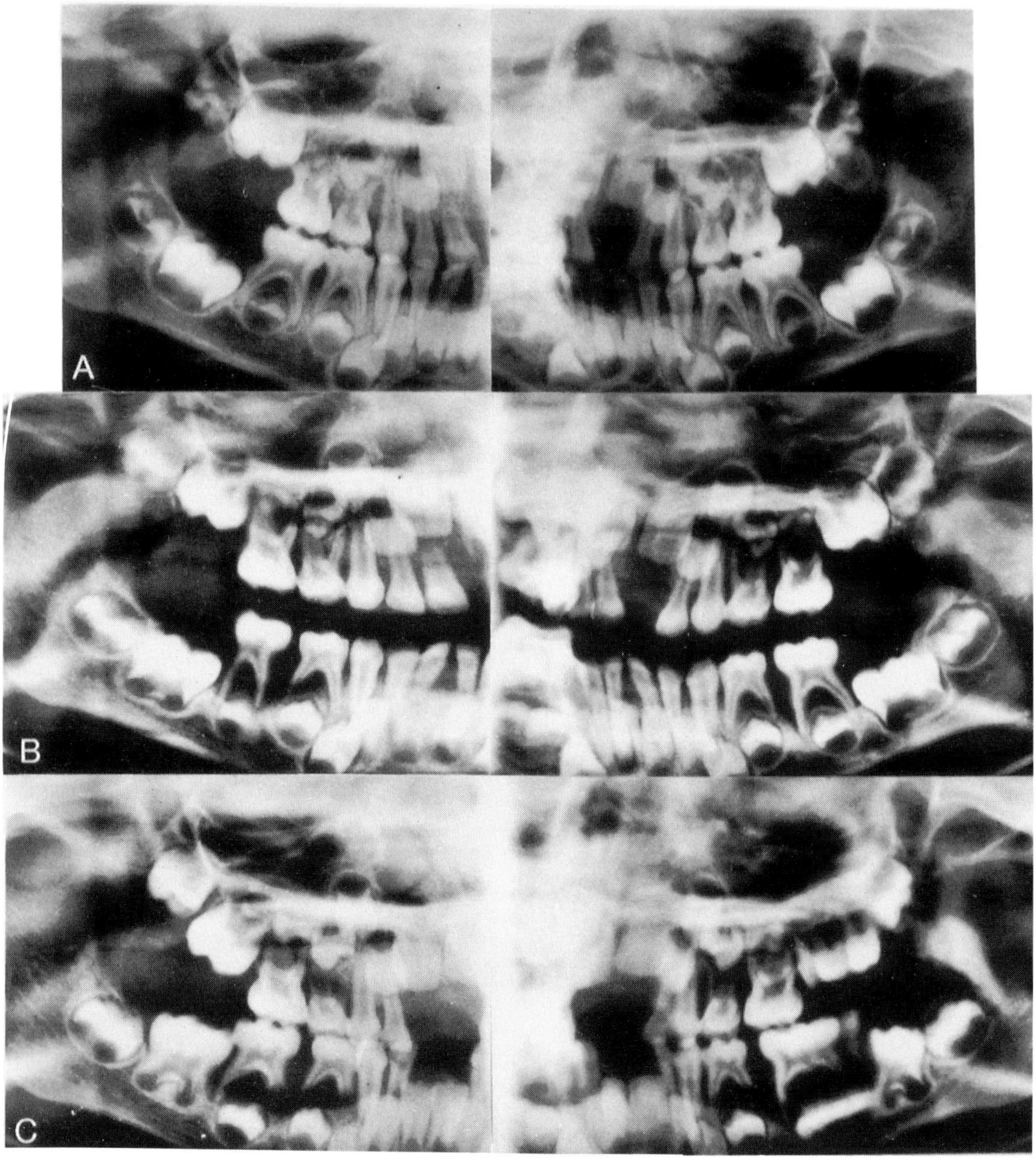

Fig. 6-2. Radiographs obtained from a Caucasian female with generalized prepubertal periodontitis: (a) in April 1978, when she was 4-5 years of age: (b) in December 1978, and (c) in August 1979. The radiographs illustrate the extent of alveolar bone loss that occurred over the 15-month period (From Page et al. 1983).

onset already at the time of the eruption of the primary dentition. The *generalized* variety of *prepubertal periodontitis* is very often a rapidly progressive disorder which not only frequently leads to an early loss of the primary dentition but may, as stated above, also spread into the permanent dentition. *Generalized prepubertal periodontitis* is associated with severe gingival inflammation, gingival tissue profileration, gingival recession or cleft formation and a widespread and rapid destruction of the alveolar bone (Figs. 6-1, 6-2). The *localized* form of *prepubertal periodontitis* is less conspicuous than the *generalized* variety. Frequently *lo-*

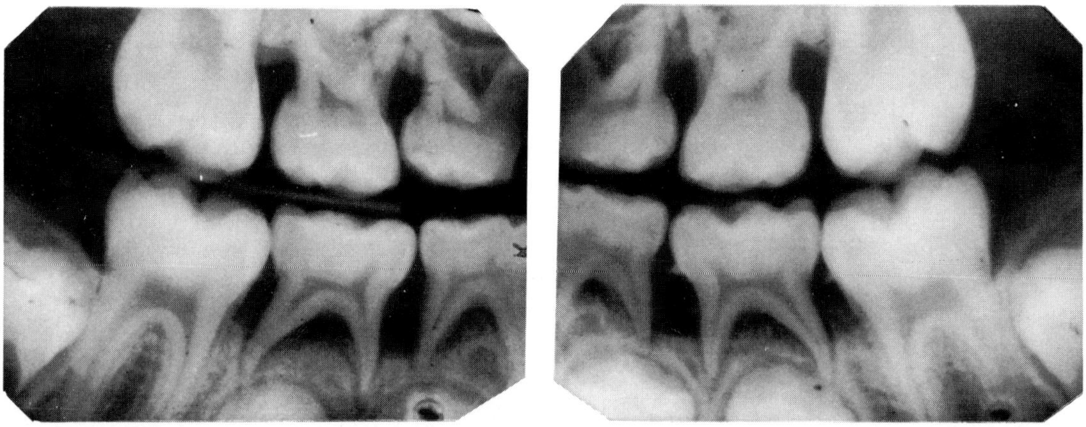

Fig. 6-3. Radiographs illustrating bone loss at deciduous molars, but no involvement of the permanent molars in a child with early onset periodontitis.

calized prepubertal periodontitis affects only the periodontal tissues at one or more of the primary molars (Fig. 6-3). According to Page et al. (1983) the gingival tissues at diseased sites in children with *localized prepubertal periodontitis* often show only moderate clinical signs of inflammation, but deep periodontal pockets and localized bone loss are dominating features of the disease. While children with *generalized prepubertal periodontitis* often have a history of recurrent otitis media and upper respiratory tract infections, children with *localized prepubertal periodontitis* seem not to be particularly sensitive to recurrent infections.

Epidemiology - prevalence

Sweeney et al. (1987) examined radiographs obtained from the primary dentition of 2,264 children, aged 5-11 years, who had been referred to the school of Dental Medicine at the University of Pennsylvania for routine dental treatment. The authors reported that less than 1% (19 subjects; 0.8%) of the children examined showed radiographic signs of distinct loss of alveolar bone at one or more primary molars. In 11 of the 19 children with *prepubertal periodontitis* the alveolar bone loss was limited to the first primary molars, while the remaining 8 children had both the first and the second primary molars involved in a periodontal disease process. Of the periodontally diseased children 10 were Black females, 6 were Black males, 2 were Caucasian males and one was an Asian male. The apparent difference in the prevalence of *prepubertal periodontitis* between the races observed in this sample may be explained by the large number of Black children that are referred to the Pedodontic Clinic of this particular dental school.

Microbiology

Table 6-1 describes findings from recent studies on the microbiology of *localized prepubertal periodontitis. Bacteroides intermedius* was found to be present at the diseased sites in 19 patients, *Actinobacillus actinomycetemcomitans* in 15 patients, *Capnocytophaga* species in 17 patients, and *Eikenella corrodens* in 10 patients. Sweeney et al. (1987) found that black-pigmented bacteroides occurred in all children with *localized prepubertal periodontitis* and, in particular, *B. intermedius* appeared to be significantly associated with the disease. These authors recovered high proportions of *A. actinomycetemcomitans* in one patient and of *Capocytophaga* in another patient. The available data indicate that *localized prepubertal periodontitis* is an infectious disease associated

Table 6-1

Microbiota of localized prepubertal periodontitis

Study	No. of individuals examined	Suspected periodontal pathogens
Blomlöf et al. (1983)	2	*A. actinomycetemcomitans*
Cogen et al. (1984)	2	*A. actinomycetemcomitans*
Nyman et al. (1985)	1	*A. actinomycetemcomitans*
Williams et al. (1985)	2	*B. intermedius* *C. ochracea* *A. actinomycetemcomitans*
Mishkin et al. (1986)	1	*B. gingivalis* *B. intermedius* *A. actinomycetemcomitans*
Baab et al. (1986)	3	*Capnocytophaga* species[a)] *B. intermedius* *B. gingivalis*[a)]
Sweeney et al. (1987)	9	*B. intermedius* *A. actinomycetemcomitans* *Capnocytophaga* species
Dalaney & Kornman (1987)	9	*A. actinomycetemcomitans* *B. intermedius* *C. sputigena* *E. corrodens*

[a)] based on serum antibody determinations

with bacteria generally regarded as major periodontal pathogens. No data have been published so far regarding the microbiology of *generalized prepubertal periodontitis*.

Host response

Localized prepubertal periodontitis has been associated with functional defects of peripheral blood neutrophils or monocytes, but apparently both types of granulocytes are not affected in the same patient (Baab et al. 1986). In contrast, in patients with the *generalized form of prepubertal periodontitis* neutrophils as well as monocytes/macrophages often have an abnormal chemotactic response (Page & Schroeder 1982). It has been suggested that improper responses of granulocytes to periodontal infections may predispose for the development of particularly severe forms of periodontal tissue destruction.

Serum antibodies to putative periodontal pa-

Table 6-2

Serum antibodies against *A. actinomycetemcomitans* in juvenile periodontitis [a]

Study	Assay	Clinical diagnosis	No. of subjects studied	Antibodies against *A. actinomycetemcomitans* [b]
Genco et al. (1980)	Immuno-precipitation	LJP[a]	52	69%[c]
		Normals	29	10%
		CJP	12	25%
		Adult periodontitis	48	15%
Listgarten et al. (1981)	Immuno-fluorescence	LJP	21	64
		Normals	21	1
		Adult periodontitis	21	4
Tsai et al. (1981)	Anti-leukotoxin antibodies	LJP+GJP	55	95%
		Normals	31	19%
		Adult periodontis	26	31%
Ranney et al. (1982)	Immuno-precipitation	LJP	22	77%
		Normals	43	2%
		GJP	35	4%
Altman et al. (1982)	ELISA	LJP	27	63%
		Prepubertal periodontitis	5	60%
		GJP	31	29%
		Adult periodontitis	21	19%
Ebersole et al. (1982)	ELISA	LJP	67	86%
		Normals	82	1%
		GJP	62	30%
		Adult periodontitis	85	11%

Continued on next page

thogens have also been examined. Williams et al. (1985) in 2 and Baab et al. (1986) in 3 patients with *localized prepubertal periodontitis* found elevated serum antibody levels to *Capnocytophaga sputigena, Capnocytophaga gingivalis* or to *Bacteroides gingivalis*. These 5 patients showed normal antibody levels to a battery of other oral bacteria. Altman et al. (1982) demonstrated elevated serum antibody levels to *A. actinomycetemcomitans* in 3 of 5 patients with *localized prepubertal periodontitis*. These findings agree with data from other studies reporting on a high recovery of Actinobacillus in patients with different forms of periodontal disease (Table 6-2).

Cementopathia

Etiologies of prepubertal periodontitis other than pathogenic bacteria and abnormalities in the granulocytes have been considered. In line with Gottlieb's (Gottlieb 1946) idea of cementum pathology, Page & Baab (1985) suggested that some cases of periodontitis in children and

Table 6-2

Serum antibodies against *A. actinomycetemcomitans* in juvenile periodontitis [a)]

Study	Assay	Clinical diagnosis	No. of subjects studied	Antibodies against *A. actinomycetemcomitans* [b)]
Taubman et al. (1982)	ELISA	LJP	38	290
		Normals	24	10
		GJP	11	100
		Adult periodontitis	38	75
Cenco et al. (1985)	ELISA	LJP	59	230
		Normals	29	15
		GJP	24	179
		Adult periodontitis	73	34
Vincent et al. (1985)	ELISA	LJP	50	76%
		Normals	35	0%
		GJP	55	25%
		Adult periodontitis	42	0%
Farida et al. (1986)	RIA	LJP	21	1,443
		Normals	14	286
		GJP	21	394
		Adult periodontitis	15	125

a) Abbreviations: ELISA = enzyme-linked immunosorbent assay; RIA = radioimmunoassay; LJP = Localized juvenile periodontitis; GJP = generalized juvenile periondontitis (includes the diagnoses early-onset severe periodontitis and rapidly progressive periodontitis)
b) Most studies include only 1 or 2 of the 3 recognized serotypes of *A. actinomycetemcomitans*
c) Titer or percent subjects with elevated antibody levels

young adults could be due to abnormal deposition or maintenance of root cementum. They furthermore proposed that a mild form of hypophosphatasia, identified by a reduced level of alkaline phosphatase in serum and the presence of phosphoethanolamine in urine, could be the underlying cause of the defective root cementum. If this assumption is valid, cementum disturbances may help to explain the site specificity for these periodontal lesions and the presence of these aggressive forms of periodontal disease in young children.

Treatment

Well-controlled treatment studies of prepubertal periodontitis have still to be carried out. However, it seems reasonable to suggest that periodontal treatment directed to reducing or eradicating the subgingival infection will help to control the disease. Treatment of prepubertal periodontitis should not include the use of drugs of the tetracycline class because of the risk of malformation and discoloration of the permanent teeth.

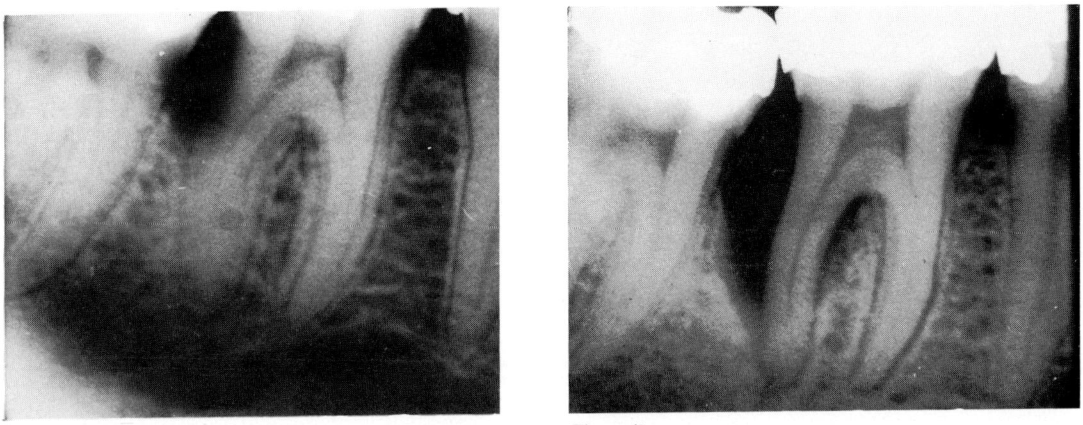

Fig. 6-4a. Fig. 6-4b.

Fig. 6-4. Radiographs illustrating bone loss at the distal aspect of the lower first molar in a 15-year-old girl (a), and progression of disease one year later (b).

Juvenile periodontitis

Periodontosis (Orban & Weinmann 1942) or *Juvenile Periodontitis* (Manson & Lehner 1974) is a disease of the periodontium which occurs in an otherwise healthy adolescent.

Clinical characteristics

Juvenile Periodontitis is characterized by a rapid loss of connective tissue attachment and alveolar bone at more than one tooth in the permanent dentition. Several classification systems have been proposed for *juvenile periodontitis* e.g. "Diffuse Bone Atrophy", "Deep Cementopathia" (Gottlieb 1923, 1928) or "Precocious Periodontitis" (Sugarman & Sugarman 1977), but a universal system has yet to be adopted. In this chapter *juvenile periodontitis* will be divided into two major subdivisions: *localized juvenile periodontitis* and *generalized juvenile periodontitis. Localized juvenile periodontitis* affects first permanent molars and incisors and not more than one or two additional permanent teeth. *Generalized juvenile periodontitis* is more extensive, affecting first permanent molars and incisors as well as several teeth in other segments of the dentition. It is still not known (see below) if *localized* and *generalized juvenile periodontitis* are separate disease entities or if the generalized form is an extension of or a more aggressive form of *localized juvenile periodontitis*.

Baer (1971) described *juvenile periodontitis* (*periodontosis*) as a well-defined, clinical entity which is different from adult periodontal disease. He stated that this particular form of periodontal disease (1) makes its debut when children are between 11 and 13 years of age, (2) affects more females than males, and (3) seems to cluster in families. Baer further stated that (4) the gingiva around the diseased teeth may have a normal texture and color, but that (5) deep periodontal pockets are present at one or more surfaces of the affected teeth. It was also claimed that (6) in the initial lesions gross deposits of subgingival calculus are uncommon and that (7) the amount of periodontal destruction observed at the disease sites is not commensurate with the amount of local irritants present. Baer argued that *juvenile periodontitis* has a typical appearance in the radiographs.

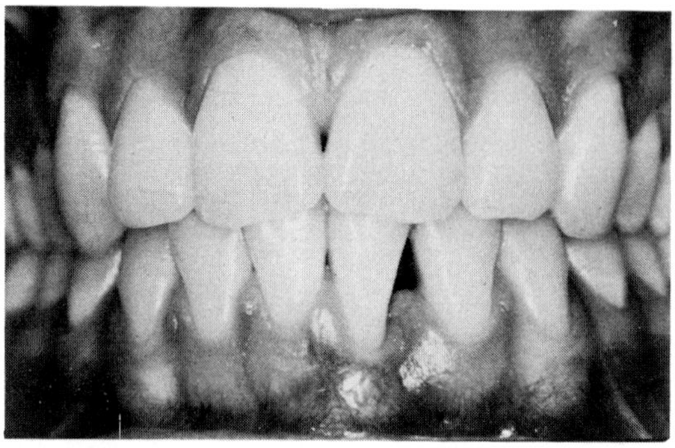

Fig. 6-5a.

Figs. 6-5a, b, c. The clinical appearance of the periodontal tissues of a 15-year-old girl suffering from juvenile periodontitis. Note the proper oral-hygiene conditions and the scalloped outline of the gingival margin. In the lower front-tooth region, the interdental papilla between teeth 31 and 32 is lost.

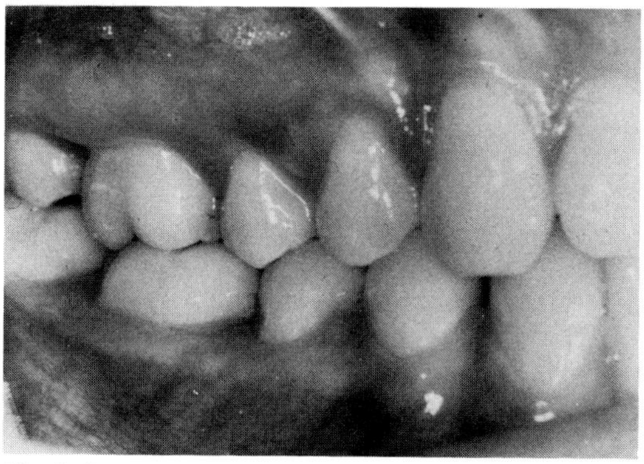

Fig. 6-5b.

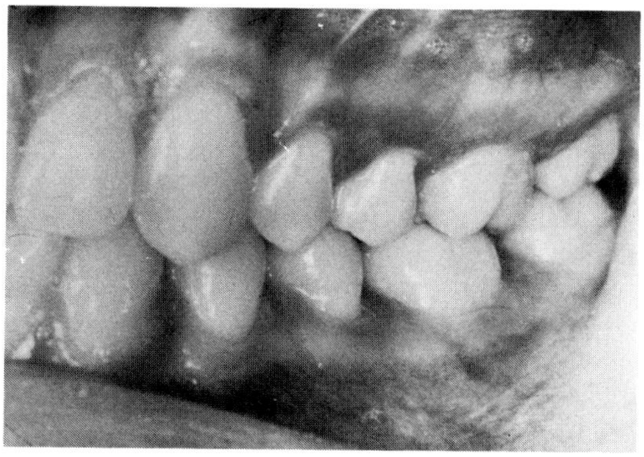

Fig. 6-5c.

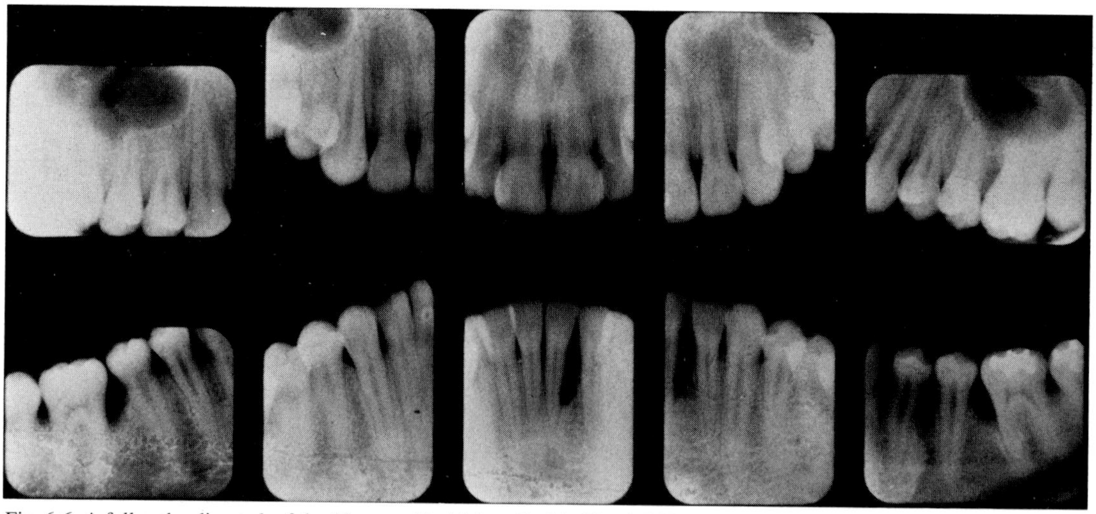

Fig. 6-6. A full oral radiograph of the 15-year-old girl described in Fig. 6-5. Note the presence of angular bony defects at the mesial aspect of tooth 46, 36 and the distal aspect of tooth 31.

Thus, (8) angular bone loss can be observed at first molars and incisors. In the molar region bone loss is frequently seen bilaterally.

Baer concluded that *juvenile periodontitis* (periodontosis) is a disease which (9) progresses rapidly, meaning that within a 4- to 5-year period after the onset between 50-75% of the attachment apparatus of the diseased tooth

Figs. 6-7a, b, c. Intraoral photographs which illustrate the clinical appearance of a 14-year-old girl. Note the excellent oral-hygiene status. Bleeding on probing has been provoked in the gingivae at the mesial aspect of teeth 16 and 26.

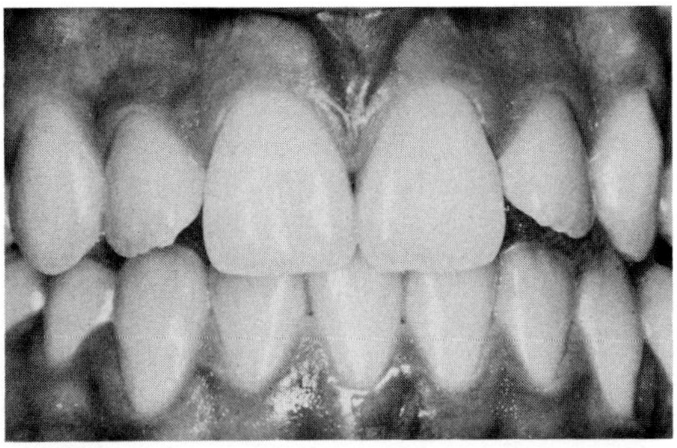

Fig. 6-7a.

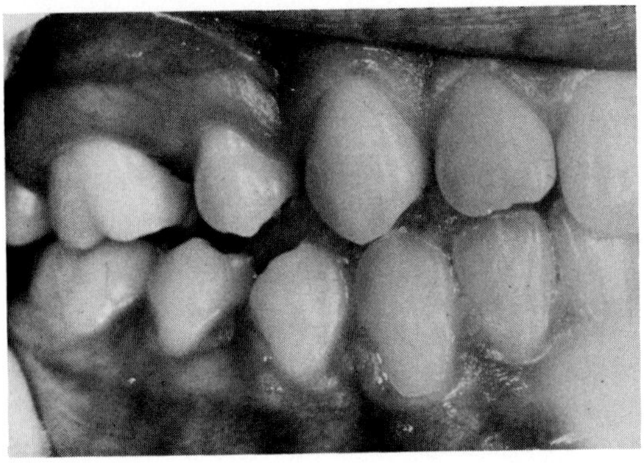

Fig. 6-7b.

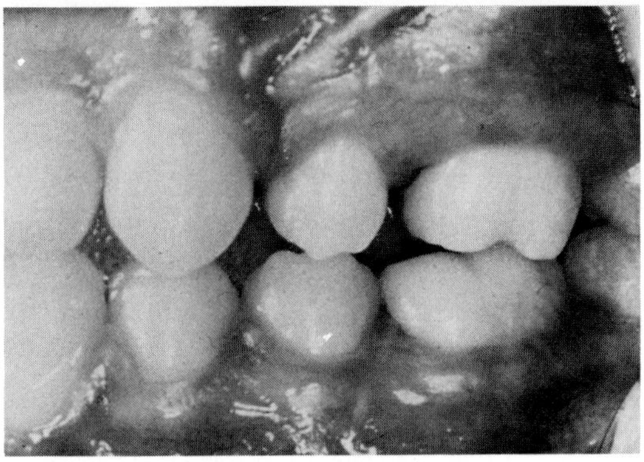

Fig. 6-7c.

regions may be involved in an inflammatory lesion. Fig. 6-4 illustrates the rate of disease progression in a 15-year-old girl. In Fig. 6-4a initial signs of bone loss can be detected at the distal aspect of 46. One year later, when the girl is 16 years of age, bone loss has progressed (Fig. 6-4b) and approximately 90% of the alveolar bone in this tooth region has been lost.

Figs. 6-5a, b and c present the clinical appearance of a 15-year-old girl with *localized juvenile periodontitis*. The interdental papilla between teeth 31 and 32 has lost some of its normal tissue volume,but the gingiva in the remaining part of the dentition is clinically normal in texture and color. Fig. 6-6 presents radiographs of the patient's dentition. Deep angular bony defects are seen at the mesial aspect of teeth 26, 36 and 46. In addition, there is a deep angular bony defect at the distal surface of 31.

Figs. 6-7a, b and c present the clinical status of her 14-year-old sister, whose gingiva in most parts of the dentition, also clinically, appears to be normal. Bleeding was provoked, however, by gentle probing in deep periodontal pockets at the mesial aspect of teeth 16, 26 and 46. Fig. 6-8a is her full-mouth radiographs. Angular bony defects can be seen at the mesial aspect of teeth 16, 26 and 46 (Fig. 6-8b).

Epidemiology

Prevalence

Findings reported from epidemiologic studies carried out in different populations have documented that advanced forms of periodontal disease in children and young adults, including *localized juvenile periodontitis*, occur at a frequency of between 0.1% and 7.6% (Table 6-3). The marked differences reported with respect to prevalence of destructive periodontal disease may be explained by (1) different clinical and

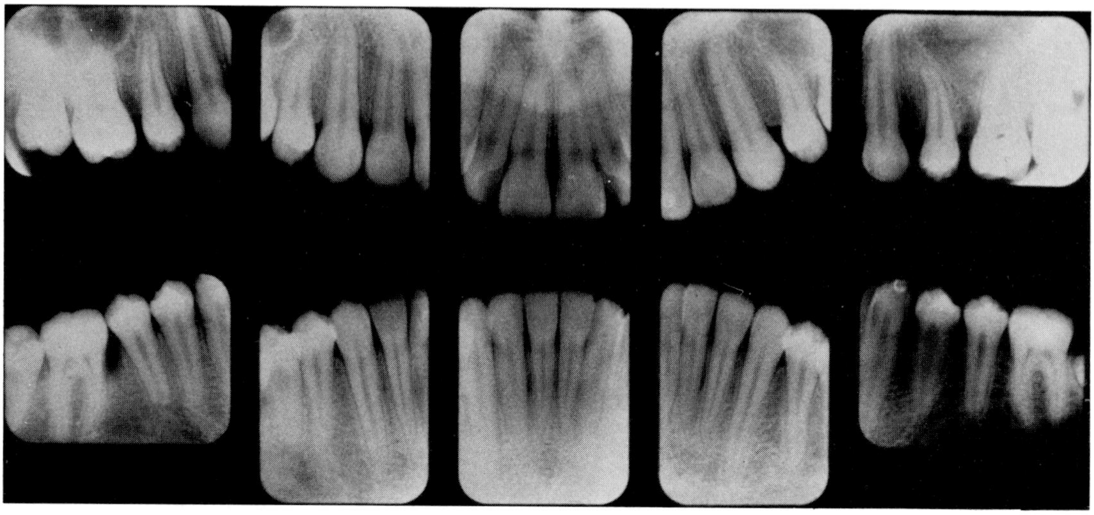

Fig. 6-8a.

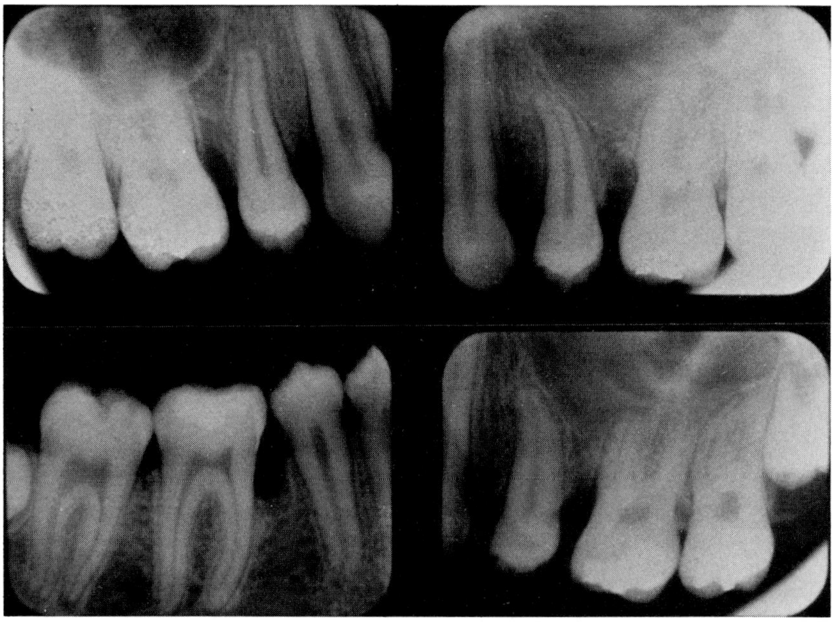

Fig. 6-8b.

Figs. 6-8a, b. Radiographs (a) of the dentition of the 14-year-old girl described in Fig. 6-5. (b) A higher magnification of the first molar regions. Note the presence of angular bony defects at the mesial aspect of 16, 26 and 46.

radiographical criteria used to define juvenile periodontitis, (2) racial and regional differences, (3) the age range of the populations studied.

In more recent years 3 epidemiological studies have been presented in which more stringent criteria for defining *localized juvenile periodontitis* have been used. In the studies by Saxén (1980a), Saxby (1984) and Kronauer et al. (1986), a subject was identified as having the disease if several of the following criteria were met:

Table 6-3

Prevalence of periodontal disease in children and young adults

Study	Geographical location	Age groups (years)	No of subjects	Prevalence
Dawson (1949)	Egypt	36-40		5.6%
Day & Shourie (1949)	India	9-60	568	17.6%
Day et al. (1955)	USA	13-65	1,269	7.0%
Ramfjord (1961)	India	11-17	1,615	2.2%
Migliani (1965)	India			0.1%
Emslie (1966)	Sudan	15-20	830	0.4%
Kaslick & Chasens (1968)	USA	16-26	3,897	0.2%
Rao & Tewani (1968)	India	15-30	1,200	0.2%
Lacy & Brasher (1977)	USA		3,235	0.4%
Saxén (1980A)	Finland	16	8,096	0.1%
Barnett et al. (1982)	USA	13-30	2,162	2.4%
Eisenmann et al. (1983)	Panama	14-19	155	7.7%
Saxby (1984)	U.K.	14-19	7,266	0.1%
Kronauer et al. (1986)	Switzerland	16	7,604	0.1%
Bial & Mellonig (1987)	USA	17-32	49,308	0.4%

1. The subject was in good health.
2. More than one tooth in the dentition was involved.
3. Alveolar bone loss of 2mm or more could be found at more than one surface of the affected teeth.
4. The probing depth at the diseased site was greater than 5mm.
5. The local irritants (calculus or overhanging margins of restorations) were not commensurate with the amount of bone loss.

In other words, in these studies the criteria proposed by Baer (1971) to identify subjects with *localized juvenile periodontitis* were more strictly adhered to.

Saxén (1980a) and Kronauer et al. (1986) examined 16-year-old subjects in Finland and Switzerland, while Saxby (1984) examined British school children aged between 14 and 19 years. In Saxén's material, which comprised about 8,000 adolescent representing a uniform Caucasian population, *localized juvenile periodontitis* lesions were found in 8 cases, i.e. at a prevalence of 0.1%. Five of the involved subjects were females and 3 were males. Saxby included in his material about 7,300 subjects representing at least four different ethnic groups: Caucasian, Black, Asian, (Indian and Pakistani) and other. He reported that the overall prevalence of *localized juvenile periodontitis* in this population was 0.1% but that there was a racial predilection for the disease. Thus, he found that the prevalence in Caucasians was 0.02%, in Blacks 0.8% and in Asians 0.2%. Kronauer et al. (1984) included in their study 7% (7,600) of all 16-year-old adolescents in Switzerland, proportionally distributed among the different ethnic groups in Switzerland, 8 subjects (4 males and 4 females) were identi-

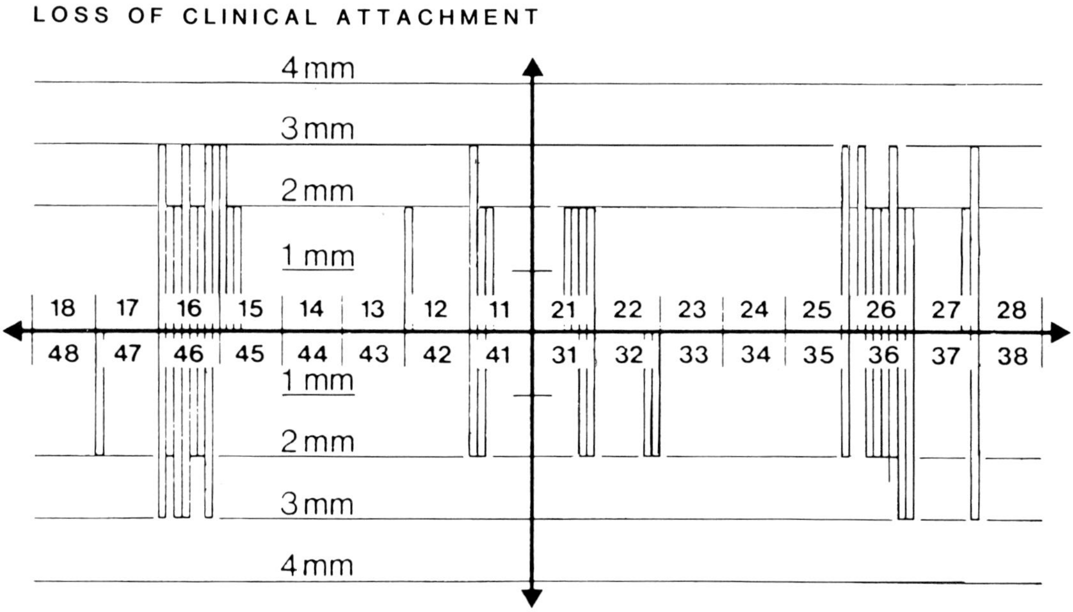

Fig. 6-9. Number and distribution of sites affected by localized juvenile periodontitis lesions (From Kronauer et al. 1986).

fied as having *localized juvenile periodontitis lesions*, i.e. a prevalence of 0.1%. The authors furthermore reported that only 3 of the 8 subjects with this disorder had lesions with attachment loss in the central incisor tooth region, thus emphasizing that the main predilection site for this disease is the first molars. Fig. 6-9 describes the number and distribution of sites affected by *localized juvenile periodontitis* in the Swiss population, as well as the amount of the attachment loss that had occurred at the various sites (Kronauer et al. 1986).

The results from the three studies referred to above, in which subjects aged between 14 and 19 years were included, clearly demonstrate that *localized juvenile periodontitis* is a rare disease in Caucasian populations of industrialized countries. In races other than Caucasian and in non-industrialized countries, however, the prevalence of the disease may be much higher (Harvey et al. 1981, Eisenmann et al. 1983, Table 6-3).

Localized to generalized periodontitis

Hörman and Frandsen (1979) examined 156 young subjects who had been referred for specialist treatment of advanced periodontal disease. They divided the patients into three age groups; 12-18 years, 19-24 years and 26-32 years, and reported that in the youngest age group few teeth were affected by deep periodontal lesions while with increasing age the number of affected teeth increased progressively. This could indicate that the more generalized form of juvenile periodontitis found in the older age groups of patients had, in fact, started as a *localized juvenile periodontitis* which, left untreated, had spread to become generalized. The hypothesis that the localized form of juvenile periodontitis may develop into a generalized form is to some extent supported by data published by Saxén (1980b), Liljenberg and Lindhe (1980) and Burmeister et al. (1984).

Burmeister and his co-workers included in their sample:

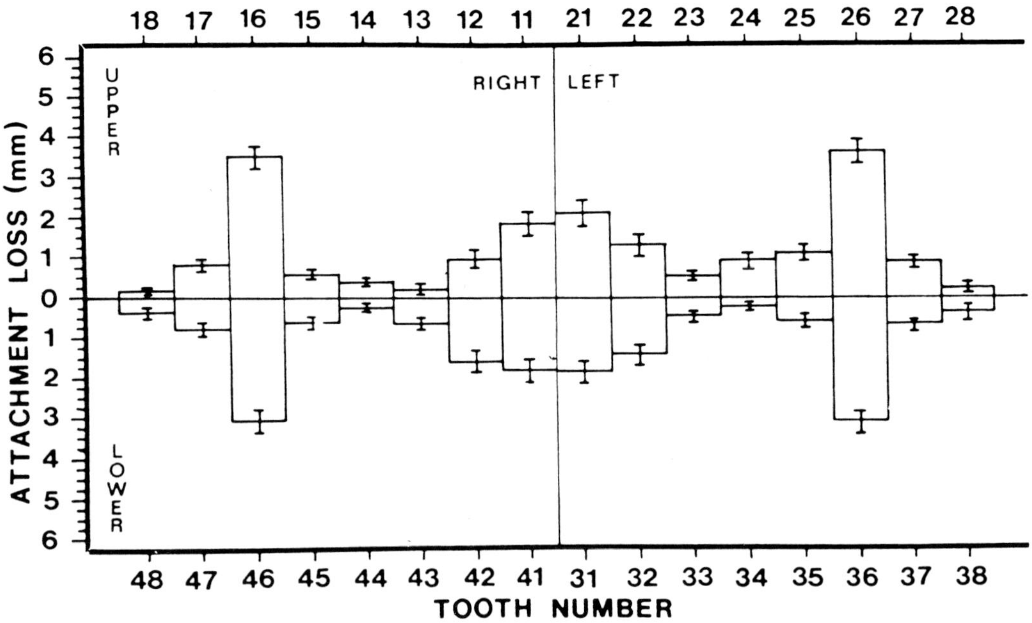

Fig. 6-10a. Periodontal attachment loss at different teeth in subjects with localized juvenile periodontitis (From Burmeister et al. 1984).

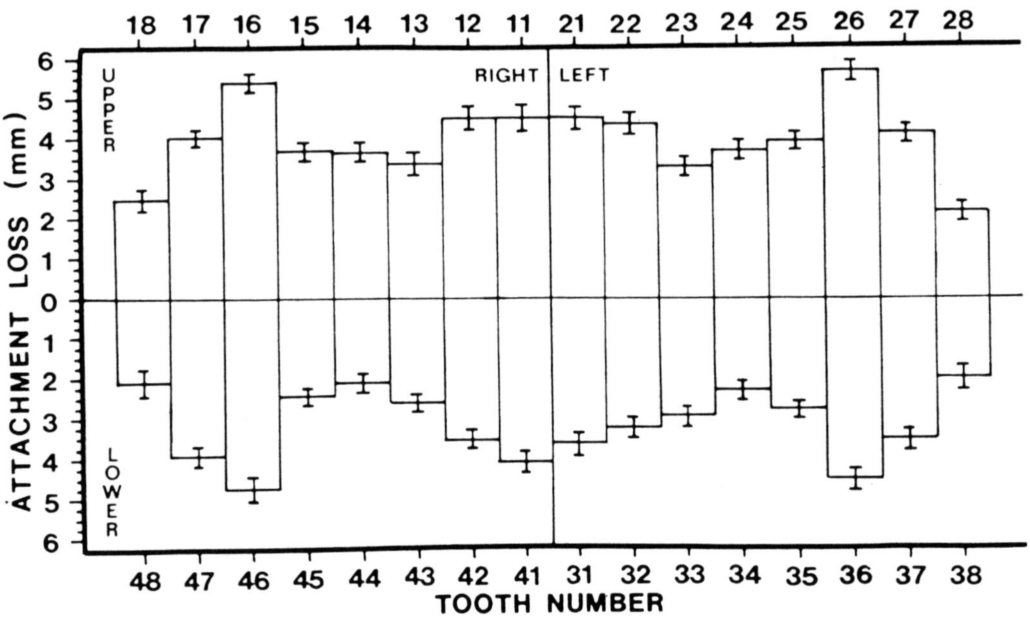

Fig. 6-10b. Periodontal attachment loss at different teeth in subjects with "severe periodontitis" (From Burmeister et al. 1984).

Group A: 46 patients aged 10-28 years (mean age 19.3 years) with localized pattern of severe periodontal destruction (limited to first molar and/or incisor teeth and not more than 2 additional teeth).

Group B: 57 patients aged 11-32 years (mean

age 25.4 years) with generalized pattern of severe periodontal destruction with attachment loss of at least 5mm at 8 or more teeth, at least 3 of which were not first molars and incisors.

The mean attachment loss per tooth observed in the 2 groups is presented in Figs. 6-10a, b. Comparisons of the attachment loss figures in the 2 groups show that the older patients (Group B) had a more generalized form of periodontal disease than the younger patients (Group A). The author concluded, "Our finding of the most severe attachment loss at first molars and incisors in (Group B) allows for the possibility of a molar-incisor-only pattern having existed previously" in some of the Group B subjects. However, since some of the subjects in Group B were in fact young individuals (12-20 years) the disease in these particular patients obviously had become widespread relatively soon after puberty. In contrast, other patients had retained the molar-incisor pattern of lesions without a tendency to spread with age. This is illustrated by the fact that 18 patients in Group A of the material reported by Burmeister et al. were older, i.e. 21-30 years of age.

In conclusion: cross-section data support the hypothesis that *localized juvenile periodontitis* may, left untreated, develop into a generalized disease. It should be emphasized, however, that verification of this hypothesis requires data from longitudinal studies.

A family tendency and a female predominance

Baer (1971) reported that juvenile periodontitis is frequently found in several members of the same families. The basis for this clustering is poorly understood, but autosomal recessive traits (Saxén 1980b) and x-linked dominance (Melnick et al. 1976) have been proposed as heritable vectors.

Baer (1971) suggested that *localized juvenile periodontitis* occurred more frequently in females than in males. This assumption was not validated by data reported in the studies by Saxén (1980a, b) Saxby (1984) and Kronauer et al. (1986).

Microbiology

Ultrastructural studies have demonstrated a sparse but relatively characteristic microbial population in deep periodontal pockets of *localized juvenile periodontitis* (Listgarten 1976, Westergaard et al. 1978). A pellicle up to 20 μm in thickness is generally present on the cementum surface (Fig. 6-11). Masses of bacteria can be attached to this pellicle, but large root surface areas with loosely attached or unattached bacteria can regularly be seen between islands of microbial plaque. A zone free of pellicle and attached bacteria is present in the most apical area of the periodontal pocket. The portion of the plaque which faces the root cementum predominantly consists of bacteria with a typical Gram positive cell wall. More superficial plaque layers (Fig. 6-12) are dominated by various Gram positive rods, and the outermost layer contains Gram negative rods, spirochetes and polymorphonuclear leukocytes. Listgarten (1976) also examined the ultrastructure of the microbiota in advanced incisor-molar lesions of individuals with postjuvenile periodontitis (generalized juvenile periodontitis). The periodontal microflora of these patients resembled that of diseased sites in adult periodontitis patients.

Early studies on cultivable microflora in localized juvenile periodontitis were carried out by Slots (1976) and Newman & Socransky (1977). In both studies, Gram negative organisms comprised approximately 2/3 of the isolates from deep periodontal pockets. In contrast, these organisms averaged only about 1/3 of the isolates in control sites with normal gingiva. The dominant Gram negative bacteria in juvenile periodontitis included *Actinobacillus actinomycetemcomitans*, *Capnocytophaga*

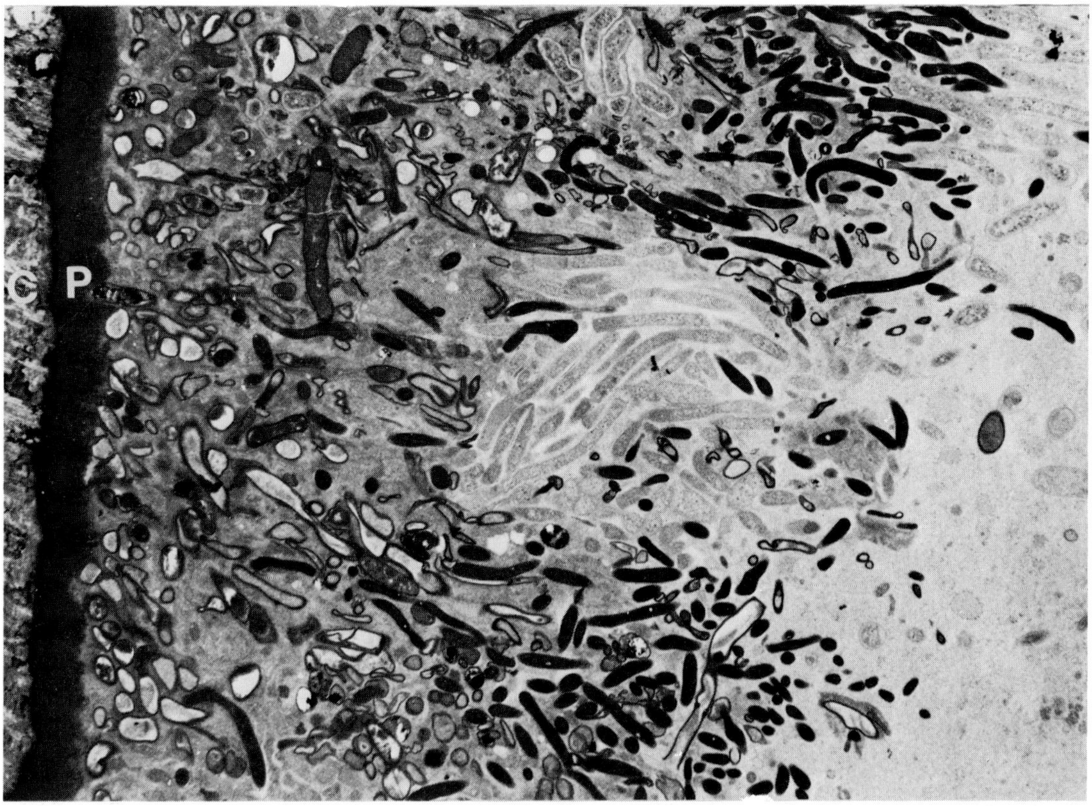

Fig. 6-11. Subgingival microbiota of a localized juvenile periodontitis lesion. Cementum (C) is covered by a pellicle (P) and bacteria, many of which exhibit degeneration in the deep plaque layer. Note the high number of rod-shaped organisms. X 5,500 (Courtesy of J. Westergaard).

species, *Eikenella corrodens, Bacteroides intermedius* and motile anaerobic rods, mainly *Wolinella recta*. Species of *Streptococcus, Actinomyces* and *Peptostreptococcus* accounted for most of the Gram positive isolates.

Recent studies have incriminated *A. actinomycetemcomitans* as the major pathogen in localized juvenile periodontitis. This organism is generally isolated from more than 90% of localized juvenile periodontitis patients and is much less frequently recovered from periodontally healthy or minimally diseased individuals (Table 6-4). Also, virtually all investigators report on significantly elevated levels of serum antibodies to *A. actinomycetemcomitans* in localized juvenile periodontitis patients (Table 6-2). Moreover, *A. actinomycetemcomitans* possesses a number of virulence factors which seem pertinent to the development of destruc-

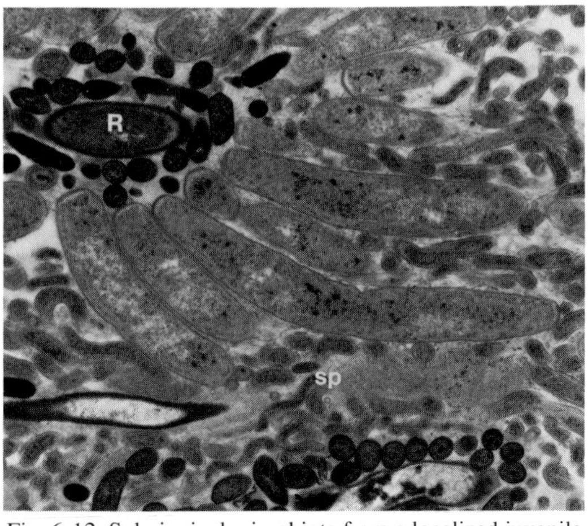

Fig. 6-12. Subgingival microbiota from a localized juvenile periodontitis lesion. Section of a rod-shaped organism (R) surrounded by cocci and long Gram negative rods (*Capnocytophaga*?). Numerous spirochetes (sp) occur peripherally to these bacteria. X 18,700 (Courtesy of J. Westergaard).

Table 6-4

The distribution of *A. actinomycetemcomitans* in localized juvenile periodontitis (LJP) gingivitis, adult periodontitis and in normal non diseased subjects.

Study	Periodontal conditions	Total no. of patients (periodontal sites) examined	% patients positive for *A. actinomy cetemcomitans*	% periodontal sites positive for *A. actinomy cetemcomitans*	Comments
Slots et al. 1980	LJP Adult periodontitis Normal juveniles Normal adults	10 (34) 12 (49) 10 (60) 11 (66)	90 50 20 36	79 35 3 17	The one LJP patient who was culture-negative exhibited serum anti-*A. actinomycetemcomitans* antibodies
Zambon et al. 1983	LJP Adult periodontitis Normal juveniles and adults	29 134 142	97 21 17	– – –	For each subject a pooled sample was obtained from 6 subgingival sites
Mandell & Socransky 1981	LJP Adult periodontitis Gingivitis	6 (18) 25 (50) 23 (46)	100 0 0	79 – –	
Mandell 1984	LJP	8 (8 progressive sites) (16 non progressive sites)	– –	– –	*A. actinomycetemcomitans* and *E. corrodens* were significantly associated with progressive sites. No association for *B. intermedius, F. nucleatum* and *C. ochracea*
Eisenmann et al. 1983	LJP Normal juveniles	12 (12) 10 (10)	100 60	100 60	Study of a mainly Black population in Panama
Moore et al. 1985	LJP	14 (31)	36	5	56 bacterial groups were statistically associated with LJP
Asikainen et al. 1986	LJP	19 (38)	89	68	Study in Finland

tive periodontal disease (see below).

Recent microscopic studies have revealed that microorganisms in localized juvenile periodontitis can invade the periodontal connective tissue (Gillett & Johnson 1982). Saglie et al. (1982, 1986), and Christersson et al. (1986) identified *A. actinimycetemcomitans* as being a prominent invading species. It is likely that

Table 6-5

Predominant microorganisms in generalized juvenile periodontitis or rapidly progressive periodontitis in adolescents or young adults (< 30 years of age)

Study	Total no. of patients (periodontal sites) examined	% of patients (sites) positive for black-pigmented *Bacteroides* spp.	Mean % recovery of black-pigmented *Bacteroides* spp. in positive patients (sites)	% of patients (periodontal sites) positive for *A. actinomycetemcomitans*	Comments
Tanner et al. 1979	4 (9)	*B. gingivalis* 75% (78%) *B. intermedius* 50% (44%)	*B. gingivalis* 26% *B. intermedius* 24%	75%	*B. gingivalis, B. intermedius* and *A. actinomycetemcomitans* were associated with disease
Loesche et al. 1981	4 (16)	100%	39%	No data	Patients ages: 17-28 Years. All black-pigmented *Bacteroides* reported were *B. gingivalis*
Moore et al. 1982	21 (34)	*B. intermedius* 4197: 35% *B. intermedius* 8944: 20%	*B. intermedius* 4197: 11% *B. intermedius* 8944: 5%	3 of 4 patients tested were positive	*B. intermedius* 4197 was associated with disease
Loesche et al. 1985	23	*B. gingivalis* 65% *B. intermedius* 78%	*B. gingivalis* 22% *B. intermedius* 14%	No data	4 lesions were sampled per patient
Wilson et al. 1985	1 (5)	*B. gingivalis* 100% *B. intermedius* 60%	*B. gingivalis* 13% *B. intermedius* 6%	100%	Site was the study unit
Williams et al. 1985	1	*B. intermedius* 100%	*B. intermedius* 11%	0%	

these bacteria, which are capable of invading the gingiva and obtaining close proximity to the periodontal ligament and the alveolar bone, may play a particularly important part in the pathogenesis of the disease.

Data concerning the microbiota of lesions of generalized juvenile periodontitis are more sparse. Table 6-5 describes 6 studies which showed *B. gingivalis*, *B. intermedius* and *A. actinomycetemcomitans* to dominate the subgingival microbiota of generalized juvenile periodontitis lesions.

Virulence factors

Several potentially tissue-destructive mechanisms have been demonstrated in juvenile periodontitis microorganisms (Slots & Genco 1984, Slots 1986).

1) Leukotoxin

Many *A. actinomycetemcomitans* strains produce a substance which can kill human polymorphonuclear leukocytes and monocytes. This leukotoxin may compromise the patient's ability to eliminate or control invading bacteria or bacterial products. On the other hand, more than 90% of patients with localized juvenile periodontitis develop neutralizing serum antibodies against the *A. actinomycetemcomitans* leukotoxin (Tsai et al. 1981). This antibody response may be of importance in controlling the effect of the leukotoxin and in modulating the progression of the disease.

A. actinomycetemcomitans and *B. intermedius* sonicates suppress the reactivity of human lymphocytes to antigens and mitogens. *B. gingivalis,* on the other hand, does not demonstrate similar immunesuppression. In *A. actinomycetemcomitans* infections the immunesuppression depends on the activation of T-suppressor cells (Shenker 1987). An increased number of T-suppressor cells may delay or decrease the humoral immune response. This may be particularly important in the early stages of localized juvenile periodontitis where high levels of protective antibodies have not yet been mounted.

2) Chemotaxis inhibition

A. actonimycetemcomitans, black-pigmented *Bacteroides,* and other Gram negative organisms found in juvenile periodontitis lesions also produce nontoxic factors which inhibit the chemotaxis of human polymorphonuclear leukocytes. These inhibitors of chemotaxis may be important determinants of virulence because they may interfere with the ability of the leukocytes to reach the infectious agents.

3) Endotoxin

The lipopolysaccharide (endotoxin) from *A. actinomycetemcomitans* can elicit pathologic phenomena similar to those characterizing a periodontal lesion. Thus, the endotoxin can induce Schwartzman reaction, macrophage toxicity, platelet aggregation, complement activation and bone resorption. In contrast, the endotoxins from black-pigmented *Bacteroides* are only weakly toxic but can stimulate bone resorption in bone culture systems.

4) Enzymes

Black-pigmented *Bacteroides* and especially *B. gingivalis* elaborate proteolytic enzymes with potential to degrade connective tissue constituents, immunoglobulins and complement proteins. Black-pigmented *Bacteroides* are some of the most proteolytic bacteria of the human oral cavity.

5) Fibroblast cytotoxicity

A. actinomycetemcomitans possesses a fibroblast growth-inhibitory factor. Inhibition of fibroblast proliferation may interfere with collagen synthesis and turn-over and result in impaired gingival healing after challenge by oral bacteria.

6) Polyclonal B-lymphocyte activation

Several periodontal bacteria possess potent polyclonal B-lymphocyte activators. These bacterial factors may contribute to periodontal disease pathogenesis by inducing B-cells to produce antibodies with determinants unrelated to the activating agents. The polyclonal B-cell activators can also induce release of cytokines, such as chemotactic factor(s) that mediate inflammatory reactions, and osteoclast-activating factor(s) which may ultimately result in bone resorption.

7) Bacteriophage - Infection

An interesting association between bacteriophage-infected *A. actinomycetemcomitans* and disease activity was made by Preus et al. (1987a,b). They found in 2 children with Papillon-Lefevre syndrome and in several subjects with localized juvenile periodontitis that actively progressing periodontal sites harbored phage-infected *A. actinomycetemcomitans* isolates, whereas non-progressing sites showed *A. actinomycetemcomitans* isolates with no phage infection. The molecular basis for an increased virulence of *A. actinomycetemcomitans* following phage infection remains to be determined.

Several potential mechanisms thus exist by which the juvenile periodontitis bacteria can cause periodontal destruction. Whether a multiplicity of pathogenic mechanisms or only a few are operative in the disease remains to be established.

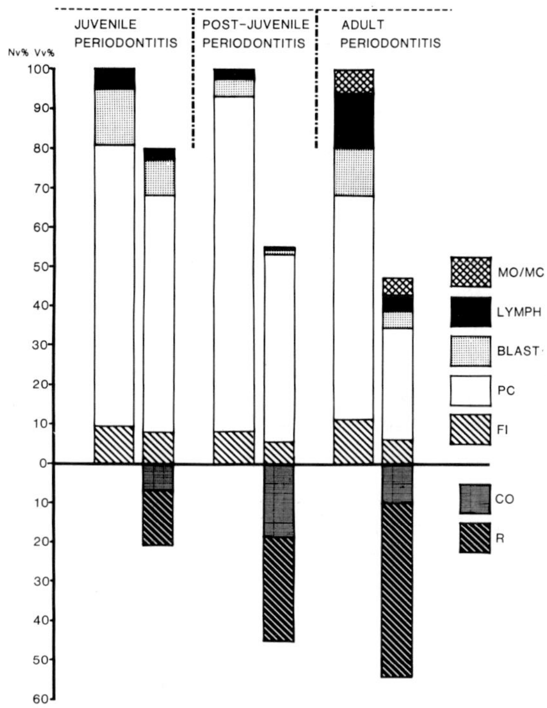

Fig. 6-13. Diagram illustrating the composition of the inflammatory cell infiltrate of periodontal lesions in patients with juvenile periodontitis, postjuvenile periodontitis and adult periodontitis. The wider bars illustrate the numerical density while the thin bars represent the volumetrical density of monocytes, macrophages, lymphocytes, blast cells, plasma cells, fibroblasts, collagen and residual tissues. (From Liljenberg & Lindhe 1980).

Host response

Recent observations have indicated that the local as well as the general host response to the bacterial infection is interfered with in juvenile periodontitis patients.

Local host response

The local host response in the gingiva to the colonization of bacteria on the tooth surface involves (1) exudation of gingival fluid, (2) migration of neutrophils and macrophages with phagocytic capability into the junctional epithelium and gingival pocket area, and (3) the establishment of inflammatory cell infiltrates in the connective tissue beneath the dentogingival epithelium.

Findings reported by Murray & Patters (1980) have indicated that in patients with juvenile periodontitis, neutrophils in the gingival lesions have a reduced phagocytic capacity when compared with cells recovered from similar lesions of common gingivitis and adult periodontitis. They also suggested that this dysfunction of the neutrophils was a localized phenomenon since only disease sites in patients with *juvenile periodontitis* showed this pathological alteration. These observations are consistent with findings by Baehni et al. (1979) Tsai et al. (1979) and McArthur et al. (1981), who demonstrated that *A. actinomycetemcomitans* has a capacity to interfere with the viability and function of neutrophils (see virulence factors).

The characteristic features of the inflammatory cell infiltrates of deep periodontal lesions in patients with juvenile periodontitis, postjuvenile periodontitis (generalized juvenile periodontitis) and adult periodontitis are illustrated in Fig. 6-13 (Liljenberg & Lindhe 1980). From the bars presented in Fig. 6-13 it can be seen that while the extracellular tissue (collagen and residual tissue) in lesions of postjuvenile periodontitis (generalized juvenile periodontitis) and adult periodontitis comprised between 50-60% of the tissue volume, in *localized juvenile periodontitis* sites, the extracellular tissue occupied only about 20% of the lesion. Since the majority of the cells in the juvenile periodontitis lesion were identified as plasma cells and blast cells, there are reasons to suggest that this particular lesion is composed of a dense accumulation of plasma cells and blast cells.

General host response

Lehner et al. (1974) examined the role of humoral and cell-mediated immunity in 34 patients with juvenile (14-21 years) and post-juvenile (22-29 years) periodontitis. They reported that the serum IgG, IgM and IgA levels were significantly higher in these patients than in healthy controls. In addition, patients in the juvenile periodontitis group showed an impaired lymphocyte blastogenic response to some selected Gram negative microorganisms but with the release of *positive* macrophage migration inhibition (MIF) activity. Studies by Ebersole et al. (1980) and Mouton et al. (1981) have confirmed the antibody data of Lehner et al. (1974) by showing that the patients with localized juvenile periodontitis frequently have increased antibody activity (serum IgG antibody) to *A. actinomycetemcomitans,* but a low titer of antibodies to *B. gingivalis*. A number of other investigations have also shown markedly elevated serum antibody levels to *A. actinomycetemcomitans* (Table 6-2). Patients with adult periodontitis or *generalized juvenile periodontitis* on the other hand were found to have a high antibody titer to *B. gingivalis* but low titers to *A. actinomycetemcomitans*. These findings together with the available microbial data imply that *localized juvenile periodontitis* on the one hand, and generalized forms of periodontitis on the other, are microbiologically different diseases.

Results reported by Cianciola et al. (1977), Clark et al. (1977), Lavine et al. (1979), van Dyke et al. (1980) and others have demonstrated that a majority of individuals with *localized juvenile periodontitis* have neutrophilic granulocytes in the circulating blood with an impaired capacity to react to chemotactic stimulus. Van Dyke et al. (1980) concluded that 26 out of 32 patients with *localized juvenile periodontitis*, but only 2 out of 23 with adult periodontitis, had neutrophils in the circulating blood with an improper ability to respond to chemotaxis. They suggested that the neutrophil dysfunction was caused by a cell-associated defect of long duration. The observation indicates that examination of children and adolescents regarding neutrophil function may be a means of discriminating children who run a risk of developing juvenile periodontitis.

Cementopathia

Gottlieb (1928) suggested that periodontitis was associated with "cementopathia". Long-term studies of early onset periodontitis by Page and co-workers (e.g. Page & Baab 1985) have recently supported this hypothesis by demonstrating that patients with prepubertal and juvenile forms of periodontitis have various degrees of hypophosphatasia, a condition known to cause a cementum aplasia. In a study by Blomlöf et al. (1986) teeth associated with localized and generalized juvenile periodontitis lesions were examined with respect to deficiencies in the root cementum: 25 teeth in 11 patients with these disorders were extracted and examined in the light and the scanning electron microscope. The patients were divided into two groups; one *localized* and one *generalized* juvenile periodontitis group: 10 extracted first molars from each of 10 patients with adult periodontitis and 5 third molars from each of 5 young patients with no disease were studied as controls. Cementum hypoplasias were found on the root surfaces of all extracted first molars from 9 patients with *localized juvenile perio-*

dontitis and on most teeth from 2 patients with *generalized* juvenile periodontitis. No hypoplasias were found on the control teeth. The hypoplasias on teeth associated with *localized juvenile periodontitis* occurred along the entire root surface, including portions that were still surrounded by alveolar bone at the time of extraction. Most hypoplasias were found on surfaces that in the radiographs were associated with extensive bone loss. The findings reported by Blomlöf et al. (1986) support observations made in a similar but preliminary study by Lindskog and Blomlöf (1983). The question still remains, however, if this deficiency in the root cementum is associated with the initiation. and progression of the inflammatory lesions in the periodontium.

Treatment

Data regarding the effect of treatment of juvenile periodontitis is sparse. Waerhaug (1977), from a retrospective study of 21 patients with juvenile periodontitis, who were monitored over a period of 8-32 years, reported that a treatment involving excision of the deepened pocket, root curettage and plaque control was effective in arresting the progression of the disorder. He stated: "the most important observation made in this material was that so-called periodontosis responds to total plaque control just as well as does ordinary advanced perio-

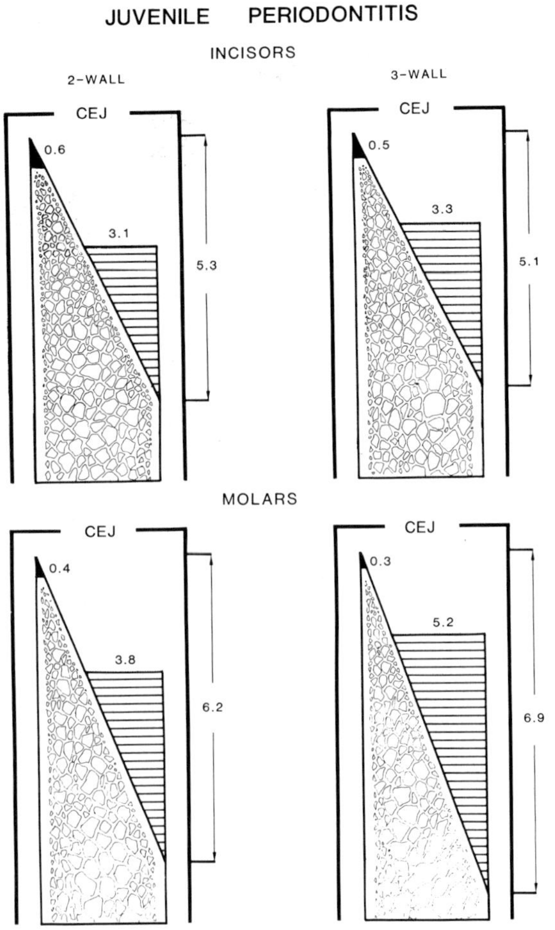

Fig. 6-14. Diagram describing the alterations of the morphology and height of angular bony defects in sites of juvenile periodontitis. In incisors as well as molars there was a slight resorption of the bone crest (0.3-0.6 mm) following therapy. Bone fill in the angular bony defects amounted to between 3.1 and 5.2 mm.

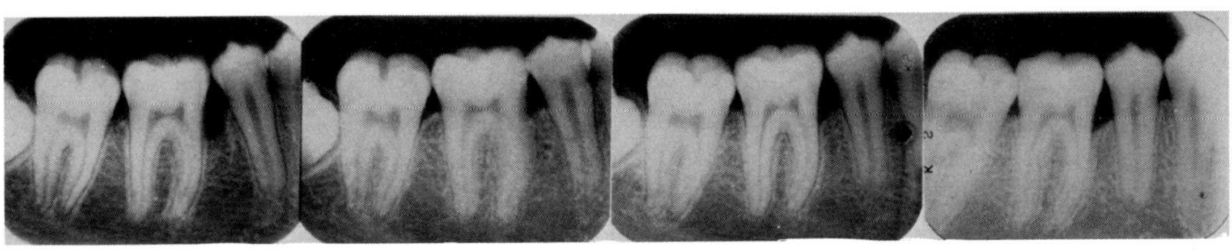

Fig. 6-15a. Fig. 6-15b. Fig. 6-15c. Fig. 6-15d.

Fig. 6-15. A localized juvenile periodontitis lesion at the mesial surface of tooth 46 before therapy (a), 2 months (b), 12 months (c) and 24 months (d) following active therapy (administration of tetracycline, flap curettage and root-surface instrumentation).

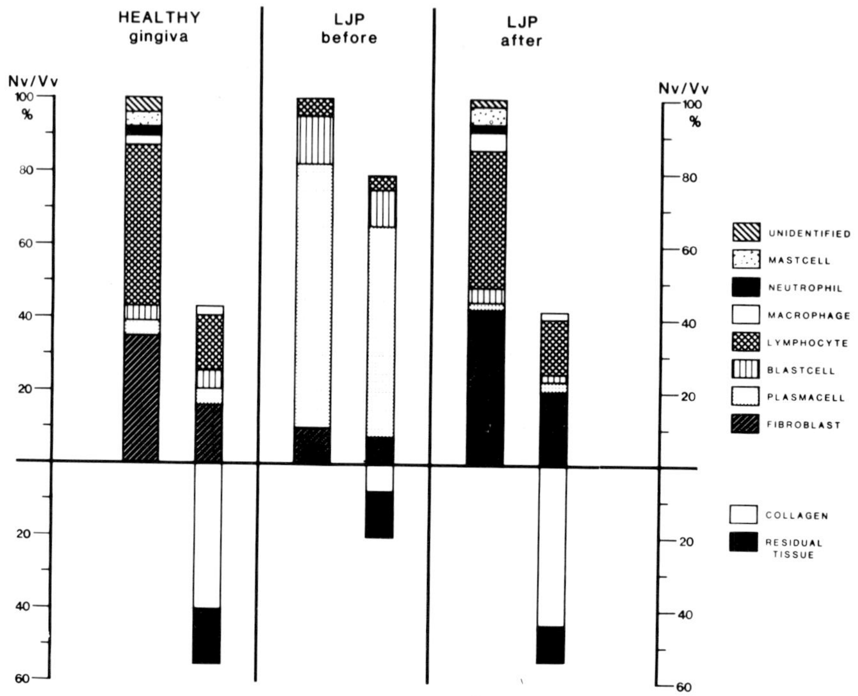

Fig. 6-16. Histogram of the composition of healthy gingival units and localized juvenile periodontitis lesions before and after therapy. The wide bars describe the numerical density and the thin bars the volumetrical density parameters. It can be seen that localized juvenile periodontitis lesions following therapy healed, i.e. tissue characteristics after treatment became similar to those of healthy gingiva. (From Lindhe 1982).

dontitis". Baer & Socransky (1979) presented a long-term follow-up history of a patient with periodontosis and suggested that antibiotics such as tetracycline and penicillin can "be a helpful adjunct to patients' managements" including "full thickness flap and curettage in affected areas".

Lindhe (1982) studied the effect on *localized juvenile periodontitis* lesions of a treatment program which included (1) systemic tetracycline, (2) surgical elimination of inflamed tissues, (3) scaling and root planing and (4) careful plaque control during healing. Treatment of *localized juvenile periodontitis* lesions was carried out on 16 individuals, aged 14-18 years. Lesions in first molars and incisors in subjects with adult periodontitis were treated in an identical manner and served as controls. A clinical examination was carried out including assessments of oral hygiene, gingival conditions, probing depths and attachment levels. Periodic reproducible radiographs were obtained from first molars and incisors to study alterations of the bony defects following treatment. After the clinical examination the patients were subjected to a treatment program involving: 1) administration of tetracycline (250mg x 4/day for 2 weeks), 2) removal of granulation tissue after flap elevation, and 3) root curettage. After surgery the patients were instructed to 4) rinse their mouths with a 0.2% chlorhexidine solution for 2 min. twice a day during the first 2 postsurgical weeks. 5) Professional tooth cleaning was carried out by a dental hygienist once every 3 months during a 2-year period. The patients were reexamined regarding their oral hygiene, gingival conditions, probing-depth attachment levels and bone-defect alterations 6, 12, 18 and 24 months following therapy.

It was observed that this treatment of *localized juvenile periodontitis* resulted in resolution of gingival inflammation, substantial gain of clinical attachment and refill of bone in the angular bony defects (Fig. 6-14). The clinical pattern of healing in the juvenile periodontitis sample was similar to that observed in patients with adult periodontitis. If anything, attachment gain and bone fill appeared to be somewhat faster in young patients with localized lesions than in older individuals (Fig. 6-15). Analysis of biopsy material obtained after therapy (Fig. 6-16) revealed that the previously diseased sites (juvenile as well as adult) had been repopulated by a tissue the composition of which was similar to that of normal gingiva.

This study, therefore, confirms the observations by Waerhaug (1977) that juvenile periodontitis lesions respond to treatment as well as do adult periodontitis lesions. It was, however, also observed that while no patient in the adult periodontitis group showed signs of *recurrent disease* during the 2 years of observation, 4 individuals and a total of 6 sites in the juvenile periodontitis group had to be retreated because of recurrence of inflammation, increasing probing depth and further loss of alveolar bone.

In a subsequent publication, Lindhe and Liljenberg (1984) described the 5-year follow-up data from the patient sample initially described by Lindhe (1982). Between the 2-year and the 5-year reexamination interval the patients were recalled for prophylaxis once every 3 months. The maintenance program prevented periodontal disease from recurring. Thus, between the 2- and 5-year examinations there was no increase of gingivitis, the probing pocket-depth of the previously diseased sites remained shallow, and the clinical attachment level remained unchanged. The authors concluded that the combined treatment program used for *localized juvenile periodontitis* lesions was highly effective but admitted that it was based more on a "clinical experience" than on scientific evidence. Tetracycline was used in order to eradicate pathogenic microorganisms associated with *localized juvenile periodontitis.* The soft tissue of the lesion was excised because it contained inflammatory cell infiltrates with large numbers of plasma cells and blast cells which may interfere with bone regrowth during heal-

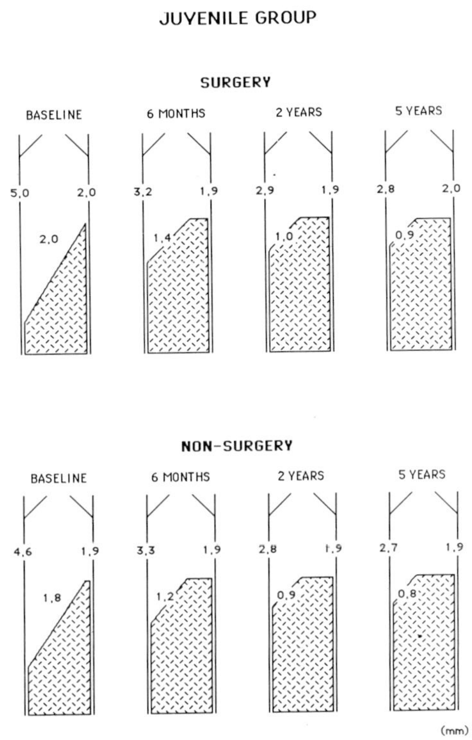

Fig. 6-17. Diagrammatic presentation of the average dimensions of the angular bony defects in the localized juvenile periodontitis group at baseline, 6 months, 2 and 5 years following treatment (from Wennström et al. 1986).

ing. The authors furthermore admitted that they had not demonstrated that each single treatment measure used in their study could be regarded as an obligatory component of therapy for *localized juvenile periodontitis.*

In another sample of 16 patients (11 with *localized juvenile periodontitis* and 5 with *generalized juvenile periodontitis*), a treatment which *did not include systemic tetracycline therapy* was delivered utilizing a split mouth design (Wennström et al. 1986). By random selection the diseased sites in one side of the jaws were treated with scaling and root planing after elevation of a modified Widman flap, while in the contralateral jaws treatment was restricted to scaling and root planing. Following active treatment the patient received a maintenance treatment which was identical to that used in

Lindhe-Liljenberg material. At 6 months, 2 and 5 years after treatment the patients were reexamined. With respect to probing pocket-depth reduction, gain of probing attachment and recession of the gingival margin, no differences could be found between the various treatment groups. In addition, the improvement of the gingival conditions was similar in the 4 groups. Fig. 6-17 demonstrates that the degree of bone fill in surgically and nonsurgically treated sites was almost identical. Since the improvement observed by Wennström et al. (1986) in *nontetracycline*-treated patients was almost identical to that reported by Lindhe & Liljenberg (1984), who utilized tetracycline, it may be suspected that neither systemic tetracycline, nor flap elevation and granulation tissue removal are obligatory components of therapy in some patients with localized juvenile periodontitis. The findings from the above studies therefore clearly indicate (1) that the crux in juvenile periodontitis, localized as well as generalized, is the infection in the periodontal pocket, and that (2) this infection in some situations may be eliminated by meticulous pocket therapy. A similar conclusion was drawn by Saxén et al. (1986) from a retrospective study on treatment of patients with juvenile periodontitis.

An alternative approach to the treatment of localized juvenile periodontitis was presented by Slots and co-workers (Slots & Rosling 1983, Christersson et al. 1985). They examined the efficacy of various treatment modalities to eliminate or markedly *suppress the pathogens,* mainly *A. actinomycetemcomitans* and capnocytophaga, from the periodontal lesions. In a first study, Slots & Rosling (1983) treated, in a sequential manner, patients with *localized juvenile periodontitis* with 1) scaling, 2) topical iodine application, and 3) systemic tetracycline administration (1 gram per day for 2 weeks). They reported that neither mechanical debridement nor topical iodine applications eradicated the infection, whereas systemic tetracycline therapy substantially reduced both *A. actinomycetemcomitans* and capnocytophaga counts in shallow as well as in deep pockets. Slots & Rosling (1983) furthermore reported that there was a clear-cut relationship between alterations of probing attachment levels and the recovery of *A. actinomycetemcomitans* after therapy. Thus, at initially deep pocket sites which lost probing attachment during therapy, *A. actinomycetemcomitans* appeared in high numbers also after treatment. In contrast, *A. actinomycetemcomitans* was not recovered from any of the deep pockets which demonstrated at least 2.5 mm of probing attachment gain. In a subsequent study Christersson et al. (1985) confirmed the findings reported by Slots & Rosling (1983) by demonstrating that gain or loss of probing attachment levels at initially diseased sites 16 weeks following therapy in patients with *localized juvenile periodontitis* was positively correlated with the presence of *A. actinomycetemcomitans.* All sites which after treatment had lost further probing attachment consistently harbored relatively high numbers of *A. actinomycetemcomitans*, while only 22% of the lesions which gained clinical attachments demonstrated small numbers of this bacterium. The authors concluded that a substantial suppression of subgingival *A. actinomycetemcomitans* is critical to the success of treatment. They also recommended that assessment of treatment efficacy should include a monitoring of subgingival *A. actinomycetemcomitans.*

Proposal for treatment of localized juvenile periodontitis

Based on the observations made in the clinical studies referred to above the following protocol for the treatment of juvenile periodontitis may be recommended:

1. Conventional periodontal therapy including thorough scaling and root planing, preferentially in conjunction with periodontal surgery to gain access to the affected root

surfaces. Carefully executed and monitored post-operative plaque control.

2. At 3 months after periodontal therapy, monitoring of the subgingival microbiota for *A. actinomycetemcomitans* and other potentially pathogenic bacteria.

3. Use of antimicrobial therapy in infected cases. Treatment with an antimicrobial agent should be short-term, intensive and aim optimally at eradicating the pathogenic components of the subgingival microbiota. Systemic Tetracycline HCI (1 g /day /21 days) may eliminate *A. actinomycetemcomitans* infections.

4. At 3 months, after termination of antimicrobial therapy, microbiological control of treatment efficacy (compliance).

References

Altman, L.C., Page, R.C., Ebersole, J.L. & Vandesteen, G.E. (1982). Assessment of host defenses and serum antibodies to suspected periodontal pathogens in patients with various types of periodontitis. *Journal of Periodontal Research* **17**, 495-497.

Asibeiner, S., Fousimies-Somer, H., Karervo, A. & Saxén, L. (1986) *Actinobacillus actinomycetemcomitans* and clinical periodontal status in Finnish juvenile periodontitis patients. *Journal of Periodontology* **57**, 91-93.

Baab, D.A., Page, P.C., Ebersole, J.L., Williams, B.L. & Scott, L.R. (1986) Laboratory studies of a family manifesting premature exfoliation of deciduous teeth. *Journal of Clinical Periodontology* **13**, 677-683.

Baab, D.A., Page, R.C. & Morton, T.H. (1985) Studies of a family manifesting premature exfoliation of deciduous teeth. *Journal of Periodontology* **56**, 403-409.

Baehni, P., Tsai, C-C., McArthur, W.P. Hammond, B.F. & Taichman, N.S. (1979) Interaction of inflammatory cells and oral microorganism. VIII. Detection of leukotoxic activity of a plaque-derived gram-negative microorganisms. *Infection and Immunity* **24**, 233-243.

Baer, P.N. (1971) The case of periodontosis as a clinical entity. *Journal of Periodontology* **42**, 516-520.

Baer, P.N. & Socransky, S.S. (1979) Periodontosis: Case report with long-term follow-up. *Periodontal Case Reports* **1**, 1-6.

Bial, J.J. & Mellonig, J.T. (1987) Radiographic evaluation of juvenile periodontitis (Periodontosis). *Journal of Periodontology* **58**, 321-326.

Bick, P.H., Beets Carpenter, A., Holdeman, L.V., Miller, G.A., Ranney, R.R., Palcanis, K.G. & Tew, J.G. (1981) Polyclonal B-cell activation induced by extracts of gram-negative bacteria isolated from periodontally diseased sites. *Infection and Immunity* **34**, 43-49.

Blomlöf, L., Hammarström, L. & Lindskog, S. (1986) Occurrence and appearance of cementum hypoplacias in localized and generalized juvenile periodontitis. *Acta Odontologica Scandinavica* **44**, 313-320.

Byström, A., Crossner, C.-G. & Unell, L. (1983) "Prepubertal" periodontitis. A case report. *Swedish Dental Journal* **7**, 254, Abstr 27.

Christersson, L.A., Slots, J., Rosling, B.G. & Genco, R.J. (1985) Microbiological and clinical effects of surgical treatment of localized juvenile periodontitis. *Journal of Clinical Periodontology* **12**, 465-476.

Cianciola, L.L., Genco, R.J., Paters, M.R., McKenna, I. & van Oss, C.J. (1977) Defective polymorphonuclear leukocyte function in a human periodontal disease. *Nature* **265**, 445-447.

Clark, R.A., Page, R.C. & Wilde, G. (1977) Defective neutrophil chemotaxis in juvenile periodontitis. *Infection and Immunity* **18**, 694-700.

Cogen, R.B., Al-Joburi, W., Caufield, P.W., Stanley, H.P. & Donaldson, K. (1984) Periodontal disease in healthy children: Two clinical reports. *Pediatric Dental* **6**, 41-45.

Delaney, J.E. & Korman, K.S. (1987) Microbiology of subgingival plaque for children with localized prepubertal periodontitis. *Oral Microbiology and Immunology* **2**, 71-76.

Ebersole, J.L., Taubman, M.A., Smith, D.J. & Socransky, S.S. (1982) Humoral immune responses and diagnosis of human periodontal disease. *Journal of Periodontal Research* **17**, 478-480.

Ebersole, J.L., Frey, D.E., Taubman, M.A., Smith,

D.J. & Genco, R.J. (1980) Serum antibody response to A. actinomycetemcomitans (Y4) in periodontal disease. *Journal of Dental Research* **59**, Special issue A, Abstr 249.

Eisenmann, A.C., Eisenmann, R., Sousa, O. & Slots, J. (1983) Microbiological study of localized juvenile periodontitis in Panama. *Journal of Periodontology* **54**, 712-713.

Farida, R., Marsh, P.D., Newman, H.N., Rule, D.C. & Ivanyi, L. (1986) Serological investigation of various forms of inflammatory periodontitis. *Journal of Periodontal Research* **21**, 365-374.

Genco, R.J., Slots, J., Mouton, C. & Murray, P. (1980) Systemic immune responses to oral anaerobic organisms. In: *Anaerobic bacterial: selected topics*, ed. Lambe, D.W. Jr., Genco, R.J. & Mayberry-Carson, K.J. pp. 277-293. New York: Plenum Press.

Genco, R.J., Zambon, J.J. & Murray, P.A. (1985) Serum and gingival fluid antibodies as adjuncts in the diagnosis of *Actinobacillus actinomycetemcomitans* - associated periodontal disease *Journal of Periodontology* **56** (special issue), 41-50.

Gibbons, R.J. & MacDonald J.B. (1961) Degradation of collagenous substrates by Bacteroides melaninogenicus. *Journal of Bacteriology* **81**, 614-621.

Gillett, R. & Johnson, N.W. (1982) Bacterial invasion of the periodontium in a case of juvenile periodontitis. *Journal of Clinical Periodontology* **9**, 93-100.

Gottlieb, B. (1923) Die diffuse astrophy des Alveolarknochens. *Zeitschrift Für Stomatologie* **21**, 195.

Gottlieb, B. (1928) The formation of the pocket: diffuse atrophy of alveolar bone. *Journal of the American Dental Association* **15**, 462.

Gottlieb, B. (1946) The new concept of periodontoclasia. *Journal of Periodontology* **17**, 7-23.

Hausmann, E., Raisz, L.G. & Miller, W.A. (1970) Endotoxin: stimulation of bone resorption in tissue culture. *Science* **168**, 862-864.

Hofstad, T. (1970) Biological activities of endotoxin from Bacteroides melaninogenicus. *Archives of Oral Biology* **15**, 343-348.

Hörmand, J. & Frandsen, A. (1979) Juvenile periodontitis. Localization of bone loss in relation to age, sex, and teeth. *Journal of Clinical Periodontology* **6**, 407-416.

Kiley, P. & Holt, S.C. (1980) Characterization of the lipopolysaccharide from Actinobacillus actinomycetemcomitans Y4 and N27. *Infection and Immunity* **30**, 862-873.

Kilian, M. (1981) Degradation of immunoglobulins A1, A2 and G by suspected principal periodontal pathogens. *Infection and Immunity* **34**, 757-765.

Laughon, B.E., Syed, S.A. & Loesche, W.J. (1982) API ZYM system for identification of Bacteroides spp., Capnocytophaga spp., and spirochetes of oral origin. *Journal of Clinical Microbiology* **15**, 97-102.

Lavine, W.S., Maderazo, E.G., Stolman, J., Ward, P.A., Cogen, R.B., Greenblatt, I. & Robertsson, P.B. (1979) Impaired neutrophil chemotaxis in patients with juvenile and rapidly progressing periodontitis. *Journal of Periodontal Research* **14**, 10-19.

Lehner, T., Wilton, M.A., Ivanyi, L. & Manson, I.D. (1974) Immunologocal aspects of juvenile periodontitis (periodontosis). *Journal of Periodontal Research* **9**, 261-272.

Liljenberg, B. & Lindhe, J. (1980) Juvenile periodontitis. Some microbiological, histopathological and clinical characteristics. *Journal of Clinical Periodontology* **7**, 48-61.

Lindhe, J. (1982) Treatment of localized juvenile periodontitis. In: *Host-Parasite Interactions in Periodontal Disease,* ed. R.J. Genco & S.E. Mergenhagen. Washington, D.C.: American Society for Microbiology.

Listgarten, M.A. (1976) Structure of the microbial flora associated with periodontal health and disease in man. A light and electron microscopic study. *Journal of Periodontology* **47**, 1-18.

Lindskog, S. & Blomlöf, L. (1983) Cementum hypoplacia in teeth affected by juvenile periodontitis. *Journal of Clinical Periodontology* **10**, 443-451.

Loesche, W.J., Syed, S.A., Laughon, B.G. & Stoll, J. (1982) The bacteriology of acute necrotizing ulcerative gingivitis. *Journal of Periodontology* **53**, 223-230.

Loesche, W.J., Syed, S.A., Morrison, E.C., Laughon, B. & Grossman, N.S. (1981) Treatment of periodontal infections due to anaerobic bacteria with short-term treatment with metronidazole. *Journal of Clinical Periodontology* **8**, 29-44.

Loesche, W.J., Syed, S.A., Morrison, E.C., Laughon, B. & Grossman, N.S. (1981) Treatment of periodontal infections due to anaerobic bacteria with short-term treatment with matronidazole. *Journal of Clinical Periodontology* **8**, 29-44.

Mandell, R.L., Siegal, M.D. & Umland, E. (1986) Localized juvenile periodontitis of the primary dentition. *Journal of Dentistry in Childhood* **53**, 193-196.

Mandell, R.L. (1984) A longitudinal microbiological investigation of *Actinobacillus actinomycetemcomitans* and *Eikenella corrodens* in juvenile periodontitis. *Infection and Immunity* **45**, 778-780.

Mandell, R.L. & Socransky, S.S. (1981) A Selective medium for Actinobacillus actinomycetemcomitans and the incidence of the organism in juvenile periodontitis. *Journal of Periodontology* **52**, 593-598.

Mansheim, B.J., Orderdonk, A.B. & Kasper, D.L. (1978) Immunochemical and biologic studies of the lipopolysaccharide of Bacteroides melaninogenicus subspecies asaccharolyticus. *Journal of Immunology* **120**, 72-78.

Manson, J.D. & Lehner, T. (1974) Clinical features of juvenile periodontitis (periodontosis). *Journal of Periodontology* **45**, 636-640.

Mishkin, D.J., Grant, N.C., Bergeron, R.A. & Young, W.L. (1986) Prepubertal periodontitis: a recently defined clinical entity. *Pediatric Dentistry* **8**, 235-238.

McArthur, W.P., Tsai, C.-C., Baehni, P.C., Genco, R.J. & Taichman, N.S. (1981) Leukotoxic effects of Actinobacillus actinomycetemcomitans. *Journal of Periodontal Research* **16**, 159-170.

Moore, W.E.C., Holdeman, L.V., Cato, E.P., Smibert, R.M., Burmeister, J.A., Palcanis, K.G. & Ranney, R.R. (1985) Comparative bacteriology of juvenile periodontitis. *Infection and Immunity* **48**, 507-519.

Moore, W.E.C., Holdeman, L.V., Smibert, R.M., Hash, D.E., Burmeister, J.A. & Ranney, R.R. (1982) Bacteriology of severe periodontitis in young adult humans. *Infection and Immunity* **38**, 1137-1148.

Mouton, C., Hammond, P.G., Slots, J. & Genco, R.J. (1981) Serum antibodies to oral Bacteroides asaccharolyticus (Bacteroides gingivalis): relationship to age and periodontal disease. *Infection and Immunity* **31**, 182-192.

Murray, P. & Patters, M. (1980) Gingival crevice neutrophil function in periodontal lesions. *Journal of Periodontal Research* **15**, 463-469.

Newman, M.G. & Socransky, S.S. (1977) Predominant cultivable microbiota in periodontosis. *Journal of Periodontal Research* **12**, 120-128.

Ngan, P.W.H., Tsai, C.-C. & Sweeney, E. (1985) Advanced periodontitis in the primary dentition: case report. *Pediatric Dentistry* **7**, 255-258.

Orban, B. & Weinmann, J.P. (1942) Diffuse atrophy of alveolar bone. *Journal of Periodontology* **13**, 31.

Page, R.C. & Baab, D.A. (1985) A new look at the etiology and pathogenesis of early onset periodontitis. Cementopathia revisited. *Journal of Periodontology* **56**, 748-751.

Page, R.C., Bowen, T., Altman, L., Vandesteen, E., Ochs, H., Mackenzie, P., Osterberg, S., Engel, D. & Williams, B. (1983) Prepubertal periodontitis. I. Definition of a Clinical Disease entity. *Journal of Periodontology* **54**, 257-271.

Page, R.C. & Schroeder, H.E. (1982) Periodontitis in man and other animals: A comparative review. Karger:Basel; New York.

Preus, H.R., Olsen, I. & Namork, E. (1987a) Association between bacteriophage-infected *Actinobacillus actinomycetemcomitans* and rapid periodontal destruction. *Journal of Clinical Periodontology* **14**, 245-247.

Preus, H.R., Olsen, I. & Namork, E. (1987b) The presence of phage-infected *A. actinomycetemcomitans* in localized juvenile periodontitis patients. *Journal of Clinical Periodontology* **14**, 605-609.

Ranney, R.R., Yanni, N.R., Burmeister, J.A. & Tew, J.G. (1982) Relationship between attachment loss and precipitating serum antibody to *Actinobacillus actinomycetemcomitans* in adolescents and young adults having severe periodontal destruction. *Journal of Periodontology* **53**, 1-7.

Rozanis, J. & Slots, J. (1982) Collagenolytic activity of *Actinobacillus actinomycetemcomitans* and black-pigmented Bacteroides. *Journal of Dental Research* **61**, Abstr 870, Annual meeting of the International Association of Dental Research.

Saglie, F.R., Carranza Jr., F.A., Newman, M.G., Cheng, L. & Lewin, K.J. (1982) Identification of tissue-invading bacteria in human periodontal disease. *Journal of Periodontal Research* **17**, 452-455.

Saxén, L. (1980) Juvenile periodontitis. *Journal of Clinical Periodontology* **7**, 1-19.

Shenker, B.J. (1987) Immunologic dysfunction in the pathogenesis of periodontal diseases. *Journal of Clinical Periodontology* **14**, 489-498.

Shenker, B.J., Kushner, M.E. & Tsai, C.-C. (1982) Inhibition of fibroblast proliferation by *Actinobacillus actinomycetemcomitans. Infection and Immunity* **38**, 986-992.

Shurin, S.B., Socransky, S.S., Sweeney, E. & Stossel, T.P. (1979) A neutrophil disorder induced by capnocytophaga, a dental microorganism. *New England Journal of Medicine* **301**, 849-854.

Slots, J. (1976) The predominant cultivable organisms in juvenile periodontitis. *Scandinavian Journal of Dental Research* **84**, 1-10.

Slots, J. (1981) Enzymatic characterization of some oral and nonoral gram negative bacteria with the API ZYM system. *Journal of Clinical Microbiology* **14**, 288-294.

Slots, J. (1986b) Virulence factors of the bacteria that cause periodontal diseases. *Compendium of Continuing Education in Dentistry* **7**, 665-671.

Slots, J. & Genco, R.J. (1984) Black-pigmented *Bacteroides* species,*Capnocytophaga* species, and *Actinobacillus actinomycetemcomitans* in human periodontal disease: virulence factors in colonization, survival, and tissue destruction. *Journal of Dental Research* **63**, 412-421.

Slots, J., Reynolds, H.S. & Genco, R.J. (1980) *Actinobacillus actinomycetemcomitans* in human periodontal disease: a cross-sectional microbiological investigation. *Infection and Immunity* **29**, 1013-1020.

Slots, J. & Rosling, B.G. (1983) Suppression of the periodontopathic microflora in localized juvenile periodontitis by systemic tetracycline. *Journal of Clinical Periodontology* **10**, 465-486.

Stevens, R.H., Sela, M.N. McArthur, W.P., Nowotny, A. & Hammond, B.F. (1980b) Biological and chemical characterization of endotoxin from Capnocytophaga sputigena. *Infection and Immunity* **27**, 246-254.

Stevens, R.H., Sela, M.N., Shapira, J. & Hammond, B.F. (1980a) Detection of a fibroblast proliferation inhibitory factor from Capnocytophaga sputigena. *Infection and Immunity* **27**, 271-275.

Sugarman, M.M. & Sugarman, E.F. (1977) Precocious periodontitis: A clinical entity and a treatment responsibility. *Journal of Periodontology* **48**, 397-409.

Sweeney, E.A., Alcoforado, G.A.P., Nyman, S. & Slots, J. (1987) Prevalence and microbiology of localized prepubertal periodontitis. *Oral Microbiology and Immunology* **2**, 65-70.

Tanner, A.C.R., Haffer, C., Bratthall, G.T., Visconti, R.A. & Socransky, S.S. (1979) A Study of the bacteria associated with advancing periodontitis in man. *Journal of Clinical Periodontology* **6**, 278-307.

Taubman, M.A., Ebersole, J.L. & Smith, D.J. (1982) Association between systemic and local antibody in periodontal disease. In: *Host-parasite interactions in periodontal diseases*, ed. Genco, R.J. & Mergenhagen, S.E., pp. 283-298. Washington, D.C.: American Society for Microbiology.

Tsai, C.-C., McArthur, W.P., Baehni, P.C., Evian, C., Genco, R.J. & Taichman, N.S. (1981) Serum neutralizing activity against Actinobacillus actinomycetemcomitans leukotoxin in juvenile periodontitis. *Journal of Clinical Periodontology* **8**, 338-348.

Tsai, C.-C., McArthur, W.P., Baehni, P.C., Hammond, B.F. & Taichman, N.S. (1979) Extraction and partial characterization of a leukotoxin from a plaque-derived gram-negative microorganism. *Infection and Immunity* **25**, 427-439.

van Dyke, T.E., Bartholomew, E., Genco, R.J., Slots, J. & Levine, M.J. (1982) Inhibition of neutrophil chemotaxis by soluble bacterial products. *Journal of Periodontology* **53**, 502-508.

van Dyke, T.E., Horoszewicz, H.U., Cianciola, L.J. & Genco, R.J. (1980) Neutrophil Chemotaxis dysfunction in human periodontitis. *Infection and Immunity* **27**, 124-132.

Vincent, J.W., Suzuki, J.B., Falkler, W.A. Jr. & Cornett, W.C. (1985) Reaction of human sera from juvenile periodontitis, rapidly progressive periodontitis and adult periodontitis patients with selected periodontopathogens. *Journal of Periodontology* **56**, 464-469.

Waerhaug, J. (1977) Plaque Control in the treatment of juvenile periodontitis. *Journal of Periodontology* **4**, 29-40.

Westergaard, J., Frandsen, A. & Slots, J. (1978) Ultrastructure of the subgingival microflora in juvenile periodontitis. *Scandinavian Journal of Dental Research* **86**, 421-429.

Williams, B.L., Ebersole, J.L., Spector, M.D. & Page, R.C. (1985) Assessment of serum antibody patterns and analysis of subgingival microflora of members of a family with a high prevalence of early-onset periodontitis. *Infection and Immunity* **49**, 742-750.

Wilson, M.E., Zambon, J.J., Suzuki, J.B. & Genco, R.J. (1985) Generalized juvenile periodontitis, defective neutrophil chemotaxis and *Bacteroides gingivalis* in a 13-year old female. A case report. *Journal of Periodontology* **56**, 457-463.

Zambon, J.J., Christersson, L.A. & Slots, J. (1983) *Actinobacillus actinomycetemcomitans* in human periodontal disease: prevalence in patient groups and distribution of biotypes and serotypes within families. *Journal of Periodontology* **54**, 707-711.

CHAPTER 7

Necrotizing Gingivitis

Definition

Necrotizing gingvitis (NG) is an inflammatory destructive gingival condition which exhibits characteristic clinical signs and symptoms, and which has been assumed to be at least partially caused by agents other than those producing common chronic marginal gingivitis. In its most typical acute form, it is characterized by interproximal necrotic ulcers. These ulcers are covered by a yellowish-white or greyish debris, they are painful to touch and bleeding is readily provoked.

Because of its relatively frequent occurrence in HIV-infected individuals, the condition has attracted renewed attention in recent years (Greenspan et al. 1986, Schiödt & Pindborg 1987, see also Chapter 10).

NG has been known under several names. "Trench mouth", "ulceromembranous gingivitis", "acute necrotizing ulcerative gingivitis" (ANUG) and "Vincent's gingivitis" or "Vincent's gingivostomatitis" are some of the terms which have been used (Pickard 1973). The designation "ulcerative" is redundant, since these superficial necrotic lesions are practically always ulcerated. The association with the name Vincent is due to the fact that he first described the particular mixed *fusospirochetal* microbiota occurring in the so-called "Vincent's angina", where the necrotic areas are typically localized in the tonsils (Vincent 1898). The same mixed microbiota is found in NG lesions. Vincent's angina and NG usually occur independently of each other, however, and should therefore be regarded as separate disease entities. Vincent's angina occurs twice as frequently in females as in males (van Cauwenberge 1976), whereas *NG* has been reported to occur more frequently in males.

NG has features in common with the far more serious *cancrum oris* or "noma". This is a necrotizing and destructive, frequently mortal stomatitis in which the same mixed fusospirochetal flora dominates. It occurs almost exclusively in certain developing countries, mostly in children and in association with systemic diseases and malnutrition (Enwonwu 1972, 1985). Some researchers have suggested that *cancrum oris* always develops from preexisting *necrotizing gingivitis* (Emslie 1963) whereas others have been unable to confirm this observation (Pindborg et al. 1966, 1967, Sheiham 1966).

Unless properly treated, *NG* has a marked tendency for recurrence (Manson & Rand 1961). For such cases the designations "recurrent" or "chronic" have been used. If this condition is allowed to persist for some time, the disease may lead to considerable loss of periodontal support.

In this chapter the acute form will be termed *acute necrotizing gingivitis (ANG)*. The chronic or recurrent form will be termed *chronic necrotizing gingivitis* (CNG). The collective term is *necrotizing gingivitis (NG)*.

Epidemiology

In industrialized countries ANG occurs particularly among young adults, 18-30 years of age. In a study conducted in the USA, Grupe & Wilder (1956) found ANG in 2.2% of 870 young military trainees. Giddon et al. (1964) found ANG in 2.5% of 326 students in their first college year. During the next year more students contracted the disease so that a total of 6.7% had encountered the disease during their first 2 college years. In a comprehensive study Pindborg (1951a) found NG in 6.0% of Danish military trainees.

ANG can be observed in all age groups, but in western countries it is practically never seen in children. In some developing countries, on the other hand, ANG is common even in early childhood and is frequently associated with malnutrition or such systemic diseases as measles and malaria (Pindborg et al. 1966, Sheiham 1966, Enwonwu 1972, 1985). Reports of epidemic-like ANG among soldiers were not uncommon some years ago. There is, however, no epidemiological or other scientific data to suggest that the disease is communicable, nor is there conclusive evidence to confirm a sex predilection in the occurrence of ANG.

While the frequency of occurrence of NG has been on the decline for some time in many industrialized countries, the disease now seems to occur more often, and, though epidemiologic data are unsatisfactory, NG is now fairly often reported in HIV-infected individuals (Greenspan et al. 1986, Silverman et al. 1986, Schiödt & Pindborg 1987, Reichart et al. 1987).

Epidemiological investigations have identified 3 factors which seem to be related to increased frequency of ANG: *Poor oral hygiene, with preexisting simple chronic marginal gingivitis* is almost always seen in individuals who develop ANG. Thus, Pindborg (1951b) found that 87 out of 91 new cases of ANG had a preexisting chronic marginal gingivitis.

Smoking shows a clear association with ANG. Very few of those who develop ANG are nonsmokers. For instance, Pindborg (1951b) found only 1 nonsmoker among 57 ANG patients. The amount smoked also appears relevant. In a population examined by Goldhaber & Giddon (1964), 41% of subjects with ANG smoked more than 20 cigarettes daily. Only 5% of controls smoked as much as this and among the controls there were significantly more nonsmokers.

The third factor which seems to be related to the occurrence of ANG is *emotional stress*. Epidemiological investigations by Pindborg (1951a, b), Giddon et al. (1963), Goldhaber & Giddon (1964) and others, seem to indicate a more frequent occurrence of ANG in periods when the individuals are exposed to psychic or emotional stress. Such periods may be related, *inter alia*, to problems in school, examinations, or with the beginning or the end of military service.

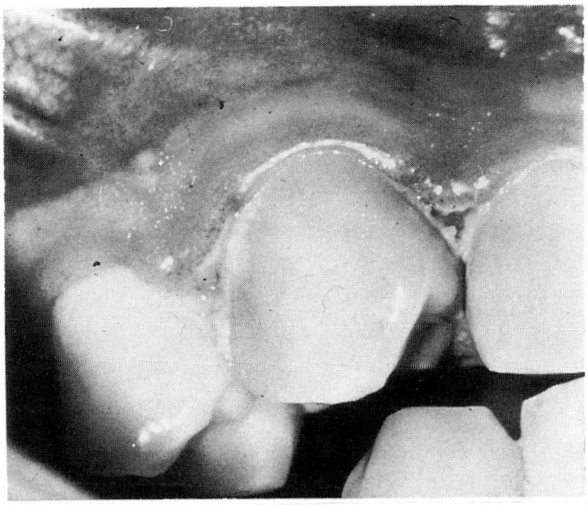

Fig. 7-1. Initial necrotic lesions in ANG. Mesial to 14 (13 is missing) initial crater formation is evident. The lesion near the tip of the interdental papilla distal to 14 is covered by a yellowish-white debris.

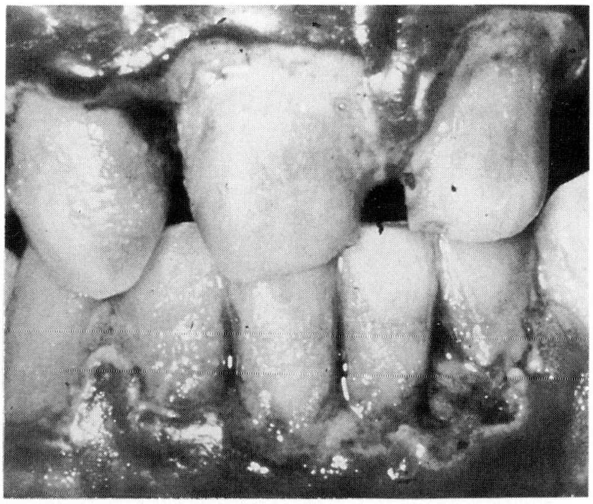

Fig. 7-2. Clinical photograph illustrating an advanced case of ANG. Confluent necrotic areas involving both the papillae and the facial gingiva are seen. Large amounts of yellowish-white soft debris cover both the necrotic zones and parts of the tooth surfaces.

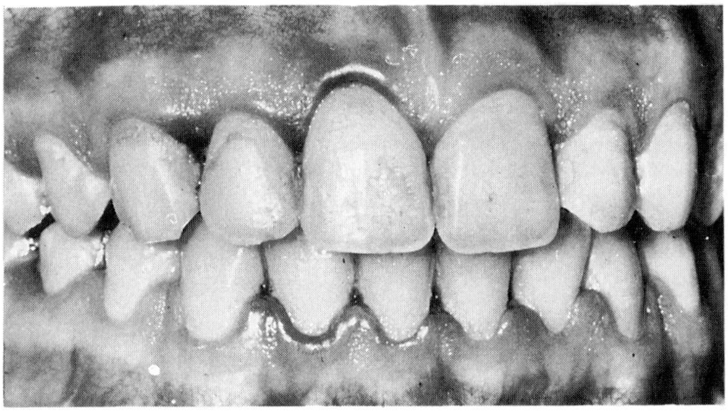

Fig. 7-3a. At this early stage of ANG, the first lesions can be seen in the lower anterior tooth region. The facial portions of the papillae are swollen and display a thickened, rounded margin. The necrotic areas are restricted to the interdental papillae and are still not very prominent.

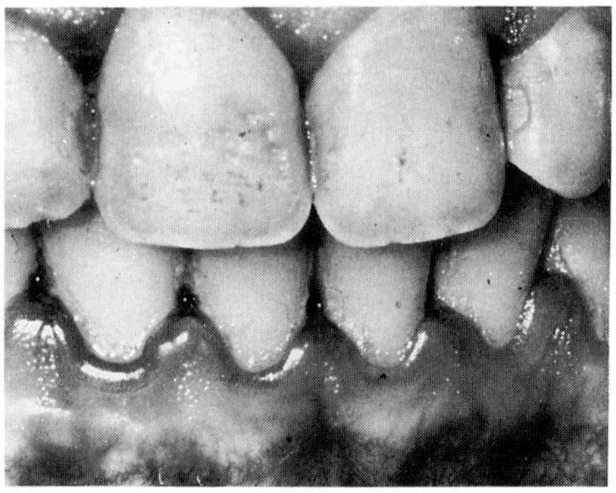

Fig. 7-3b. Higher magnification of the incisor regions from the patient shown in Fig. 7-3a.

Clinical characteristics

Acute necrotizing gingivitis (ANG)

Marginal necrosis

The most characteristic finding in ANG is necrotic lesions of the marginal gingiva. In the early stages, destruction is almost always localized to one or more interdental papillae. The first lesions are often seen interproximally in the lower anterior region, but they may occur in any interproximal space (Figs. 7-1, 7-3). In regions where lesions first appear there are usually also signs of preexisting chronic marginal gingivitis. The process commonly manifests itself with the occurrence of a necrotic ulcer on the tip of the papilla. The facial part tends to swell and becomes thickened with a rounded contour. The papillae do not always appear edematous at this stage; on the contrary, they may have a relatively firm consistency and gingival stippling is often maintained.

Necrosis develops rapidly. Within a few days

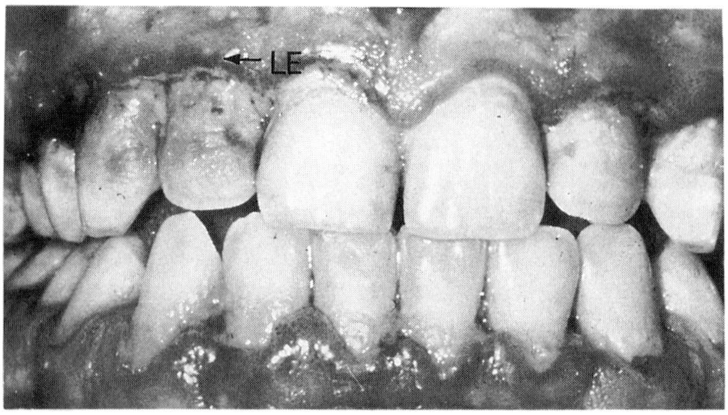

Fig. 7-4a. A typical case of ANG. In the lower anterior tooth region, necrotic areas are limited to the interproximal spaces where they are mostly hidden by the swollen interdental papillae. In the upper anterior tooth region, necrotic areas can be seen both facially and approximally. At teeth 13, 12 and partially at 11, the necrotic areas form a continuous zone covered by large amounts of soft yellowish-white debris. The linear erythema (LE) is the relatively well-delineated red zone separating the marginal necrotic areas from the rest of the gingiva. In the upper anterior tooth region white debris covers most of the free and attached gingiva.

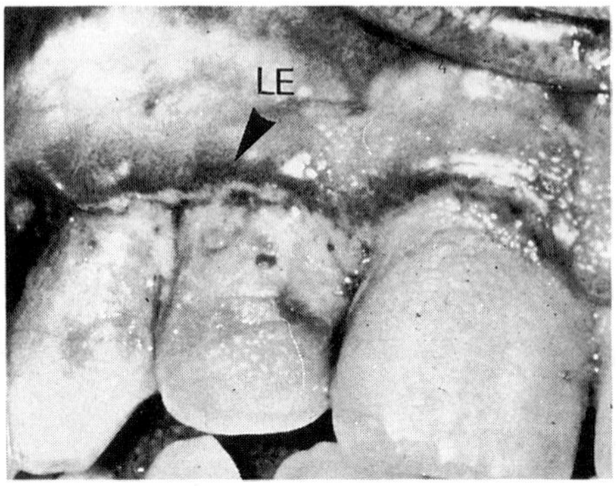

Fig. 7-4b. Higher magnification of teeth 11, 12 and 13, shown in Fig. 7-4a. Note the linear erythema (LE).

the involved papillae are separated into one facial and one lingual portion with an interposed necrotic depression between them. In this central depressed portion, the necrosis produces considerable tissue destruction and a crater is formed. The necrosis may also extend laterally to the marginal gingiva along the oral or facial surfaces of the teeth. Necrotic zones originating from neighboring interproximal spaces may merge and form a continuous necrotic area (Figs. 7-2, 7-4). These superficial necrotic lesions in ANG are primarily limited to the gingiva and only rarely do they cover the entire width of the attached gingiva. Usually only a relatively narrow zone of the marginal gingiva is afflicted.

The palatal and lingual marginal gingiva is less frequently involved than the corresponding facial area. If other parts of the oral mucosa are involved in the process, the simultaneous occurrence of ANG and another disease should be suspected. The most likely systemic condition to be involved in such instances is herpetic gingivostomatitis (see under *Differential diagnosis*).

Yellowish-white debris

The soft yellowish-white or greyish material which covers the necrotic zones has been termed "pseudomembrane". This is not a good term since the soft material bears little resemblance to a true membrane. It consists primarily of leukocytes, erythrocytes, fibrin, necrotic tissue remnants and masses of bacteria, and can not be removed as a continuous membrane. Attempts to remove this material will cause it to break up, and the bleeding, ulcerated connective tissue becomes exposed. The soft deposits also often cover subgingival calculus which is frequently found in large amounts on approximal surfaces of teeth next to the necrotic areas.

Personal oral hygiene in patients who contract ANG is usually poor. Moreover, brushing of teeth and contact with the acutely inflamed gingiva is painful. There are therefore frequently large amounts of plaque on the teeth, especially along the gingival margin. A thin whitish film of bacteria and debris may even cover the entire attached gingiva (Fig. 7-4). This film is composed of desquamated epithelial cells and some bacteria in a meshwork of salivary pro-

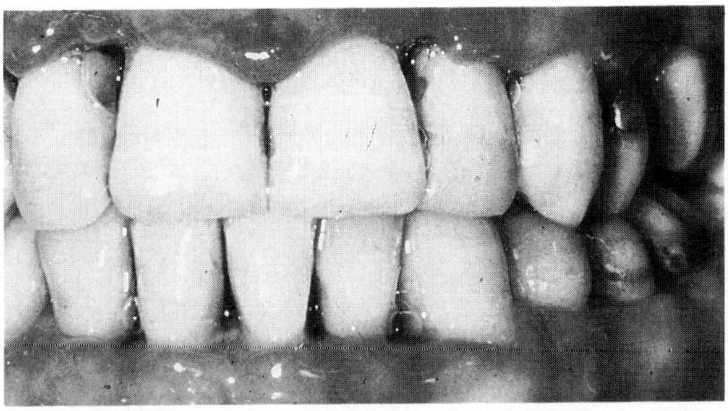

Fig. 7-5. In chronic necrotizing gingivitis (CNG) tenderness and pain may be relatively mild and the patient may therefore be able to maintain a better oral hygiene than in ANG. A thick, gingival margin exhibiting so-called "reverse gingival architecture" is characteristic.

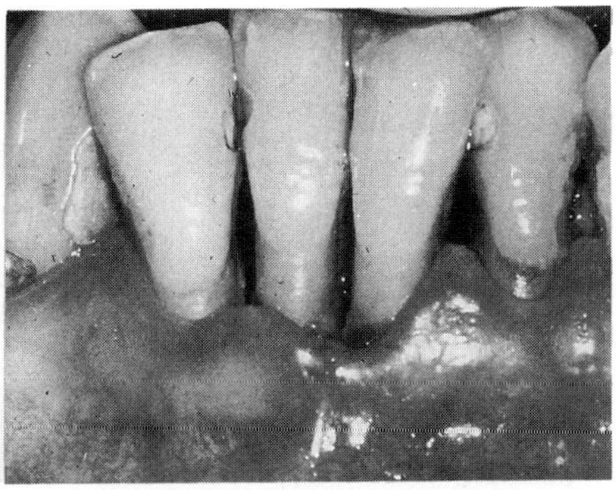

Fig. 7-6. The area around the lower incisors exhibits several findings of CNG: A thick rounded gingival margin, concave papillae, craters filled by subgingival calculus, and a relatively firm attached gingiva without obvious signs of acute lesions. The patient's oral hygiene is better than in most cases of ANG.

teins and, possibly, fibrin deposits from the inflammatory exudate. It can be readily removed by a water spray.

Linear erythema

The zone between the marginal necrosis and the relatively unaffected gingiva usually exhibits a well-demarcated narrow erythematous zone. This zone is called the linear erythema. It is caused by hyperemia of the vessels of the gingival connective tissue peripherally to the necrotic lesions (Fig. 7-4).

Bleeding

Acute inflammation and necrosis with exposure of the underlying connective tissue in ANG produces a marked tendency to bleeding. Bleeding may start spontaneously as well as in response to even gentle touch.

Pain

In the initial stages, when necrotic lesions in ANG are relatively few and small, pain is usually moderate. In more advanced cases the pain may be considerable and may be associated with a markedly increased salivary flow.

Foetor ex ore

A characteristic and pronounced foetor ex ore is often noticed in ANG, but can vary in intensity and in some cases is not very noticeable. It should further be noted that strong foetor ex ore can also be found in such other pathological conditions of the oral cavity as chronic destructive disease. Strong foetor ex ore is, therefore, not pathognomonic for ANG.

Lymphadenitis

Swelling and tenderness of the regional lymph nodes may occur in ANG, particularly in advanced cases. Such lymphadenitis is usually confined to the submandibular lymph nodes, but the cervical lymph nodes may also be involved. In children with ANG, Jiménez & Baer (1975) found that lymphadenitis and increased bleeding tendency were the most pronounced clinical findings. Others, like Grupe & Wilder (1956), have not found lymphadenitis clearly characteristic of ANG.

Fever and malaise

There is no general agreement concerning the occurrence of fever and malaise in ANG. Investigations by Grupe & Wilder (1956), Goldhaber & Giddon (1964) and by Shields (1977)

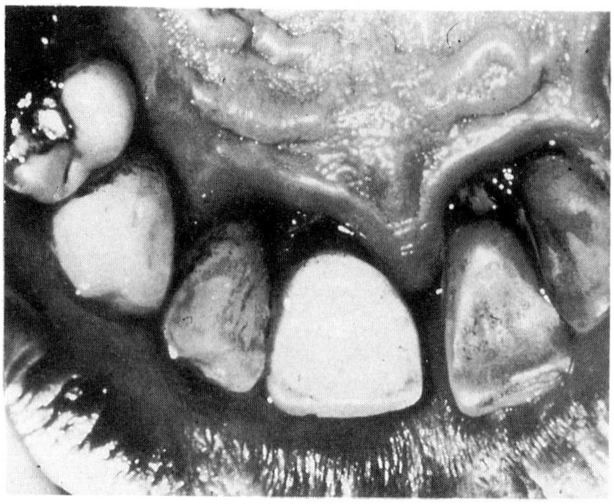

Fig. 7-7a. CNG with wide crater formation in the upper anterior tooth region. The patient's history and the clinical picture indicated that the formation of the defects had started several years earlier during an episode of ANG. The acute inflammation was not properly treated and later passed to a chronic stage with continuous tissue destruction in the interproximal craters.

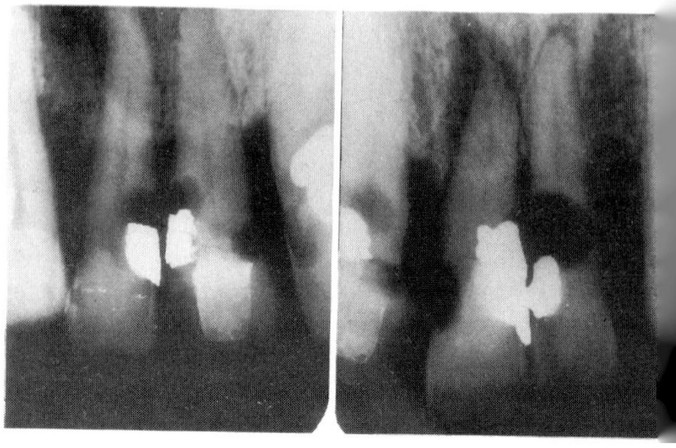

Fig. 7-7b. Radiographs of the interproximal areas of the upper anterior teeth of the patient shown in Fig. 7-7a. Note advanced interproximal osseous destruction and extensive caries lesions on root surfaces adjoining the interproximal craters.

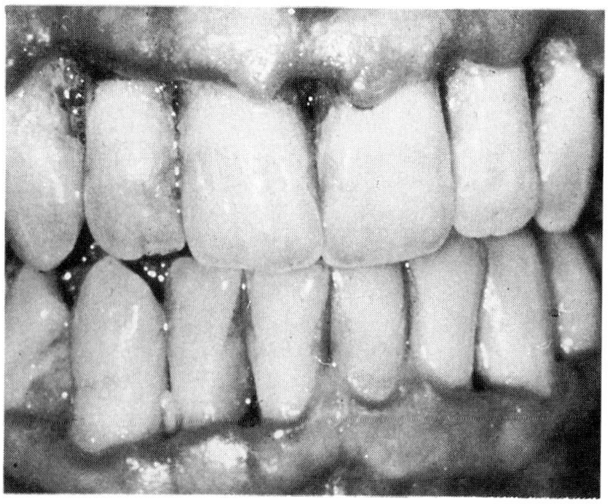

Fig. 7-8a. By local application of astringent medication a necrotizing gingivitis may be converted from acute to chronic form. This patient has been treated over a period of 14 months by repeated application of carbolfuchsin without institution of proper cause-related treatment. Note the characteristic "reverse gingival architecture".

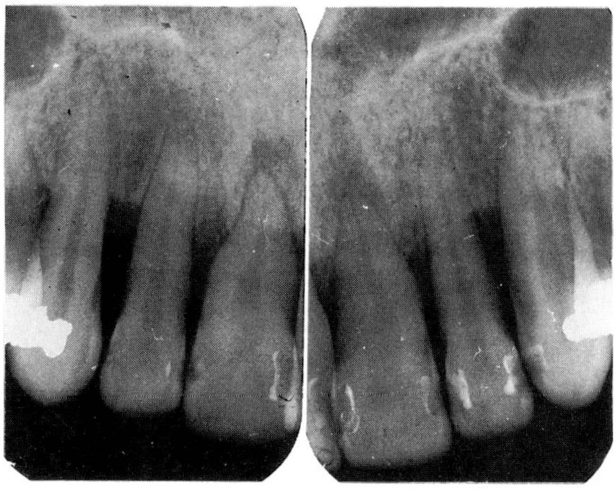

Fig. 7-8b. Radiographs from the patient shown in Fig. 7-8a exhibit advanced loss of alveolar bone. The tissue destruction has continued particularly in the interproximal areas. The "treatment" of the original condition only masked the tissue destruction by alleviating the acute symptoms.

indicate that elevated body temperature is not common in ANG and that, when present, the elevation of body temperature is usually moderate. Even a small decrease in body temperature in ANG has been described. The reason for disagreement on this point is thought to stem from a tendency to misdiagnose primary herpetic gingivostomatitis as ANG when it occurs in youths or young adults.

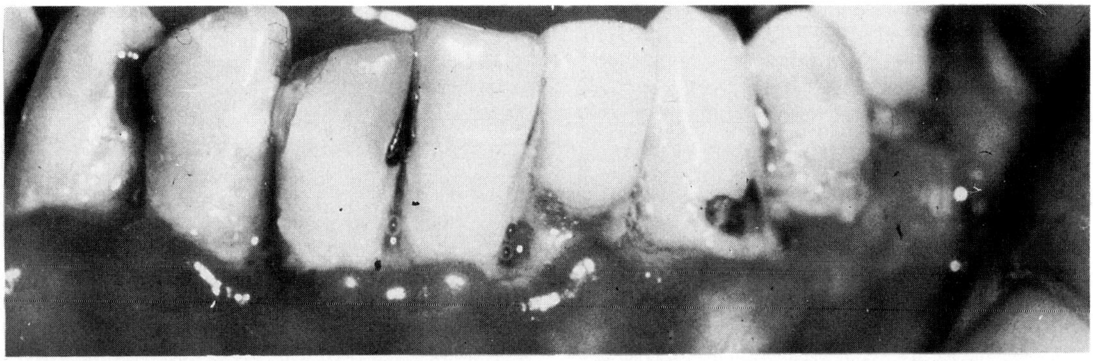

Fig. 7-9. CNG with recurrence or exacerbation of acute symptoms. This condition has sometimes been called recurrent necrotizing gingivitis. Necrosis, pain, increased bleeding tendency, etc. have recurred. The patient's history will assist the therapist to differentiate this condition from primary ANG. The necrotic lesions are localized to preexisting craters and the gingival contour is typical of CNG.

Chronic necrotizing gingivitis (CNG)

If inadequately treated or untreated, the acute phase of ANG will gradually subside. The condition becomes less unpleasant to the patient. The necrotic tissues do not, however, heal completely. The destruction of periodontal tissue continues, although at a slower rate and with less dramatic symptoms. This condition has been termed chronic necrotizing gingivitis (CNG) (Figs. 7-5, 7-6). The necrotizing lesions persist as open craters, frequently filled by subgingival calculus and bacterial plaque. The characteristic yellowish-white, necrotic areas of the acute phase usually disappear. Acute exacerbations with intervening quiescent periods may occur. In recurrent acute phases, subjective symptoms again become more noticeable and necrotic ulcers with masses of yellowish-white deposits reappear (Fig. 7-9). These masses are, however, frequently less conspicuous than in ANG, because they are located in preexisting interdental craters and are therefore not always readily detected.

A characteristic feature of CNG is a thickened and rounded gingival margin, which may give the impression of "reversed gingival architecture" (Figs. 7-5, 7-6, 7-8, 7-9). Adjoining interdental craters may fuse into one continuous trough-like crater which contains large amounts of calculus and plaque.The facial and oral gingivae in such areas may be entirely separated and form two distinct flaps or "lips".

CNG may produce considerable destruction of supporting tissues. The most pronounced tissue loss usually occurs in association with the interproximal craters. Furthermore, carious lesions may be found on the exposed root surfaces (Fig. 7-7).

Histopathology

The histopathologic picture of characteristic NG lesions reveals a nonspecific, acute necrotizing inflammation. The necrosis involves both the epithelium and the superficial layers of the connective tissue (Fig. 7-10). Normal tissue has been replaced by a meshwork of fibrin with degenerated epithelial cells, leukocytes and erythrocytes, and by bacteria and cellular debris. This layer corresponds to the yellowish-white debris which can be observed clinically. The viable connective tissue exhibits dilated and proliferating vessels and dense infiltrates of neutrophilic polymorphonuclear leukocytes. In the deeper layers, at some distance from the necrotic areas, the tissue exhibits signs of chronic inflammation and contains many plasma cells and monocytes. The ne-

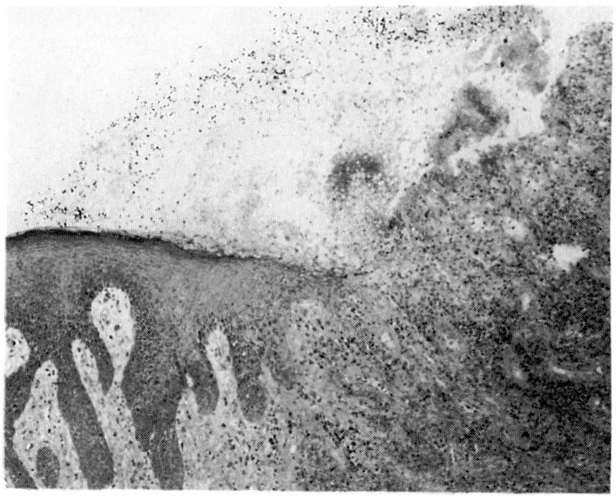

Fig. 7-10a. Interdental gingiva with necrotic defect from an ANG patient. The illustration shows the transition from the facial part of the gingival papilla to the interdental necrotic areas. The lesion is covered by a thick layer of fibrin, leukocytes, erythrocytes and bacteria (X 43).

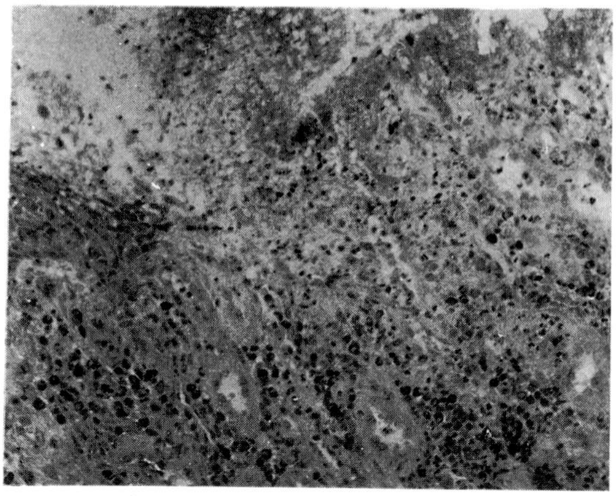

Fig. 7-10b. Section taken from the necrotic lesion near the intact epithelium. The sulcus and junctional epithelia are completely necrotized, only a small residue is visible to the left, and on top, bacterial masses with cellular debris. The necrotic part of the connective tissue and the region immediately subjacent to this area contains many polymorphonuclear leukocytes. In the deeper portion there is a dense infiltration of lymphocytes and particularly plasma cells, and the tissue contains many dilated vessels (X 115).

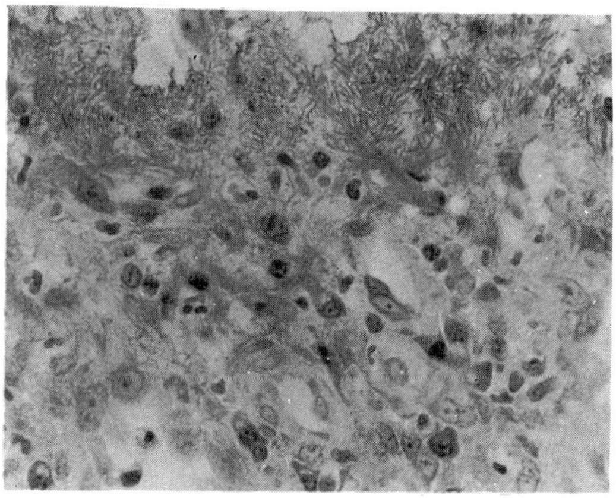

Fig. 7-10c. The section from the necrotic and spirochete infiltrated zones exhibits direct contact between bacteria and connective tissue. The tissue architecture is characterized by necrotic cells, disorganized collagen structures and accumulations of leukocytes. Several vessels are in close relation to the necrotic tissue. Among the bacteria, fusobacteria and spirochetes dominate, and close to the connective tissue practically only spirochetes are present (X 360).

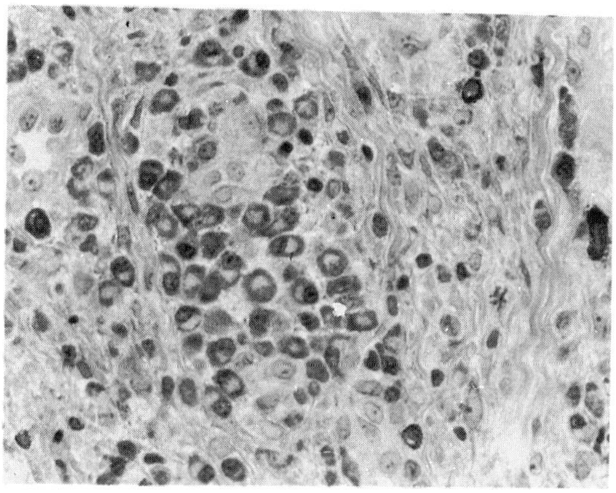

Fig. 7-10d. A viable connective tissue is seen peripherally to the necrotic lesion. This tissue is dominated by proliferating vessels, plasma cells and some monocytes forming a dense infiltrate. Intercellular collagen fibers can also be seen (X 360).

crotic area and the zone between this and the viable tissue contain large amounts of bacteria, particularly fusobacteria and spirochetes (Figs. 7-11, 7-12, 7-13). Spirochetes have been reported to penetrate the superficial layers of the viable connective tissue. Listgarten (1965) in an electron microscopic investigation found large and medium-sized spirochetes located as

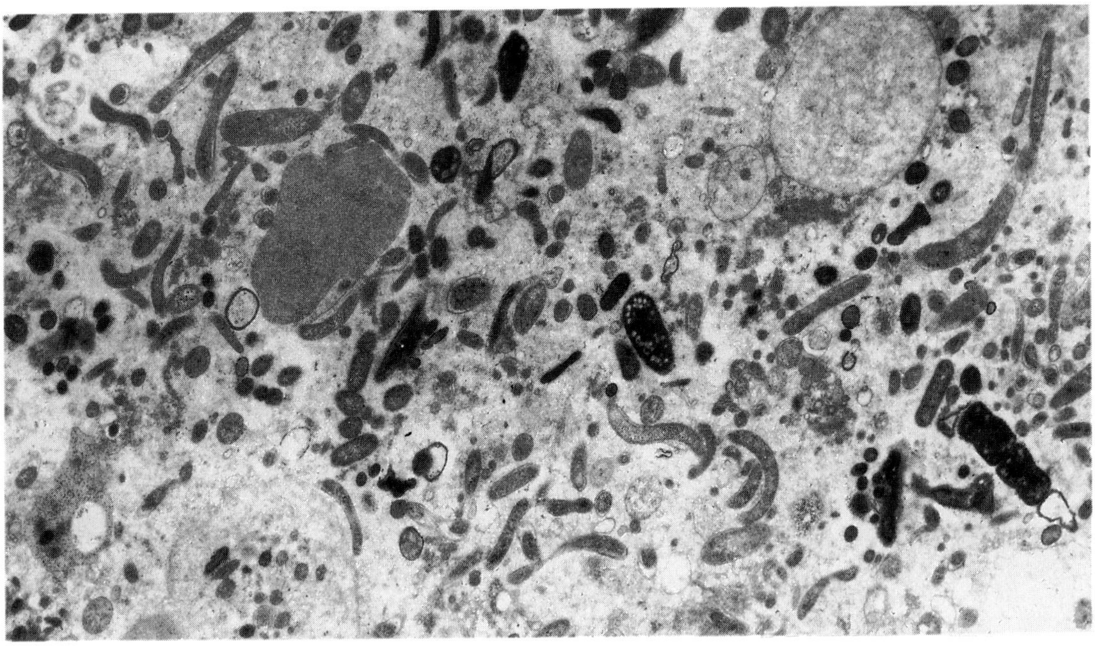

Fig. 7-11. Electron microscopic picture exhibiting the heterogeneous mixture of bacteria, cells and degenerated tissue components near the surface of the ulcerated connective tissue (X 7,500).

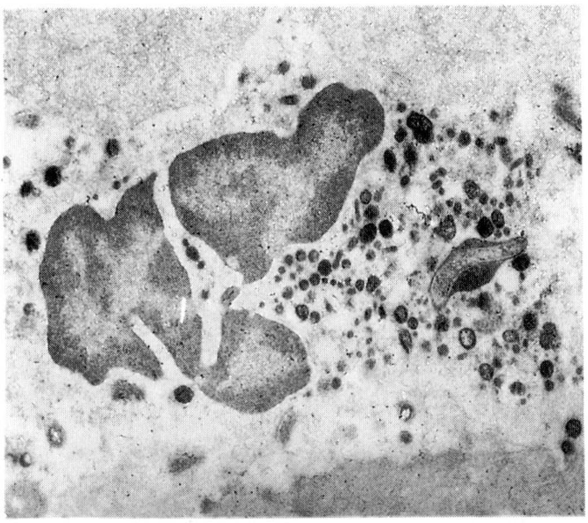

Fig. 7-12. Polymorphonuclear neutrophilic granulocyte from bacteria infiltrated area. Intracellularly, between the characteristic granulae, a phagocytosed spirochete is seen (X 8,400).

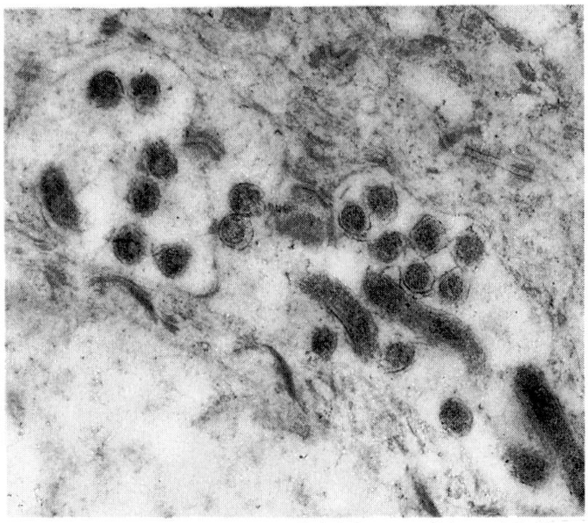

Fig. 7-13. Section from superficial layers of the epithelium near the periphery of the necrotic lesion. Spirochetes have invaded the widened intercellular spaces between the epithelial cells (X 15,000).

much as 0.25 mm below the necrotic surface. No other microorganisms were found to penetrate as deeply as this. Listgarten (1965) and Heylings (1967) also demonstrated compact masses of spirochetes and short, fusiform rods intercellularly in a presumably vital epithelium.

According to Listgarten (1965) the electron microscopic picture of the necrotic lesions in ANG exhibits 4 zones starting from the surface:

1. *The bacterial zone,* which consists of bacteria of varying sizes and forms including small, medium-sized and large spirochetes.
2. *The neutrophil rich zone,* which contains many leukocytes with a dominance of neutrophilic granulocytes. Between these cells bacteria are observed, including many spirochetes.
3. *The necrotic zone,* containing disintegrated cells, many large and medium-sized spirochetes, and other bacteria which, judging from their size and shape, may be fusobacteria.
4. *The spirochetal infiltration zone,* where the tissue components appear intact, the tissue is infiltrated by large and medium-sized spirochetes, but no other microorganisms can be seen.

Microbiology and host response

ANG is commonly regarded as an endogenous, opportunistic infection caused by a combined influence of several microorganisms. It has been suggested that ANG lesions may develop only if predisposing alterations in the resistance to infection of the host tissues have occurred. The most important predisposing conditions are *preexisting gingivitis, smoking and emotional/psychic stress.* Systemic diseases and malnutrition are of minor importance in industrialized countries but may play an important role as ANG predispositional factors in developing countries.

Several observations support the concept that a particular microbiota plays a decisive role in the development of ANG. The condition shows a dramatic improvement when the patient is given such antibiotics as penicillin or tetracycline. A characteristic bacterial flora of fusobacteria and spirochetes is always present. Spirochetes and fusiform bacteria can invade the epithelium (Heylings 1967). The spirochetes can also invade the vital connective tissue (Listgarten 1965). Both fusobacteria and spirochetes can liberate endotoxins (Mergenhagen et al. 1961, Kristoffersen & Hofstad 1970). Experiments have shown that these organisms possess biological activities which may contribute to the pathogenesis of ANG. Nevertheless, the exact role of the various microorganisms has not been clarified (Johnson & Engel 1986), and the fact that they are present in large numbers does not necessarily mean that they are of primary etiologic importance. Their presence could equally well result from secondary overgrowth (See Chapter 4).

Attempts to transmit the disease from one animal to another, or to produce necrotic lesions in experimental animals, have failed to yield conclusive results (MacDonald et al. 1963). Several suspect microorganisms and several combinations of microorganisms can produce similar lesions in experimental animals. MacDonald et al. (1956) found that a combination of 4 different bacteria, none of them fusobacteria or spirochetes, had such properties. Further experiments gave indications that among the 4 bacterial species, *Bacteroides melaninogenicus* was the true pathogen (MacDonald et al. 1963). *B. melaninogenicus* may, under certain conditions, produce an enzyme which degrades native collagen (Gibbons & MacDonald 1961). It is still not clear, however, whether this microorganism is of particular importance in the pathogenesis of ANG. More recently, Mikx & van Campen (1982) induced NG lesions in dogs pretreated with steroids and inoculated with a fusiform-spirochete culture from dogs which had gingival lesions similar to the NG lesions seen in humans. The lesions produced in experimental animals may not be identical to those which occur in humans. It is also important to note that even if necrotic lesions can be transmitted by transmission of infectious material or bacterial cultures, this does not necessarily mean that the disease is truly contagious.

Loesche et al. (1982) in plaque samples from 22 ulcerated sites in 8 patients with NG by quantitative anaerobic cultivation and direct microscopic analysis found that the samples contained a "constant flora" and a "variable flora". The "constant flora" contained *Treponema sp.*, *Selenomonas sp.*, *Fusobacterium sp.* and *B. intermedius*, and the "variable flora" consisted of a heterogeneous array of bacterial types. Experimental tratment with 250 mg of metronidazole 3 times daily for 7 days caused a prompt resolution of clinical symptoms, coinciding with a significant reduction of the plaque proportions of *Treponema sp.*, *B. intermedius* and *Fusobacterium sp.* The findings are taken as a support of the role of these specific anaerobes in the lesions, without demonstrating that they initiated the infection. Though not confirmed by their data, the authors proposed that if a particular constellation of these organisms already existed in the plaque, the corticosteroids associated with stress might provide them with a selective nutrient advantage.

An important role for *Treponema sp.* and *B. intermedius* was also suggested by studies of antibodies in NG patients to such bacteria, compared to levels in age- and sex-matched controls with healthy gingiva or with simple gingivitis (Chung et al. 1983).

Our knowledge of the pathogenic mechanisms by which the bacterial flora produces the tissue changes characteristic of ANG is limited, particularly since it has been difficult to establish an acceptable animal experimental model. It seems reasonable to believe that several of the pathogenic mechanisms which have been associated with chronic gingivitis and periodontitis may also be of etiologic importance in ANG (see also Chapters 4 and 5).

Several observations indicate that the effects of endotoxins are more prominent in ANG than in chronic gingivitis and periodontitis. The large masses of Gram negative bacteria liberate endotoxins in close contact with connective tissue. Endotoxins may produce tissue destruction both by direct toxic effects and indirectly, by activating and modifying tissue responses of the host (Wilton & Lehner 1980). Through direct toxic effect, endotoxins may lead to damage of cells and vessels. Necrosis is a prominent feature in the so-called "Shwartzman-reaction", which is caused by endotoxins. Indirectly, endotoxins can contribute to tissue damage in several ways: they can function as antigens and elicit immune reactions, they can activate complement directly through the alternative pathway and thereby liberate chemotoxins, they can also activate macrophages and, acting as mitogens on B and T-lymphocytes, may influence the host's immune reactions. To what extent such reactions contribute to host defence or to tissue damage is not known. In addition, it has been shown, in *in vitro* experiments, that endotoxins can stimulate bone resorption.

Wilton et al. (1971) investigated the cellular and humoral immune responses in both necrotizing and chronic gingivitis. Titers of antibodies to *Actinomyces viscosus, Fusobacterium fusiforme* and *Veillonella alcalescens* were similar in patients with ANG and chronic gingivitis. This observation invalidates the theory that ANG is the result of a specific infection by one of these microorganisms. On the other hand, it supports the clinical finding that ANG always develops from a preexisting chronic gingivitis. Cellular immune responses were in accordance with these observations, but a stronger reaction to fusobacteria was taken as an indication that these microorganisms could be involved in the transition from chronic to acute gingivitis.

A further indication of the importance of the immune system in the etiology of NG is the relatively frequent and early occurrence of NG in many HIV-infected individuals. HIV infection attacks the T-helper cells of the body, causing a drastic change in the T-helper/T-suppressor ratio with severe impairment of the host's resistance to infection (Reichart et al. 1987).

Predisposing factors

Preexisting gingivitis

Whether or not ANG may occur at all without preexisting gingivitis is uncertain. Clinical observation and histopathologic evidence (Hooper & Seymour 1979) suggest that NG is superimposed on chronic marginal gingivitis lesions. The mechanisms by which chronic gingivitis may predispose to the occurrence of ANG remain obscure. Several hypotheses have been advanced, among them changes in leukocyte function (Cogen et al. 1983) and changes in immune response (Johnson & Engel 1986). Wilton et al. (1971) found reduced levels of IgG and increased levels of IgM in serum from ANG patients, and suggested that this might be an endotoxin effect, possibly also influencing the cellular immune response. Whether such changes predispose to development of ANG, or in fact reflect a response to ANG, remains to be determined.

Smoking

Smoking may predispose to ANG in several ways. Smokers in general have poorer oral hygiene than do nonsmokers, and with increasing tobacco consumption the oral hygiene status tends to deteriorate further. Smoking may also influence tissue reaction to irritation. It is known that smoking leads to contraction of peripheral vessels and this phenomenon has been suggested as one mechanism by which smoking could predispose to ANG (Schwartz & Baumhammers 1972, Bergström & Preber 1986). Smoking also influences polymorphonuclear leukocytes. Kenney et al. (1977) found the oral leukocytes from smokers were less effective in phagocytosis than leukocytes from nonsmokers. The calcium concentration in dental plaque of smokers is significantly higher than in nonsmokers (Macgregor et al. 1985). This might influence the rate of calculus formation and thereby contribute to a further deterioration of the oral hygiene.

Emotional stress

The role of anxiety and psychic stress in the pathogenesis of ANG has been borne out by both psychiatric and biochemical investigations (Moulton et al. 1952, Shannon et al. 1969, Maupin & Bell 1975). Goldhaber & Giddon (1964) and Manhold et al. (1971) have discussed various mechanisms through which stress may influence the gingival tissues. During periods of stress, actions and habits which are under the control of the patient may be influenced. Both the oral hygiene and the nutrition of the patient may suffer, and smoking habits may start or alter. In addition, host tissue resistance may be changed by mechanisms acting through the autonomic nervous system and endocrine glands, so that gingival circulation and salivary flow become affected. Loesche et al. (1982) further suggested that the corticosteroids associated with stress might provide specific parts of the bacterial flora with a nutrient advantage, helping these bacteria to gain ascendency in the plaque.

Diagnosis

The diagnosis of NG should primarily be based on clinical signs and symptoms as described above. The patient's past history may also give valuable information. The patient has frequently noticed pain and bleeding from the gingiva, particularly upon touch. Fever and malaise may occur even though this is not characteristic of NG. Smoking and emotional or psychic stress predispose to the disease.

A bacterial smear which shows a dominance of fusobacteria and spirochetes may confirm the diagnosis, but in such smears a great var-

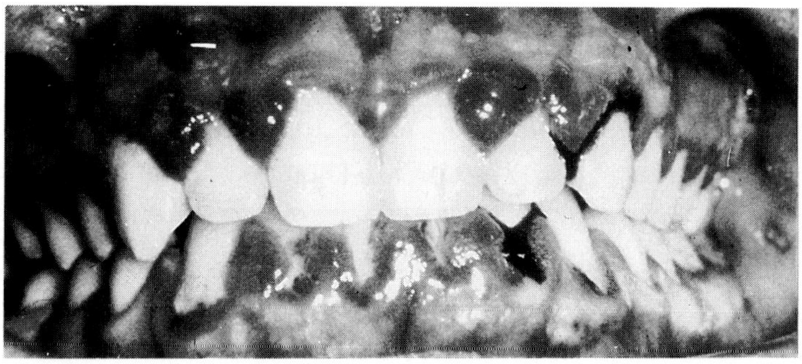

Fig. 7-14a. Primary herpetic gingivostomatitis in an 18-year-old male. The edematous swelling of the interproximal papillae may produce an interdental morphology similar to approximal craters. These interdental areas may also be covered by a moderate amount of yellowish-white debris. Marked color changes involving both oral mucosa and wide areas of the attached gingiva can be seen as well as increased bleeding tendency. A small round ulcer is visible in the buccal mucosa. The patient was a mouth breather.

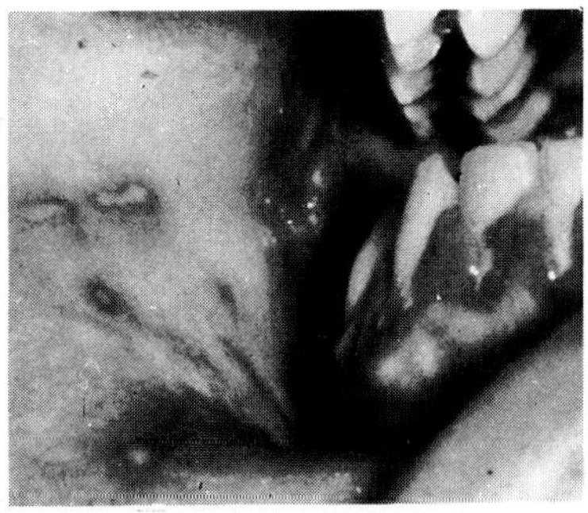

Fig. 7-14b. Buccal mucosa from the right side of the mouth of the patient shown in Fig. 7-14a. There are characteristic herpetic lesions. They are flat, painful and covered by a greyish membraneous debris, surrounded by an elevated margin with a diffuse erythematous zone.

iety of microorganisms may be found, and in some areas the fusospirochetal mixed flora may be less dominant. A biopsy will reveal superficial tissue necrosis with nonspecific inflammatory changes. The histopathological picture is not pathognomonic for NG, and biopsy is not usually indicated.

Due to the relatively frequent reports on NG in HIV-infected patients the following procedure is recommended:

a. Have all patients who present with a history suggestive of NG follow the hygienic regimen recommended for HIV-infected patients (Greenspan et al. 1986, Barr & Marder 1987). Many national health authorities have issued guidelines and recommendations.
b. Establish whether the patient may be at high risk to attract HIV-infection.
c. Inspect the entire oral cavity, looking particularly for signs of fungal infections such as candidiasis and for "hairy leukoplakia", possible Kaposi's tumor etc. (Greenspan et al. 1986).
d. Take a blood sample for immunologic (and hematologic) tests.
e. Until results of these tests are available, proceed as if the patient is HIV-positive. (Cfr. sections on "Diagnosis and Treatment" below).

NG occurring as a complication to HIV-infection apparently does not present clinical features which distinguish it from NG in "ordinary" patients, but a history of frequent relapses and poor response to traditional or drug therapy may be suggestive (Greenspan et al. 1986).

Differential diagnosis

ANG may be confused with other diseases of the oral mucosa. Primary herpetic gingivostomatitis (PHG) is not infrequently mistaken for ANG (Fig. 7-14) (Klotz 1973). The important differential diagnostic criteria for the two diseases have been listed in Table 7-1. It should be noted that in the USA and in northern Europe, ANG occurs very rarely in children, whereas PHG is most commonly found in children. If the body temperature is markedly raised, to 38°C or more, PHG should be suspected. ANG has a marked predilection for the interdental papillae, while PHG shows no such limitation and may occur anywhere on the free or the attached gingiva, or in the alveolar mucosa. In PHG the erythema is of a more diffuse charac-

Table 7-1

Clinical criteria for the differential diagnosis between acute necrotizing gingivitis (ANG) and primary herpetic gingivostomatitis (PHG)

	ANG	PHG
Occurrence	Rare in children (in Europe, USA)	Most frequently seen in children
Fever, malaise	May occur, but is usually moderate	Temperature elevation, frequently marked, is characteristic
Sites of predilection	Preferentially occurs interdentally, penetrates deeply and spreads laterally. Rarely lesions outside the gingiva	No definite intraoral predilection sites. Diffusely spread over the entire gingiva. Lesions are frequently seen on lip and tongue, in the buccal and other sites in the oral mucosa
Lesion and erythema	Necrotic ulcers with yellowish-white debris and a narrow, linear erythema which sharply separates the lesions from the adjoining mucosa	Round, greyish small vesicles which disrupt and leave small ulcers without appreciable tissue destruction. Diffuse erythema
Foetor ex ore	Characteristic foetor has been reported as typical of the disease. May not always be pronounced and is not pathognomonic	Foetor may be present, but is not regarded as being typical of this condition

ter and may comprise the entire gingiva and parts of the alveolar mucosa. The vesicular lesions in PHG which disrupt and produce small ulcers surrounded by diffuse erythema, occur both on the lips and tongue as well as on the buccal mucosa. PHG and ANG may occur simultaneously in the same patient, and in such cases there may be mucosal lesions outside the gingiva, and fever and general malaise tend to occur more frequently than with ANG alone.

Among oral mucosal diseases that have been confused with ANG are desquamative gingivitis, benign mucous membrane pemphigoid, erythema multiforme exudativum, streptococcal gingivitis, gonococcal gingivitis, and others. All of these are described in Chapter 10 and are clinically quite distinct from ANG.

In some forms of leukemia, especially acute leukemia, necrotizing ulcers may occur in the oral mucosa and are not infrequently seen in association with the gingival margin, apparently as an exacerbation of an existing chronic inflammatory condition. The clinical appearance can resemble ANG lesions, and the symptoms they produce may be the ones that first make the patient seek professional consultation. In acute leukemia the gingiva often appears bluish-red and swollen with edema. Varying degrees of ulceration and necrosis occur, sometimes with formation of a "pseudomembrane". Generally, the patient has more marked systemic symptoms than with ordinary ANG, but can for a while feel relatively healthy. The dentist should be aware of the possibility that leukemias present such oral manifestations. Hematologic examination of the patient's blood may be indicated, whereas biopsy usually is not.

Treatment

In spite of the characteristic clinical and bacteriologic findings in NG, therapy should follow the same principal guidelines as for treatment of chronic gingivitis and periodontitis. Practical implementation of treatment may necessitate certain modifications, particularly because of the nature of the lesions, including pain and bleeding in the acute phase and great loss of interdental supporting tissues by crater formation.

Cause-related treatment

Bleeding and sensitivity to touch may complicate both debridement and personal oral hygiene. Nevertheless, scaling should be attempted, as thoroughly as conditions will allow, even during the first consultation. Ultrasonic scaling may be preferable to the use of hand instruments. With minimal pressure against the soft tissues, ultrasonic cleaning may accomplish the removal of soft and mineralized deposits. The continuous water spray combined with adequate suction will allow good visibility. How far it is possible to proceed with debridement during the first visit will usually depend on the intensity of pain and the patient's tolerance of instrumentation.

Patients with ANG are not easily motivated to carry out a proper program of oral hygiene. They frequently have poor oral hygiene habits and possibly a negative attitude to dental treatment in general. As a result, some patients discontinue treatment as soon as pain and other acute symptoms are alleviated. Motivation and instruction should be planned to prevent this happening, and should be reinforced during later visits.

Instruction in tooth brushing and approximal cleaning should largely follow the recommendations of ordinary periodontal therapy. Some clinicians have emphasized the importance of gentle and light brushing during initial phases of ANG treatment. However, patients themselves generally apply oral hygiene measures with sufficient leniency because of bleeding and pain. If the dentist overemphasizes the importance of gentle brushing and interdental cleaning, it can result in unnecessarily inefficient oral hygiene. Clinical experience does, however, indicate that soft toothbrushes are preferable.

To support the patient's oral hygiene during the initial phase of treatment, frequent rinsing with a mixture of equal parts 3% H_2O_2 and lukewarm water is regarded by some as a useful aid. Twice daily rinses with a 0.2% chlorhexidine solution (e.g. Corsodyl®, Hibitane®) is a very effective adjunct to self-performed oral hygiene during the first 2 weeks of treatment.

Further treatment in ANG must be adapted to the individual case. The efficiency of the patient's oral hygiene efforts and the reduction of pain and bleeding will determine the progression of therapy. The patient should be seen at least once a week as long as the acute symptoms persist. Systematic subgingival scaling with curettes, correction of restoration margins and polishing of restorations and root surfaces should be performed during these visits in addition to supplementary oral hygiene instruction and patient motivation.

Cause-related treatment in CNG does not differ appreciably from treatment of ordinary chronic periodontitis. Symptoms do not complicate scaling and self-performed oral hygiene measures to the same extent as in ANG. On the other hand, there are often large amounts of subgingival calculus present in CNG, and scaling may require considerable effort.

Surgical treatment

When the cause-related phase of treatment has been completed, necrosis and other acute symptoms in ANG will have disappeared. The formerly necrotic areas have healed and the gingival craters are reduced in size, although as a rule some defects persist. In such areas bacterial plaque readily accumulates, and the craters, therefore, predispose to recurrence of NG or the further destruction because of a persisting chronic inflammatory process, or both; these sites require surgical correction.

In CNG, the soft-tissue defects are usually pronounced. The surrounding tissues are often firm and fibrous and a gradual change towards a more favorable topography in response to treatment is less likely to occur than in ANG. Surgical treatment therefore is almost always necessary in CNG.

Shallow craters can be removed by simple gingivectomy, while the elimination of deep defects may require flap surgery. Thinning of thick flap margins and correction of form to achieve optimal interproximal coverage and contour are important and may be technically demanding. Treatment of necrotizing gingivitis has not been completed until all gingival defects have been eliminated and optimal conditions for future plaque control have been established.

Drugs in treatment of NG

Miller & Greene (1958) have reported that more than 100 different drugs have been suggested for the treatment of NG. This illustrates the uncertainty and confusion associated with treatment of this periodontal disease.

Escharotics such as chromic acid and silver nitrate or substances with an *astringent* and possibly some *antibacterial effect* such as gentian violet and carbolfuchsin, have been widely used in the treatment of ANG (Fig. 7-8). The rationale for using such substances was probably that they appeared to alleviate acute symptoms such as bleeding and pain when applied to the inflamed gingiva. The effect of escharotics is, however, extremely difficult to control. The etching may penetrate deep into the periodontium and contribute to permanent destruction of healthy or potentially healthy periodontal tissues. There is considerably less danger of such undesired effects associated with the use of astringent substances. On the other hand, some of these are regarded as potentially carcinogenic. The effects of escharotics and astringents are purely symptomatic and they should therefore be avoided in the treatment of NG. Recurrences are frequently seen (Manson & Rand 1961) since such "therapy" will only mask the destructive inflammatory process, permitting it to continue into the deeper portions of the periodontium.

Hydrogen peroxide and other oxygen-releasing agents also have a long-standing tradition in the treatment of ANG. Hydrogen peroxide has been used as a caustic or etching substance (30%), for debridement (3%) and as a mouthrinse (equal portions 3% H_2O_2 and warm water). For debridement in necrotic areas and as a mouthrinse, hydrogen peroxide is still used. It has been thought that the apparently favorable effects of hydrogen peroxide may be due to mechanical cleaning, and the influence on anaerobic bacterial flora of the liberated oxygen (Wennström & Lindhe 1979, MacPhee & Cowley 1981).

Chlorhexidine, 0.2% solution is marketed in several European countries as a mouthrinse. Its effect is discussed elsewhere in this textbook. Chlorhexidine is useful as a supplement to the patient's personal oral hygiene measures during the acute phase of ANG (see above). For an optimal effect of this medicament, it should be used only in conjunction with and in addition to systematic scaling and root planing. The chlorhexidine solution does not penetrate well subgingivally and the preparation is readily inactivated by exudates, necrotic tissues and masses of bacteria (Gjermo 1974). The effectiveness of chlorhexidine mouthrinses therefore is dependent upon a simultaneous, thorough mechanical debridement.

Antibiotics and chemotherapeutics are aimed directly at the bacteria which are the direct cause of the inflammatory process in ANG. Penicillins and other broad-spectrum antibiotics such as tetracyclines are most effective. However, the important role of such medication in the treatment of other, more serious infectious diseases, calls for a restrictive attitude towards their use in less serious conditions such as ANG. Only in rare cases of ANG is the patient's general health affected to such an extent that the use of antibiotics is indicated. *Topical application* of broad-spectrum antibiotics is strictly contraindicated in the treatment of ANG.

Metronidazole (e.g. Flagyl®, Rhodia), *e.g.* 250 mg 3 times daily for 7 days, has been found effective against spirochetes and has been used both locally and systemically in the treatment of ANG (Proctor & Baker 1971, Shinn 1976, Loesche 1982).

In conclusion, drugs are of limited usefulness in the treatment of NG, and only those producing improved plaque control in the cause-related therapy phase should be used.

Modifications for suspected or verified HIV-positive patients

In HIV-positive individuals, treatment with antibiotics or chemotherapeutics (such as metronidazole) may cause overgrowth of opportunistic microorganisms, such as fungi. In patients with uncompromised immune responses such conditions can be readily controlled, but in HIV-infected persons they may cause serious or even life threatening complications. If the dentist decides to start the treatment of an NG patient with an antimicrobial such as metronidazole before the results of immunologic tests are available, or if the patient has been found to be HIV-positive, one should anticipate such responses and should prescribe an antimyotic or fungicidal drug as well, for instance amphotericine lozenges or nystatin.

For HIV-positive patients it has been recommended to prescribe chlorhexidine mouthrinses for some days before starting cause-related treatment. The patient should be referred for further medical diagnosis and treatment, while dental treatment may usually continue.

It should be understood that the amount of clinical experience in this field is still limited. It is important that the dental team stays informed about the most recent developments.

References

Barr, C.E. & Marder, M.Z. (1987) *Aids: A guide for dental practice.* Chicago: Qiuntessence books.

Bergström, J. & Preber, H. (1986) The influence of cigarette smoking on the development of experimental gingivitis. *Journal of Periodontal Research* **21**, 668-676.

Chung, C.P., Nisengard, R.J., Slots, J. & Genco, R.J. (1983) Bacterial IgG and IgM antibody titers in acute necrotizing ulcerative gingivitis. *Journal of Periodontology* **54**, 557-562.

Cogen, R.B., Stevens, A.W., Cohen-Cole, S.et al. (1983) Leukocyte function in the etiology of acute necrotizing gingivitis. *Journal of Periodontology* **54**, 402-407.

Emslie, R.D. (1963) Cancrum oris. *Dental Practitioner* **13**, 481-485.

Enwonwu, C.O. (1972) Epidemiological and biochemical studies of necrotizing ulcerative gingivitis and noma (cancrum oris) in Nigerian children. *Archives of Oral Biology* **17**, 1357-1371.

Enwonwu, C.O. (1985) Infectious oral necrosis (cancrum oris) in Nigerian children: a review. *Community Dentistry and Oral Epidemiology* **13**, 190-194.

Gibbons, R.J. & MacDonald, J.B. (1961) Degradation of collagenous substrates by *Bacteroides melaninogenicus. Journal of Bacteriology* **81**, 614-621.

Giddon, D.B., Goldhaber, P. & Dunning, J.M. (1963) Prevalence of reported cases of acute necrotizing ulcerative gingivitis in a university population. *Journal of Periodontology* **34**, 366-371.

Giddon, D.B., Zackin, S.J. & Goldhaber, P. (1964) Acute necrotizing ulcerative gingivitis in college students. *Journal of the American Dental Association* **68**, 381-386.

Gjermo, P. (1974) Chlorhexidine in dental practice. *Journal of Clinical Periodontology* **1**, 143-152.

Goldhaber, P. & Giddon, D.B. (1964) Present concepts concerning the etiology and treatment of acute necrotizing ulcerative gingivitis. *International Dental Journal* **14**, 468-496.

Greenspan, D., Greenspan, J.S., Pindborg, J.J. & Schiödt, M. (1986) *Aids and the Dental Team.* Copenhagen: Munksgaard.

Grupe, H.E. & Wilder, L.S. (1956) Observations of necrotizing gingvititis in 870 military trainees. *Journal of Periodontology* **27**, 255-261.

Heylings, R.T. (1967) Electron microscopy of acute ulcerative gingivitis (Vincent's type). *British Dental Journal* **122**, 51-56.

Jiménez, M.L. & Baer, P.N. (1975) Necrotizing ulcerative gingivitis in children: A 9-year clinical study. *Journal of Periodontology* **46**, 715-720.

Johnson, B.D. & Engel, D. (1986) Acute necrotizing ulcerative gingivitis. A review of diagnosis, etiology and treatment. *Journal of Periodontologyl* **57**, 141-150.

Kenney, E.B., Kraal, J.H., Saxe, S.R. & Jones, J. (1977) The effect of cigarette smoke on human oral polymorphonuclear leukocytes. *Journal of Periodontal Research* **12**, 227-234.

Klotz, H. (1973) Differentiation between necrotic ulcerative gingivitis and primary herpetic gingivostomatitis. *New York State Dental Journal* **39**, 283-294.

Kristoffersen, T. & Hofstad, T. (1970) Chemical composition of lipopolysaccharide endotoxins from oral fusobacteria. *Archives of Oral Biology* **15**, 909-916.

Listgarten, M.A. (1965) Electron microscopic observations on the bacterial flora of acute necrotizing ulcerative gingivitis. *Journal of Periodontology* **36**,328-339.

Loesche, W.J., Syed, S.A., Laughon, B.E. & Stoll, J. (1982) The bacteriology of acute necrotizing ulcerative gingivitis. *Journal of Periodontology* **53**, 223-230.

MacDonald, J.B., Sutton, R.M., Knoll, M.L., Medlener, E.M. & Grainger, R.M. (1956) The pathogenic components of an experimental fusospirochaetal infection. *Journal of Infectious Diseases* **98**, 15-20.

MacDonald, J.B., Socransky, S.S. & Gibbons, R.J. (1963) Aspects of the pathogenesis of mixed anaerobic infections of mucous membranes. *Journal of Dental Research* **42**, 529-544.

Macgregor, I.D.M., Edgar, W.M. & Greenwood, A.R. (1985). Effects of cigarette smoking on the rate of plaque formation. *Journal of Clinical Periodontology* **12**, 35-41.

MacPhee, T. & Cowley, G. (1981) *Essentials of Periodontology.* 3rd ed., pp. 157-177. Oxford: Blackwell Scientific Publications.

Manhold, J.H., Doyle, J.C. & Weisinger, E.H. (1971) Effects of social stress on oral and other tissues. II. Results offering to a hypothesis for the mechanism of formation of periodontal pathology. *Journal of Periodontology* **42**, 109-111.

Manson, J.D. & Rand, H. (1961) Recurrent Vincent's disease. A survey of 61 cases. *British Dental Journal* **110**, 386-390.

Maupin, C.C. & Bell, W.B. (1975) The relationship of 17-hydroxycorticosteroid to acute necrotizing ulcerative gingivitis. *Journal of Periodontology* **46**, 721-722.

Mergenhagen, S.E., Hampp, E.G. & Scherp, H.W. (1961) Preparation and biological activities of endotoxin from oral bacteria. *Journal of Infectious Diseases* **108**, 304-310.

Mikx, F.H.M. & van Campen, G.J. (1982) Microscopical evaluation of the microflora in relation to necrotizing ulcerative gingivitis in the beagle dog. *Journal of Periodontal Research* **17**, 576-584.

Miller, S.C. & Greene, H.I. (1958) A world-wide survey of acute necrotizing ulcerative gingivitis: A preliminary report. *Journal of Dental Research* **13**, 66-81.

Moulton, R., Ewen, S. & Thieman, W. (1952) Emotional factors in periodontal disease. *Oral Surgery, Oral Medicine and Oral Pathology* **5**, 833-860.

Pickard, H.M. (1973) Historical aspects of Vincent's Disease. *Proceedings of the Royal Society of Medicine* **66**, 695-698.

Pindborg, J.J. (1951a) Gingivitis in military personnel with special reference to ulceromembranous gingivitis. *Odontologisk Revy* **59**, 407-499.

Pindborg, J.J. (1951b) Influence of service in armed forces on incidence of gingivitis. *Journal of the American Dental Association* **42**, 517-522.

Pindborg, J.J., Bhat, M., Devanath, K.R., Narayana, H.R. & Ramachandra, S. (1966) Occurrence of acute necrotizing gingivitis in South Indian children. *Journal of Periodontology* **37**, 14-19.

Pindborg, J.J., Bhat, M. & Roed-Petersen, B. (1967) Oral changes in South Indian children with severe protein deficiency. *Journal of Periodontology* **38**, 218-221.

Proctor, D.B. & Baker, C.G. (1971) Treatment of acute necrotizing ulcerative gingivitis with metronidazole. *Journal of the Canadian Dental Association* **37**, 376-380.

Schiödt, M. & Pindborg, J.J. (1987) Aids and the oral cavity. *International Journal of Maxillofacial Surgery* **16**, 1-14.

Schwartz, D.M. & Baumhammers, A. (1972) Smoking and periodontal disease. *Periodontal Abstracts* **20**, 103-106.

Shannon, I.L., Kilgore, W.G. & O'Leary, T.J. (1969) Stress as a predisposing factor in necrotizing gingivitis. *Journal of Periodontology* **40**, 240-242.

Sheiham, A., (1966) An epidemiological survey of acute ulcerative gingivitis in Nigerians. *Archives of Oral Biology* **11**, 937-942.

Shields, W.D. (1977) Acute necrotizing ulcerative gingivitis. A study of some of the contributing factors and their validity in an army population. *Journal of Periodontology* **48**, 346-349.

Shinn, D.L. (1976) Vincent's disease and its treatment. In *Metronidazole*. Proceedings of the International Metronidazole Conference. pp. 334-340. Montreal, Quebec, Canada, May 26-28.

Silverman, S., Migliorati, C.A., Lozada-Nur, F. et al. (1986) Oral findings in people or at high risk for AIDS: A study of 375 homosexual males. *Journal of the American Dental Association* **112**, 187-192.

Van Cauwenberge, P. (1976) De betekenis van de "fusospirillaire associatie" (Plaut-Vincent). *Acta Otorhinolaryngologica Belgica* **30**, 334-345.

Vincent, H. (1898) Sur une forme particulière d'engine différoide (engine à bacilles fusiformes). *Archives Internationales de Laryngologie* **11**, 44-48.

Wennström, J. & Lindhe, J. (1979) Effect of hydrogen peroxide on developing plaque and gingivitis in man. *Journal of Clinical Periodontology* **6**, 115-130.

Wilton, J.M.A., Ivanyi, L. & Lehner, T. (1971) Cell-mediated imunity and humoral antibodies in acute ulcerative gingivitis. *Journal of Periodontal Research* **6**, 9-16.

Wilton, J.M.A. & Lehner, T. (1980) Immunological and microbial aspects of periodontal disease. In *Recent Advances in Clinical Immunology,* No. 2, ed. Thompson, R.A., pp. 145-181. Edinburgh: Churchill Livingstone.

CHAPTER 8

Trauma From Occlusion

Definition and terminology

Trauma from occlusion is a term used to describe pathological alterations or adaptive changes which develop in the periodontium as a result of undue force produced by the masticatory muscles. *Trauma from occlusion* is only one of many terms that have been used to describe such alterations in the periodontium. Other terms often used are: *traumatizing occlusion, occlusal trauma, traumatogenic occlusion, periodontal traumatism, overload,* etc. In addition to producing damage in the periodontal tissues excessive occlusal force may also cause injury in e.g. the temporomandibular joint, the masticatory muscles, the pulp tissue. This chapter deals exclusively with the effects of *trauma from occlusion* on the periodontal tissues.

Trauma from occlusion was defined by Stillman (1917) as "a condition where injury results to the supporting structures of the teeth by the act of bringing the jaws into a closed position". WHO in 1978 defined *trauma from occlusion* as "damage in the periodontium caused by stress on the teeth produced directly or indirectly by teeth of the opposing jaw". In "Glossary of Periodontic Terms" (American Academy of Periodontology, 1986), *Occlusal Trauma* was defined as "An injury to the attachment apparatus as a result of excessive occlusal force".

Traumatizing forces may act on an individual tooth or on groups of teeth in premature contact relationship; may occur in conjunction with parafunctions such as clenching and bruxism, in conjunction with loss or migration of premolar and molar teeth with an accompanying, gradually developing spread of the anterior teeth of the maxillary jaw, etc.

In the literature, the tissue injury associated with *trauma from occlusion* is often divided into *primary* and *secondary*. The *primary* form includes a tissue reaction (damage), which is elicited around a tooth with normal height of the periodontium, while the *secondary* form is related to situations in which occlusal forces cause injury in a periodontium of reduced height. The distinction between a *primary* and a *secondary* form of injury - *primary* and *secondary occlusal trauma* - serves no meaningful purpose, since the alterations which occur in the periodontium as a consequence of trauma from occlusion are similar and independent of the height of the target tissue, i.e. the periodontium. It is, however, important to understand that symptoms of *trauma from occlusion* may develop only in situations when the magnitude of the load elicited by occlusion is so high that the periodontium around the exposed tooth cannot properly withstand and distribute the resulting force with unaltered position and stability of the tooth involved. This means that in cases of severely reduced height of the periodontium even comparatively small forces may produce traumatic lesions or adaptive changes in the periodontium.

Trauma from occlusion and plaque-associated periodontal disease

Ever since Karolyi (1901) postulated that an interaction may exist between "*trauma from occlusion*" and "*alveolar pyrrohea*" different opinions have been presented in the literature regarding the validity of this claim. Already in the 1930's Box (1935) and Stones (1938) reported experiments in sheep and monkeys, the result of which seemed to indicate that "trauma from occlusion is an etiologic factor in the production of that variety of periodontal disease in which there is vertical pocket formation associated with one or a varying number of teeth" (Stones 1938). The experiments by Box and Stones, however, have been criticized because they lacked proper controls and because the experimental design of the studies did not justify the conclusions drawn.

The interaction between *trauma from occlusion* and plaque-associated periodontal disease in humans was in the period 1955-1970 frequently discussed in connection with "report of a case", "in my opinion statements", etc. Even if such anecdotal data may have some value in clinical dentistry, it is obvious that conclusions drawn from research findings are much more pertinent. The research-based conclusions are not always indisputable but they invite the reader to a critique which anecdotal data do not. In this chapter, therefore, the presentation will be limited to findings collected from research endeavors involving: (1) human autopsy material, (2) clinical trials, and (3) animal experiments.

Analysis of human autopsy material

Results reported from carefully performed research efforts involving examinations of human autopsy material have been difficult to interpret. In the specimens examined (1) the histopathology of the lesions in the periodontium have been described, as well as (2) the presence and apical extension of microbial deposits at adjacent root surfaces, (3) the mobility of the teeth involved and (4) "the occlusion" of the sites under scrutiny. It is obvious that assessments made in specimens from cadavers have a limited to questionable value when "cause-effect" relationships between occlusion, plaque and periodontal lesions are to be described. It is not surprising, therefore, that *conclusions* drawn from this type of research can be controversial. This can best be illustrated if "Glickman's concept" is compared with "Waerhaug's concept" of what autopsy studies have revealed regarding trauma from occlusion and periodontal disease.

Glickman's concept

Glickman (1965, 1967) claimed that the pathway of the spread of a plaque-associated gingival lesion can be changed if forces of an abnormal magnitude are acting on teeth harboring subgingival plaque. This would imply that the

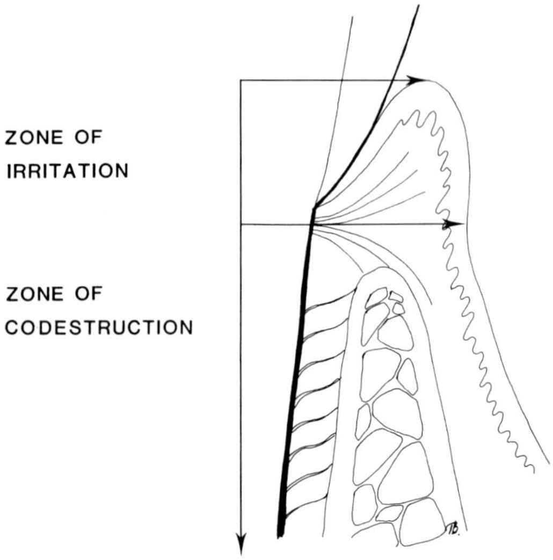

Fig. 8-1. Schematic drawing of the zone of irritation and the zone of codestruction according to Glickman.

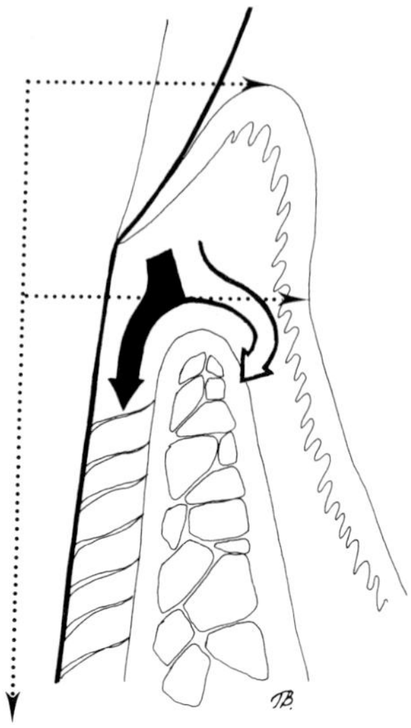

Fig. 8-2. The inflammatory lesion in the zone of irritation can, in teeth not subjected to trauma, propagate into the alveolar bone (open arrow), while in teeth also subjected to trauma from occlusion, the inflammatory infiltrate spreads directly into periodontal ligament (filled arrow).

character of the progressive tissue destruction of the periodontium at a "traumatized tooth" will be different from that characterizing a "non-traumatized" tooth. Instead of an even destruction of the periodontium and alveolar bone (suprabony pockets and horizontal bone loss), which according to Glickman occurs at sites with uncomplicated plaque-associated lesions, sites which are also exposed to abnormal occlusal force will develop angular bony defects and infrabony pockets.

Since the concept of Glickman regarding the effect of *trauma from occlusion* on the spread of the plaque-associated lesion is often cited, a more detailed presentation of his theory seems pertinent:

The periodontal structures can be divided into two zones:

1. the *zone of irritation* and
2. the *zone of codestruction* (Fig. 8-1).

The *zone of irritation* includes the marginal and interdental gingiva. The soft tissue of this zone is bordered by hard tissue (the tooth) only on one side and is not affected by forces of occlusion. This means that gingival inflammation cannot be induced by *trauma from occlusion* but is the result of irritation from microbial plaque. The plaque-associated lesion at a "non-traumatized" tooth propagates in apical direction by first involving the alveolar bone and only later the periodontal ligament area. The progression of this lesion results in an even (horizontal) bone destruction.

The zone of *codestruction* includes the periodontal ligament, the root cementum and the alveolar bone and is coronally demarcated by the transseptal (interdental) and the dentoalveolar collagen fiber bundles (Fig. 8-1). The tissue in this zone may become the seat of a lesion caused by *trauma from occlusion*.

The fiber bundles which separate the zone of codestruction from the zone of irritation can be affected from two different directions:

1. from the inflammatory lesion maintained by plaque in the *zone of irritation*.
2. from trauma-induced changes in the *zone of codestruction*.

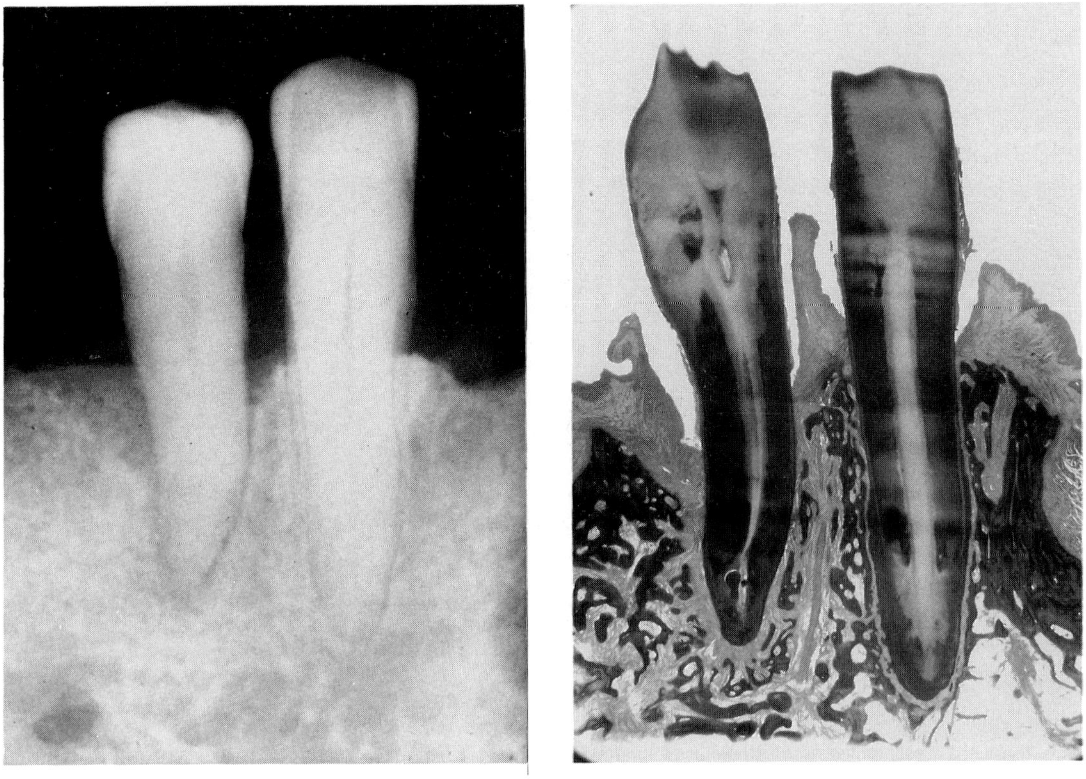

Figs. 8-3 a, b. Fig. a represents a radiograph of a mandibular premolar region. Note the angular bony defect at the distal aspect of the premolar.

Fig. b represents a histological mesio-distal section of the specimen illustrated in Fig. 8 a. Note the infrabony pocket at the distal aspect of the premolar (From Glickman & Smulow 1965).

Through this exposure from two different directions the fiber bundles may become dissolved and/or oriented into a direction parallel to the root surface. The spread of an inflammatory lesion from the *zone of irritation* directly down into the periodontal ligament (i.e. not via the interdental bone) may hereby be facilitated (Fig. 8-2). This alteration of the "normal" pathway of spread of the plaque-associated inflammatory lesion results in the development of angular bony defects. Glickman (1967) in a review paper stated that *trauma from occlusion* is an etiological factor (codestructive factor) of importance in situations where angular bony defects combined with infrabony pockets are found at one or several teeth (Fig. 8-3).

Waerhaug's concept

Waerhaug (1979) examined similar autopsy specimens (Fig. 8-4) as Glickman, but measured in addition the distance between the subgingival plaque and (1) the periphery of the associated inflammatory cell infiltrate in the gingiva and (2) the surface of the adjacent alveolar bone. He concluded from his analysis that angular bony defects and infrabony pockets occur equally often at periodontal sites of teeth which are not affected by trauma from occlusion as in traumatized teeth. In other words, he refuted the hypothesis that *trauma from occlusion* played a role in the spread of a gingival lesion into the "zone of co-destruction". The loss of connective attachment and the resorption of

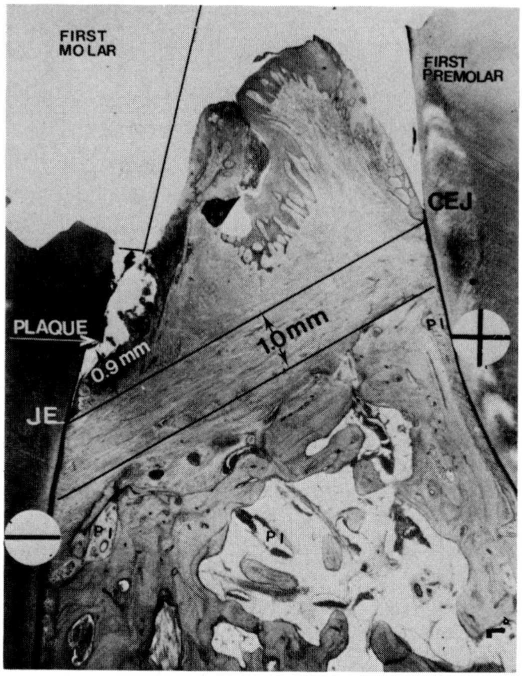

Fig. 8-4a.

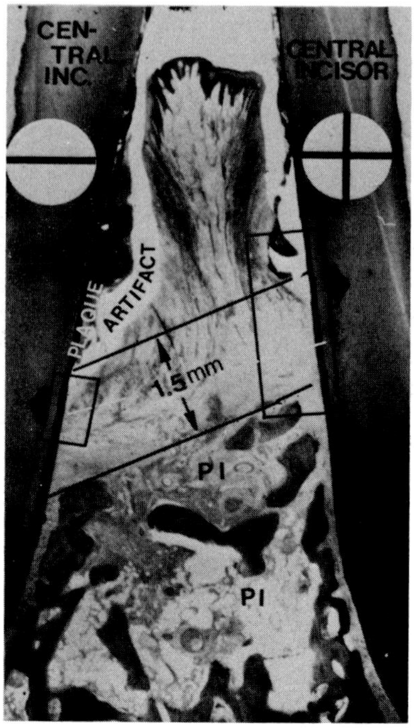

Fig. 8-4b.

Figs. 8-4a, b. Microphotographs illustrating two interproximal areas with angular bony defects. ⊖ denotes a tooth not subjected and ⊕ denotes a tooth subjected to trauma from occlusion. In categories ⊖ and ⊕ the distance between the apical cells of the junctional epithelium and the supporting alveolar bone is about 1-1.5 mm, and the distance between the apical extension of plaque and the apical cells of the junctional epithelium about 1 mm. Since the apical cells of the junctional epithelium are located at different levels on the two adjacent teeth, the outline of the bone crest becomes oblique. A radiograph from such a site would disclose the presence of an angular bony defect at a nontraumatized ⊖ tooth.

bone around teeth are, according to Waerhaug, exclusively the result of inflammatory lesions associated with subgingival plaque. Waerhaug concluded that angular bony defects and infrabony pockets occur when the subgingival plaque of one tooth has reached a more apical level than the microbiota on the neighboring tooth, and when the volume of the alveolar bone surrounding the roots is comparatively large. Waerhaug's observations support findings presented by Prichard (1965) and Manson (1976) which imply that the pattern of loss of supporting structures is the result of an interplay between the form and volume of the alveolar bone and the apical extension of the microbial plaque on the adjacent root surfaces.

It is obvious, as stated above, that examinations of autopsy material have a limited value when "cause-effect" relationships with respect to trauma and progressive periodontitis are to be determined. As a consequence, the conclusions drawn from this field of research have not been generally accepted. A number of authors tend to accept Glickman's conclusions that trauma from occlusion is an aggravating factor in periodontal disease (e.g. Macapanpan & Weinman 1954, Posselt & Emslie 1959, Glickman & Smulow 1962, 1965) while others accept Waerhaug's concept, i.e. that there is no relationship between occlusal trauma and the degree of periodontal tissue breakdown (e.g. Lovdahl et al. 1959, Belting & Gupta 1961, Baer et al. 1967, Waerhaug 1979).

Clinical trials

In addition to the presence of angular bony defects, and infrabony pockets, *increased tooth mobility* is frequently listed as an important sign of occlusal trauma. For details regarding tooth mobility see Chapter 21 "Occlusal Therapy". Conflicting data have been reported also regarding the periodontal conditions of mobile teeth. In one clinical study by Rosling et al. (1976) patients with advanced periodontal disease associated with multiple angular bony defects and mobile teeth were exposed to antimicrobial therapy (i.e. subgingival sealing after flap elevation). Healing was evaluated by probing attachment level measurements and radiographic monitoring. The authors reported that "the infrabony pocket located at hypermobile teeth exhibited the same degree of healing as those adjacent to firm teeth".

In another study, however, Fletzar et al. (1980) reported on the influence of tooth mobility on healing following periodontal therapy including both root debridement and occlusal adjustment. They concluded that "pockets of clinically mobile teeth do not respond as well to periodontal treatment as do those of firm teeth exhibiting the same disease severity".

A third study (Pihlstrom et al. 1986) studied the association between *trauma from occlusion* and periodontitis by assessing a series of clinical and radiographic features at upper first molars. Parameters included in this study were: probing depth, probing attachment level, tooth mobility, wear facets, plaque and calculus, bone height, widened periodontal space, etc. Pihlstrom and his associates concluded from their measurements and examinations that teeth with increased mobility and widened periodontal ligament space had, in fact, deeper pockets, more attachment loss and less bone support than teeth without these symptoms.

Provided that the resistance offered by the periodontal tissues to probing (see Chapter 12) is similar for nonmobile and mobile teeth - and this has not been determined - the findings from the studies by Fletzar and Pihlstrom lend some support to the concept that *trauma from occlusion* (and increased tooth mobility) may have a detrimental effect on the periodontium. On the other hand, the study by Rosling et al. supports Waerhaug's concept that progressive periodontitis is caused by plaque and that occlusal trauma or tooth hypermobility fails to contribute to disease progression.

Since neither analysis of autopsy material nor data from clinical trials can be used to properly determine the role *trauma from occlusion* may play in periodontal pathology, it is necessary to describe the contributions made by means of animal research in this particular field. Results from such experiments, describing the reactions of the normal and subsequently the diseased periodontium to occlusal forces, are presented below.

Animal experiments

Orthodontic type trauma

The reaction of the periodontal tissues to traumatic forces initiated by occlusion has been studied principally in animal experiments. In early experiments the reaction of the normal periodontium was studied following the application of forces which were inflicted on teeth in one direction only. Biopsies including tooth and periodontium were harvested after varying experimental time intervals and prepared for histologic examinations. Analysis of the tissue sections (Häupl & Psansky 1938, Reitan 1951, Mühlemann & Herzog 1961, Ewen & Stahl 1962, Waerhaug & Hansen 1966, Karring et al. 1982) revealed the following: when a tooth is exposed to unilateral forces of a magnitude, frequency or duration that its periodontal tissues are unable to withstand and distribute while maintaining the stability of the tooth, certain well-defined reactions develop in the periodontal ligament, eventually resulting in an adaptation of the periodontal structures to the

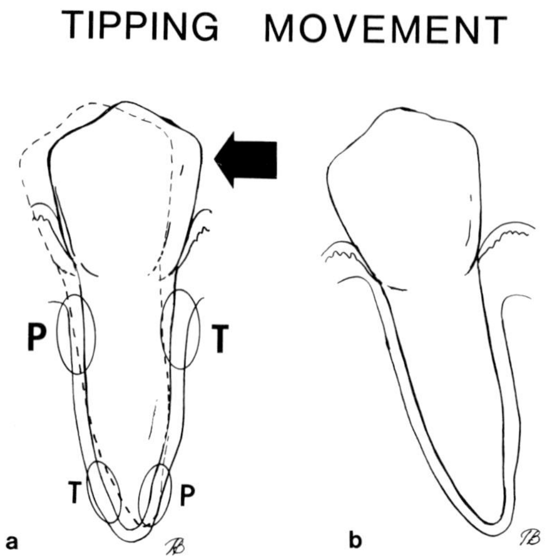

Figs. 8-5a, b. If the crown of a tooth is exposed to excessive, horizontally directed forces (arrow), pressure (P) and tension (T) zones will develop within the marginal and apical parts of the periodontium (a). The supraalveolar connective tissue remains unaffected by force application. Within the pressure and tension zones tissue alterations take place which eventually allow the tooth to tilt in the direction of the force. When the tooth has escaped the trauma complete regeneration of the periodontal tissues takes place (b). There is no apical downgrowth of the dentogingival epithelium.

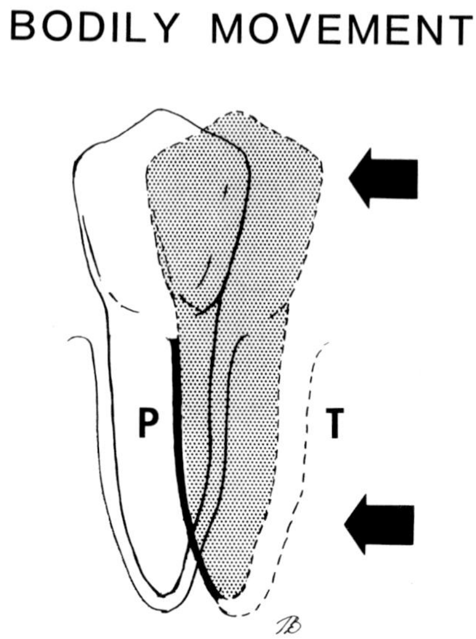

Fig. 8-6. When a tooth is exposed to forces which produce "bodily tooth movement", e.g. in orthodontic therapy, the pressure (P) and tension (T) zones, depending on the direction of the force, are extended over the entire tooth surface. Neither in conjunction with tipping nor in conjunction with bodily movements of teeth is the supraalveolar connective tissue affected. Forces of this kind, therefore, will not induce inflammatory reactions in the gingiva. No apical downgrowth of the dentogingival epithelium occurs.

altered functional demand. If the crown of a tooth is affected by such horizontally directed forces, the tooth tends to tilt (tip) in the direction of the force (Fig. 8-5). This tilting force results in the development of *pressure* and *tension zones* within the marginal and apical parts of the periodontium. The tissue reactions which develop in the *pressure zone* are characterized by increased vascularization, increased vascular permeability, vascular thrombosis, and disorganization of cells and collagen fiber bundles. If the magnitude of forces is within certain limits allowing the maintenance of the vitality of the periodontal ligament cells, bone-resorbing osteoclasts soon appear on the bone surface of the alveolus in the *pressure zone*. A process of bone resorption is initiated. This phenomenon is called "*direct bone resorption*".

If the force applied is of higher magnitude, the result may be necrosis of the periodontal ligament tissue in the *pressure zone*, i.e. decomposition of cells, vessles, matrix and fibers, (*hyalinization*). "Direct bone resorption" therefore cannot occur. Instead, osteoclasts appear in marrow spaces within the adjacent bone tissue where the stress concentration is lower than in the periodontal ligament and a process of undermining or "*indirect bone resorption*" is initiated. Through this reaction the surrounding bone is resorbed until there is a breakthrough to the hyalinized tissue within the *pressure zone*. This breakthrough results in a reduction of the stress in this area, and cells from the neighboring bone or adjacent areas of the periodontal ligament can proliferate into the *pressure zone* and replace the previously hyalinized tissue, thereby reestablishing prerequisites for "direct bone resorption". Irrespective of whether the bone resorption is of a direct or an indirect nature the tooth moves (tilts) further in the direction of the force.

Concomitant with the tissue alterations in the *pressure zone*, apposition of bone occurs in the *tension zone* in order to maintain the normal width of the periodontal ligament in this area. Because of the tissue reactions in the *pressure* and *tension* zones the tooth becomes, temporarily, hypermobile. When the tooth has moved (tilted) to a position where the effect of the forces is nullified, healing of the periodontal tissues takes place in both the *pressure* and the *tension zones* and the tooth becomes stable in its new position. In orthodontic tilting (tipping) movements, neither gingival inflammation nor loss of connective tissue attachment will occur in a healthy periodontium, and - as long as the tooth is not moved through the envelop of the alveolar process - there is no apical migration of the dentogingival epithelium. In other words, since the supraalveolar connective tissue is only bordered by hard tissue (the tooth) on one side (in the direction of the force), this structure remains unaffected by tipping forces.

These tissue reactions do not differ fundamentally from those which occur as a consequence of *bodily tooth movement* in orthodontic therapy (Reitan 1951). The main difference is that the *pressure* and *tension zones*, depending on the direction of the force, are more extended in apical-coronal direction along the root surface than in conjunction with tipping movement (Fig. 8-6). Neither in conjunction with tipping nor in conjunction with bodily movements of the tooth is the supraalveolar connective tissue affected by the *force*. Unilateral forces directed to the crown of teeth, therefore, will not induce inflammatory reactions in the gingiva or cause loss of connective tissue attachment.

Recent studies (Steiner et al. 1981, Wennström et al. 1987) have demonstrated, however, that orthodontic forces producing bodily (or tipping) movement of teeth may result in gingival recession and loss of connective tissue attachment. This breakdown of the attachment apparatus occurred at sites with gingivitis when, in addition, the tooth was moved through the envelope of the alveolar process. At such sites a bone dehiscence becomes established and, if the covering soft tissue is thin (in the direction of the movement of the tooth), recession (attachment can) may occur.

Criticism has been directed, however, to experiments in which only unilateral trauma is exerted on teeth (Wentz et al. 1958). It has been suggested that in humans, unlike in the animal experiments described above, the occlusal forces act alternately in one and then in the opposite direction. Such forces have been termed *jiggling forces.*

Jiggling-type trauma

Healthy periodontium with normal height

Experiments have been reported in which traumatic forces were exerted on the crowns of the teeth, alternately in buccal and lingual or mesial and distal directions, and in which the teeth were not allowed to move away from the force (e.g. Wentz et al.1958, Glickman & Smulow 1968, Svanberg & Lindhe 1973, Meitner 1975, Ericsson & Lindhe 1982). In conjunction with so-called *"jiggling-type trauma"* no clearcut *pressure* and *tension zones* can be identified but rather a combination of pressure and tension occurs on both sides of the jiggled tooth (Fig. 8-7).

The tissue reactions in the periodontal ligament provoked by the combined *pressure* and *tension* forces were found to be similar, however, to those reported for the pressure zone at orthodontically moved teeth, with the one difference that the periodontal ligament space at jiggling gradually increased in width on both sides of the tooth. During the phase when the periodontal space gradually increased in width 1) inflammatory changes were present in the ligament tissue, 2) active bone resorption oc-

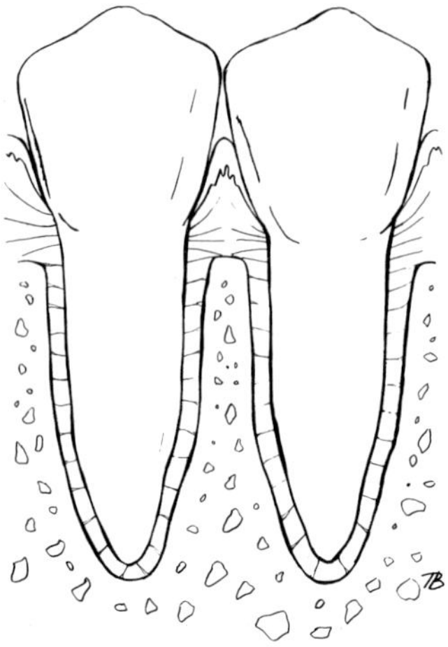

Fig. 8-7a.

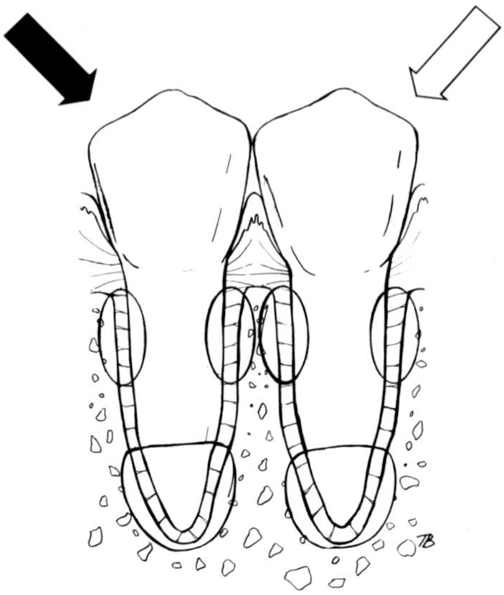

Fig. 8-7b.

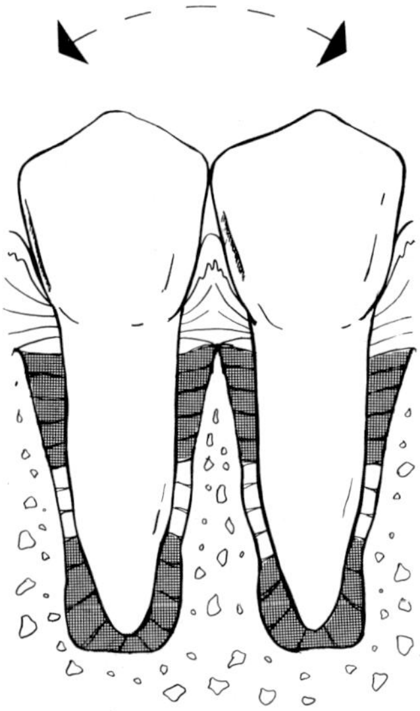

Fig. 8-7c.

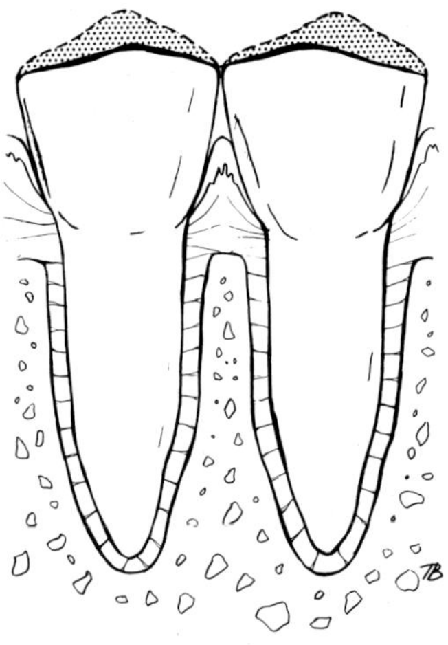

Fig. 8-7d.

Figs. 8-7a-d. Two mandibular premolars with normal periodontal tissues (a) are exposed to jiggling forces (b) as illustrated by the two arrows. The combined tension and pressure zones (encircled areas) are characterized by signs of acute inflammation including collagen resorption, bone resorption and cementum resorption. As a result of bone resorption the periodontal ligament space gradually increases in size on both sides of the teeth as well as in the periapical region. When the effect of the force applied has been compensated for by the increased width of the periodontal ligament space (c), the ligament tissue shows no sign of inflammation. The supraalveolar connective tissue is not affected by the jiggling forces and there is no apical downgrowth of the dentogingival epithelium. After occlusal adjustment the width of the periodontal ligament becomes normalized (d) and the teeth are stabilized.

curred, and 3) the tooth displayed signs of gradually increasing (*progressive*) mobility. When the effect of the forces applied had been compensated for by the increased width of the periodontal ligament space, the ligament tissue showed no signs of increased vascularity or ex-

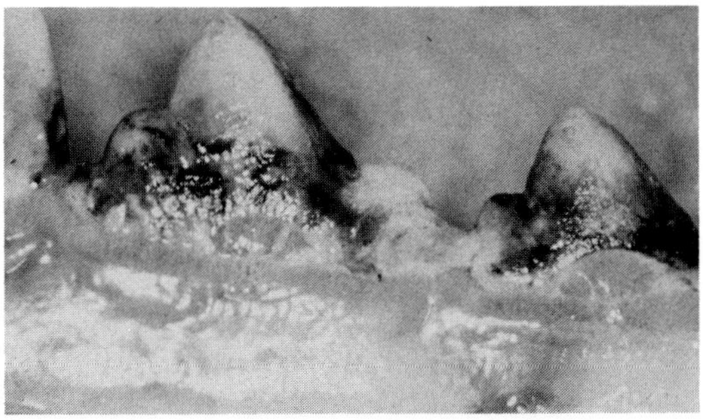

a

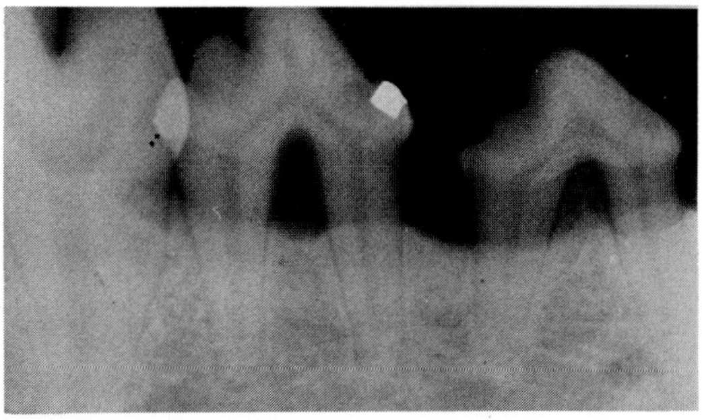

b

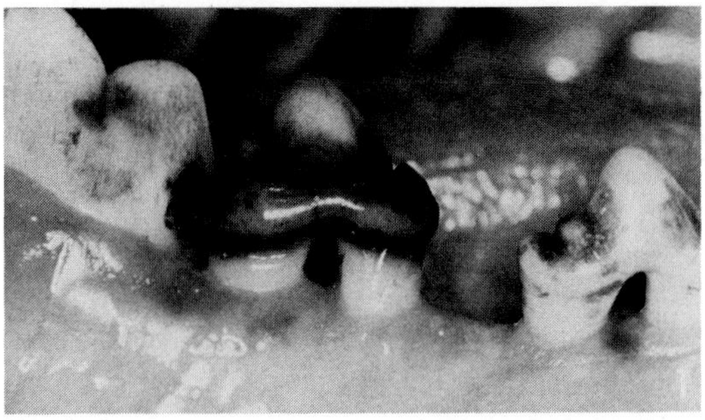

c

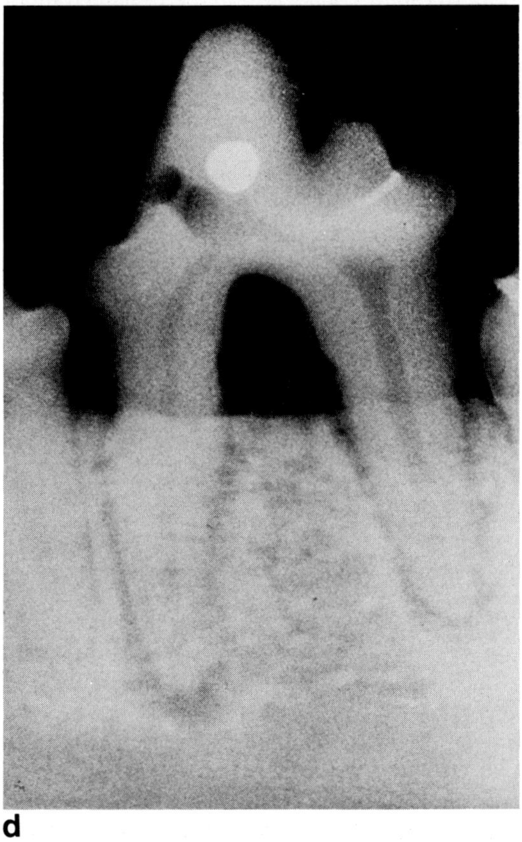

d

Figs. 8-8a-e. Dogs were allowed to accumulate plaque and calculus in the lower premolar regions (a). When around 50% of the periodontal tissue support had been lost (b) the animals were treated by scaling, root planing and pocket elimination. During surgery a notch was prepared in the root at the level of the bone crest. The dogs were subsequently placed on a plaque control program and 8 months later the teeth were surrounded by a healthy periodontium with reduced height (c). The lower fourth premolar in one side of the jaw was exposed to jiggling forces. As a consequence, a widened periodontal ligament and increased tooth mobility resulted (d). This increase in tooth mobility and the development of widened periodontal ligament space did not, however, result in apical downgrowth of the dentogingival epithelium (e). The arrow indicates the apical extension of the junctional epithelium (JE) coinciding with the apical border of the notch (N), prepared in the root surface prior to jiggling.

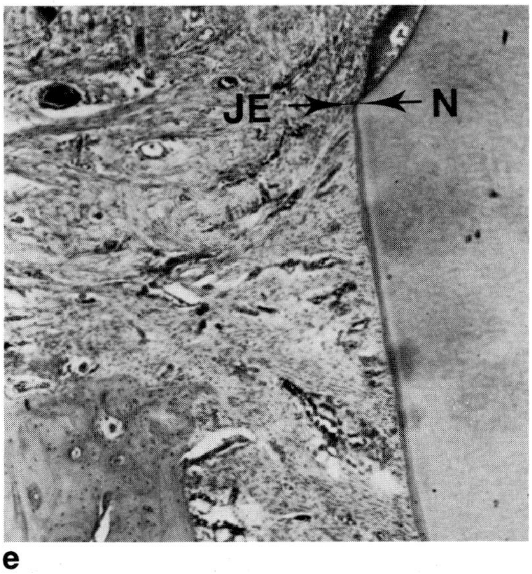

e

udation. The tooth was hypermobile but the mobility was no longer *progressive* in character. Distinction should thus be made between *progressive* on the one hand, and *increased* tooth mobility on the other.

In "*jiggling-type trauma*" experiments, performed on animals with a normal periodontium, the supraalveolar connective tissue was not influenced by the occlusal forces, the reason being that this tissue compartment is bordered on one side only by hard tissue. This means that a gingiva which was noninflamed at the start of the experiment remained noninflamed, but also that an overt inflammatory lesion residing in the supraalveolar connective tissue was not aggravated by the jiggling forces.

Healthy periodontium with reduced height

Progressive periodontal disease is characterized by gingival inflammation and a gradually developing loss of connective tissue attachment and alveolar bone. Treatment of periodontal disease, i.e. removal of plaque and calculus and elimination of pathologically deepened pockets, will result in the reestablishment of a healthy periodontium but with reduced height. The question is whether a healthy periodontium with reduced height has a capacity similar to that of the normal periodontium to adapt to traumatizing occlusal forces (secondary occlusal trauma).

This problem has also been examined in animal experiments (Ericsson & Lindhe 1977). Destructive periodontal disease was initiated in dogs by allowing the animals to accumulate plaque and calculus for a period of 6 months (Fig. 8-8). When around 50% of the periodontal tissue support had been lost (Figs. 8-8a, b), the progressive disease was subjected to treatment by scaling, root planing and pocket elimination (Fig. 8-8c). The animals were subsequently, during an 8-month period, enrolled in a careful plaque control program. During this period certain premolars were exposed to traumatizing jiggling forces. The periodontal tissues in the combined *pressure* and *tension zones* reacted to the forces by vascular proliferation, exudation and thrombosis, as well as by bone resorption. In radiographs, widened periodontal ligaments (Fig. 8-8d) could be found around the traumatized teeth which at clinical examination displayed sign of *progressive* tooth mobility. The gradual increase in the width of the periodontal ligament and the resulting progressive increase in tooth mobility took place during a period of several weeks but eventually terminated. The active bone resorption ceased and the markedly widened periodontal ligament tissue regained its normal composition; healing had occurred (Fig. 8-8e). The teeth were hypermobile but surrounded by periodontal structures which had adapted to the altered functional demands.

During the entire experimental period the supraalveolar connective tissue remained unaffected by the jiggling forces. There was no further loss of connective tissue attachment and no further downgrowth of dentogingival epithelium (Fig. 8-8e). The results from this study clearly reveal that within certain limits a healthy periodontium with reduced height has a capacity similar to that of a periodontium with normal height to adapt to altered functional demands (Fig. 8-9).

Plaque-associated periodontal disease

Experiments carried out on humans and animals have demonstrated that *trauma from occlusion* cannot induce pathological alterations in the supraalveolar connective tissue, i.e. cannot produce inflammatory lesions in a normal gingiva or aggravate a gingival lesion associated with plaque and cannot induce loss of connective tissue attachment. The question remains if abnormal occlusal forces can influence the spread of the plaque-associated lesion and enhance the rate of tissue destruction in periodontal disease. This has been studied in animal experiments (Lindhe & Svanberg 1974, Meit-

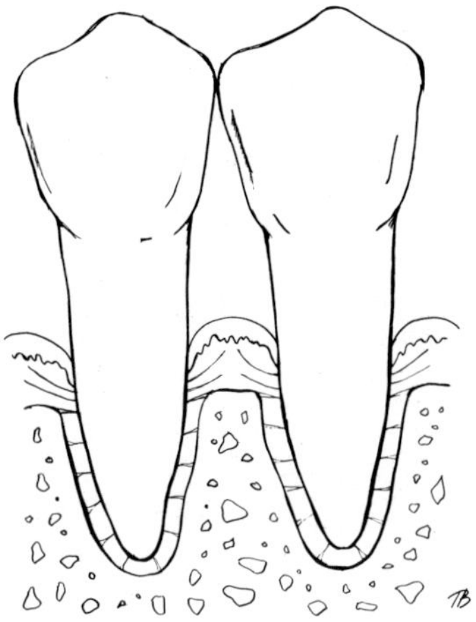

Fig. 8-9a.

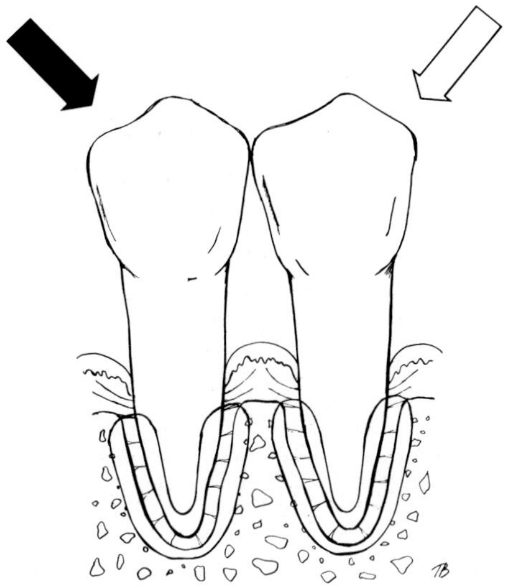

Fig. 8-9b.

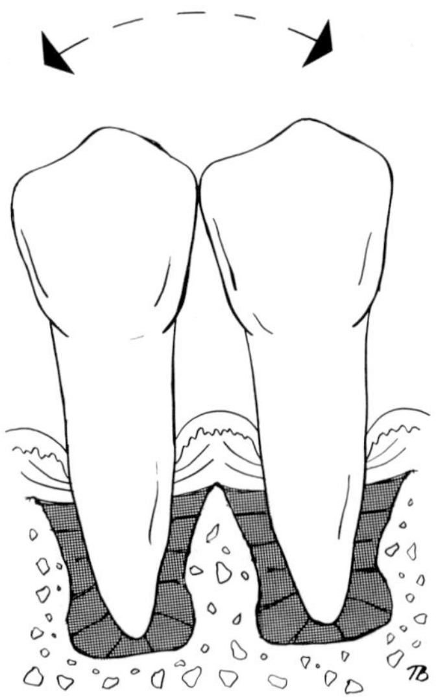

Fig. 8-9c.

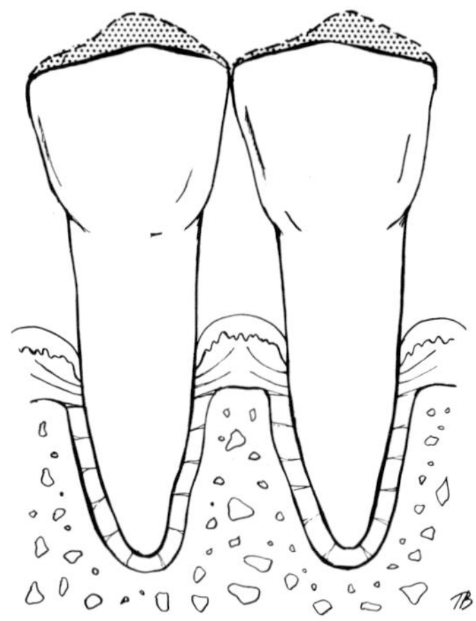

Fig. 8-9d.

Figs. 8-9a-d. Two lower premolars are surrounded by a healthy periodontium with reduced height (a). If such premolars are subjected to traumatizing forces of the jiggling type (b) a series of alterations occurs in the periodontal ligament tissue (encircled areas). These alterations result in a widened periodontal ligament space (c) and in an increased tooth mobility but do not lead to further loss of connective tissue attachment. After occlusal adjustment (d) the width of the periodontal ligament is normalized and the teeth stabilized.

ner 1975, Nyman et al. 1978, Ericsson & Lindhe 1982, Polson & Zander 1983). In these experiments progressive and destructive periodontal disease was first initiated in dogs or monkeys by allowing the animals to accumulate plaque and calculus. Teeth thus involved in a progressive periodontal disease process were also subjected to trauma from occlusion.

Jiggling forces were (Lindhe & Svanberg 1974) exerted on premolars and were found to

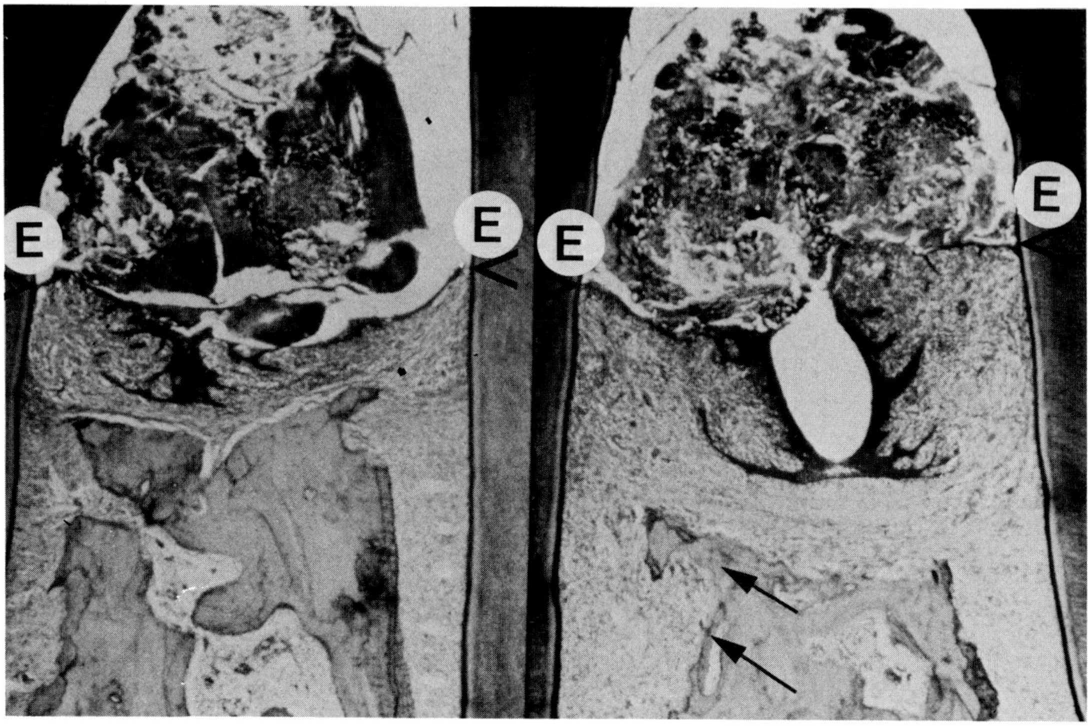

Fig. 8-10a. Fig. 8-10b.

Figs. 8-10a, b. A composite photomicrograph illustrating the interdental space between two pairs of teeth. The teeth have been subjected to experimental, ligature-induced periodontitis and the teeth in (b) also to repetitive mechanical injury. In (b), there is considerable loss of alveolar bone and an angular widening of the periodontal ligament space (arrows). However, the apical downgrowth of the dentogingival epithelium in the two areas (a and b) is similar. E indicates the apical level of the dentogingival epithelium. (Courtesy of Dr. Meitner).

induce certain tissue reactions in the combined *pressure/tension zones.* The periodontal ligament tissue in these zones, within a few days of the onset of the jiggling forces, displayed signs of inflammation, had increased numbers of vessels, showed increased vascular permeability and exudation, thrombosis, as well as retention of neutrophils and macrophages. On the adjacent bone surfaces there was a large number of osteoclasts. Since the teeth could not orthodontically move away from the jiggling forces, the periodontal ligament of both sides of the tooth gradually increased in width, the teeth became hypermobile (*progressive* tooth mobility) and angular bony defects could be detected in the radiographs. The forces were eventually nullified by the increased width of the periodontal ligament.

If the forces applied were within a magnitude to which the periodontal structures could adapt, the *progressive* increase of the tooth mobility terminated within a few weeks. The active bone resorption ceased but the angular bone destruction persisted as well as the increased tooth mobility. The periodontal ligament had an increased width but a normal tissue composition. Histological examination of biopsies revealed that this adaptation had occurred with no greater apical proliferation of the dento-gingival epithelium than was caused by the plaque-associated lesion (Figs. 8-10a,b; Meitner 1975). This means that occlusal forces which allow adaptive alterations to develop in the *pressure/tension* zones of the periodontal ligament will not aggravate a plaque-associated periodontal disease (Fig. 8-11).

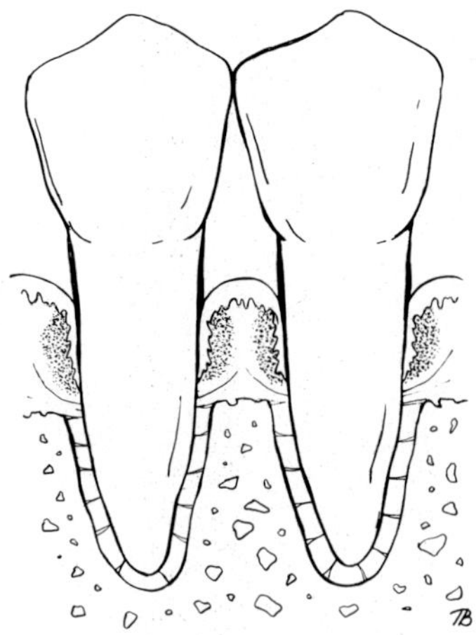

Fig. 8-11a.

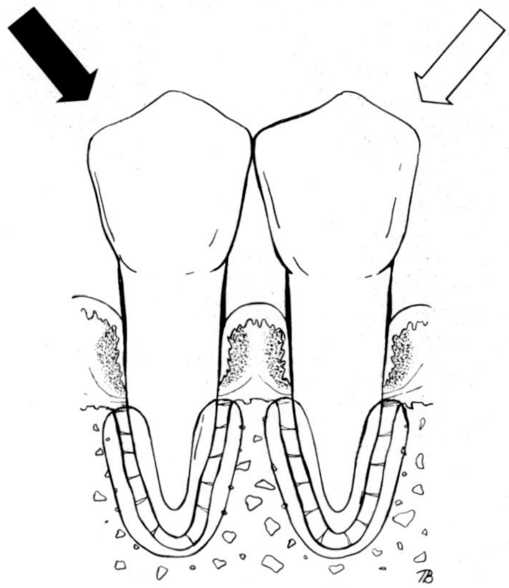

Fig. 8-11b.

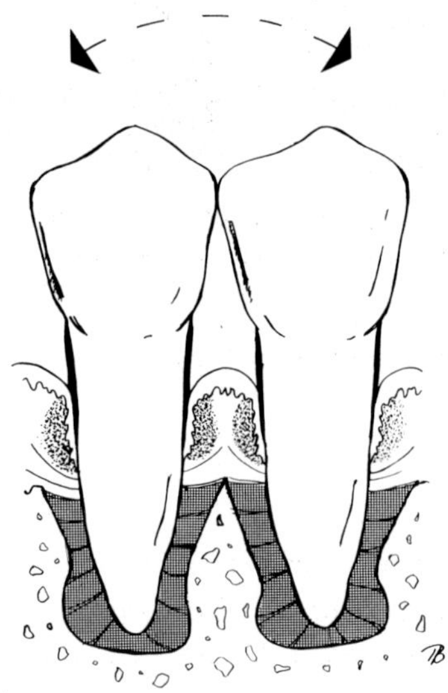

Fig. 8-11c.

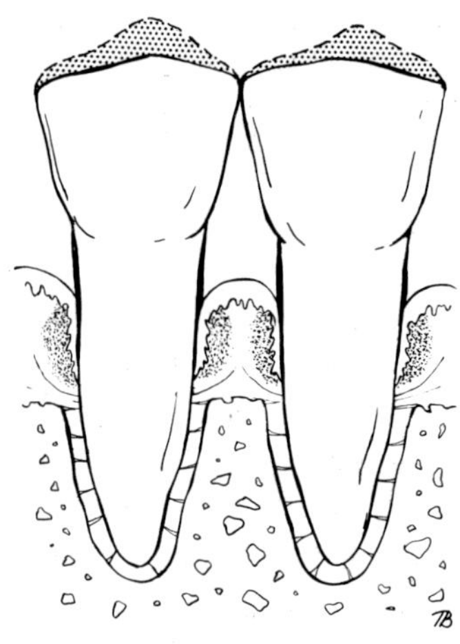

Fig. 8-11d.

Figs. 8-11 a-d. Two lower premolars with supra- and subgingival plaque, advanced bone loss and periodontal pockets of a suprabony character (a). Note the connective tissue infiltrate (shadowed areas) and the noninflamed connective tissue between the alveolar bone and the apical portion of the infiltrate. If these teeth are subjected to traumatizing forces of the jiggling type (b), pathological and adaptic alterations occur within the periodontal ligament space (encircled areas). These tissue alterations which include bone resorption result in a widened periodontal ligament space increased tooth mobility but no further loss of connective tissue attachment (c). Occlusal adjustment results in a reduction of the width of the periodontal ligament (d) and in less mobile teeth.

If, however, the jiggling forces had such a magnitude and direction that during the course of the study (6 months) the tissues in the *pressure/tension* zones could nor become adapted, the injury in the *zones of codestruction* had a more permanent character. The periodontal ligament in the *pressure/tension* zones displayed for several months signs of inflammation (vas-

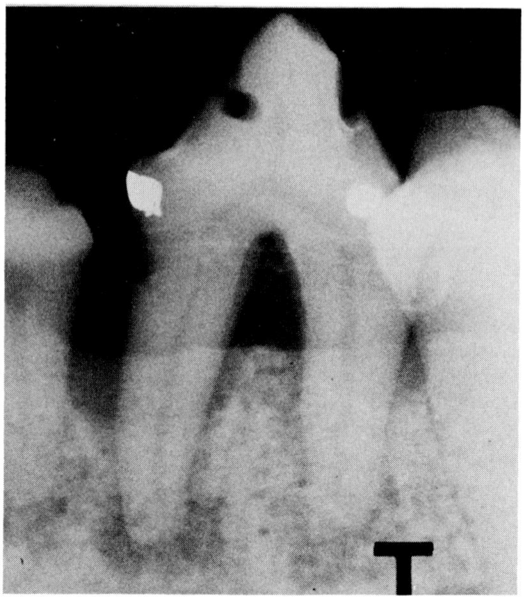

Fig 8-12. Radiographic appearance of one test tooth (T) at the termination of an experiment in which periodontitis was induced by ligature placement and plaque accumulation and in which trauma of the jiggling type was induced. Note angular bone loss particularly around the mesial root of the lower premolar. (From Lindhe & Svanberg 1974).

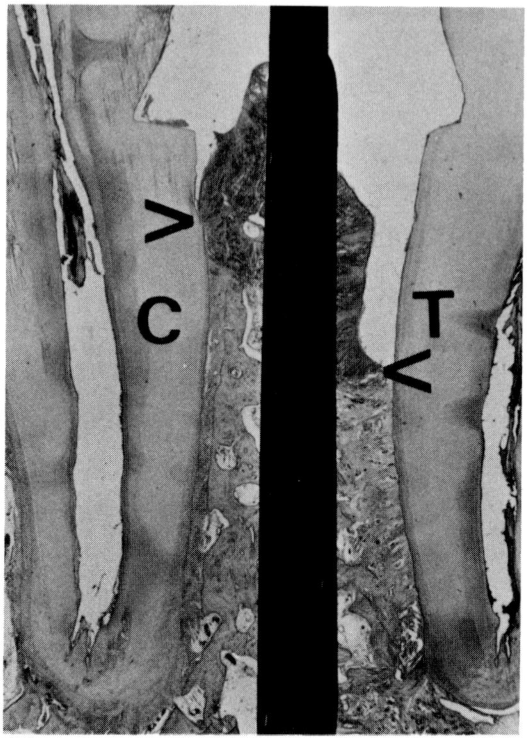

Fig. 8-13. Microphotographs from one control (C) and one test (T) tooth after 240 days of experimental periodontal tissue breakdown and 180 days of trauma from occlusion of the jiggling type (T). The arrowheads denote the apical position of the dentogingival epithelium. The attachment loss is more pronounced in T than in C. (From Lindhe & Svanberg 1974).

cular proliferation, exudation, thrombosis, retention of neutrophils and macrophages, collagen destruction). Osteoclasts residing on the walls of the alveolus maintained the bone-resorptive process which resulted in a gradual widening of the periodontal ligament in the *pressure/tension* zones (Fig. 8-12). As a consequence, the resulting angular bone destruction was continuous and the mobility of the teeth remained progressive. The plaque-associated lesion in the "zone of irritation" and the inflammatory lesion in the "zone of codestruction" merged; the dentogingival epithelium proliferated in an apical direction and periodontal disease was aggravated (Figs. 8-13, 8-14; Lindhe & Svanberg 1974).

Similar findings were reported from another experiment in the dog (Ericsson & Lindhe 1982) in which the effect was assessed of a *prolonged* period of jiggling force application on the rate of progression of plaque-associated, marginal periodontitis. Thus, in dogs with continuing periodontal disease, certain teeth were exposed to jiggling forces during a period of 10 months. Control teeth were not jiggled. Fig. 8-15a illustrates the marked periodontal tissue breakdown around a tooth which for several months was exposed to plaque infection combined with jiggling trauma and Fig. 8-15b illustrates a control tooth which was exposed to plaque infection only.

On the other hand, more short-term experiments in the monkey (Polson & Zander 1983), evaluating the effect of *trauma from occlusion* on teeth involved in an ongoing process of periodontitis, failed to support the findings by

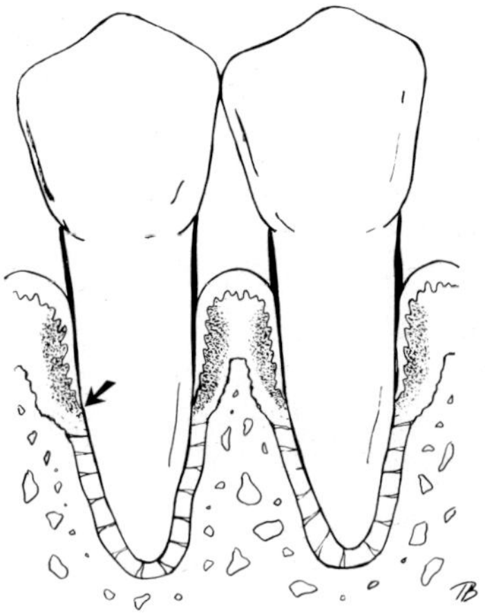

Fig. 8-14a.

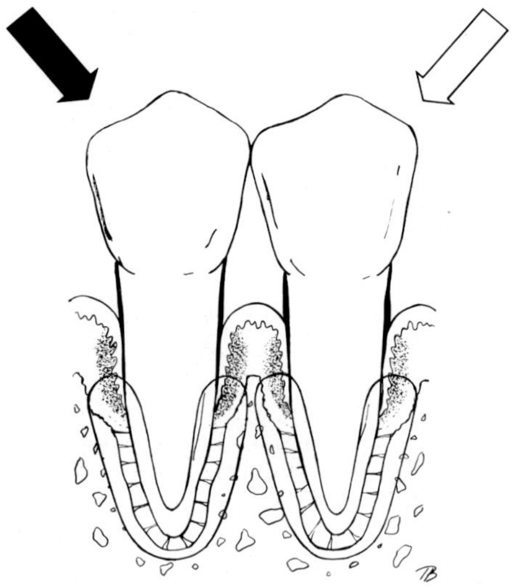

Fig. 8-14b.

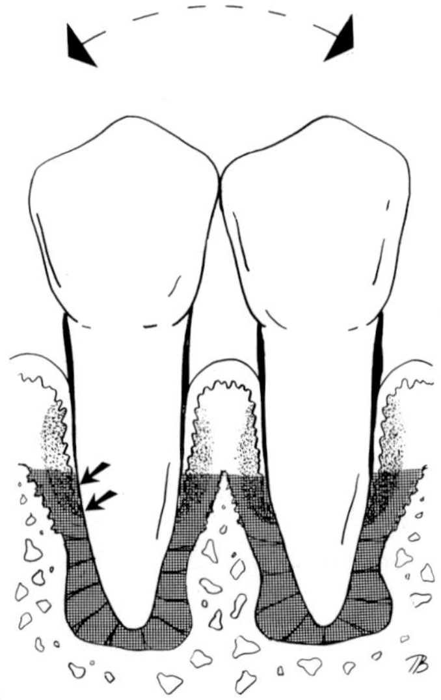

Fig. 8-14c.

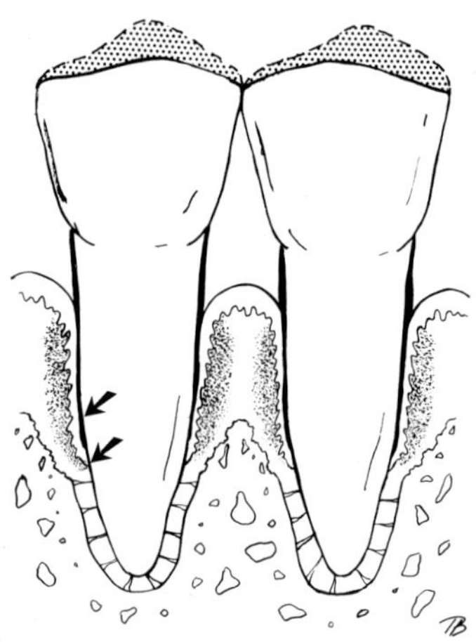

Fig. 8-14d.

Fig. 8-14. Illustration of a tooth where subgingival plaque has mediated the development of an infiltrated soft tissue (shadowed area) and an infrabony pocket (a). When trauma from occlusion of the jiggling type is inflicted (arrows) on the crown of this tooth (b), the associated pathological alterations occur within a zone of the periodontium (encircled area) which is also occupied by the inflammatory cell infiltrate (shadowed area). In this situation the increasing tooth mobility may also be associated with an enhanced loss of connective tissue attachment and further downgrowth of dentogingival epithelium; compare arrows (c). Occlusal adjustment will result in a narrowing of the periodontal ligament, less tooth mobility, but no improvement of the attachment level (Lindhe & Ericsson 1982).

Lindhe & Svanberg (1974) and Ericsson & Lindhe (1982). Polson & Zander (1983) observed that trauma superimposed on periodontal lesions associated with angular bony defects (1) caused increased loss of alveolar bone but (2) failed to produce additional loss of connective tissue attachment.

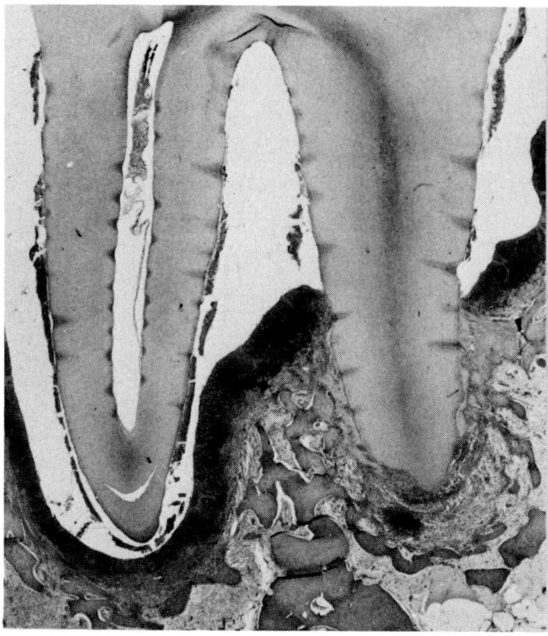

Fig. 8-15a.

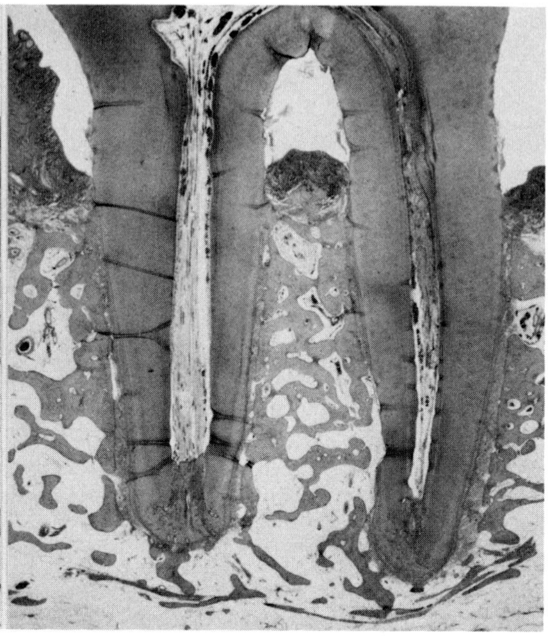

Fig. 8-15b.

Figs. 8-15a-b. Fig. a illustrates the periodontal conditions around a tooth which has been exposed to trauma from occlusion (of the jiggling type) for 300 days in combination with plaque-associated experimental periodontitis. Fig. b illustrates the condition of a control tooth from the same dog in which experimental periodontitis but no jiggling trauma had been in operation. Note the difference between (a) and (b) regarding the degree of bone destruction and loss of connective tissue attachment. Note also in (a) the location of the subgingival plaque at the apex of the root. (From Ericsson & Lindhe 1982).

Conclusions

Experiments, carried out in humans as well as animals, have produced convincing evidence that neither unilateral forces nor jiggling forces, applied to teeth with a healthy periodontium, result in pocket formation or in loss of connective tissue attachment. *Trauma from occlusion cannot induce periodontal tissue breakdown.* Trauma from occlusion does, however, result in resorption of alveolar bone leading to an increased tooth mobility which can be of transient or permanent character. This bone resorption with resulting increased tooth mobility should be regarded as a physiologic adaptation of the periodontal ligament and surrounding alveolar bone to the traumatizing forces, i.e. to altered functional demands.

In teeth with progressive, plaque-associated periodontal disease, trauma from occlusion may, however, under certain conditions enhance the rate of progression of the disease, i.e. act as a cofactor in the destructive process. From the clinical point of view, this knowledge strengthens the demand for proper treatment of plaque associated with periodontal disease. This treatment will arrest the destruction of the periodontal tissues even if the occlusal trauma persists. A treatment directed towards the trauma alone, i.e. occlusal adjustment or splinting, may reduce the mobility of the traumatized teeth, result in some regrowth of bone but will not arrest the rate of further breakdown of the supporting apparatus caused by plaque. (For detailed discussion on treatment of teeth exhibiting increased mobility see Chapter 21).

References

Baer, P., Kakehashi, S., Littleton, N.W., White, C.L. & Lieberman, J.E. (1963) Alveolar bone loss and occlusal wear. *Periodontics* **1**, 91.

Belting, C.M. & Gupta, O.P. (1961) The influence of psychiatric disturbances on the severity of periodontal disease. *Journal of Periodontology* **32**, 219-226.

Box, H.K. (1935) Experimental traumatogenic occlusion in sheep. *Oral Health* **25**, 9-25.

Ericsson, I. & Lindhe, J. (1977) Lack of effect of trauma from occlusion on the recurrence of experimental periodontitis. *Journal of Clinical Periodontology* **4**, 115-127.

Ericsson, I. & Lindhe, J. (1982) The effect of long-standing jiggling on experimental marginal periodontitis in the beagle dog. *Journal of Clinical Periodontology* **9**, 497-503.

Ewen, S.J. & Stahl. S.S. (1962) The response of the periodontium to chronic gingival irritation and long-term tilting forces in adult dogs. *Oral Surgery, Oral Medicine and Oral Pathology* **15**, 1426-1433.

Glickman, I. (1965) Clinical significance of trauma from occlusion. *Journal of the American Dental Association* **70**, 607-618.

Glickman, I. (1967) Occlusion and periodontium. *Journal of Dental Research* **46**, Supplement 1, 53.

Glickman, I. & Smulow, J.B. (1962) Alterations in the pathway of gingival inflammation into the underlying tissues induced by excessive occlusal forces. *Journal of Periodontology* **33**, 7-13.

Glickman, I. & Smulow, J.B. (1965) Effect of excessive occlusal forces upon the pathway of gingival inflammation in humans. *Journal of Periodontology* **36**, 141-147.

Glickman, I. & Smulow, J.B. (1968) Adaptive alteration in the periodontium of the Rhesus monkey in chronic trauma from occlusion. *Journal of Periodontology* **39**, 101-105.

Haupl, K. & Psansky, R. (1938) Histologische Untersuchungen der Wirdungsweise der in der Funktions-Kiefer-Orthopedie verwendeten Apparate. *Deutsche Zahn-, Mund- und Kieferheikunde* **5**, 214.

Karolyi, M. (1901) Beobachtungen über Pyorrhea alveolaris. *Osterreichisch-Ungarische Viertel jahresschrift für Zahnheilkunde* **17**, 279.

Karring, T., Nyman, S., Thilander, B. & Magnusson, I. (1982) Bone regeneration in orthodontically produced alveolar bone dehiscences. *Journal of Periodontal Research* **17**, 309-315.

Knowles, J.W. (1967) Occlusal interferences and loss of periodontal attachment. *IADR Abstract* No. 517.

Lindhe, J. & Ericsson, I. (1982) The effect of elimination of jiggling forces on periodontally exposed teeth in the dog. *Journal of Periodontology* **53**, 562-567.

Lindhe, J. & Svanberg, G. (1974) Influences of trauma from occlusion on progression of experimental periodontitis in the Beagle dog. *Journal of Clinical Periodontology* **1**, 3-14.

Lovdahl, A., Schei, O., Waerhaug, J. & Arno, A. (1959) Tooth mobility and alveolar bone resorption as a function of occlusal stress and oral hygiene. *Acta Odontologica Scandinavica* **17**, 61-77.

Macapanpan, L.C. & Weinmann, J.P. (1954) The influence of injury to the periodontal membrane on the spread of gingival inflammation. *Journal of Dental Research* **33**, 263-272.

Manson, J.D. (1976) Bone morphology and bone loss in periodontal disease. *Journal of Clinical Periodontology* **3**, 14-22.

Meitner, S.W. (1975) *Co-destructive Factors of Marginal Periodontitis and Repetitive Mechanical Injury.* Thesis. Rochester, USA: Eastman Dental Center and The University of Rochester, USA: Eastman Dental Center and The University of Rochester.

Muhlemann, H.R. & Herzog, H. (1961) Tooth mobility and microscopic tissue changes reproduced by experimental occlusal trauma. *Helvetica Odontologia Acta* **5**, 33-39.

Nyman, S., Lindhe, J. & Ericsson, I. (1978) The effect of progressive tooth mobility on destructive periodontitis in the dog. *Journal of Clinical Periodontology* **7**, 351-360.

Polson, A. & Zander, H. (1983) Effect of periodontal trauma upon infrabony pockets. *Journal of Periodontology* **54**, 586-591.

Posselt, U. & Emslie, R.D. (1959) Occlusal disharmonies and their effect on periodontal diseases. *International Dental Journal* **9**, 367-381.

Prichard, J.F. (1965) *Advanced Periodontal Disease.* Philadelphia: W.B. Saunders.

Reitan, K. (1951) The initial tissue reaction incident to orthodontic tooth movement as related to the influence of function. *Acta Odontologica Scandinavica* **10**, Supplement 6.

Stillman, P.R. (1917) The management of pyorrhea. *Dental Cosmos* **59**, 405.

Stones, H.H. (1938) An experimental investigation into the association of traumatic occlusion with periodontal disease. *Proceedings of the Royal Society of Medicine* **31**, 479-495.

Steiner, G.G., Pearson, J.K. & Ainamo, J. (1981) Changes of the marginal periodontium as a result of labial tooth movement in monkeys. *Journal of Periodontology* **56**, 314-320.

Svanberg, G. & Lindhe, J. (1973) Experimental tooth hypermobility in the dog. A methodological study. *Odontologisk Revy* **24**, 269-282.

Waerhaug, J. (1979) The infrabony pocket and its relationship to trauma from occlusion and subgingival plaque. *Journal of Periodontology* **50**, 355-365.

Waerhaug, J. & Hansen, E.R. (1966) Periodontal changes incident to prolonged occlusal overload in monkeys. *Acta Odontologica Scandinavica* **24**, 91-105.

Wennström, J., Lindhe, J., Sinclair, F. & Thilander, B. (1987) Some periodontal tissue resections to orthodontic tooth movement in monkeys. *Journal of Clinical Periodontology* **14**, 121-129.

Wentz, F.M., Jarabak, J. & Orban, B. (1958) Experimental occlusal trauma imitating cuspal interferences. *Journal of Periodontology* **29**, 117-127.

CHAPTER 9

Interrelationships between Periodontics and Endodontics

Clinical and radiographic symptoms of inflammatory disease in the periodontium such as periodontal pockets, suppuration from periodontal pockets, swelling of the marginal gingiva, fistulae, tenderness to tooth percussion, increased tooth mobility and angular bone defects may not exclusively be the result of plaque-associated periodontal disease. Such symptoms may also be the results of irritants present in the root canal system of the affected tooth.

The differential diagnosis between an endodontic lesion* and a periodontal lesion** is seldom difficult, since endodontic lesions most often induce symptoms from the apical periodontium, while symptoms of periodontal disease usually are confined to the marginal periodontium. However, the clinical symptoms may sometimes be confusing and their etiology misinterpreted. What may appear as a marginal lesion may actually be a pulpal problem and *vice versa*. The establishment of a correct diagnosis may also be complicated by the fact that both marginal and endodontic lesions can simultaneously affect the same tooth. In such a situation, one of the lesions may either be the result of, or the cause of, the other, or the two lesions may constitute two separate processes, which have developed independently.

Proper diagnosis of the various disorders affecting the pulpal and periodontal tissues is important to establish in order to preclude un-

* The term *endodontic lesion* is used to denote an inflammatory process in the periodontal tissues resulting from noxious agents present in the root canal system of the tooth, usually a root canal infection.

** The term *periodontal lesion* is used to denote an inflammatory process in the periodontal tissues resulting from dental plaque accumulation on the external tooth surfaces.

necessary and even detrimental treatment. The clinician should, therefore, be well acquainted with the mechanisms involved in disease development in these tissues as well as with available diagnostic measures.

The purpose of this chapter is to describe possible interrelationships between disease processes in the dental pulp and in the periodontium. Emphasis will be placed upon diagnosis and treatment. Since, in addition, endodontic treatment measures may induce alterations in the periodontium, and periodontal treatment measures may provoke alterations in the pulp, such complications will also be addressed.

Influence of pathologic conditions in the pulp on the periodontium

Vital pulp - pulpitis

Inflammatory alterations in the vital pulp seldom cause lesions in the periodontal tissues that can be detected by clinical means. In other words, rarely will the inflamed pulp produce sufficient amounts of irritants to sustain distinct inflammatory lesions in the adjacent periodontium. Teeth with pulpitis may occasionally be associated with radiographic signs of inflammation, i.e. disruption of the apical lamina dura with widening of periodontal ligament space or a minor periapical radiolucency. In such cases, clinical symptoms of spontaneous pain, thermal sensitivity or tenderness to percussion may or may not be present. Hence, it is important to understand that as long as the pulp is vital, although inflamed, it is not likely that pronounced destruction of the periodontal tissues is caused by this condition.

Nonvital pulp - necrosis

Asymptomatic apical periodontitis (periapical lesion)

Involvement of the periodontal tissue is frequently a result of bacterial infection of a necrotic pulp. In the necrotic pulp microorganisms originating from the oral microbiota find conditions which favor their growth. Bacteria may grow in necrotic debris and exudates as well as on the root canal walls (Nair 1987). Root canal bacteria frequently enter the dentinal tubules. Only occasionally will they overcome the host defense and invade the periodontal tissue (Sundqvist & Reuterving 1980, Nair & Schroeder 1984, Byström et al. 1987, Haapasalo et al. 1987, Tronstad et al. 1987).

The microbiota in infected necrotic pulps has many features in common with the microbiota which is associated with periodontal disease (see Chapter 4). However, the endodontic microflora is not as complex as the microbiota in periodontitis and it is usually composed of a limited number of bacterial species. The majority of microorganisms found in necrotic pulp tissue are anaerobes. *Bacteroides, Fusobacterium, Peptostreptococcus, Eubacterium* and *Arachnia* belong to genera that are most frequently isolated (Sundqvist 1976). Also spirochetes and a variety of motile organisms reside in infected root canals (Thilo et al. 1986).

Upon growth and disintegration in the root canal, bacteria will release various substances (enzymes, metabolites, antigens, etc.) that will emerge into the periodontium through canals and foramina that connect the pulp chamber with the periodontal ligament. Once in the periodontium, the bacterial products will induce inflammatory alterations resulting in destruction of periodontal tissue fibers and adjacent alveolar bone (Fig. 9-1). Apical root resorption may occur. Most frequently, inflammatory lesions will develop around the apex of the tooth (Fig. 9-1).

The extension of the periodontal tissue de-

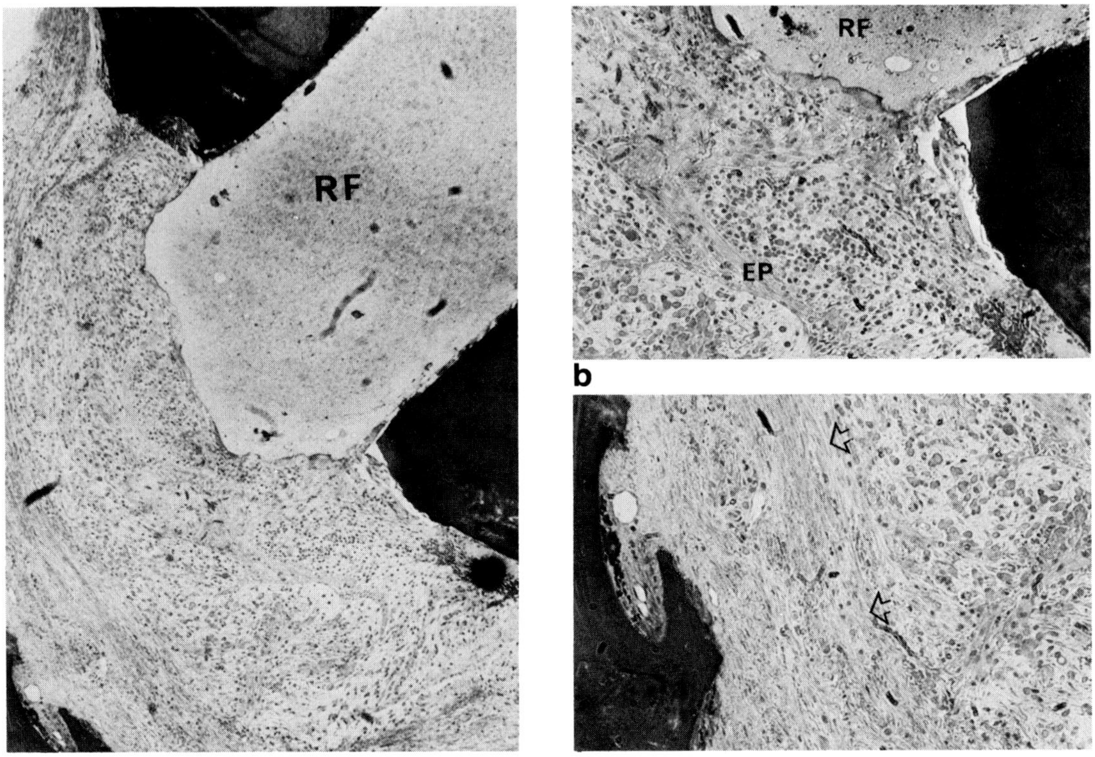

a b c

Fig. 9-1. Light-microscopic demonstration of a small inflammatory lesion associated with a root-filled tooth (a). Close to the root-filling (RF); numbers of plasma cells and lymphocytes have infiltrated the connective tissue. Epithelium (EP) has proliferated through the lesion (b). In peripheral parts only few inflammatory cells are seen and collagen-rich connective tissue (arrows) adjacent to bone tissue circumscribes the lesion (c). (From Bergenholtz et al. 1983).

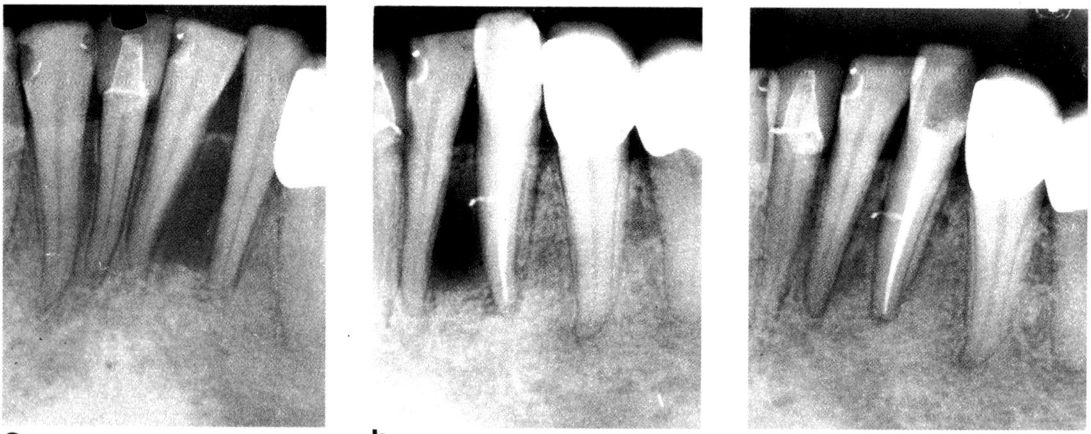

a b c

Fig. 9-2. Destruction of alveolar bone is observed between the roots of 31 and 32 (a). Vitality test indicated that 32 was non-vital. Endodontic treatment was performed (b). On condensing gutta percha into the canal, an accessory canal communicating with the bone defect was filled. Recall 2 years after treatment (c) demonstrated an obvious reduction of the bone lesion. (Courtesy of Dr. Conrad Jacobsson).

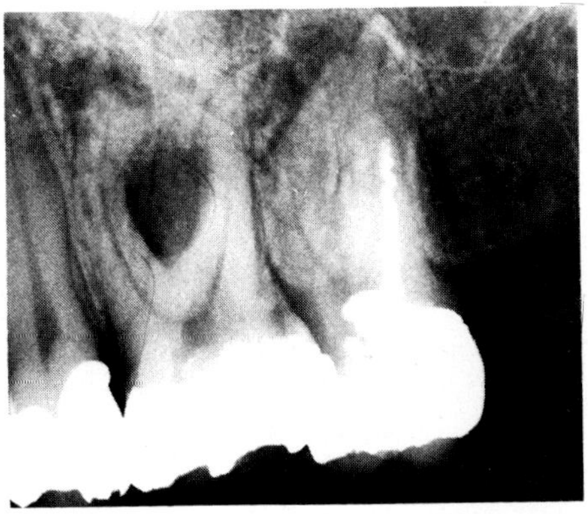

a

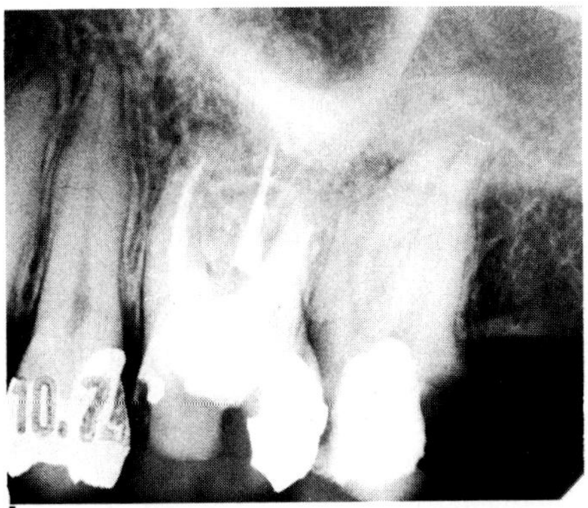

b

Fig. 9-3. Loss of interradicular bone of an upper molar simulating a periodontal lesion (a). The process, however, had no marginal genesis as indicated by the following findings: (1) periodontal probing failed to identify a periodontal pocket, (2) the pulp was nonvital, (3) endodontic treatment resulted in complete resolution of the lesion (b). (Courtesy of Dr. Björn Ödesjö).

struction which develops as a result of root canal infection is largely dependent on the quality and quantity of the bacteria present in the root canal and the capacity of the host defense to confine and neutralize the bacterial products released into the periodontium. If a balanced host-parasite relationship is established the inflammatory process may remain unchanged in size for years. Cyst transformation of the lesion may occasionally occur and result in extensive destruction of the alveolar bone.

Histopathologically, the periapical inflammatory lesion is characterized by a richly vascularized, granulation tissue which, to a varying degree, is infiltrated by inflammatory cells (Fig. 9-1). The inflammatory cell composition of these lesions may vary, probably depending on the intensity and nature of the bacterial irritants affecting the periodontal tissues. Neutrophilic granulocytes may be present in large numbers close to apical foramina, while more peripheral portions of the lesion contain increasing numbers of plasma cells, macrophages, lymphocytes and fibroblasts (Yanagisawa 1980, Bergenholtz et al. 1983, Stern et al. 1981, Nielsen et al. 1984).

Lateral lesion

Inflammatory processes in the periodontium occurring as a result of root canal infection may not only be localized at the tooth apex but may also appear along the lateral aspects of the root (Fig. 9-2) and in furcation areas of 2- and 3-rooted teeth (Fig. 9-3). In such cases the inflammatory process may be induced and maintained by bacterial products which reach the periodontium through accessory canals.

Accessory canals normally harbor vessels which connect the circulatory system of the pulp with that of the periodontal ligament. Such anastomoses are formed during the early phases of tooth development. During the completion of root formation several anastomoses become blocked and reduced in width by continuous deposition of dentin and root cementum. However, patent communications of varying size, number and location in the root, between the pulp and the periodontal ligament, may remain in the adult dentition. Accessory canals can be observed in all groups of teeth. The majority are found in the apical portion of the root. In the middle and cervical portions the prevalence is small. In a study of 1140 extracted teeth from adult human subjects, DeDeus (1975) reported a prevalence of accessory root canals of 27%. The canals were distributed

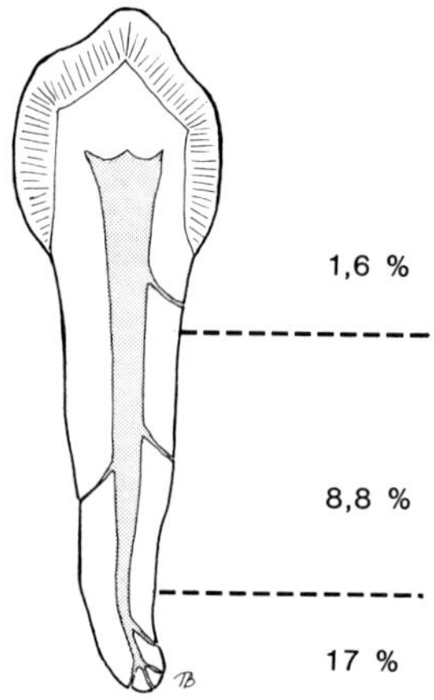

Fig. 9-4. Frequency of accessory canals at different levels of the root. The data are average values obtained from De-Deus (1975). Observations were made after the teeth had been rendered transparent and the root-canal system filled with China ink. The figures for the vertical portion of the root include those of the bi-and trifurcations.

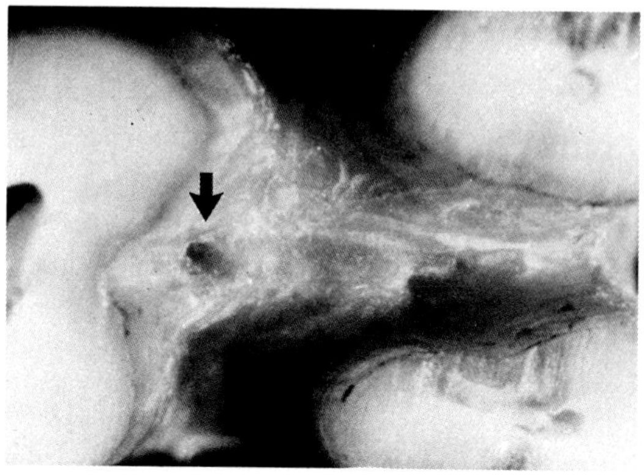

Fig. 9-5. Photograph of the furcation area of an extracted maxillary molar with cut roots demonstrating the opening of an accessory canal (arrow). Scanning electron microscopic observations indicate that the frequency of such furcation foramina is great (Burch & Hulen 1974, Koenigs et al. 1974), whereas the number of openings at the pulpal floor is small (Perlich et al. 1981). This suggests that furcation foramina at the external surface of the root do not necessarily represent patency to the pulpal chamber. (Courtesy of Dr. Robert C. Bowers).

at various levels of the root as depicted in Fig. 9-4.

The frequency of accessory canals in the furcation area of 2- and 3-rooted teeth has been determined in numerous studies of extracted human teeth (Fig. 9-5). A variety of techniques have been used, which may explain the divergent results obtained. Some studies report furcation canals in between 20% and 60% of examined teeth (Lowman et al. 1973, Vertucci & Williams 1974, Gutmann 1978), whereas others have failed to demonstrate the presence of such canals at furcation sites (Pineda & Kuttler 1972, Hession 1977).

Clinically, it is seldom possible to identify accessory canals unless they have been filled with a contrasting root-filling material following endodontic therapy (Fig. 9-2b). A lateral position of a radiolucency associated with a pulpless tooth may also indicate the possibility of the presence of an accessory canal (Fig. 9-2a).

The clinical significance of accessory canals in spreading infectious products from necrotic pulp to the periodontium is not clear, and no scientific documentation is yet available concerning the prevalence of endodontically derived lesions in the marginal periodontium. Clinical observations demonstrate that such lesions may occur (Fig. 9-2), but the rate of occurrence is low.

No evidence has yet been presented indicating that infectious products from a necrotic pulp can affect the periodontal tissues through normal walls of dentin and cementum. Even if the width of the dentinal tubules is large enough for the passage of both bacteria and bacterial products, an intact layer of cementum evidently acts as an effective barrier against such a penetration occurring into the periodontal structures. Armitage et al. (1983) reported on the presence of structural changes in the cementum of teeth with necrotic pulps containing massive numbers of root canal bacteria. The significance of this finding is not yet understood.

Symptomatic apical periodontitis

Inflammatory lesions in the periodontal tissues,

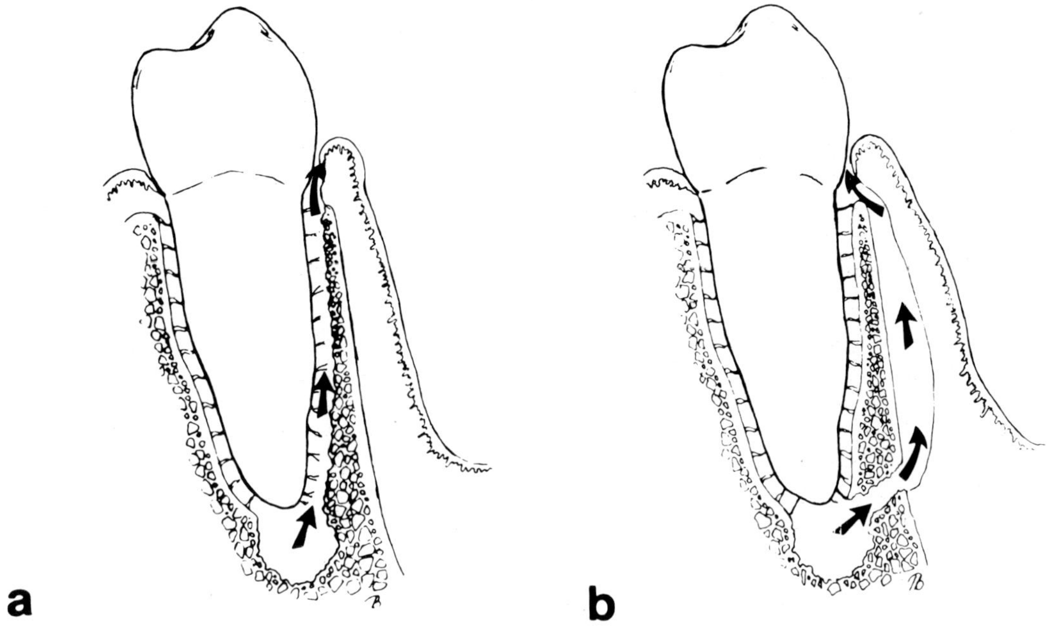

Fig. 9-6. Schematic illustration of drainage of a periapical abscess into the gingival sulcus/pocket. a = periodontal ligament fistulation. b = extraosseous fistulation.

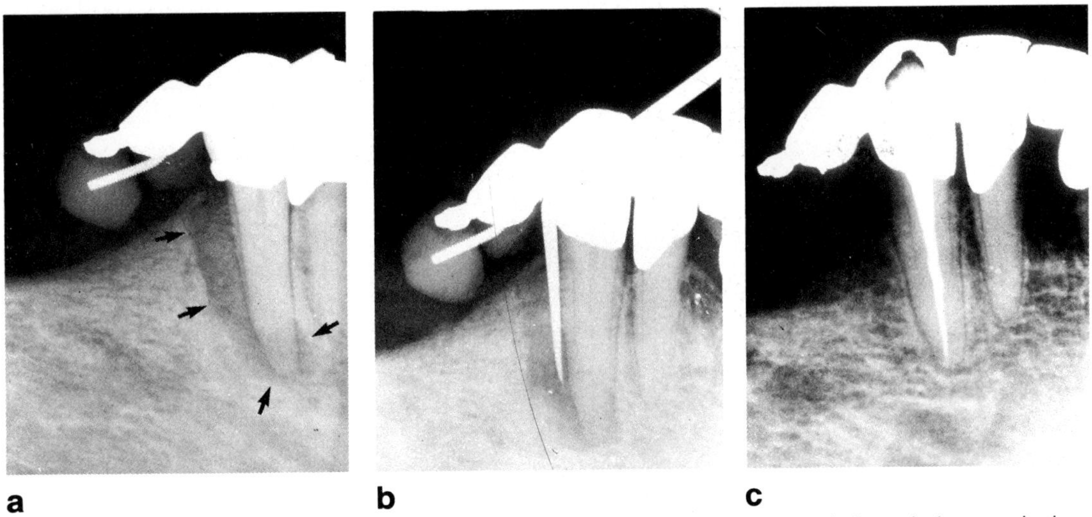

Fig. 9-7. Angular bone defect is observed along the distal root surface of a lower canine (a). Apical-marginal communication was confirmed by periodontal probing (b). Endodontic treatment resulted in complete reestablishment of the periodontal structures demonstrating that the periodontal defect in this case was the result of endodontic infection only. (Courtesy of Dr. Ralph Milthon).

induced and maintained by root canal infection, often have a limited extension around the apex of the tooth or at the orifice of a lateral canal. Following exacerbation and abscess formation, rapid and extensive destruction of the supporting tissues can occur.

Abscesses derived from a periapical lesion drain in different directions, of which drainage

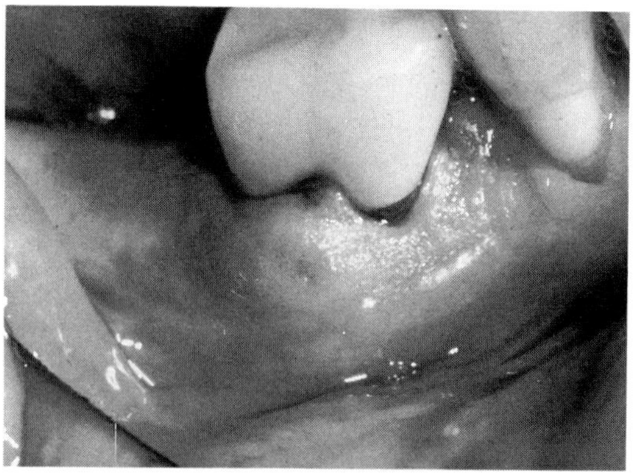

Fig. 9-8a.

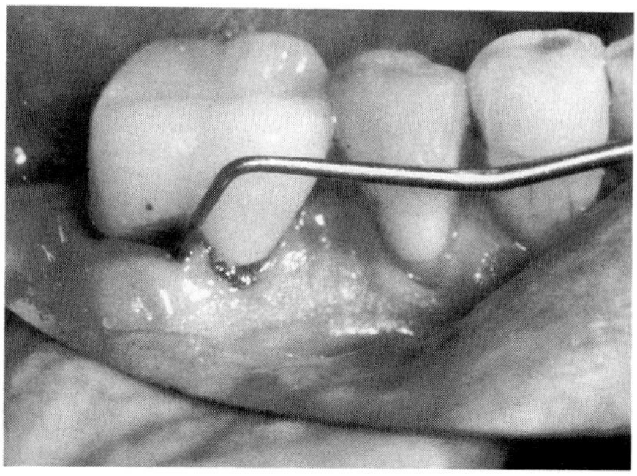

Fig. 9-8b.

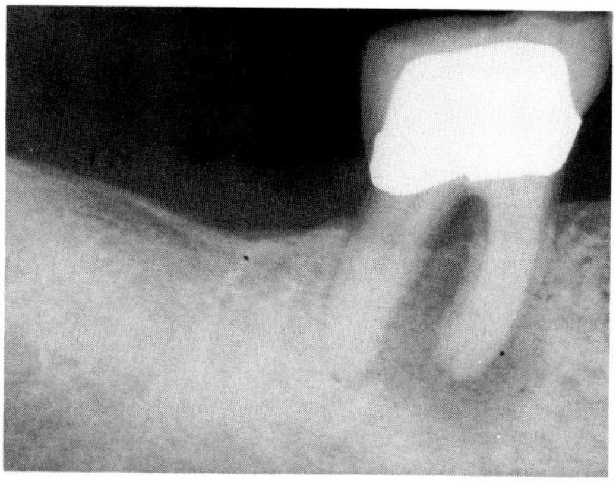

Fig. 9-8c.

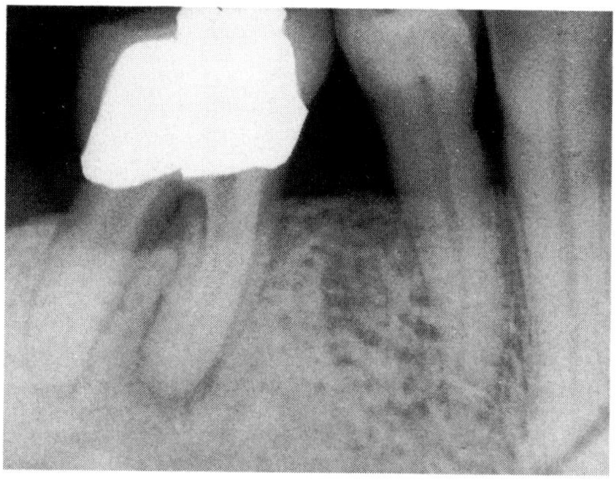

Fig. 9-8d.

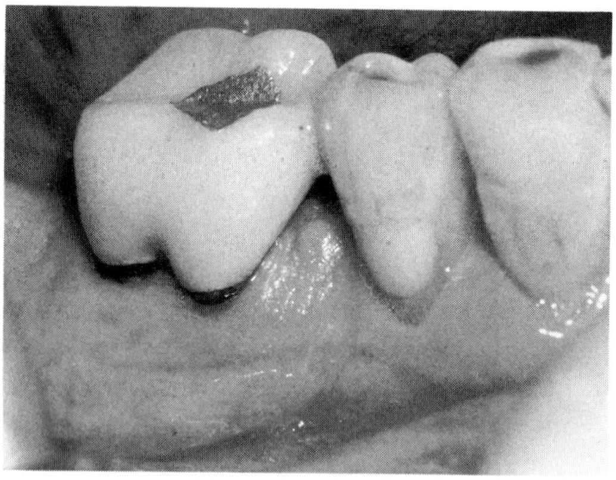

Fig. 9-8e.

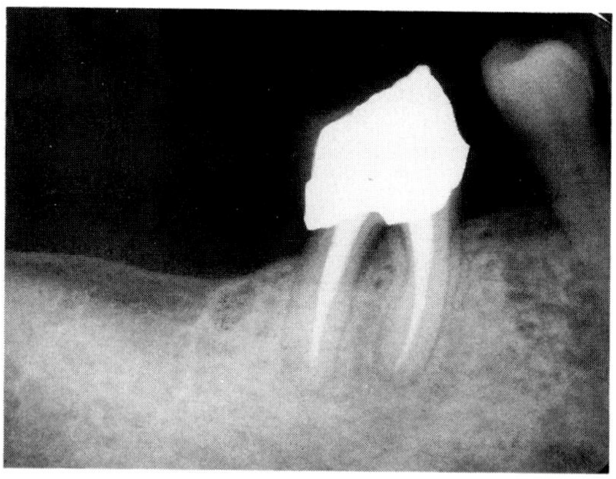

Fig. 9-8f.

Fig. 9-8. Facial swelling associated with tooth 46 as a result of symptomatic apical periodontitis (a). Patient had experienced pain and tenderness in the area for one week. Periodontal probing disclosed a deep facial pocket along the mesial root (b). Radiographically, the lesion circumscribed the mesial root with marginal extension in the furcation (c). It was not possible to determine the condition of the pulp by conventional pulp-vitality tests. Test cavity preparation revealed a necrotic pulp that was endodontically treated, including intracanal dressing with calciumhydroxide. Obvious reduction in lesion size is observed 3 months after treatment (d). Gingival lesion resolved leaving no abnormal probing depth (e). Endodontic treatment was completed by obturation of the root canals with gutta-percha. Twelve months after root filling complete resolution of the bone defect has occurred (f). Diagnosis and treatment of this case was carried out in collaboration with Dr. David Simpson.

into the gingival sulcus/pocket is of particular interest with respect to its effect on the periodontal tissues. The process may or may not be associated with clinical signs of acute inflammation including throbbing pain, tenderness to pressure and percussion, increased tooth mobility, and swelling of the marginal gingiva. These symptoms also are typical of periodontal abscesses (see Fig. 9-20).

In general, drainage of periapical abscesses into the sulcus/pocket follows 1 of 2 routes (Fig. 9-6):

1. The suppurative lesion may produce a sinus tract along the periodontal ligament space (periodontal ligament fistulation; Fig. 9-6a). This usually results in only a narrow opening of the fistula into the gingival sulcus/pocket. *Such a fistula can readily be probed down to the apex of the tooth* (Fig. 9-7), *where no increased probing depth otherwise exists around the tooth.* In multi-rooted teeth a periodontal ligament fistulation can drain in the furcation area. The resulting lesion often resembles a "through and through" furcation defect from a periodontal lesion (Fig. 9-8).
2. A periapical abscess can also perforate the cortical bone close to the apex, elevating the soft tissue including the periosteum from the bone surface, and drain into the gingival sulcus/pocket (Fig. 9-6b). This type of drainage will result in a wide opening of the fistula into the sulcus/pocket (extraosseous fistulation), and is most often seen at the buccal aspect of the tooth. Since this type of fistula is not associated with loss of bone tissue at the inner walls of the alveolus, a periodontal probe cannot penetrate into the periodontal ligament space.

It is essential to be aware that both types of lesions described are strictly of endodontic origin. Therefore, following proper endodontic treatment, both types of fistulae can be expected to heal rapidly without a persistent periodontal defect (Figs. 9-7, 9-8, 9-9); there is generally no need for adjunctive periodontal therapy. The endodontic treatment of the involved tooth should be performed without delay to prevent repeated exacerbations and the establishment of a permanent apical-marginal communication. If a periodontal ligament fistulation passes undetected or is left untreated, the potential exists for downgrowth of plaque and epithelium along the involved root surface. In this situation endodontic treatment might have less chance of success and will possibly have to be supplemented with adjunctive periodontal treatment.

a

b

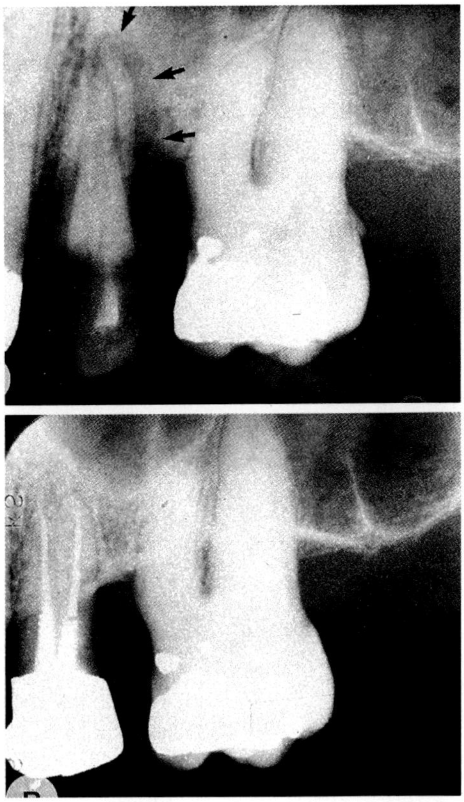

Fig. 9-9. Radiolucent area along the distal root surface of tooth 25 combined with a horizontal marginal-bone destruction (a). The tooth pulp was nonvital. Six months after endodontic treatment normal periodontal structures had reformed in the previous area of angular bone destruction. (Courtesy of Dr. Conrad Jacobsson).

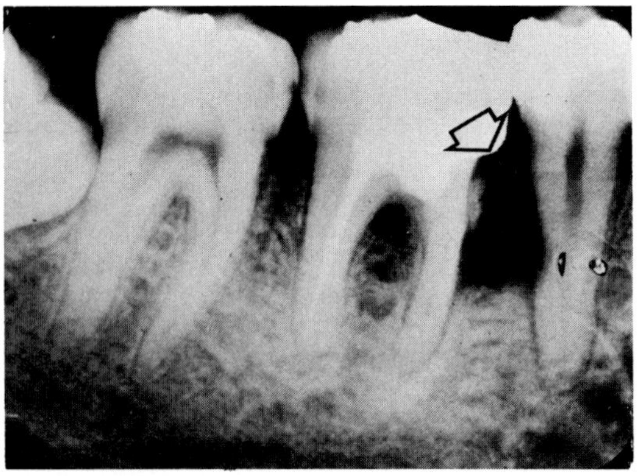

Fig. 9-10. Destruction of alveolar bone between tooth 45 and tooth 46 as a result of leakage of paraformaldehyde applied in order to devitalize the pulp of tooth 46. A bone sequestrum has formed (arrow).

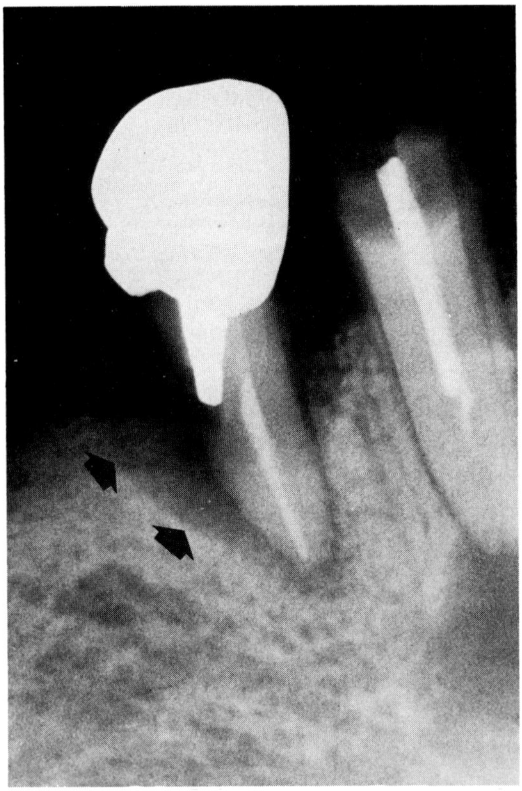

Fig. 9-11. Angular bone defect at the distal root surface of a mandibular premolar (arrows). The root is perforated. Conceivably, this occurred in conjunction with preparation of the root canal for insertion of the dowel. Clinical symptoms involved drainage of pus from the pocket and increased tooth mobility. The tooth was extracted.

Influence of endodontic treatment measures on the periodontium

When the beakdown of the periodontal tissues is associated with a root-filled tooth, endodontic etiology should be considered, particularly if the root filling is defective. Infectious products may leak through apical or accessory canals to the periodontium from unfilled spaces in the root canal. In addition, periodontal lesions may be caused by infectious products released from sites of root perforations or root fractures. Periodontal inflammatory lesions may also result from mechanical as well as chemical irritation initiated in conjunction with root canal preparation in endodontic therapy. Medication for canal irrigation and disinfection and materials for obturation used in modern endodontics, however, are comparatively well tolerated by the connective tissue of the periodontium, even if, during treatment, they are forced into the periodontal ligament. On the other hand, strong antiseptic drugs used for root canal disinfection and pulp devitalization can cause severe damage if they leak into the periodontium. (Fig. 9-10).

Root perforation

During endodontic treatment, and in conjunction with preparation of root canals for insertion of posts, instrumentation can accidentally cause perforation of the root and wounding of the periodontal ligament. Perforations can be made through the lateral walls of the root or through the pulpal floor in multirooted teeth. At the site of such perforations, an inflammatory reaction will develop in the periodontium. If the perforation is located close to the gingival margin, the developing lesion can result in the

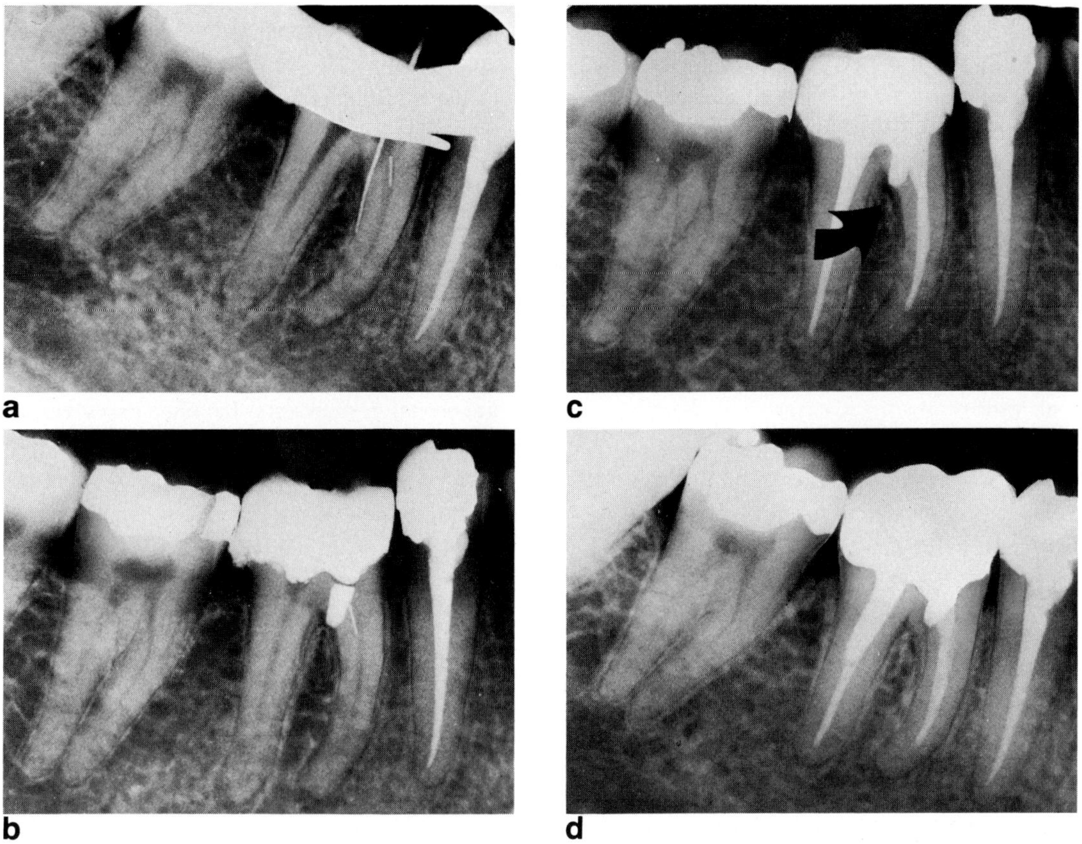

Fig. 9-12. In conjunction with search for root canal openings, perforation of the pulpal floor of the first mandibular molar occurred (a). The perforation was immediately obturated with gutta-percha (b). One month after treatment a slight radiolucency appeared at the perforation site on the periodontium (c). After an observation period of 2 years normal periodontal conditions had been reestablished both clinically and radiographically (d). (Courtesy of Dr. Gunnar Heden).

formation of a periodontal pocket. Other complications can involve exacerbation of a preexisting periodontal inflammatory lesion and development of clinical symptoms, similar to those of a periodontal abscess: acute pain, swelling, drainage of pus through the pocket, increased tooth mobility and further loss of fibrous attachment (Fig. 9-11).

Root perforations are identified by the occurrence of sudden pain and bleeding during preparation of root canals coronal to the working length. These symptoms, however, are not necessarily seen if the perforation is made in conjunction with pulpectomy performed under local anesthesia. In such cases the perforation may be detected during later treatment of the root canal by the presence of coagulated blood or granulation tissue which has proliferated into the root canal from the site of perforation. Elimination of such granulation tissue is frequently accompanied by bleeding which can be difficult to stop.

As soon as a root perforation has been detected, treatment should be initiated. Fig. 9-12 demonstrates the successful result of treatment of a perforation made in the furcation of a mandibular molar. Healing of lesions in the periodontium depends largely on whether bacterial infection can be excluded from the wound area by tight obturation of the perforation site (Beavers et al. 1986). For various reasons this may be difficult to accomplish. If the perforation is made at an oblique angle in the lateral wall of the root and if it has been produced by a reamer or a root canal file, the artificial canal has an oval-shaped orifice into the periodontium. Obturation of such perforations with gutta percha can result in a defective seal and subsequent bacterial irritation of the periodontal tissues. Because of the internal sealing difficulties of lateral preforations, healing is unpredictable. Therefore, a questionable prognosis of such treatments should be anticipated (Petersson et al. 1986).

The use of calcium hydroxide has been suggested for the treatment of root perforations, since this chemical promotes the healing of wounds in the dental pulp with the formation of new hard tissue adjacent to the capping material. Experiments in monkeys (Beavers et al. 1986) have demonstrated that healing of perforations into the periodontium also can occur following sealing with a hard-setting calcium hydroxide compound. However, healing was not characterized by the closure of the perforation with new hard tissue but with a layer of uninflamed connective tissue and alveolar bone which formed adjacent to the medicament.

If a perforation is located in the cervical part of the root, a surgical approach may be attempted. After elevating a flap and exposure of the perforation site, amalgam may be used to obturate the defect.

Vertical root fracture

Clinical symptoms typical of endodontic and periodontal lesions may also be detected at teeth with vertical root fractures. A vertical root fracture is defined as a fracture of the root that is longitudinally oriented at a more or less oblique angle towards the long axis of the tooth. It can traverse the root in different directions mesially/distally or facially/lingually and may or may not involve the pulpal chamber. A vertical root fracture can extend the entire length of a root and involve the gingival sulcus/pocket area but may also be incomplete and confined to the alveolus area. Furthermore, it should be noted that vertical root fractures usually involve both sides of the root. Occasionally, only one side can be involved.

The etiology and prevalence of vertical root fractures is not well established. In some situations the cause of the fracture may be iatrogenic from pin and post placements, root canal obturation procedures, and seating of intracoronal restorations. In other cases vertical root fractures seem to occur spontaneously without any obvious reason. Since vertical root fractures more often are associated with root-filled teeth than teeth with vital pulps, the assumption has been made that root-filled teeth, with time, become more brittle and less resistant to mastication forces. This hypothesis appears to be supported by observations that root fractures are often detected several years after the completion of endodontic treatment and final restoration of the tooth. In a study comprising 32 root fractures, the average time between the completion of the endodontic treatment and the detection of root fracture was 3.25 years with a range varying between 3 days and 14 years (Meister et al. 1980).

Clinical symptoms associated with vertical root fractures often show a varying character. In some situations, the symptoms are pronounced and include pain, tenderness and abscess formation - symptoms similar to those of a periodontal abscess or symptomatic apical periodontitis. In other instances, a narrow, local deepening of a periodontal pocket associated with the fracture is the only clinical finding. Other clinical symptoms occurring in conjunction with root fractures are tenderness to mastication, fistulous tract, mild pain and dull discomfort.

The diagnosis of a vertical root fracture is often difficult to make because the fracture is usually not readily detectable by clinical inspection and radiographic examination unless

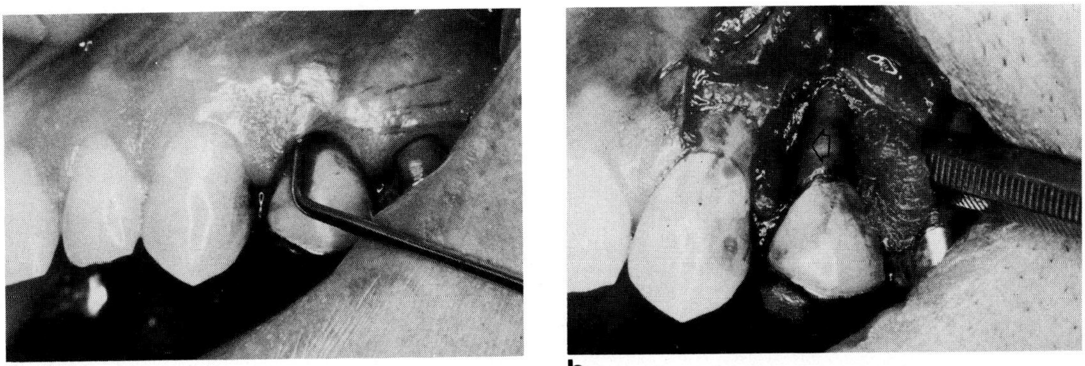

a b

Fig. 9-13. Clinical photographs of a maxillary premolar with a longitudinal root fracture. A deep periodontal pocket was probed at the buccal aspect of the tooth (a). No other clinical symptoms were present. The elevation of a mucoperiosteal flap (b) revealed extensive loss of marginal bone at the buccal aspect of the root and a thin root fracture (arrow). (Courtesy of Dr. Claes Reit).

there is a clear separation of the root fragments. It has been demonstrated that only when the central x-ray beam catches the fracture plane is there a chance of radiographic detection of the fracture line (Rud & Omnell 1970). The suspicion of a vertical root fracture is often inferred from clinical symptoms that cannot readily be explained by either an endodontic or periodontal lesion.

A number of diagnostic procedures can be undertaken to confirm the diagnosis. Application of iodine tincture onto the crown and the root surface can sometimes be helpful. The iodine will enter the fracture space, which will show up as a dark line against the surrounding tooth substance. Indirect illumination of the root using fiberoptic light can also be a valuable diagnostic aid. The fiberoptic probe should be placed at various positions on the crown or the root, whereby the fracture line may clearly present itself. In premolars and molars the diagnosis may be supported from observation of varying pain sensations elicited by loading facial and lingual cusps. This can be done by asking the patient to bite down on a Burlew wheel or a wooden stick wrapped with cotton. Often the diagnosis of a vertical fracture has to be confirmed by a surgical exposure of the root that allows direct visual examination (Walton et al. 1983; Fig. 9-13).

As a result of bacterial growth in the fracture space, the adjacent periodontal ligament will become the seat of an inflammatory lesion causing breakdown of connective tissue fibers and alveolar bone. This breakdown can manifest itself radiographically in a number of different ways. The radiographic defect may be similar to those found at endodontic and periodontal lesions (Fig. 9-14). In other situations the appearance may be atypical of these disorders. A diffuse widening of the periodontal ligament space along both or one of the lateral root surfaces may indicate the presence of a root fracture. A thin halo-like apical radiolucency is another example of a radiographic lesion suggestive of a vertical root fracture (Pitts & Natkin 1983).

Vertical root fractures that involve the gingival/sulcus area usually have a hopeless prognosis due to continuous bacterial invasion of the fracture space from the oral environment. A single-rooted tooth will have to be extracted. In a multirooted tooth hemisection and extraction of the fractured root may be considered as a treatment alternative.

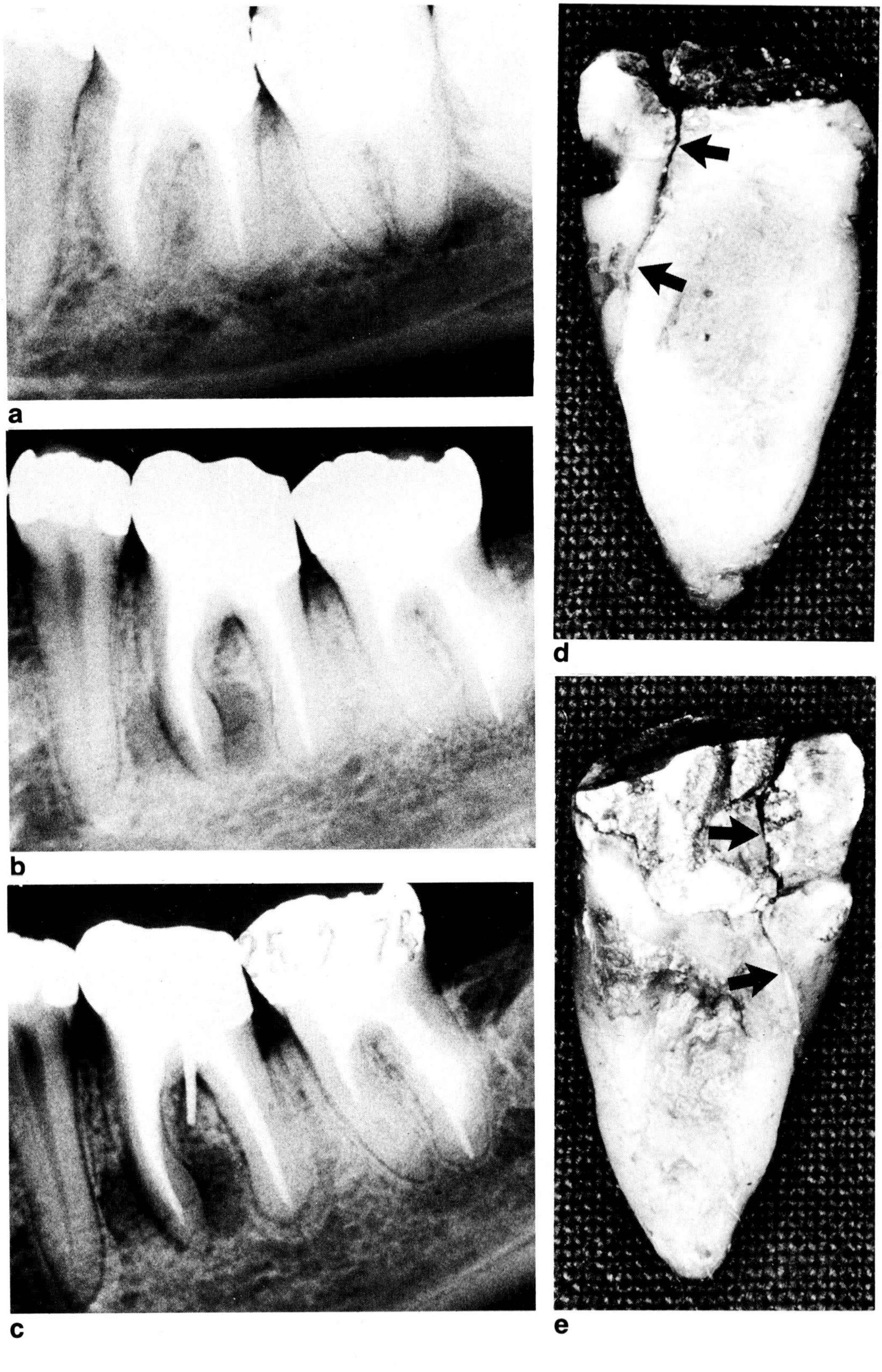
a
b
c
d
e

Influence of periodontal disease on the condition of the pulp

The progressive breakdown of the attachment apparatus in periodontal disease and the formation of bacterial plaque on the detached root surfaces can occasionally induce pathologic changes in the pulp tissue. Bacterial products and substances released by the inflammatory process in the periodontium may gain access to the pulp via exposed accessory canals, apical and furcal foramina, and dentinal tubules in a way similar to spread of infectious products in the opposite direction from necrotic pulp to periodontal tissue.

Inflammatory alterations as well as localized necrosis of pulp tissue have been reported adjacent to accessory canals exposed by periodontal disease (Seltzer et al. 1963, Rubach & Mitchell 1965). Severe breakdown of pulp, however, presumably does not occur until the periodontal disease process has reached a terminal state, i.e. when bacterial plaque involves the main apical foramina (Langeland et al. 1974). This observation demonstrates that the pulp has a good capacity for defense against the injurious elements released by plaque bacteria and the lesion in the periodontium as long as the blood supply through the apical foramen is intact.

A clear-cut relationship between progressive periodontal disease and pulpal involvement does not invariably exist (Mazur & Massler 1964, Czarnecki & Schilder 1979). In an experiment in monkeys, Bergenholtz & Lindhe (1978) studied the nature and frequency of tissue changes in the pulp of teeth with moderate breakdown of the attachment apparatus. The majority of the roots examined (70%) exhibited no pathologic tissue changes in the pulp, despite the fact that approximately 30-40% of the periodontal attachment was lost. The remaining roots (30%) displayed small inflammatory cell infiltrates and/or formations of irregular secondary dentin in an area of the pulp subjacent to root areas exposed through periodontal tissue destruction. These tissue changes in pulp were frequently associated with root surface resorption (Fig. 9-15), suggesting that the irritation of the pulp had been transmitted through exposed dentinal tubules. This observation further suggests that the presence of an intact cementum layer may be important to the protection of pulp from injurious elements produced by the plaque microbiota.

In the study by Bergenholtz & Lindhe (1978), destructive periodontal disease was produced experimentally during a comparatively short period (5-7 months), while in humans a similar degree of destruction of the periodontal tissues normally requires several years. It has been reported that the pulp of teeth with longstanding periodontal disease can develop changes such as fibrosis and dystrophic calcifi-

Fig. 9-14. A typical case of root fracture. The first mandibular molar had been asymptomatic for 15 years after completion of endodontic treatment. Fig. 9-14a shows normal periapical conditions in a radiograph taken 2 years after treatment. For a month the patient had slight pain and a tenderness on mastication that could not be relieved by occlusal adjustment. Radiographic examination (b) revealed an apical bone destruction adjacent to the mesial root. Within a narrow zone at the lingual aspect of the tooth, a deep periodontal pocket (10 mm) could be probed. A gutta-percha point inserted into the pocket indicated marginal communication with the apical lesion (c). Clinical examination could not confirm the presence of a fracture. However, the findings that clinical and radiographic symptoms suddenly developed 15 years after therapy, and that a localized narrow pocket was found at a single tooth in a dentition otherwise free from periodontal disease, strongly suggested the presence of a root fracture. The tooth was extracted and the diagnosis confirmed. Fig. 9-14d shows the fracture line at the mesial aspect of the root and Fig. 9-14e at the distal aspect.

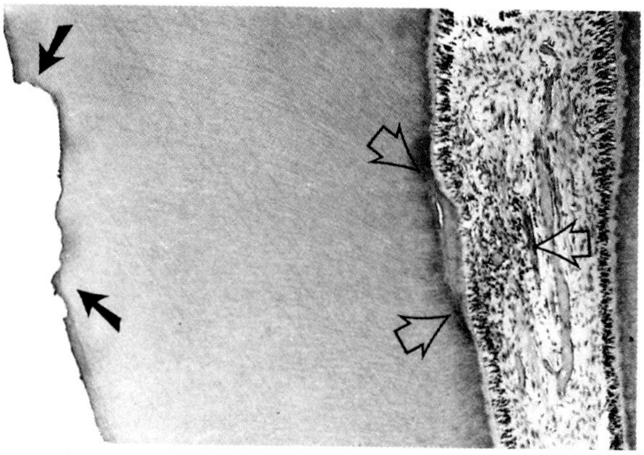

Fig. 9-15. Histologic section of a monkey tooth exposed to experimental periodontal tissue breakdown. Beneath resorptive defects in the external root surface a slight infiltrate of inflammatory cells and a small rim of irregular secondary dentin are observed in the pulp. (From Bergenholtz & Lindhe 1978).

cations (Bender & Seltzer 1972; Fig. 9-16). The number of blood vessels and nerve fibers can also be reduced. It seems reasonable that tissue changes of this nature represent the accumulated response of pulp to relatively weak, but repeatedly occurring, insults to the pulp tissue via accessory canals and dentinal tubules.

It is important to remember that periodontal disease rarely produces significant pathologic changes in the pulp. In teeth with moderate breakdown of the attachment apparatus, the pulp is usually vital and in proper function. The vitality of the pulp is usually not lost until the periodontal lesion has reached the apical foramen and impaired pulpal blood circulation.

Influence of periodontal treatment measures on the pulp

Scaling and root planing

Scaling and root planing not only remove bacterial deposits from the root surface but also

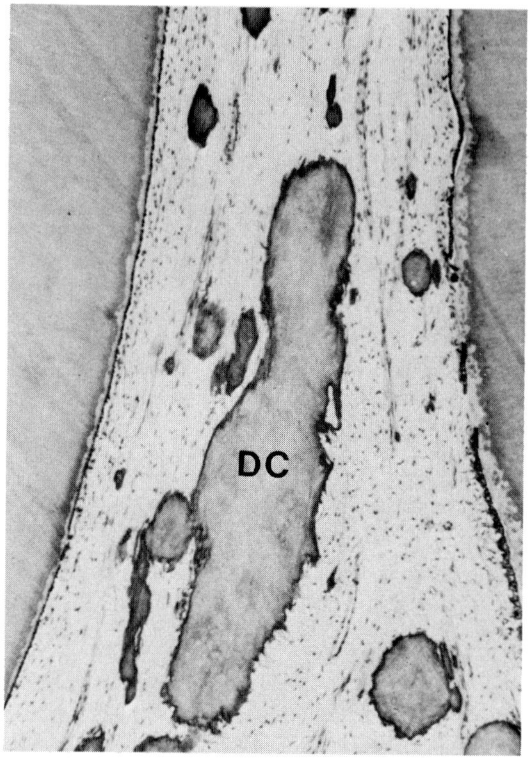

Fig. 9-16. Histological preparation of the palatal root of a first maxillary molar exposed to extensive periodontal breakdown, showing numerous dystrophic calcifications in the pulp (DC). The pulp tissue is noninflamed.

cementum and superficial parts of dentin. Therefore, by this instrumentation, dentinal tubules will be exposed to the oral environment. Subsequent microbial colonization of the exposed root dentin may result in bacterial invasion of the dentinal tubules (Adrians et al. 1985). As a consequence inflammatory lesions can be induced in the pulp (Bergenholtz & Lindhe 1978). The risk of bacterial penetration and pulpal injury is further enhanced by an injudicious use of citric acid for conditioning of root surfaces. A greater frequency and severity of adverse pulpal responses have been observed in citric acid-treated teeth following periodontal surgery than in teeth subjected to surgery alone (Ryan et al. 1984).

The vitality of pulp does not seem to be jeopardized by scaling procedures, even though

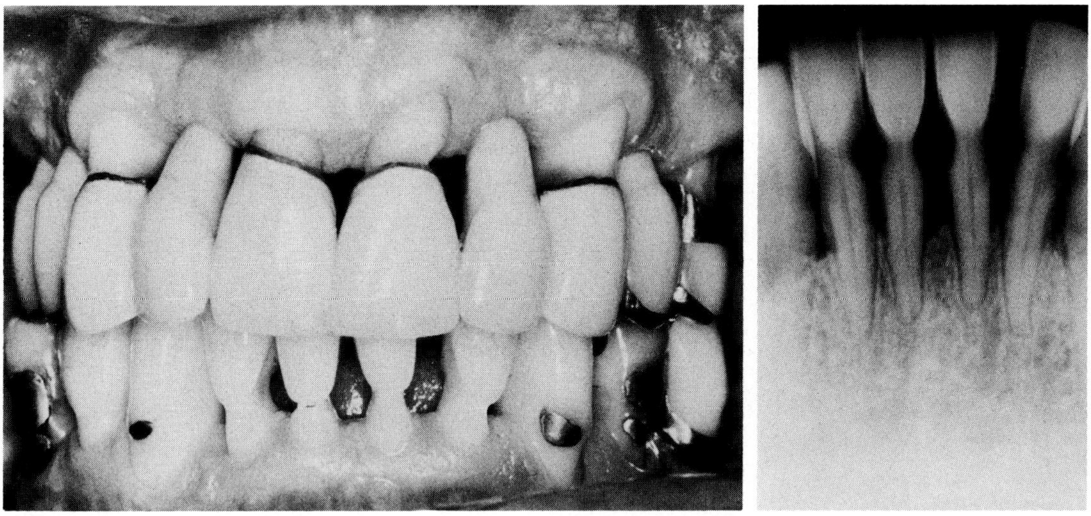

Fig. 9-17. Hourglass-shaped teeth in the mandibular front region resulting from improper use of interdental toothbrushes (a). The coronal portions of the pulp chamber are filled with hard tissue (b). One of the teeth (42) later had a crown fracture due to the weakening of tooth substance, but without clinical exposure of the pulp. (Courtesy of Dr. Sture Nyman).

clinical symptoms of pulpitis may follow such measures (see below). In studies in experimental animals (Bergenholtz & Lindhe 1978, Hattler & Listgarten 1983, Nilvéus & Selvig 1983) scaling and root planing did not result in severe pathological tissue changes in the pulp. In pulp tissue adjacent to scaled root surfaces, localized inflammatory alterations and irregular secondary dentin formation (reparative dentin) were observed in some teeth while other teeth displayed normal pulp tissue morphology even though dental plaque had been allowed to accumulate on the scaled root surfaces.

During the maintenance phase of periodontal therapy (see Chapter 13) scaling and planing of roots are frequently repeated procedures. At each recall session, the root surfaces are debrided and some dentin is removed. This therapy can result not only in weakening of the tooth but also in extensive irregular secondary dentin formation in the pulp (Fig. 9-17).

Root hypersensitivity

Following periodontal treatment, including scaling and root planing, patients not infrequently complain of increased sensitivity of the treated roots to thermal, osmotic, and mechanical stimuli. Usually, the symptoms develop and peak during the first week after treatment. In most cases the symptoms are transitory and will subside or disappear within a few weeks. Occasionally root hypersensitivity may become a serious problem which may persist for months and years. In such severe cases shorter or longer periods of lingering pain are often provoked. Even minimal contact between a toothbrush and the root dentin may result in intense pain - a condition not only uncomfortable but one likely to make proper oral hygiene measures difficult.

The etiology of root hypersensitivity and its underlying mechanisms are not well understood (Dowell & Addy 1983). Several hypotheses have been forwarded and are based on the fact that dentinal tubules remain open to the oral environment subsequent to treatment (Absi et al. 1987). It is well known that a variety of stimuli, including tactile, thermal and pharmacological, elicit pain sensations when applied on exposed dentin. The transmission of dentinal pain is best explained by the hydrodynamic theory (Brännström 1966). This theory implies that a sudden shift of the dentinal tubular content resulting from the insult will stimulate pulpal pain receptors. However, this theory cannot account for the increasing sensitivity that patients experience over time. In other words, movement of tubular content cannot be the only factor that explains why stimuli that normally cause a slight pain sensation, in hypersensitive teeth cause a much more severe pain response.

It is conceivable that the problem of root hypersensitivity involves alterations in pulpal sensory nerve activity (Kim 1986). The pain threshold levels of local sensory nerves can be affected by the release of inflammatory mediators (Närhi 1985). Keeping in mind that exposure of dentin may result in pulpal inflammation from permeation of bacterial components in saliva and in dental plaque (Bergenholtz & Lindhe 1975, 1978), root hypersensitivity may be mediated by the following three mechanisms: (1) patency of involved dentinal tubules, (2) localized pulpal inflammation, and (3) lowered pain threshold of pulpal nociceptors.

The role of patent dentinal tubules appears to be best established (Pashley 1986, Absi et al. 1987). It has been observed that exposed dentin which is nonsensitive to touch and thermal changes frequently shows surface occlusions of the dentinal tubules by mineralized material (Hiatt & Johansen 1972). The tubules are occluded only for a short distance (5-10 microns; Mendis & Darling 1979). The origin of the mineralized material is not known. The finding of tubular occlusion of dentin pieces worn by patients in partial dentures suggests precipitation of minerals originating from the oral fluids (Brännström & Garberoglio 1980).

The surface occlusion of dentinal tubules in exposed root dentin may be removed easily by repeated scaling. Experimental data also suggest that certain dietary factors, in particular wines, fruit juices and yogurt, can produce etching effects and maintain tubular patency (Addy et al. 1987).

In cases of severe root hypersensitivity, active treatment is urgent. However, remedy is not always possible with methods presently available. Most therapeutic methods proposed are designed to cause a surface occlusion of dentinal tubules by either an astringent or coagulating effect. Common methods involve:

1. *topical application of chemical substances* to the dentin surface; examples of such agents are strontium chloride, sodium monofluorophosphate, sodium fluoride, calcium hypophosphate, calcium hydroxide, potassium nitrate, potassium oxalate, formaldehyde, stannous fluoride etc.,
2. *electric deposition of chemical substances* with the use of iontophoresis,
3. *use of dentifrices containing "active substances"* (Sr Cl_2Na_2, PO_3F, SnF_2), and
4. *resin impregnation of exposed dentin.* Unfortunately none of these methods has been proven to result in a predictable therapeutic effect (Addy & Dowell 1983, McFall 1986).

Meticulous plaque control can lead to reduction of root hypersensitivity. It has been observed clinically that with time teeth in patients with proper oral-hygiene habits develop hard, smooth and insensitive root surfaces. Electron microscopic examination of the dentin of such root surfaces has revealed that the tubular openings are obliterated by mineral deposits (Hiatt & Johansen 1972).

When severe symptoms of root sensitivity have emerged it is difficult to motivate the patient to maintain a degree of plaque control necessary to allow for a natural occlusion of the dentinal tubules. In such situations an agent should be used which has a reasonable capacity to block the tubular openings, at least temporarily, so that proper oral-hygiene measures can be reinforced. Promising therapeutic techniques have been reported following treatment of hypersensitive root dentin with waterpastes of calcium hypophosphate (Hiatt & Johansen 1972) or calcium hydroxide (Levin et al. 1973, Green et al. 1977). When $Ca(OH)_2$ is used, it should be applied on the dentin surface for 5 min. During application the gingiva must be protected to avoid soft-tissue damage occurring as a result of the high alkalinity displayed by the compound. Immediate relief is often obtained by this treatment and a long-term effect has been demonstrated in controlled clinical studies (Levin et al. 1973, Green et al. 1977). The mode of action of this type of treatment is not clear. It has been assumed that the chemical agent denatures the organic contents of the tubules in the superficial part of the dentin, thus inducing the formation of a surface protein plug (Bergenholtz & Reit 1980). It is also possible that the compound during the application procedure is forced into the tubular openings and in this way creates a surface block. There is a need for further documentation regarding the efficacy and mode of action of this and other methods of treatment of dentin hypersensitivity.

As a part of the treatment, dietary advice should be given to patients who admit excessive consumption of citrus or apple fruits or any other food or drinks that are acid by nature. In severe cases, where no remedy is achieved with any advice or treatment, pulpectomy of the vital pulp tissue and root filling may be considered.

Endodontic considerations in root resection of multirooted teeth in periodontal therapy

Treatment of periodontally diseased, multirooted teeth may involve separation and extraction of one or two roots (see Chapters 13 and 20). As a rule, endodontic treatment of the root to be retained should be performed prior to surgery. Information will thus be gained regarding the effect of the endodontic measures before alternative roots are extracted. This rule should be followed for both vital and nonvital teeth. The root canals of molars are sometimes difficult to prepare, in particular when the tooth has been exposed to long-standing periodontal disease. As previously mentioned, such teeth can harbor both dystrophic calcifications and irregular secondary dentin formations that jeopardize proper endodontic treatment.

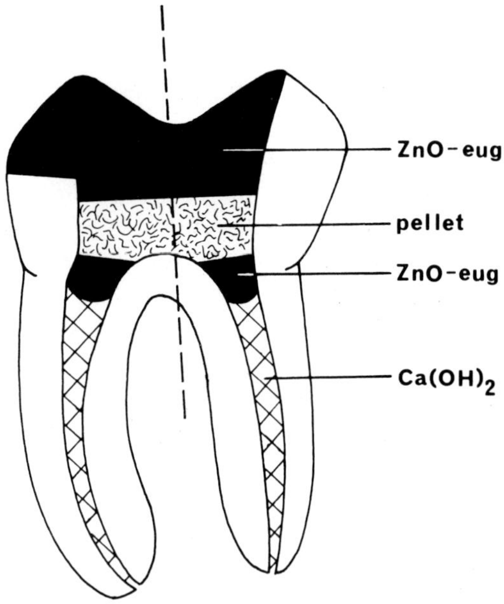

Fig. 9-18. Endodontic procedure prior to root resection. Root canals are filled with $Ca(OH)_2$ after canal preparation. The canal openings are sealed with zinc oxide-eugenol cement. A cotton pellet and temporary cement are placed for removal in conjunction with surgery to facilitate the separation procedure.

In multirooted teeth with advanced periodontal destruction it is not always possible to decide before surgery which root(s) can be preserved. As an alternative to permanent filling of all root canals in such teeth, pulpectomy can be performed and the canals temporarily filled with calcium hydroxide (see Fig. 9-18). Each of the canal openings is sealed with a zinc oxide eugenol cement. Root separation can then be performed without bacterial contamination of the root canals. Permanent root filling of the root(s) retained is performed after surgery.

Instead of endodontic treatment, capping of the pulp exposed by the root separation has been advocated (Haskell et al. 1980). Sufficient documentation of the long-term result of such treatment is lacking.

Differential diagnostic considerations

It is clear from the previous text that during treatment of periodontal disease one is not infrequently challenged with the dilemma of accurately assessing the contribution of an endodontic infection to deep periodontal pockets. In this chapter, several examples of lesions in the periodontium have been presented which are not associated with plaque accumulation on the root surfaces (see Figs. 9-7, 9-8, 9-9, 9-11, 9-12, 9-15). Two cases are presented below showing clinical and radiographic symptoms similar to those of symptomatic apical lesions, endodontic perforations or root fractures. The cases demonstrate that diagnostic entities such as location, form and extension of radiolucencies, clinical symptoms of pain or swelling, increased probing depths, etc., are not always effective diagnostic parameters for differentiating a periodontal lesion from an endodontic disorder.

The clinical photograph in Fig. 9-19a shows swelling of the marginal gingiva on the buccal aspect of tooth #11. This swelling had for a few days been preceded by severe throbbing pain. Radiographic examination (Fig. 9-19b) disclosed the presence of an angular bone defect that involved the apical portions of the tooth. In this case the pulp responded vital to testing, indicating that the pathologic condition was not of endodontic etiology. Pocket debridement

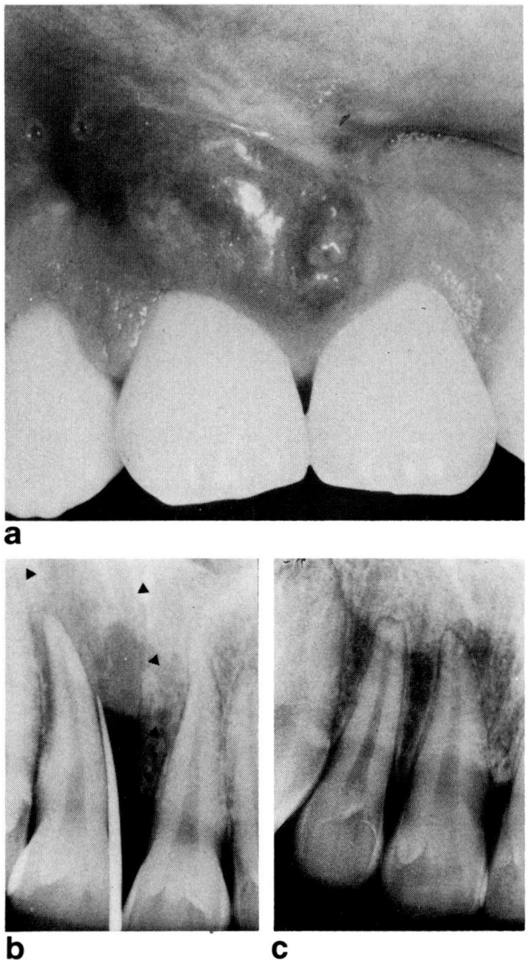

Fig. 9-19. Fig. 9-19a demonstrates a gingival swelling at the buccal aspect of tooth 11. Fig. 9-19b shows the radiographic appearance of the area. Note the advanced destruction of alveolar bone along the mesial aspect of the root (arrow heads). Fig. 9-19c shows healing of the area 7 months following periodontal treatment. (Courtesy of Dr. Harald Rylander).

was combined with irrigation with 0.2% chlorhexidine digluconate solution and systemic administration of antibiotics. The lesion healed rapidly. Seven months following treatment new bone had formed around the apex and along the mesial root surface (c). This case demonstrates that the periodontal destruction observed was caused by periodontal disease.

Fig. 9-20 illustrates another case of differential diagnostic interest. A radiograph taken of

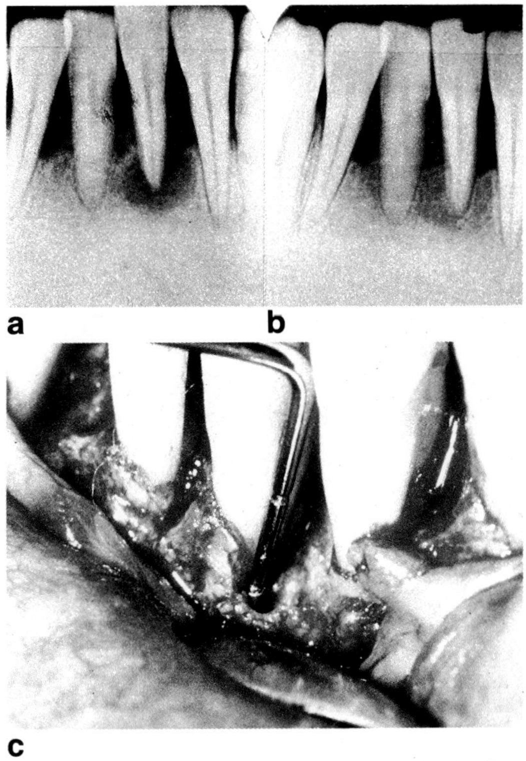

Fig. 9-20a. Demonstrates advanced destructions of alveolar bone including an angular bone defect simulating an endodontic periapical lesion around tooth 31. The pulp responded vital and the tooth was therefore periodontally treated with the use of a flap procedure (b). Fig. 9-20c (radiograph obtained 6 months after treatment) shows healing of the lesion. (Courtesy of Dr. Ingvar Magnusson).

the front tooth region of the mandibular jaw demonstrates bone loss around the apex of tooth #31 in addition to a generalized horizontal loss of alveolar bone (Fig. 9-20a). The form and the extension of the apical radiolucency around tooth 31 are similar to those resulting from an endodontic lesion. Clinically, a deep periodontal pocket could be probed along the distobuccal root surface. Vitality tests indicated that the tooth pulp was vital. Therefore, endodontic treatment was not performed. Following elevation of a mucoperiosteal flap, an angular bone defect was found at the buccal aspect of the root but without involving the apex. The wound area was debrided and the root surface infection was eliminated by scaling. Rapid bone fill followed treatment surgery (Fig. 9-20c) and the pulp of the tooth maintained its vitality.

The two cases described (Figs. 9-19, 9-20) demonstrate that neither clinical symptoms nor radiographic findings invariably lead to the correct diagnosis. The only significant observation for the differential diagnosis was the pulp vitality.

Pulp vitality means that the pulp chamber is occupied by connective tissue supplied by nerves and blood vessels. Sensory nerve function is normally present. Vital pulp tissue may or may not be subjected to inflammatory and degenerative tissue changes.

In most situations pulp vitality must be determined by indirect means and such measures are based on the assumption that a vital pulp is able to respond to sensory stimuli such as mechanical, thermal and electric stimulation. This means that the *sensitivity* of the pulp is tested rather than the *vitality* of the pulpal tissue. There is extensive documentation to support the concept that a tooth which responds to sensory stimuli is vital. Conversely, if a tooth does not respond to sensory stimuli, the pulp may be nonvital. It must be recognized that both false positive and false negative readings occur. Therefore, a combination of various test methods should be used to ensure a correct diagnosis.

Pulpal sensitivity can be examined by thermal stimulation with the use of ethyl chloride, carbon dioxide snow, ice, or heated gutta-percha sticks and by the use of electric stimulation with a pulp tester. Another testing method is mechanical stimulation by, for example, preparing a test cavity in dentin.

It is important to remember that the recognition of pulp vitality is essential for a differential diagnosis and for the selection of primary measures for treatment of inflammatory lesions in the marginal and apical periodontium. Deep restorations, dental trauma, endodontic treat-

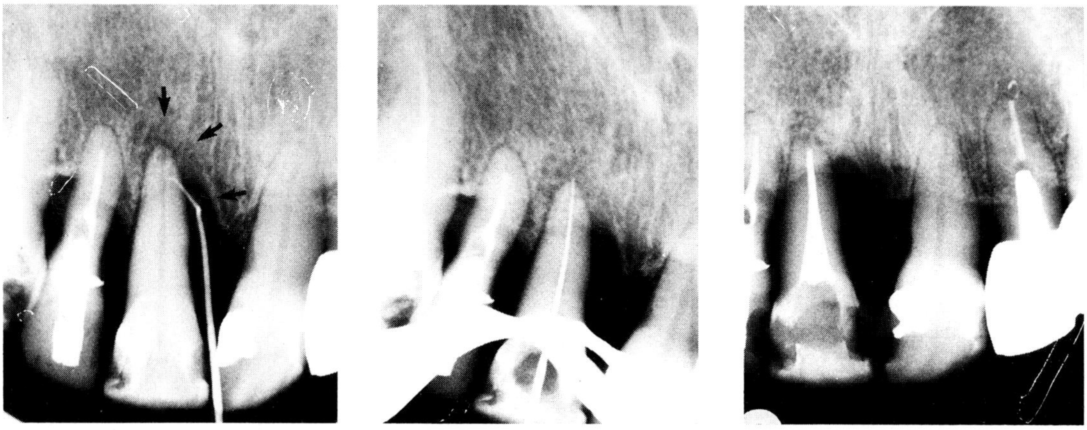

a b c

Fig. 9-21. At the mesial root surface of tooth 11 a deep, angular, bone defect extends to the apical level of the tooth. A gutta-percha cone has been inserted into the gingival pocket as an indicator of its depth (a). The tooth exhibited markedly increased mobility in both horizontal and vertical direction. No other clinical symptoms of inflammation were present. Vitality tests indicated that the pulp was nonvital, suggesting the diagnosis of a combined lesion. A combined endodontic and periodontal treatment was attempted since extraction of the tooth would have resulted in extensive prosthetic treatment. Endodontic treatment (b) was instituted followed by scaling and root planing in conjunction with flap surgery. Treatment resulted in healing of the apical part of the lesion (c) and in the arrest of the progression of periodontal disease. However, the marginal part of the angular defect failed to heal with bone fill.

ment, previous pulp capping, etc., are factors to consider when assessing the need for endodontic treatment as a part of the overall periodontal therapy. Location, form and extension of radiolucencies, as well as clinical symptoms of pain, tenderness, abscess formation, increased probing depth, etc., may not invariably distinguish a periodontal from an endodontic lesion.

Treatment strategies for combined endodontic and periodontal lesions

Occasionally, endodontic and periodontal lesions may occur in one and the same tooth. Lesions may be totally separated from each other and present no extraordinary therapeutic considerations. In other situations there is no obvious demarcation between the two lesions, which both radiographically and clinically appear as one lesion (Fig. 9-21). This type of combined lesion defect may be identified by probing along the root to the apical region of the tooth (Fig. 9-21a).

Treatment of combined endodontic and periodontal lesions does not differ from treatment given when the two disorders occur separately. The part of the lesion sustained by the root canal infection can usually be expected to resolve after proper endodontic treatment (Fig. 9-21c). The part of the lesion caused by the plaque infection may also heal following periodontal therapy, although little or no regeneration of the attachment apparatus can be expected (see Chapter 13). This suggests that the prognosis for regeneration of the attachment apparatus seems to be the more favorable the larger the part of the lesion that is caused by pulpal infection. It is important to realize that it is clinically not possible to determine to what extent one or the other of the two disorders (endodontic or periodontal) has affected the supporting tissues. Therefore, the treatment strategy must be to first focus on the pulpal infection and perform debridement and disinfection of the root canal system. The second phase includes a period of observation whereby the extent of periodontal healing that resulted from the endodontic treatment is determined. Reduced probing depth can usually be expected within a couple of weeks while bone regeneration may require several months before it can be detected in radiographs. Thus, periodontal therapy including deep scaling with and without periodontal surgery should be postponed until the result of the endodontic treatment can be properly evaluated (see Fig. 9-8).

It should be understood that periodontal disease may be responsible for the entire loss of the supporting apparatus around a tooth and in addition be the cause of the breakdown of the pulpal tissue. In such cases endodontic treatment will not contribute to periodontal healing and the problem will have to be solved by a periodontal treatment approach.

When there is doubt as to whether a lesion in the periodontium is of endodontic or periodontal origin, or both, the following treatment strategy may be followed:

Cause	**Condition of the pulp**	**Treatment**
Endodontic	Non-vital	Endodontic
Periodontal	Vital	Periodontal
Endodontic/ Periodontal	Non-vital	Endodontic- first observe the result of this therapy and institute periodontal therapy if necessary.

References

Absi, E.G., Addy, M. & Adams, D. (1987) Dentine hypersensitivity. A study of the patency of dentinal tubules in sensitive and non-sensitive cervical dentin. *Journal of Clinical Periodontology* **14**, 280-284.

Addy, M., Absi, E.G. & Adams, D. (1987) Dentine hypersensitivity. The effects in vitro of acids and dietary substances on root-planed and burred dentine. *Journal of Clinical Periodontology* **14**, 274-279.

Addy, M. & Dowell, P. (1983) Dentine hypersensitivity - A review. Clinical and *in vitro* evaluation of treatment agents. *Journal of Clinical Periodontology* **10**, 351-363.

Adrians, P. & Loesche, W.J. (1985) Bacterial invasion of the radicular dentin of periodontally involved caries-free human teeth. *Journal of Dental Research* (IADR Abstract) **64**: 354.

Armitage, G.C., Ryder, M.I. & Wilcox, S.E. (1983) Cemental changes in teeth with heavily infected root canals *Journal of Endodontics* **9**, 127-130.

Beavers, R.A., Bergenholtz, G. & Cox, C.F. (1986) Periodontal wound healing following intentional root perforations in permanent teeth of Macaca mulatta. *International Journal of Endodontics* **19**, 36-44.

Bender, I.B. & Seltzer, S. (1972) The effect of periodontal disease on the pulp. *Oral Surgery* **33**, 458-474.

Bergenholtz, G., Lekholm, U., Liljenberg, B. & Lindhe, J. (1983) Morphometric analysis of chronic inflammatory periapical lesions in root-filled teeth. *Oral Surgery* **55**, 295-301.

Bergenholtz, G. & Lindhe, J. (1975) Effect of soluble plaque factors on inflammatory reactions in the dental pulp. *Scandinavian Journal of Dental Research* **83**, 153-158.

Bergenholtz, G. & Lindhe, J. (1978) Effect of experimentally induced marginal periodontitis and periodontal scaling on the dental pulp. *Journal of Clinical Periodontology* **5**, 59-73.

Bergenholtz, G. & Reit, C. (1980) Reactions of the dental pulp to microbial provocation of calcium hydroxide treated dentin. *Scandinavian Journal of Dental Research* **88**, 187-192.

Brännström, M. (1966) Sensitivity of dentine. *Oral Surgery* **21**, 517-526.

Brännström, M. & Garberoglio, R. (1980) Occlusion of dentinal tubules under superficial attried dentin. *Swedish Dental Journal* **4**, 87-91.

Burch, J.G. & Hulen, S. (1974) A study of the

presence of accessory foramina and the topography of molar furcations. *Oral Surgery* **38**, 451-455.

Byström, A., Happonen, R.-P., Sjögren, U. & Sundqvist, G. (1987) Healing of periapical lesions of pulpless teeth after endodontic treatment with controlled asepsis. *Endodontics and Dental Traumatology* **3**, 58-63.

Czarnecki, R.T. & Schilder, H. (1979) A histological evaluation of the human pulp in teeth with varying degrees of periodontal disease. *Journal of Endodontics* **5**, 242-253.

DeDeus, Q.D. (1975) Frequency, location, and direction of the lateral, secondary and accessory canals. *Journal of Endodontics* **1**, 361-366.

Dowell, P. & Addy, M. (1983): Dentine hypersensitivity - A review. Aetiology, symptoms, and theories of pain production. *Journal of Clinical Periodontology* **10**, 341-350.

Green, B.W., Green, M.L. & McFall, W.T. (1977) Calcium hydroxide and potassium nitrate as desensitizing agents for hypersensitive root surfaces. *Journal of Periodontology* **48**, 667-672.

Gutmann, J.L. (1978) Prevalence, location and patency of accessory canals in the furcation region of permanent molars. *Journal of Periodontology* **49**, 21-26.

Haapasalo, M., Ranta, K. & Ranta, H. (1987) Mixed anaerobic periapical infection with sinus tract. *Endodontic and Dental Traumatology* **3**, 83-85.

Haskell, E.W., Stanley, H.E. & Goldman, S. (1980) A new approach to vital root resection. *Journal of Periodontology* **51**, 217-224.

Hattler, A.B. & Listgarten, M.A. (1984) Pulpal response to root planing in a rat model. *Journal of Endodontics* **10**, 471-476.

Hession, R.W. (1977) Endodontic morphology. A radiographic analysis. *Oral Surgery* **44**, 610-620.

Hiatt, W.H. & Johansen, E. (1972) Root preparation. I. Obturation of dentinal tubules in treatment of root hypersensitivity. *Journal of Periodontology* **43**, 373-380.

Kim, S. (1986) Hypersensitive teeth: Desensitization of pulpal sensory nerves. *Journal of Endodontics* **12**: 482-485.

Koenigs, J.F., Brilliant, J.D. & Foreman, D.W. (1974) Preliminary scanning electron microscope investigations of accessory foramina in the furcation areas of human molar teeth. *Oral Surgery* **38**, 773-782.

Langeland, K., Rodrigues, H. & Dowden, W. (1974) Periodontal disease, bacteria and pulpal histopathology. *Oral Surgery* **37**, 257-270.

Levin, M.P., Yearwood, L.L. & Carpenter, W.N. (1973) The desensitizing effect of calcium hydroxide and magnesium hydroxide on hypersensitive dentin. *Oral Surgery* **35**, 741-746.

Lowman, J.V., Burke, R.S. & Pelleu, G.B. (1973) Patent accessory canals: incidence in molar furcation region. *Oral Surgery* **36**, 580-584.

Mazur, B. & Massler, M. (1964) Influence of periodontal disease on the dental pulp. *Oral Surgery* **17**, 592-603.

McFall, W.T. (1986): A review of the active agents available for treatment of dentinal hypersensitivity. *Endodontic and Dental Traumatology* **2**, 141-149.

Meister, F., Lommel, T.J. & Gerstein, H. (1980) Diagnosis and possible causes of vertical root fractures. *Oral Surgery* **49**, 243-253.

Mendis, B.R.N. & Darling, A.I. (1979) A scanning electron microscope and microradiographic study of closure of human coronal dentinal tubules related to occlusal attrition and caries. *Archives of Oral Biology* **24**, 725-733.

Nair, P.N.R. (1987) Light and electron microscope studies of root canal flora and periapical lesions. *Journal of Endodontics* **13**, 29-39.

Nair, P.N.R. & Schroeder, H.E. (1984) Periapical actinomycosis. *Journal of Endodontics* **10**, 567-570.

Närhi. M.V.O. (1985) The characteristics of interdental sensory units and their responses to stimulation. *J Dent Res* 64 (special issue), 564-571.

Nielsen, R., Johannessen, A.C., Skaug, N. & Matre, R. (1984) In situ characterization of mononuclear cells in human dental periapical inflammatory lesions using monoclonal antibodies. *Oral Surgery* **58**: 160-165.

Nilvéus, R. & Selvig, K.A. (1983) Pulpal reactions to the application of citric acid to root-planed dentin in beagles. *Journal of Periodontal Research* **18**: 420-428.

Pashley, D.H. (1986): Dentin permeability, dentin sensitivity, and treatment through tubule occlusion. *Journal of Endodontics* **12**, 465-474.

Perlich, M.A., Reader, A. & Foreman, D.W. (1981) A scanning electron microscopic investigation of accessory foramens on the pulpal floor of human molars. *Journal of Endodontics* **7**, 402-406.

Petersson, K., Hasselgren, G. & Tronstad, L. (1986) Endodontic treatment of experimental root perforations in dog teeth. *Endodontics and Dental Traumatology* **1**: 22-28.

Pineda, F. & Kuttler, Y. (1972) Mesiodistal and buccolingual roentgenographic investigation of 7,275 root canals. *Oral Surgery* **33**, 101-110.

Pitts, D.L. & Natkin, E. (1983): Diagnosis and treatment of vertical root fractures. *Journal of Endodontics* **9**, 338-346.

Rubach, W.C. & Mitchell, D.F. (1965) Periodontal disease, accessory canals and pulp pathosis. *Journal of Periodontology* **36**, 34-38.

Rud, J. & Omnell, K.Å. (1970) Root fractures due to corrosion: diagnostic aspects. *Scandinavian Journal of Dental Research* **78**, 397-403.

Ryan, P.C., Newcomb, G.M., Seymour, G.J. & Po-well, R.N. (1984) The pulpal response to citric acid in cats. *Journal of Clinical Periodontology* **11**, 633-643.

Seltzer, S., Bender, I.B. & Ziontz, M. (1963) The interrelationship of pulp and periodontal disease. *Oral Surgery* **16**, 1474-1490.

Stern, M.H., Dreizen, S., Mackler, B.F., Selbst, A.G. & Levy, B.M. (1981) Quantitative analysis of cellular composition of human periapical granuloma. *Journal of Endodontics* **7**, 117-122.

Sundqvist, G. (1976) Bacteriologic studies of necrotic dental pulps. Umeå University Odontological Dissertation #7.

Sundqvist, G. & Reuterving, C-O. (1980) Isolation of Actinomyces israeli from periapical infection. *Journal of Endodontics* **6**, 602-606.

Thilo, B., Baehni, P.& Holz, J. (1986) Dark-field observation of the bacterial distribution in root canals following pulp necrosis. *Journal of Endodontics* **12**, 202-205.

Tronstad, L., Barnett, F., Riso, K. & Slots, J. (1987) Extraradicular endodontic infections. *Endodontics and Dental Traumatology* **3**, 86-90.

Walton, R.E., Michelich, R.J. & Smith, G.N. (1983) The histopathogenesis of vertical root fractures. *Journal of Endodontics* **10**, 48-56.

Vertucci, T.J. & Williams, R.G. (1974) Furcation canals in the human mandibular first molar. *Oral Surgery* **38**, 308-314.

Yanagisawa, S. (1980) Pathologic study of periapical lesions. I. Periapical granulomas: clinical, histopathologic and immunohistopathologic studies. *Journal of Oral Pathology* **9**, 288-300.

CHAPTER 10

Manifestation of Systemic Disorders in the Periodontium

Infectious diseases

Herpetic gingivostomatitis

Fig. 10-1. When the herpes simplex virus affects the oral mucosa it results in a herpetic gingivostomatitis, usually seen in children between the ages of 2 and 4, but in recent years also diagnosed in a number of older age groups. After an incubation period of 1 week, the patients develop fever, swollen submandibular lymph nodes and a diffuse gingivitis. Fig. 10-1 is a typical example of herpetic gingivostomatitis in a 12 year old boy. There is marked edema of the marginal gingiva and occurrence of vesicles on the interdental papillae of 12,11 and 42,41. On the interdental papilla between 22,12 and on the labial mucosa there are burst vesicles covered by fibrin.

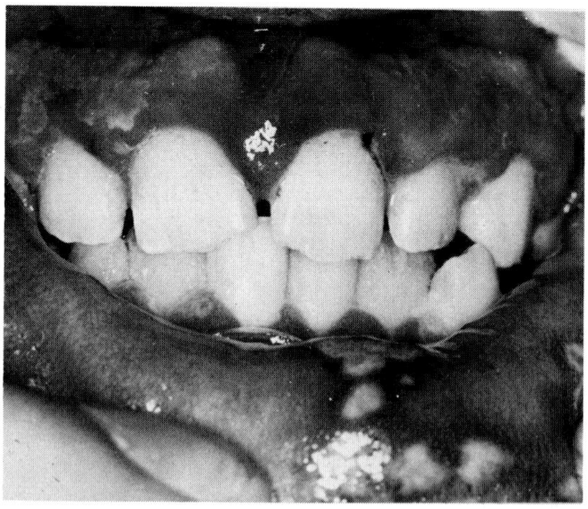

Fig. 10-1.

Verucca vulgaris

Fig. 10-2 shows, in a 12 year old boy, a gingival change in the form of a small, white, elevated lesion which was clinically diagnosed as a papilloma. It is easy to understand why confusion between a papilloma and a verruca may occur as they are very similar from a clinical point of view. In the verucca it is possible, by means of electron microscopy, to demonstrate virus particles in the epithelial cells. Virus is transferred to the mouth from verrucae (warts) on the hands when they are chewed. Oral verrucae are seen mainly in children, the favorite location being the mucosa of lip and tongue. In recent years it has been found that patients infected with HIV have an increased frequency of oral verrucae vulgaris sometimes located to the gingiva.

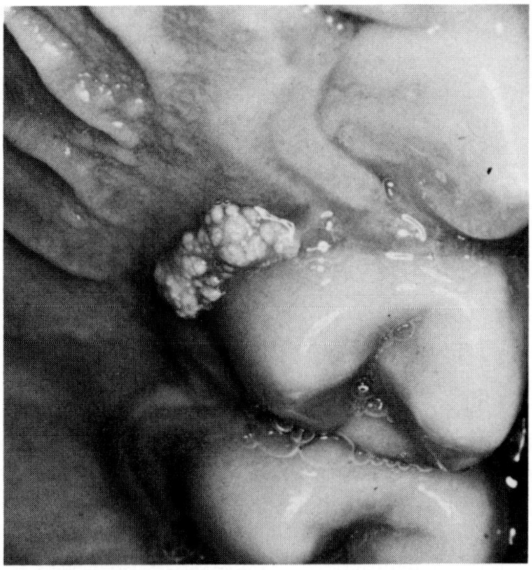

Fig. 10-2.

Condyloma acuminatum

Fig. 10-3 illustrates, in a 44 year old man, a lesion which at first glance looks like an epulis of a papillomatous type. It is characterized by its cauliflower-like appearance, typical of condyloma acuminatum. The patient has condylomas on the penis and the histologic examination of the removed "epulis" reveals structures characteristic of condyloma acuminatum. The rarity of oral condylomas in the literature may be due to such lesions usually being diagnosed as papillomas, verrucae vulgares or fibroepithelial hyperplasias. In most patients with oral condylomas an orogenital contact is revealed, together with genital condylomas of the partner. Oral condylomas are found with greater frequency in patients infected with HIV.

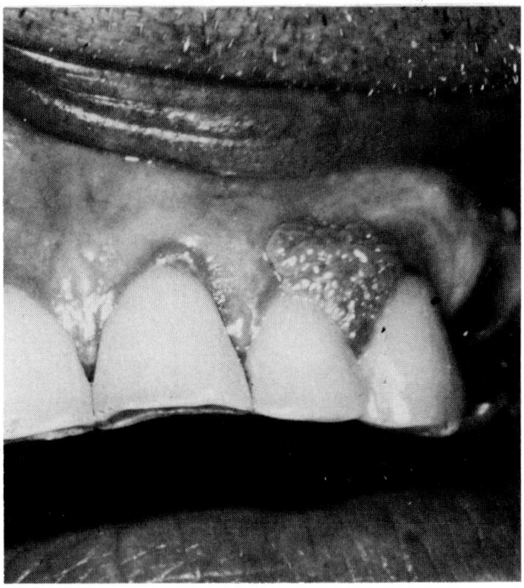

Fig. 10-3.

Human immunodeficiency virus

The first report indicating an association between HIV infection and periodontal lesions came in 1985 from Houston (Dennison et al.). One year later, a report from San Francisco (Silverman et al.) showed that premature and advanced periodontal disease, as demonstrated by gingivitis, gingival recession and loss of alveolar bone was frequent in a sample of 375 homosexual men (136 with AIDS). Another report from San Francisco (Winkler et al. 1986) described 4 patients with hairy leukoplakia and 3 AIDS patients, all having foetor ex ore, necrotizing gingivitis and interproximal loss of bone (ANUG). In all cases, the healing re-

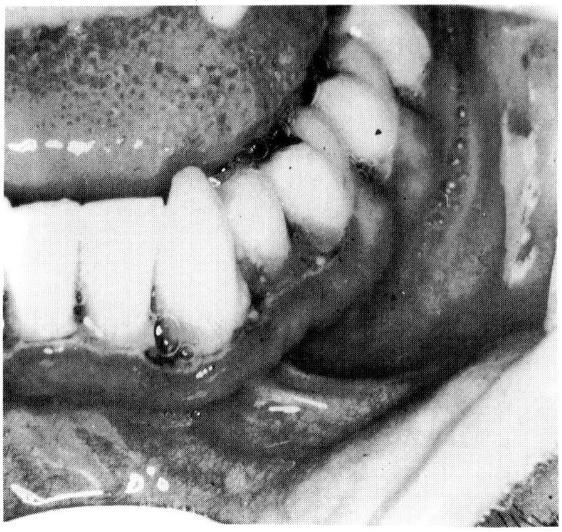

Fig. 10-4.

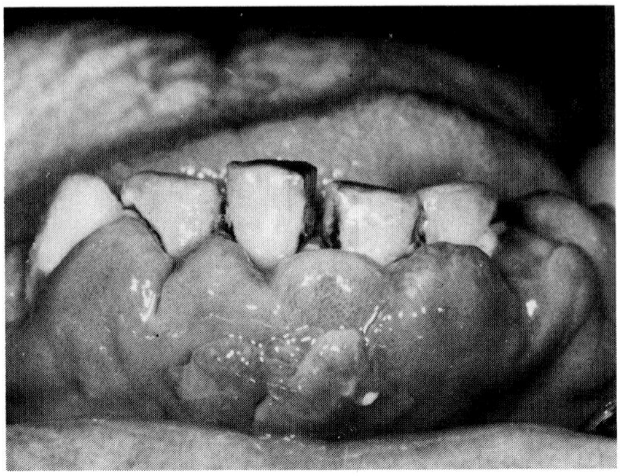

Fig. 10-5.

sponse to traditional ANUG treatment was very slow. The authors suggested that the necrotizing lesion in the HIV infected patients was an atypical form of ANUG. From Copenhagen came a report in 1987 on 3 patients with necrotizing gingivitis, who had antibodies to the HIV but no AIDS (Pindborg & Holmstrup). Fig. 10-4 illustrates a typical example of such a necrotizing gingivitis with extensive loss of interdental papillae.

Malignant systemic diseases

Acute monocytic leukemia

Whereas chronic leukemia only rarely causes oral lesion, the acute forms are often associated with oral manifestations, which may be pronounced and quite disturbing. Fig. 10-5 demonstrates a very marked increase in gingival volume in a 32 year old woman who suddenly experienced pain in the gingiva, enlarged lymph nodes of the neck and later an increase in temperature. The gingiva has lost its normal stippling and has a spongy appearance. There are very deep pseudopockets and the teeth are loose. The patient was referred to a department of internal medicine where the tentative diagnosis of leukemia was confirmed. Two weeks later the patient died.

Endocrinopathies

Diabetes mellitus

Diabetes mellitus is a syndrome characterized by insufficient secretion of insulin, decreased glucose tolerance and a tendency for development of microangiopathy, neuropathy and arteriosclerosis.

Diabetically conditional periodontal changes have often been discussed in the literature, and it has been postulated that diabetes does not predispose to periodontal disease. Several studies in recent years have demonstrated, however, that there is a causal relationship.

It has been demonstrated that child-diabetics with well controlled disease had more gingivitis than age matched controls without diabetes; both groups had the same plaque score (Faulconbridge et al. 1981).

In adults it had been shown, in a longitudinal

study, that even patients with controlled diabetes, have more gingivitis and loss of epithelial attachment than nondiabetics (Cohen et al. 1970).

Data indicate that altered neutrophil function may be responsible for accelerated periodontal tissue breakdown in poorly controlled diabetics. An impaired chemotactic and phagocytic activity of the polymorphonuclear leukocytes has been found in diabetics.

Fig. 10-6 demonstrates the periodontal conditions in a 56 year old man suffering from diabetes mellitus. Along the marginal gingiva are some limited granulomatous changes particularly at 21. The periodontal tissue around most of his teeth is the seat of advanced periodontal disease. The asymmetric location of the gingival changes should arouse suspicion of systemic disease.

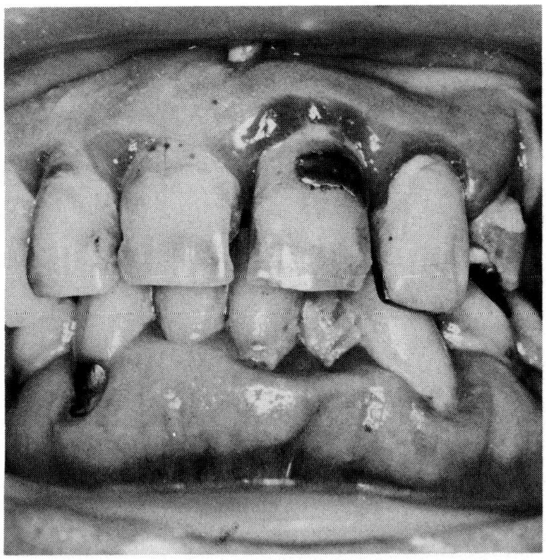

Fig. 10-6.

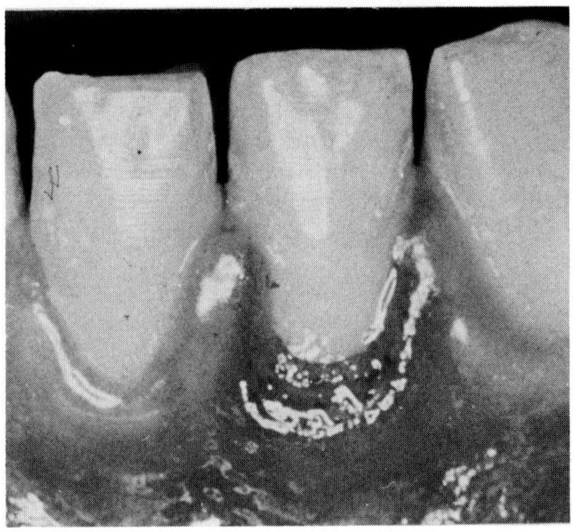

Fig. 10-7.

Blood diseases

Cyclic neutropenia

In 1949 it was recognized that neutropenia, in some patients, had a cyclic course and the term cyclic neutropenia was introduced for a disease characterized by a dramatic fall in the number of circulating neutrophil leukocytes at 3 week periodic intervals. After 5-8 days the number of leukocytes increases, but it never reaches the normal level. The etiology of cyclic neutropenia is unknown. In the periods with a low number of leukocytes, the patient suffers from fever and general malaise. At the same time, changes occur on the skin and in the mouth. The oral lesions consist of a subacute gingivitis and/or aphthae-like ulcerations very often localized to the marginal gingiva, where recurrent aphthae are rarely seen. Furthermore, the neutropenic ulcerations have a punch-out appearance as can be seen in Fig. 10-7, from an 8 year old boy whose cyclic neutropenia was identified through his gingival lesions.

A very characteristic change, in both idiopathic and cyclic neutropenia, is sharply demarcated, hyperemic zones along the marginal gingiva.

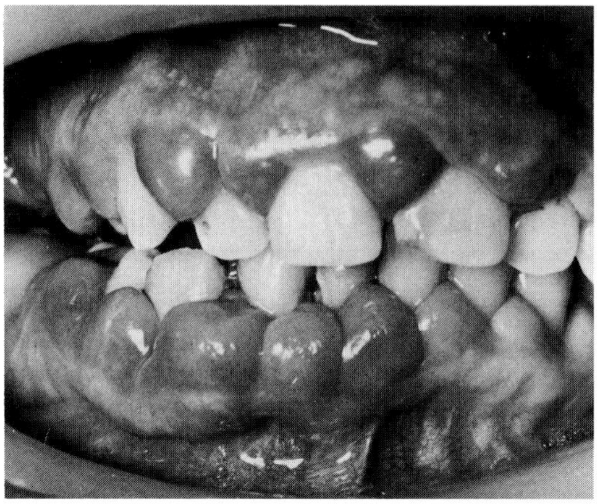

Fig. 10-8.

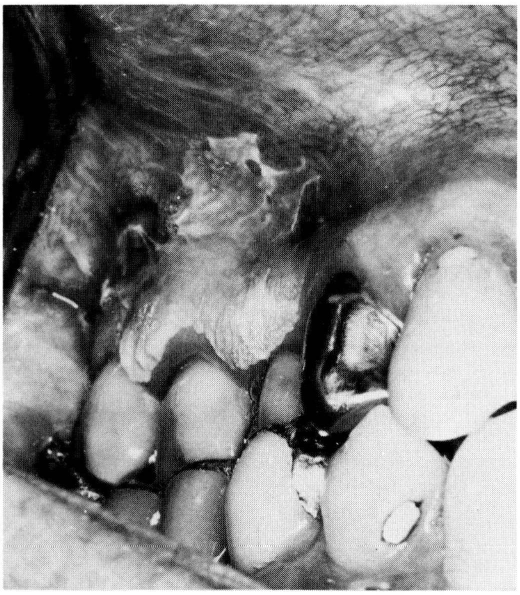

Fig. 10-9.

Diseases of the digestive system

Idiopathic gingival fibromatosis

Fig. 10-8 illustrates a very pronounced swelling of the gingiva, mostly affecting the interdental papillae, in a 26 year old woman, who has for many years suffered from gingival enlargement. In the premolar and molar areas the enlargement is so marked that the teeth are covered to the occlusal surfaces. There is no history of phenytoin medication, so the lesion can only be classified as an idiopathic gingival fibromatosis. The molars were extracted because of extensive bone loss. The patient discloses that she suffers from hypertrichosis, a phenomenon reported to occur in a number of cases of idiopathic gingival fibromatosis.

Frictional keratosis

Fig. 10-9 shows a white patch combined with leukoplakia limited to the areolar and alveolar gingivae and parts of the buccal groove. A mild gingival retraction points at energetic tooth brushing, which, however, is not enough to cause such an intense hyperkeratosis beyond the gingiva. Another etiologic factor is the 20 cigarettes the patient smokes daily. It is peculiar that the leukoplakia has spared the marginal gingiva of 16. It is rather rare to observe leukoplakias on the gingiva, which may be explained by the fact that the marginal and alveolar gingivae are normally keratinized, apparently by a protective structure.

Diseases related to pregnancy, menstruation, and oral contraceptives

Pregnancy gingivitis

It seems beyond any doubt that pregnancy may cause gingival changes. However, the reported frequency of so-called "pregnancy gingivitis" varies between 30-100%, reflecting the diversity of opinion which exists. According to studies using well defined indices, a gingival change is noticeable in pregnant women from the 2nd month of gestation, reaching a maximum in the 8th month. During the last month of gestation a definite decrease occurs. Furthermore, it has been found that the state of gingiva immediately after parturition is similar to that at the 2nd month of pregnancy (Löe & Silness 1963). The same investigators also found that, although the gingiva of the molar teeth showed the highest scores thoughout pregnancy, the greatest relative increase was observed around the anterior teeth. The interproximal areas are by far the most frequent sites of gingival inflammation both during pregnancy and after parturition.

Several studies have suggested that gingivitis during pregnancy is a result increased levels of progesterone and its effect on the microvasculature (Hugoson 1970). It has also been proposed that exaggeration of the gingival inflammatory response during pregnancy could be due to hormonal charges altering tissue metabolism (Löe & Silness 1963).

The prevalence of gingivitis in pregnancy seems to be offset to some degree by a concomitant decrease in debris accumulation (Adams et al. 1974). During pregnancy both the gingival-periodontal index and horizontal tooth mobility are increased (Cohen et al. 1971).

Clinically, the gingival changes in pregnancy are characterized by a fiery red color of the marginal gingiva and interdental papillae. At the same time, the gingiva becomes enlarged, with the swelling mainly affecting the interdental papillae. The gingiva shows an increased tendency to bleed, and, in advanced cases, the patients sometimes even experience slight pain. Fig. 10-10 shows the increased volume of the marginal gingiva and the interdental papillae in a 20 year old woman in the 5th month of pregnancy. The gingival changes have been present from the 3rd month.

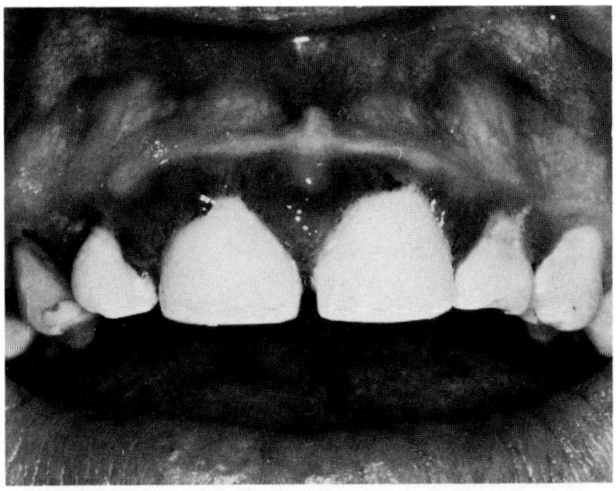

Fig. 10-10.

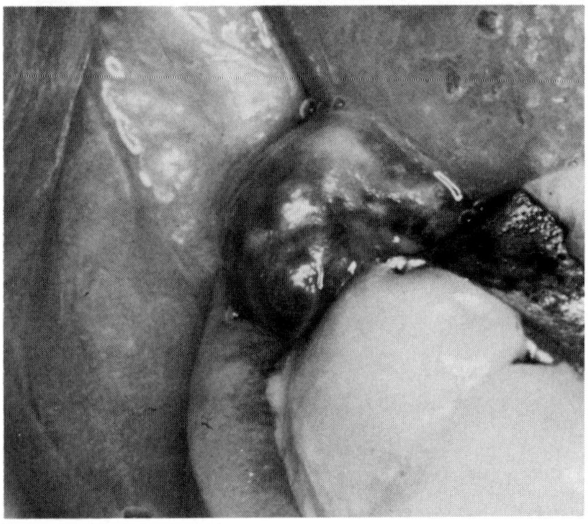

Fig. 10-11.

Pregnancy granuloma

Apart from the generalized gingival changes, pregnancy may also give rise to the formation of tumor-like growths, epulides, along the gingival margin, so-called pregnancy granulomas. The reported frequency of pregnancy granuloma varies from 0-5%. Occurring more frequently in the maxilla, favoring the vestibular aspect of the anterior region, it usually arises during the second trimester, though occasionally earlier, and often shows rapid growth, although seldom becoming larger than 2 cm in diameter. After parturition, the granuloma begins to regress spontaneously and sometimes

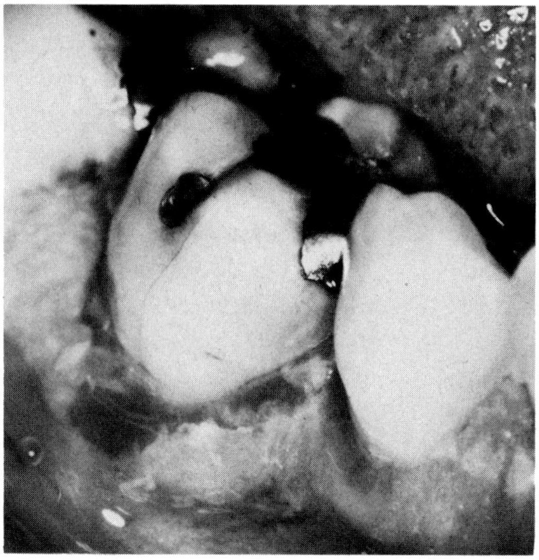

Fig. 10-12.

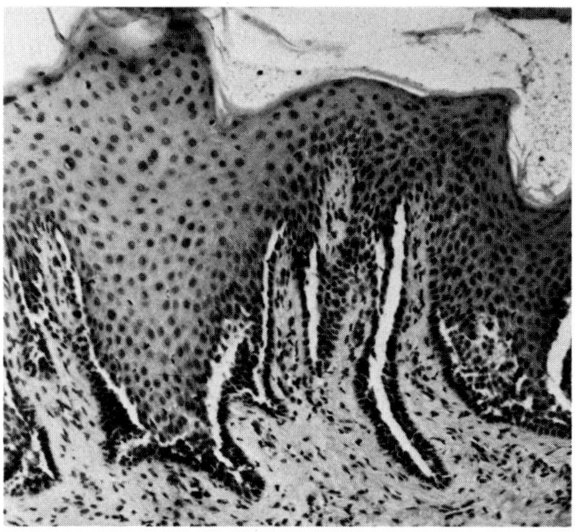

Fig. 10-13.

disappears entirely. Pregnancy granuloma is mostly a pedunculated soft growth of interdental origin with a fiery red color and often with small fibrin covered areas like those seen in Fig. 10-11, from a 31 year old woman in the 8th month of pregnancy. Pregnancy granulomas have a structure similar to the structure in pyogenic granulomas.

Effect of oral contraceptives

Several studies have shown that women taking hormonal contraceptives have an increased prevalence of gingivitis accompanied by a higher gingival fluid flow. Recent studies have confirmed these observations and have demonstrated that there is a statistically significant increase in gingival inflammation related to the duration of drug therapy (Pankhurst et al. 1981).

Diseases of the skin

Pemphigus vulgaris

Fig. 10-12 shows gingival change in a 43 year old woman who has had increasing oral mucosal trouble. The changes, consisting of blisters which burst during eating, began in the palate, later spreading to the entire oral mucosa. The gingival change in Fig. 10-12 is erythematous with focal spots of fibrin. In the periphery of the lesion there are flakes of epithelium. A biopsy from the palate shows an intraepithelial bulla in its early stage of development (Fig. 10-13). Pemphigus is a chronic bulla forming disease of skin and mucous membranes with a severe prognosis and autoimmune pathogenesis. All patients will show oral lesions in the course of the disease, and in approximately 60% the oral manifestations are its first indication. Because of the humid environment and trauma, the bullae of the oral mucosa will rupture shortly after formation, leaving a nonspecific ulceration, which sometimes makes it very difficult to arrive at a correct diagnosis. Pemphigus vegetans is another type of pemphigus having a milder course than the vulgaris type. It is characterized by fungus-like proliferations in areas where a bulla has developed. Like the vulgaris type, pemphigus vegetans often has its debut in the mouth.

Benign mucous membrane pemphigoid

Fig. 10-14 shows a bulla on the alveolar gingiva of 44 and a burst bulla at 43. It is from a 55 year old man who for 6 months had an itching, burning sensation of the gingiva and other areas of the mouth. Besides the changes mentioned above, the gingiva was the seat of erythema and there was total loss of normal stippling. The fluid filled bulla was excised and studied histologically. The bulla proved to be subepithelial, thus compatible with the diagnosis of benign mucous membrane pemphigoid. Further confirmation of the diagnosis was found in the presence of bullae on the conjunctiva.

It is rare to find the disease in men, the patients are usually women over the age of 50. In several areas, flakes of epithelium can be seen. Histologic examination of a biopsy, from an area where the epithelium is intact, showed subepithelial fluid accumulation which has caused an atrophy of the overlying epithelium. There is marked chronic inflammation of both the fluid and the connective tissue (Fig. 10-15). By means of immunofluorescence microscopy it can be demonstrated that the basement membrane area is the seat of an accumulation of immunoglobulins, which is the result of an antibody reaction against antigens in the basement membrane. There is no doubt that most of the cases of so-called "desquamative" gingivitis are benign mucous membrane pemphigoid. A smaller number can be identified as erosive lichen planus. Pemphigoid is classified into bullous pemphigoid and benign mucous membrane pemphigoid, both characterized by subepithelial bulla formation and identical oral lesions. However, the latter are more rare in bullous pemphigoid, which is dominated by skin changes.

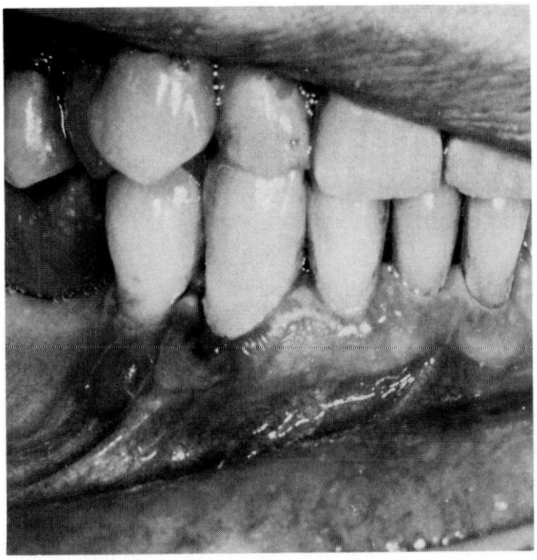

Fig. 10-14.

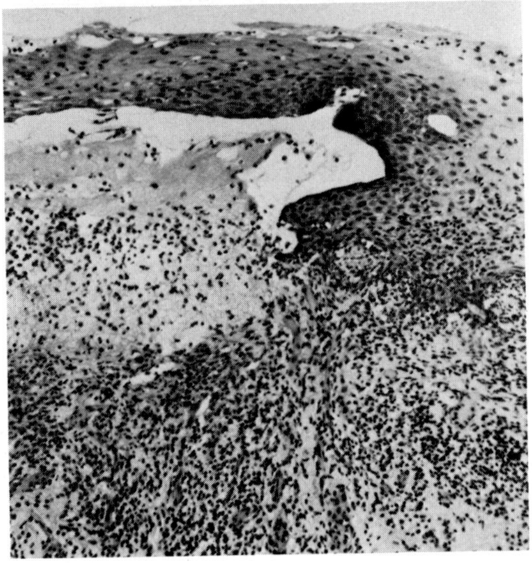

Fig. 10-15.

Erythema multiforme exudativum

Fig. 10-16 illustrates gingival changes in the form of small ulcerated lesions in a 28 year old man with erythema multiforme exudativum. For some days the patient had influenza-like

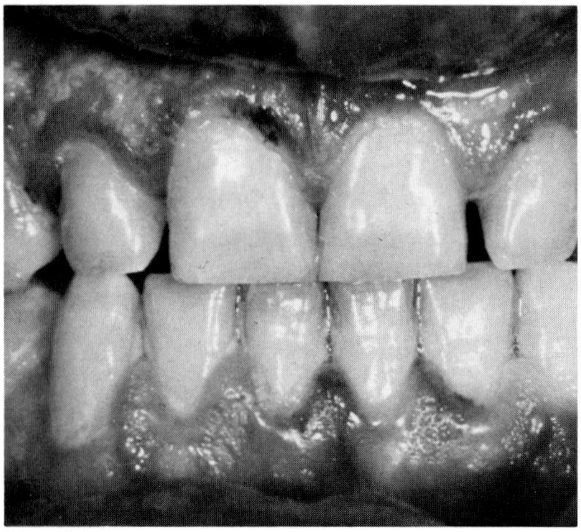

Fig. 10-16.

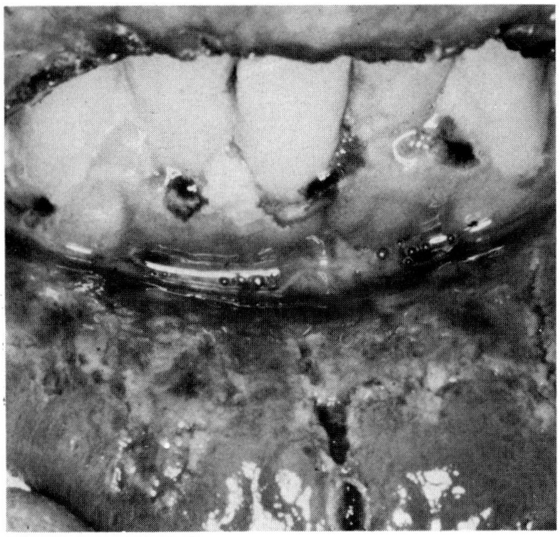

Fig. 10-17.

symptoms and oral discomfort. Such symptoms are typical of erythema multiforme exudativum. The disease is characterized by stomatitis, conjunctivitis, balanitis, and skin changes. It occurs especially in the young and more frequently in men. The course of the disease is acute and may sometimes be dramatic with a high temperature and general malaise. The patients are often disturbed by a pronounced crust formation on the lips. Not all patients have gingival changes. When present they are not diagnostic for the disease, as can be seen from Fig. 10-16. The picture, however, demonstrates an asymmetry of the gingival lesions which points towards a systemic background. Fig. 10-17 illustrates marked mucosal changes in a 23 year old man, who, shortly after angina, experienced blisters on the labial mucosa. Within 6 days fever, red eyes and labial affections appeared. Although the disease is vesiculo-bullous, it is rare to see fluid filled blisters; they burst quickly and become covered by fibrin. Note also the gingival changes in Fig. 10-17; they are asymmetric and nonspecific. Further, the gingiva is the seat of accumulation of desquamated epithelial cells caused by lack of mastication and tooth brushing.

Lichen planus

Lichen planus is a relatively common chronic, inflammatory skin disease of unknown etiology accompanied by small (flat), polygonal, red-brown papules, the surface of which is characterized by fine, small, and keratinized lines, the so-called "Wickham's striae". Lichen is often associated with oral manifestations. The prevalence of oral lichen planus is approximately 2%, and slightly higher in women. Among patients with oral lichen planus only 30% will show skin lesions. The oral manifestations present a rather varied picture. Usually the oral lesions are classified into reticular, papular, plaque, atrophic-ulcerative, and bullous types. It should not, however, be forgotten that two or more types can be found in the same patient. The gingival mucosa is often affected in patients with oral lichen planus. The appearance of the lesions is dependent upon the location in the mouth. Thus, physiologically keratinized mucosa, i.e. palate and gingiva, will not exhibit such well defined Wickham striae as non-keratinized mucosa. This fact is clearly illustrated in Fig. 10-18, a 45 year old woman with lichen planus lesions on the interdental papillae. Although the Wickham's striae are wider and less well defined than usual, they can still be identified. A histologic examination will in most cases confirm a clinical suspicion of lichen planus. Fig. 10-19 is a photomicrograph of a biopsy which contained a stria of Wickham. All features characteristic of lichen planus can be seen in the picture. There is hyperorthokeratosis and hyperplasia of the epithelium corresponding to Wickham's striae. Furthermore, there is a "sawtooth" appearance of the rete ridges, which are also marked by degenerative changes in connection with the band-like accumulation of lymphocytes in the juxtaepithelial connective tissue. A more diffuse type of gingival manifestation of lichen planus is seen in Fig. 10-20, a 46 year old woman who for 1 year had cutaneous lichen planus affections. The gingival lesion is quite similar to the gingival lesion caused by discoid lupus erythematosus. In the patient of Fig. 10-2, both sides of the buccal mucosa showed typical reticular elements. On the picture both confluent striae of Wickham and a red atrophic area are visible. An accentuation of the atrophic element can be seen in Fig. 10-21, a 43 year old woman who for 1 month had itching sensations in the gingiva. Clinically, the changes are characterized by alternating white and red (erythematous) areas all over the gingiva. The erythematous areas, caused by atrophic epithelium and subepithelial inflammation, appear dark on the illustration. Sometimes strong symptoms of disturbance were experienced after toothbrushing or eating spicy food. The patient also reported aggravation in periods of psychic stress. In some pa-

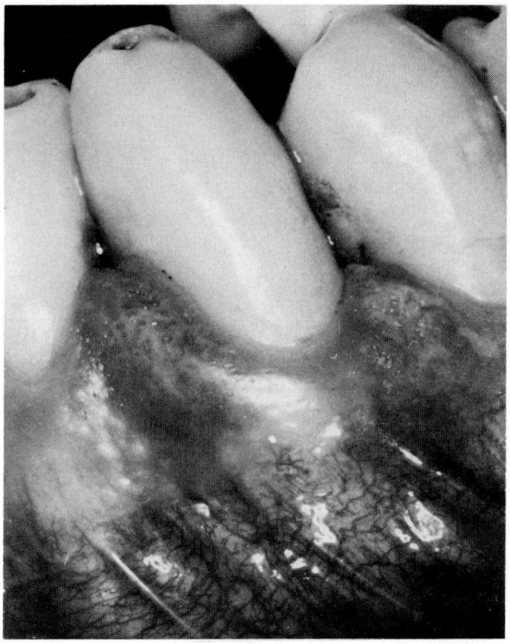

Fig. 10-18.

Fig. 10-19.

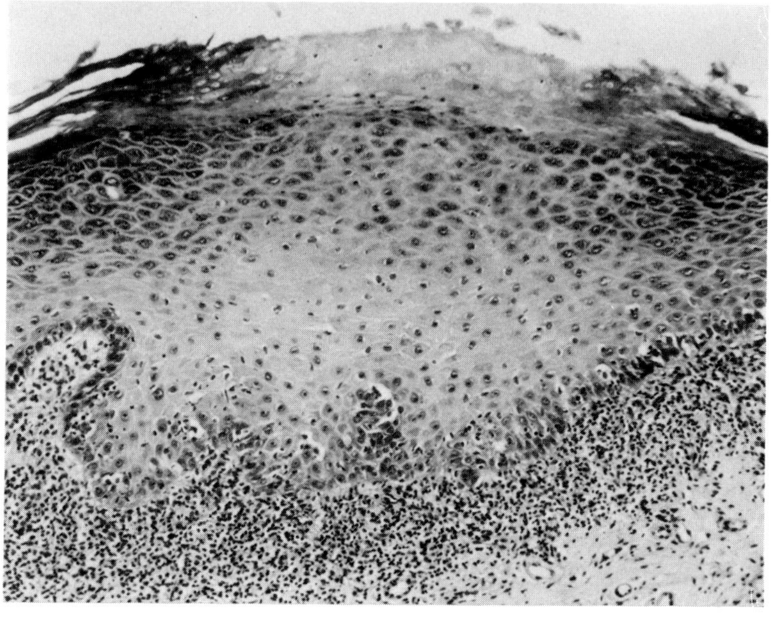

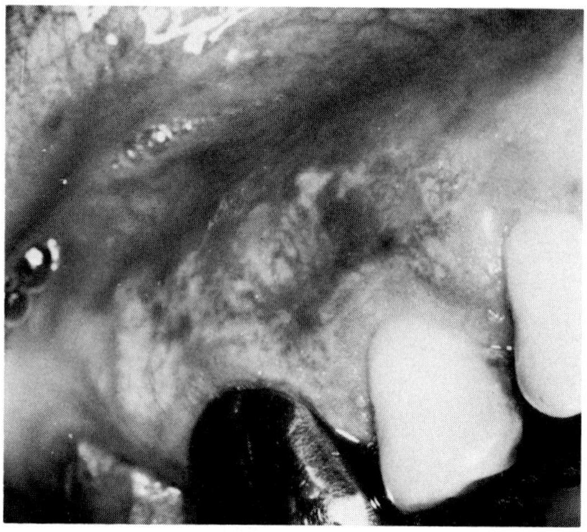

Fig. 10-20.

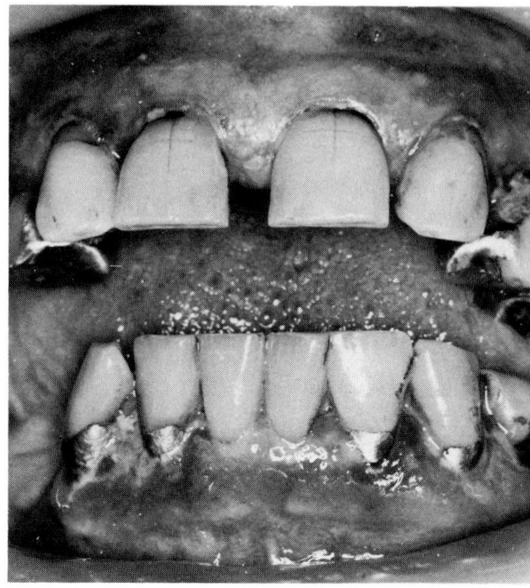

Fig. 10-21.

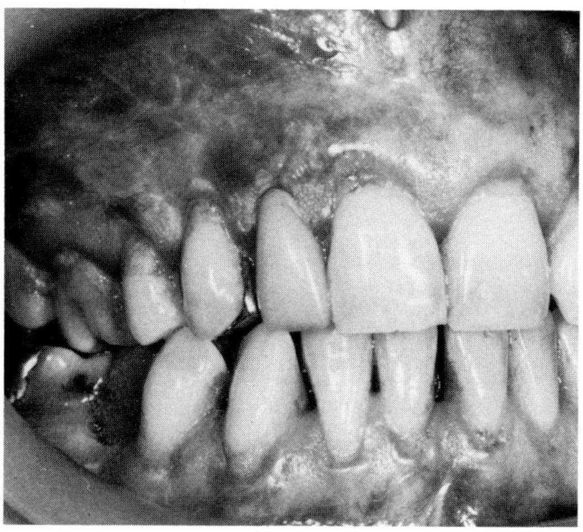

Fig. 10-22.

tients, the epithelium becomes so atrophic that it bursts spontaneously or by a light trauma, giving rise to an ulcerative (erosive) type of oral lichen planus. This condition is illustrated in Fig. 10-22 from a 50 year old woman. In both maxilla and mandible there is diffuse involvement of the entire gingival mucosa. There are areas of erythema and areas of ulcerations covered by fibrin, especially in the mandible. These clinical manifestations are similar to those observed in patients with benign mucous membrane pemphigoid. The atrophic (ulcerative) lichen planus is histologically characterized by a very thin epithelium. Often the epithelium is only 1/5 of its normal thickness, and it is easy to understand that the mucosa in these areas assumes a red color, as the many small vessels from the inflamed areas shine through. The bullous type is very seldom met with and rarely affects the gingiva. The plaque type may also involve the gingiva. Clinically it appears as white, homogenous areas which in a number of cases may be conceived as a superimposed leukoplakia as these patients frequently smoke. The atrophic and ulcerative types of lichen planus, also including the gingival manifestations, are often accompanied by marked pain, which necessitates treatment. An influence from corroded metal restorations ought to be excluded first. As most of the patients with ulcerative lesions have a superimposed *Candida albicans* infection, this complication should be treated either before or at the same time as the steroid treatment of the lichen planus is carried out. It is often necessary to treat a patient for several months in order to arrive at a satisfactory result.

Diseases of the musculoskeletal system

Scleroderma

Fig. 10-23 is a radiograph of 16, 15, 14 in a 21 year old man, suffering from diffuse scleroderma. He experienced toothache-like symptoms from 15, which is intact, but in traumatic occlusion and articulation. Radiography disclosed a marked widening of the periodontal membrane of 15 and most of the other teeth. Concurrently with the widening of the periodontal membrane there is a thickening of the lamina dura of the alveolar bone. Widening of the periodontal membrane in patients with scleroderma has been reported by several investigators, but the frequency of the changes varies from 7-40%. Diffuse scleroderma is a chronic disease characterized by diffuse fibrosis of the skin and other organs. The etiology is unknown, but immunologic factors appear to play a part. In the present case the toothache-like symptoms are explicable by the traumatic load which 15 has been exposed to, due to extrusion of the tooth resulting from the edema of the periodontal membrane. When the tooth was relieved by grinding, the symptoms disappeared. Fig. 10-24 shows the histologic changes in the widened periodontal membrane of 24 in a 43 year old woman with diffuse scleroderma. The normal straight course of the Sharpey's fibers is replaced by a collagenous tissue without orientation of the fibers and with focal hyalinization.

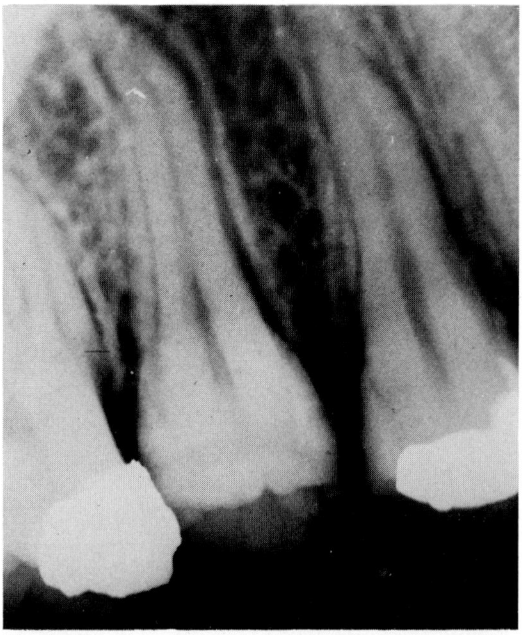

Fig. 10-23.

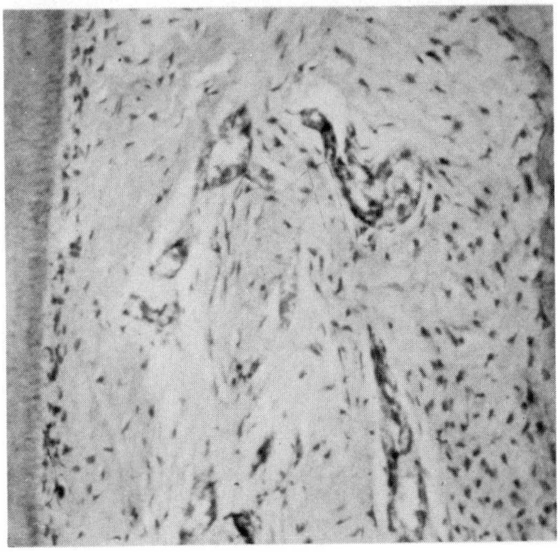

Fig. 10-24.

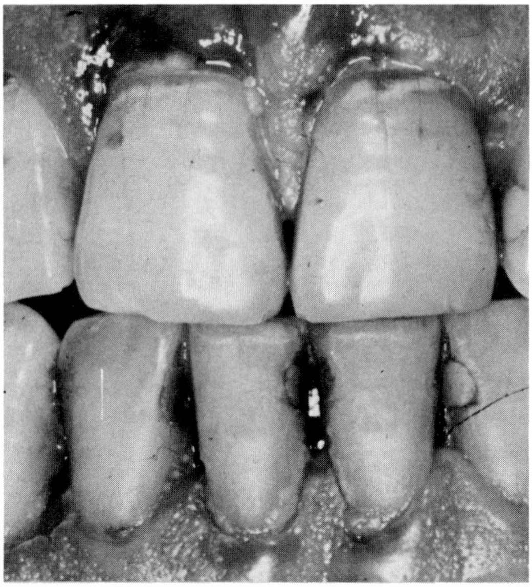

Fig. 10-25.

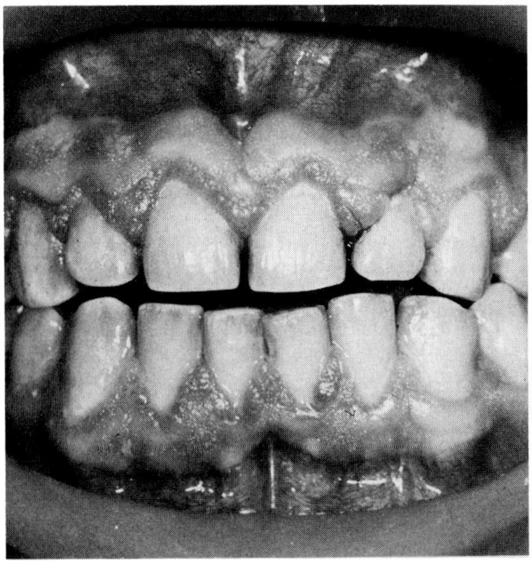

Fig. 10-26.

Drug stomatitis

Cytostatics

Fig. 10-25 illustrates some irregular and asymmetric gingival lesions in the form of small localized necroses at 11, 21 and 43, 42, 41 and 31 in a 42 year old man, who received immunosuppressive treatment with azathioprine in connection with a kidney transplantation. Azathioprine belongs to the group of cytostatics which are also being used in the treatment of malignant systemic diseases. Some patients treated with these compounds develop a drug stomatitis characterized by erythemas and ulcerations.

Hydantoin derivatives

For 40 years phenytoin (5.5-diphenylhydantoin (DPH), Dilantin®, Epanutin®) has been the preferred medication for epilepsy. However, in the last 10 years phenytoin has to a certain extent been replaced by carbamazepine because it has fewer side effects.

The side effects of phenytoin are varied and comprise, besides the well known gingival enlargement, disturbances of the nervous system, blood forming tissues, bone, skin, liver, endocrine glands and the immune system.

The gingival enlargement has been designated as hyperplasia gingivae diphenyl hydantoinea, diphenylhydantoin gingival overgrowth, Dilantin® hyperplasia, etc. The gingival enlargement in phenytoin treatment is not due to either hypertrophy or hyperplasia of fibroblasts and/or collagenous fibers. The number of these elements per unit tissue is normal, but the growth is uncontrolled, consequently the term gingival overgrowth. The reported incidence of gingival hyperplasia in patients receiving phenytoin varies from 3-62%; there is no sex predilection.

A number of histologic studies have tried to elucidate the pathogenesis of the gingival enlargement. By means of autoradiography an increased mitotic activity has been demonstrated in fibroblasts from biopsies from phenytoin conditioned gingival changes. Tissue cultures of fibroblasts have been treated with phenytoin and an increased mitotic activity was found. However, the activity decreased under the influence of ascorbic acid. The pathogenesis is still an unsolved problem. An excellent review is provided by Hassell (1981).

A characteristic feature of the fibrous overgrowth is hyperplasia of the covering squamous cell epithelium, which sends long and slender projections into the connective tissue. The gingival enlargement begins as an overgrowth of the interdental papillae followed by a spreading in the other regions of the gingiva. Fig. 10-26, from an 18 year old man, shows a slight increase in volume of several interdental papillae. This epileptic patient was treated with phenytoin for several years. Fig. 10-27 illustrates an enlargement which is quite monstrous. The patient, a 15 year old boy, received 300 mg phenytoin daily for 2 years on account of epileptic seizures. Despite the marked enlargement, the gingiva has maintained its normal stippling and color in contrast to idiopathic gingival fibromatosis, where the color is red and the surface glossy. In later stages, where the fibrous overgrowth has led to the formation of deep pseudopockets, an inflammation develops whereby the stippling is lost.

There is a correlation between degree of gingival enlargement and daily dosage of phenytoin, oral hygiene and other local irritants. The incidence of gingival enlargement is higher in younger persons. Although the increase in volume affects the vestibular as well as the lingual gingivae, the vestibular changes are the most pronounced. Inexplicable is the definite predilection for the anterior gingiva. It is characteristic that the fibrous overgrowth does not appear on the edentulous alveolar ridge.

The most severe cases of gingival enlargement must be treated by gingivectomy. Several studies have demonstrated that it is possible to prevent the development of marked lesions by an intense effort comprising removal of calculus and plaque every 3rd month, combined with careful toothbrushing and use of dental floss. Despite these precautions a small increase in gingival volume may develop in the anterior segment within the first 6 months, a change which is not aggravated in the following months.

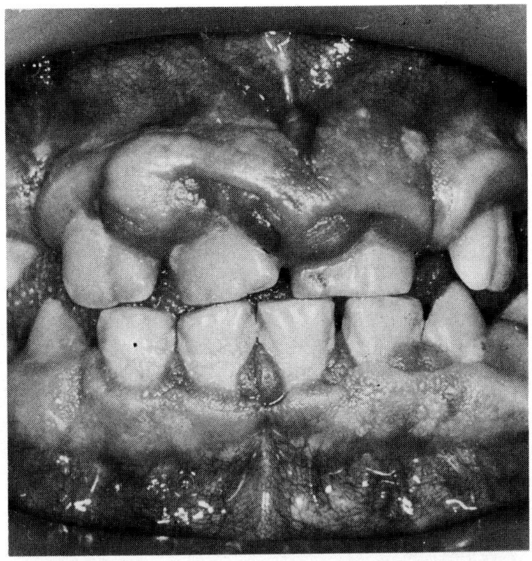

Fig. 10-27.

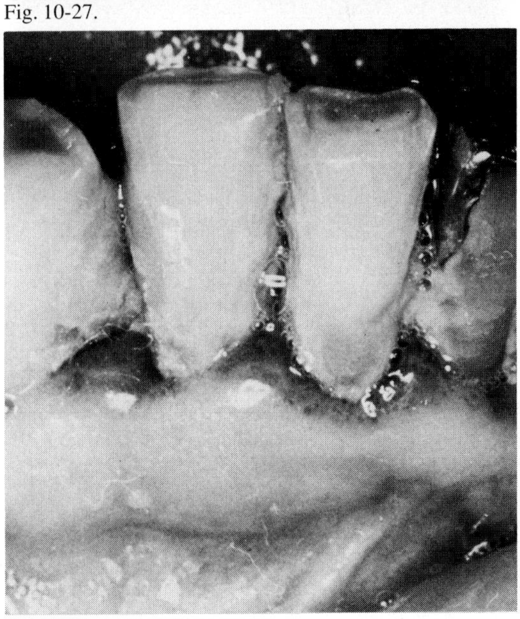

Fig. 10-28.

Gingival enlargement has recently been reported in patients receiving treatment with cyclosporin or nifedipine.

Industrial intoxication

Lead

Fig. 10-28 shows a typical lead line in a 45 year old man who worked in a battery plant for many years. Besides the gingival lead line (halo saturninus) the patient suffers from fatigue, lead colic, and a grayish color of the skin, characteristic symptoms of lead intoxication. As lead is widely used in industry, lead intoxication is still an important industrial hazard. In a number of cases lead intoxication has been recognized by a gingival lead line. The line is bluish-black, a few mm wide and follows the marginal gingiva. The lead line is due to deposits of insoluble lead sulfide in the endothelial cells of the capillaries and in the histiocytes. In some cases it may be difficult to distinguish between a lead line and subgingival calculus.

References

Aas, E. (1963) Hyperplasia gingivae diphenylhydantoniea. *Acta Odontologica Scandinavica*, Supplement 34.

Adams, D., Carney, J.S. & Dicks, D.A. (1974) Pregnancy gingivitis: a survey of 100 antenatal patients. *Journal of Dentistry* **2**, 106-110.

Bernick, S.M., Cohen, D.W., Baker, L. & Laster, L. (1975) Dental disease in children with diabetes mellitus. *Journal of Periodontology* **46**, 241-246.

Cohen, W.D., Friedman, L.A., Shapiro, J., Kyle, C.G. & Franklin, S. (1970) Diabetes mellitus and periodontal disease: two year longitudinal observations. I. *Journal of Periodontology* **41**, 709-712.

Cohen, W.D., Shapiro, J., Friedman, L., Kyle, C.G. & Franklin, S. (1971) A longitudinal investigation of the periodontal changes during pregnancy and fifteen months postpartum, II. *Journal of Periodontology* **42**, 653-657.

Dennison, D.K., Smith, B., Newland, J.R. (1985) Immune responsiveness and ANUG. *Journal of Dental Research* **64**, Spec. Issue, Abstr.No. 204.

Faulconbridge, A.R., Bradshaw, W.C.L., Jenkins, P.A. & Baum, J.D. (1981) The dental status of a group of diabetic children. *British Dental Journal* **151**, 253-255.

Hassell, T.M. (1981) *Epilepsy and the oral manifestations of phenytoin therapy*. Monographs in Oral Science. New York: S. Karger.

Hugoson, A. (1970) Gingival inflammation and female sex hormones. A clinical investigation of pregnant women and experimental studies in dogs. *Journal of Periodontal Research* **5**, Supplement 5.

Lindhe, J. & Attström, R. (1967) Gingival exudation during the menstrual cycle. *Journal of Periodontal Research* **2**, 194-198.

Löe, H. & Silness, J. (1963) Periodontal disease in pregnancy. I. Prevalence and severity. *Acta Odontologica Scandinavica* **21**, 533-551.

Pankhurst, C.L., Waite, I.M., Hicks, K.A., Allen, Y. & Harkness, R.D. (1981) The influence of oral contraceptives therapy on the periodontium - duration of drug therapy. *Journal of Periodontology* **52**, 617-620.

Pindborg, J.J. (1985) *Atlas of diseases of the oral mucosa*. 4th ed. Copenhagen: Munksgaard.

Pindborg, J.J. & Holmstrup, P. (1987) Necrotizing gingivitis related to human immunodeficiency & virus (HIV) infection. *African Dental Journal* **1**, 5-8.

Silverman, S. Jr., Migliorati, C.A., Lozadanur, F., Greenspan, D. & Conant, M.A. (1986) Oral findings in people with or at high risk for AIDS: a study of 375 homosexual males. *Journal of the American Dental Association* **112**, 187-192.

Winkler, J.R., Murray, R.A., Greenspan, D. & Greenspan, J.S. (1986) AIDS virus associated periodontal disease. *Journal of Dental Research* **65**, Spec. Issue, Abstr. No. 139.

CHAPTER 11

Tumors and Tumor-like Lesions Originating from the Periodontium

The present descriptions of tumors and tumor-like lesions do not pretend to be a complete account of such lesions related to the periodontal tissues. They should serve as characteristic examples and emphasize partly that the periodontal tissues may be the origin of such lesions and partly that the reaction of these tissues may differ from reactions observed at other locations. The author distinguishes between a tumor and a neoplasm.

Epulides

Peripheral giant cell granuloma

Fig. 11-1 shows a rather large tumor between 22 and 23, which have become separated by the pressure exerted by the tumor. It is from a 58 year old man who for 6 months has had a swelling between 22 and 23. The tumor, which is bluish in color, is soft, well defined and the seat of an ulceration. Tumor-like lesions, originating from the gingiva, are called epulides, a term which is occasionally conceived as a synonym for a giant cell-containing process. This

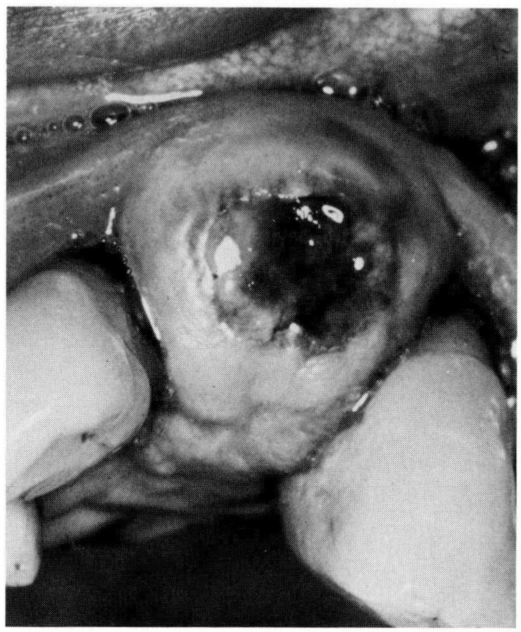

Fig. 11-1.

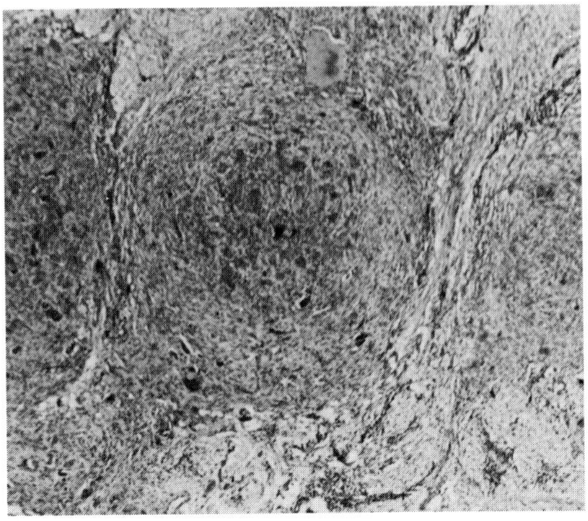

Fig. 11-2.

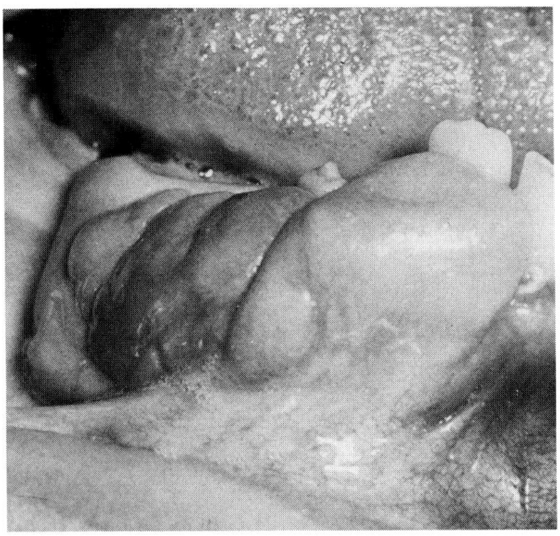

Fig. 11-3.

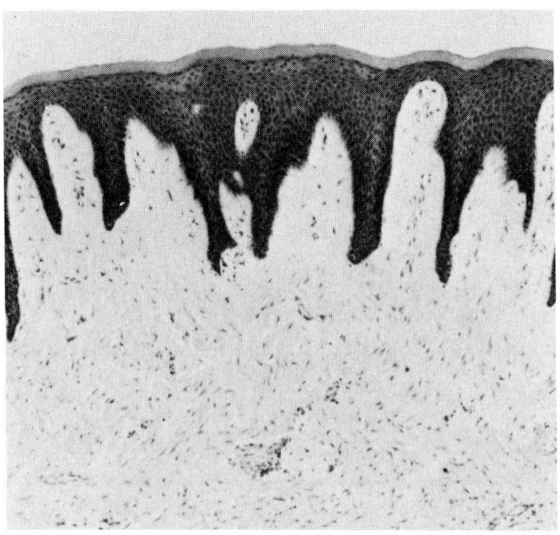

Fig. 11-4.

is an erroneous concept, as the term epulis, literally translated from Greek, only means "arisen from the gingiva". Many different pathologic processes may appear clinically as epulides. The peripheral giant cell granuloma, most often seen in younger individuals, is more frequent in women than in men, and the mandible is more often affected than the maxilla. The predominant location is facially in the anterior regions. Fig. 11-2 is a photomicrograph of the peripheral giant cell granuloma in Fig. 11-1. In the low power magnification, numerous giant cells can be identified. They occur in granuloma-like formations separated by septae of collagenous fibers. At the bottom of the picture osteoid tissue can be noticed. These two features: connective tissue septae and osteoid are characteristic of giant cell granulomas. Between the giant cells there is a vivid proliferation of endothelial cells leading to the formation of numerous small capillaries. In these areas many hemorrhages are seen, causing the typical color of the lesion. The giant cell granuloma has great growth potential as can be observed from Fig. 11-1. It is characteristic that the giant cell granuloma has a marked tendency for recurrence.

Gingival fibroma

Fig. 11-3 is from a 25 year old man who lacks the molars in the right side of the mandible. In contrast to the giant granuloma, the lesion illustrated in Fig. 11-3 is firm and of the same color as the adjacent mucosa. As the lesion contains fibrous tissue, it is often called a "fibrous epulis", a term which should be replaced by "gingival fibroma". These fibromas may vary in size, although it is quite rare to see such a large lesion as in Fig. 11-3. The fibroma occurs more often in women than in men and more frequently in the maxilla than in the mandible. The majority of these lesions is found in the anterior region. The gingival fibroma possesses considerable force and is able to separate the teeth from each other. Chronic irritation may play a part in the development of a gingival fibroma. Fig. 11-4 is a photomicrograph of such a fibroma, which is covered by squamous cell epithelium, slightly keratinized and shows some variations in the length of the epithelial ridges. The major part of the lesions consists of cell poor, collagenous tissue where the fiber bundles can be recognized. As the histologic structure is the same as in fibromas at other locations of the oral mucosa it is difficult to understand why the gingival fibroma is associated with a high rate of recurrence, not found at other locations.

Pyogenic granuloma

Fig. 11-5 illustrates a lesion in a 30 year old woman, between 22 and 21, which have become separated due to pressure from the lesion which is fiery red with small ulcerations. The appearance is characteristic of a pyogenic granuloma, sometimes called a telangiectatic granuloma. The pyogenic granuloma may occur in all areas of the oral mucosa, but is most frequently found on the marginal gingiva. The granuloma may be conceived as an exaggerated reaction to minor trauma without it having been possible to demonstrate a definite infectious organism. Due to its red color, which may sometimes turn to a cyanotic hue, the pyogenic granuloma may be mistaken for a giant cell granuloma. Fig. 11-6 is a photomicrograph of the lesion shown in Fig. 11-5. To the right in the picture there is a squamous cell epithelium; the rest of the surface is a fibrin covered ulceration. Just below the surface there is heavy acute inflammation. After that follows massive proliferation of endothelial cells characterized by numerous, very small and thin walled lumina. The content of erythrocytes in these luminae is responsible for the red color of the lesion. As is the case with the giant cell granuloma and the gingival fibroma, the pyogenic granuloma has a high potential for recurrence.

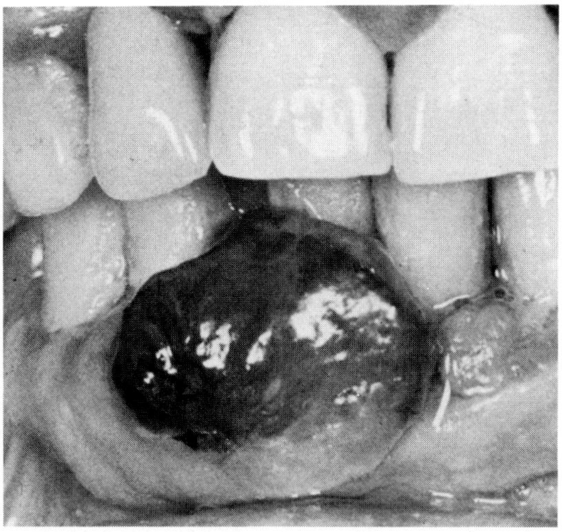

Fig. 11-5.

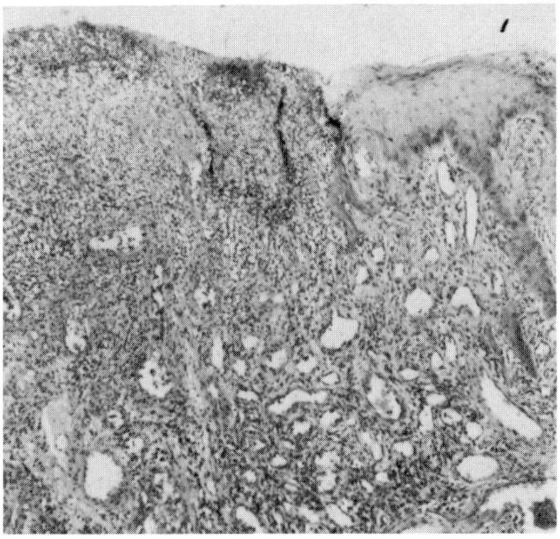

Fig. 11-6.

Benign neoplasms of oral mucosa

Neurilemoma

Fig. 11-7 shows an epulis (i.e. a tumor originating from the gingiva) in a 19 year old man who has had the lesion for the past 6 months. It originated suddenly as a soft, well defined tumor in the gingiva of 43. Since then, the lesion has become somewhat harder and two

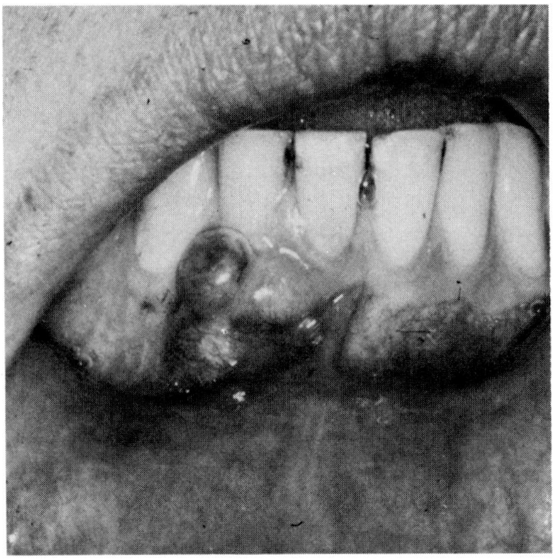

Fig. 11-7.

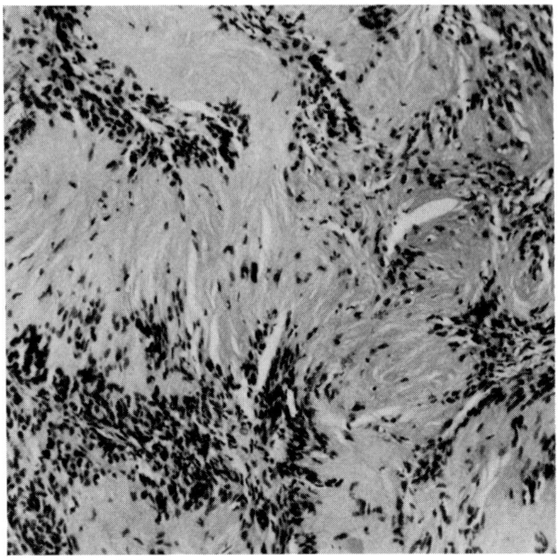

Fig. 11-8.

more lesions have appeared as can be seen in the illustration. The tumor extends down to the bottom of the labial groove. A radiographic examination does not reveal any osseous destruction. The "epulis" is surgically removed and the histologic examination shows a well encapsulated neoplasm. The fine structure is characterized by fusiform cells arranged as palisades and a cell free zone with delicate fibers as seen in Fig. 11-8. The neurilemoma is a benign tumor arising from the sheaths of peripheral nerves. When the neoplasm occurs in the mouth it is supposed to stem from branches of the fifth cranial nerve, the trigeminal. Clinically, the neoplasm is found in the superficial soft tissues as a firm, nodular tumor. The consistency may be softer when a cystic degeneration has taken place.

Capillary hemangioma

After fibromas, pyogenic granulomas and verruca vulgaris, hemangiomas are the most frequent tumors of the oral mucosa. Several authors doubt whether hemangiomas are true neoplasms and suggest they be classified as developmental anomalies. That may apply for the capillary type, but not for the cavernous hemangiomas. The latter are the second type of hemangiomas to be found in the mouth.

Fig. 11-9 shows a capillary hemangioma which not only affects the gingiva but also the corresponding area of the upper lip. The patient is a 20 year old man who has had the lesion as long as he can remember. It is deep red in color, slightly lobulated and often causes bleeding at toothbrushing. Fig. 11-10 is a photomicrograph of the hemangioma from Fig. 11-9. Two areas of intense endothelial proliferation can be seen with formation of small, thin walled vessels. Between the two areas there is a band of cell poor collagenous tissue. When Fig. 11-10 is compared with Fig. 11-16, depicting a pyogenic granuloma, it is evident that the endothelial proliferation of the pyogenic granuloma is complicated by a strong inflammatory reaction which is not observed in the capillary hemangioma.

Calcifying epithelial odontogenic tumor

Odontogenic tumors seldom originate from the periodontal tissues. It is often debated whether gingival fibromas with islands of odontogenic epithelium should be classified as odontogenic

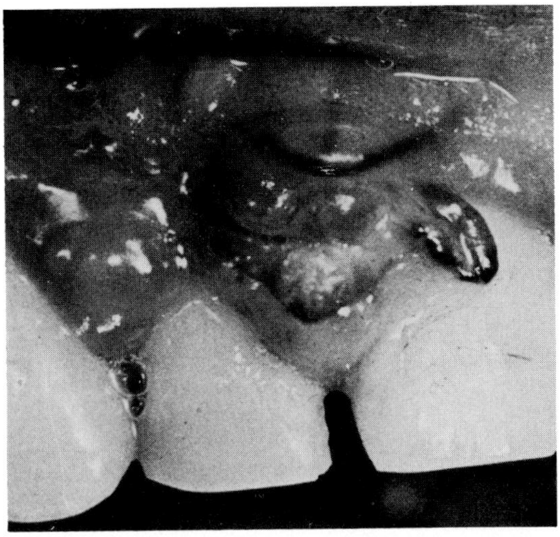

Fig. 11-9.

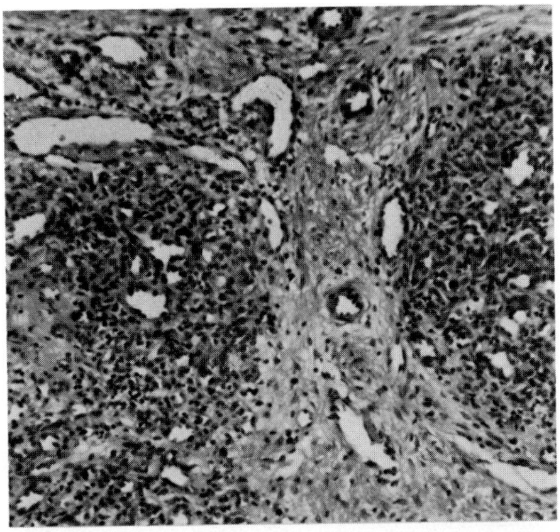

Fig. 11-10.

tumors. Some authors call these lesions odontogenic epithelial hamartomas. The following entities may occur as an "epulis": ameloblastoma, dentinoma, adenomatoid odontogenic tumor, calcifying odontogenic cyst and calcifying epithelial odontogenic tumor. The peripheral ameloblastoma presenting as a gingival tumor is by some authors conceived as the so-called "gingival basal cell carcinoma".

Fig. 11-11 is an example of a peripheral type of calcifying epithelial odontogenic tumor found in a 29 year old woman. The tumor manifests itself as a gingival swelling, firm and well demarcated. The lesion does not arise from the marginal gingiva for which reason it is not a true "epulis". The lesion has been present for 5 years and has not caused any symptoms. There are no osseous changes. Fig. 11-12 is a photomicrograph of the neoplasm in Fig. 11-11. The picture is dominated by large island of epithelium with odontogenic intracellular degeneration with swelling of the cytoplasm. In the illustration there are no calcifications, but these were found in other sections. An extraosseous location of the calcifying epithelial odontogenic tumor is rare; in an analysis of 113 cases only 5 were extraosseous.

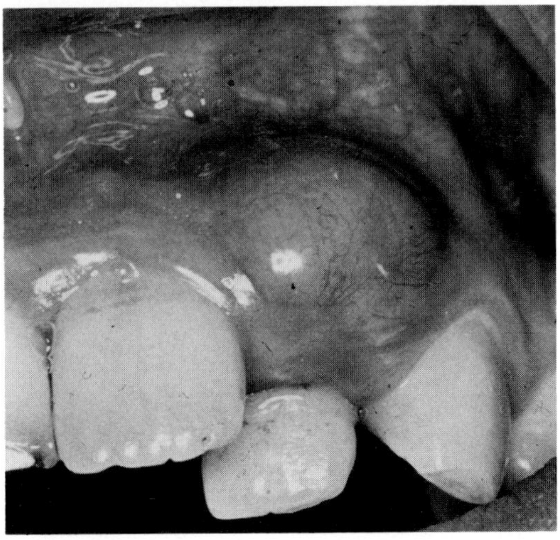

Fig. 11-11.

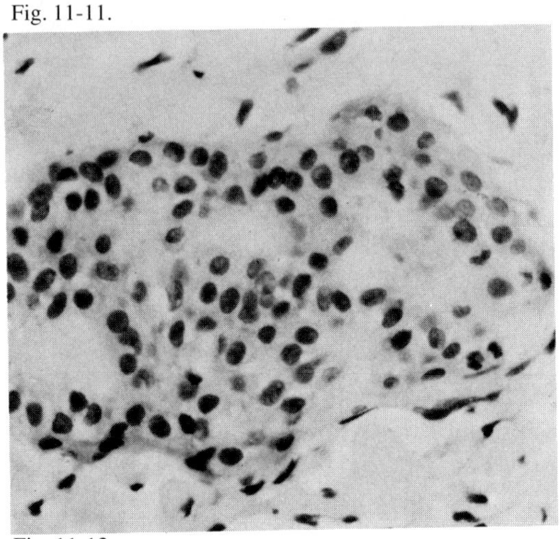

Fig. 11-12.

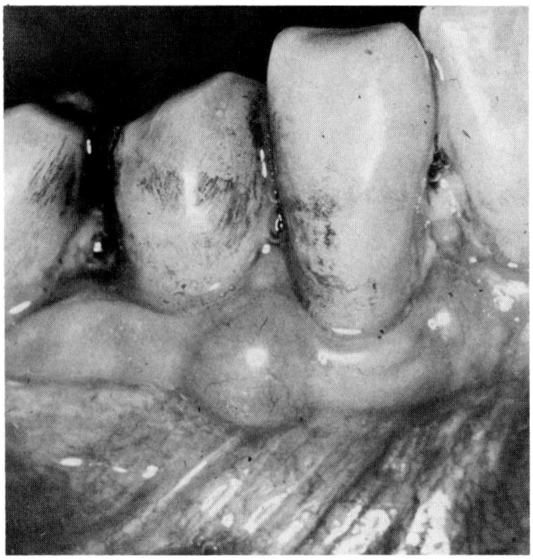

Fig. 11-13.

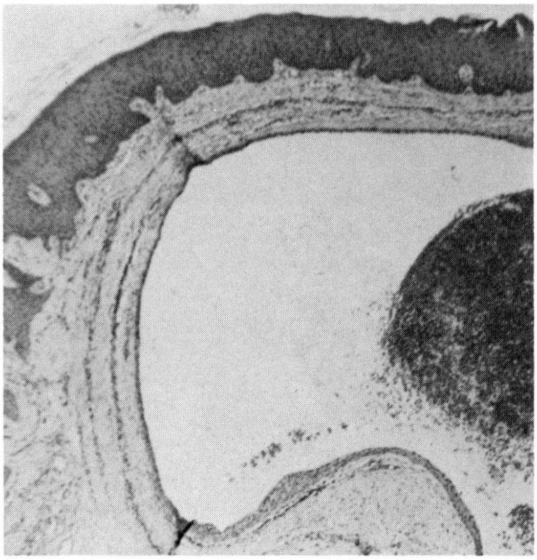

Fig. 11-14.

Cysts

Gingival cyst

Fig. 11-13 shows a well demarcated, soft and fluctuating swelling on the alveolar gingiva between 44 and 43 in a 75 year old woman. The presumed cyst is surgically removed and studied histologically. Fig. 11-14 illustrates a cyst, partially filled with erythrocytes. The wall of the cyst is a very thin, squamous cell epithelium, often only two layers thick, and nonkeratinized. Gingival cysts are most often found between the lateral incisor and first premolar on the facial aspect. Some cases are diagnosed clinically, whereas some are recognized histologically in biopsies from the gingiva. Clinically recognizable cysts are most frequent in the mandible. A gingival cyst may arise from (1) rests of the dental lamina, enamal organ, or the islands of Malassez, (2) degenerative, cystic changes in proliferating epithelial ridges from the gingival epithelium, or (3) from traumatic implantation of surface epithelium into the connective tissue. Gingival cysts are more prevalent than was hitherto thought.

Malignant tumors

Squamous cell carcinoma

Fig. 11-15 shows an ulcerated neoplasm in a 79 year old man, an ardent smoker, who for 1 month experienced symptoms from the gingiva. The neoplasm extends from 46 to 32 and is characterized by indurated margins and a fibrin covered ulceration appearing red on the picture. All four mandibular incisors are very loose and a radiograph reveals destruction of the osseous part of the periodontium. A biopsy (Fig. 11-16) shows a highly differentiated squamous cell carcinoma with horn pearl formation. The carcinoma is infiltrating the cross striated muscles at the bottom of the picture. The carcinoma has elicited a strong immunologic reaction illustrated by a massive accumulation of lymphocytes. In the literature it is rare to see a distinction maintained between a gingival cancer and a cancer developed on the edentulous alveolar ridge. Thus, many reports deal with cancer of the "gums". In most of these cases men have dominated, and only older people are affected. In recent years a marked shift in male/female ratio has been observed. In England the ratio was 5:1 in 1932-39, but in

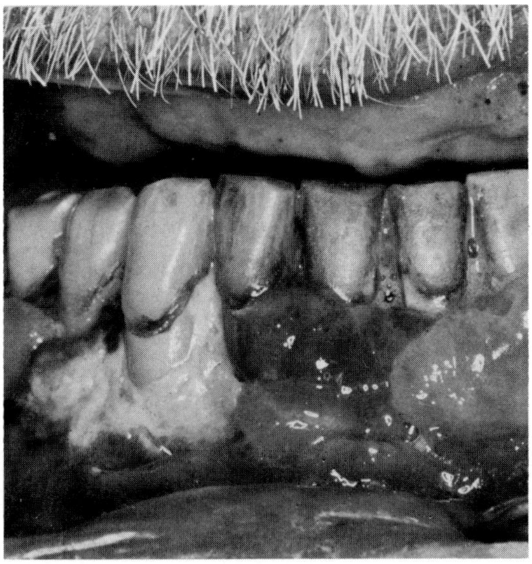

Fig. 11-15.

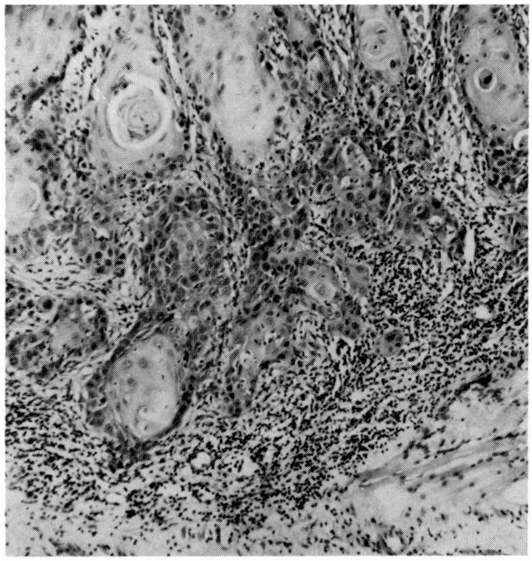

Fig. 11-16.

1960-69 it was 1:1. Most gingival cancers affect the maxilla and 60% are located posteriorly to the premolars. In an American study it has been shown that dentists play an important part in the early recognition of gingival cancer; 60% of these patients are first seen by a dentist. Gingival cancer begins as an ulceration, often associated with leukoplakia, and infiltrates rapidly in depth, with osseous involvement. In another American study gingival cancer had exceeded 3 cm at admission in 44% of the referred cases.

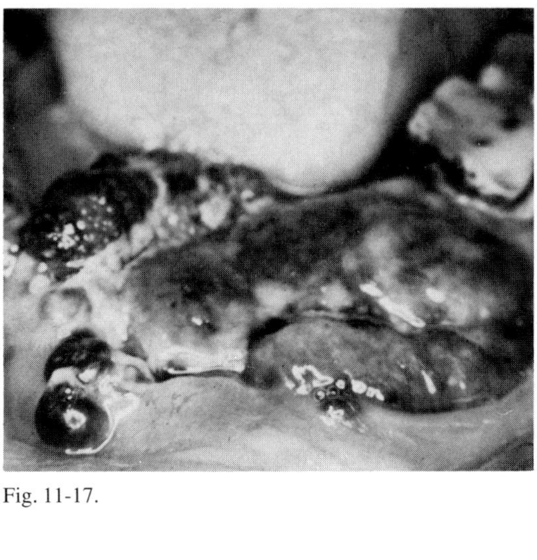

Fig. 11-17.

Malignant melanoma

Fig. 11-17 shows a large malignant melanoma originating from the gingiva in a dark skinned individual from Kerala in South India. Because of the growth of the neoplasm, the teeth in the affected area have been lost. In contrast to the carcinoma there is no induration at the periphery of the melanoma. Fig. 11-18 is a photomicrograph of a biopsy from a malignant melanoma similar to the neoplasm seen in Fig. 11-17. The surface epithelium is atrophic and a direct transition from epithelium to tumor tissue

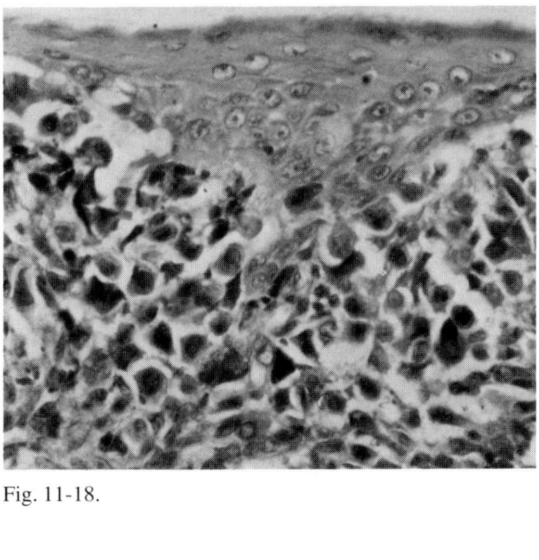

Fig. 11-18.

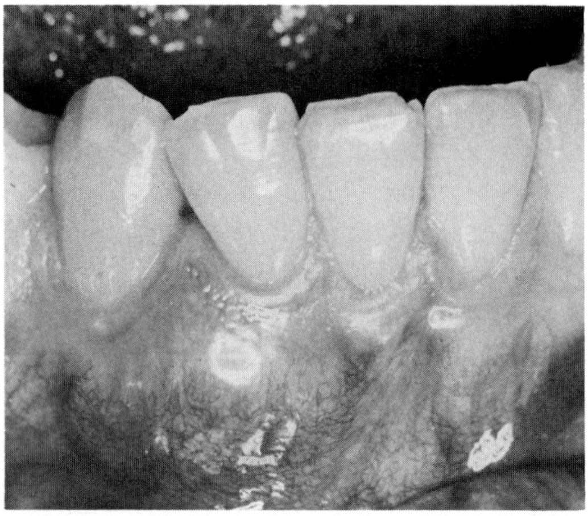

Fig. 11-19.

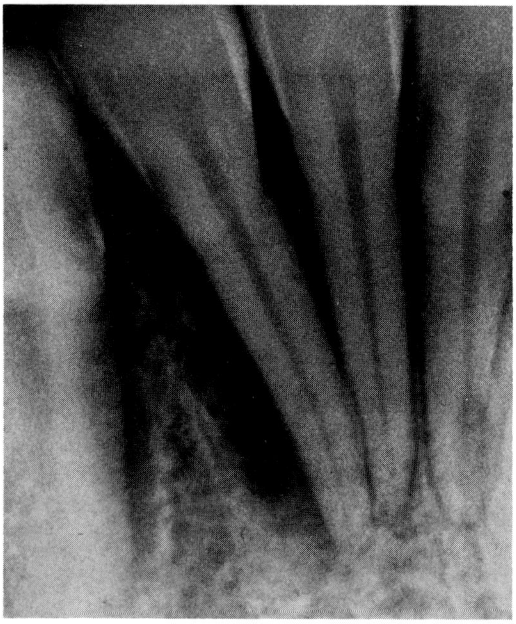

Fig. 11-20.

can be seen in the form of junctional activity. The tumor cells are large and very irregular in shape. There are many cells with abnormal accumulation of chromatin, and the mitotic activity is high. The black and white reproduction does not allow the recognition of the many melanin granules which are present in the cytoplasm of the tumor cells. The tumor originates from the melanocytes present in the basal layer of the oral epithelium.

Both sexes appear to be equally affected. The palatal mucosa is the favorite site for development of melanomas, followed by gingiva and tongue. The degree of pigmentation varies a great deal; in some cases the tumor is colorless, an amelanotic melanoma. Usually, the tumor is recognizable by a swelling which bleeds easily even after small traumas. The prognosis is worse for oral melanomas than for cutaneous melanomas. The 5 year survival rate is only 20% for oral melanomas. The prognosis is most severe in cases where the tumor arises suddenly and becomes substantial within a few weeks. In the early stages of a melanoma an amalgam tattoo and a blue nevus may be relevant in the differential diagnostic considerations.

Osteoblastic osteosarcoma

Fig. 11-19 shows a round, well demarcated, firm swelling on the alveolar gingiva between 43 and 42 in a 26 year old woman. It is also evident that 42 is tilted against 43. Two months before admission, the patient noticed soreness of 42, and for 5 days there had been a feeling of swelling in the affected region. A radiograph (Fig 11-20) reveals that the periodontal membrane distally to 42 is much widened. Mesially on 43 there is a lesser, but evident, widening of the periodontal membrane. As thcsc changes have only been reported in patients with osteosarcoma this diagnosis appears likely. A biopsy shows a typical osteoblastic osteosarcoma (Fig 11-21), to the right in the picture, the root surface of 42 can be seen. The periodontal membrane is very wide and most of the Sharpey's fibers are replaced by tumor tissue which consists partly of cellular tissue with tumor cells, partly of bone produced by the tumor cells. As these are similar to osteoblasts the tumor is designated as an osteoblastic osteosarcoma. In a 10 year follow-up period there has been no recurrence.

Fig. 11-21.

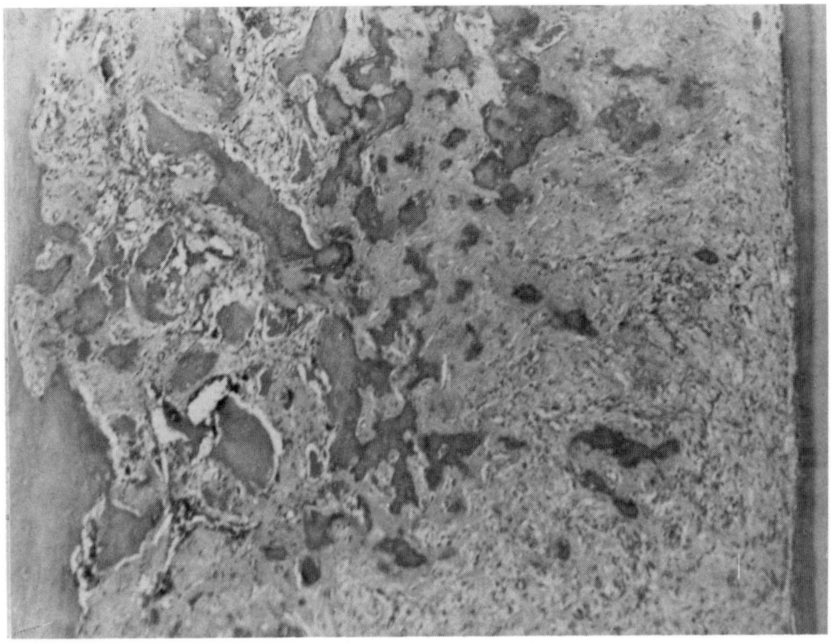

Chondroblastic osteosarcoma

Fig. 11-22 is a radiograph of the area between 21 and 22 in a 26 year old woman who 3 months before admission noticed a swelling of the affected region. Clinically, there is an elongation of 21, which is slightly tilted. There is a marked widened periodontal membrane with an irregular contour comprising small radiopaque bodies. A biopsy shows that the lesion is a chondroblastic osteosarcoma. After resection of the area containing the tumor the patient was followed for 11 years without any signs of recurrence. A Danish study has shown that there is one jaw osteosarcoma per year per million population. A U.S. study has found 0.07 cases of jaw osteosarcoma per 100,000 population per year. 1/6 of the jaw sarcomas encountered are osteosarcomas. In recent years it has been recognized that a number of jaw osteosarcomas will have, as their first manifestation, a widening of the periodontal membrane as described in the 2 cases above. When the first symptoms of a jaw osteosarcoma appear the patients are, on average, 30 years old, a decade older than for osteosarcomas in other bones. The mandible is more often affected than the maxilla. Although trauma may occasionally be present in the case history, the majority of patients give no information of trauma. In contrast to carcinomas, swellings associated with osteosarcomas are rarely ulcerated.

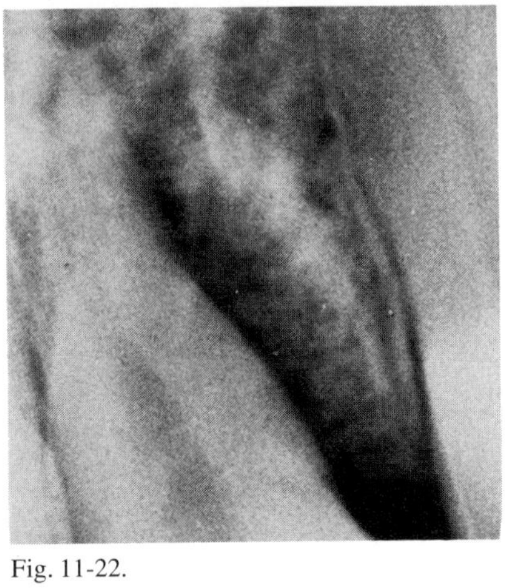

Fig. 11-22.

Metastasis from an adenocarcinoma of colon

Fig 11-23 is a radiograph of the area 43-31 in a 60 year old man who has an indolent swelling

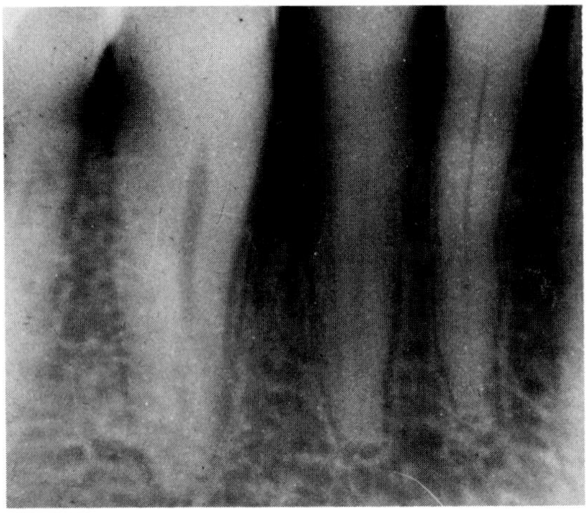

Fig. 11-23.

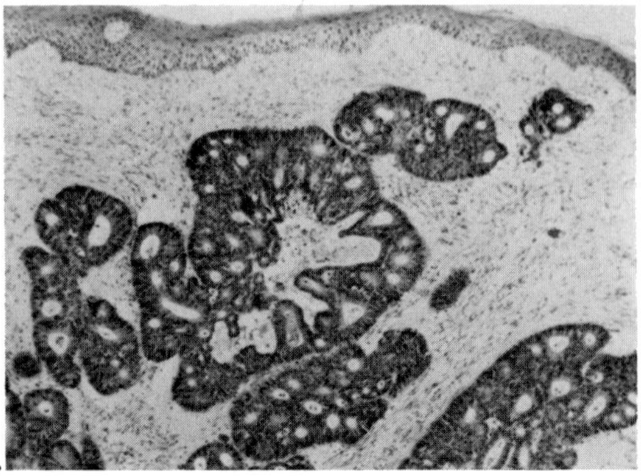

Fig. 11-24.

of the gingiva, an "epulis", corresponding to 43-31, recognized by the patient 2 weeks before admission. The radiograph reveals an osseous destruction between 43 and 42. Two weeks later the two teeth are extracted due to a marked purulent exudation from the pockets. As the swelling has not disappeared 3 weeks after the extractions, a biopsy is taken showing an adenocarcinoma. The past history of the patient reveals that 5 years ago he was operated on for an adenocarcinoma of the colon. Three years later there are lung metastases and then, after a further 2 years, the gingival metastasis develops. Four months after gingival biopsy the patient dies from extensive metastases. The histologic picture is typical of an adenocarcinoma (Fig 11-24). In a Finnish analysis of 331 metastases to the oral tissues 8% were from carcinoma of the colon and rectum. Of the 26 cases, 22 were found in the mandible and only 3 in the maxilla. In 2 cases, metastases to the soft tissue of the mouth could be demonstrated.

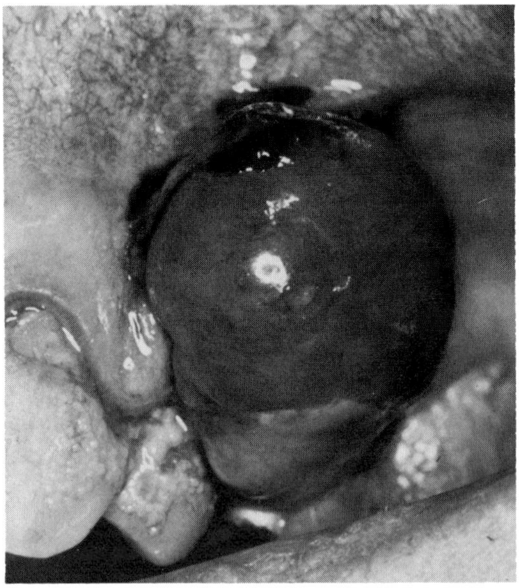

Fig. 11-25.

Metastasis from lung carcinoma

Fig. 11-25 shows a large "epulis" originating from the gingiva between 24 and 25 in a 65 year old woman who, for 4 months, has had a pain in the left side of the mandible. Two

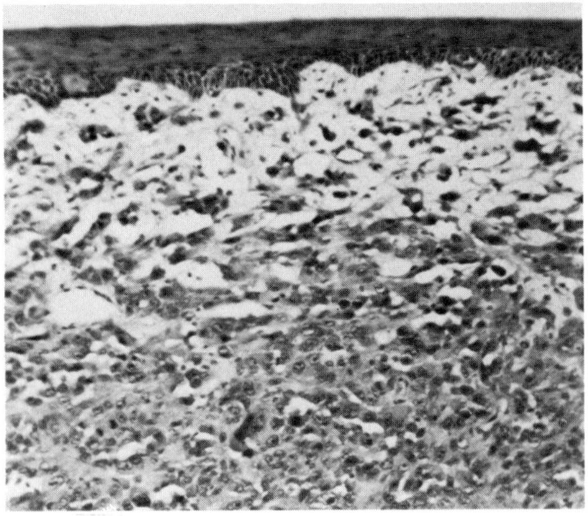

Fig. 11-26.

weeks before admission the patient noticed a swelling of the gingiva corresponding to the premolars in the left side of the maxilla. The tumor is soft, fiery red and, in the incisal third, the seat of a fibrin covered ulceration. The entire tumor is removed surgically and studied histologically (Fig 11-26). The microscopic diagnosis is a low differentiated carcinoma with suspected metastasis. As the patient has been operated on 3 months previously for a lung carcinoma, it is concluded that the "epulis" most likely is a metastasis from primary lung tumor. The photomicrograph shows that the surface is covered by an atrophic epithelium. Just below the surface epithelium, tumor tissue is present without a capsule. A certain nuclear pleomorphism can be recognized even at the low power magnification. Among the metastases to the oral regions, lung cancer occupies the second place after metastases from mammary cancers. Whereas the majority of metastases are to the osseous part of the mandible, a number of lung metastases will occur in the form of an "epulis", a fact which emphasizes the need for a histologic examination of all "epulides". In a recent study of metastases to the oral regions it turned out that there is an increase in a number of reported cases of metastases from lung tumors, due most likely to the explosive increase of smoking related lung cancers. In an analysis

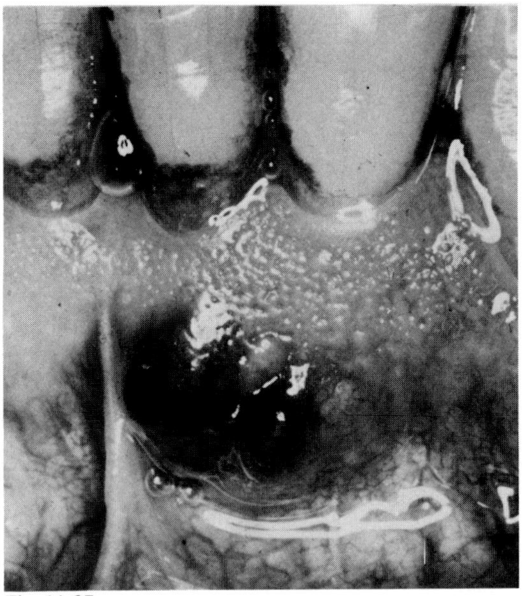

Fig. 11-27.

of 18 cases of metastases to the soft tissues of the mouth, not less than 50% occur as an "epulis". In a Finnish analysis of soft tissue metastases to the mouth, 30% were localized to the gingiva.

Kaposi's sarcoma

In 1872 Kaposi described what he called "multiple idiopathic hemorrhagic sarcoma"

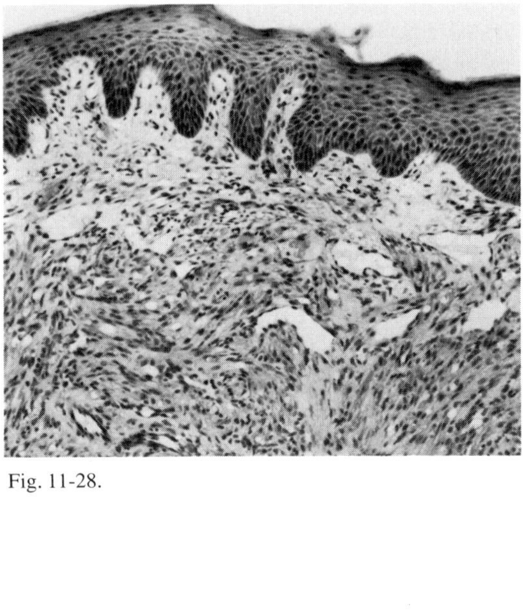

Fig. 11-28.

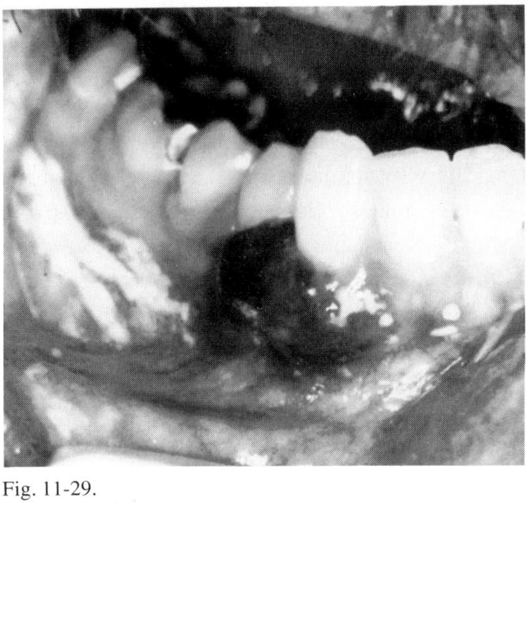

Fig. 11-29.

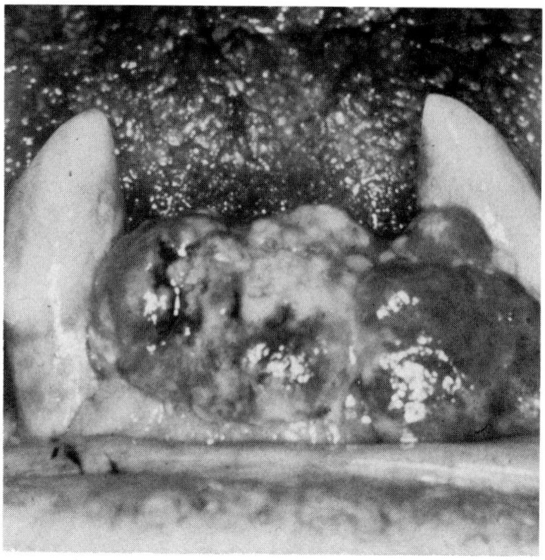

Fig. 11-30.

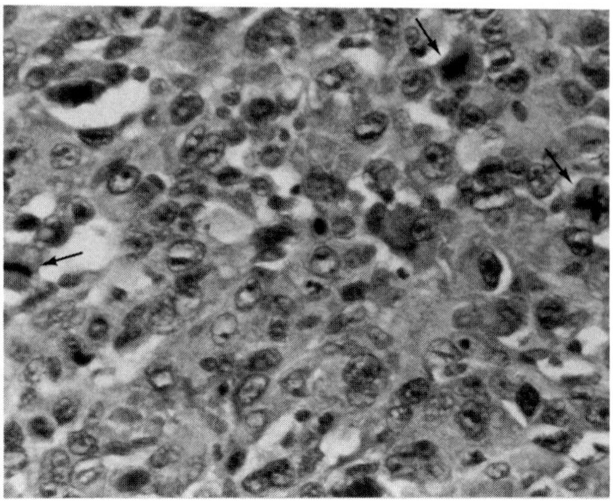

Fig. 11-31

which later came to bear his name. Most of his patients were Jews, especially Ashkenazim. Later it was reported that Kaposi's sarcoma occurred among people living around the Mediterranean.

Then, in the middle of the 50's, reports came from Sub-Saharan Africa that Kaposi's sarcoma was a prevalent malignant tumor in that area. It is characteristic that oral manifestations of Kaposi's sarcoma in Jews and Africans are rare.

The next phase in the occurrence of Kaposi's sarcoma was the recognition of the disease in individuals who had had a kidney transplantation and had been treated with immunosuppressive drugs. Related to the immunosuppressive therapy, the patient illustrated in Fig. 11-27 first developed a herpetic gingivostomatitis with manifestations in several areas of the oral mucosa. Some weeks after that attack, Kaposi's sarcoma was diagnosed on the left crus and a few days later oral lesions appeared in the same areas which had been affected by the herpetic infection. The oral Kaposi sarcoma lesions were red, elevated, angioma-like and well demarcated. Fig. 11-27 illustrates the gingival lesion, which was removed and subjected to histologic examination. Fig. 11-28 shows the typical features of the tumor: a cell rich lesion containing many thin walled vascular luminae. There is an increased number of mitoses of which some are atypical.

The last phase, so far, in the occurrence of Kaposi's sarcoma is among homosexual men suffering from the acquired immunodeficiency syndrome (AIDS). The appearance of a Kaposi's sarcoma is one of the criteria for the development of AIDS in patients infected with human immunodeficiency virus (HIV). In most instances the Kaposi's sarcoma will first appear as skin lesions followed by oral lesions. In rare cases oral manifestations may be the first sign of Kaposi's sarcoma. The frequency of oral manifestations is high, varying from 70 to 100%. The site of predilection in the mouth is the palate, but gingiva is often the seat of the lesions. Fig. 11-29 illustrates a typical manifestion appearing as an "epulis" in a 39 year old homosexual man with AIDS. A biopsy revealed the same histologic structure as illustrated in Fig. 11-28. There is agreement that the cell of origin for all the four types of Kaposi's sarcoma is the endothelial cell.

Histiocytic lymphoma

Previously, histiocytic lymphoma was called reticulosarcoma. It is a malignant tumor consisting of large cells with rather bright nuclei.

Many mitoses are present and in a number of cases a reticulum stain will disclose fine argyrophilic fibrils around the tumor cells. Fig. 11-30 shows a large and soft tumor in the incisor region of a 73 year old man, who 3 years previously has been operated on for a histiocytic lymphoma in the stomach. The tumor is ulcerated but not indurated. Fig. 11-31 is a photomicrograph of an oral histiocytic lymphoma. The arrows indicate three mitotic figures. The primary histiocytic lymphoma is rare in the oral cavity. When it occurs, the diagnosis may be quite difficult to arrive at as the first manifestations may resemble a nonspecific periodontal disease or a pericoronitis.

In HIV infected patients non-Hodgkin's lymphomas occur with increased frequency. Occasionally an "epulis" may be the first manifestation of a non-Hodgkin's lymphoma in an HIV infected patient (Fig. 11-32).

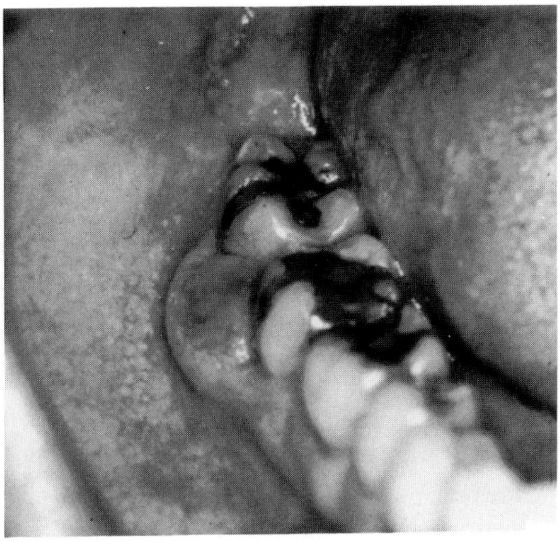

Fig. 11-32.

References

Cawson, R.A. & Eveson, J.W. *Oral pathology and diagnosis*. London: William Heinemann Medical Books.

Lucas, R.B. (1984). *Pathology of tumors of the oral tissues*. Edinburgh: Churchill, Livingstone.

Pindborg, J.J. (1985). *Atlas of diseases of the oral mucosa*. Copenhagen: Munksgaard.

CHAPTER 12

Examination of Patients with Periodontal Disease

Symptoms of periodontal disease

Clinically, periodontal disease is characterized by color and texture alterations of the gingiva, e.g. redness and swelling, as well as an increased tendency to bleeding on probing in the gingival sulcus/pocket area (Figs. 12-1 a-c). In addition, the periodontal tissues may exhibit a reduced resistance to probing (increased depth of the clinical pocket) and/or tissue recession. Advanced stages of the disease are also frequently associated with increased tooth mobility and drifting of teeth.

In the radiograph, periodontal disease may be recognized by reduced height of the alveolar bone (Fig. 12-2). If bone loss has progressed at a similar rate in a certain part of the dentition, the crestal contour of the remaining bone in the radiograph is even: "horizontal" bone loss. Angular bony defects are the result of bone loss which has developed at different rates around different teeth/tooth surfaces: "vertical" bone loss.

In the histological section, periodontal disease is characterized by the presence of an inflammatory cell infiltrate (Fig. 12-3) within an area of the gingival connective tissue adjacent to the bacterial deposits on the tooth. Within the infiltrated area there is a pronounced loss of collagen. In more advanced forms of periodontal disease, loss of connective tissue attachment and apical downgrowth of dentogingival epithelium are important findings.

Results from clinical and animal research have demonstrated that periodontal disease

1. affects different parts of the dentition to a varying degree,
2. is often progressive in character and, if left untreated, may result in tooth loss,
3. can be arrested or even cured following proper therapy. In order to arrive at a meaningful treatment plan, periodontal disease has to be recognized and its involvement in various parts of the dentition identified.

Examination of a patient with respect to perio-

Fig. 12-1 a-c. Clinical status of a patient suffering from advanced periodontal disease. Note the presence of different signs of periodontal disease such as texture alterations of the gingiva, gingival recessions (in the region of teeth 23 and 31), crowding of teeth (the mandibular front teeth), pus formation (tooth 14) and drifting of the premolars and molars.

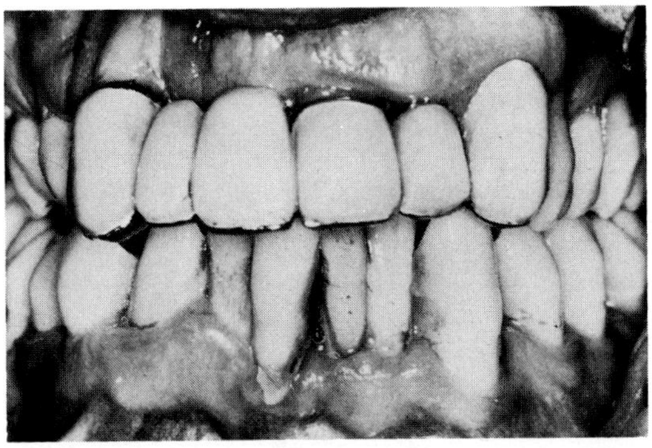

Fig. 12-1a.

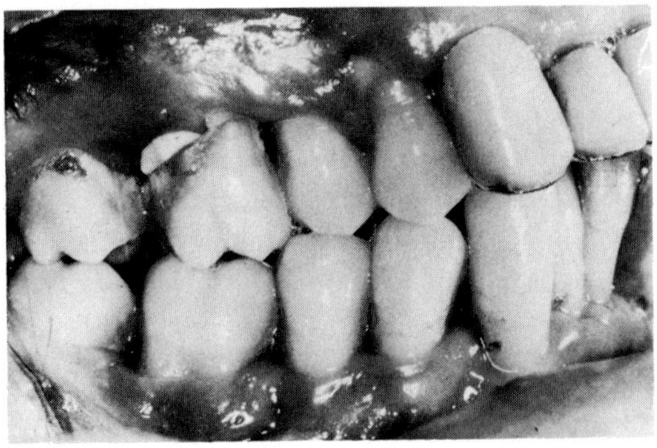

Fig. 12-1b.

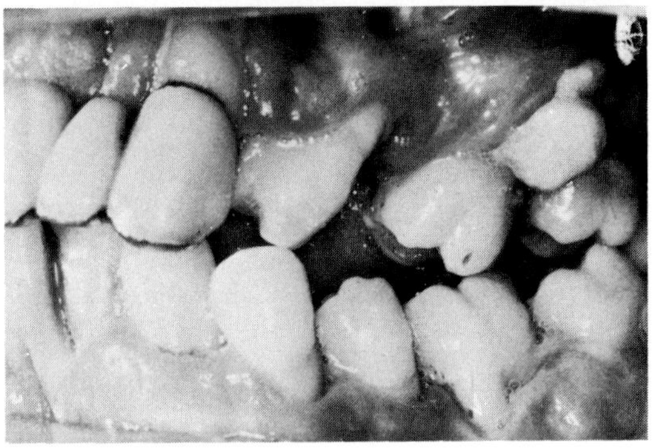

Fig. 12-1c.

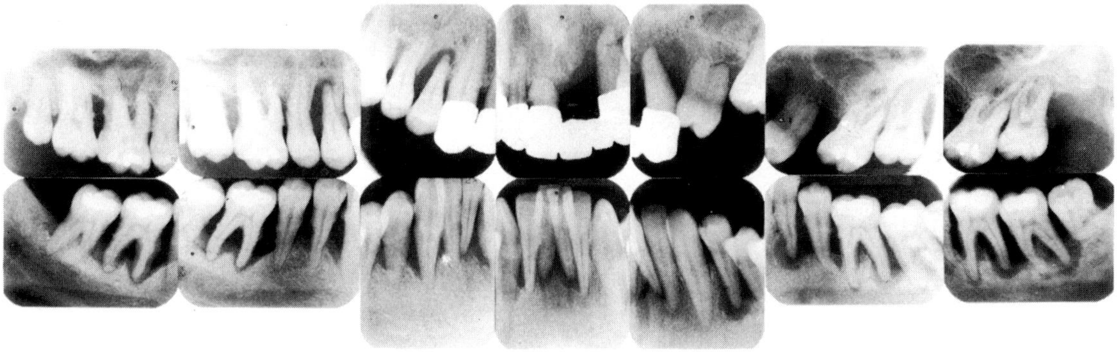

Fig. 12-2. Radiographic status of the patient described in Figs. 12-1 a-c.

dontal disease must not only identify sites with inflammatory alterations in the dentition but also the extent of tissue breakdown in these sites. The examination should therefore include all parts of the dentition and describe the periodontal conditions at all buccal, lingual and approximal tooth surfaces. Since periodontal disease includes inflammatory alterations of the gingiva and a progressive loss of periodontal ligament and alveolar bone, the examination must include measures describing such pathological alterations.

Fig. 12-4 a-c illustrates the clinical status of a 55-year-old male with periodontal disease. The examination procedures used in evaluating the location and extension of periodontal disease will be demonstrated by using this case as an example.

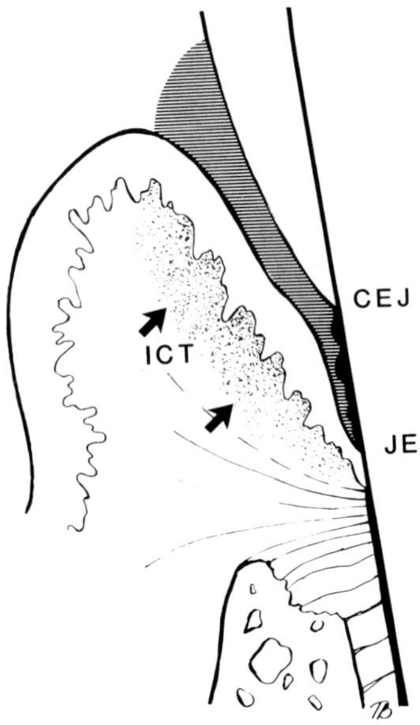

Fig. 12-3. Schematic drawing illustrating the histological features of periodontal disease. Note the infiltrated connective tissue area (ICT).

The gingiva

Clinical signs of gingival inflammation include changes in color and texture of the soft marginal tissue and an increased tendency for bleeding on probing.

Various index systems have been developed to describe gingivitis in epidemiological and clinical research (for a detailed presentation of these indices the reader is referred to Chapter 2). In the individual patient, refined and qualitative distinctions between various forms of gingivitis, i.e., initial, early and established gingival lesions (Page & Schroeder 1976), serve no meaningful purpose since the correct diagnosis of the gingival lesion can be made only in the histological section. Since, however, the symptom "bleeding on probing" to the bottom of the gingival sulcus/pocket is associated with the presence of an inflammatory cell infiltrate in this area, the occurrence of such bleeding is an important indicator of disease. The identification of the apical extent of the gingival lesion

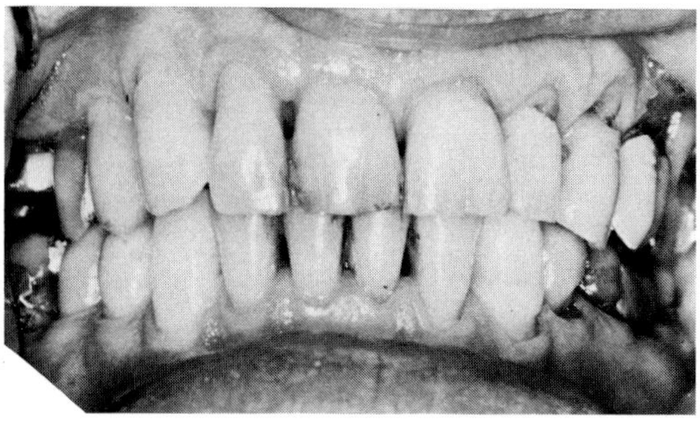

Fig. 12-4a.

Fig. 12-4 a-c. Clinical status of a 55-year-old male with periodontal disease.

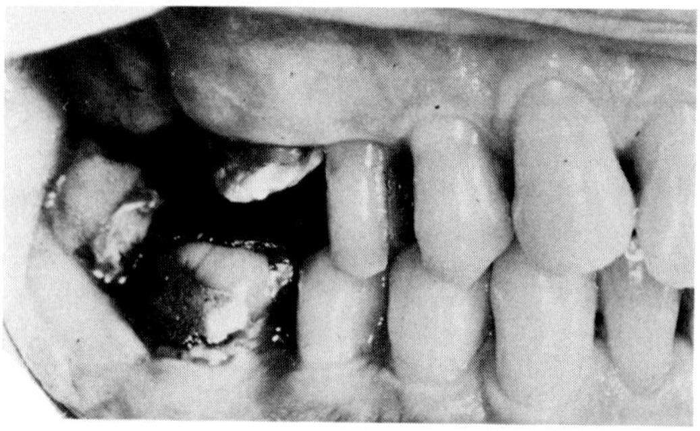

Fig. 12-4b.

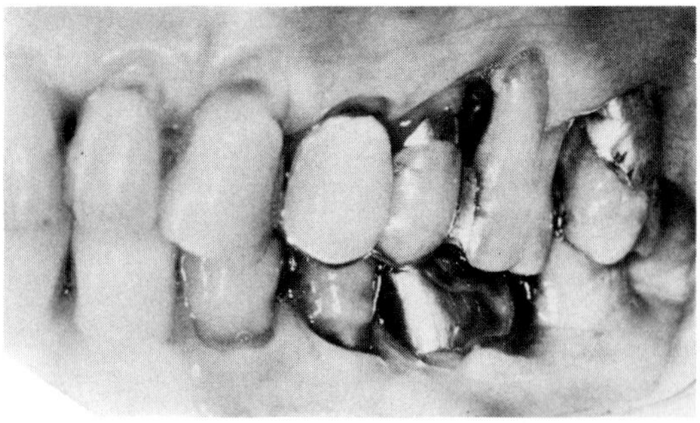

Fig. 12-4c.

is made in conjunction with *pocket depth measurements*. This means that in sites where "shallow" pockets are present, inflammatory lesions residing in the overt portion of the gingiva are distinguished by probing in the superficial marginal tissue. When the infiltrate resides in sites with deepened pockets and attachment loss, the inflammatory lesion in the apical part of the pocket should be identified by probing to the bottom of the deepened pocket and not by probing in the marginal portion of the gingiva.

Bleeding on probing: a blunt periodontal probe is inserted to the "bottom" of the gingival pocket and is moved gently along the tooth (root) surface (Fig. 12-5). If bleeding is provoked by this instrumentation, the site examined is considered inflamed.

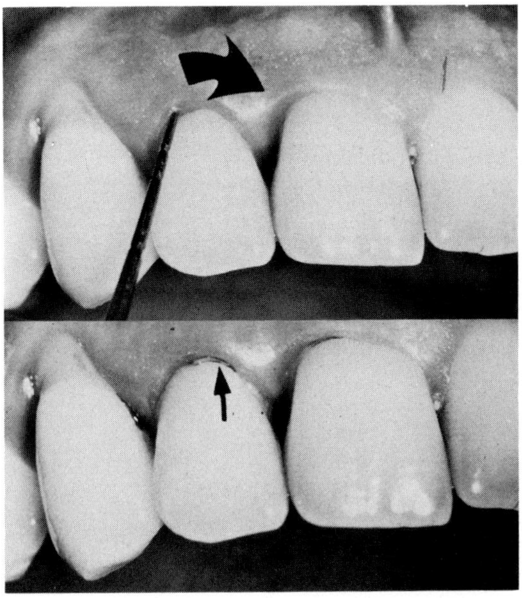

Fig. 12-5. Pocket probing used to identify gingival inflammation. A site is considered inflamed if bleeding is provoked by gentle probing to the bottom of the pocket.

Fig. 12-6 illustrates the chart used to identify gingival sites which at the initial examination of the 55-year-old patient referred to above were found to bleed on probing. Each tooth in the chart is represented by a square and each tooth surface by a triangle. The upper triangle represents the buccal gingival unit, the bottom triangle the lingual unit and the remaining fields the 2 approximal gingival units. A cross is inserted in the fields of the chart which corresponds to the inflamed gingival units. The mean gingivitis score is given as a percentage figure. In the present patient (Fig. 12-4 a-c) 27 out of a total number of 52 gingival units in the maxilla bled on probing. The gingivitis score for the maxillary dentition is thus 50%. The corresponding score for the mandibular dentition is 59%. This method of charting not only serves as a means of documenting areas of health and disease in the dentition but similar charting during the course of therapy will disclose sites which remain inflamed.

Sites with gingivitis

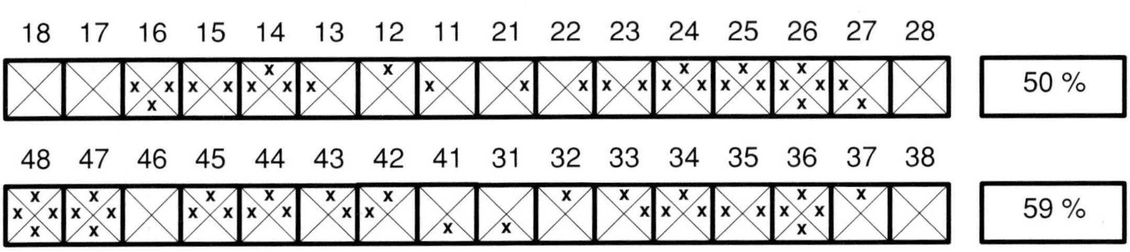

Fig. 12-6. The gingivitis chart of the patient seen in Fig. 12-4.

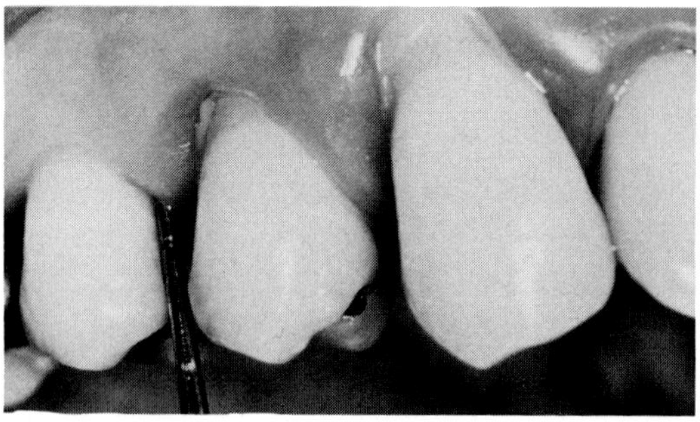

Fig. 12-7. Measurement of probing depth. Note the gingival recession at the buccal aspect of teeth 14 and 13.

The periodontal ligament - the root cementum

In order to evaluate the amount of tissue lost in periodontal disease and also to identify the apical extension of the inflammatory lesion the following parameters should be recorded:

a. pocket depth (probing depth)
b. attachment level (probing attachment level)
c. furcation involvement
d. tooth mobility

Assessment of pocket depth

The pocket depth, i.e. the distance from the gingival margin to the bottom of the gingival pocket, is measured by means of a graduated probe (Fig. 12-7). The pocket depth should be assessed at each surface of all teeth in the dentition. In the periodontal chart (Fig. 12-10) it may be sufficient to identify only the deepest value recorded at each tooth surface. Pocket depth values of < 4 mm may be excluded from the chart since such pockets can be regarded as falling within normal variations.

Results from pocket depth measurements only in rare situations (when the gingival margin coincides with the cementoenamel junction) give proper information regarding the extent of loss of attachment. For example, an inflammatory edema may cause a swelling of the free gingiva resulting in a coronal displacement of the gingival margin without a concomitant migration of the dentogingival epithelium to a level apical to the cementoenamel junction. In such a situation a pocket depth exceeding 3-4 mm represents a so-called "pseudopocket". In other situations, an obvious loss of attachment may have occurred without a concomitant increase of the pocket depth. A situation of this kind is shown in Fig. 12-7 at the buccal aspect of teeth 14 and 13 (two-digit systems; FDI 1970) where recessions of the gingiva can be seen.

Assessment of attachment level

Attachment levels may be assessed by means of a graduated probe and expressed as the distance in mm from the cemento-enamel junction to the bottom of the gingival pocket. The longest distance for each tooth surface is recorded and may be included in the periodontal chart.

Errors inherent in periodontal probing

The distances recorded in a periodontal examination using a periodontal probe have generally been assumed to represent a fairly accurate estimate of the pocket depth or attachment level at a given site. In other words, the tip of the probe has been assumed to identify the level of the most apical cells of the dentogingival epithelium. Results from research published in the 1970s have demonstrated, however, that this is seldom the case (Saglie et al. 1975, Listgarten et al. 1976, Armitage et al. 1977, Ezis & Burgett 1978, Spray et al. 1978, Robinson & Vitek 1979, van der Velden 1979, Magnusson & Listgarten 1980, Polson et al. 1980). Listgarten (1980) listed a variety of factors which influence the result of a measurement made

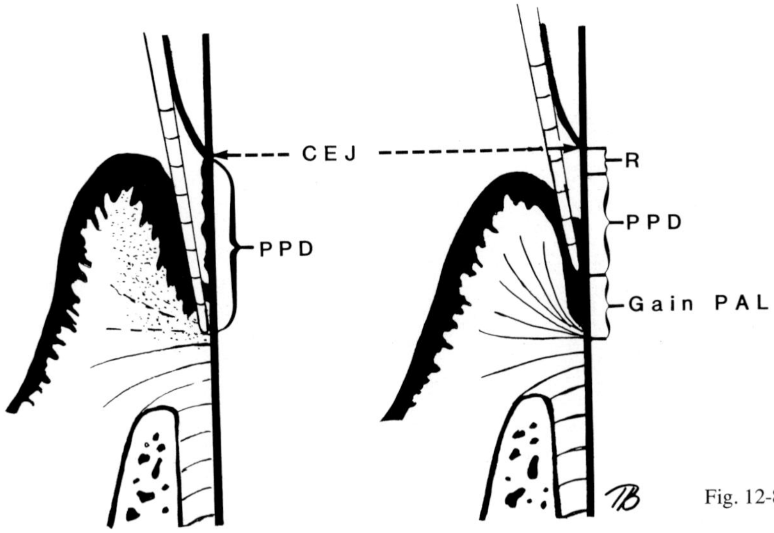

Fig. 12-8a. Fig. 12-8b.

Fig. 12-8. In the presence of gingivitis the probe penetrates apically to the bottom of the histological pocket (a). Following successful therapy the gingival infiltrate is replaced by collagen (b); The probe fails to reach the apical part of the dento-gingival epithelium. CEJ = cementoenamel junction. PPD = probing pocket depth, PAL = probing attachment level, R = recession.

with a periodontal probe. These factors include 1) the thickness of the probe used, 2) malposition of the probe due to anatomic features such as the contour of the tooth surface, 3) the pressure applied on the instrument during probing, 4) the degree of inflammatory cell infiltration in the soft tissue and accompanying loss of collagen, etc. Listgarten suggested that "a distinction should be made between the histological and the clinical pocket depth to differentiate between the depth of the actual anatomic defect and the measurement recorded by the probe".

Measurement errors depending on factors such as the thickness of the probe, the contour of the tooth surface and improper angulation of the probe can be reduced or avoided by the selection of a proper instrument and careful management of the examination procedure. More difficult to avoid, however, are errors resulting from variations in probing force and the extent of inflammatory alterations of the periodontal tissues. As a rule, the greater the probing force, the deeper is the penetration of the probe into the tissue. In this context it should be realized that, in investigations designed to disclose the force used by different clinicians, the probing force was found to range from 3-130 g (Gabathuler & Hassell 1971, Hassell et al. 1973), and also to differ by as much as 2:1 for the same dentist from one examination to another. In order to exclude measurement errors related to the effect of variations in probing force, so-called pressure sensitive probes have been developed. Such probes will enable the examiner to probe with a predertermined force (van der Velden & de Vries 1978, Vitek et al. 1979, Polson et al. 1980). However, over- and underestimation of the "true" pocket depth or attachment level may occur also when this type of probing device is employed (Armitage et al. 1977, Robinson & Vitek 1979, Polson et al. 1980). Thus, when the connective tissue subjacent to the pocket epithelium is infiltrated by inflammatory cells, the periodontal probe will most certainly penetrate beyond the apical termination of the dentogingival epithelium. This results in an overestimation of the "true" depth of the pocket. Conversely, when the inflammatory infiltrate decreases in size following successful periodontal treatment, and a concomi-

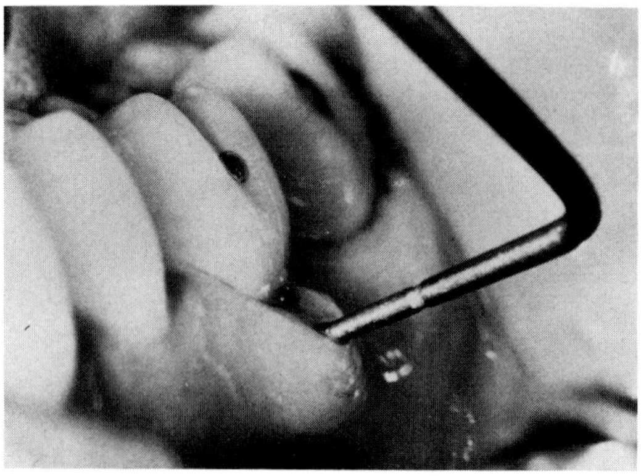

Fig. 12-9. A periodontal probe inserted into the buccal furcation area of a mandibular molar. A furcation involvement of degree 2 was found.

tant deposition of new collagen takes place within the previously inflamed tissue area, the dentogingival tissue will become more resistant to penetration by the probe. The probe may now fail to reach the apical termination of the epithelium. This results in an underestimation of the "true" pocket depth or attachment level. The magnitude of the difference between the probing measurement and the histologic "true" pocket depth may range from fractions of a millimeter to several millimeters (Listgarten 1980).

From this discussion it should be understood that reduction of pocket depths following periodontal treatment and/or gain of attachment, assessed by periodontal probing, are not necessarily signs of formation of a new connective tissue attachment in the bottom of the previous pocket. Rather, such a change may merely represent a resolution of the inflammatory process without an accompanying attachment gain (Fig. 12-8). In this context it should be realized that the terms "pocket depth" and "gain and loss of attachment" in modern literature have often been changed to the more exact terms "probing depth" and "gain and loss of clinical attachment" or "probing pocket depth" and "probing attachment level".

Current knowledge of the histopathology of periodontal lesions and healing of such lesions has thus resulted in an altered concept regarding the validity of periodontal probing. However, despite difficulties in interpreting the proper significance of pocket depth and attachment level measurements, such determinations still give the clinician a useful estimation of the degree of disease involvement and particularly so when the information obtained is related to other findings of the examination procedures such as "bleeding on probing", alveolar bone height alterations, etc.

Assessment of furcation involvement

In progression of periodontal disease around multirooted teeth the destructive process may involve the supporting structures of the furcation area (Fig. 12-9). Elaborate therapeutic techniques must often be used to properly treat such *furcation involvements*. Therefore, the precise identification of the presence and extension of periodontal tissue breakdown within the furcation area of each multirooted tooth is of importance for proper diagnosis and treatment planning.

Furcation involvements may be classified into:

Degree 1: horizontal loss of supporting tissues not exceeding 1/3 of the width of the tooth.

Degree 2: horizontal loss of supporting tissues exceeding 1/3 of the width of the tooth, but not encompassing the total width of the furcation area.

Degree 3: horizontal "through-and-through" destruction of the supporting tissues in the furcation.

The degree of furcation involvement is presented in the periodontal chart (Fig. 12-10) together with a description of which tooth surface the involvement has been identified on (e.g. tooth 26: 2m,b,d; tooth 48: 2b; tooth 36: 2b,1 etc.). A detailed discussion regarding diagnosis of furcation involvements and treatment of furcation-involved teeth is presented in Chapter 20.

Assessment of tooth mobility

The continuous loss of the supporting tissues in progressive periodontal disease may result in increased tooth mobility. Increased tooth mobility may be classified in the following way:

Degree 1: Movability of the crown of the tooth 0.2-1 mm in horizontal direction

Degree 2: Movability of the crown of the tooth exceeding 1 mm in horizontal direction

Degree 3: Movability of the crown of the tooth in vertical direction as well.

In this context it should be realized that plaque-associated periodontal disease is not the only cause of increased tooth mobility. For instance, overloading of teeth and trauma may result in tooth hypermobility. Increased tooth mobility can frequently be observed also in conjunction with periapical lesions, immediately following periodontal surgery, etc. From a therapeutic point of view it is important not only to assess the degree of increased tooth mobility but also the cause of the observed hypermobility (see Chapters 8 and 21).

All data collected in conjunction with measurements of pocket depths and attachment levels and from the assessments of furcation involvements and tooth mobility are included in the periodontal chart (Fig. 12-10). The various teeth in this chart are denoted according to the two-digit system adopted by FDI in 1970.

Periodontal chart							Diagnosis
							Gingivitis Parodontitis levis Parodontitis gravis et complicata
Tooth	Pocket depth M	B	D	L	Furcation involvement	Tooth mobility	
~~18~~							
~~17~~							
16	4	4	4		3		
15	4		6			1	
14	5		6	4			
13	4		4				
12	4		6	6			
11							
21			6	5			
22	6		7	4			
23	4		8	5			
24	6						
25		4	7			1	
26	6		4		m,b,d 2		
27	4	4	8	8	3		
~~28~~							
48	8	8	4	4	b 2	2	
47	6	14	8	4	3	1	
~~46~~							
45	4		6	4			
44			6	4			
43			4				
42	6						
41			4				
31			4				
32			4				
33	6						
34			4				
35	5		6	6		1	
36	10		8		b, 1 2		
37	6	4	10	6	b 2		
~~38~~							

Fig. 12-10. Periodontal chart including the data obtained from the examination of the patient presented in Fig. 12-4.

The alveolar bone

Radiographic analysis

The height of the alveolar bone and the outline of the bone crest are examined in the radiographs (Fig. 12-11). The radiographs provide information of the height and configuration of the interproximal alveolar bone. Covering structures (bone tissue, teeth) often make it difficult to properly identify the outline of the buccal and lingual alveolar bone crest. The analysis of the radiographs must therefore be combined with a detailed evaluation of the pocket depth and attachment level data in order to arrive at a correct diagnosis concerning "horizontal" and "vertical" bone loss.

Following active treatment, patients must be enrolled in a follow-up and maintenance care program aimed at preventing recurrence of periodontal disease. This program includes regular reexaminations to study the periodontal conditions. Such reexaminations often require repeated radiographic analysis of teeth and

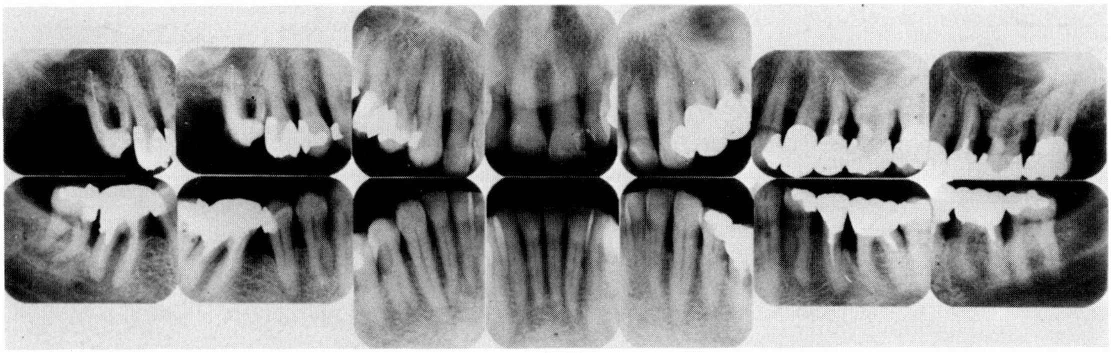

Fig. 12-11. Radiographic status of the patient presented in Fig. 12-4.

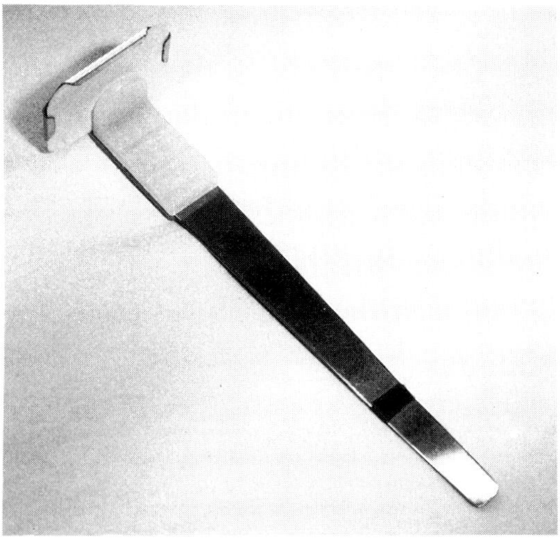

Fig. 12-12. The Eggen device for obtaining "standardized" radiographs.

jaws at given time intervals. To enable meaningful comparative analysis, a radiographic technique should be used which produces periodic reproducible roentgenograms. A technique of this kind has been described by e.g. Eggen (1969) (Fig. 12-12).

Sounding

In order to arrive at a correct diagnosis with respect to the alveolar bone level, the presence of angular bony defects and interdental osseous craters etc., an additional method, called "sounding", may be used. Following local anesthesia the periodontal probe is inserted into the pocket. The tip of the probe is forced through the supraalveolar connective tissue to make contact with the bone and the distance from the cementoenamel junction to the bone level is assessed in mm.

Diagnosis of the periodontal lesions

The information regarding the condition of the various periodontal structures (the gingiva, the periodontal ligament - the root cementum and the alveolar bone) which has been obtained through the examination procedures presented above should form the basis for the diagnosis of periodontal disease (Fig. 12-13). It is advantageous to give each tooth in the dentition an individual diagnosis. Four different diagnoses may be used:

Gingivitis

This diagnosis is used when one or several gingival units around a particular tooth are found to bleed on probing. Pocket depth and attachment level measurements and the radiographic analysis *must fail* to indicate loss of supporting tissues. "Pseudopockets" may be present.

Diagnosis of the periodontal lesion

Diagnosis	**Criteria** *Periodontal charting* *Radiographic analysis*	*Miscellaneous*
Gingivitis	No loss of supporting tissues (pseudo-pockets)	Bleeding on probing
Periodontitis levis	Horizontal loss of supporting tissues < 1/3 of the root length	Bleeding on probing
Periodontitis gravis	Horizontal loss of supporting tissues > 1/3 of the root length	Bleeding on probing
Supplementary diagnosis		
...et complicata	Angular bony defects: interdental craters infrabony pockets	
	Furcation involvement 2,3	

Fig. 12-13. The conditions of the periodontal tissues around each individual tooth in the dentition are described using different criteria (periodontal charting, radiographic analysis) and diagnosis.

Periodontitis levis (overt periodontitis)

The pocket depth and attachment level measurements and radiographic analysis indicate an even ("horizontal") loss of supporting tissues not exceeding 1/3 of the length of the root. Inflammation must be present, i.e. "bleeding on probing" will occur when the site is probed to the "bottom of the pocket".

Periodontitis gravis (advanced periodontitis)

Pocket depth and attachment level measurements and the radiographic analysis indicate an even ("horizontal") loss of supporting tissues exceeding 1/3 of the length of the root. "Bleeding on probing" to the "bottom of the pocket" must be present.

A supplementary diagnosis *periodontitis complicata* is used

1. when an angular bony defect (infrabony pocket, interdental osseous crater) is present adjacent to a tooth, and
2. for a multirooted tooth in which furcation involvements of degree 2 or 3 have been identified.

When an angular bony defect is present, the level of the adjacent bone of the affected tooth should also be described. Hence, a tooth with an angular bony defect is given a combined diagnosis: *periodontitis levis et complicata* when the apical bone level of the defect is located on the "gravis level" but the overall bone loss of the tooth is at the "levis" level.

A chart of diagnosis is shown in Fig. 12-14. This particular chart refers to the patient whose clinical status is shown in Figs. 12-4 a-c, periodontal chart in Fig. 12-10 and radiographic status in Fig. 12-11. The various teeth have received the diagnoses described in Fig. 12-14.

Tooth	Symptom	Diagnosis	Tooth	Symptom	Diagnosis
			48	furcation involvement (2)	gravis et complicata
			47	furcation involvement (3)	gravis et complicata
16	furcation involvement (3)	gravis et complicata			
15	“horizontal” loss of supporting tissues > 1/3 of the root length	gravis	45	“horizontal” loss of supporting tissues > 1/3 of the root length	gravis
14	“horizontal” loss of supporting tissues > 1/3 of the root length	gravis	44	“horizontal” loss of supporting tissues < 1/3 of the root length	levis
13	“horizontal” loss of supporting tissues < 1/3 of the root length	levis	43	“horizontal” loss of supporting tissues < 1/3 of the root length	levis
12	angular bony defect (bottom of the defect located on “gravis level”)	gravis et complicata	42	“horizontal” loss of supporting tissues < 1/3 of the root length	levis
11	“horizontal” loss of supporting tissues < 1/3 of the root length	levis	41	“horizontal” loss of supporting tissues > 1/3 of the root length	gravis
21	“horizontal” loss of supporting tissues > 1/3 of the root length	gravis	31	“horizontal” loss of supporting tissues > 1/3 of the root length	gravis
22	“horizontal” loss of supporting tissues > 1/3 of the root length	gravis	32	“horizontal” loss of supporting tissues < 1/3 of the root length	levis
23	“horizontal” loss of supporting tissues < 1/3 of the root length	levis	33	“horizontal” loss of supporting tissues < 1/3 of the root length	levis
24	“horizontal” loss of supporting tissues < 1/3 of the root length	levis	34	“horizontal” loss of supporting tissues < 1/3 of the root length	levis
25	angular bony defect (bottom of the defect located on “gravis level”	gravis et complicata	35	“horizontal” loss of supporting tissues > 1/3 of the root length	gravis
26	furcation involvement (2)	gravis et complicata	36	angular bony defect (bottom of the defect located on “gravis level”) furcation involvement (2)	levis et complicata
27	furcation involvement (3)	gravis et complicata	37	angular bony defect (bottom of the defect located on “gravis level”) furcation involvement (2)	levis et complicata

← Fig. 12-14. Chart of diagnosis describing the patient in Fig. 12-4. ↓

DIAGNOSIS	~~18~~	~~17~~	16	15	14	13	12	11	21	22	23	24	25	26	27	~~28~~
Gingivitis																
Parodontitis levis						X		X			X	X				
Parodontitis gravis			X	X	X		X		X	X			X	X	X	
et complicata			X										X	X	X	
	48	47	~~46~~	45	44	43	42	41	31	32	33	34	35	36	37	~~38~~
Gingivitis																
Parodontitis levis					X	X	X			X	X	X		X	X	
Parodontitis gravis	X	X		X				X	X				X			
et complicata	X	X												X	X	

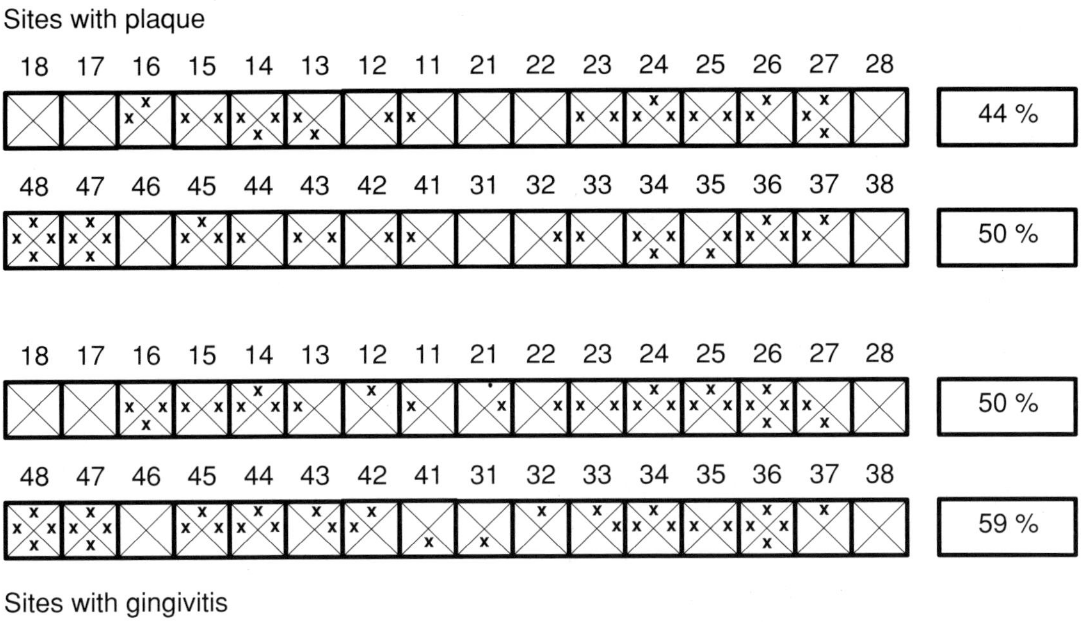

Fig. 12-15. The plaque and gingivitis chart of the patient presented in Fig. 12-4.

Oral hygiene status

In conjunction with examination of the periodontal tissues, the patient's oral hygiene must also be evaluated. Absence or presence of plaque on each tooth surface in the dentition is recorded. The bacterial deposits may be stained with a disclosing solution to facilitate their detection. The presence of plaque is marked in appropriate fields in the plaque chart shown in Fig. 12-15. The mean plaque score for the dentition is given as a percentage value in correspondence with the system used for gingivitis.

Alterations with respect to the presence of plaque and gingival inflammation are illustrated in a simple way by the repeated use of the combined plaque and gingivitis chart (Fig. 12-15) during the course of treatment.

In addition to the assessment of plaque, retention factors for plaque, such as supra- and subgingival calculus, defective margins of dental restorations, etc., should also be identified and included in the periodontal chart.

The methods described above for the examination of patients with respect to periodontal disease provide a thorough analysis of the presence, extent and severity of the disease in the dentition. The correct diagnosis for each individual tooth should form the basis for the treatment planning of the individual case.

References

Armitage, G.C., Svanberg, G.K. & Löe, H. (1977) Microscopic evaluation of clinical measurements of connective tissue attachment level. *Journal of Clinical Periodontology* **4**, 173-190.

Eggen, S. (1969) Standardisered intraoral röntgenteknik. *Sveriges Tandläkareförbunds Tidning* **17**, 867-872.

Ezis, I. & Burgett, F. (1978) Probing related to attachment levels on recently erupted teeth. *Journal of Dental Research* **57**, Special Issue A 307, Abstract No. 932.

Gabathuler, H. & Hassell, T. (1971) A pressure sensitive periodontal probe. *Helvetica Odontologica Acta* **15**, 114-117.

Hassell, T.M., Germann, M.A. & Saxer, V.P. (1973) Periodontal probing: investigator discrepancies and correlations between probing force and recorded depth. *Helvetica Odontologica Acta* **17**, 38-42.

Listgarten, M.A. (1980) Periodontal probing: What does it mean? *Journal of Clinical Periodontology* **7**, 165-176.

Listgarten, M.A., Mao, R. & Robinson, P.J. (1976) Periodontal probing and the relationship of the probe tip to periodontal tissues. *Journal of Periodontology* **47**, 511-513.

Magnusson, I. & Listgarten, M.A. (1980) Histological evaluation of probing depth following periodontal treatment. *Journal of Clinical Periodontology* **7**, 26-31.

Page, R.C. & Schroeder, H.E. (1976) Pathogenesis of chronic inflammatory periodontal disease. A summary of current work. *Laboratory Investigations* **33**, 235-249.

Polson, A.M., Caton, J.G., Yeaple, R.N. & Zander, H.A. (1980) Histological determination of probe tip penetration into gingival sulcus of humans using an electronic pressure-sensitive probe. *Journal of Clinical Periodontology* **7**, 479-488.

Robinson, P.J. & Vitek, R.M. (1979) The relationship between gingival inflammation and resistance to probe penetration. *Journal of Periodontal Research* **14**, 239-243.

Saglie, R., Johansen, J.R. & Flötra, L. (1975) The zone of completely and partially destructed periodontal fibers in pathological pockets. *Journal of Clinical Periodontology* **2**, 198-202.

Spray, J.R., Garnick, J.J., Doles, L.R. & Klawitter, J.J. (1978) Microscopic demonstration of the position of periodontal probes. *Journal of Periodontology* **49**, 148-152.

van der Velden, U. (1979) Probing force and the relationship of the probe tip to the periodontal tissues. *Journal of Clinical Periodontology* **6**, 106-114.

van der Velden, U. & de Vries, J.H. (1978) Introduction of a new periodontal probe: The pressure probe. *Journal of Clinical Periodontology* **5**, 188-197.

Vitek, R.M., Robinson, P.J. & Lautenschlager, E.P. (1979) Development of a force-controlled periodontal instrument. *Journal of Periodontal Research* **14**, 93-94.

CHAPTER 13

Treatment Planning

Introduction

Caries and periodontal disease, the most prevalent disorders of the dentition, have until recently been treated mainly by symptomatic (reparative) measures. This mode of treatment could be considered appropriate as long as the etiology of these two disorders remained obscure. At the present time, however, important aspects of the etiology and pathogenesis of both caries and periodontal disease are understood and therapeutic methods are available by which the causative factors can be eradicated or controlled and their recurrence prevented.

Caries and periodontal disease are infectious disorders associated with bacterial colonization of the surfaces of teeth. Factors such as bacterial specificity and pathogenicity as well as the disposition of the individual for the disease, e.g. local and general resistance, may influence the initiation, rate of progression and clinical character of the plaque-associated dental disorders. Findings from animal experiments and longitudinal studies in humans, however, have demonstrated that treatment including the elimination or control of the plaque infection and the introduction of careful plaque control measures in most, if not all, cases results in dental and periodontal health. Even if health cannot always be achieved and maintained, the arrest of disease progression following treatment must be the goal of modern dental care.

Treatment of patients suffering from caries and periodontal disease including symptoms of associated pathological conditions such as pulpitis, periapical periodontitis, marginal abscess, tooth migration, etc., should from a didactic point of view be divided into 3 different categories:

Cause-related measures

The objective of this treatment is the removal or control of the various plaque infections.

Corrective measures

Including traditional therapeutic measures such as periodontal surgery, endodontic therapy, restorative and prosthetic treatment. The volume of corrective therapy required and the selection of means for the restorative and prosthetic therapy should be determined only when the level of success of the causative therapy can be properly evaluated. The patients' ability to cooperate in the overall therapy must determine the content of the corrective treatment. If this ability is failing or lacking it is often not worth

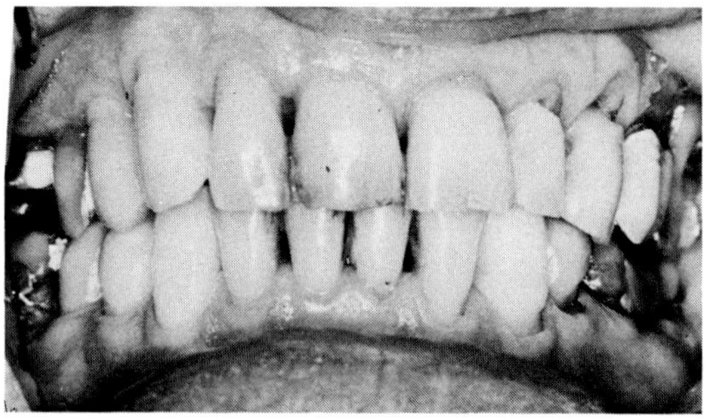
Fig. 13-1a.

Figs. 13-1 a-c. Clinical status of a 55-year-old male patient (U.N.) with periodontal disease.

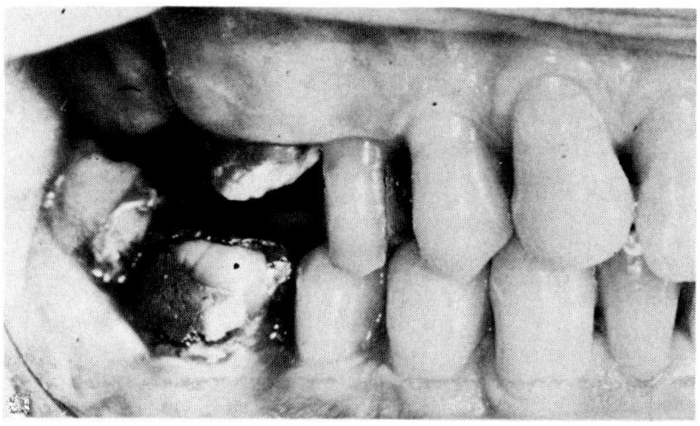
Fig. 13-1b.

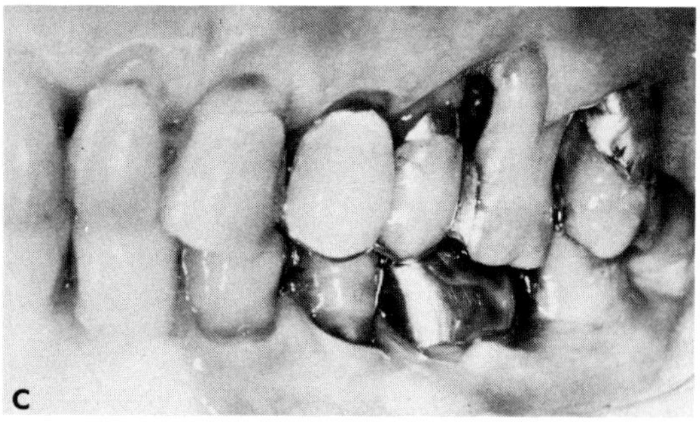

Fig. 13-1c.

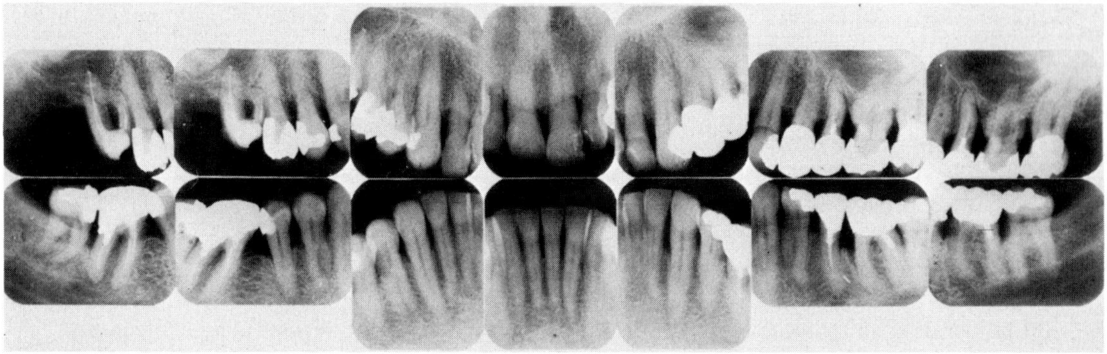
Fig. 13-2. Periodontal chart and radiographs relating to patient U.N. described in Fig. 13-1.

initiating treatment procedures which only in the fully cooperative patient will improve the results of therapy. The validity of this statement can be exemplified by the results of studies aimed at assessing the relative value of different types of surgical methods in the treatment of periodontal disease. Thus, a number of clinical trials (Lindhe & Nyman 1975, Nyman et al. 1975, 1977, Rosling et al. 1976 a, b, Nyman & Lindhe 1979) have demonstrated that gingivectomy and flap procedures performed in patients with proper plaque control levels often result in gain of alveolar bone and clinical attachment, while surgery in plaque-infected dentitions may cause additional destruction of the periodontium.

Maintenance measures

The aim of this treatment is the prevention of disease recurrence. For each individual patient a recall system must be designed which includes 1) the outline of selfperformed but pro-

Periodontal chart							Diagnosis		
Tooth	Pocket depth M	B	D	L	Furcation involvement	Tooth mobility	Parodontitis gravis et complicata	Parodontitis levis	Gingivitis
~~18~~									
~~17~~									
16	4	4	4		3		X	X	
15	4		6			1		X	
14	5		6	4				X	
13	4		4						X
12	4		6	6			X	X	
11									X
21			6	5				X	
22	6		7	4				X	
23	4		8	5					X
24	6								X
25		4	7			1	X	X	
26	6		4		m,b,d 2		X	X	
27	4	4	8	8	3		X	X	
~~28~~									
48	8	8	4	4	b 2	2	X	X	
47	6	14	8	4	3	1	X	X	
~~46~~									
45	4		6	4				X	
44			6	4					X
43			4						X
42	6								X
41			4					X	
31			4					X	
32			4						X
33	6								X
34			4						X
35	5		6	6		1		X	
36	10		8		b, 1 2		X		X
37	6	4	10	6	b 2		X		X
~~38~~									

fessionally monitored plaque control programs, 2) scaling and root planing measures, 3) fluoride application, etc. In addition, this treatment involves the regular control of fillings and other restorations made during the corrective phase of therapy.

In a textbook chapter it is obviously impossible to discuss all the different symptoms of disease which may be encountered in each individual patient. The aim of this presentation is to explain the overall objectives of the treatment planning for patients with moderately advanced and advanced periodontal disease and to describe the logical order of the use of different means of therapy.

Examination

of

Periodontal disease
Caries
Endodontic problems
Occlusal problems
Temporomandibular dysfunction
Etc.

} Diagnoses

Fig. 13-3.

Diagnosis

The basis for the treatment planning described in this chapter is established by the clinical data collected from the examination of the patient presented in Chapter 12. This particular patient (U.N., male, 55 years of age) was examined with respect to his periodontal conditions, i.e. gingival sites displaying signs of *bleeding on probing* were assessed, *pocket depths* and *furcation involvements* were measured and graded, *tooth mobility* was assessed and the radiographs were analyzed to determine the *height* and *outline* of the *alveolar bone crest.*

The clinical characteristics of the dentition of this patient are shown in Figs. 13-1 a-c. The periodontal chart and the radiographs are presented in Fig. 13-2. Based on these findings, each tooth in the dentition was given a proper periodontal diagnosis (Fig. 13-2). In addition to the examination of the periodontal conditions, detailed assessments of primary and recurrent *caries* were made for all tooth surfaces in the dentition. Furthermore, the patient was also examined with respect to endodontic problems, occlusal problems, temporomandibular joint dysfunction, etc. (Fig. 13-3).

The present patient exhibited signs of secondary caries lesions adjacent to several restorations, particularly in the molar regions (Fig. 13-1b), and root caries in the distal surface of 25 (Fig. 13-2) and mesial surface of 26 (Fig. 13-1c). It should be observed that in a patient with a large number of caries lesions an additional number of examination procedures, e.g. assessments of secretion rate and buffering capacity of the saliva, number of lactobacilli, *Streptococcus mutans*, etc., will facilitate the selection of therapeutic measures. In addition a periapical lesion was diagnosed in 47 and several defective root fillings were found (Fig. 13-2).

Treatment planning

Initial treatment plan

Not until a detailed diagnosis of all pathological conditions has been made, have proper prerequisites been established for an appropriate tentative treatment plan. At this early stage in the management of a patient it is in most instances impossible to make a definite decision regarding all aspects of the corrective therapy, because:

1. *The degree of success of the cause-related treatment remains unknown*: the result of the cause-related treatment of an individual case forms the basis for the selection of means for corrective therapy. The degree of disease elimination that can be reached depends on the efficacy of e.g. subgingival scaling and root planing, but also to a certain extent on the patient's ability to adopt proper dietary habits and plaque control techniques.
2. The patient's *"subjective" need for treatment is not known*: when the dentist has completed the examination of the patient and an inventory has been made regarding periodontal disease, caries, pulpal disease, temporomandibular joint disease, etc., he/she presents "the case" for his/her patient. During the case presentation session it is important to find out if the patient's subjective need for dental therapy coincides with the dentist's professional appreciation of the kind of therapy required. It is important that the dentist understands that the main objective of dental therapy, besides *elimination of pain, is to satisfy the patient's demands regarding esthetics and chewing function (comfort)*, demands which certainly vary considerably from one individual to another.
3. *The result of certain parts of the treatment cannot be predicted:* in patients exhibiting advanced forms of caries and periodontal disease it is often impossible to anticipate if all teeth which are present at the initial examination can be successfully treated or to predict the result of certain parts of the intended therapy. In other words, critical and difficult parts of the treatment must be performed first and the result must be evaluated before all aspects of the definitive corrective treatment can be properly anticipated and described.

Case presentation

The "Case presentation" is an essential component of the initial treatment and must include a description for the patient of different therapeutic goals available. At the case presentation for the present patient the following treatment plan was described:

> The teeth in the dentition from 15 to 24 and from 45 to 35 may probably not present the dentist with any major therapeutic challenges. For the remaining teeth in the dentition, however, the treatment may involve several complicated measures.

The following scenario was presented to the patient:

48 *and* 47 extraction: cannot be treated due

to the advanced loss of supporting tissue at the buccal aspect of the teeth in combination with deep furcation involvements and periapical periodontitis as far as 47 is concerned (Fig. 13-2).

16 extraction: even if it is possible, from a therapeutic point of view, to preserve the palatal root, the maintenance of this root does not improve esthetics or chewing comfort; the tooth has no antagonist after extraction of 47 (Fig. 13-2).

25 *and* 27 extraction: 25 cannot be treated due to advanced root caries in combination with advanced loss of periodontal tissue support at the distal aspect of the tooth; 27 has a periodontal pocket communicating with periapical lesions in combination with furcation involvement of degree 3 (Fig.13-2).

26, 36 *and* 37 present a number of difficult problems from a therapeutic point of view: 26 shows signs of deep and extended root caries on the mesiobuccal root in combination with furcation involvement of degree 2 m,b,d (Figs. 13-1 c and 13-2). Note also the unfavorable root- and root canal anatomy of the buccal roots with respect to endodontic treatment. However, the palatal root of 26 can be maintained; in 36 there is a deep angular bony defect on the mesial aspect and furcation involvement of degree 2 b,1; 37 has a deep infrabony pocket at the distal surface (10 mm, see the periodontal chart) and furcation involvement of degree 2 b. The distal root 36 or the mesial root 37 (or both) are available for treatment.

Two different *alternatives for treatment* were presented to the patient:

Alternative 1. Extraction of 25 and all molars and the maintenance of a dentition comprising 15-24 and 45-35. This alternative may be adequate with respect to "chewing comfort" but may be questionable from an esthetic point of view.

Alternative 2. Extraction of the molars in the right side of the upper and lower jaws (16, 48, 47) and also of 25 and 27; root separation of 26 with the maintenance of the palatal root to be used as abutment for a 3-unit bridge to replace the extracted 25; root separation of one of the molars 36 or 37 with the maintenance of one root to be used as abutment for a 3-unit bridge to obtain occlusal contact with the maxillary bridge.

It should be observed that *alternative 2* involves a considerably larger volume of therapy than *alternative 1*. In a situation like this, expected benefits inherent in a certain treatment versus obvious disadvantages should always be explained to and discussed with the patient. His/her attitude to the alternatives presented must guide the dentist in the design of a proper plan for the overall treatment. In the present case the patient preferred the treatment described as *alternative 2*.

Initial (cause-related) therapy

The treatment was initiated and included the following measures to eliminate or control the plaque infection:

1. *Instruction* in oral hygiene measures with subsequent check-ups and reinstruction.
2. *Scaling and root planing* in combination with removal of retention factors for plaque.
3. *excavation and restoration* of carious lesions.
4. *Endodontic treatment* 26 (palatal root) and 37 (mesial root). Endodontic treatment was carried out at an early stage to allow a proper evaluation of healing before the restorative treatment was initiated.

5. *Extraction* of 16, 48, 47. Temporary prosthetic replacement (for esthetic and functional reasons) of teeth which, during this initial phase of the treatment, have to be extracted should preferably be made in the form of removable partial dentures. The use of a removable prosthesis allows the dentist to eventually choose between a removable partial denture and a fixed bridge as permanent prosthetic therapy. If, on the other hand, the temporary prosthetic reconstruction is made in the form of a fixed bridge, the permanent prosthetic therapy must inevitably include fixed bridgework. Such an alternative may, however, during the course of treatment appear to be contraindicated. In the present case a temporary prosthesis was not made.

Reexamination

The initial phase of therapy is terminated with a thorough analysis (reexamination) of the results obtained with respect to the elimination or degree of control of the dental diseases. This implies that a reevaluation of the patient's caries activity must be performed as well as new assessments of gingival conditions, pocket depths, tooth mobility, etc. The result of this reevaluation forms the basis for the selection of corrective measures which should be included in the phase of definite treatment.

Planning of corrective therapy (definitive treatment plan)

If the results from the reexamination, made at the termination of the initial treatment phase, show that caries and periodontal disease have been brought under proper control, the corrective treatment may be carried out in the following sequence:

1. *Extractions* of teeth that cannot be maintained. If such extractions include teeth which must be replaced for esthetic or functional reasons, a temporary removable partial denture or a temporary fixed brigde must be inserted.
2. *Additional endodontic treatment*
3. *Periodontal surgery:* The planning of the type and extent of surgical treatment should be based on the pocket depth and "bleeding on probing" measurements made at the end of the initial phase of treatment. Periodontal surgery should be limited to those areas of the dentition where the inflammatory lesions in pockets of > 4 mm had not been resolved by scaling and root planing.
4. *Definitive restorative and prosthetic treatment* including permanent restorative therapy (crown and bridge, removable partial dentures, etc.).

Corrective therapy

The present patient after initial therapy displayed low plaque and gingivitis values (5-10%) and no active carious lesions. The corrective treatment therefore included the following components:

1. *Periodontal surgery* around teeth, where pockets (> 4 mm) persisted which bled on probing.
2. *Root separation* 37 and extraction of the distal root. *Root separation* 26 and extraction of the buccal roots.
3. *Extraction* 36, 25 and 27.
4. Preparation and installation of *fixed bridges* 24, 25, 26 (palatal root) and 35, 36, 37 (mesial root).

The result of the overall treatment is shown in Figs. 13-4 a-c and Fig. 13-5.

Figs. 13-4 a-c. Clinical status of patient U.N. after periodontal and restorative treatment. Compare with Fig. 13-1.

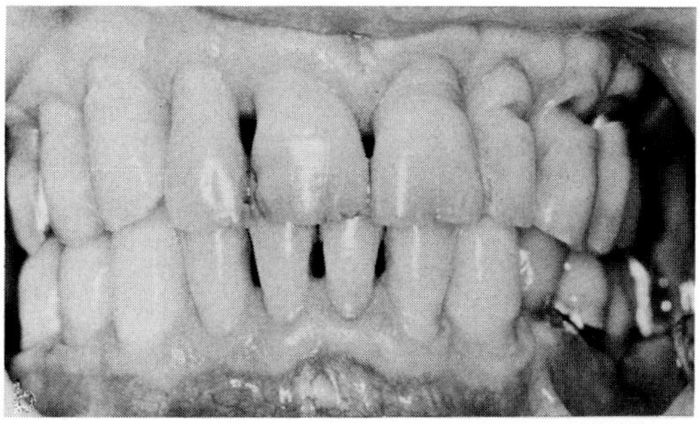

Fig. 13-4a.

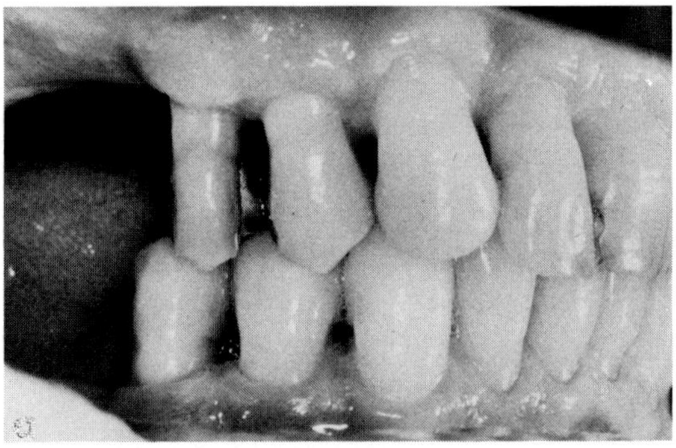

Fig. 13-4b.

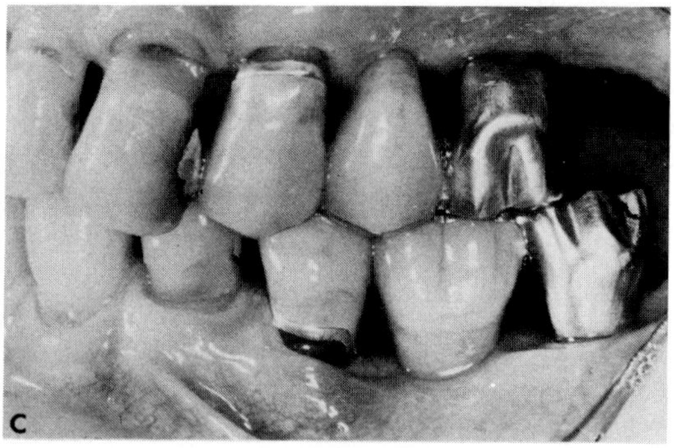

Fig. 13-4c.

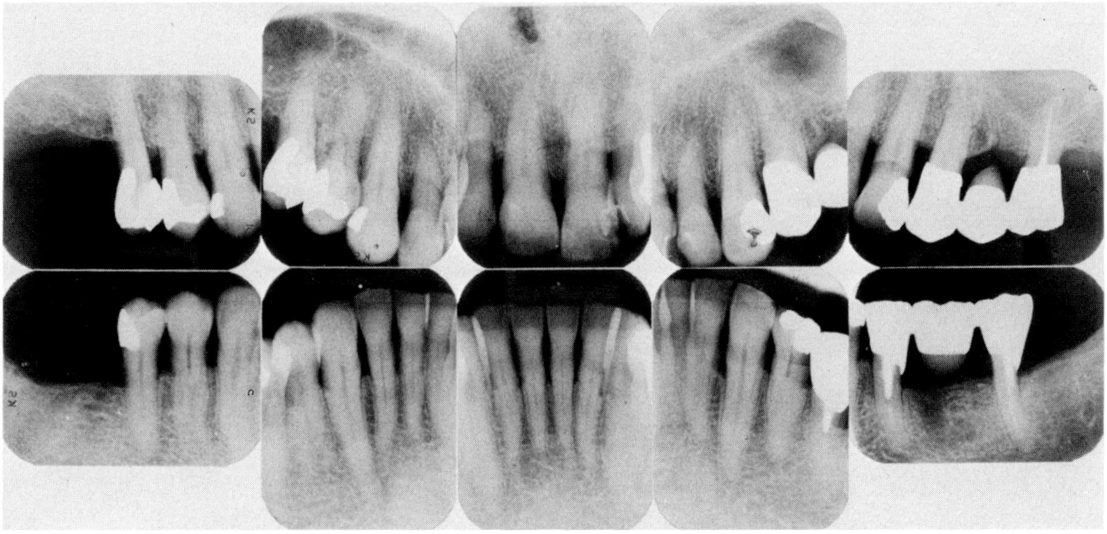

Fig. 13-5. Radiographs of patient U.N. after periodontal and restorative treatment. Compare with Fig. 13-2.

Planning of maintenance therapy

Following completion of *cause-related and corrective therapy* the patient must be enrolled in a recall system which aims at preventing the recurrence of disease. The time interval between the recall appointments should always be related to the ability of the patient to maintain a proper oral hygiene standard. Findings reported from several long-term clinical trials have suggested that a maintenance program based on recall appointments once every 3 months is, for most patients, effective in preventing disease recurrence. It is important to emphasize, however, that the recall program must be designed to meet the individual patient's need. Some patients must be recalled every month, while other patients may have to be checked only once a year.

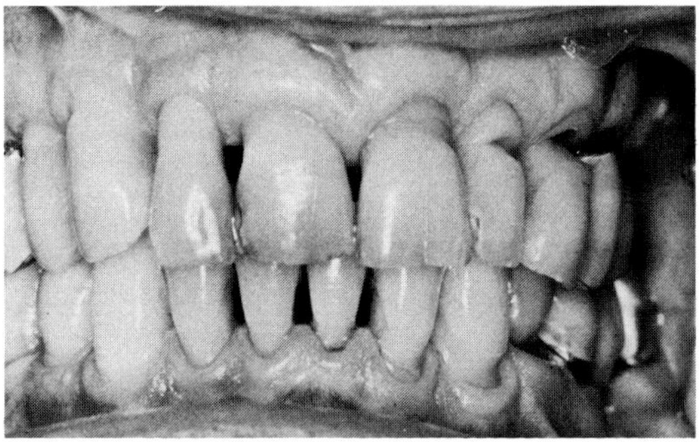

Fig. 13-6. Clinical status of patient U.N. 8 years after active treatment.

At the various recall visits the following procedures should be carried out:

1. Evaluation of the oral hygiene standard.
2. Scaling and polishing of the teeth (if indicated).

At least once a year an examination should be performed including assessments of 1) caries surfaces, 2) gingivitis, 3) pathologically deepened pockets, 4) furcation involvements, 5) tooth mobility and 6) alterations of the alveolar bone level.

The patient used in this chapter to describe the guiding principles of treatment planning was, during the first 6 months after the active treatment, recalled once every 2 months, during the next 6 months once every 3 months, and subsequently only once every 6 months. The clinical and radiographic status 8 and 11 years after active treatment are shown in Fig. 13-6 and 13-7. In the course of this 11-year period

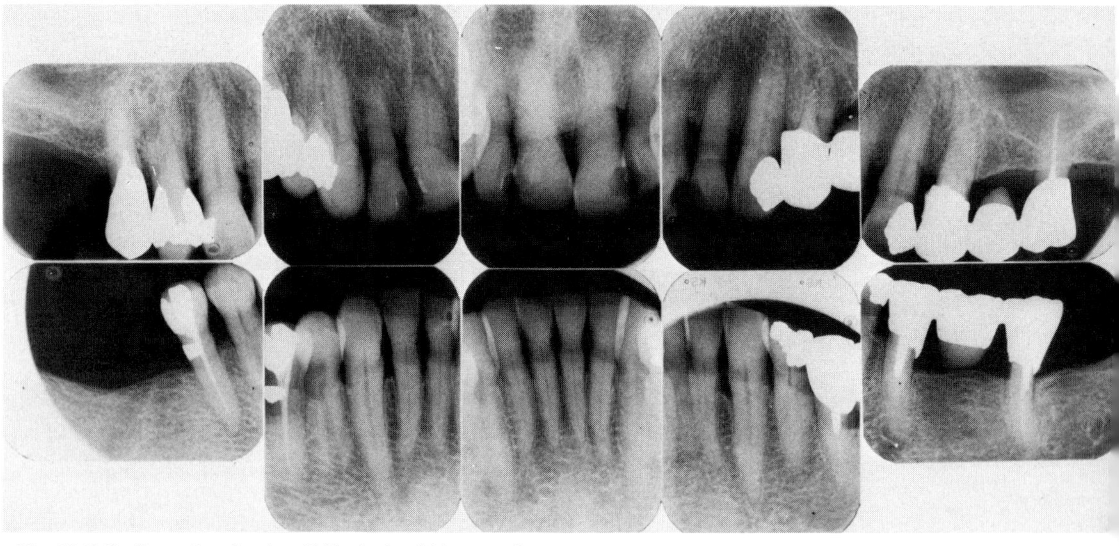

Fig. 13-7. Radiographs of patient U.N. obtained 11 years after treatment.

Examination I →	Diagnoses
	↓
of dental disorders and dysfunctions	Initial treatment plan Case presentation
	↓
	Cause related therapy 1. Periodontal treatment 2. Caries treatment 3. Endodontic treatment 4. Extractions (temporary prosthetic reconstructions)
Reexamination →	↓
Plaque and Gingivitis Pocket depth Reevaluation of caries activity	Cooperation ↓ Definitive treatment plan Corrective therapy 1. Extractions 2. Temporary prosthetic reconstructions 3. Periodontal surgery 4. Definitive restorative therapy
	↓
Periodic recall	Maintenance therapy

Fig. 13-8. Flow chart describing the sequence of delivery of various treatment procedures in the overall therapy.

there were no signs of recurrence of caries or periodontal disease. The buccal cusp of the crown of the tooth 15 was fractured approximately 5 years after active therapy and the tooth restored with a gold crown with a porcelain facing.

The large variety of treatment problems that different patients may present may obviously require that deviations are made from the sequence of treatment steps (initial therapy, corrective therapy, maintenance therapy, etc.) discussed above. Such deviations may be accepted as long as the fundamental principles regarding the overall therapy are understood (Fig. 13-8: flow chart).

Three patients will be presented below together with a brief description of their specific dental problems and the treatment delivered in order to demonstrate the rationale behind such variations in the sequence of therapy.

Case reports

Patient K.A. (female, 29 years old)

Initial examination

The periodontal status (pocket depths, furcation involvements, tooth mobility, radiographs and diagnoses) from the initial examination of patient K.A. is shown in Fig. 13-9. The data obtained from this examination disclosed the presence of an advanced destruction of the supporting tissues in most parts of the dentition and the presence of a large number of angular bony defects. The teeth 14, 12, 11, 21, 22, 23, 24, 25, 43, 42, 41, 31, 32, 33, 37 exhibited increased mobility. The plaque and gingivitis scores were 75 and 70% respectively.

Treatment planning

In the planning of the treatment of this case it seemed reasonable to anticipate the extraction of some teeth in this severely diseased dentition, namely 14, 11, 21 and 31 (see radiograph: Fig. 13-9). The extraction of these teeth calls for extensive prosthetic therapy. Should additional teeth be scheduled for extraction on "prosthetic" indications? The neighboring teeth of 11, 21, 31, also exhibited advanced loss of supporting structures and showed signs of increased mobility. It could be questioned, therefore, if these teeth (12, 22, 41, 32) could serve as proper abutments for fixed bridge reconstructions. The extraction of tooth 31 would most likely motivate the extraction of the remaining 3 mandibular incisors too, and consequently a therapy could be anticipated which included the preparation and installation of a fixed bridge from tooth 44 to tooth 34. Extraction of 11 and 21 would motivate the extraction of 12, 22, 14 and 24 as well, and call for a bridge construction from tooth 16 to 25 or 26. The prerequisites for a proper prognosis for the prosthetic therapy described above are 1) optimal self-performed oral hygiene, 2) proper healing of the periodontal tissues following

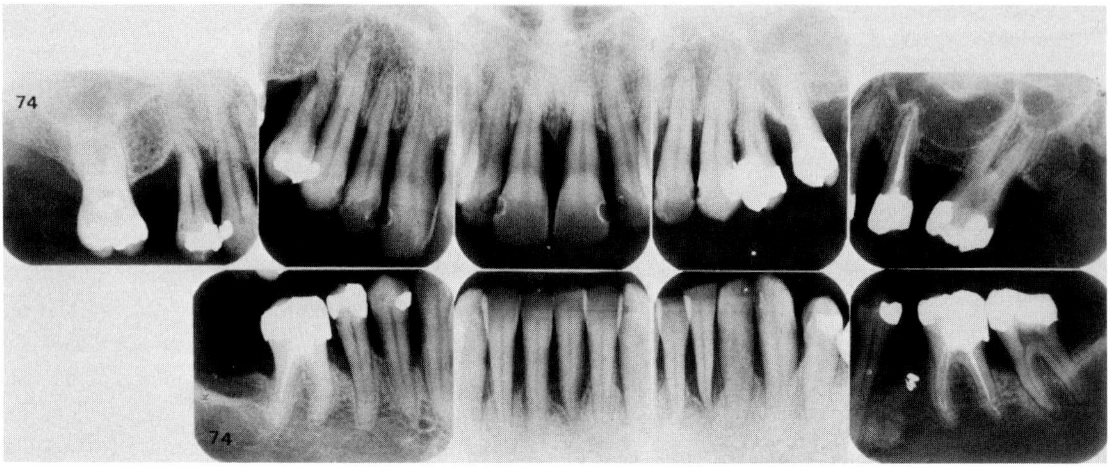

Fig. 13-9. Case K.A. (29-year-old female patient). Periodontal chart and radiographs prior to therapy.

Periodontal chart — Diagnosis

Tooth	Pocket depth M	B	D	L	Furcation involvement	Tooth mobility	Gingivitis	Parodontitis levis	Parodontitis gravis et complicata
~~18~~									
~~17~~									
16					b 1		X		
~~15~~									
14	8		8	7	m,d 1	2		X	X
13			5	5				X	
12	8		5			1		X	
11	8		5	5		2		X	X
21	8		7	6		2		X	X
22	6		6	5		1		X	
23			4	5		1		X	
24	6		8	4	m,d 1	1		X	X
25			5					X	
~~26~~									
27			6		b,d 1			X	
~~28~~									
~~48~~									
~~47~~									
46	5		5		b 1			X	
45			7					X	X
44	8		8	4				X	X
43	8		6	6		1		X	X
42	6		5			1		X	
41	4					1		X	
31	6		6	6		2		X	X
32	4		5			1		X	
33	8		7	5		1		X	X
34								X	X
~~35~~									
36			5		b 1			X	
37	7		7	6	b 1	1		X	
38									

cause-related and corrective therapy, and 3) a carefully monitored maintenance care program. If these prerequisites can be met, it may, on the other hand, be possible to avoid all anticipated tooth extractions in this patient. If this attempt is successful, prosthetic therapy can be entirely avoided. As stated above most of the teeth had increased mobility. This mobility, however, did not disturb the chewing comfort of this patient. The tooth mobility per se, therefore, was not regarded as an indication for splinting.

Conclusions: In a case of this character extensive efforts should be made to properly treat inflammatory periodontal disease in the entire dentition *before* decisions are made to extract one or several teeth. Decisions regarding possible extractions should, if possible, not be made until after the healing of periodontal surgery.

Treatment

Subsequent to initial examination, the patient was given a detailed "Case presentation" and information regarding alternative goals of and prerequisistes for the overall treatment. This information included a description of the role of dental plaque in the etiology of periodontal disease and the significance of optimal plaque control for a successful therapeutic result. A treatment program was subsequently planned

Figs. 13-10 a-c. Case K.A. Clinical status 5 years after initial treatment.

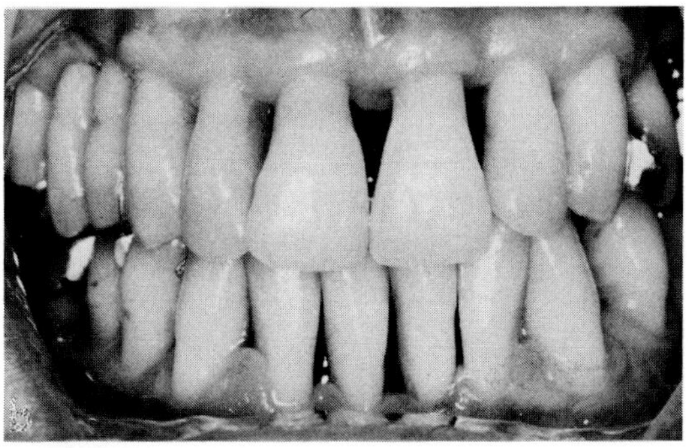

Fig. 13-10a.

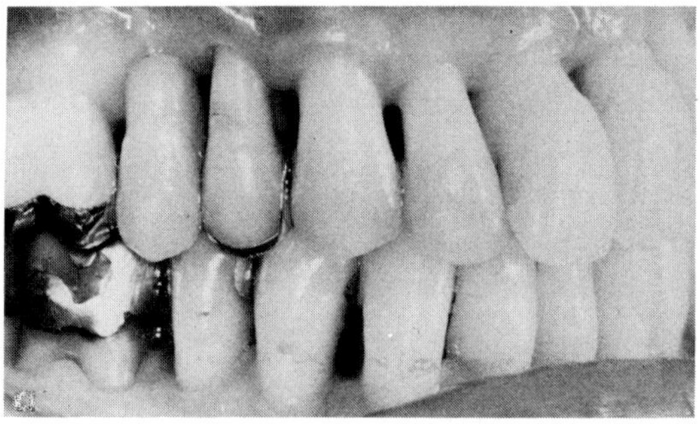

Fig. 13-10b.

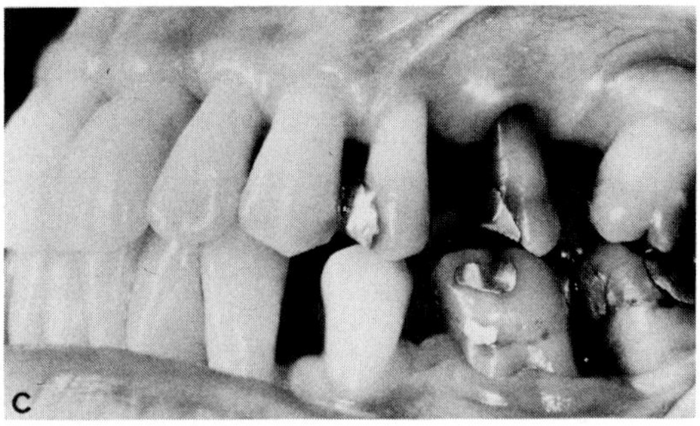

Fig. 13-10c.

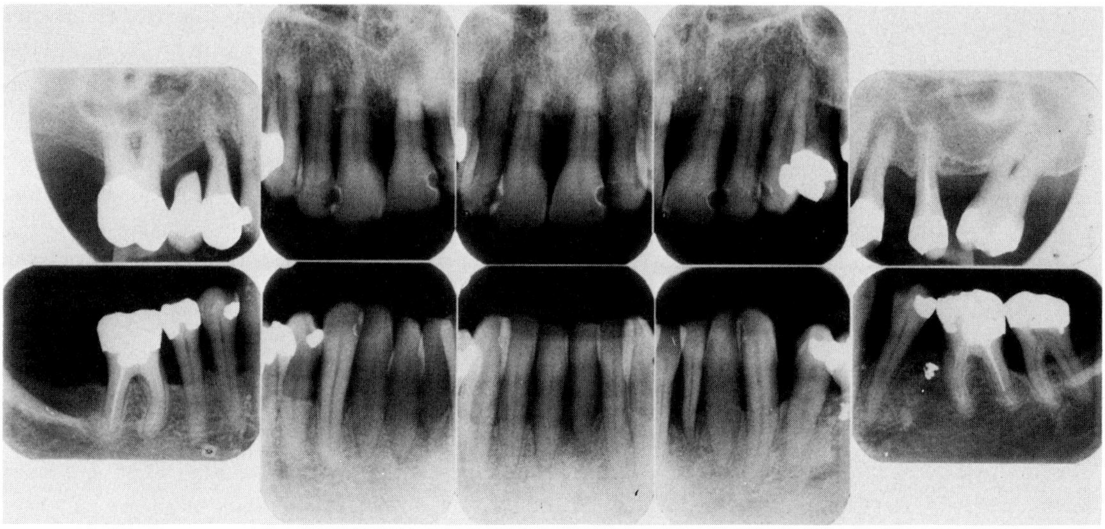

Fig. 13-11. Case K.A. Radiographs obtained 8 years after treatment.

which aimed at maintaining all teeth, thereby avoiding extensive prosthetic therapy. The overall treatment was performed in the following sequence:

Initial therapy

Oral hyiene instruction and plaque control evaluation. Scaling and root planing. Adjustment of improper amalgam restorations.

Periodontal chart

Tooth	Pocket depth M B D L	Furcation involvement	Tooth mobility	
~~18~~				
~~17~~				
16				
~~15~~				
14				
13				
12			1	
11				
21			1	
22			1	
23				
24				
25				
~~26~~				
27				
~~28~~				
~~48~~				
~~47~~				
46				
45				
44				
43				
42			1	
41			1	
31			2	
32			1	
33				
34				
~~35~~				
36				
37				
~~38~~				

Fig. 13-12. Case K.A. Periodontal chart from recordings made 8 years after treatment.

Corrective therapy (following evaluation at reexamination)

Periodontal surgery involving careful removal of subgingvial soft and hard deposits and root planing. All teeth in the dentition could be maintained and the furcation involvements in the premolar and molar areas could be treated successfully with furcation plasty (see chapter 20). After healing, a fixed bridge (16, 15, 14) was fabricated and inserted on esthetic indications.

Maintenance therapy

During the first 6 months after completion of the initial and corrective therapy the patient was recalled for maintenance care every 3 weeks. This interval between the recall appointments was then gradually extended to 3 months.

Concluding remarks

The result of the treatment is shown in Figs. 13-10 a-c (clinical status 5 years after initial treatment), Fig. 13-11 (radiographs 8 years after treatment) and Fig. 13-12 (periodontal chart 8 years after treatment).

There has been no recurrence of periodontal disease during the period of maintenance.

The planning of the overall treatment and the sequence of the different treatment procedures used in this case were selected for presentation in order to illustrate the following principle: In patients exhibiting a generalized advanced breakdown of the periodontal tissues, but with an intact number of teeth, considerable efforts should be made to maintain all teeth if this is technically possible. Extraction of one single tooth in such a dentition will frequently also mean the extraction of several others for "prosthetic reasons". The end result could be an extensive prosthetic rehabilitation which would have been entirely unneccessary if the treatment planning had been properly done.

Patient B.H. (female, 40 years old)

Initial examination

The periodontal status (pocket depths, furcation involvements, tooth mobility, radiographs) from the initial examination is shown in Fig. 13-13. The data obtained from this examination disclosed essentially shallow pockets in most parts of the dentition except for isolated areas (the region 11-24) where some pockets exhibited probing depths varying between 4 and 7 mm. It should be observed that, particularly in the maxillary front region, pronounced gingival recessions prevailed. This means that even the

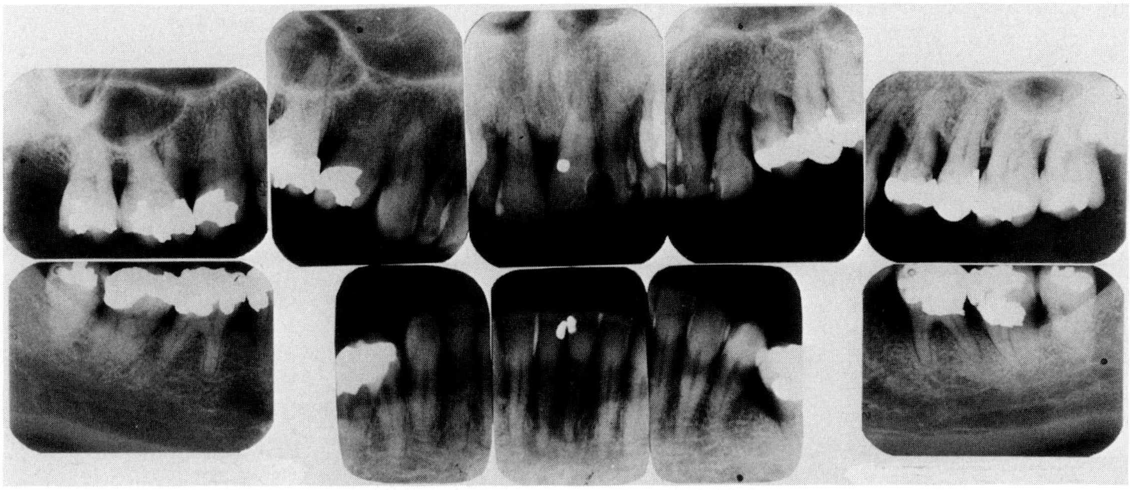

Fig. 13-13. Case B.H. (40-year-old female patient). Periodontal chart and radiographs from the initial examination.

moderate probing depth values obtained reflected advanced loss of the supporting tissues. This was further confirmed by the severe loss of alveolar bone (see radiographs: Fig. 13-13) in this region where some of the teeth exhibited increased mobility (tooth 11: degree 2 in combination with elongation; tooth 23: degree 3 and tooth 24: degree 2). In the posterior tooth regions there was a loss of the periodontal tissues varying between ⅓ and ½ of the length of the roots. In the mandibular front tooth region the destruction was severe, particularly around tooth 31. This tooth was found to be non-vital and exhibited a mobility of degree 2. The plaque and gingivitis scores were 25 and 30% respectively.

Treatment

In discussing with the patient different alternatives of treatment it was first suggested that tooth 23 had to be extracted. Not more than 2-3 mm of the apical portion of the root was still invested in supporting bone. The tooth exhibited a degree 3 mobility in conjunction with premature occlusal contact in the intercuspal position and on laterotrusive movement of the mandible. The question arose, however, of

Periodontal chart

Tooth	Pocket depth M	B	D	L	Furcation involvement	Tooth mobility
~~18~~						
17	4					
16	4			4		
~~15~~						
14			4			
13				4		
12						
11	6			4		2
21	4					
22			4			
23	5		6	5		3
24	4		7			2
25						
26			5		d 1	
27	6	4				
~~28~~						
48						
47						
46						
45	4		4			
44			4			
43						
42						
41						
31						2
32						
33	4					
34	4					
~~35~~						
36	4				b 1	
37	4				b 1	
38						

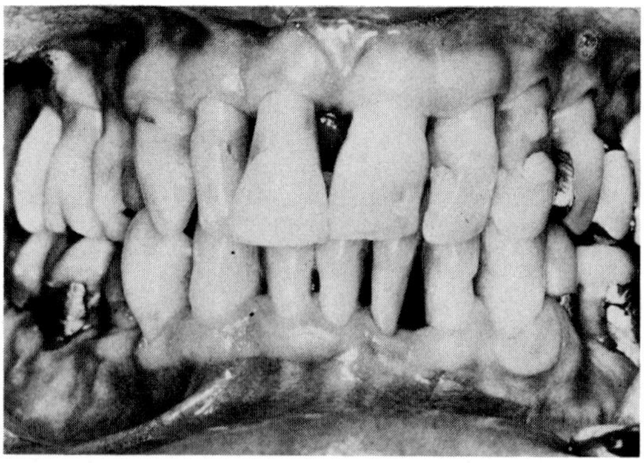

Fig. 13-14a.

Figs. 13-14 a-c. Case B.H. Clinical status 12 years after treatment.

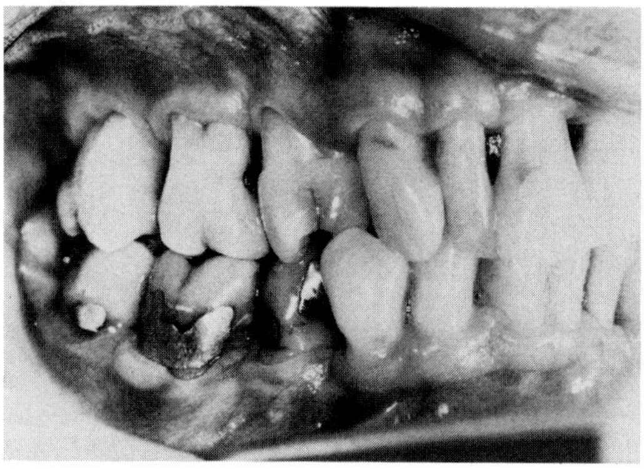

Fig. 13-14b.

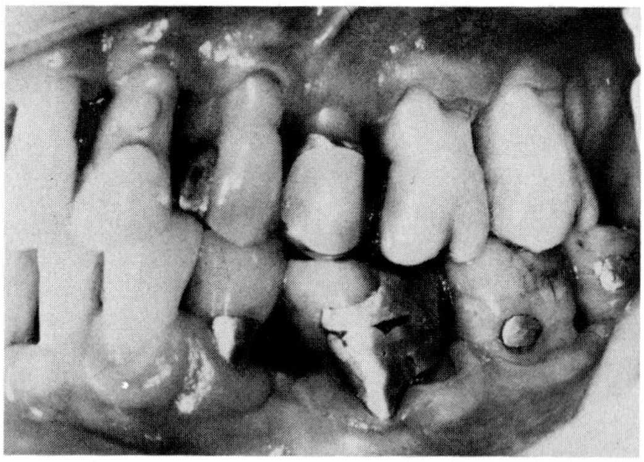

Fig. 13-14c.

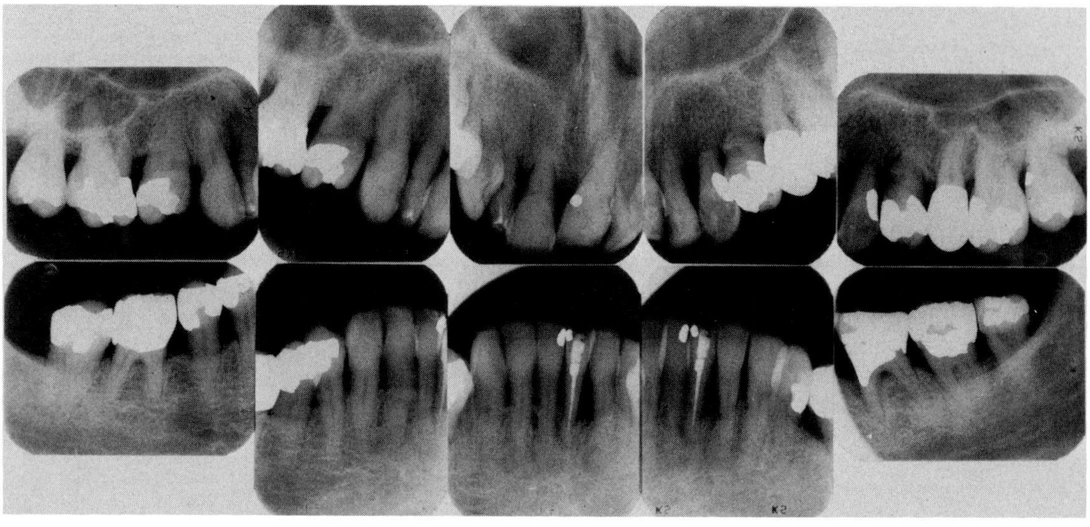

Fig. 13-15. Case B.H. Radiographs obtained 12 years after active therapy. Note that no loss of alveolar bone has occurred during the 12 years of maintenance. Compare with Fig. 13-13.

what consquences extraction of tooth 23 would have on the overall therapy. For instance: the neighboring teeth (22 with advanced periodontal destruction at the distal aspect, and 24 with severe loss of supporting tissue including increased mobility) could not be considered as proper abutment teeth for a 3-unit bridge replacing tooth 23. The demand for proper abutment teeth would therefore require a further extension of the bridge restoration to include teeth 21 and 25 (following extraction also of 24). This extension of the bridge construction implies, however, that tooth 11 will be the first nonsplinted neighboring tooth. Considering the small amount of periodontium which persisted around this tooth, possible recurrence of disease following treatment would almost certainly result in loss of tooth 11. It may, therefore, appear to be necessary to extract 11 as well, and to extend the bridge to tooth 13, since tooth 12 may also be considered improper as the terminal abutment tooth on the right side of the jaw.

From this discussion it is apparent that extraction of one single tooth (23) in this dentition will lead to extraction of a number of additional teeth to exclude their incorporation in the permanent reconstruction. The result is, thus, an extensive bridge therapy which can be avoided if only the critical tooth (23) can be maintained. Therefore it was decided to treat all teeth and postpone the decision of tooth extractions until the result of the periodontal treatment could be properly evaluated.

Initial therapy

Oral hygiene instruction and plaque control evaluation. Scaling and root planing. Occlusal adjustment of 11, 23 and 24. Correction of improper amalgam restorations.

Corrective therapy (following evaluation at reexamination)

Periodontal surgery in the region of 11-24. Extraction of 28 and 48 (semi-impacted molars). Endodontic treatment of 31.

Six months following this part of the corrective treatment, a new evaluation including measurements of tooth mobility showed that no pathologically deepened pockets were present and that the mobility had decreased in all initially hypermobile teeth (11: from degree 2 to 2; 23: from degree 3 to 2; 24: from degreee 2 to 0; 31 from degree 2 to 1). All teeth could thus be maintained and there were no indications for additional tooth extractions. The treatment was completed by preparation and insertion of a crown restoration in tooth 25.

Maintenance therapy

During the first year after completion of the corrective therapy the patient was enrolled in a maintenance care program with recall appointments once every 3 months and thereafter once every 6 months.

The result of the treatment (12 years after) is shown in Figs. 13-14 a-c (clinical status) and Fig. 13-15 (radiographs). No further loss of supporting tissues had occurred during this observation period.

Patient P.O.S (male, 30 years old)

Initial examination

The clinical status of this patient is illustrated in Figs. 13-16 a-c and the periodontal status (pocket depths, furcation involvements, tooth mobility, radiographs and diagnoses) from the initial examination in Fig. 13-17. The dentition was characterized by severe destruction of the supporting apparatus, including advanced loss of the interradicular periodontal tissues in all molars and the 2 first maxillary premolars. Most teeth were markedly mobile, particularly the incisors in both jaws. The plaque and gingivitis scores were 100%.

Treatment planning

A thorough analysis of the periodontal conditions in this patient revealed that certain teeth could no longer be treated and maintained but had to be extracted. Hence, it was decided to extract teeth 14 and 24 (furcation involvement of degree 2 from both mesial and distal aspects) and 12, 11, 21, 22 (loss of the supporting tissues to a level close to or beyond the apices in combination with a mobility of degree 3). In

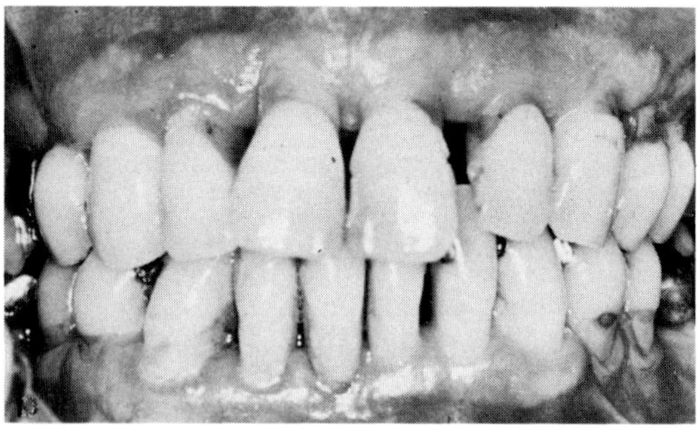

Fig. 13-16a.

Fig. 13-16 a-c. Case P.O.S. (30-year-old male patient). Clinical status prior to surgery.

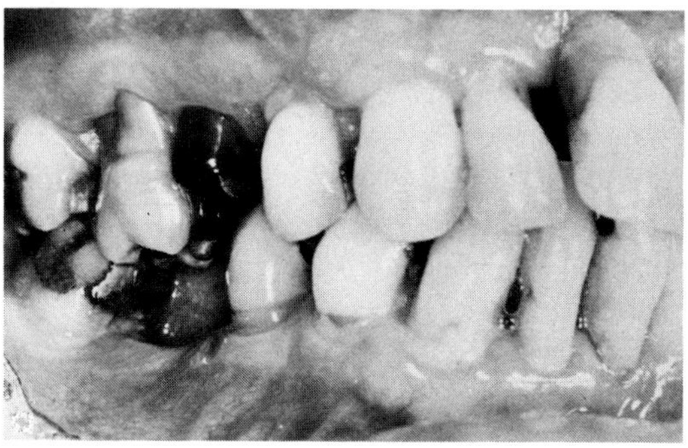

Fig. 13-16b.

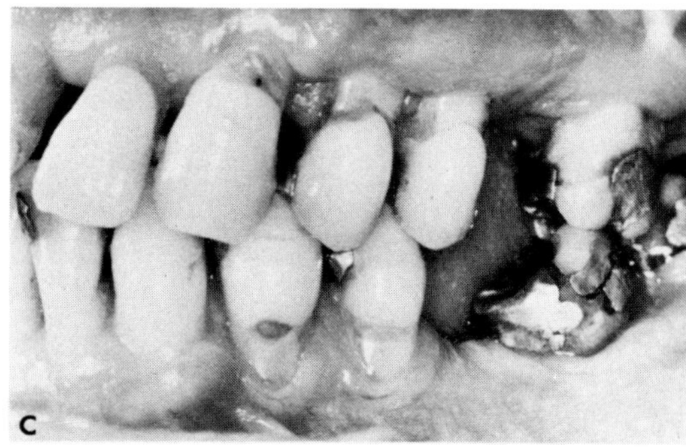

Fig. 13-16c.

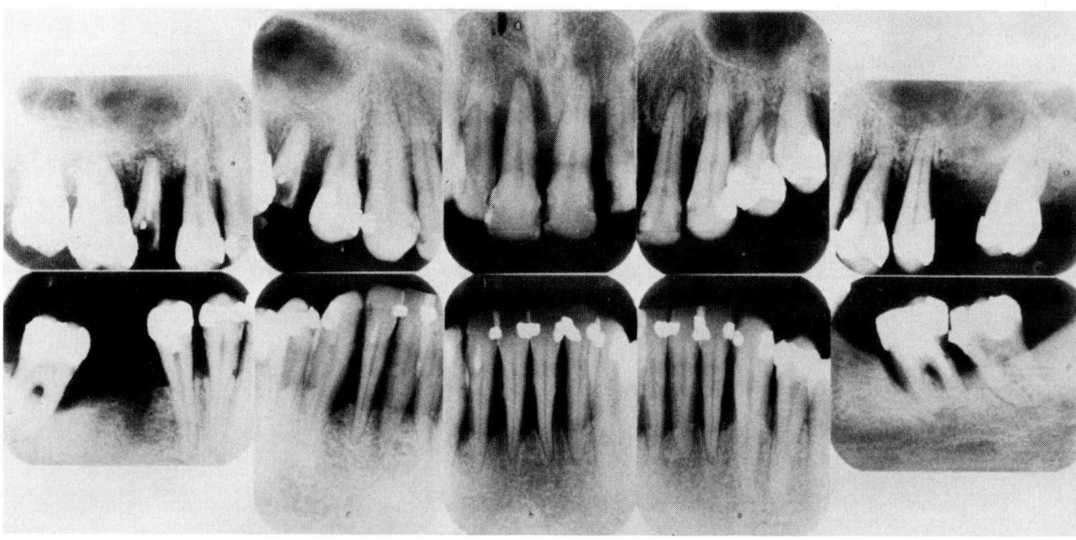

Fig. 13-17. Case P.O.S. Periodontal chart and radiographs from the initial examination.

the mandible, 42, 41, 31, 32 and 37 could not be maintained. The overall treatment of this patient, therefore, had to include prosthetic replacement of a number of teeth.

Alternative 1

Mandible: In the planning phase it was anticipated that the prosthetic rehabilitation of the mandibular dentition ought not to involve any technical difficulties since 33 and 43 as well as

Periodontal chart

Diagnosis: Gingivitis; Parodontitis levis; Parodontitis gravis et complicata

Tooth	Pocket depth M	B	D	L	Furcation involvement	Tooth mobility	Diagnosis	
~~18~~								
17	9		8	6	m,d 2	1	X	X
16	8		8		m,b,d 2	2	X	X
15	8		7	4		1		X
14	8	4	8	5	m,d 2	2	X	X
13	6		5	4		1		X
12	8	4	7	8		3	X	X
11	10	8	10			3	X	X
21	7		10	8		3		X
22	8	5	7	5		3		X
23	8		10	6		2	X	X
24	9		10	7	m,d 2	2	X	X
25	8	6	8	7		2		X
~~26~~								
27	10	8	8	4	m,d 2, d 1	2	X	X
~~28~~								
~~48~~								
47	10	5	8	7	3	1	X	X
~~46~~								
45	8		7	5				X
44	8		8	7		1		X
43	7		8	5		1	X	X
42	7	4	7	7		3	X	X
41	7	4	7	7		3	X	X
31	7	4	7	7		3		X
32	7	4	7	7		3		X
33	8		5	6		1		X
34	10		6	7		1	X	X
35	5		4					X
~~36~~								
37	10	7	8	7	3	2	X	X
38	6	8	9	8	b, 1 2	2	X	X

34, 35 and 44, 45 were available for periodontal therapy and, hence, could be used as abutment teeth for a cross-arch fixed bridge. It did not seem reasonable to maintain the furcation-involved molars 47 and 38, so these teeth were also scheduled for extraction. In this context it should be understood that if 47 and 38 were maintained, the treatment would have included not only endodontic measures but also root separation and periodontal surgery, production of posts and cores, and the incorporation of the preserved roots as abutments in the cross-arch bridge construction.

Maxilla: The maxillary dentition presented more difficult therapeutic problems. If the patient was to be restored with a fixed bridge, it was considered pertinent to maintain the 2 maxillary canines (teeth 13 and 23) and at least 1 tooth in the premolar (molar) regions on both sides of the jaw (15 and 25) and/or more roots of 17,16 and 27. *Definitive* prosthetic treatment of the maxillary dentition by means of a removable, partial denture was not considered appropriate since the various abutment teeth for such a denture displayed a markedly increased mobility. For the same reason it was considered inappropriate to *temporarily* replace the extracted teeth by means of a provisional, removable partial denture. The provisional prosthesis has to be fabricated in the form of a fixed bridge in order to enable proper stabilization (splinting) of the hypermobile 13, 23 and 25 prior to periodontal surgery. In the present case the temporary bridge should not include tooth 15 and the maxillary molars. Tooth 15 was to be left uncovered in order to facilitate endodontic therapy and the preparation and insertion of a post and core. In addition, the maxillary molars had to be accessible for periodontal therapy including endodontic treatment and root separation. In order to facilitate the surgical procedures and also to avoid the risk of a further increase of the tooth mobility, the extraction of 14, 12, 11, 21 and 22 and the insertion of the temporary bridge had to be carried out prior to the start of the surgical phase of treatment.

Alternative 2

The alternative treatment to the one outlined above is a complete denture in the maxillary jaw and a removable partial denture in the mandible with the use of 45, 44, 43 and 33, 34, 35 as abutment teeth.

Treatment

The clinical and radiographical symptoms of the advanced disease present as well as the therapeutic alternatives were thorougly discussed with the patient. This discussion included a detailed explanation of the role of op-

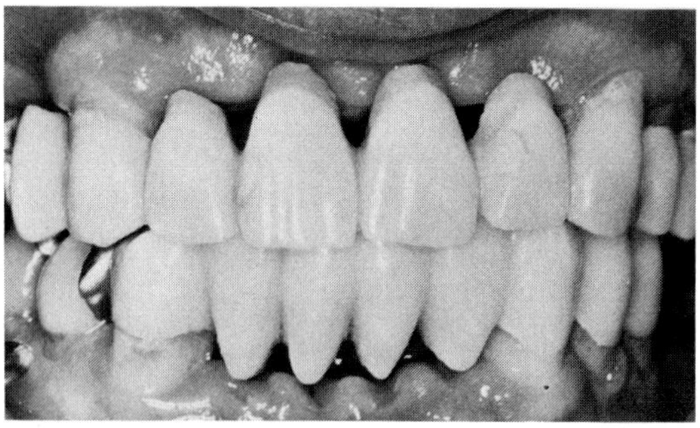

Fig. 13-18. Case P.O.S. Clinical status of the front tooth region at completion of the initial, cause-related treatment.

timal plaque control for the long-term good prognosis. The treatment was performed according to *alternative 1* and in the following sequence:

Initial therapy
Instruction regarding oral hygiene measures. Scaling and root planing. Evaluation of the ability of the patient to maintain a high standard of oral hygiene.

Extraction of 14, 12, 11, 21, 22. Temporary acrylic bridge 14, 13, 12, 11, 21, 22, 23, 24, 25; (24 was temporarily maintained in order to ensure proper stability of the temporary bridge).

Extraction of 47, 42, 41, 31, 32, 37, 38. Temporary acrylic bridge 44, 43, 42, 41, 31, 32, 33, 34, 35; (45: because the tooth was non-vital it was not incorporated in the temporary bridge; this to facilitate endodontic treatment). Endodontic treatment 15, 45. The clinical status at the completion of the initial treatment is seen in Fig. 13-18.

Corrective therapy
Periodontal surgery around the teeth which at the reevaluation of the case after initial therapy still exhibited pathologically deepened pockets which bled on probing. The palatal roots of 17 and 27 were maintained and the buccal roots were extracted following separation.

Extraction of 16 and 24.

Following healing after surgery, posts and cores were inserted in 17, 15, 27 and 45 (Figs. 13-19 a,b) and permanent fixed bridges were designed and fabricated with the following outline:

Maxilla: 17 (palatal root), 16, 15, 14, 13, 12, 11, 21, 22, 23, 24, 25, 26, 27 (palatal root).

Mandible: 46, 45, 44, 43, 42, 41, 31, 32, 33, 34, 35, 36.

Maintenance therapy
After completion of active treatment this patient was enrolled in a maintenance care program including recall appointments once every 3 months. Clinical photographs (Figs. 13-20 a-c) and radiographs (Fig. 13-21) illustrate the result of the treatment at the 8-year control. No further loss of supporting tissues occurred during the maintenance period.

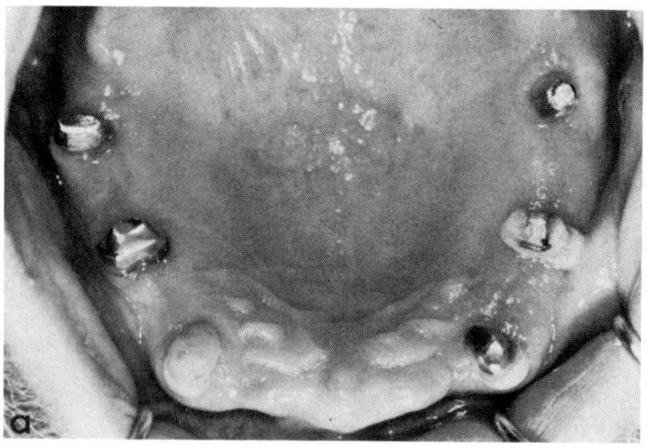

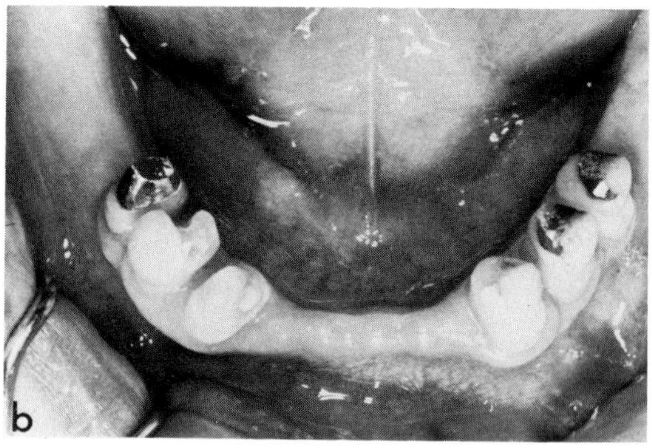

Figs. 13-19 a,b. Case P.O.S. The abutment teeth used for a maxillary (a) and a mandibular (b) bridge.

Figs. 13-20 a-c. Case P.O.S. Clinical photographs illustrating the result of treatment after 8 years of maintenance.

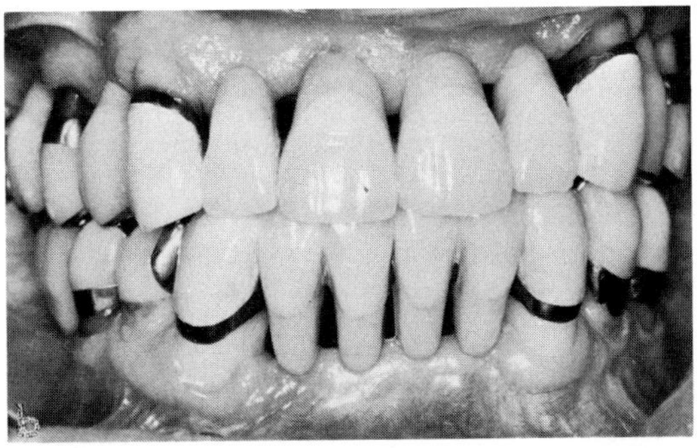

Fig. 13-20a.

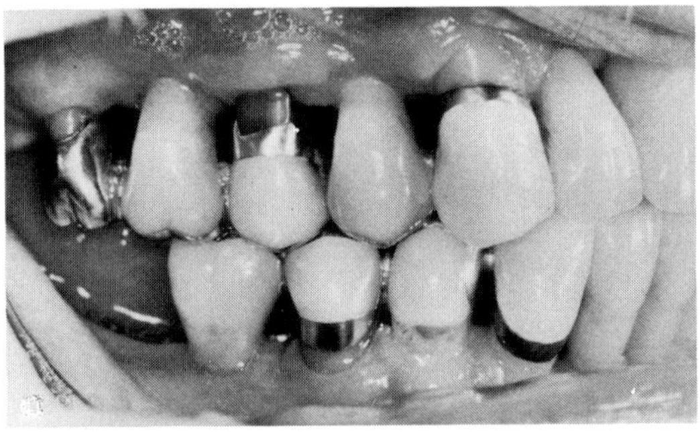

Fig. 13-20b.

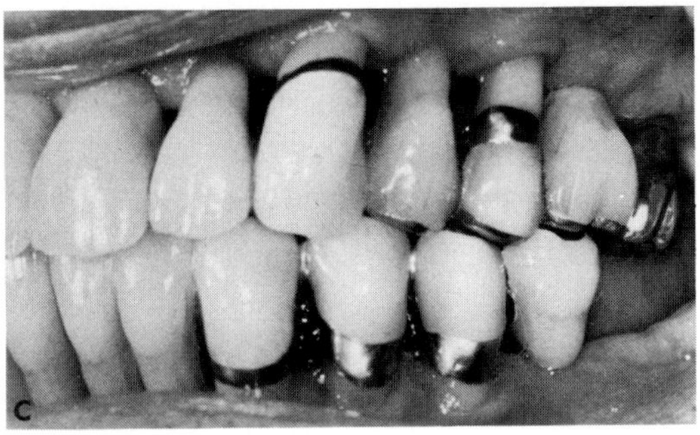

Fig. 13-20c.

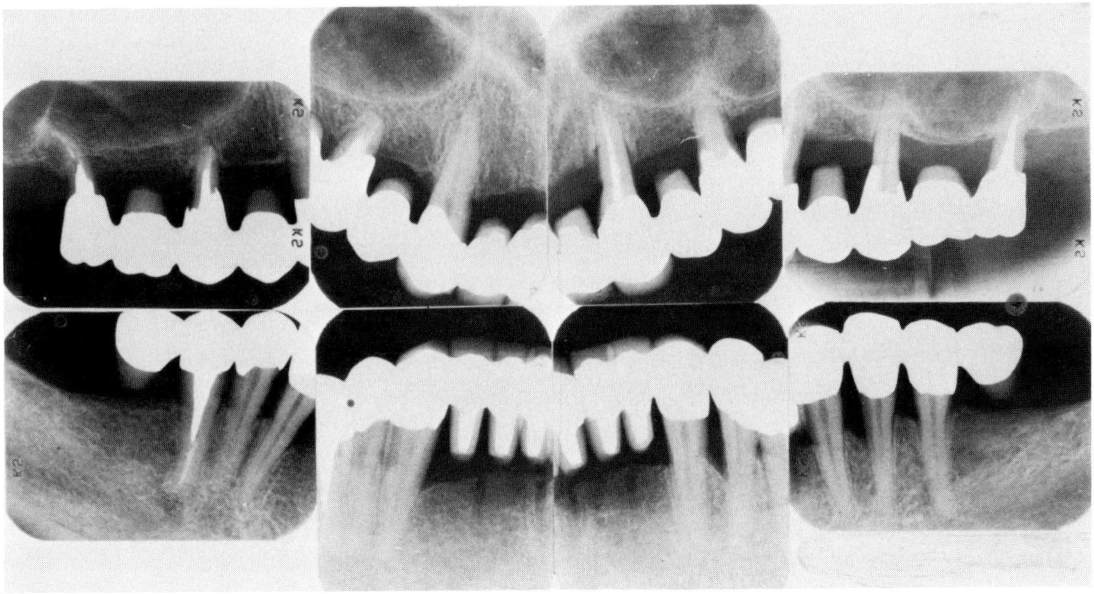

Fig. 13-21. Case P.O.S. Radiographs obtained 8 years after completion of active therapy. Note that no further loss of alveolar bone has occurred during the 8 years of maintenance.

References

Lindhe, J. & Nyman, S. (1975) The effect of plaque control and surgical pocket elimination on the establishment and maintenance of periodontal health. A longitudinal study of periodontal therapy in cases of advanced disease. *Journal of Clinical Periodontology* **2**, 67-79.

Nyman, S. & Lindhe, J. (1979) A longitudidinal study of combined periodontal and prosthetic treatment of patients with advanced periodontal disease.*Journal of Periodontology* **50**, 163-169.

Nyman, S., Lindhe, J. & Rosling, B. (1977) Periodontal surgery in plaqueinfected dentitions.*Journal of Clinical Periodontology* **4**, 240-249.

Nyman, S., Rosling, B. & Lindhe, J. (1975) Effect of professional tooth cleaning on healing after periodontal surgery. *Journal of Clinical Periodontology* **2**, 80-86.

Rosling, B., Nyman, S. & Lindhe, J. (1976a) The effect of systematic plague control on bone regeneration in infrabony pockets. *Journal of Clinical Periodontology* **3**, 38-53.

Rosling, B., Nyman, S., Lindhe, J. & Jern, B. (1976b) The healing potential of the periodontal tissues following different techniques of periodontal surgery in plague-free dentitions. A 2-year clinical study. *Journal of Clinical Periodontology* **3**, 233-250.

CHAPTER 14

The Cause-Related Phase of Periodontal Therapy

The overall treatment of patients suffering from periodontal disease and caries including associated pathologic conditions (e.g., pulpitis, periapical lesions, tooth migration, tooth loss) can, for didactic purposes, be divided into three different but frequently overlapping phases (see Chapter 13).

1. *The cause-related* (initial) *phase*; the objective of which is to control or eliminate gingivitis and to arrest the progression of further periodontal tissue destruction by the removal (or control) of the microbial plaques.
2. *The corrective phase*; the main objective of which is to restore function and esthetics.
3. *The maintenance phase*, which is aimed at preventing recurrence of periodontal disease.

In this chapter measures will be described which are commonly used in the cause-related (initial) phase of therapy.

Objectives of cause-related therapy

The measures used in the cause-related phase of therapy with respect to *periodontal disease* aim at the elimination and the prevention of recurrence of supra- and subgingivally located bacterial deposits from the tooth surfaces. This is accomplished by:

- Motivating the patient to combat dental disease (*patient information*)
- Giving the patient *instruction* in proper oral hygiene techniques (*self-performed plaque control methods*)
- *scaling and root planing.*
- *removal* of additional *retention factors* for plaque such as overhanging margins of restorations, ill-fitting crowns etc.

Means of cause-related therapy

Patient information

Most individuals brush their teeth at fairly regular intervals but do not clean their teeth thoroughly enough to effectively prevent plaque accumulation on the tooth surfaces. A common reason for the inadequate standard of self-performed oral hygiene is lack of adequate knowledge of periodontal disease and caries and thus proper motivation to combat oral diseases.

In most cases, therefore, the cause-related phase of therapy must be initiated by a demonstration to the patient of symptoms of dental disease found in her/his mouth. This can be accomplished by allowing the patient to participate in the professional examination of her/his oral cavity (e.g. by the use of a magnifying handmirror). Areas of the dentition exhibiting health should be identified by the dentist as well as sites displaying symptoms of disease. The patient should be instructed to recognize a carious lesion, to distinguish between a healthy and inflamed gingival unit and to appreciate the difference between a normal and an increased probing depth.

The *Bleeding Index* chart illustrating the patient's gingival conditions as well as the Probing depth chart showing the result of the probing depth examinations should be presented and explained (see Chapter 12). The result of the radiographic examination should also be reported; areas of the dentition with normal height of alveolar bone should be outlined, as well as sites with varying degrees of bone loss. The findings from the radiographic examination can subsequently be compared with the probing depth data and the relationship between the two parameters explained. In other words, the patient must be given the opportunity to familiarize him/herself with his/her own dentition.

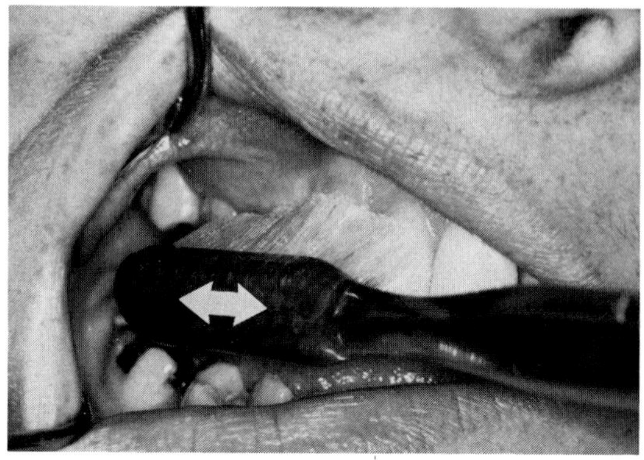

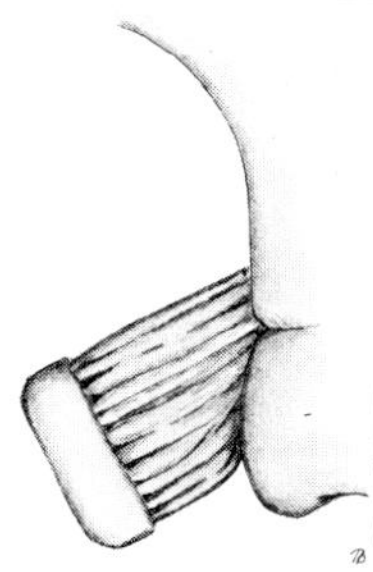

45°

Fig. 14-1. The Bass'method of toothbrushing. The head of the toothbrush is in this illustration placed against the buccal surfaces of the posterior teeth of the right maxilla. Note the angulation of the bristles against the tooth and the direction (arrows) of the motion.

The *second stage* of this information may include a description of the reasons for the presence and the particular location in the dentition of disease. It is important that the dentist emphasizes that bacteria which colonize the tooth surfaces are the main cause of both periodontal disease and caries. The patient should be informed that bacteria which have formed dental plaques can reducc not only the plaque pH - and produce caries lesions - but also release substances which initiate and maintain inflammatory alterations of the gingiva and cause destruction of the attachment apparatus.

The *third stage* may involve the illustration of the location of the plaques in the dentition. First the plaque is stained with a disclosing solution. Then the patient and the dentist in collaboration examine the tooth surfaces, one by one, for presence of plaque. Areas in the dentition without plaque and without signs of pathology should be identified, as well as sites with plaque and associated signs of periodontal disease and caries. The patient should now be made aware that his/her active participation in

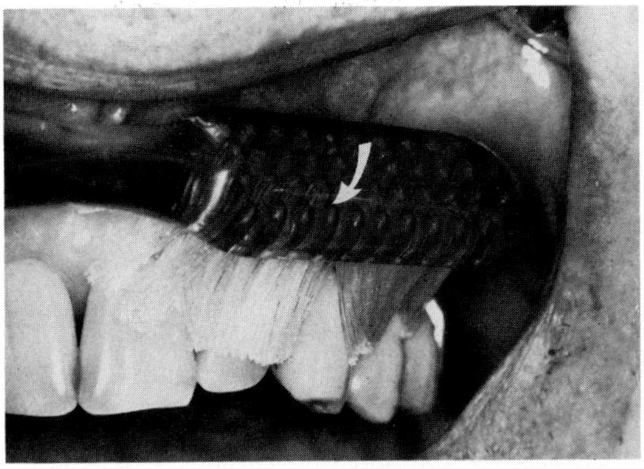

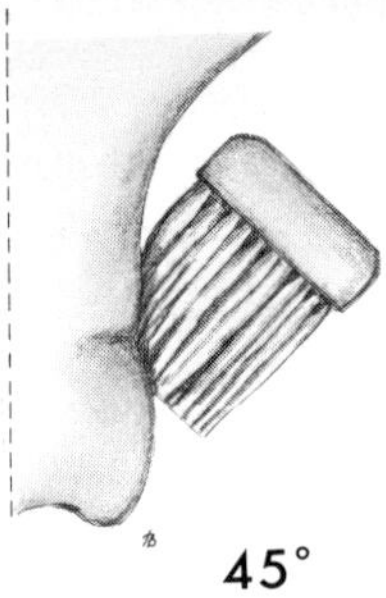

Fig. 14-2a. The Charters' method of toothbrushing. The head of the toothbrush is placed in the left maxilla. Note the angulation of the bristles against the buccal tooth surfaces. The bristles are forced into the interproximal areas.

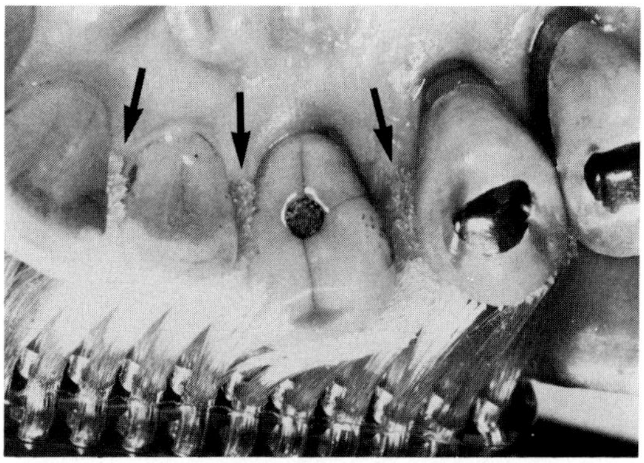

Fig. 14-2b. The palatal aspect of the incisor region in the maxilla illustrating the penetration of the bristles through the interproximal spaces (arrows).

the treatment is essential for a successful outcome.

In summary: detailed information must be given to the patient regarding his/her dental status and the relationship between the presence of dental plaque and calculus in the mouth and the location of sites showing dental disease. This information is aimed at motivating the patient to cooperate in the treatment. The subsequent instruction in proper oral hygiene techniques will only be meaningful and effective if the patient recognizes oral health as a valuable asset or goal of therapy. The information that patients must receive concerning the cause and symptoms of periodontal disease can be delivered in many different ways. The "step by step system" described above has been used for many years and in a large number of clinical trials performed at the department of Periodontology, University of Gothenburg, Sweden (Lindhe & Nyman 1975, Rosling et al. 1976, Lindhe et al. 1982).

Self-performed controls methods

Toothbrushing methods

A variety of toothbrushing methods or techniques have been described in the literature. These methods can be classified into different categories with respect to the pattern of motion that the brush performs:

roll: "Rolling Stroke", "Modified Stillman"
vibratory: "Stillman", "Charters", "Bass"
circular: "Fones"
vertical: "Leonard"
horizontal; "Scrub-brush".

A number of studies have been carried out in order to compare the tooth cleaning effect accomplished by brushing using some of the above-mentioned techniques. So far, however, no method of toothbrushing has been shown to be *clearly* superior to the others. However, Sagnes (1974) in children and Rugg-Gunn et al. (1979) in adolescents reported that the horizontal scrub-technique had a somewhat better plaque-removing potential than the roll technique.

More important than the selection of a certain method of toothbrushing for the establishment of proper home care habits is the *willingness*, and to some extent the *ability* of the individual patient to properly clean his/her

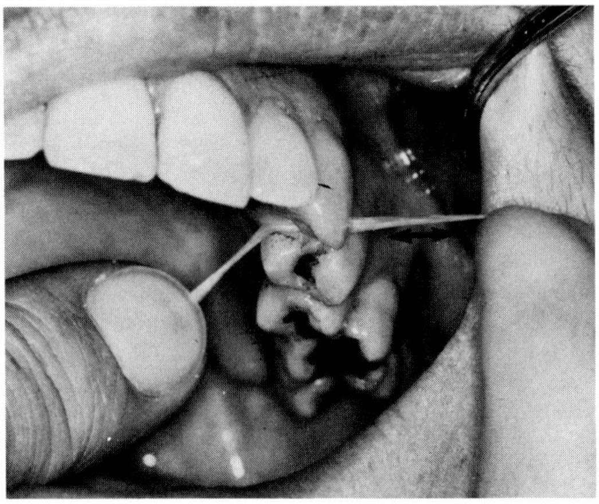

Fig. 14-3a. Dental floss is used for interproximal cleaning. The floss is carefully guided through the contact point between teeth 23 and 24. When contact has been established between the floss and the distal/mesial tooth surface the floss is moved, by minute sawing movements, against the surface for cleaning.

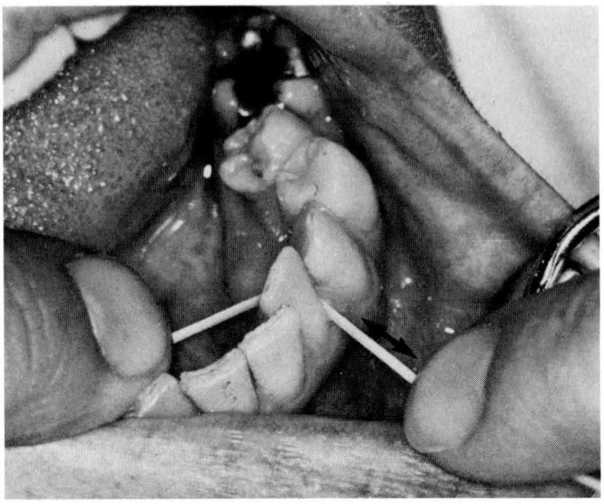

Fig. 14-3b. The dental floss is guided through the interdental contact point between teeth 33 and 32 by the two *index* fingers.

teeth. The control of the result of the self-performed tooth cleaning, preferably with the use of *plaque-disclosing agents* (see below) is also more important for the institution of proper home-care techniques than the instruction and practice in a particular method of brushing.

Since, however, the Bass' (Bass 1954) and the Charters' (Chartes 1948) methods of toothbrushing probably are the most commonly recommended techniques in dental practice, a description of these methods seems justified:

1. The Bass' method.
A soft, multitufted brush is applied with its head at an angle of 45° to the long axis of the teeth (Fig. 14-1) and pressed in an apical direction against the gingival margin. The brush is moved in an anterior-posterior direction with short strokes as in a vibrating motion. When the lingual surfaces of the anterior teeth are cleaned, the brush has to be turned to a vertical position to obtain proper access to the gingival area of the teeth. The Bass' method, properly used, is effective for the removal of soft deposits located immediately above and below the gingival margin.

2. The Charters' method.
The head of the brush is applied to the teeth at an angle of approximately 45° to the occlusal plane (Fig. 14-2). The bristles of the toothbrush are directed towards the occlusal/incisal surfaces and the brush is moved back and forth in a rotatory motion. This method of tooth cleaning is effective particularly in cases with receded interdental papillae, i.e. when the interdental spaces are open and thus accessible to the penetration of the brush bristles.

Interdental cleaning

Tooth cleaning using an ordinary toothbrush will not properly eliminate plaque in the interdental areas (Lövdal et al. 1958). Adjunctive devices therefore have to be used for interproximal plaque removal. Depending upon the shape of the interproximal space *dental floss* or *tape, toothpicks, interproximal brushes* and/or *single-tufted brushes* should be used.

Dental floss and tape
In cases where the interdental papillae completely fill the interdental spaces, effective removal of plaque from the interproximal tooth surfaces may be accomplished by flossing. In

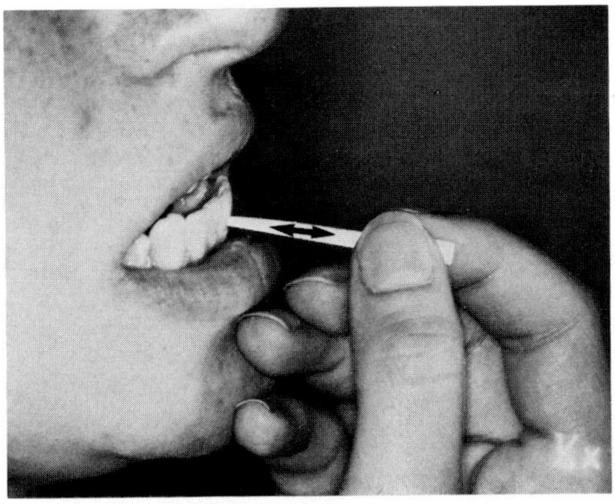

Fig. 14-4a. A triangular toothpick is used for interproximal tooth cleaning. The toothpick is secured in its position with "finger rest" on the cheek for stabilization of movements.

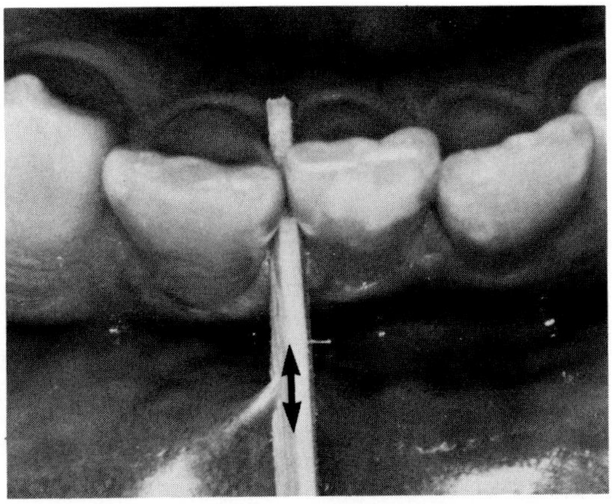

Fig. 14-4b. The toothpick is properly inserted in an interproximal site in the lower front tooth region.

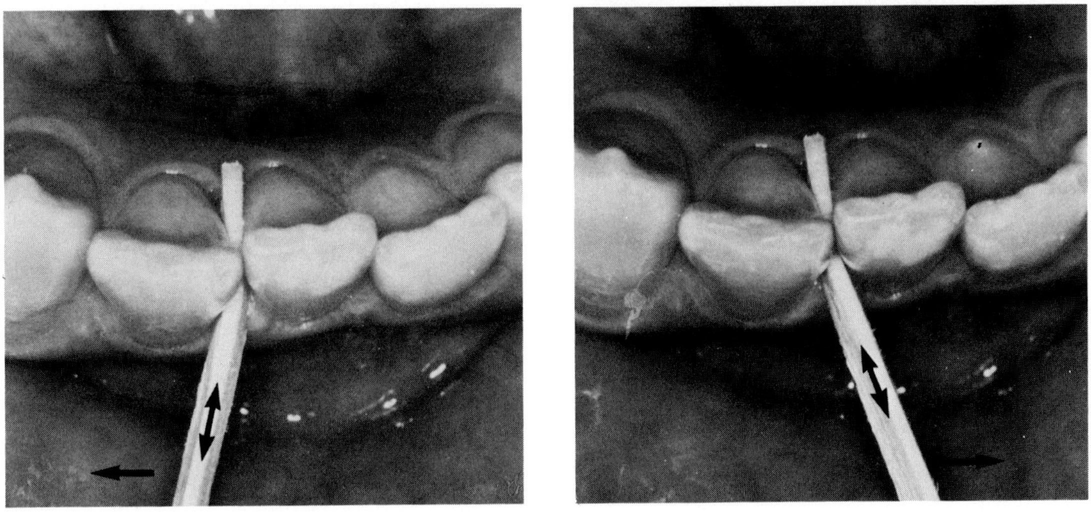

Fig. 14-4c. By changing the direction of insertion of the toothpick the two proximal tooth surfaces are properly cleaned.

the daily plaque-control program the dental floss can, without causing damage to the gingiva and periodontal ligament, be brought 2-3.5 mm below the tip of the papilla (Waerhaug 1981). Several types of floss (waxed, unwaxed) have been introduced, but no clear-cut differences in the cleansing potential of different brands of floss have so far been reported (Keller & Manson-Hing 1969). The correct technique for applying the dental floss is illustrated in Fig. 14-3. When properly used, almost all parts of the interproximal surfaces can be cleaned with the floss (O'Leary 1970). However, this method of interdental cleaning has some limitations:

1. For some patients with inadequate dexterity the technique is difficult to master
2. Flossing may be more time-consuming than interproximal cleansing with toothpicks (Gjermo & Flötra 1970)
3. Improper use of the floss can cause damage to the interdental gingival tissues (Thoma & Goldman 1960).

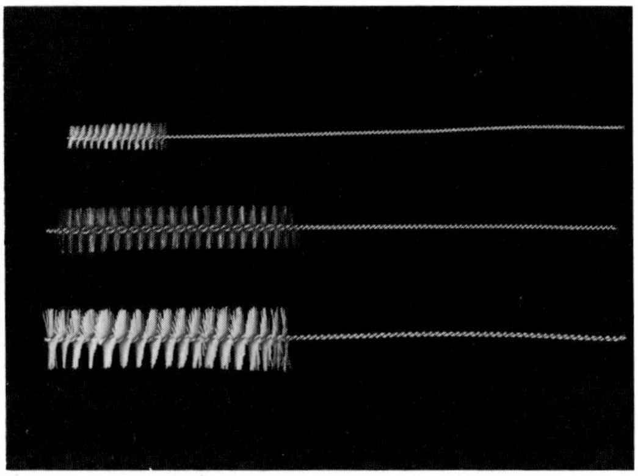

Fig. 14-5. Interproximal brushes of three different sizes.

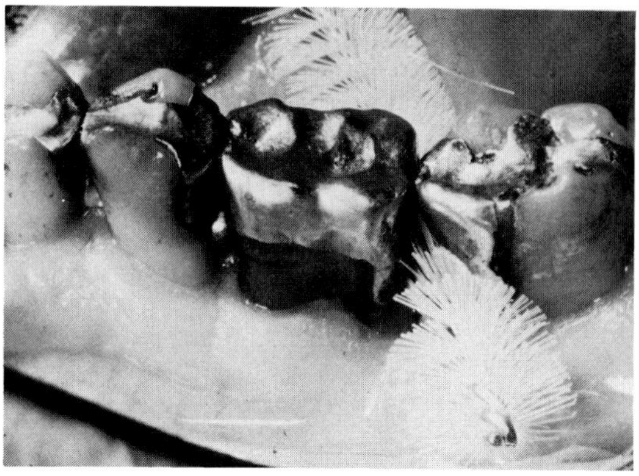

Fig. 14-6. An interproximal brush has been inserted in a wide interdental space between teeth 46 and 47. Lingual view.

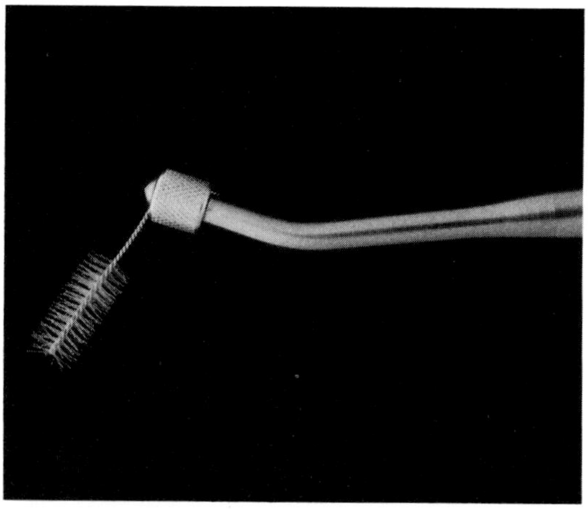

Fig. 14-7. A small interproximal brush inserted in a custom-made handle.

Toothpicks

In sites where the interdental papillae are receded the toothpick is an excellent substitute for dental floss for inter-proximal cleaning. The toothpick should be made of soft wood, have a triangular shape, to fit the interdental space (Waerhaug 1959). The proper use of toothpicks is illustrated in Fig. 14-4.

Interproximal brush

In cases with wider interdental spaces an interproximal brush (bottle neck brush) is often effective for the removal of plaque from the approximal surfaces. The interproximal brushes are manufactured in different sizes (Fig. 14-5) and should be selected to fit, as closely as possible, the individual interdental space (Fig. 14-6). Small interproximal brushes can be inserted into handles (Fig. 14-7) which may facilitate the cleaning of the interproximal areas in the posterior parts of the dentition. The interproximal brush is also the aid of choice in approximal areas where the surfaces have a concave outline or where rootfurrows are present. In "through and through" furcation defects the use of an interproximal brush is suitable for proper cleaning and can also be used as a carrier of antimicrobial agents, i.e. chlorhexidine.

Single-tufted brush

A single-tufted brush can be recommended to be used in regions of the dentition which are not easily reached with other oral hygiene devices, e.g. furcation areas, distal surfaces of the most posterior molars and buccal or lingual tooth surfaces with an irregular gingival margin (Fig. 14-8).

Electric brushes

The electric toothbrush may be a valuable alternative or supplement to manual brushes, e.g. for handicapped persons and in the dental care of hospitalized individuals. Also some patients will be more motivated to improve their oral

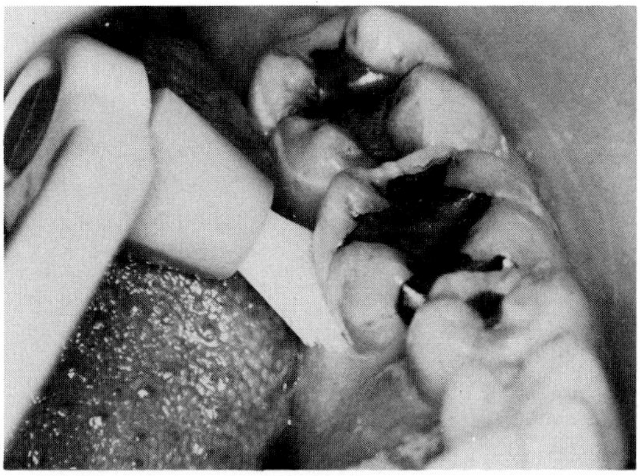

Fig. 14-8a. A single-tufted toothbrush is used in tooth regions where cleaning by the use of an ordinary tooth brush is difficult to master. The lingual surfaces of lower molars are cleaned.

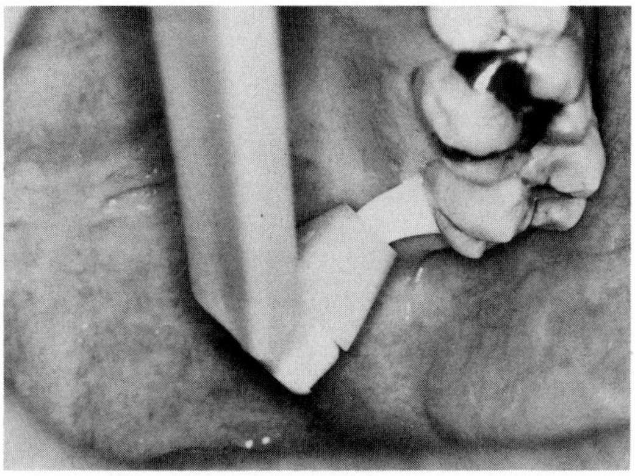

Fig. 14-8b. The palatal and distal surfaces of maxillary molars are cleaned by means of a single-tufted toothbrush.

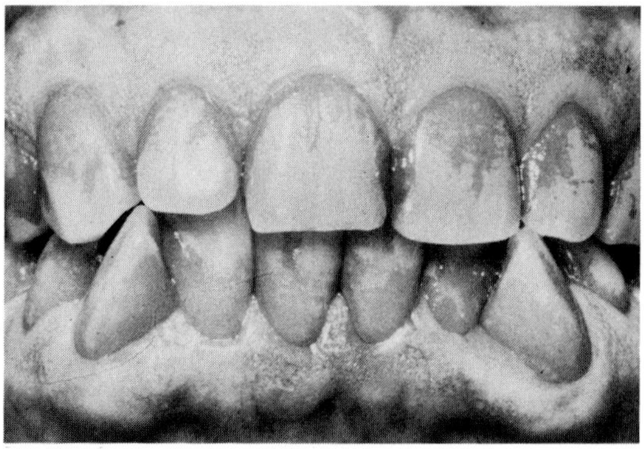

Fig. 14-9a. Disclosing agents are used to disclose the presence of dental plaque. Note remaining dental plaque on the buccal tooth surfaces after staining.

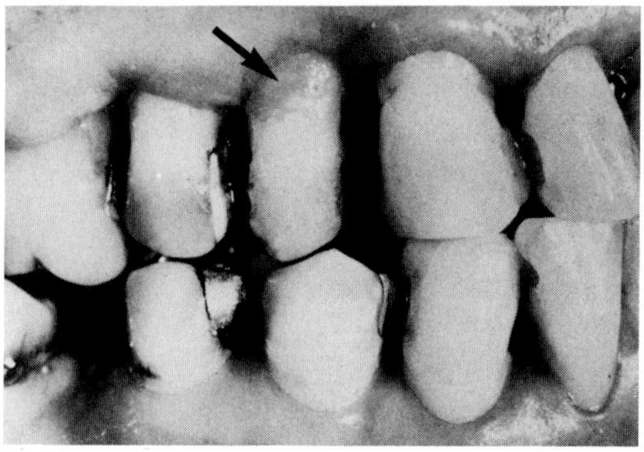

Fig. 14-9b. After self-performed tooth cleaning, remaining plaque can be identified by the patient following rinsing with a disclosing solution (arrow).

hygiene when recommended to use an electric toothbrush. A certain type of electric brush (Rotadent®) which in design and function resembles rotating instruments used by professionals for tooth cleaning has recently been introduced and its effectiveness assessed in a clinical study performed by Glavind & Zeuner (1986). The authors concluded that the use of this single type of rotating electric toothbrush for self-performed plaque control was equally effective as a more comprehensive set of oral hygiene devices (toothbrush, toothpick etc.) in the hands of the patients.

Adjunctive aids

Disclosing agents

Dental plaque is difficult to detect, particularly to the untrained eye. Disclosing agents should be used, therefore, to demonstrate the presence and location of plaque and to evaluate the efficacy of the patient's home care technique (Fig. 14-9). As a rule, the disclosing agent should be applied after toothbrushing and interdental cleaning. The patient can hereby identify sites at which the oral hygiene efforts have been inadequate. Substances aimed at staining dental plaque have been used in dentistry for many years (Arnim 1963, Ten 1981). Examples of such substances are *erythrocin*, *fuchsin* and more recently a *fluorescein-containing* dye for

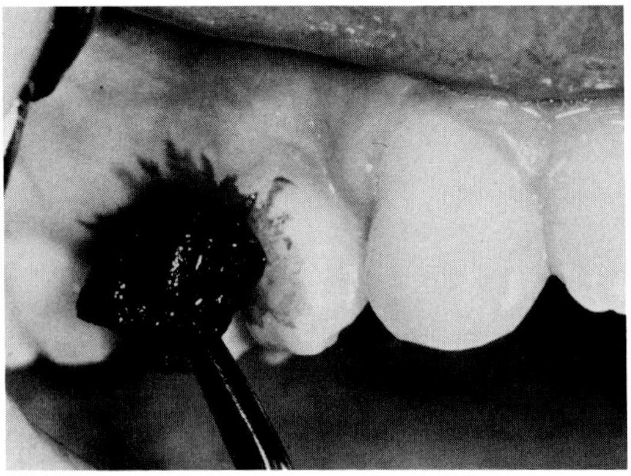

Fig. 14-10. Wafers containing disclosing solutions are often used to identify plaque.

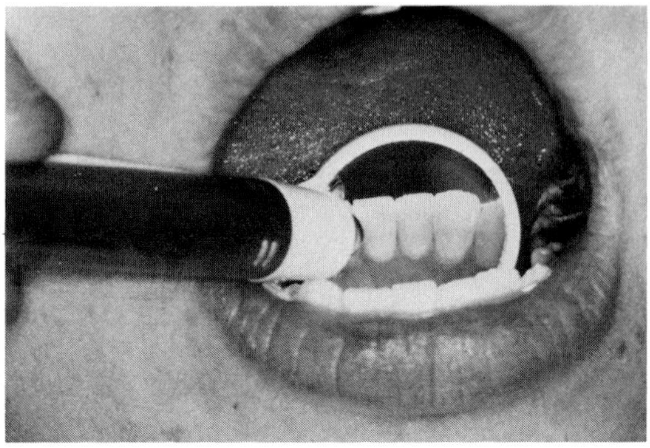

Fig. 14-11. A mirror-light combination may facilitate for the patient the detection of plaque on the lingual tooth surfaces.

visualization of plaque when exposed to an ultraviolet light (Plack-lite®). Erythrosin containing *tablets* or *wafers* are available as "over the counter products". The disclosing tablets should be used by the patient in the home care program and the wafers by the dentist for plaque assessments (Fig. 14-10).

Intraoral mirror

As stated above, an important step in the patient's self-performed home care is the nonprofessional control of the efficacy of the toothcleaning procedures. Bathroom lights are often inadequate for intraoral illumination, which is why a mirrorlight combination for some patients can be a useful adjunct for the detection of remaining plaque (Fig. 14-11).

Irrigation devices

The use of water-irrigating devices has been recommended as a valuable supplement to mechanical plaque control measures. Many investigators have tried to determine the potential of such devices to assist in the removal of dental plaque, but the findings reported from such clinical trials are inconclusive. Studies by Matsuzaki et al. (1974) an Hugoson (1978) failed to demonstrate significant reduction of plaque and gingivitis scores in patients using water irrigators. However, in special cases the use of a device for the irrigation of antiseptics (chlorhexidine) may be an excellent adjunct to mechanical tooth cleaning for the removal of both food debris and plaque (Lang & Räber 1982).

Dentifrices

A dentifrice should be used in combination with toothbrushing for the purpose of 1) facilitating plaque removal and 2) applying agents to the tooth surfaces for therapeutic or preventive purposes. The abrasive material of the dentifrice should have a particle size and composition which prevents wear of tooth substances but facilitates plaque removal. The question remains how abrasive a dentifrice should be to assist in the removal of plaque without causing damage. Studies comparing the effect of abrasive and non-abrasive dentifrices regarding their potential as adjuncts for plaque removal have failed to disclose an obvious benefit of abrasive toothpastes. The establishment of a stained pellicle seems, however, to be favored in subjects using non-abrasive dentifrices (Bergenholtz et al. 1971). The dentifrice is also an excellent vehicle for the administration of substances to the tooth surfaces such as *fluorides, antiseptics* (e.g. chlorhexidine), *enzymes* (e.g. amyloglucosidase, glucose oxidase) or other substances (e.g. for desensitization of hypersensitive tooth surfaces and to retard the development of supragingival calculus).

Plaque control program for the periodontal patient

The system used to teach the patient a proper tooth-cleaning technique may of course vary from one dentist/dental hygienist to another. Below is presented one system which has been used in clinical trials by Lindhe & Nyman 1975, Rosing et al. 1976, Lindhe et al. 1982.

First session

1. Ask the patient to clean the teeth using her/his traditional technique.
2. Explain to the patient the use of disclosing agents to identify plaque at sites where the tooth-cleaning technique has been inadequate. Apply the disclosing solution to the teeth. Use disclosing wafers. Demonstrate the result for the patient; use a hand mirror and ask the patient to identify all sites where plaque remains.
3. Ask the pateint to clean the teeth once more and stress the importance of removing plaque from the stained sites. Discuss the possibility of altering her/his traditional toothbrushing technique.
4. Check the result of the second tooth-cleaning practice together with the patient. Are there still areas which harbor stained material? Discuss the need for adjunctive devices for interproximal brushes.
5. Allow the patient under careful supervision to practice the use of dental floss or toothpick. Discuss the result obtained.

Second session (2-4 days later)

1. Apply the disclosing solution on the teeth and ask the patient to evaluate the result of her/his home-care program. All sites harboring stained material should be identified on a chart.
2. Discuss the result and adjust, if necessary, the technique.

Third session (1-2 weeks later)

Apply the disclosing solution to the teeth and evaluate the result of the home-care program. All sites harboring stained material should be identified on a chart. Discuss the result of the self-performed tooth cleaning with the use of a plaque chart (Fig. 14-12) and, if needed, adjust the technique and the armamentarium.

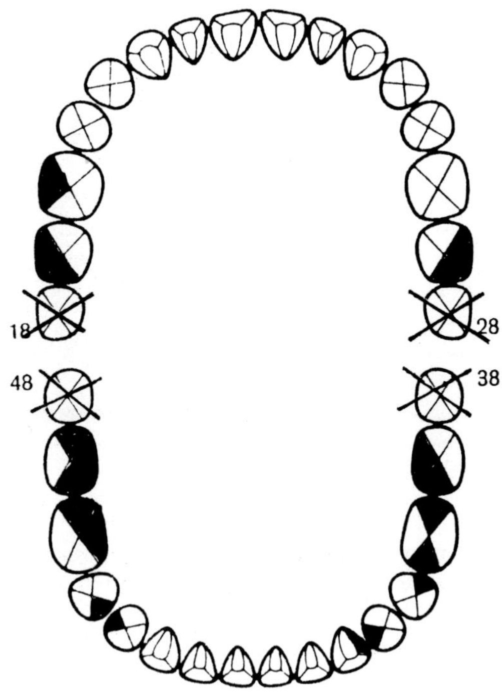

Fig. 14-12. A chart illustrating the teeth and tooth surfaces in the upper and lower jaws. The distribution of tooth surfaces with dental plaque (shadowed areas) is identified. In this case the plaque score is 17%.

Depending on the ability of the patient to learn how to practise proper oral hygiene measures, the time required for the instruction may vary considerably. Thus, additional oral hygiene sessions may be required. It is important, however, to point out that the efficacy of self-performed plaque control should be evaluated and presented to the patient at each appointment during both active and maintenance phases of therapy (see Chapter 25).

Lesions produced by oral hygiene measures

Damage of hard and soft tissues caused by extensive toothbrushing or the use of adjunctive

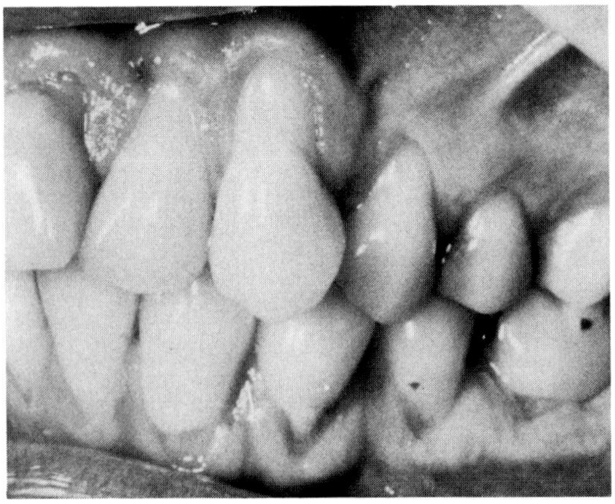

Fig. 14-13a. Soft-tissue damage as a result of extensive tooth brushing. Note gingival recession on the buccal gingival surface of e.g. tooth 23.

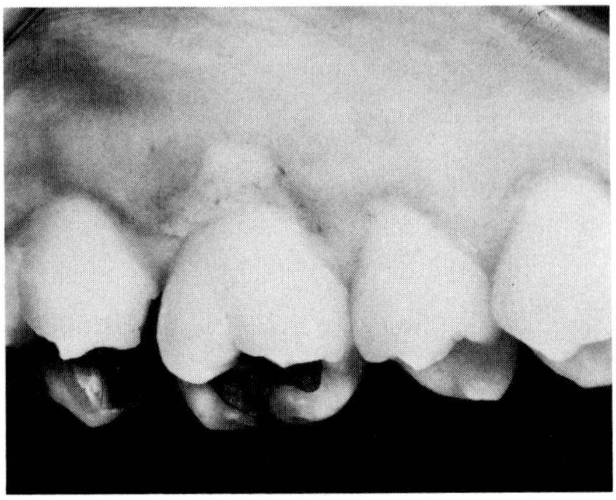

Fig. 14-13b. Note multiple ulcerations of the buccal gingival margin in the right maxilla.

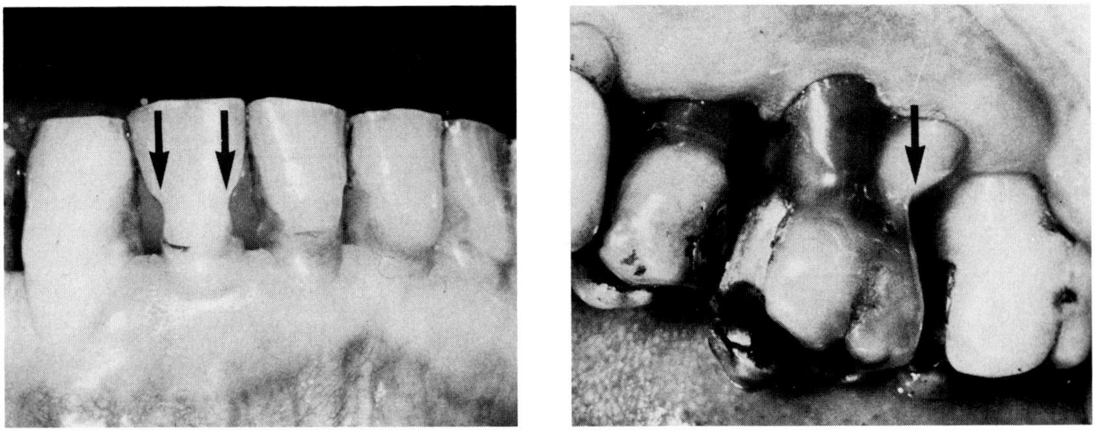

Fig. 14-13c,d. Hard-tissue damage (arrows) has resulted after extensive use of interdental brushes.

oral hygiene aids are sometimes seen in periodontal patients. In rare cases the damage may be extensive. The buccal aspects of canines and premolars and the approximal surfaces of lower incisors are sites at which this type of damage is most common (Fig. 14-13). Factors contributing to such damages can include 1) too stiff bristles of the toothbrush, 2) too extensive toothbrushing and interdental instrumentation and 3) the use of a highly abrasive dentifrice during brushing and interdental cleaning.

Findings from clinical and laboratory research have demonstrated that damage of *hard tissue* is mainly due to the abrasive component of the dentifrice used, while lesions in the gingiva can be produced by toothbrushing or flossing also without the use of a dentifrice. It is important to realize that as soon as soft and/or hard tissue damage is identified, the oral hygiene technique has to be changed in order to arrest the progression of the lesions.

Scaling and root planing

Definitions

Scaling is a procedure which aims at the removal of plaque and calculus from the tooth surface. Depending on the location of the deposits scaling has to be performed by supragingival or subgingival instrumentation. The objective of supragingival scaling is the removal of deposits from the clinical crown of the teeth. *Root planing* denotes a technique of instrumentation by which the "softened" cementum is removed and the root surface is made "hard" and "smooth". Subgingival scaling and root planing (root curettage) are performed as either closed or open procedures. The *closed* procedure implies subgingival instrumentation without intentional displacement of the gingiva, i.e. the root surface is not accessible for direct visual inspection. The *open* procedure calls for exposure of the affected root surface by measures which displace the gingival tissue. The gingivae are thus incised and reflected to facilitate access for the instrument and visibility for the operator in the field of operation.

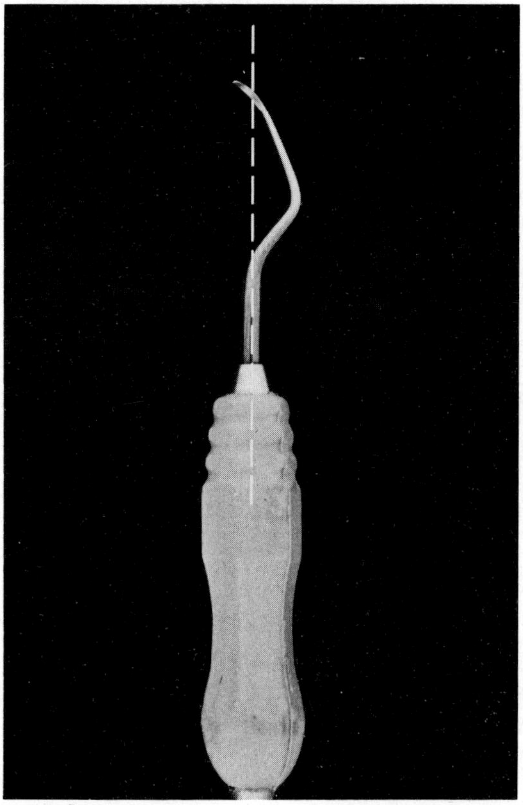

Fig. 14-14. A double-ended hand instrument with col-grip. The cutting edges of the blades are centered over the long axis of the handle.

Instruments and instrumentation
Instruments used for scaling and root planing are classified as:

1. Hand instruments
   Curettes, Sickels, Hoes, Chisels, Files
2. Ultrasonic and sonic instruments
3. Rotating instruments

Hand instruments
A hand instrument is composed of three parts: The *working part* (the blade), the *shank* and the *handle*. The cutting edges of the blade are centered over the long axis of the handle in order to obtain proper balance of the instrument (Fig. 14-14). The blade is often made of *carbon steel, stainless steel* or *tungsten carbide*.

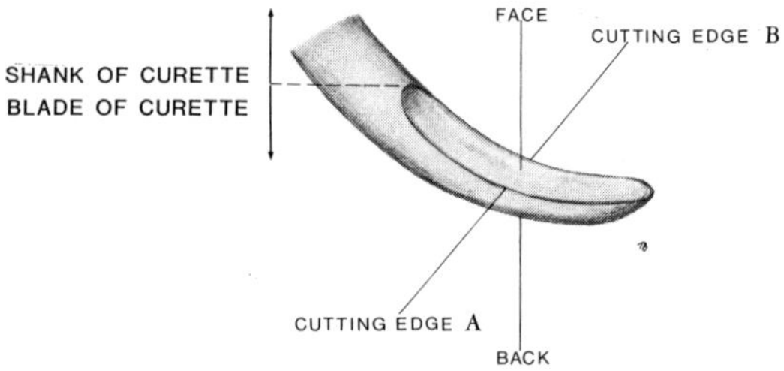

Fig. 14-15. Schematic illustration of the design of the blade of a curette.

Curettes (Fig. 14-15)
Curettes are instruments used for both supra- and subgingival scaling and root planing. The working part of the curette is the spoon-shaped blade which has two curved cutting edges. The two edges are united by the rounded toe. The curettes are usually made "double-ended" with mirror-turned blades. The length and angulation of the shank as well as the dimensions of the blade differ between different brands of the instrument (Fig. 14-16).

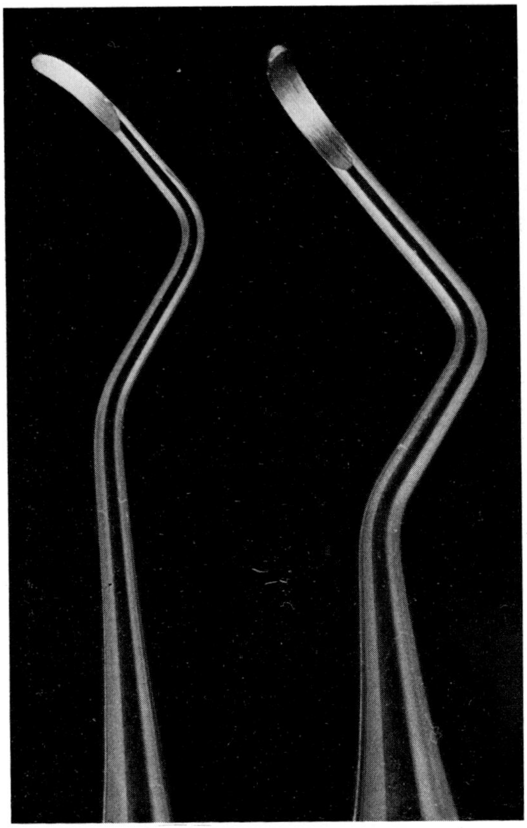

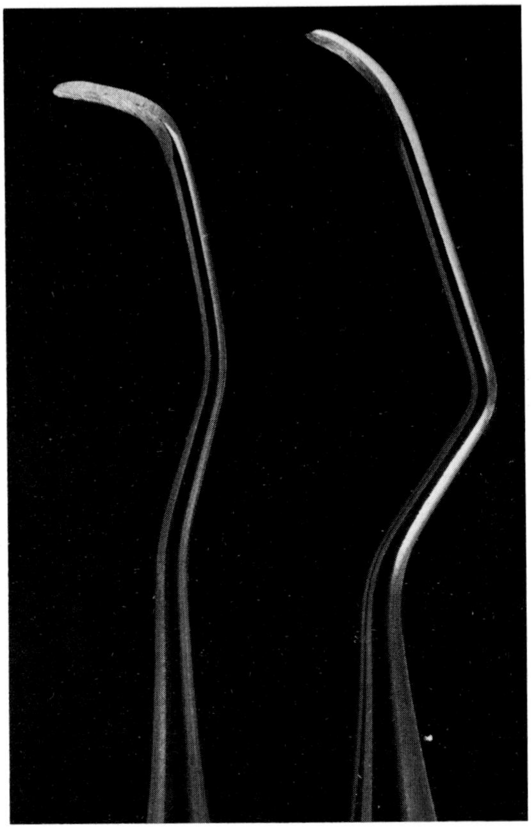

Fig. 14-16. Curettes with different lengths and angulations of the shank. (a) and (b) are curettes used for supragingival and (c) and (d) curettes for subgingival instrumentation. Increased angulation of the shank (b and d) of the curettes permits proper instrumentation in posterior tooth regions.

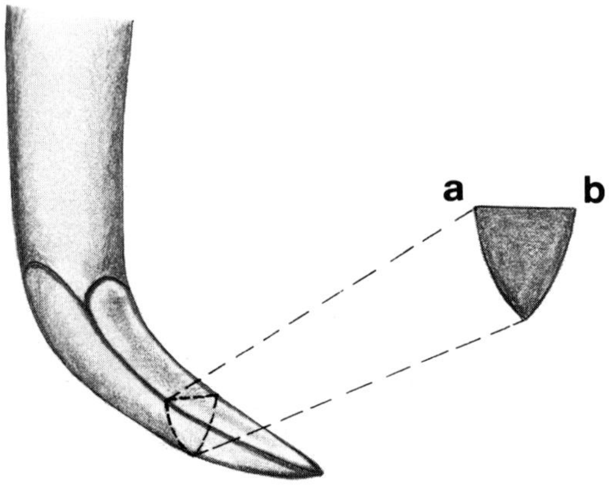

Fig. 14-17. Schematic illustration of the cross section of the blade of a sickle. The cutting edges are positioned at (a) and (b).

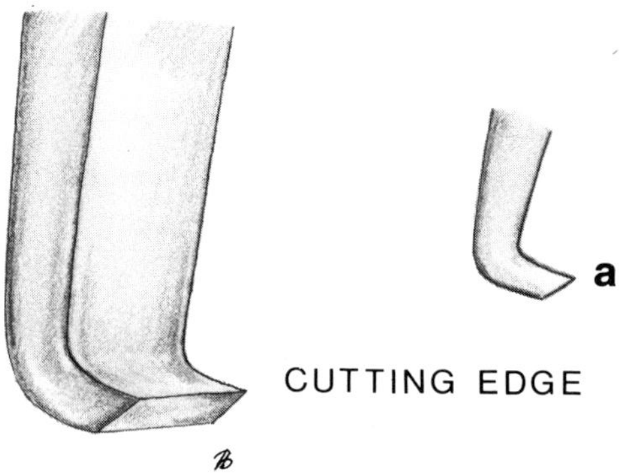

Fig. 14-18. The cross section of a hoe. Note the position of the cutting edge (a).

Sickles (Fig. 14-17)

The sickle is manufactured with either a curved or a straight blade which has a triangular cross section and two cutting edges. The "facial" surface between the two cutting edges is flat in

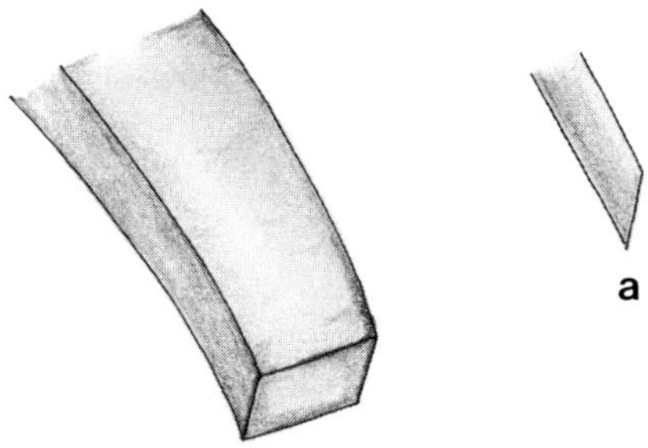

Fig. 14-19. The cross section of a chisel. Note the position of the cutting edge (a).

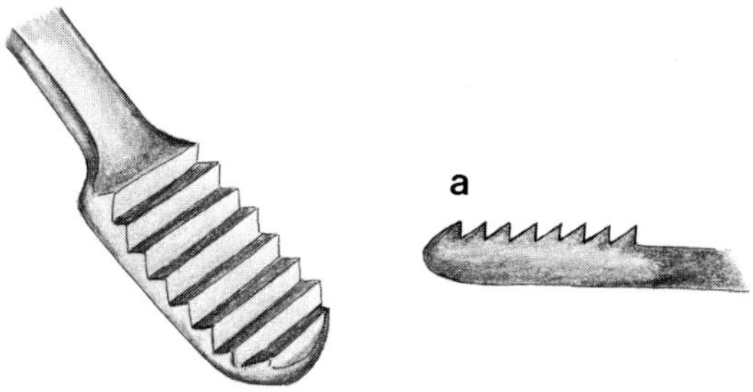

Fig. 14-20. The cross section of a file. Note the position of the cutting edges (a).

Fig. 14-21a. Photograph illustrating the lingual aspect of the mandibular front tooth region with supragingival plaque and calculus.

Fig. 14-21b. The same tooth region 3 weeks after supragingival scaling and institution of proper oral hygiene.

Fig. 14-21c. Radiographs of the maxillary left jaw before and after removal of calculus and amalgam overhangs.

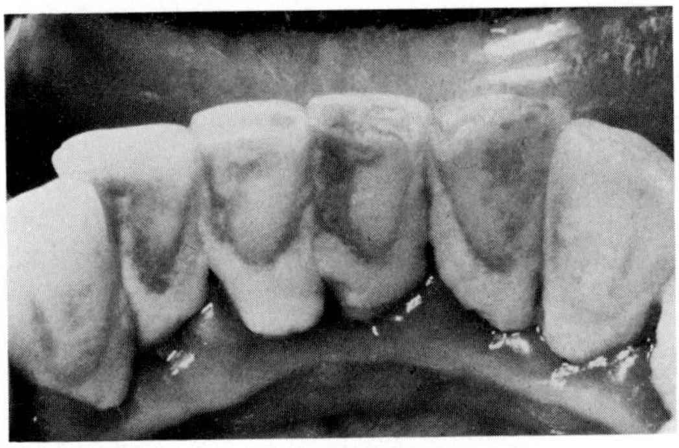

Fig. 14-21a.

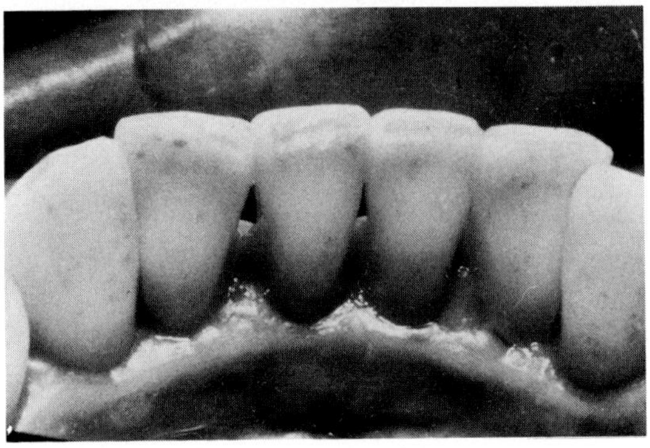

Fig. 14-21b

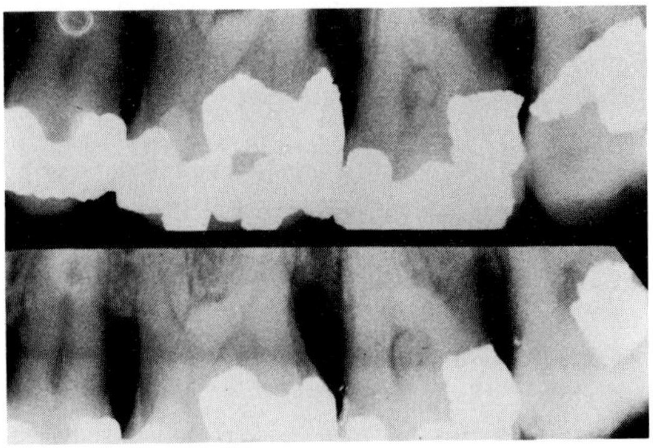

Fig. 14-21c.

lateral direction but may be curved in the direction of its long axis. The "facial" surface converges with the two lateral surfaces of the blade. The sickles are mainly used for supragingival debridement or scaling in shallow pockets.

Hoes (Fig. 14-18)
The hoe has only one cutting edge. The blade is turned at a 100-degree angle to the shank with the cutting edge bevelled at a 45-degree angle. The blade can be positioned at four different inclinations in relation to the shank: facial, lingual, distal and mesial. The hoe is mainly used for supragingival scaling but is an excellent instrument for root planing during periodontal surgery.

Chisels (Fig. 14-19)
The periodontal chisel is nowadays probably

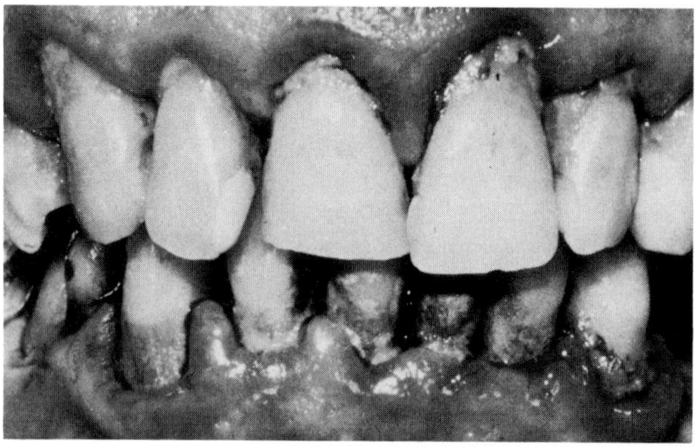

Fig 14-22a.

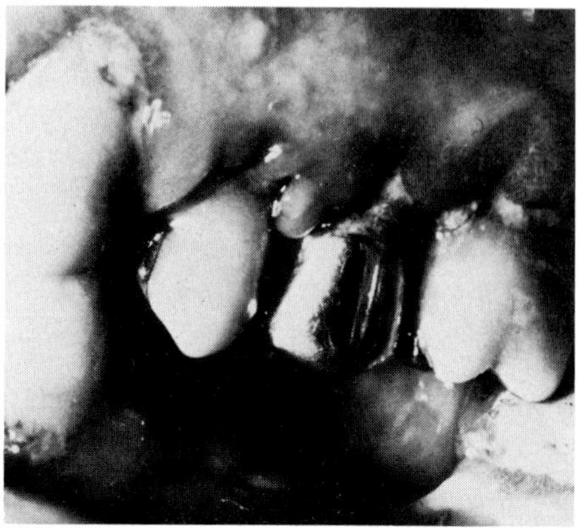

Fig 14-22b.

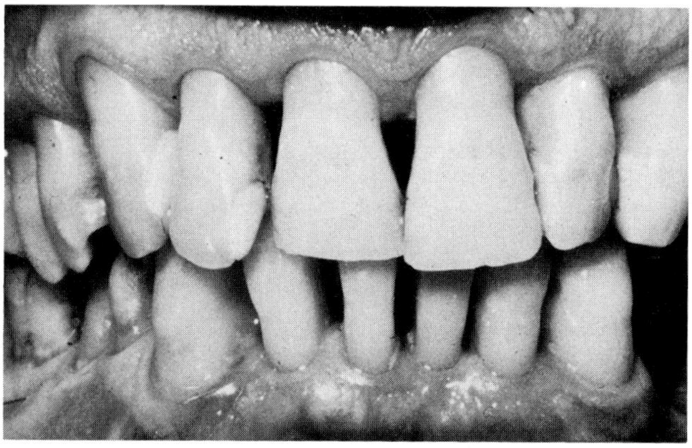

Fig 14-22c.

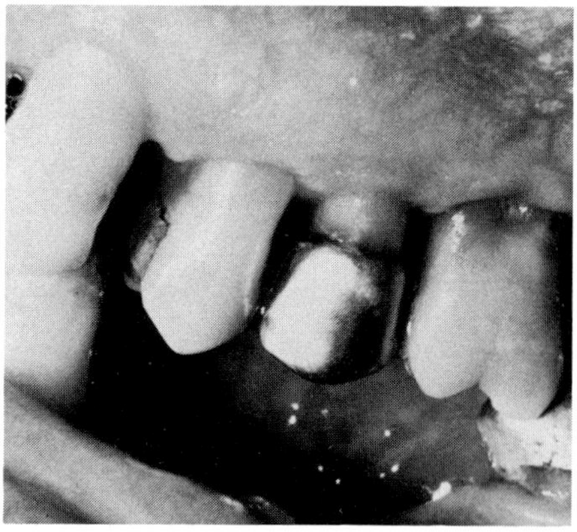

Fig 14-22d.

Fig. 14-22a-d. Photographs illustrating the effect of scaling, root planing and proper self-performed plaque control on the gingival tissues. Note gingival recession and the stippled outer surface of the gingiva after treatment (c,d) compared to the status before treatment (a,b).

not commonly used. The straight or bent chisel may be used for the rapid dislodgement of heavy masses of calculus, located on the approximal and lingual surfaces of mandibular anterior teeth.

Files (Fig. 14-20)

A periodontal file has multiple cutting edges lined up as a series of miniature hoes on a round or rectangular base. A flat and small file can be used for planing root surfaces in narrow pockets or furcation areas which may be inaccessible with other instruments.

Instrumentation

Supragingival scaling

The debridement of the dentition of a patient with periodontal disease is almost always initiated with supragingival scaling. To facilitate subgingival instrumentation supragingival calculus and gross overhangs of amalgam restorations or metal crowns should first be removed (see below; Fig. 14-21). This initial phase of the debridement can be performed with the use of hand instruments or ultrasonic instruments (see below). When hand instrumentation is preferred for the initial debridement a curette, a sickle, or a chisel may be used to split off calculus from its attachment to the enamel and/or the exposed part of the root. Following hand instrumentation the clinical crowns should be polished with rubber cups and first pumice and subsequently more finegrained (2-3 μm) polishing pastes. In many cases the *supragingival scaling* effort can be completed in one session. This will allow the patient without further delay to start exercising the "improved" self-performed plaque control program.

Subgingival scaling and root planing
Performed with hand instruments, these treatment procedures aim at removing not only soft and hard deposits from the root surface but also small amounts of tooth substance. Root cementum and dentine are removed in the shape of small chips which carry the deposits and which during the cutting operation are curled up at the front side (in the cutting direction) of the blade of the instrument. This method of instrumentation is denoted "orthogonal cutting", which implies the removal of tooth substance by means of an edge which to a varying extent penetrates the hard substance of the root. The result of the cutting operation is dependent on the material and geometry of the edge, the sharpness of the edge and the forces used during instrumentation (Lindhe 1964). Even if subgingival scaling and root planing often are regarded as two separate procedures with different objectives (see definition) in clinical work, they cannot always be separated from one another. As stated above subgingival instrumentation aims at resolving the inflammation in the gingiva and arresting the progressive destruction of the attachment apparatus by removing the microbiota of the gingival pocket. Coupled with supragingival plaque control, therefore, subgingival debridement is the most important measure in the treatment of plaque-associated periodontal disease. As a matter of fact, in many patients who adopt proper self-performed plaque control habits subgingival instrumentation results in gingival health (Fig. 14-22).

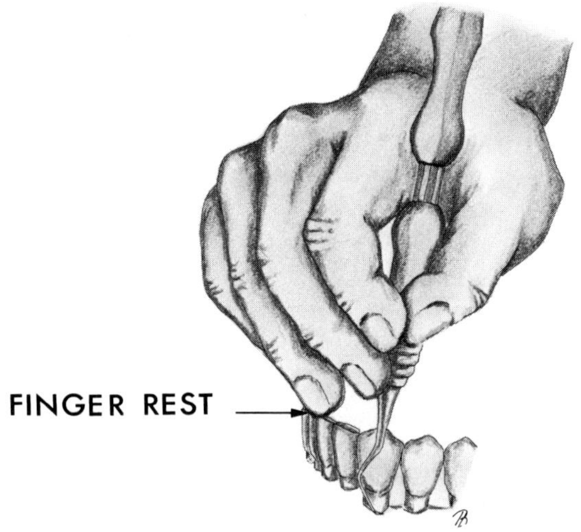

Fig. 14-23. Schematic illustration demonstrating the proper "third finger rest" using a modified pen grasp in the molar region in the right lower jaw.

Prior to the start of the subgingival instrumentation the degree of gingival inflammation and breakdown of the supporting apparatus in all parts of the dentition must have been properly assessed (see Chapter 12). Depending on the severity of the case and the skill of the operator the number of teeth that may be included in each session of subgingival scaling and root planing varies. As a general rule, however, each session should not involve the treatment of more than 4-6 teeth.

The subgingival instrumentation is often performed under local anesthesia. The root surface of the diseased site is first explored with a probe to identify 1) the probing depth 2) the anatomy of the root surface (irregularities, root furrows, open furcation etc). 3) the location of the calcified deposits.

When the characteristics of all surfaces selected for treatment have been assessed, the instrument, almost always a curette, is inserted into the first pocket. The instrument is held in a so-called *modified pen grasp* and with a *finger rest* - fourth finger rest or third finger rest - with the face of the blade parallel to but in only light contact with the root surface (Fig. 14-23).

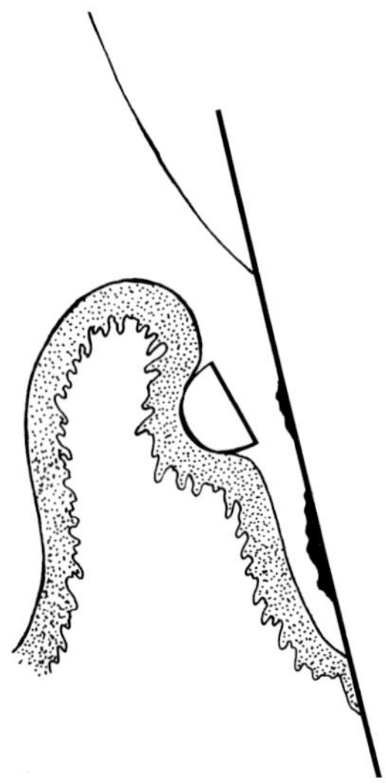

Fig. 14-24a. The curette is inserted into the periodontal pocket. Note the close-to-zero degree angulation of the face of the curette against the root surface.

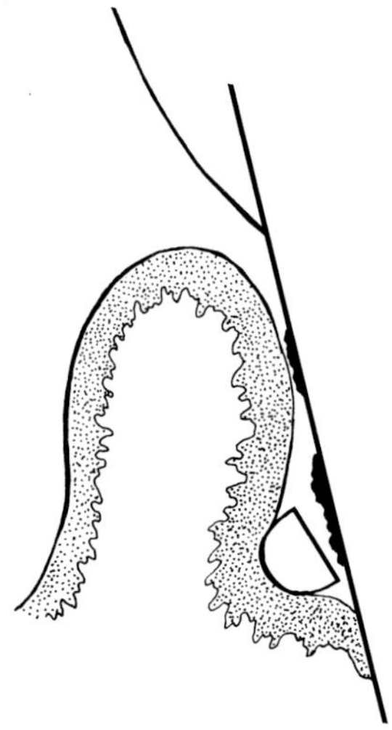

Fig. 14-24b. The bottom of the periodontal pocket is identified with the distal edge of the blade of the curette.

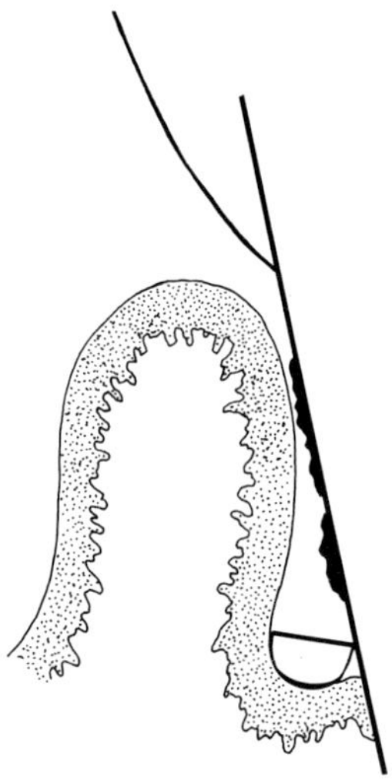

Fig. 14-24c. The curette is turned to a cutting position for scaling.

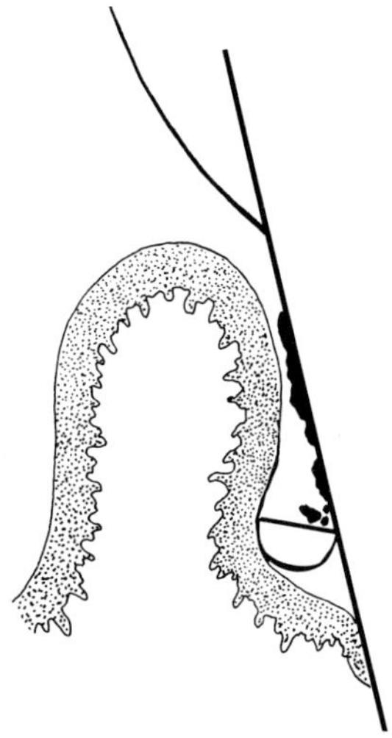

Fig. 14-24d. The blade is moved along the root surface in a scaling stroke to remove calculus.

It is important that all root surface instrumentation is performed with a proper finger rest. This implies that one finger - the third or the fourth- should act as a fulcrum for the movement of the blade of the instrument. A proper finger rest should fulfill the following requirements: 1) provide a stable fulcrum, 2) permit optimal angulation of the blade, 3) enable the use of wrist-forearm motion. In addition, the finger rest should be secured as close as possible to the particular root surface selected for treatment to enable careful instrumentation.

After the base of the periodontal pocket has been identified with the distal edge of the blade, the instrument is turned into a proper "cutting" position (Fig. 14-24). The grasp of

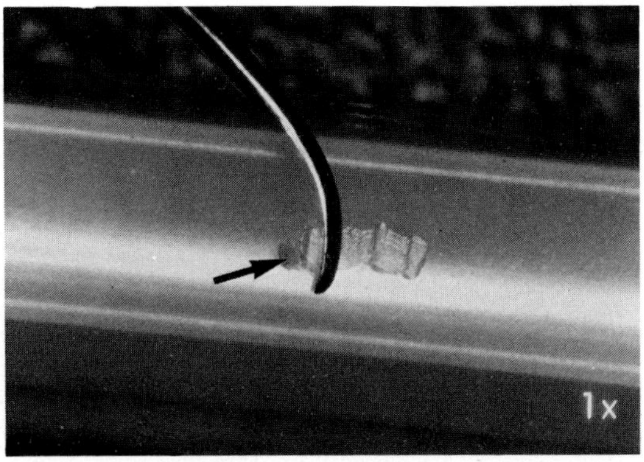

Fig. 14-25. The sharpness of a curette is tested on a plastic stick. A chip (arrow) is easily produced by a sharp instrument.

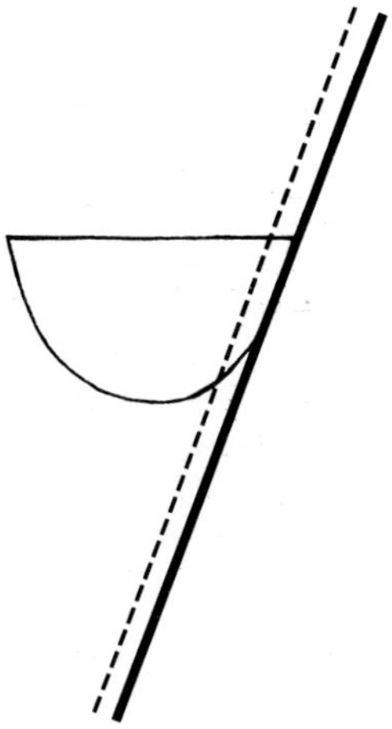

Fig. 14-26. Schematic drawing illustrating the sharpening of a curette. The original geometry of the cutting edge must be maintained during the sharpening procedure.

the instrument is tightened, the force between the cutting edge and the root surface is increased, and the blade is moved in a firm stroke (working stroke) in coronal direction. Due to the structural and chemical composition of root cementum and dentine, the cutting operation *should always be initiated at the bottom of the pocket and be guided in coronal direction.* In this movement the edge penetrates, to some extent, the root surface and removes, in the form of a chip, root substance with attached calculus. The working stroke is followed by a finishing stroke the objective of which is to produce a smooth root surface (root planing). After the *working* and *finishing strokes* have been made, the probe is inserted in the pocket again and the surface characteristics of the root surface assessed anew. Working and finishing strokes must be made in different directions to cover all aspects of the selected root surface (crosswise, back and forth) but, as stated above, the strokes should always start from an apical position and be guided in coronal direction. The root surface should not be considered properly treated until the operator, using a periodontal probe, finds the surface "smooth" and "hard".

Instrument sharpening

The hand instruments must have proper cutting edges in order to make subgingival instrumentation a precise and efficient procedure. In order to remove calculus and tooth substance a curette with *a blunt cutting edge* must be *pressed* against the root surface with a larger force than is required with a sharp instrument. The tactile sensitivity is hereby impaired. Scaling with instruments with blunt cutting edges often results in an incomplete removal of calculus but in the establishment of a "smoothened" root surface. Remaining calculus on such a "smoothened" root surface is difficult to detect even with a periodontal probe. The cutting edge of the hand instrument, therefore, has to be controlled repeatedly during scaling, by testing it on e.g. a plastic stick (Fig. 14-25). During the course of the scaling session sharpened stones should therefore be frequently used to maintain the cutting edges in proper condition.

The sharpening of hand instruments can be performed by the use of either "rotating" (cylindrical or coneshaped) stones or "plain" stones (India or Arkansas stones). Curettes and sickles are sharpened by grinding the lateral surfaces and/or the face of the blade. It is important that the original geometry of the instrument is not changed by the sharpening procedure (Fig. 14-26).

It is not the intention of this textbook chapter to describe in detail the technique for subgingi-

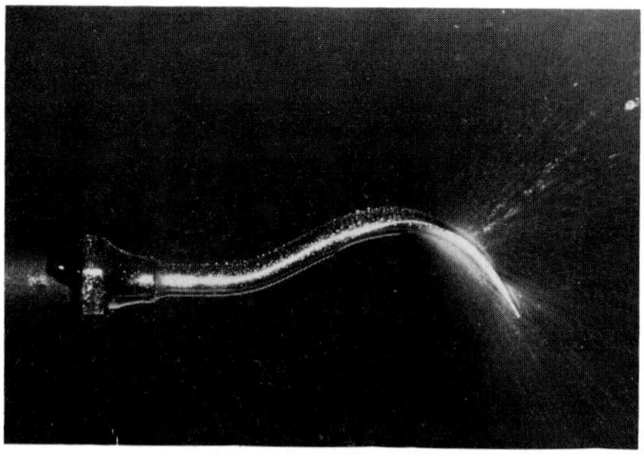

Fig. 14-27. The tip of the ultrasonic instrument. Note the spraying and cavitation of the fluid used for cooling.

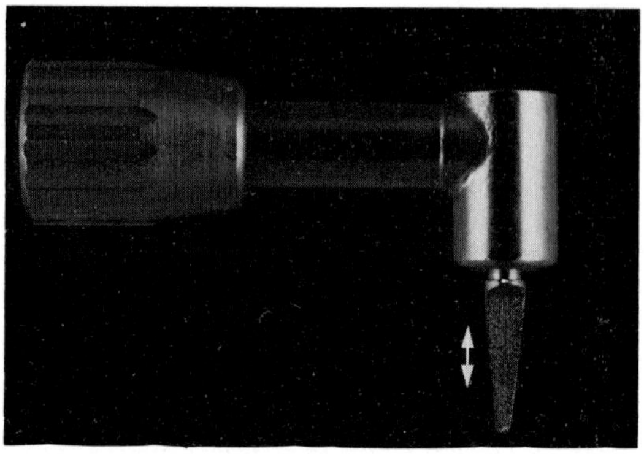

Fig. 14-28. A triangular diamond tip inserted in a handpiece. Arrows indicate the directions of the movement.

val instrumentation. Clinical training under careful supervision is the only way by which the proper technique for subgingival scaling and root planing can be learned.

Ultrasonic and sonic instruments

For many years ultrasonic scalers (e.g. Cavitron®, Amdent®, Odontoson®) have been used for removal of plaque, gross deposits of calculus and stain. Scaling with ultrasonic instruments often results in the establishment of an uneven root surface. It has been suggested, therefore, that ultrasonic scaling should be supplemented by hand instrumentation to establish a smooth root surface (Björn & Lindhe 1962). Recent clinical studies have evaluated the effect of scaling using ultrasonic or hand instruments (Torafson et al. 1979, Badersten et al. 1981). The authors found that debridement of 4-7 mm pockets with ultrasonic instrumentation was as successful for healing of diseased periodontal sites as was scaling with hand instruments (curettes). It has also been questioned whether indeed *a smooth* root surface after treatment in subgingival areas is important for successful healing (Rosenberg & Ash 1974). Waerhaug (1956) found that a junctional epithelium readapted and formed a normal "epithelial cuff" also on uneven root surfaces. Properly used, therefore, ultrasonic instrumentation must be regarded as a valuable substitute for (not only as an adjunct to) conventional scaling with hand instruments and may even be the best instrument for scaling at furcation areas (Leon & Vogel 1987). Recently a new type of instrument for tooth debridement has been introduced - the sonic scaler (e.g. Titan-S®, Micro-Mega Air Scaler®). This instrument is air-driven and produces vibrations in the instrument tip in the sonic range 2,300-6,300 cycles per second). In an *in vitro* study (Lie & Leknes 1985) and in a clinical study (Loos et al. 1987) it was shown that the sonic scaler was as efficient for calculus removal as the ultrasonic instrument and, besides, the sonic scaler caused less root surfaces roughness than did the ultrasonic device.

Instrumentation

The removal of plaque and calculus by ultrasonic and sonic instrumentation is accomplished by a) the vibration of the tip of the instrument, b) the spraying and cavitation effect of the fluid coolant.

The vibrations (amplitude ranging from 0.006-0.1 mm) in the ultrasonic instruments are produced by a metal core which can change its dimension in an electromagnetic field with an operating frequency between 25,000 and 42,000 cycles per second. In the sonic instruments, the vibrations are generated mechanically. During the generation of the ultrasonic vibrations heat is produced, which is why the tip during instrumentation always has to be ir-

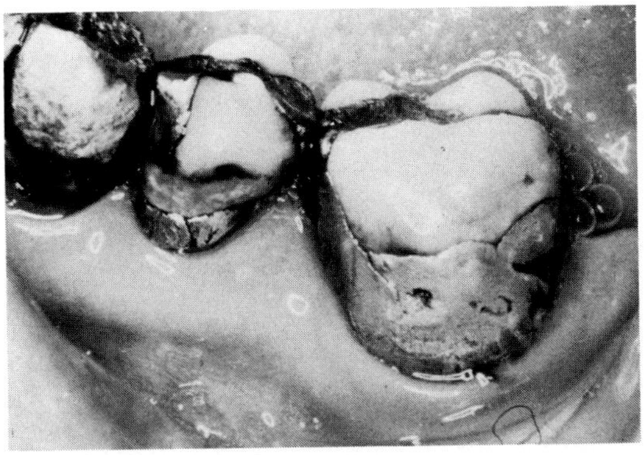

Fig. 14-29a.

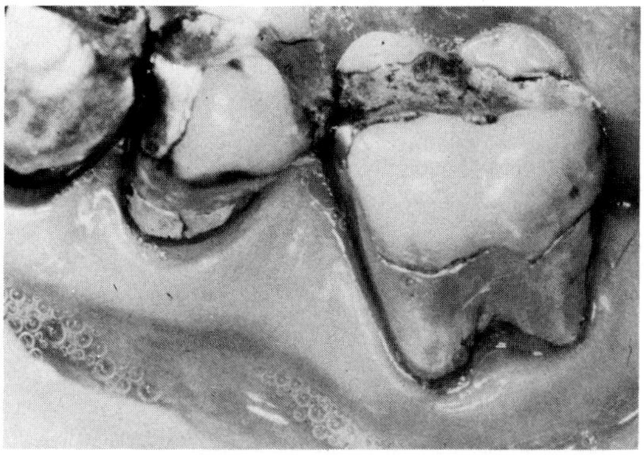

Fig. 14-29b.

Fig. 14-29a-b. Amalgam restorations before (a) and after (b) the adjustment of the overhangs. The buccal restoration in tooth 36 is prepared in order to reduce the degree of furcation involvement.

rigated with water or saline.

Before use, the ultrasonic instrument must be adjusted regarding the power (tuning) and waterspray according to the manual (Fig. 14-27). The tip should be applied to the tooth surface with very light pressure and be moved back and forth over the surface in sweeping movements and in such a way that its pattern of vibration is orientated parallel to the tooth surface to prevent damage to the root. A periodontal probe should always be used to check the root surface characteristics after instrumentation.

Rotating instruments

Root furrows, furcation areas and root surfaces in deep narrow pockets are difficult to properly debride with the use of hand instruments. At such sites, therefore, rotating instruments like fine-grained diamonds are often used. Care should be taken, however, to avoid excessive removal of tooth substance with this cutting operation.

Removal of plaque-retention factors

In an epidemiological study, Björn et al. (1969, 1970) observed that ill-fitting artificial crowns and fillings were associated with a reduced height of the periodontal bone level. Jeffcoat & Howell (1980) reported that marginal bone loss was more pronounced around teeth with overhanging amalgam restorations than around teeth without restorations. Rodrigues-Ferrer et al. (1980) concluded that "the presence of a subgingival overhanging defective margin may be the only important clinically significant feature of an amalgam restoration related to the pathogenesis of chronic inflammatory periodontal disease". It is not the overhang of the restoration *per se*, however, which causes or maintains periodontal disease. Waerhaug (1960) pointed out that the more advanced gingival inflammation observed in sites with ill-fitting restorations, was the result of extensive plaque accumulation and not of mechanical irritation by the filling material. Thus, overhangs of restorations must be removed to 1) facilitate the removal of plaque and calculus and 2) to establish an anatomy of the restoration which facilitates self-performed tooth cleaning.

Overhanging margins of dental restorations can be removed using a flame-shaped diamond stone mounted on a handpiece for rotatory movements or a flat diamond stone mounted on a handpiece for horizontal reciprocal movements (Eva-system®, Fig. 14-28). The overhang should be removed and the restoration should be given a proper form and surface. The

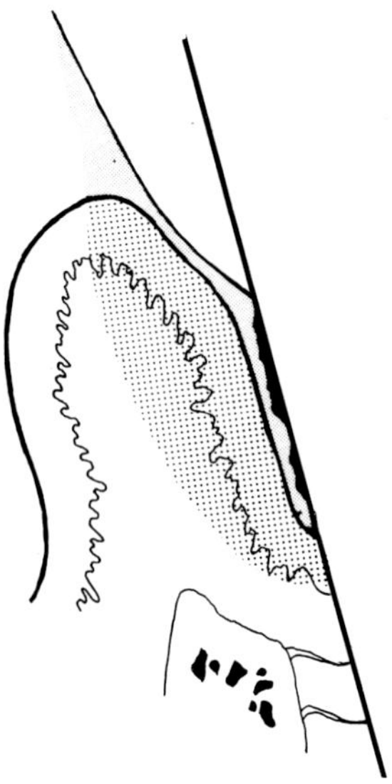

Fig. 14-30a.

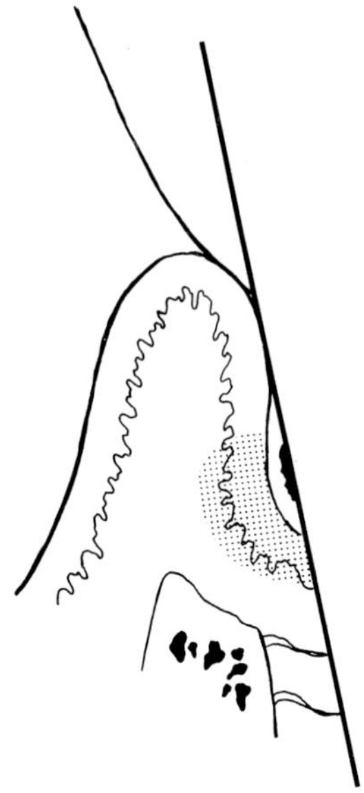

Fig. 14-30b.

Fig. 14-30a-b. Schematic drawing illustrating a gingival unit before (a) and after (b) cause-related therapy. Clinical signs such as reduced plaque and gingivitis scores and reduced probing depth values as a result of recession indicate healing after the cause-related therapy. Remaining plaque and calculus in the apical part of the root surface of the pocket area (b) may, however, maintain the inflammatory lesion (shadowed area) in the apical part of the pocket. Probing to the bottom of the pocket will result in bleeding.

instrumentation should always be completed by the use of flame-shaped finish burs and a polishing paste (grain size 40-2 μm). After polishing, fluorides should be applied (in solutions or in a varnish) in order to reinstitute the fluoride concentration of the adjacent tooth surface.

The adjustment of an improperly designed filling or artificial crown is often a difficult and time-consuming procedure. It is often more convenient to remove the improper filling (crown) and insert a new one with a proper marginal fit. Fig. 14-29 illustrates the effect on the periodontal tissues of the adjustment of amalgam overhangs.

Evaluation of the effect of the cause-related therapy

Since cause-related therapeutic measures constitute the most significant part of the overall treatment of periodontal disease, the meticulous assessment of the result obtained by these measures is of utmost importance. Hence, the clinical examination performed towards the end of this phase of treatment must include assessments of the effect of the professional procedures as well as of the patient's home-care standard. The result of the therapeutic measures should be described in terms of 1) degree of resolution of gingival inflammation, 2) degree of reduction of probing depth and alterations of clinical attachment levels, 3) degree of reduced improvement of tooth mobility, and 4) improvement of the self-performed oral hygiene.

The findings made at this reexamination form the basis for the selection of therapeutic measures which should be included in the corrective phase of treatment. It is usually possible, with the data obtained from this reexamination, to classify the patient into one of the following categories:

1. The data from the reexamination may de-

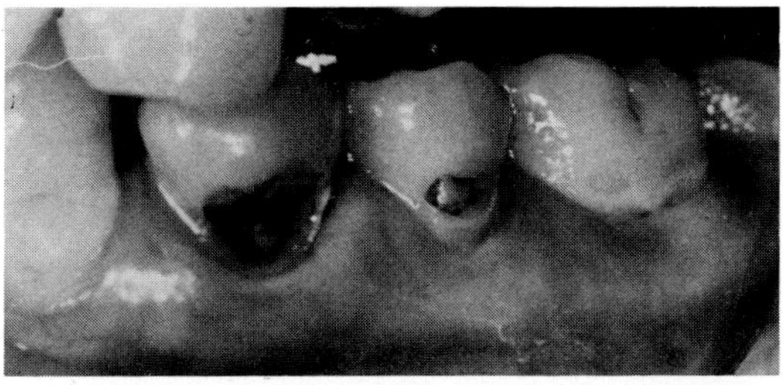

Fig. 14-31a.

	33	34	35	36	37
Mesial	6	8	7	8	10
Buccal			5	5	4
Distal	8	6	8	9	6
Lingual	4	5	6	6	5

Fig. 14-31b.

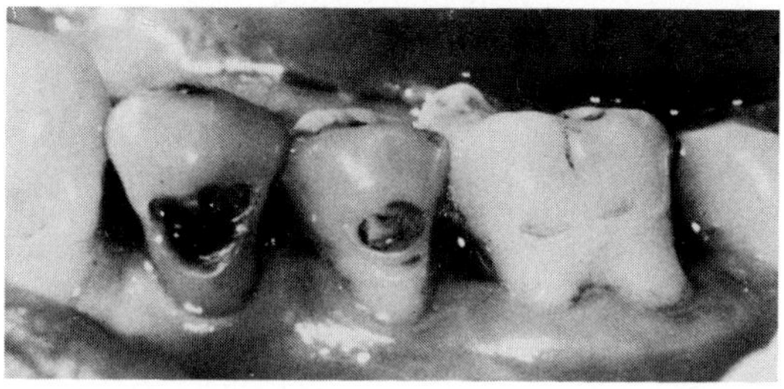

Fig. 14-31c.

	33	34	35	36	37
Mesial				4	4
Buccal					
Distal					4
Lingual					

Fig. 14-31d.

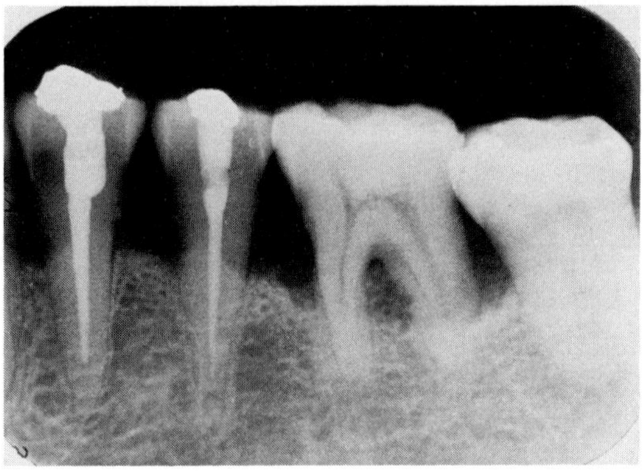

Fig. 14-31e.

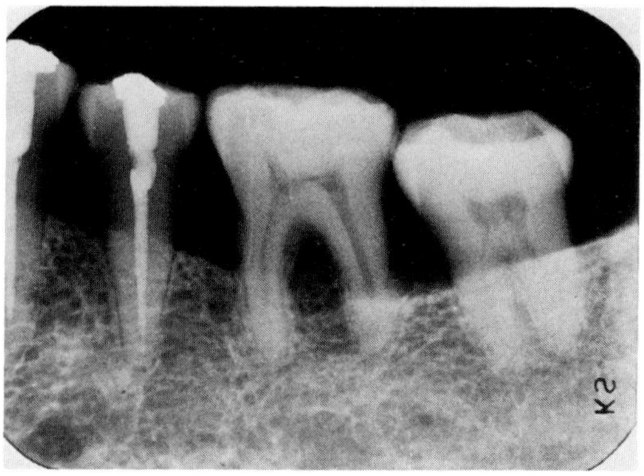

Fig. 14-31f.

Fig. 14-31a-f. Photographs illustrating the buccal surfaces of premolars and molars before (a) and 1 year after cause-related periodontal therapy (c). Note the recession of the gingival margin following therapy. The reduction of probing depths and absence of bleeding on probing from the bottom of the pockets after treatment (b,d) indicate resolution of gingivitis. A comparison between the radiographs obtained before (e) and after (f) scaling and root planing demonstrates that treatment has also changed the outline of the alveolar bone crest.

scribe a patient who has a proper standard of oral hygiene, but in whom a number of gingival sites still bleed on probing, and in whom a significant reduction of the probing depths at these sites has not been achieved. In such a patient the phase of corrective treatment should include periodontal surgery in order to gain access to root surfaces on which subgingival scaling and root planing evidently failed to remove plaque and calculus (Fig. 14-30).

2. The reexamination may describe a patient with a proper oral hygiene standard, no gingival inflammation (no bleeding on probing), in whom the probing depths have been markedly reduced and the clinical attach-

ment levels improved. In such a patient, no further periodontal treatment may be indicated even if, in some areas, deepened pockets may exist (Fig. 14-31).

3. The reexamination may recognize a patient who, despite repeated instructions in self-performed plaque control, has a poor standard of oral hygiene. This patient evidently lacks motivation or ability to exercise proper home care and should not be regarded as a candidate for periodontal surgery. The patient must be made aware of the fact that even though the professional part of the cause-related therapy has been performed to perfection, reinfection of the periodontal pockets may in his/her case sooner or later result in recurrence of destructive periodontal disease.

References

Arnim, S.S. (1963) The use of disclosing agents for measuring tooth cleanliness. *Journal of Periodontology*, **34**, 227-245.

Badersten, A., Nilvéus, R. & Egelberg, J. (1981) Effect of nonsurgical periodontal therapy. I. Moderately advanced periodontitis. *Journal of Clinical Periodontology* **8**, 57-72.

Bass, C.C., (1954) An effective method of personal oral hygiene. *Journal of Louisiana Medical Society* **106**, 100-112.

Bergenholtz, A., Lignell, L. & Öberg, G. (1971) *Quantitative evaluation of the plaque-removing ability of four commercial dentifrices.* (In preparation).

Björn, H. & Lindhe, J. (1962) The influence of periodontal instruments on the tooth surface. A methodological study. *Odontologisk Revy* **13**, 355-369.

Björn, A-L., Björn, H. & Grkovic, B. (1969) Marginal fit of restorations and its relation to periodontal bone level. Part I: Metal fillings. *Odontologisk Revy* **20**, 311-322.

Björn, A-L., Björn, H. & Grkovic, B. (1970) Marginal fit of restorations and its relation to periodontal bone level. Part II: Crowns. *Odontologisk Revy* **21**, 337-346.

Charters, W.J. (1948) Proper home care of the month. *Journal of Periodontology* **19**, 136-139.

Gjermo, P. & Flötra, L. (1970) The effect of different methods of interdental cleaning. *Journal of Periodontal Research* **5**, 230-236.

Glavind, L. & Zeuner, E. (1986) The effectiveness of a rotary electric toothbrush on oral cleanliness in adults. *Journal of Clinical Periodontology* **13**, 135-138.

Hugoson, A. (1978) Effect of the Water Pik® device on plaque accumulation and development of gingivitis. *Journal of Clinical Periodontology* **5**, 95-104.

Jeffcoat, M.K. & Howell, T.H. (1980) Alveolar bone destruction due to overhanging amalgam in periodontal disease. *Journal of Periodontology* **51**, 599-602.

Keller, S.E. & Manson-Hing, L.R. (1969) Clearence studies of proximal tooth surfaces. Part III and IV: In vivo removal of interproximal plaque. *Alabama Journal of Medical Science* **6**, 399-405.

Lang, N.P. & Räber, K. (1982) Use of oral irrigators as vehicle for the application of antimicrobial agents in chemical plaque control. *Journal of Clinical Periodontology* **8**, 177-188.

Leon, E.L. & Vogel, R.I. (1987) A comparison of the effectiveness of hand scaling and ultrasonic debridement in furcations as evaluated by differential dark-field microscopy. *Journal of Periodontology* **58**, 86-94.

Lie, T. & Leknes, K.N. (1985) Evaluation of the effect on root surfaces of air turbine scalers and ultrasonic instrumentation. *Journal of Periodontology* **56**, 522-531.

Lindhe, J. (1964) Orthogonal cutting of dentine. *Odontologisk Revy* **15**, suppl. 8.

Lindhe, J. & Nyman, S. (1975) The effect of plaque control and surgical pocket elimination on the establishment and maintenance of periodontal health. A longitudinal study of periodontal therapy in cases of advanced disease. *Journal of Clinical Periodontology* **2**, 67-79.

Lindhe, J., Westfelt, E., Nyman, S., Socransky, S.S., Heijl, L. & Bratthall, G. (1982) Healing following surgical/non-surgical treatment of periodontal disease. *Journal of Clinical Periodontology* **9**, 115-128.

Loos, B., Kieger, R. & Egelberg, J. (1987) An evaluation of basic periodontal therapy using sonic and ultrasonic scalers. *Journal of Clinical Periodontology* **14**, 29-33.

Lövdal, A., Arnö, A. & Waerhaug, J. (1958) Incidence of clinical manifestations of periodontal disease in light of oral hygiene and calculus formation. *Journal of the American Dental Association* **56**, 21-23.

Matsuzaki, A., Sugano, K., Tachibana, T., Katano, Y. & Nahamura, J. (1974) The effects of toothbrushing and water jetting on oral hygiene. *The Japanese Journal of Conservative Dentistry* **17**, 150-153.

O'Leary, T. J. (1970) Oral hygiene agents and procedures. *Journal of Periodontology* **41**, 625-629.

Rodriguez-Ferrer, H.J., Strahan, J.D. & Newman, H.N. (1980) Effect on gingival health of removing overhanging margins of interproximal subgingival amalgam restorations. *Journal of Clinical Periodontology* **7**, 457-462.

Rosenberg, R.M. & Ash Jr., N.N. (1974) The effect of root roughness on plaque accumulation and gingival inflammation. *Journal of Periodontology* **45**, 146-150.

Rosling, B., Nyman, S. & Lindhe, J. (1976) The effect of systematic plaque control on bone regeneration in infrabony pockets. *Journal of Clinical Periodontology* **3**, 38-53.

Rugg-Gunn, A., MacGregor, I., Edgar, W. & Ferguson, M. (1979) Toothbrushing behaviour in relation to plaque and gingivitis in adolescent schoolchildren. *Journal of Periodontal Research* **14**, 231-238.

Sagnes, G. (1974) Effectiveness of vertical and horizontal toothbrushing techniques in the removal of plaque. *Journal of Dentistry for Children* **41**, 39-43.

Ten, A. (1981) Disclosing agents in plaque control. *The Journal of Western Society of Periodontology*, Periodontal abstracts 29, 81-86.

Thoma, K.H. & Goldman, H.M. (1960) *Oral pathology.* The C.V. Mosby Co., St. Louis, Ed. 5, p. 209.

Torafson, T., Kiger, R., Selvig, K.A. & Egelberg, J. (1979) Clinical improvement of gingival conditions following ultrasonic versus hand instrumentation of periodontal pockets. *Journal of Clinical Periodontology* **6**, 165-176.

Waerhaug, J. (1956) Effect of rough surfaces upon gingival tissue. *Journal of Dental Research* **35**, 323-325.

Waerhaug, J. (1959) Periodontiddprofylaxe. *Nordisk Klinisk Odontologi*, kap 14/11:1. A/S Forlaget for Faglitteratur, Copenhagen.

Waerhaug, J. (1960) Histologic considerations which govern where the margin of restorations should be located in relation to the gingiva. *Dental Clinics of North America* 167-176.

Waerhaug, J. (1981) Healing of the dento-epithelial junction following the use of dental floss. *Journal of Clinical Periodontology* **8**, 144-150.

CHAPTER 15

Antiseptics and Antibiotics in Periodontics

The accumulation of bacterial plaque on teeth and in the gingival sulcus elicits an inflammatory response in the marginal gingiva (Löe et al. 1965) which may spread and result in loss of connective fiber attachment and alveolar bone (Lindhe et al. 1975).

Individuals vary considerably, however, in their response to plaque (Löe et al. 1965, Van der Velden et al. 1985). In order to prevent the development of periodontal disease, therefore, oral hygiene measures must aim at 1) inhibiting plaque *formation*, or if that is not possible, 2) reducing, at regular intervals, the amount of plaque *formed* to a level at and below which no destructive inflammatory disease develops.

Plaque control based on mechanical means is laborious and time-consuming. Löe (1973) therefore suggested the use of chemicals as adjuncts to mechanical means to facilitate patient maintenance of a proper standard of oral hygiene. The objectives of such chemical plaque control measures may include:

1. inhibition of microbial colonization on tooth surfaces;
2. inhibition of plaque growth;
3. elimination or alteration of existing plaque.

The rationale for chemical plaque control

Non-specific plaque concept

It has not yet been possible to identify *one particular microorganism or a well-defined group of microorganisms* which can be held responsible for the initiation and progression of periodontal disease. Mechanical debridement , i.e. oral hygiene instruction, scaling and root planing, as methods of periodontal therapy were developed from a "non-specific" plaque theory. If this concept is adhered to, chemical plaque control used as a substitute for or an adjunct to mechanical methods must aim at the prevention and elimination of the entire plaque mass.

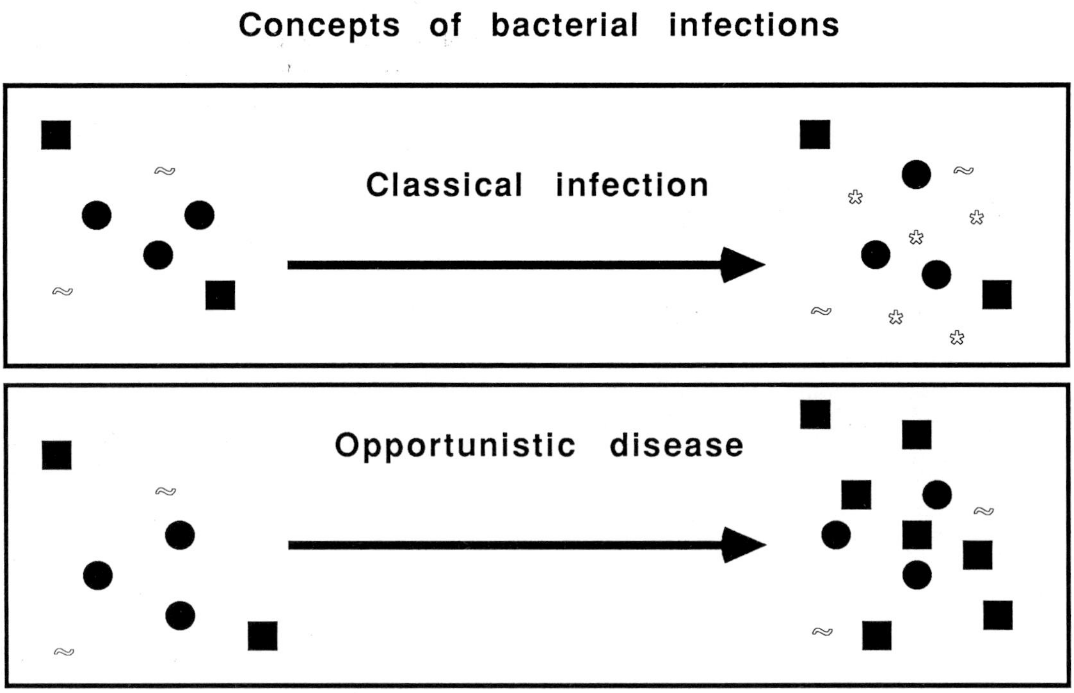

Fig. 15-1. Concepts of bacterial infection. In a classical infection, an exogenous pathogen (asterisk) colonizes the host. In an opportunistic disease, a commensal with pathogenic potential (■) proliferates as a result of a favorable change in the ecosystem.

Specific plaque concept

In disagreement with the "non-specific" plaque concept, Loesche (1976) presented the "specific plaque hypothesis" and suggested that *one or only a few types of microoroanisms* within the bacterial mass constitute the *dental plaque infection, i.e. the etiological factor* in gingivitis and periodontitis. A periodontal or prevention program based on the concept of a specific plaque infection must include a proper microbiological diagnosis. Based on this diagnosis, an antimicrobial compound may be selected which has the potential to eliminate the pathogens, but leave the non-pathogenic bacteria unaffected.

Findings from different research laboratories suggest that, in many situations, periodontal disease may develop and progress in response to rather well-defined plaque infections (see Chapter 4). The clinical application of this knowledge requires more testing, however, before drugs are introduced in periodontal therapy to combat "specific" infections.

Opportunistic plaque infection

In *classic infection* an exogenous pathogen enters the host in large numbers to elicit an inflammatory response. In a disease caused by an *opportunistic infection*, on the other hand, the environment in an ecological niche must change to allow for the establishment of a microbiota which elicits an inflammatory response (Fig. 15-1).

Essential prerequisites for the development of an opportunistic plaque infection include:

1. the presence of microorganisms in an ecological niche;

2. the establishment of an environment in the niche which favors the multiplication and proliferation of certain segments of the microbiota;
3. the development of an altered host-resistance which makes the host incapable of coping with the microbiota present in the ecological niche.

The gingival sulcus of a healthy periodontium may harbor Gram-negative anaerobic bacteria, microorganisms which in experimental animals have a potential to induce destructive periodontal disease (Slots 1977, Slots et al. 1978). This suggests that the infection associated with periodontal disease may be of the "opportunistic" type. Findings from experimental studies have confirmed this hypothesis. Thus, Kornman et al. (1981) and Slots et al. (1979) placed ligatures in the gingival sulcus of monkeys. Ligature placement "opened the pocket", changed the environment in the ecological niche and allowed for subgingival plaque formation. The authors reported that, following ligature placement, there was a significant increase in *B. gingivalis* and that this increase occurred concomitant with tissue changes such as loss of connective tissue attachment and alveolar bone.

Several factors may act to modify the environment in the gingival sulcus (the ecological niche):

1. increase of the amount or alteration of the composition of the supragingival plaque (Kornman 1986a);
2. the calcification of the bacterial plaque (Waerhaug 1955);
3. the placement of resorations with overhangs (plaque retention) (Lang et al. 1983);
4. hormonal changes during pregnancy and puberty (Kornman & Loesche 1980, Mombelli et al. 1987).

Since the supragingival plaque obviously may contribute to a change of the environment in the ecological niche, there are reasons to suggest that prevention of periodontal disease may be based on methods, mechanical or chemical, which inhibit the formation of or eliminate already-formed supragingival plaque.

Principles for chemoprevention and therapy

While chemical methods, i.e. the use of antibiotics, are effective in the treatment of a classical infection (Fig. 15-2), such treatment methods may have a limited value in an opportunistic infection. The use of antimicrobial agents in an opportunistic infection may result in a limited, but transient suppression of the microbiota. Regrowth of the residual microbiota in the unchanged environment of the ecological niche is inevitable. Treatment of an opportunistic infection, therefore, should aim at altering the environment and turning the gingival sulcus/pocket into an unfavorable habitat for periodontal pathogens.

Basic approaches to prevent gingivitis and to prevent the conversion of gingivitis to periodontitis

1. To completely eliminate all clinically detectable plaque

Regularly repeated, meticulous tooth cleaning is an effective means to prevent gingivitis (Löe et al. 1965, Lang et al. 1973). Also, the progression of periodontal disease can be inhibited during extended periods in individuals who, following treatment, are maintained in a proper plaque control regimen (Axelsson & Lindhe 1978, Knowles et al. 1979, Lindhe & Nyman 1984).

It may be anticipated that non-selective, supragingival plaque control based on chemical methods is as effective as preventive methods based on mechanical plaque removal.

2. To reduce plaque below certain threshold levels

It may not be necessary in all subjects to completely remove all plaque, since in some subjects a relatively non-pathogenic microflora may constitute the bulk of the plaque mass. A reasonable second preventive approach, therefore, includes the reduction of plaque below the threshold level at which the individual host develops disease. This threshold level must be assessed in the individual patient. It should be emphasized, however, that the plaque level at which health is maintained may vary considerably with time in the same individual.

3. To attempt to alter the microbial composition of plaque

A much more selective approach would be required if the *composition* of the bacterial plaque was to be altered to the extent that periodontitis would not occur. Data from animal experiments suggest that such selective alterations of the subgingival microbiota may prevent a gingival lesion from converting into periodontitis (Kinder et al. 1984). In the study referred to, non-virulent antagonists to the subgingival pathogens were introduced. The innocuous microorganisms colonized the gingival pocket and became established in the ecological niche. The virulent strains were thereby replaced. This principle for disease prevention, albeit promising, has not yet been studied in a systematic way and is consequently not yet clinically applicable (Hammond 1986).

4. To prevent the adhesion of bacteria to the tooth surface

Another "futuristic" approach to prevent plaque from forming involves the interference with the formation of the pellicle and the initial adherence of bacteria to the tooth surface (Glantz & Attström 1986). By changing the surface chemistry of the tooth surface, a firm attachment of the bacteria to the tooth may be prevented. Studies by Attström et al. (1983) and Brecx et al. (1987) demonstrated that Octapinol, a substituted aminoalcohol, when used as a mouth rinse, almost completely inhibited the formation of bacterial plaque. Although promising, this approach to dental disease prevention is still at an early stage of development.

Evaluation of antimicrobial agents

Numerous chemical agents have been evaluated for their ability to influence plaque development, (for review, see Lang 1980, Kornman 1986b). According to Loesche (1976) several basic criteria must be discussed when considering a chemical plaque control agent:

1. Specificity

Antimicrobial substances, reserved for the treatment of serious medical infections, must as a rule not be used to control plaque locally. Systemically administered antibiotics may be used in rare situations in patients with aggressive and refractory forms of periodontal disease, but only after an accurate microbiological diagnosis.

2. Efficacy

The antimicrobial agent selected must be effective against microorganisms implicated in the etiology of gingivitis and periodontitis.

In the "experimental gingivitis model" (Löe et al. 1965), a chemical agent, chosen to control plaque formation on the basis of the non-specific plaque concept (Loesche 1976), should either completely inihibit or significantly delay the development of gingivitis.

3. Substantivity

Substantivity is a measure of the contact time that connects a substance and a substrate in a given medium. For any degree of substantivity, adherence of a substance to a substrate should

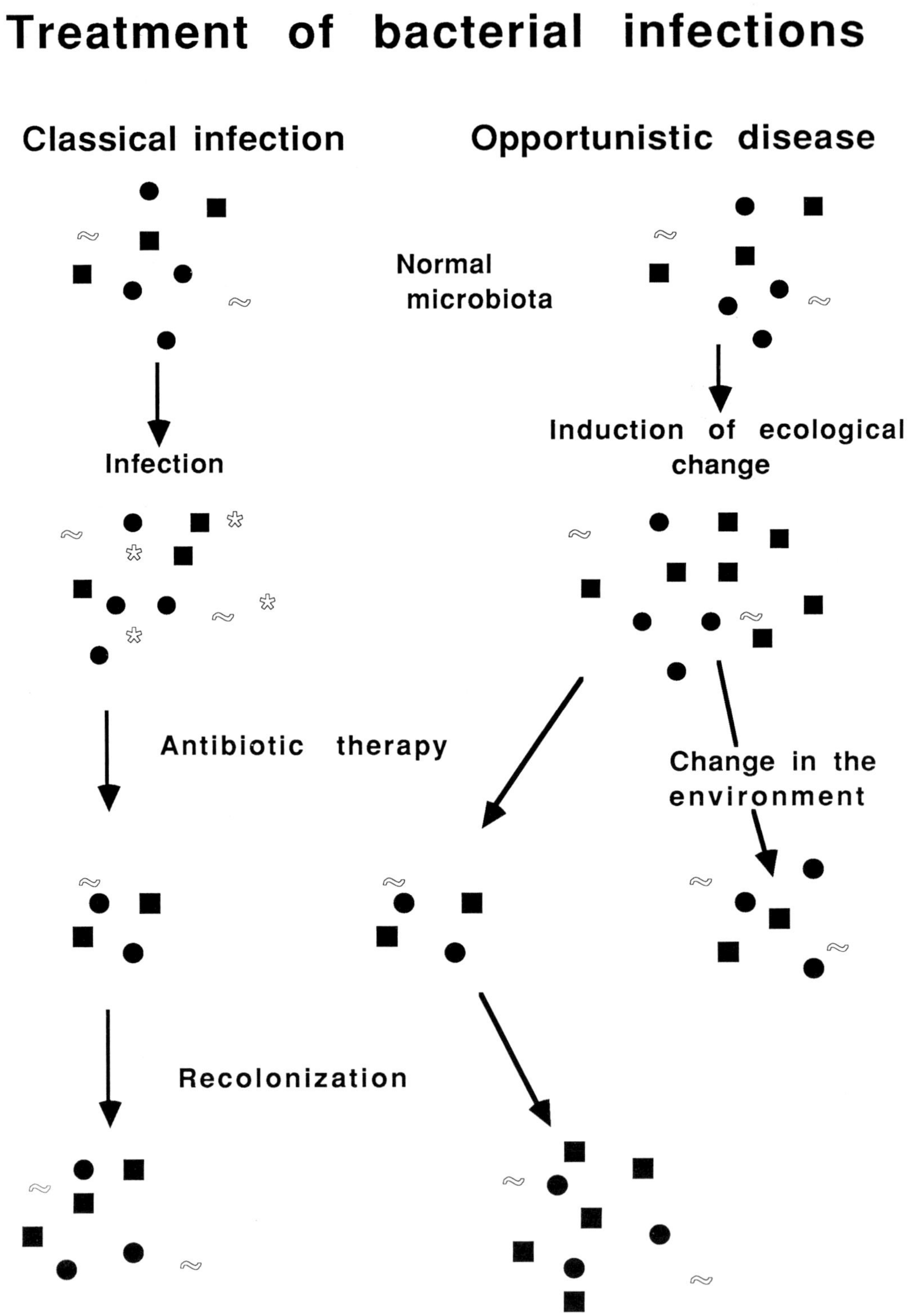

Fig. 15-2. Treatment concepts for classical and opportunistic infections. Antibiotic therapy is only effective in classical infections. Treatment of the opportunistic infection requires a change in the ecosystem as well.

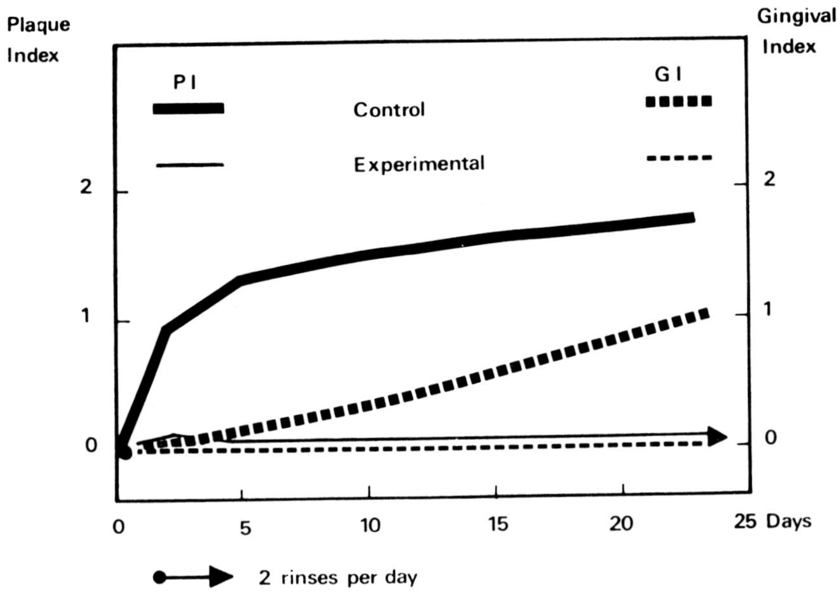

Fig. 15-3. Mean Plaque Index and Gingival Index scores of 5 individuals during a control period of 24 days without active oral hygiene and during an equally long experimental period in which active oral hygiene was substituted with two daily 1-minute rinses with 0.2% chlorhexidine digluconate (Löe & Schiött 1970a, In *Dental Plaque*, (ed.) Mc Hugh, W.D., p. 249. Edinburgh: Livingstone).

be greater or more extended than would occur following simple mechanical deposition (von Abbé 1974). In treating dental plaque infections, the substantivity of the antimicrobial agent is of the utmost importance, since the agent needs a certain amount of contact time in order to inhibit or kill a microorganism.

4. Safety
The safety of an antimicrobial substance should be tested in animal studies prior to its clinical use. Side effects should be carefully investigated in human studies.

5. Stability
Antimicrobial agents should be stable at room temperature for a considerable time. Most antiseptics used to prevent plaque formation are stable (Gjermo & Eriksen 1974).

Disinfectants and antibacterial agents

The use of disinfectants to control plaque dates back to Miller (1890), who suggested that caries could be prevented by antimicrobial therapy. However, since the disinfectants of that time were toxic and showed too many side effects, the concept of chemical plaque control was abandoned for many years.

In a recent state-of-the-art review (Kornman 1986b) chemical agents were categorized according to their substantivity. Certain antibiotics, quaternary ammonium compounds, phenolic compounds, oxidizing agents, fluorides, and plant alkaloids have a weak substantivity and are referred to as first generation antimicrobials. Second generation antimicrobials have a high substantivity. Included in this group are the bisbiguanides. Substances interfering with or preventing bacterial adhesion to tooth surfaces are referred to as third generation antimicrobial agents These latter compounds have not yet been properly or extensively tested. For the time being, therefore, the second generation antimicrobials appear to be the agents of choice in preventive dentistry.

Clinical efficacy

A short-term experiment of Löe & Schiött (1970b) showed that topical application of a second generation antimicrobial, chlorhexidine digluconate, leads to successful plaque control. Plaque formation and the development of gingivitis were inhibited in human volunteers by five or two daily rinses (Fig. 15-3) with a 10 ml aqueous solution of 0.2% chlorhexidine digluconate. The same effect was achieved by one daily topical application of a 2% solution (Löe et al. 1971). The development of caries could also be prevented by this plaque control regimen (von der Fehr, Löe & Theilade 1970, Löe, von der Fehr & Shiött 1972).

In order to compare the efficacy of other antiseptics with that of chlorhexidine on plaque and gingivitis, studies have been conducted using the model of experimental gingivitis (Löe et al. 1965). In separate studies, the effect of two daily rinses with 0.12% chlorhexidine digluconate solution was compared with rinsing with solutions of a quaternary ammonium compound (cetyl pyridinium chloride) (Lang & Briner 1984), a phenolic compound (Listerine), a plant alkaloid (sanguinarine) (Siegrist et al. 1986) and hydrogen peroxide (Gusberti et al. 1988). Compared to a placebo control group, two daily rinses with the chlorhexidine solution gave a plaque reduction of 75%. The quaternary ammonium compound reduced mean plaque scores by 8%, the phenolic compound by 25%, the plant alkaloid by 30% and hydrogen peroxide by 28% (Fig. 15-4). Only rinsing with chlorhexidine maintained the Gingival Index scores at the pre-experimental levels throughout the 21 days of experiment. Almost identical results have been obtained in a 6-month longitudinal trial (Manhart et al. 1988).

Chlorhexidine digluconate

Although the initially tested concentration of chlorhexidine digluconate amounted to 0.2% (Löe & Schiött 1970a,b), recent studies have documented that two daily rinses with 15 ml of a 0.12% solution provide clinical benefits almost identical to the 0.2% solution (Segreto et al. 1986). However, when lower concentrations of the compound are used in oral rinses, less potent clinical effects can be anticipated (Fig. 15-5) (Lang et al. 1986).

The excellent results achieved in short-term clinical trials with chlorhexidine were also observed in several long-term studies. In the first of these studies (Löe et al. 1976), 150 medical students rinsed daily for 2 years with a solution of 0.2% chlorhexidine digluconate. Although interaction with a flavoring agent reduced the effective concentration of chlorhexidine, significant reductions in plaque, gingivitis, total numbers of facultative and anaerobic bacteria and *Streotococcus mutans* in the saliva were observed (Schiött et al. 1976a). In the same clinical trial, several medical tests, such as blood count, urine analysis and sedimentation rate were carried out at regular invervals. No significant differences were observed between test and control subjects for any of the parameters evaluated (Schiött et al. 1976b). Based on these data, it seems reasonable to claim that chlorhexidine can safely be used for extended periods of time. A potential danger of prolonged application of an antimicrobial agent is the possibility of developing resistant mutants. In an animal study (Briner & Wunder 1977), in which three daily applications of chlorhexidine were given for 4 years, no reduced sensitivity to chlorhexidine was found to occur among any of the bacteria tested.

In a 6-month study (Lang et al. 1982), the effects of supervised rinsing with chlorhexidine

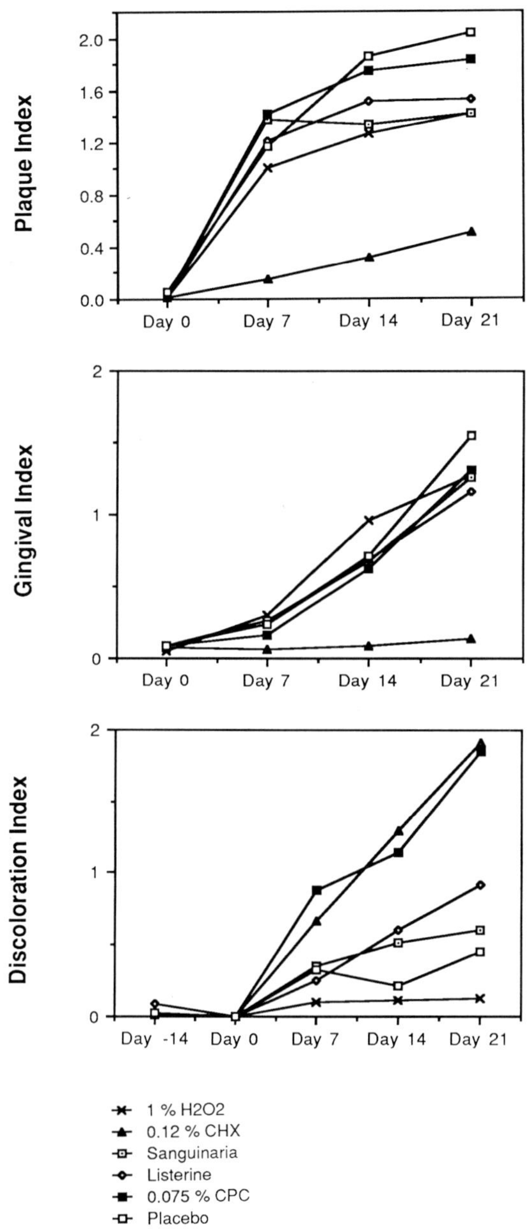

Fig. 15-4. Mean Plaque, Gingival and Discoloration Indices in six groups of 8 individuals refraining from oral hygiene for 21 days rinsing with either 0.12% chlorhexidine digluconate, 0.075% cetylpyridinium chloride, Listerine® sanguinarine, 1% H_2O_2 or placebo.

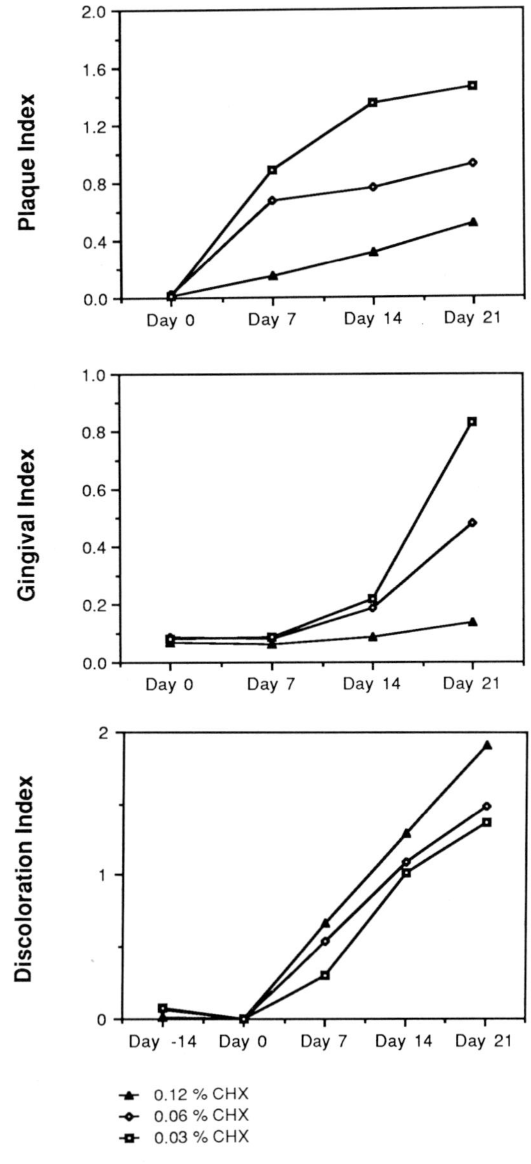

Fig. 15-5. Mean Plaque, Gingival and Discoloration Indices in three groups of 8 individuals refraining from oral hygiene for 21 days rinsing with either 0.12%, 0.06% or 0.03% chlorhexidine digluconate.

in 158 schoolchildren were evaluated. The children were divided into three test groups and one control group. The first test group rinsed with a 0.2% solution of chlorhexidine 6 times a week, the second with the same concentration, but only twice a week. The third test group

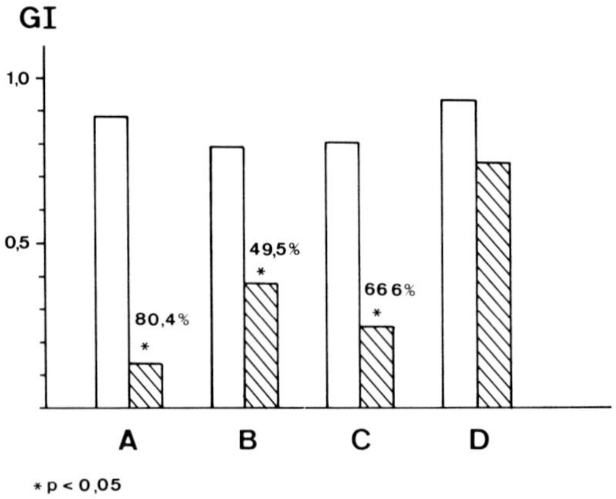

Fig.15-6. Mean Gingival Index in four groups of schoolchildren rinsing with chlorhexidine digluconate (CHX) or placebo solution for 6 months under supervision.

A. 0.2% CHX 6 times weekly

B: 0.2% CHX 2 times weekly

C: 0.1% CHX 6 times weekly

D: Placebo 6 times weekly

rinsed 6 times a week with a 0.1% solution and the control group 6 times a week with a placebo. No attempt was made to change the children's own oral hygiene habits. After 6 months, the group that had rinsed 6 times a week with a 0.2% solution of chlorhexidine had an 88% reduction of the mean Gingival Index (GI 0.13, Fig. 15-6). The group that had rinsed only twice a week with an identical solution had a 50% reduction, and the group rinsing 6 times a week with the 0.1% solution had a 66% reduction of the gingivitis score. It was concluded that gingivits can indeed be controlled successfully and over extended periods by the regular use of 0.1% or 0.2% chlorhexidine mouth rinses.

In another long-term (6 months) study, carried out in 430 adults, similar reductions of the gingivitis scores were reported (Grossman et al. 1986).

Substantivity and mechanisms of action

Chlorhexidine adsorbs to the surfaces of oral tissues including the teeth, and is then slowly released in active form (Lang & Brecx 1986). The kinetic mechanisms of chlorhexidine adsorption from mouthwashes and its slow release into the saliva have been tested with radioactively labeled chlorhexidine (Gjermo 1974, Bonesvoll, Lökken & Rölla 1974a). Approximately 30% of a 10 ml solution of 0.2% chlorhexidine will bind to the oral surfaces.

A solution of 0.2% chlorhexidine digluconate will significantly reduce the number of bacteria adhering on plastic films placed on smooth tooth surfaces during the first hours of plaque accumulation (Brecx & Theilade 1984). The cationic chlorhexidine molecule binds to anionic compounds such as free sulfates, carboxyl and phosphate groups of the pellicle, and salivary glycoproteins (Rölla & Melsen 1975) and will thereby reduce the adsorption of proteins to the tooth surface required for the formation of dental pellicle. Coating salivary bacteria with chlorhexidine molecules also alters the mechanisms of adsorption of bacteria to the tooth (Rölla & Melsen 1975). Chlorhexidine molecules bound to salivary proteins will be released in active form in 8-12 hours (Bonesvoll et al. 1974b). Low concentrations of chlorhexidine can still be recovered after 24 hours.

Chlorhexidine is active against Gram-positive and Gram-negative microorganisms and yeast cells. Because of its high cationic nature, chlorhexidine has a great affinity for the cell wall of microorganisms and changes the surface structures. Osmotic equilibrium is lost and, as a consequence, the cytoplasmic membrane is extruded, vesicles are formed, and the cytoplasm precipitates (Davies 1973, Brecx & Theilade 1984). These precipitations inhibit the repair of the cell wall, and the bacteria are no longer able to recover.

Side effects

The most common side effect of chlorhexidine is the formation of an extrinsic yellow-brown stain on teeth and tongue (Löe & Schiött

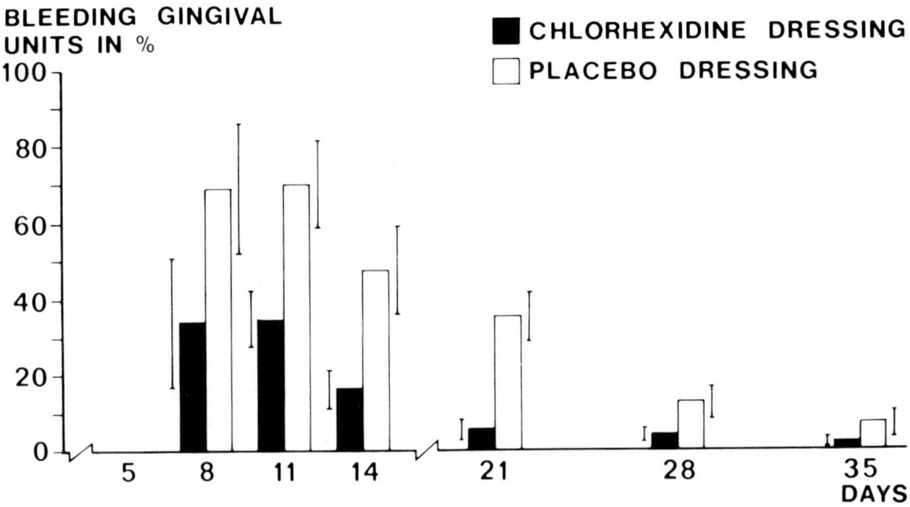

Fig. 15-7. Mean Plaque Index in 11 groups of 10 subjects refraining from oral hygiene but using an Oral Irrigator System with various dosages and concentrations of chlorhexidine digluconate.

1970a). The degree of staining seems to depend on the concentration of the compound and varies greatly from one individual to another (Heyden 1973). Stain can appear on natural teeth, artificial teeth and composite restorations. *In vitro* (Addy et al. 1979) and *in vivo* (Prayitno et al. 1979) studies have demonstrated that tannin-containing substances such as tea, red wine, and port wine will increase the level of chlorhexidine discoloration. However, also other antiseptics will induce varying degrees of discoloration. Discoloration by the five antiseptics in the comparative studies already referred to (Lang & Briner 1984, Siegrist et al. 1986, Gusberti et al. 1988) are illustrated in Figs. 15-4 and 15-5.

Desquamations and painful lesions occurred in some subjects using a 0.2% chlorhexidine digluconate solution in a 4-month clinical study (Flötra et al. 1972). However, such lesions have not been found in studies using concentrations of less than 0.2%. Furthermore, a quality-specific impairment for salty taste perception which appear to be short-lasting has been found (Lang et al. 1988), indicating that chlorhexidine rinses should be applied after meals or before retiring at night.

Metabolism and toxicology

Animal experiments using radiolabelled chlorhexidine have indicated that the primary route of excretion is through the feces. There is minimal metabolic cleavage, and no evidence has been reported for the formation of carcinogenic substances (Winrow 1973). Because chlorhexidine is poorly absorbed in the gastrointestinal tract, it is not surprising that the compound displays low toxicity (Faulkes 1973).

Clinical applications

Mouthrinses

The application of chlorhexidine digluconate as a mouthrinse is the method most commonly studied in the literature (Lang & Brecx 1986). Two daily rinses (for 30-45 seconds) with 10 ml of an aqueous solution of 0.2% will assure complete plaque inhibition (Löe & Schiött 1970a), but discolorations on teeth and dental restorations may occur within a few weeks.

Since such side effects seem to depend on the concentrations used (Heyden 1973), several researchers have attempted to achieve satisfactory (but not complete) plaque inhibition using lower concentrations. They found that desirable plaque reductions can be achieved by one or two daily rinses with 10 ml of a 0.1% chlorhexidine solution.

Irrigators

If the concentration of chlorhexidine in a rinse is diluted in order to reduce the amount of stain, the plaque inhibiting potential is also reduced. This reduction is especially pronounced in the interproximal areas (Lang & Räber 1981). The reduced clinical effects may be compensated for by increasing the dose and, therefore, oral irrigators may represent an ideal vehicle for the application of antimicrobial agents (Cumming & Löe 1973, Agerbaek, Melsen & Rölla 1975, Lang & Räber 1981). Studies have demonstrated that 400 ml of a 0.02% solution of chlorhexidine digluconate (80 mg), applied once daily in an oral irrigator, will give complete plaque inhibition (Lang & Ramseier-Grossman 1981) (Fig. 15-7).

Gels

Chlorhexidine digluconate has also been incorporated in a gel. Gels applied for a period of 5 minutes once or twice a day in individual trays or acrylic stents have proved to be effective in the treatment of denture stomatitis (Budtz-Jörgensen & Löe 1972) and oral candidiasis (Budtz-Jörgensen 1977). Three daily applications of a 1% gel reduced the severity as well as the duration of aphthous ulcerations (Addy 1977).

Chlorhexidine incorporated in a gel and used in individual trays improved the oral hygiene condition of handicapped children (Usher 1975) more than when nurses brushed the children's teeth with chlorhexidine solutions (Storhaug 1977).

Sustained release devices

In order to affect the subgingival microbiota, sustained release devices (SRD) were developed. Such devices used ethyl cellulose and polyethylene glycol as polymers and chlorhexidine and ethanol as solvents (Friedman & Golomb 1982). The SRD's which contained 30% of the dry weight of chlorhexidine were placed in periodontal pockets. Over a period of 6 days approximately 50% of the chlorhexidine was released into the subgingival area, thereby reducing the relative proportions of the motile organisms, including spirochetes, to negligible levels (Soskolne et al. 1983, Stabholz et al. 1986).

Other possible agents for chemical plaque control

Most other antiseptics or topically used antibiotic compounds belong to the group of first-generation agents. They clearly demonstrate antibacterial capability *in vitro*, but have minimal substantivity. However, a brief review appears appropriate for better understanding of our current concepts.

Enzymes

A series of pancreatic enzyme preparations containing trypsin, chemotrypsin, carboxypeptidases, amylases, lipases, elastases and esterases, as well as several nucleases, have been tested for a possible effect on plaque and calculus development (Jensen 1959, Bauhammers, Landay & Pinkus 1968, Ennever & Sturzenberger 1961, Packman et al. 1963). Unfortunately, the results reported are not very convincing. Other authors have tested the incorporation of mucinases into toothpastes and attempted with this enzyme to affect the intermicrobial substance of plaque in order to inhibit calculus formation (Stewart 1952, Aleece & Forscher 1954). Belting & Gordon (1966) added concentrations of urea to mouthwashes and toothpastes with the same intention. A calcification inhibition of 30% could be achieved. Almost all of the results of studies with proteolytic enzymes and urea indicate a successful inhibition of calculus formation, but no inhibition of dental plaque.

Gibbons & Bannhardt (1967) demonstrated that certain oral streptococci produce a great amount of extracellular dextrans with low solubility. The theory of the importance of these substances for the adhesion of plaque to the tooth surface and the cohesion of plaque components led to extensive studies of the enzyme dextranase with regard to plaque inhibition. Although the results from animal experiments looked promising (König & Guggenheim 1968), these tests were not successful in humans (Lobene 1971). Attempts to reduce the formation of dental plaque and, consequently, the development of gingivitis in humans with the use of a crude mutanase (α-1, 3 glucanohydrolase) (Kelstrup et al. 1978), incorporated in a chewing gum, resulted (in comparison to placebo controls) in a slightly lower plaque accumulation and in some retardation of gingivitis development. However, bacteriologic studies of interproximal plaques failed to show differences between the groups which could have explained the clinical findings. Similar studies, performed in the Netherlands and in Switzerland failed to confirm Kelstrup's observation. A major problem in the use of enzymes for chemical plaque control lies with the mode of application. It appears that enzymes which are distributed through mouthwashes or chewing gums may not act long enough to be effective against plaque formation (Ennever & Sturzenberger 1961).

Surface active substances

Fluorides have proven to be effective in caries prevention.

Although several mechanisms of action have been described for fluorides, the accurate protective mode of action against dental caries still remains unknown. Fluorides may be exchanged with hydroxyl groups in the apatite crystals and thus decrease the solubility of enamel (Posner 1969). Fluorides may also be incorporated in the space between the hydroxyapatite crystals, reinforce the crystal structure (Young & Elliott 1966) and increase the threshold level for acid solubility of enamel. However, laboratory investigations have also demonstrated that low concentrations of fluorides have an antimicrobial activity (Bibby & Van Kesteren 1940). Animal experiments have confirmed that frequent topical application of fluorides will result in reduced plaque formation (Keyes et al. 1966). Fluorides may reduce the surface energy of the teeth (Glantz 1969) or may reduce the potential of the enamel surface to adsorb proteins (Ericsson & Ericsson 1967).

In recent years, stannous fluorides have been tested as antimicrobial agents. Partial plaque inhibition could be achieved with low pH solutions of stannous fluorides (Tinanoff 1977, Tinanoff et al. 1979). However, heavy yellow-brown stains were observed as a side effect. The fact that two daily toothbrushings with a 0.4% SnF_2 gel reduced plaque and gingivits dramatically in a 6-month clinical trial (Tinanoff et al. 1988) makes this compound a good candidate for future research.

Antibiotics

Penicillin

Penicillin has shown good results in inhibiting plaque formation in animal experiments. The antibiotics have either been added to the diet (Fitzgerald 1955, Mühlemann et al. 1961, Larson et al. 1963) or applied topically (Keyes 1966). In treating acute necrotizing ulcerative gingivitis in humans, the use of penicillin in chewing gums has shown a certain degree of success (Emslie et al. 1962).

Even though penicillin might successfully inhibit plaque formation, this antibiotic should not be used for plaque control purposes.

Vancomycin

This antibiotic is a non-absorbable polypeptide effective against Gram-positive organisms. Topical application of vancomycin inhibited plaque formation in the hamster. An adhesive paste containing 1% vancomycin reduced plaque development in children (Mitchell & Holmes 1965). Jensen et al. (1968) demonstrated, however, that three daily rinses with an aqueous solution of vancomycin did not successfully inhibit plaque formation at the gingival margin. Obviously, the data on vancomycin are controversial and the compound should not be used in the clinic.

Kanamycin

Kanamycin, a broad spectrum antibiotic, is a non-absorbable aminoglycan without special taste and with a very high stability. Although the topical application of a 5% kanamycin paste was successful in reducing plaque accumulation in children, the antibiotic was not successful in treating already existing gingivitis (Loesche & Nafe 1973).

Spiramycin

Spiramycin as well as erythromycin are macrolide antibiotics. Spiramycin has the unique property of giving higher salivary than serum levels (Harvey 1961). In rodents, spiramycin is stored in the salivary glands from which it is slowly released in the saliva (Yankell et al. 1971). By virtue of this feature, spiramycin would be an ideal antibiotic to use in the prevention and treatment of dental plaque infections. Unfortunately, there are only few studies available to confirm this hypothesis. Harvey (1961) presented a poorly controlled clinical trial in which the use of spiramycin in cases with periodontitis was reported to improve the clinical condition. The systemic application of four daily doses of 250 mg spiramycin for 5 days significantly reduced gingival index values in patients with gingivitis and periodontitis (Mills et al. 1979). However, the greatest effect was established by using the antimicrobial compound in advanced periodontal disease patients, where parameters describing gingival inflammation were significantly reduced. Also, the average probing depth was reduced by approximately 30% in advanced cases. From this study, it appears that more well controlled clinical trials should be performed to explore the potential use of spiramycin in routine periodontal treatment.

Tetracycline

Tetracyclines have been applied systemically on a large scale to patients with refractory periodontal disease and have also been tested in some animal (Williams et al. 1979a) as well as human studies (Österberg et al. 1979, Listgarten et al. 1978). The results of these studies are controversial. Using the Beagle dog model, Williams et al. (1979b) demonstrated that systemic administration of tetracyclines caused arrest of bone loss and a slight alteration of the composition of the pocket microbiota. When treating periodontal pockets in the human with systemic administration of tetracyclines, the same clinical microbiological and histological changes were observed as when the pockets were debrided mechanically (Listgarten et al. 1978). The discontinuation of treatment with tetracycline led to an immediate return of microbial and histological parameters characterizing disease. In a single case report, Österberg et al. (1979) demonstrated that the microbiota could be altered significantly when systemic tetracyclines were applied. Asaccharolytic bacterial strains were almost eliminated from the subgingival plaque. Recolonization of these pockets with suspected pathogenic organisms occurred within 6 to 16 weeks following cessation of antimicrobial treatment. Furthermore, a high level of tetracycline-resistant, predominantly Gram-positive cocci were found as a result of the tetracycline administration. When tetracycline was applied locally in hollow fiber devices (Goodson et al. 1979), spirochetes could practically be eliminated from infected sites and did not rapidly recolonize.

From these studies, it appears that systemic administration of tetracyclines has no advantage over local debridement and mechanical plaque control. This has been confirmed in several studies of long- and short-term character (Lindhe et al. 1979, Slots et al. 1979, Cinacio et a1 1982, Kornman & Karl 1982).

Metronidazole

Metronidazole is a nitroimidazole which bears the nitro group that has been associated with the occurrence of blood dyscrasias such as neutropenia. Although it has been claimed that metronidazole is carcinogenic for rodents and mutagenic in bacteria (Roe 1977), well-controlled studies in humans (Beard et al. 1979) failed to detect a carcinogenic effect of the drug. The material of this study was based on 771 women given mitronidazole for treatment of vaginal trichomoniasis. No appreciable increase in cases of cancer was observed.

Metronidazole, which is normally used in the treatment of protozoal infections, particularly trichomoniasis and amebiasis, has been found to be effective in the treatment of acute necrotizing ulcerative gingivitis (Shinn 1962, Lozdan et al. 1971). The drug is highly effective against Gram-negative anaerobic bacteria and spirochetes. This would suggest that it could be successful in treating cases of advanced periodontal disease, rapidly progressive periodontitis, and acute necrotizing ulcerative gingivitis. Heijl and Lindhe (1979) demonstrated that 20 mg/kg body weight per day of metronidazole, administered systemically during a 28-day period, can effectively reduce plaque and gingivitis development in Beagle dogs. The bacterial microbiota from subgingival sites of healthy gingiva was dominated in this study by coccoid cells and straight rods. During the phase of developing gingivitis, the percentage of coccoid cells and rods tended to decrease, while motile rods and spirochetes increased. During the 28 days of metronidazole treatment, the subgingival plaque microbiota maintained its "healthy" composition, i.e. a gradual influx of motile rods and spirochetes was prevented.

The data reported from clinical trials on the effects of systemic metronidazole therapy as an adjunct to scaling and root planing have been inconsistent. 16 weeks following this combined antibiotic / mechanical therapy, significantly greater pocket reductions were observed (Joyston-Bechal et al. 1984), an effect which was no longer detectable after 3 years of observation (Joyston-Bechal et al. 1984)

After having demonstrated beneficial clinical and microbiological effects using metronidazole in patients with advanced periodontitis (Loesche et al. 1981), Loesche et al. (1984) staged a double-blind clinical trial to test the effect of mechanical debridement with or without adjunctive administration of metronidazole. Significant gain of probing attachment was noted 30 weeks following the combined antibiotic/mechanical therapy. Significant reductions in presumptive periodontopathogenic bacteria, such as *B. gingivalis* and large spirochetes were noted, while intermediate spirochetes, *B. intermedius* and *Capnocytophaga* were not affected to the same extent.

A well-controlled study in 16 humans showed that the administration of 200 mg metronidazole, 4 times daily for 3 periods of 2 weeks each, separated by 8-week intervals additional to scaling and root planing resulted in the disappearance of clinical and histopathological signs of periodontal disease (Lindhe et al. 1982, 1983). Similar results were obtained by van Oosten et al. (1987).

Ornidazole

Ornidazole is another nitroimidazole derivative with an antibiotic efficacy spectrum similar to that of metronidazole (Wüst 1977). However, its absorptive capacity in the intestinal tract, as well as its improved kinetics offer some advantages over other nitroimidazoles (Schwartz & Jeunet 1976, Schwartz et al. 1979). In a study on the treatment of recurrent periodontal disease by scaling and root planing, adjunctive systemic administration of 1 g of ornidazole (Tibera®) for 10 days, a prolonged interval was noted for the reestablishment of a subgingival microbiota which may be conducive to periodontal disease (Mombelli et al. 1988). In a double-blind study on combined ornidazole and mechanical therapy of advanced periodontitis in 14 patients (Gusberti et al. 1986, 1987), significantly reduced frequencies for bleeding on probing, reduced probing depth, and reduced levels of spirochetes and Gram-negative anaerobic rods such as *Bacteroides* species were maintained for 4-6 months. These studies indicated that, similar to the adjunctive therapy with metronidazole, adjunctive ornidazole therapy offers additional microbiological and clinical benefits in well-selected groups, such as very advanced periodontitis patients or patients with previously treated, but reinfected periodontal sites. It is understood that a microbiological diagnosis should complement the clinical diagnosis prior to using nitroimidazoles in order to assure that the subgingival microbiota is susceptible to the drug.

Summary

In summarizing the use of antibiotics in periodontal therapy it should be stated (Van Palenstein Helderman 1986) that:

1. Adult periodontitis can successfully be treated by mechanical debridement followed by plaque control. Systemically administrated adjunctive antibiotics offer no significant benefits. In very advanced or rapidly progressing periodontitis, the additional use of nitroimidazoles, such as metronidazole and ornidazole may be successful in eradicating periodontal pathogens. A microbiological diagnosis is a prerequisite for this treatment approach.
2. In juvenile periodontitis and in patients with sites with recurrent periodontitis the use of adjunctive antibiotics to mechanical debridement may offer some advantage. Antibiotics in sustained release devices, or topically administered, also lack the proof of superiority over mechanical debridement and meticulous plaque control.
3. So far, no specific group or strain of microorganism has been identified as the responsible etiologic pathogen in periodontal diseases. Therefore, the use of antibiotics can only represent a supplement to a non-specific treatment approach.

References

Addy, M. (1977) Hibitane in the treatment of aphthous ulceration. *Journal of Clinical Periodontology* **4**, 108-116.

Addy, M., Prayitno, S., Taylor, L. & Cadogan, S. (1979) An in vitro study of the role of dietary factors in the etiology of tooth staining associated with the use of chlorhexidine. *Journal of Periodontal Research* **14**, 403-410.

Agerbaek, N., Melsen, B. & Rölla, G. (1975) Application of chlorhexidine by oral irrigation systems. *Scandinavian Journal of Dental Research* **83**, 284-287.

Aleece, A.A. & Forscher, B.K. (1954) Calculus reduction with mucinase dentifrice. *Journal of Periodontology* **25**, 122-125.

Attström, R., Matsson, L., Edwardsson, S., Willard, L.-O. & Klinge, B. (1983) The effect of octapinol on dento-gingival plaque and development of gingivitis. III. Short-term studies in humans. *Journal of Periodontal Research* **18**, 445-451.

Bauhammers, A., Landay, M.A. & Pinkus, D.T. (1968) Dental calculus inhibition in rats through pancreatin applications. *Archives of Oral Biology* **13**, 353-356.

Beard, C.M., Noller, K.L., O'Fallon, W.O., Kurland, L.T. & Dockerty, M.B. (1979) Lack of evidence for cancer due to use of metronidazole. *New England Journal of Medicine* **301**, 519-522.

Belting, C.M. & Gordon, D.L. (1966) In vivo effect of a urea-containing dentifrice on dental calculus formation.

Bibby, B.G. & von Kestern, M. (1940) The effect of fluorine on mouth bacteria. *Journal of Dental Research* **19**, 391.

Bonesvoll, P., L¢kken, P. & Rölla, G. (1974a). Influence of concentration, time, temperature and pH on the retention of chlorhexidine in the human oral cavity after mouth rinses. *Archives of Oral Biology* **19**, 1025-1029.

Bonesvoll, P., L¢kken, P., Rölla, G. & Paus, P.N. (1974b). Retention of chlorhexidine in the human oral cavity after mouth rinses. *Archives of Oral Biology* **19** 209-212.

Brecx, M.C. & Theilade, J. (1984) Effect of chlorhexidine rinses on the morphology of early dental plaque formed on plastic films. *Journal of Clinical Periodontology* **11**, 553-564.

Brecx, M.C., Theilade, J., Attström, R. & Glantz, P.-O. (1987) The effect of chlorhexidine and octapinol on early human plaque formation. A light and electron microscopic study. *Journal of Periodontal Research* **22**, 290-295.

Briner, W.W. & Wunder, J.A. (1977) Sensitivity of dog plaque microorganisms to chlorhexidine during longitudinal studies. *Journal of Periodontal Research* **12**, 135-139.

Budtz-Jørgensen, E. (1977) Hibitane in the treatment of oral candidiasis. *Journal of Clinical Periodontology* **4**, Supplement 117-128.

Budtz-Jørgensen, E. & Löe, H. (1972) Chlorhexidine as a denture disinfectant in the treatment of denture stomatitis. *Scandinavian Journal of Dental Research* **80**, 457-463.

Ciancio, S.G., Slots, J., Reynolds, H.S., Zambon, J.J. & Mc Kenna, J.D. (1982) The effect of short-term administration of minocycline HCI on gingival inflammation and subgingival microflora. *Journal of Periodontology* **53**, 557-561.

Cumming, B.R. & Löe, H. (1973) Optimal dosage and method of delivering chlorhexidine solutions for the inhibition of dental plaque. *Journal of Periodontal Research* **8**, 57-62.

Davies, A. (1973) The mode of action of chlorhexidine. *Journal of Periodontal Research* **8**, Supplement 12:68-75.

Emslie, R.D., Cross, W.G. & Blake, G.C. (1962) A clinical trial of an ascorbic acidperoxide preparation and penicillin chewing-gum in the treatment of acute ulcerative gingivitis. *British Dental Journal* **112**, 320-323.

Ennever, J. & Sturzenberger, O.P. (1961) Inhibition of dental calculus formation by use of an enzyme chewing gum. *Journal of Periodontology* **32**, 331-333.

Ericsson, T. & Ericsson, Y. (1967) The effect of partial fluorine substitution of the phosphate change and protein adsorption of hydroxylapatite. *Helvetica Odontologica Acta* **11**, 10-14.

Faulkes, E. (1973) Some toxicological observations in chlorhexidine. *Journal of Periodontal Research* **8**, Supplement 12:55-57.

Fitzgerald, R.J. (1955) Influence of antibiotics on experimental rat caries. *Science* **187**.

Flötra, L., Gjermo, P., Rölla, G. & Waerhaug, J. (1972) A 4-month study on the effect of chlorhexidine mouth washes on 50 soldiers. *Scandinavian Journal of Dental Research* **80**, 10-17.

Friedman, M. & Golomb, G. (1982) New sustained release dosage form of chlorhexidine for dental use. I. Development and kinetics of release. *Journal of Periodontal Research* **17**, 323-328.

Gibbons, R.J. & Banghardt, S.B. (1967) Synthesis of extracellular dextran by cariogenic bacteria and its presence in human dental plaque. *Archives of Oral Biology* **12**, 11-24.

Gjermo, P. (1974) Chlorhexidine in dental practice. *Journal of Clinical Periodontology* **1**, 143-152.

Gjermo, P. & Eriksen, H.M. (1974) Unchanged plaque inhibiting effect of chlorhexidine in human subjects after 2 years of continuous use. *Archives of Oral Biology* **19**, 317-319.

Glantz, P.O. (1969) On wettability and adhesiveness.

A study of enamel, dentine, some restorative materials and dental plaque. *Odontologisk Revy* **20**, Supplement 17.

Glantz, P.-O. & Attström, R. (1986) Tooth-surface alteration agents. State-of-the-science review. In: Löe, H. & Kleinman, D.V., (eds). *Dental plaque control measures and oral hygiene practices.* Washington, D.C.: IRL Press, 7:185-194.

Goodson, J.M., Haffajee, A. & Socransky, S.S. (1979) Periodontal therapy by local delivery of tetracycline. *Journal of Clinical Periodontology* **6**, 83-92.

Grossman, E., Reiter, G., Sturzenberger, O.P., de la Rosa, M., Dickinson, T.D., Ferretti, G.A., Ludlam, G.E. & Meckel, A.H. (1986) Six-month study of the effects of a chlorhexidine mouthrinse on gingivitis in adults. *Journal of Periodontal Research* **21**, Supplement 16:33-43.

Gusberti, F.A., Sampathkumar, P., Siegrist, B.E. & Lang, N.P. (1988) Microbiological and clinical effects of chlorhexidine digluconate and hydrogen peroxide mouthrinses on developing plaque and gingivitis. *Journal of Clinical Periodontology* **15**, 60-67.

Gusberti, F.A., Syed, S.A., Gusberti, R. & Lang, N.P. (1987) Effects of ornidazole and mechanical debridement on periodontitis and subgingival plaque. IADR Abstract No. 1994. *Journal of Dental Research* **66**, 356.

Gusberti, F.A., Syed, S.A. & Lang, N.P. (1986) Klinische und mikrobiologische Effekte einer zehntägigen oralen Verabreichung von Ornidazol (Tiberal®) nach der mechanischen Behandlung der Paradontitis marginalis. *Acta Parodontologica,* In: *Schweizerische Monatsschrift für Zahnmedizin* **96**, 893-907.

Hammond, B. (1986) Ecology alteration. State-of-the-science review. In: Löe, H. & Kleinman, D.V., (eds). *Dental plaque control measures and oral hygiene practices,* Washington D.C. : IRL Press 8:197-212.

Harvey, R.F. (1961) Clinical impressions of a new antibiotic in periodontics: Spiremycine. *Journal of the Canadian Dental Association* **27**, 576-580.

Heijl, L. & Lindhe, J. (1979) The effect of metronidazole on the development of plaque and gingivitis in the beagle dog. *Journal of Clinical Periodontology* **6**, 197-209.

Heyden, G. (1973) Relation between locally high concentration of chlorhexidine and staining as seen in the clinic. *Journal of Periodontal Research* **8**, Supplement 12:76-80.

Jensen, A.L. (1959) Use of dehydrated pancreas in oral hygiene. *Journal of the American Dental Association* **59**, 923-930.

Jensen, S.B., Löe, H., Schiött, C.R. & Theilade, E. (1968) Experimental gingivitis in man. IV. Vancomycin induced changes in bacterial plaque composition as related to development of gingival inflammation. *Journal of Periodontal Research* **3**, 284-293.

Joyston-Bechal, A., Smales, F.C. & Duckworth, R. (1984) Effect of metronidazole on chronic periodontal disease subjects using a topically applied chlorhexidine gel. *Journal of Clinical Periodontology* **11**, 53-62.

Kelstrup, J., Holm-Pedersen, P. & Poulsen, S. (1978) Reduction of the formation of dental plaque and gingivitis in humans by crude mutanase. *Scandinavian Journal of Dental Research* **86**, 93-102.

Keyes, P.H. (1966) Evaluation of two topical application methods used to assess the antidental caries potential of drugs in hamsters. *Journal of Oral Therapeutics and Pharmacology* **2**, 285-294.

Keyes, P.H. Rowberry, S.A., Englander, H.R. & Fitzgerald, R.J. (1966) Bio-assays for medicaments for the control of dentobacterial plaque, dental caries, and periodontal lesions in Syrian hamsters. *Journal of Oral Therapeutics and Pharmacology* **3**, 157-173.

Kinder, S.A., Kornman, K.S. & Holt, S.C. (1984) Selective alteration of the subgingival microbiota prevents induction of periodontitis. IADR Abstract No. 1535. *Journal of Dental Research* **63**, 341.

König, K.G. & Guggenheim, B. (1968) In vivo effects of dextranase on plaque and caries. *Helvetica Odontologica Acta* **12**, 48-54.

Kornman, K.S. (1986a) The role of supragingival plaque in the prevention and treatment of periodontal diseases. *Journal of Periodontal Research* **21**, Supplement 16:5-22.

Kornman, K.S. (1986b) Antimicrobial agents, State-of-the-science review. In: Löe, H. & Kleinman, D.V., (eds). *Dental plaque control measures and oral hygiene practices.* Washington, D.C.:IRL Press, 5:121-142.

Kornman, K.S. & Karl, E.H. (1982) The effect of long-term low-dose tetracycline therapy on the subgingival microflora in refractory adult periodontitis. *Journal of Periodontology* **53**, 604-610.

Lang, N.P. (1980) The implications of antiseptics, antibiotics, enzymes and vaccines in plaque control. In: Shanley, D., ed. *Efficacy of Treatment Procedures in Periodontics* pp. 57-76. Chicago, Berlin, Rio de Janeiro & Tokyo: Quintessence Publishing Co.

Lang, N.P. & Briner, W.W. (1984) Chemical control of gingivitis in man. *Journal of the American Dental Association* **109**, 223.

Lang, N.P. & Brecx, M.C. (1986) Chlorhexidine digluconate - an agent for chemical plaque control and prevention of gingival inflammation. *Journal of Periodontal Research* **21**, Supplement 16:74-89.

Lang, N.P., Catalanotto, F.A., Knöpfli, R.U. & Antczak, A.A.A. (1988) Quality-specific taste impairment following the application of chlorhexidine digluconate mouthrinses. *Journal of Clinical Periodontology* **15**, 43-48.

Lang, N.P., Hotz, P., Graf, H., Geering, A.H. & Saxer, U.P. (1982) Longitudinal effects of supervised chlorhexidine mouthrinses in children. *Journal of Periodontal Research* **17**, 101-111.

Lang, N.P. & Räber, K. (1981) The use of oral irrigators as a vehicle for the application of antimicrobial agents in chemical plaque control. *Journal of Clinical Periodontology* **8**, 177-188.

Lang, N.P. & Ramseier-Grossmann, K. (1981) Optimal dosage of chlorhexidine digluconate in clinical plaque control when applied by the oral irrigator. *Journal of Clinical Periodontology* **8**, 189-202.

Lang, N.P., Weber, H.P. & Witt, J.J. (1986) Clinical effects of varying concentrations of chlorhexidine digluconate formulated into a mouthwash. AADR Abstract No 689. *Journal of Dental Research* **65**, 246.

Larson, R.H., Zipkin, I. & Fitzgerald, R.J. (1963) Effect of dehydroacetic acid and tetracycline on caries activity and its transmission in the rat. *Journal of Dental Research* **42**, 95-102.

Lindhe, J., Hamp, S.-E. & Löe, H. (1975) Plaque induced periodontal disease in beagle dogs - a 4-year clinical roentgenographical and histometris study. *Journal of Periodontal Research* **10**, 243-255.

Lindhe, J., Hejil, L., Goodson, J.M. & Socransky, S.S. (1979) Local tetracycline delivery using hollow fiber devices in periodontal therapy. *Journal of Clinical Periodontology* **6**, 141-149.

Lindhe, J., Liljenberg, B., Adielson, B. & Börjesson, I. (1982) The effect of metronidazole therapy on human periodontal disease. *Journal of Periodontal Research* **17**, 534-536.

Lindhe, J., Liljenberg, B., Adielson , B. & Börjesson, I. (1983) Metronidazole as a probe in the study of human periodontal disease. *Journal of Clinical Periodontology* **10**, 100-112.

Listgarten, M.A., Lindhe, J. & Helldén, L. (1978) Effect of tetracycline and/or scaling on human periodontal disease. Clinical, Microbiological and histological observations. *Journal of Clinical Periodontology* **5**, 246-271.

Lobene, R.R. (1971) A clinical study on the effect of dextranase on human dental plaque. *Journal of the American Dental Association* **82**,132-135.

Löe, H. (1973) Does chlorhexidine have a place in the prophylaxis of dental diseases? *Journal of Periodontal Research* **8**, Supplement 12:93-99.

Löe, H., Mandell, M., Derry, A. & Schiött, C.R. (1971) The effect of mouth rinses and topical application of chlorhexidine on calculus formation in man. *Journal of Periodontal Research* **6**, 312-314.

Löe, H. & Schiött, C.R. (1970a) The effect of suppression of the oral microflora upon the development of dental plaque and gingivitis. In: McHugh, W.E., ed. *Dental PlaqueL pp, 247-255. Edinburgh:E & S Livingston.*

Löe, H. & Schiött, C.R. (1970b) The effect of mouthrinses and topical application of chlorhexidine on the development of dental plaque and gingivitis in man. *Journal of Periodontal Research* **5**, 79-83.

Löe, H., Schiött, C.R., Glavind, L. & Karring, T. (1976) Two years oral use of chlorhexidine in man. I. General design and clinical effects. *Journal of Periodontal Research* **11**, 135-144.

Löe, H., Theilade, E. & Jensen, S.B. (1965) Experimental gingivitis in man. *Journal of Periodontology* **36**, 177-187.

Löe, H., von der Fehr, F. & Schiött, C.R. (1972) Inhibition of experimental caries by plaque prevention. The effect of chlorhexidine mouthrinses. *Scandinavian Journal of Dental Research* **80**, 1-9.

Loesche, W.J. & Nafe, D. (1973) Reduction of supragingival plaque accumulations in institutionalized Down's Syndrome patients by periodic treatment with topical Kanamycin. *Archives of Oral Biology* **18**, 1131-1143.

Loesche, W.J. (1976) Chemotherapy of dental plaque infections. In: Melcher, A.H. & Zarb, G.H. (eds). *Oral Sciences Reviews* **9** Copenhagen: Munksgaard, 65-107.

Loesche, W.J., Syed, S.A., Morrison, E.C., Kerry, G.J., Higgins, T. & Stoll, J. (1984) Metronidazole in periodontitis. I. Clinical and bacteriological results after 15 to 30 weeks. *Journal of Periodontology* **55**, 325-335.

Loesche, W.J., Syed, S.A., Morrison, E.C., Laughon, B. & Grossman, N.S. (1981) Treatment of periodontal infections due to anaerobic bacteria with short-term treatment with metronidazole. *Journal of Clinical Periodontology* **8**, 29-44.

Lozdan, J., Sheiham, A., Pearlman, B.A., Keiser, B., Rachanis, C.C. & Meyer, P. (1971) The use of nitrimidazine in the treatment of acute ulcerative gingivitis. A double blind controlled trial. *Beitish Dental Journal* **130**, 294.

Manhart, M.D., Grossman, E., Sturzenberger, O.P., Vick, V.C., Bollmer, B.W. & Moore, D.J. (1988) Efficacy of chlorhexidine digluconate in comparison to phenolic and plant alkaloid compound. IADR Abstract No. 570. *Journal of Dental Research* **67**, 184.

Miller, W.D. (1890) The microorganisms of the mouth. *(Die Mikroorganismen der Mundhöhle).* Leipzig: Georg Thieme, 447p.

Mills, W.H., Thompson, G.W. & Beagrie, G.S. (1979) Clinical evaluation of Spiramycin and Erythromycin in control of periodontal disease. *Journal of Clinical Periodontology* **6**, 308-316.

Mitchell, D.F. & Holmes L.A. (1965) Topical antibiotic control of dentogingival plaque. *Journal of Periodontology* **36** 202-208.

Mombelli, A., Gusberti, F.A. & Lang, N.P. (1988) Treatment of recurrent periodontal disease by root planing and ornidazole (Tiberal®). Clinical and microbiological findings. IADR Abstract No. 762. *Journal of Dental Research* **67**, 208.

Mühlemann, H.R., Meyer, R.W., König, K.G. & Marthaler, T.M. (1961) The cariostatic effect of antibacterial compounds in animal experimentation. *Helvetica Odontologica Acta* **5**, 18-22.

Österberg, S.K.-Å., Williams, B.L. & J¢rgensen, J. (1979) Long-term effects of tetracycline on the subgingival microflora. *Journal of Clinical Periodontology* **6**, 133-140.

Packman, E.W., Abbot, D.D., Harrison, J.W.E. & Salisbury, G.B. (1963) Effect of enzyme chewing gums upon oral hygiene. *Journal of Periodontology* **34**, 255-258.

Posner, A.S. (1969) Chrystal chemistry of bone mineral. *Physiological Review* **49**, 760-764.

Prayitno,S., Taylor, L., Cadogen, S. & Addy, M. (1979) An in vivo study of dietary factors in the etiology of tooth staining associated with the use of chlorhexidine. *Journal of Periodontal Research* **14**, 411-417.

Roe, F.J.C. (1977) Metronidazole: review of uses and tixicity. *Journal of Antimicrobial Chemotherapy* **3**, 205-212.

Rölla, G. & Melsen, B. (1975) On the mechanism of the plaque inhibition by chlorhexidine. *Journal of Dental Research* **54**, Special Issue B, 57-62.

Schiött, C.R., Briner, W.W., Kirkland, J.J. & Löe, H. (1976a) Two years oral use of chlorhexidine in man. III. Changes in sensitivity of the salivary flora. *Journal of Periodontal Research* **11**, 153-157.

Schiött, C.R., Löe, H. & Briner, W.W. (1976b) Two years oral use of chlorhexidine in man. Effect on various medical parameters. *Journal of Periodontal Research* **11**, 158-164.

Schwartz, D.E. & Jeunet, F. (1976) Comparative pharmacokinetic studies of ornidazole and metronidazole in man. *Chemotherapy* **22**, 19-29.

Schwartz, D.E., Jordan, J.-C., Vetter, W. & Oesterhelt, G. (1979) Metabolic studies of ornidazole in the rat, in the dog and in man. *Xenobiotica* **9**, 571-581.

Segreto, V.A., Collins, E.M., Beiswanger, B.B., de la Rosa, M., Isaacs, R.L., Lang, N.P., Mallatt, M.E. & Meckel, A.H. (1986) A comparison of mouthrinses containing two concentrations of chlorhexidine. *Journal of Periodontal Research* **21**, Supplement 16:23-32.

Shinn, D.L.S. (1962) Metronidazole in acute ulcerative gingivitis. *Lancet* **1**, 1191.

Siegrist, B.E., Gusberti, F.A., Brecx, M.C., Weber, H.P. & Lang, N.P. (1986) Efficacy of supervised rinsing with chlorhexidine digluconate in comparison to phenolic and plant alkaloid compounds. *Journal of Periodontal Research* **21**, Supplement 16:60-73.

Slots, J., Hausman, E. & Gibbons, R.J. (1979) Longitudinal study of experimentally induced periodontal disease in Macaca arctoides: Relationship between microflora and alveolar bone loss. *Infection and Immunity* **23**, 260-269.

Soskolne, A., Golomb, G., Friedman, M. & Sela. M.N. (1983) New sustained release dosage form of chlorhexidine for dental use. II. Use in periodontal therapy. *Journal of Periodontal Research* **18**, 330-336.

Stabholz, A., Sela, M.N., Friedman, M., Golomb, G. & Soskolne, A. (1986) Clinical and microbiological effects of sustained release chlorhexidine in periodontal pockets. *Journal of Clinical Periodontology* **13**, 783-788.

Stewart, G.G. (1952) Mucinase - a possible means of rêducing calculus formation. *Journal of Periodontology* **23**, 85-90.

Storhaug, K. (1977) Hibitane in oral disease in handicapped patients. *Journal of Clinical Periodontology* **4**, Supplement 102-107.

Tinanoff, N. (1977) Screening of nine fluoride mouthrinses for antiplaque properties. IADR Abstracts No. 382. *Journal of Dental Research* **56**, Special issue A 138.

Tinanoff, N., Hock, j., Camosci, D. & Helldén, L. (1979) Clinical trial to test antiplaque effect of SnF_2 mouthrinse. IADR Abstract No768. *Journal of Dental Research* **58**, Special issue A 284.

Tinanoff, N., Manwell, M.A., Zameck, R. & Grasso, J.E. (1988) Daily use of stannous fluoride gel reduces plaque and gingivitis in adults. IADR Abstract No. 770. *Journal of Dental Research* **67**, 209.

Usher, P.J. (1975) Oral hygiene in mentally handicapped children. A pilot study of the use of chlorhexidine gel. *British Dental Journal* **138**, 217-221.

Van Oosten, M.A.C., Mikx, F.H.M. & Renggli, H.H. (1987) Microbial and clinical measurements of periodontal pockets during sequential periods of non-treatment, mechanical debridement and metronidazole therapy. *Journal of Clinical Periodontology* **14**, 197-204.

Van Palenstein Helderman, W.H. (1986) Is antibiotic therapy justified in the treatment of human chronic inflammatory periodontal disease? *Journal of Clinical Periodontology* **13**, 932-938.

Van der Velden, U., Abbas, F. & Hart. A.A.M. (1985) Experimental gingivitis in relation to susceptility to periodontal disease (I) Clinical observations. *Journal of Clinical Periodontology* **12**, 61-68.

Von Abbé, N.J. (1974) The substantivity of cosmetic ingredients to the skin, hair and teeth. *Journal of the Society of Cosmetic Chemists* **25**, 23.

Von der Fehr, F.R., Löe, H. & Theilade, E. (1970) Experimental caries in man. *Caries Research* **4**, 131-148.

Williams, B.L., ¥sterberg, S.K.-Å. & J¢rgensen, J. (1979a) Subgingival microflora of periodontal patients on tetracycline therapy. *Journal of Clinical Periodontology* **6**,210-221.

Williams, R.C., Sandler, M.B., Aschaffenburg, P.H. & Goldhaber, P. (1979b) Preliminary observations on the inhibitory effect of tetracycline on alveolar bone loss in Beagle dogs. *Journal of Periodontal Research* **14**, 341-351.

Winrow, M.J. (1973) Metabolic studies with radiolabelled chlorhexidine in animals and man. *Journal of Periodontal Research* **8**, Supplement 12:45-48.

Wüst, J. (1977) Susceptibility of anaerobic bacteria to metronidazole, ornidazole and tinidazole, and routine susceptibility testing by standardized methods. *Antimicrobial Agents and Chemotherapy* **11**, 631-637.

Yankell, S.L., Lenug, F.C., Gardner, J.M. & Paor, W.S. (1971) Spiramycin excretion in animals: I. A single oral dose in rats. *Journal of Dental Research* **50**, 1359.

Young, R.A. & Elliot, J.C. (1966) Atomic scale bases for several properties of apatites. *Archives of Oral Biology* **11**, 699-707.

CHAPTER 16

Periodontal Surgery

Over the years, several different surgical techniques have been described and used in periodontal therapy. A superficial review of the literature in this area may give the reader a somewhat confusing picture of the specific objectives and indications relevant for various surgical techniques. It is a matter of historical interest that the first surgical techniques used in periodontal therapy were described as means of gaining access to diseased root surfaces. Such access could be accomplished without excision of the soft tissue pocket ("open-view operations"). Later, procedures were described by which the "diseased gingiva" was excised (gingivectomy procedures).

The concept that not only inflamed soft tissue but also "infected and necrotic bone" had to be eliminated called for the development of surgical techniques by which the alveolar bone could be exposed and resected (flap procedures). Other concepts such as 1) the importance of maintaining the muco-gingival complex (i.e. a wide zone of keratinized and attached gingiva) and 2) the possibility for regeneration of periodontal tissues have also prompted the introduction of "tailor-made" surgical techniques.

Since most forms of periodontal disease are plaque-associated disorders it is obvious that surgical treatment can only be considered as adjunctive to cause-related therapy. Therefore, the various surgical methods should be evaluated on the basis of their potential to facilitate plaque control and thereby to enhance the long-term preservation of the periodontium.

Objectives of periodontal surgery

Traditionally, *pocket elimination* has been the main objective of periodontal therapy. The removal of the pocket by surgical means served two purposes: 1) the pocket, which established an environment for events leading to progression of periodontal disease, was eliminated and 2) the root surface was made accessible for scaling and, after healing, for self-performed tooth cleaning.

While these objectives cannot be entirely discarded today, the necessity for pocket elimination in periodontal therapy has been challenged. During recent years our understanding of the biology of the periodontal tissues, the pathogenesis of periodontal disease and the healing capacity of the periodontium has markedly increased. This new information has thus formed the basis for a more broadly differentiated understanding of the role played by periodontal surgery in the preservation of teeth.

In the past, *increased pocket depth* was the main indication for periodontal surgery. However, pocket depth is no longer as unequivocal a concept as it used to be. The *probeable depth*, i.e. the distance from the gingival margin to the point where the periodontal probe is stopped by tissue resistance, may only rarely correspond to the "true" depth of the pocket (e.g. Listgarten 1980). Furthermore, regardless of the accuracy with which pockets can be measured, there is no established correlation between probeable pocket depth and the presence or absence of active disease. This means that symptoms other than increased probing depth should be present to justify surgical therapy. These include clinical signs of inflammation, especially exudation and bleeding on probing (to the bottom of the pockets), as well as suspect gingival morphology. Finally, the fact that proper plaque control, maintained by the patient, is a decisive factor for a good prognosis (Rosling et al. 1976a, Nyman et al. 1977) must be considered prior to the initiation of surgery.

In conclusion, the main objective of periodontal surgery is to contribute to the preservation of the periodontium by facilitating plaque removal and plaque control, and periodontal surgery can serve this purpose by

1. creating accessibility for proper professional scaling and root planing
2. establishing a gingival morphology which facilitates the patient's self-performed plaque control

In addition to this, periodontal surgery may aim at the

3. regeneration of periodontal attachment lost due to destructive disease. (New attachment procedures in periodontal therapy are discussed in Chapter 18).

General guidelines for periodontal surgery

The overall treatment of periodontal disease can be divided into different phases (see Chapter 13):

– Examination including medical and dental

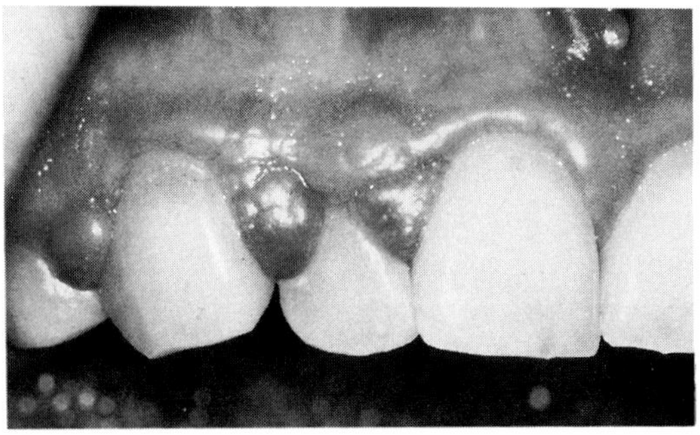

Fig. 16-1a.

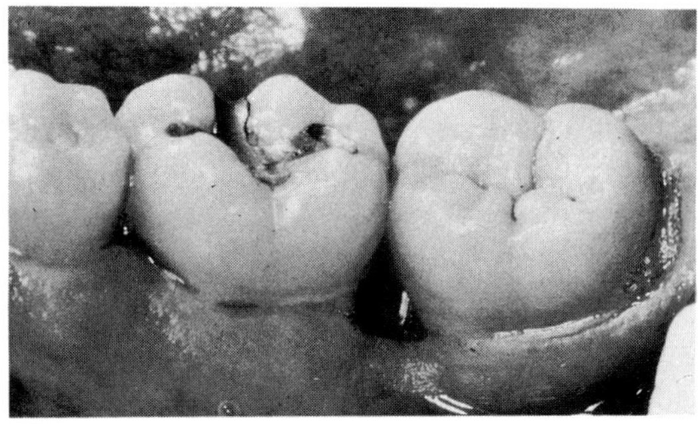

Fig. 16-1b.

Fig. 16-1. Examples of gingival aberrations which favor plaque retention and thereby impede the patient's plaque control. (a) Gingival hyperplasia. (b) Gingival crater.

history, *temporary treatment planning*, and treatment of acute conditions when indicated.

- *Cause-related phase*; comprising removal of tooth deposits, and establishing of proper home care techniques. Tooth extractions, placement of temporary fillings and prostheses, endodontic treatment (when indicated).
- *Evaluation of patient cooperation and tissue response*. The time lapse between termination of the cause-related phase of therapy and this evaluation may vary from 1 to 6 months.
- *Definitive treatment phase;* periodontal surgery, restorative/functional treatment.
- *Maintenance phase.*

In accordance with this sequence, the final decision concerning type and extent of periodontal surgery to be performed should be made after the effect of cause-related measures has been evaluated. This practice has the following advantages:

1. the removal of calculus and bacterial plaque has eliminated or markedly reduced the inflammatory cell infiltrate in the gingiva (edema, hyperemia, flabby tissue consistency), thereby making assessment of the "true" gingival contours and pocket depths possible
2. the resolution of gingival inflammation has made the tissue firmer, which facilitates the surgical treatment. The propensity for bleeding is reduced, making inspection of the field of operation easier
3. a better basis for the prognosis has been established. The effectiveness of the patients' home care is of decisive importance for the long-term prognosis. Lack of effective home care will often mean that the patient should be excluded from surgical treatment.

Indications for surgical treatment

Impaired access for scaling and root planing

Scaling and root planing are methods of therapy which are difficult to master. The difficulties in accomplishing proper debridement increase with 1) increasing depth of the periodontal pockets, 2) increasing width of the tooth surfaces, 3) the presence of root fissures, root concavities, furcations, and defective margins of dental restorations in the subgingival area.

Provided a correct technique and suitable instruments are used (Chapter 14), it is usually possible to properly debride pockets up to 5 mm deep (Waerhaug 1978, Caffesse et al.

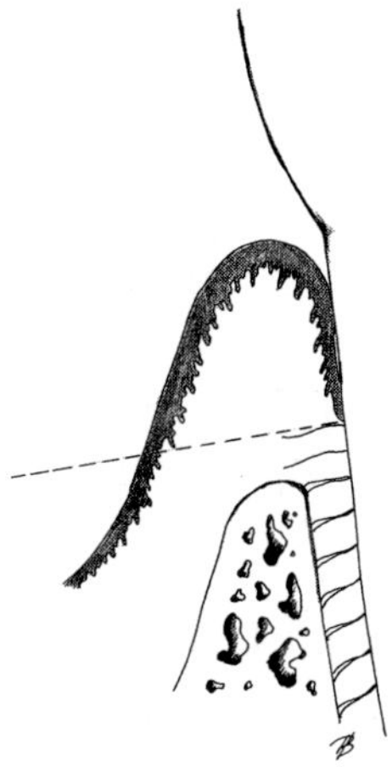

Fig. 16-2a.

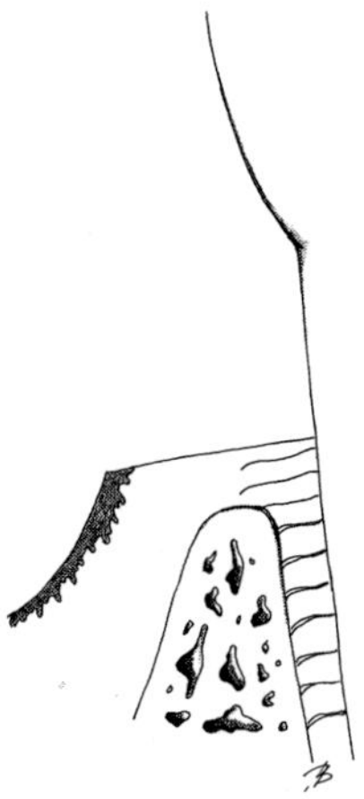

Fig. 16-2b.

Fig. 16-2. *Gingivectomy.* The incision is directed towards the bottom of the pocket (a) and the part of the gingiva enclosing the pocket is removed (b).

1985). However, this mm limit cannot be used as a universal rule-of-thumb. Reduced accessibility and the presence of one or several of the above-mentioned impeding conditions may prevent proper debridement of shallow pockets whereas at sites with good accessibility and favorable root morphology proper debridement can be accomplished even in deeper pockets (Badersten et al. 1981, Lindhe et al. 1982).

It is often difficult to ascertain by clinical means whether subgingival instrumentation has been properly performed. Following scaling, the root surface should be smooth and hard - roughness will often indicate the presence of remaining subgingival calculus. It is also important to monitor carefully the gingival reaction to subgingival debridement. If inflammation persists and if bleeding is elicited by gentle probing in the subgingival area, the presence of subgingival deposits should be suspected. If such symptoms are not resolved by repeated subgingival instrumentation, surgical treatment should be performed and the root surfaces exposed for proper cleaning.

Impaired access for self-performed plaque control

The level of plaque control which can be maintained by the patient is determined not only by their interest and dexterity but also, to some extent, by the morphology of the dentogingival area.

The patients' responsibility in a plaque control program must obviously include the cleansing of the supragingival tooth surfaces and the marginal part of the gingival sulcus. This means that the tooth area coronal to the gingival margin and at the entrance to the gingival sulcus should be the target for the patients' home care efforts.

Pronounced gingival hyperplasia and gingival craters (Fig. 16-1) are examples of morphological aberrations which may impede proper home-care. Likewise, the presence of restorations with defective marginal fit or adverse contour and surface characteristics at the gingival margin may seriously compromise plaque removal.

By the professional treatment of periodontal disease, the dentist prepares the dentition in

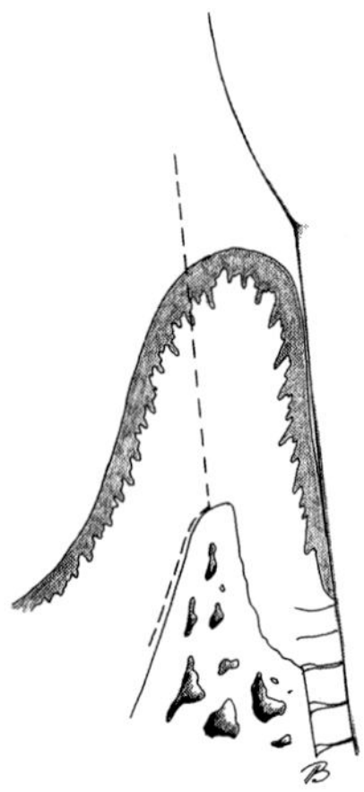

Fig. 16-3a.

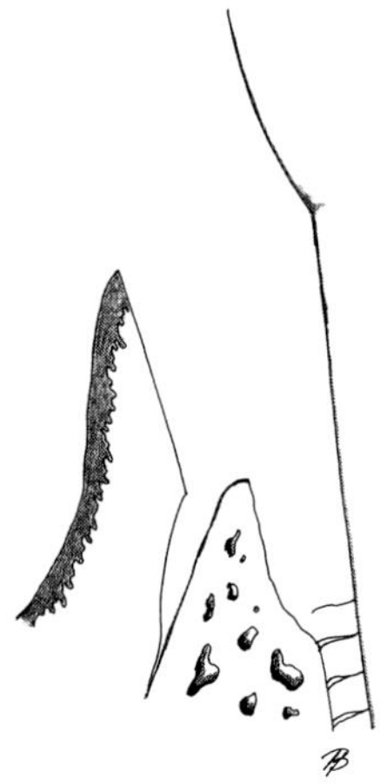

Fig. 16-3b.

Fig. 16-3. *Flap operation.* (a) Incision from the gingival margin to the crest of the alveolar bone. (b) Deflection of the flap and removal of the pocket epithelium and the inflamed connective tissue.

such a way that home care can be effectively managed. At the completion of treatment, the following objectives should have been met:

- no sub- or supragingival dental deposits
- no pathological pockets (no bleeding on probing to the bottom of the pockets)
- no plaque-retaining aberrations of gingival morphology
- no plaque-retaining parts of restorations in relation to the gingival margin

These requirements lead to the following indications for periodontal surgery:
- accessibility for proper scaling and root planing
- establishment of a morphology of the dentogingival area conducive to plaque control
- pocket depth reduction
- correction of gross gingival aberrations
- shift of the gingival margin to a position apically to plaque retaining restorations
- facilitate proper restorative therapy.

Indications for various surgical techniques

Attempts have been made to classify different surgical modalities used in the treatment of periodontal disease. Distinctions between methods involving the marginal tissues and those involving the muco-gingival area have been made and, further, between tissue eliminating/resective varieties and tissue preserving/reconstructive types. Such classifications appear less than precise since several techniques are often combined in the treatment of individual cases, and since there is no clear-cut relationship between disease characteristics and selection of surgical methods.

In the following, the general *indications* for the various surgical methods will be presented.

Curretage

Curretage, which was formerly used extensively, is defined as the removal, by the use of a curette, of the inner surface of the soft tissue wall of the pocket. The rationale behind this includes that:

- the removal of pocket epithelium and inflamed connective tissue results in new attachment of connective tissue and/or epithelium to the tooth surface (see Chapter 18)
- tissue shrinkage following curettage contributes to pocket reduction.

The reasons for curettage no longer being frequently used are:

- the procedure is technically difficult to master and is time-consuming
- the complete removal of subgingival deposits by scaling and root planing results in optimal healing without curettage
- if removal of pocket epithelium and adjacent connective tissue is to be attempted, more effective methods are available (reverse bevel incision).

Gingivectomy

The obvious indication for gingivectomy is the presence of deep supraalveolar pockets (Fig. 16-2). In addition, the gingivectomy technique can be used to reshape abnormal gingival contours such as gingival craters and gingival hyperplasias (Fig. 16-1). In such cases the technique is often termed *gingivoplasty*. Gingivectomy is not considered suitable in situations where the incision will lead to the removal of the entire zone of keratinized gingiva. This is the case when the bottom of the probeable pocket to be excised is located at or below the mucogingival junction. Furthermore, since the gingivectomy procedure is aimed at the complete elimination of the periodontal pocket, this procedure cannot be used in periodontal sites when infrabony lesions or bony craters are present.

These limitations, combined with the development in recent years of surgical methods which have a broader field of application, have led to less frequent use of gingivectomy.

Flap operation with or without osseous surgery

Flap operations can be used in all cases where surgical treatment of periodontal disease is indicated. Flap procedures are particularly useful at sites where pockets extend beyond the mucogingival border and/or where treatment of bony lesions and furcation involvements is required (Fig. 16-3).

The principles of osseous surgery in periodontal therapy were outlined by Schluger (1949) and Goldman (1950). They pointed out that alveolar bone loss caused by inflammatory periodontal disease often results in an uneven outline of the bone crest. Since, according to these authors, the gingival contour is closely dependent on the contour of the underlying bone as well as the proximity and anatomy of adjacent tooth surfaces, the elimination of soft tissue pockets often has to be combined with osseous reshaping and the elimination of osseous craters and angular bony defects to establish and maintain shallow pockets and optimal gingival contour after surgery. As a general rule, however, care must be exercised when supporting bone, i.e. bone directly involved in the attachment of the tooth, is to be removed.

The advantages of flap operations include:

- existing keratinized gingiva is preserved
- the marginal alveolar bone is exposed whereby the morphology of bony defects can be identified and the proper treatment rendered
- furcation areas are exposed, the degree of involvement and the “tooth - bone” relationship can be identified
- the flap can be repositioned at its original level or shifted apically, thereby making it possible to adjust the gingival margin to the local conditions
- the flap procedure preserves the oral epithelium and often makes the use of surgical dressing superfluous

- the postoperative period is usually less unpleasant to the patient when compared to gingivectomy.

Contraindications for periodontal surgery

Patient cooperation

Since optimal postoperative plaque control is decisive for the success of periodontal treatment (Rosling et al. 1976 b, Nyman et al. 1977, Axelsson & Lindhe 1981), a patient who fails to cooperate during the cause-related phase of therapy should not be exposed to surgical treatment.

Even though short-term postoperative plaque control entails frequent professional treatments, the long-term responsibility for maintaining good oral hygiene must rest with the patient. Theoretically, even the poorest oral hygiene performance by a patient may be compensated for by frequent recall visits (e.g. once a week), but it is unrealistic to consider larger groups of patients being maintained in this manner. A typical recall schedule for periodontal patients involves professional consultations once every 3 months. Patients who cannot maintain satisfactory oral hygiene over such a 3-month period should normally be considered unsuited for periodontal surgery.

Cardiovascular disease

Arterial hypertension does not normally preclude periodontal surgery. The patient's medical history should be checked for previous untoward reactions to local anesthesia. Local anesthetics free from or low in adrenaline may be used and an aspirating syringe should be adopted to safeguard against intravascular injection.

Angina pectoris does not normally preclude periodontal surgery. The drugs used and the number of episodes of angina may indicate the severity of the disease. Premedication with sedatives and the use of local anesthesia low in adrenaline are often recommended. Safeguards should be adopted against intravascular injection.

Heart infarction-patients should not be subjected to periodontal surgery in the months immediately following hospitalization, and thereafter only in cooperation with the physician responsible for the patient.

Anticoagulant treatment implies increased propensity for bleeding. Periodontal surgery should be scheduled after consultation with the physician. Salicylates should not be used for postoperative pain control since they increase bleeding tendency.

Rheumatic endocarditis, congenital heart lesions and heart and vascular implants involve risk for transmission of bacteria to heart tissues and heart implants during the transient bacteremia which follows manipulation of infected periodontal pockets. Treatment of patients with these conditions should be preceded by antiseptic mouthrinsing (0.2 % chlorhexidine) and an appropriate antibiotic should be prescribed and administered a few hours before surgery.

Blood disorders

If the medical history includes blood disorders, the exact nature of these should be ascertained.

Patients suffering from acute leukemias, agranulocytosis and lymphogranulomatosis must *not* be subjected to periodontal surgery.

Anemias in mild and compensated forms do not preclude surgical treatment. More severe and less compensated forms may entail lowered resistance to infection and increased propensity for bleeding. In such cases, periodontal surgery should only be performed after consultation with the patient's physician.

Hormonal disorders

Diabetes mellitus entails lowered resistance to infection, propensity for delayed wound healing and predisposition for arteriosclerosis. Well compensated patients may be subjected to periodontal surgery provided precautions are taken not to disturb dietary and insulin routines.

Adrenal function may be impeded in patients receiving large doses of corticosteroids over an extended period. These conditions involve reduced resistance to physical and mental stress, and the doses of corticosteroid may have to be altered during the period of periodontal surgery. The patient's physician should be consulted.

Neurological disorders

Multiple sclerosis and Parkinson's disease may in severe cases make ambulatory periodontal surgery impossible. Paresis, impaired muscular function, tremor, and uncontrollable reflexes may necessitate treatment under general anesthesia.

Epilepsy is often treated with *phenytoin* which, in approximately 50% of cases, may mediate the formation of gingival hyperplasia. These patients may, without special restrictions, be subjected to periodontal surgery for correction of the hyperplasia. There is, however, a strong propensity for recurrence of the hyperplasia, which in many cases can be countered by intensifying the plaque control.

Local anesthesia in periodontal surgery

The pain experienced by the periodontal patient during the surgical procedure may be caused not only by the mechanical instrumentation in the preparation of the wound area, but may also emanate from the teeth. Thus, pain of varying intensity can be elicited from the teeth, especially in cases of exposed root dentin, by factors such as cold, heat, vibration, drying etc.

In order to prevent pain during the course of surgical treatment, the entire area of the dentition scheduled for surgery, the teeth as well as the periodontal tissues, should be properly blocked by a locally applied anesthetic drug.

Local anesthesia in the maxilla

The presence of porosities in the external lamina of the alveolar bone of the maxilla allows an anesthetic solution, deposited in the buccal oral mucosa, to penetrate the alveolar bone and reach the apex of the target tooth. Thus, local analgesia of the pulp and buccal periodontal tissues of the maxillary dentition can easily be accomplished by a series of injections in the muco-gingival fold of the treatment area.

After the administration of 0.5 to 1 ml of the anesthetic solution as a deposit in the buccal fold, pulpal analgesia will be accomplished in the tooth close to the injection site and, in some 80% of cases, also in the neighboring teeth. Thus, if larger areas of the dentition are scheduled for treatment, repeated injections (in the buccal fold) have to be performed at, e.g., the central incisor, canine, second premolar and second molar.

In the posterior maxillary regions the number of injection sites may be reduced by using a tuberosity injection which is made to block the superior alveolar branches of the maxillary nerve as they descend on the zygomatic surface of the maxilla and which, consequently, provides analgesia in a larger area. Because of the risk of intravascular injections, however, in most instances this type of block anesthesia should be avoided.

The palatal nerves are blocked by an injection made at right angles to the mucosal surface and placed around 10 mm apical to the gingival margin. If the treatment area on the palatal aspect of the jaw is wide in the apicocoronal direction, about 1 ml of the anesthesia solution should be placed close to the major palatine foramen. This injection will block the anterior and accessory palatine nerves and produce analgesia of all soft and hard tissues from the area of the third molar to the canine. Analgesia of the palatal tissues of the front tooth region is accomplished by an injection made at the site of the incisive papilla. In order to prevent unnecessary pain from this injection, and to avoid a deposition of the anesthesia solution in the vessels emerging from the incisor canal, a lateral injection approach should be preferred. The pain produced by injections into the non-resilient palatal tissue can, in cases of advanced bone loss, be minimized if the injections are performed from the buccal aspect, i.e. through the interdental gingiva.

In order to obtain proper ischemia in the gingival tissues small amounts of the anesthesia solution can also be injected into the interdental papillae. Such injections should be performed after proper analgesia has been accomplished by buccal and palatal infiltration.

If the anesthetic solution (2% solution of lidocaine, containing 10-12.5 μg adrenaline/ml) is distributed in the upper jaw in the way proposed above, in the vast majority of the cases proper analgesia will be accomplished for a period of at least 60 minutes.

Local anesthesia in the mandible

In the front tooth region of the lower jaw an infiltration with an anesthetic solution in the buccal fold will produce proper analgesia in many cases, especially in young patients. The anesthetic effect is the result of the penetration of the drug through porosites in the mandible, similar to those present in the maxilla. In older patients, however, such pores often have reduced dimensions. Consequently, the rate and degree of penetration of the anesthetic solution towards the apices of the mandibular front teeth are reduced and the anesthetic effect obtined by injections in the buccal fold is therefore insufficient. As a rule, analgesia of the teeth and the soft and hard tissues of the mandible should be obtained by a mandibular blockade injection made at the site of surgery, supplemented by an infiltration anesthesia at the mental foramin of the contralateral side.

The periodontal tissues on the buccal side of the mandible are anesthetized by blocking the buccal nerve with an injection made at the lateral side of the mandible, preferably at the level of the second or third molar. The lingual periodontal tissues are anesthetized by blocking the lingual nerve, either by a blockade close to the mandibular foramen, often made in connection with the mandibular blockade, or by an injection in the floor of the mouth close to the site of operation. Supplementary injections to obtain proper ischemia of the gingival tissues may be made in the interdental papillae. It should be noted that the lagtime between the injection and the establishment of proper analgesia after a mandibular blockade is significantly longer (about 3 to 5 minutes) than following infiltration injections in the maxillary jaw.

Local anesthetic solutions used in periodontal surgery

All local anesthetic procedures should aim at the use of the lowest dose of the least concentrated solution. Proper analgesia for periodontal treatment procedures can almost always be obtained with the use of a 2% solution of lidocaine containing 10-12.5 μg adrenaline/ml. Some clinicians may advocate the use of a

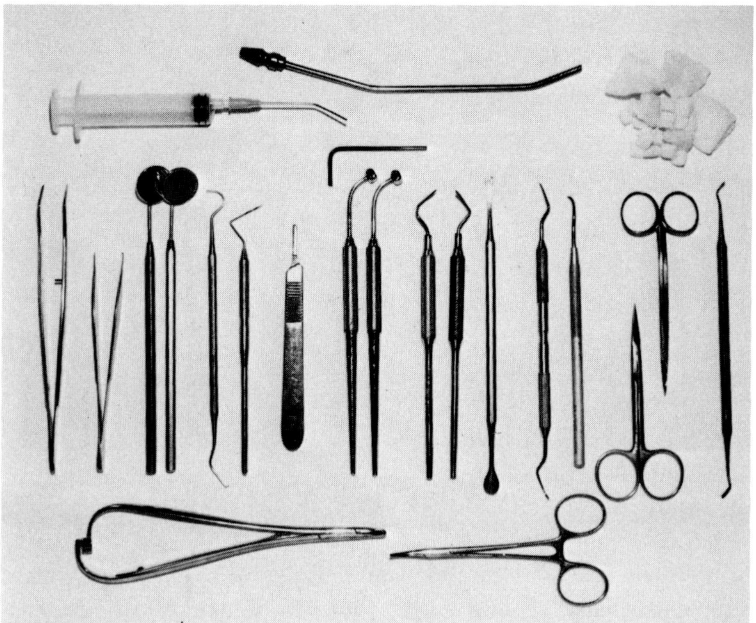

Fig. 16-4. Instruments used for periodontal surgery; included in a standard tray.

higher epinephrine concentration (20 µg/ml) but such a highly concentrated solution may only result in a marginal increase of the duration of the analgesia. The high epinephrine content may, however, increase the risk of side effects, especially if the solution is inadvertently injected intravascularly in a patient with circulatory disorders.

Provided proper *lege artis* measures are followed, a 2% lidocaine solution (epinephrine concentration 10-12.5 µg/ml) can be safely used in all healthy patients. Prior to injection of any anesthetic solution, careful aspiration must be performed. The injections must be administered slowly so that any adverse systemic effects induced by the drug can be observed and counteracted before the entire dosage has been administered.

Instruments used in periodontal surgery

General considerations

Surgical procedures used in periodontal therapy often involve the following measures:

- Incision and excision
- Deflection and readaptation of mucosal flaps
- Removal of adherent fibrous and granulomatous tissue
- Scaling and root planing
- Removal of bone tissue
- Root sectioning
- Suturing
- Application of wound dressing

Instruments used for these purposes include:

- Periodontal knives
- Periosteal elevators
- Tissue scissors
- Soft tissue and bone rongeurs
- Scalers and curettes
- Bone chisels and files
- Burs
- Sutures and needle holders
- Suture scissors
- Plastic instruments

The set of instruments used for the various periodontal surgical procedures should have a

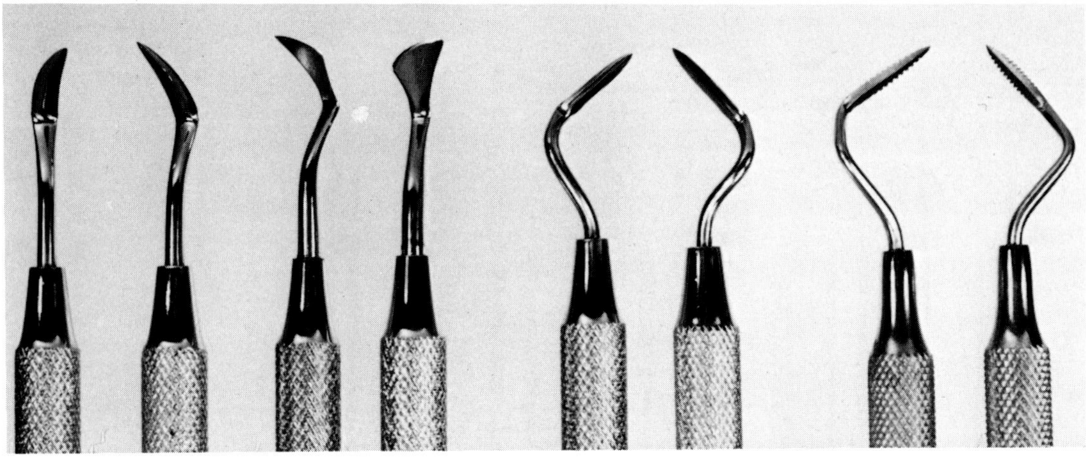

Fig. 16-5. Examples of paired gingivectomy knives. From left to right: Crane-Kaplan 3/4, Kirkland 15/16, Orban 1/2, Waerhaug 1/2.

comparatively simple design. As a general rule, the number and varieties of instruments should be kept to a minimum. In addition to particular instruments used for periodontal treatment modalities, equipment and instruments generally used in oral surgery are often needed.

Within each category of surgical instruments used for periodontal therapy there are usually several brands available, varying in form and quality, leaving ample room for individual preferences.

In the selection of instruments, e.g. scalers and curettes, with blades of different sizes, it should be realized that the accessibility to the root surfaces of deep pockets is often limited. In such sites gracile instruments are therefore to be preferred.

The instruments should be stored in sterile "ready-to-use" packs or trays. Handling, storing and labelling of surgical instruments and equipment must be managed in such a way that interchanging of sterile and non-sterile items is prevented.

It is also important that the instruments are kept in good working condition. The maintenance routine should ensure that scalers, curettes, knives with fixed blades etc. are sharp and the hinges of scissors, rongeurs and needle holders are properly lubricated. Spare instruments (sterile) should always be available to replace instruments found to be defective or accidentally contaminated.

The instrument tray

Instrument trays for periodontal surgery may be arranged in several ways. Different trays can be used for different procedures or a standard tray can be used for all procedures supplemented with the particular instruments that are needed for a specific procedure.

A commonly used standard tray combines the basic set of instruments used in oral surgery and a few periodontal instruments. The instruments listed below are often found on such a standard tray (Fig. 16-4):

Cotton pliers
Tissue pliers (a.m. Ewald)
Mouth mirrors
Explorer (a.m. Maillefer)
Graduated periodontal probe
Handles for disposable surgical blades
  a. Bard-Parker handle
  b. Blakes handles with screw-key
Waerhaug knives (No. 1 and 2)
Mucoperiosteal elevator
Curettes (e.g. Columbia No. 2R/2L,
  Sandviken Coromant No. 2)

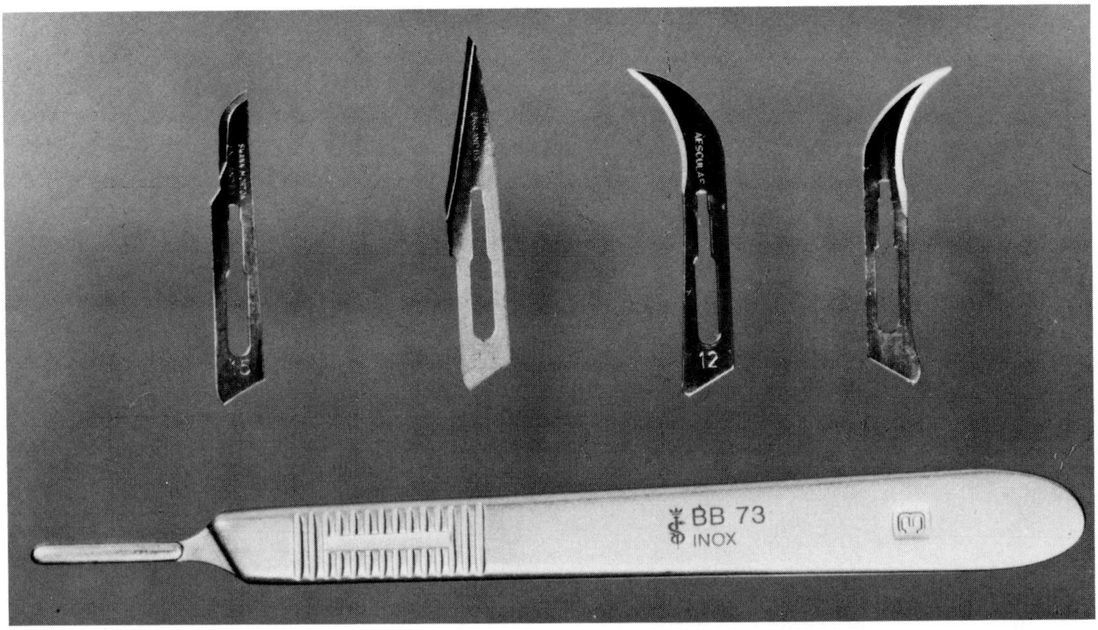

Fig. 16-6. Disposable blades and a Bard-Parker handle. The shape of the blades are from left to right: No. 15, No. 11, No. 12, No. 12d

Suture scissors
Tissue scissors
Plastic instrument
Hemostat
Needle holder
Syringe for irrigation
Aspirator tip

Additional equipment may include:
Drapings for the patient
Rubber gloves
Physiological saline
Syringe for local anesthesia

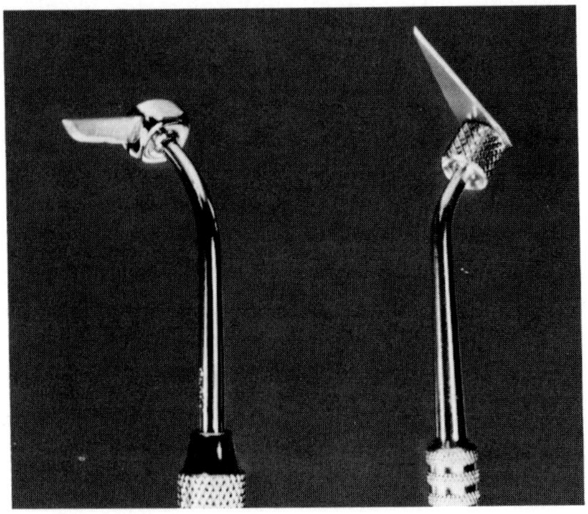

Fig. 16-7. Special handles for disposable blades.
Left: Blake handle.
Right: Detsch handle.

Surgical instruments

Knives

Knives are available with fixed or replaceable blades. The advantage of the fixed blade versions is that the blade can be given any desired shape and orientation in relation to the handle. A disadvantage is that such instruments need frequent resharpening. Fig. 16-5 shows examples of knives with fixed blades.

New disposable blades are always sharp. They can be rapidly replaced if found defective. The cutting edge of the blades normally follows the long axis of the handle, a fact which limits their use. However, knives with disposable blades fitted in angulation in rela-

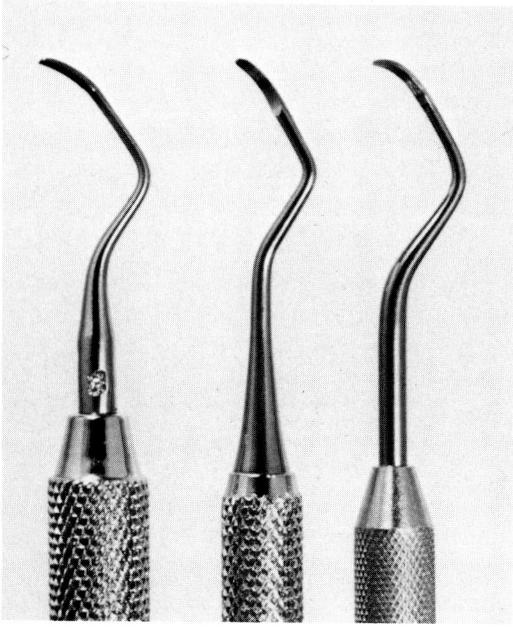

Fig. 16-8. Curettes which may be used in conjunction with periodontal surgery.

From left to right:

Tungsten-carbide curette (Ash 13/14),

Goldman-Fox 3/4,

Columbia 13/14.

These instruments are double ended. Only one end of each instrument is illustrated.

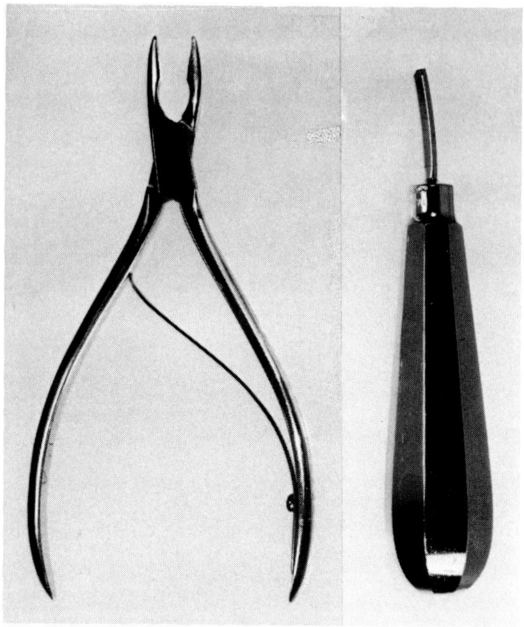

Fig. 16-9. Bone rongeur and bone chisel.

tion to the handle are also available.

The disposable blades are manufactured in different shapes (Fig. 16-6). When mounted in ordinary handles (Bard-Parker®), they are used for releasing incisions in flap operations and mucogingival surgery and for reverse bevel incisions where access is obtainable. Special handles (Fig. 16-7) make it possible to mount blades in positions which facilitate the use of such knives for both gingivectomy excisions and reverse bevel incisions.

Scalers and curettes

Scaling and root planing in conjunction with periodontal surgery take place on exposed root surfaces. Therefore access to the root surfaces for debridement may be obtained also with the use of comparatively sturdy instruments (Fig. 16-8). Tungsten carbide curettes and scalers with durable cutting edges are often used when "access" is not a problem. Rotating diamond stones (fine-grained) may be used within infrabony pockets, root concavities and entrances to furcations.

Instruments for bone removal

Sharp bone chisels or bone rongeurs (Fig. 16-9) cause the least tissue damage and should be employed whenever access permits. With reduced access, surgical burs or files may be used. The burs should operate at low speed and ample rinsing with sterile physiological saline should ensure cooling and removal of tissue remnants.

Instruments for handling flaps

The proper healing of the periodontal wound is critical for the success of the operation. It is therefore important that the manipulations of the soft tissue flaps are performed with the minimum of tissue damage. Thus, care should be exercised in the use of periosteal elevators when flaps are deflected. Plastic instruments may be used as periosteal elevators and tissue retractors. Surgical pliers and tissue retractors which pierce the tissues should not be applied in the marginal area of the flaps. Needle holders with small beaks and atraumatic sutures should be used.

Additional equipment

Hemorrhage is rarely a problem in periodontal surgery. The characteristic oozing type of bleeding can normally be controlled by a pressure pack (sterile gauze moistened with saline). Bleeding from small vessels can be stopped by clamping and tying using a hemostat and resorbable sutures. If the vessel is surrounded by bone, bleeding may be stopped by crushing the nutrient canal in which the vessel runs with a blunt instrument.

Sterile physiological saline is used for rinsing and moistening the field of operation and for cooling when burs are employed. The saline solution may be kept in a sterile metal cup on the instrument tray and may be applied to the wound by means of a sterile disposable plastic syringe and a needle with rounded tip.

Visibility in the field of operation is secured by using effective suction. The lumen of the aspirator tip should have a smaller diameter than the rest of the tube, in order to prevent clogging.

The patient's head may be covered by autoclaved cotton drapings or sterile disposable plastic/paper drapings. The surgeon and all assistants should wear sterile rubber gloves.

Techniques in periodontal pocket surgery

In the following, surgical procedures will be described which represent important steps in the development of the surgical component of periodontal therapy.

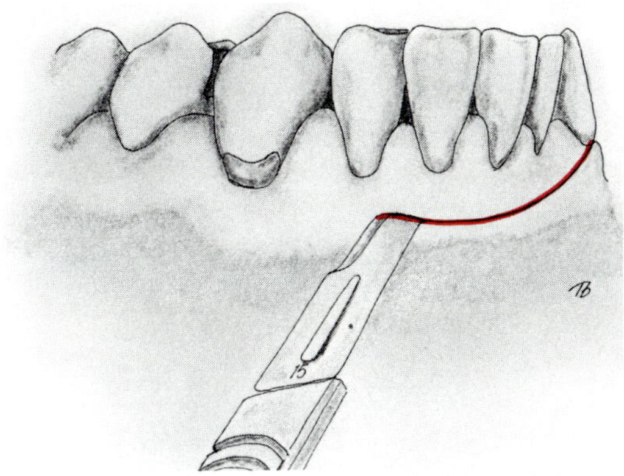

Fig. 16-10. *Gingivectomy.* The straight incision technique.

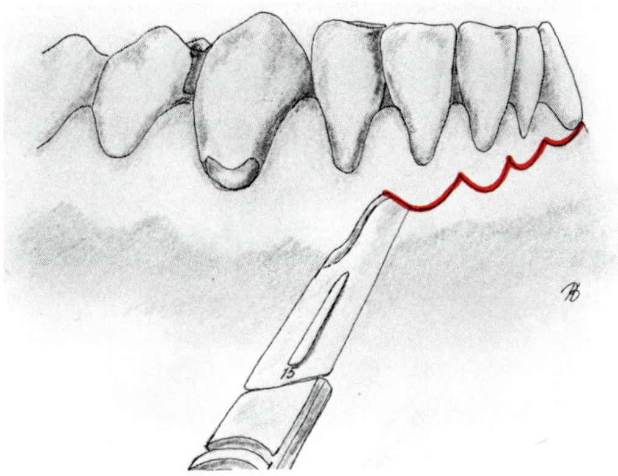

Fig. 16-11. *Gingivectomy.* The scalloped incision technique.

Gingivectomy procedures

The surgical approach as an alternative to subgingival scaling for pocket therapy was already recognized in the latter part of the 19th century, when Robicsek (1884) pioneered the so-called *gingivectomy* procedure. Gingivectomy was later defined by Grant et al. (1979) as being "the excision of the soft tissue wall of a pathologic periodontal pocket". The surgical procedure which aimed at "pocket elimination" was usually combined with recountering of the diseased gingiva to restore physiological form.

Robicsek (1884) and, later, Zentler (1918) described the gingivectomy procedure in the following way:

The line to which the gum is to be resected is determined first. Following a straight (Robicsek; Fig. 16-10) or scalloped (Zentler; Fig. 16-

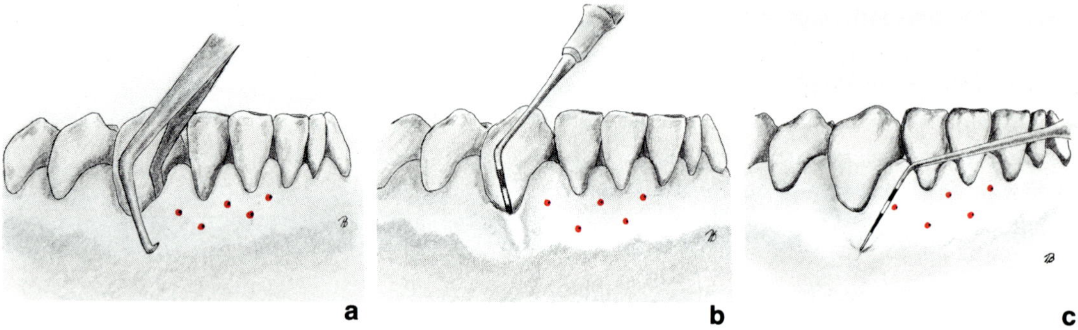

Fig. 16-12. *Gingivectomy.* Pocket-marking. (a) When a pocket marking forceps is used the probing beak of the instrument is placed parallel to the long axis of the tooth. This gives a correct orientation for the perforating beak to indicate the "bottom" of the pocket. (b) An ordinary periodontal probe can also be used to identify the bottom of the deepened pocket. (c) When the depth of the pocket has been assessed an equivalent distance is delineated on the outer aspect of the gingiva. The tip of the probe is then turned horizontally and used to produce a bleeding point at the level of the pocket bottom.

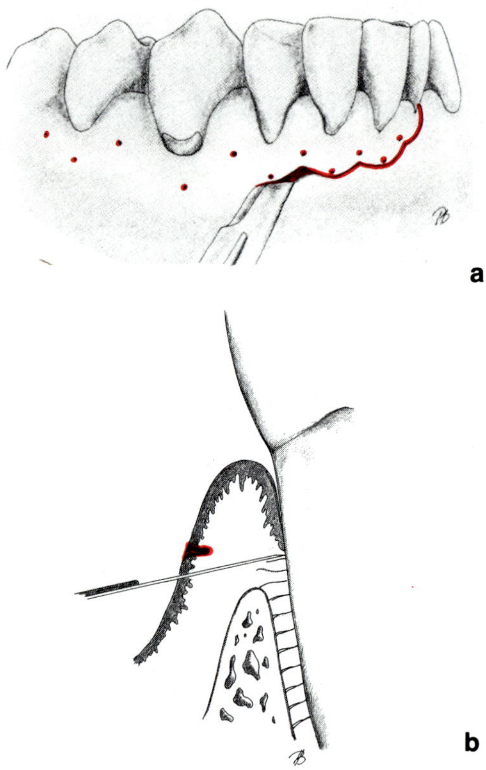

Fig. 16-13. *Gingivectomy.* (a) The primary incision. (b) The incision is terminated at a level apical to the "bottom" of the pocket and is angulated to give the cut surface a distinct bevel.

11) incision, first on the labial and then on the lingual surface of each tooth, the diseased tissue should be loosened and lifted out by means of a hook-shaped instrument. After elimination of the soft tissue, the exposed alveolar bone should be scraped. The area should then be covered with some kind of antibacterial gauze or be painted with disinfecting solutions. The result obtained should include eradication of the deepened periodontal pocket and a local condition which could be kept clean more easily.

Technique

The gingivectomy procedure as it is employed today was described 1951 by Goldman. When the dentition in the area scheduled for surgery has been properly anesthesized, the depths of the pathological pockets are identified either with a pocket marking forceps (e.g. ad modum Crane-Kaplan; Fig. 16-12a) or by means of a conventional periodontal probe (Figs. 16-12b, c). At the level of the bottom of the pocket, the gingiva is pierced with the blade of the forceps (probe) and a bleeding point is produced on the outer surface of the soft tissue. The pockets are probed and bleeding points produced at several location points around each tooth in the area. The series of bleeding points produced describes the depth of the pockets in the area scheduled for treatment and is used as a gui-

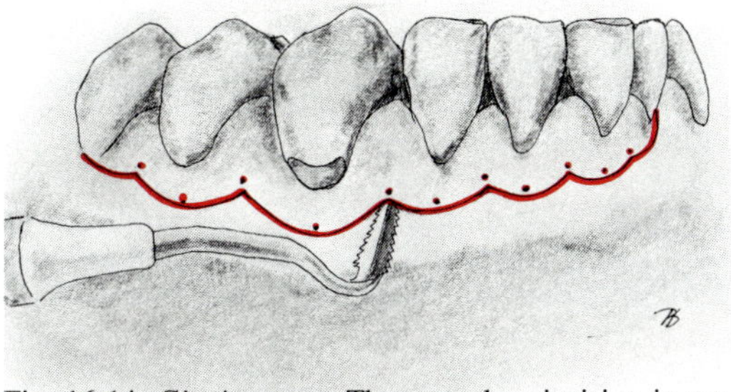

Fig. 16-14. *Gingivectomy.* The secondary incision is performed with the use of a Waerhaug knife.

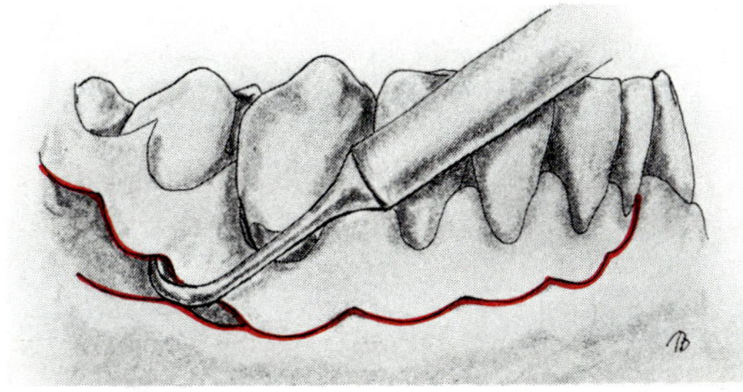

Fig. 16-15. *Gingivectomy.* The detached gingiva is removed with a scaler.

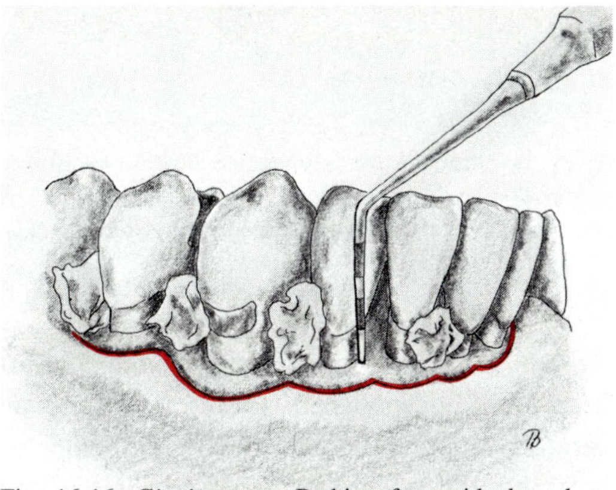

Fig. 16-16. *Gingivectomy.* Probing for residual pockets. Note that gauze packs have been placed in the interproximal spaces to control bleeding.

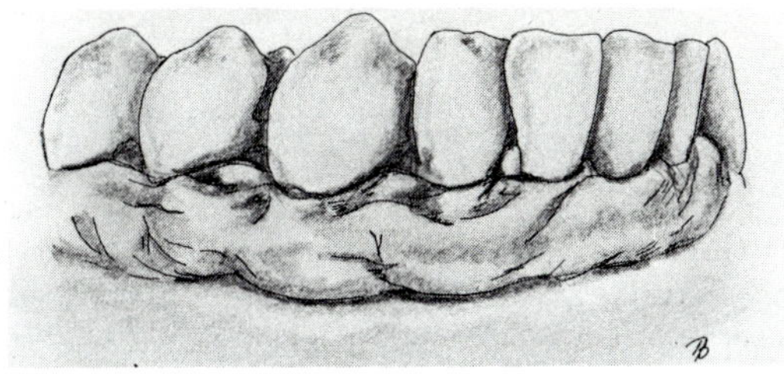

Fig. 16-17. *Gingivectomy.* The periodontal dressing has been applied and properly secured.

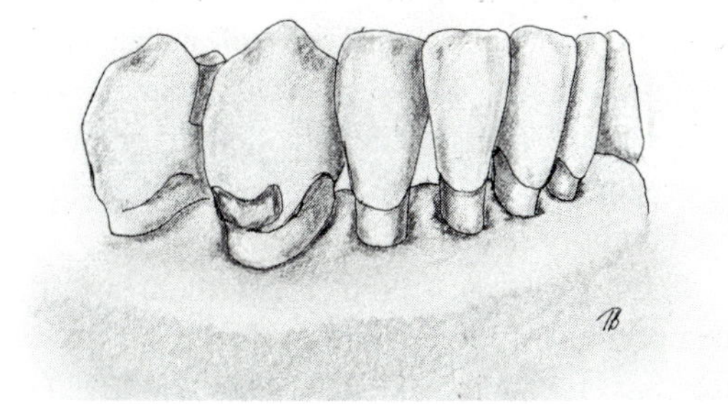

Fig. 16-18. *Gingivectomy.* The postoperative appearance of the surgically treated area.

deline for the incision.

The primary incision (Fig. 16-13), which may be made by a scalpel (blade No. 12B or 15; Bard-Parker®) in either a Bard-Parker handle or a Blake's handle, or a Kirkland knife No. 15 or 16, should be planned to give a thin and properly festooned margin of the remaining gingiva. Thus, in areas where the gingiva is bulky, the incision must be placed at a level more apical to the level of the bleeding points than in areas with a thin gingiva, where a less accentuated bevel is needed. The beveled incision is directed towards the base of the pocket or to a level slightly apical to the apical extension of the junctional epithelium. In areas where the interdental pockets are deeper than the buccal or lingual pockets, additional amounts of buccal and/or lingual (palatal) gingiva must be removed in order to establish a "physiologic" contour of the gingival margin. This is often accomplished by initiating the incision at a more apical level.

Once the primary incision is completed on the buccal and lingual aspects of the teeth, the interproximal soft tissue is separated from the interdental periodontium by a secondary incision using an Orban knife (No. 1 or 2) or a Waerhaug knife (No. 1 or 2; a saw-toothed modification of the Orban knife; Fig. 16-14).

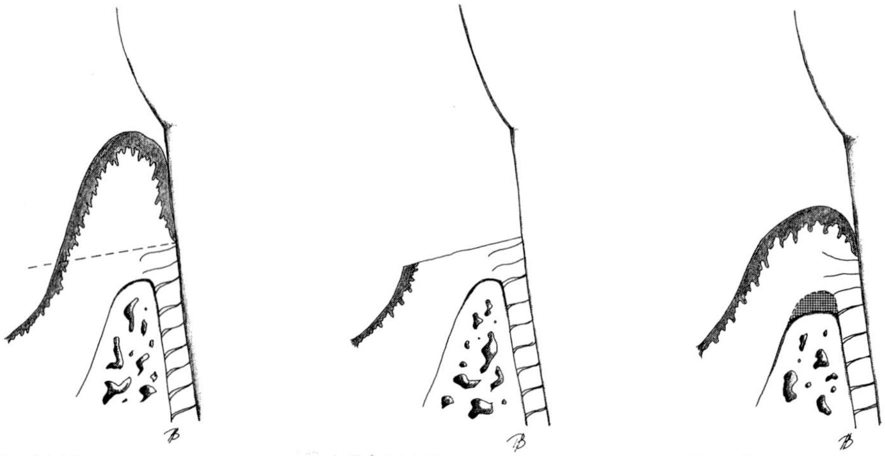

Fig. 16-19a. Fig. 16-19b. Fig. 16-19c.

Fig. 16-19. *Gingivectomy.* Dimensional changes as a result of therapy. (a) Illustrates the preoperative dimensions. Broken line indicates the location of the primary incision. (b) The suprabony pocket has been eliminated. (c) Dimensions following proper healing. Minor resorption (shadowed area) of the alveolar bone crest as well as some loss of connective tissue attachment has occurred.

The incised tissues are carefully removed by means of a curette or a scaler (Fig. 16-15). Remaining tissue tabs are removed with a curette or a pair of scissors. Pieces of gauze packs often have to be placed in the interdental areas to control bleeding. When the field of operation is properly prepared, the exposed root surfaces are carefully scaled and planed.

Following meticulous debridement the dento-gingival regions are probed again to detect any remaining pockets (Fig. 16-16). The gingival contour is checked and, if necessary, corrected by means of knives or rotating diamond burs.

To protect the incised area during the period of healing, the wound surface must be covered by a periodontal dressing (Fig. 16-17). The dressing should be closely adapted to the buccal and lingual wound surfaces as well as to the interproximal spaces. Care should be taken not to allow the dressing to become too bulky, since this is not only uncomfortable for the patient, but also facilitates the dislodgement of the dressing. The dressing should remain in position for 10 to 14 days.

After removal of the dressing, the teeth must be cleaned and polished. The root surfaces are carefully checked and remaining calculus removed with a curette. Excessive granulation tissue is eliminated with a curette. The patient is instructed to properly clean the operated segments of the dentition which now have a different morphology as compared to the preoperative situation (Fig. 16-18).

Healing and dimensional changes following gingivectomy

Within a few days following excision of the inflamed gingival soft tissues coronal to the base of the periodontal pocket, epithelial cells start to migrate over the wound surface. The epithelialization of the gingivectomy wound is usually complete within 7 to 14 days following surgery (Engler et al. 1966, Stahl et al. 1968). During the following weeks a new dento-gingival unit is formed (Fig. 16-19). The fibroblasts in the supraalveolar tissue adjacent the tooth surface proliferate (Waerhaug 1955) and new connective tissue is laid down. If this regeneration occurs in the vicinity of a plaque-free tooth surface, a free gingival unit will form which has all the characteristics of a normal free gingiva (Hamp et al. 1975). This regeneration occurs in a coronal direction and appears clinically as a gain in marginal height (Fig. 16-19c). The height of the newly formed free gingival unit may vary not only between different parts of the dentition but also from one tooth surface to another.

The reestablishment of a new, free gingival unit by coronal regrowth of tissue from the line of the "gingivectomy" incision implies that sites with so-called "zero pockets" only occasionally occur following gingivectomy. Complete healing of the gingivectomy wound takes 4 to 5 weeks, although the surface of the gingiva may appear by clinical inspection to be healed already after approximately 14 days (Ramfjord et al. 1966). Minor remodelling of the alveolar bone crest may also occur during the healing phase.

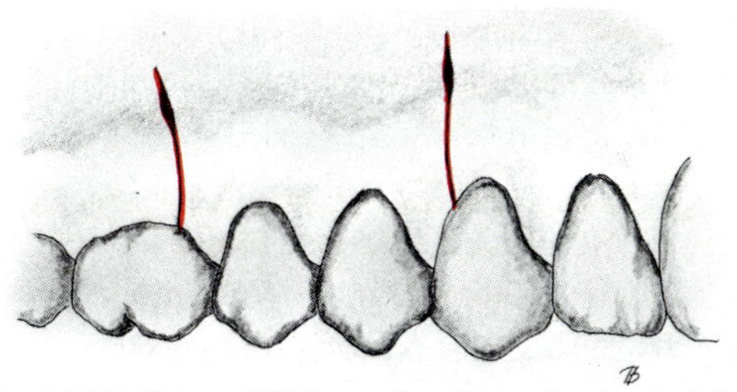

Fig. 16-20. *Original Widman flap.* Two releasing incisions demarcate the area scheduled for therapy.

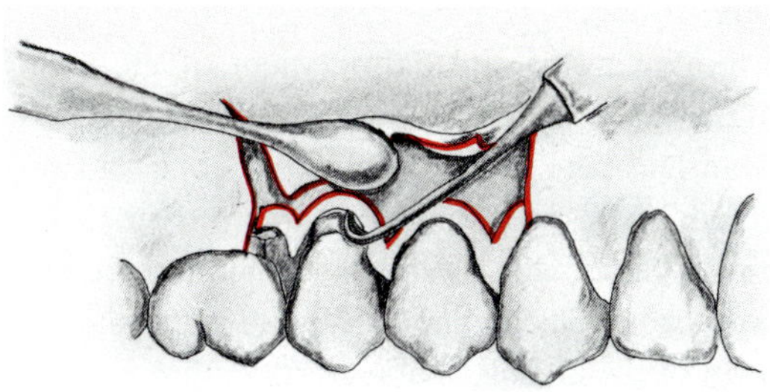

Fig. 16-21. *Original Widman flap.* The collar of inflamed gingival tissue is removed following the elevation of a mucoperiosteal flap.

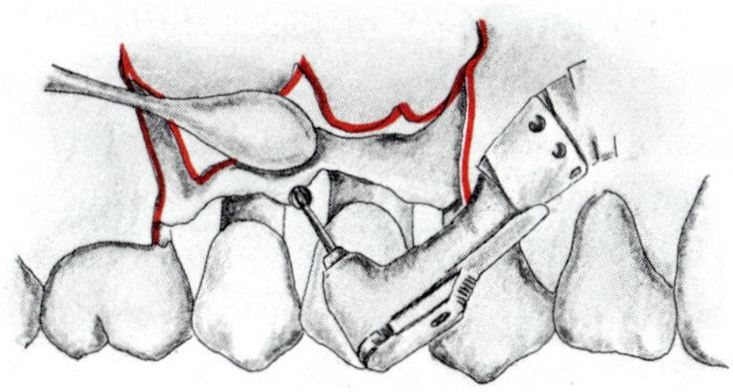

Fig. 16-22. *Original Widman flap.* By bone recontouring, a "physiologic" contour of the alveolar bone may be reestablished.

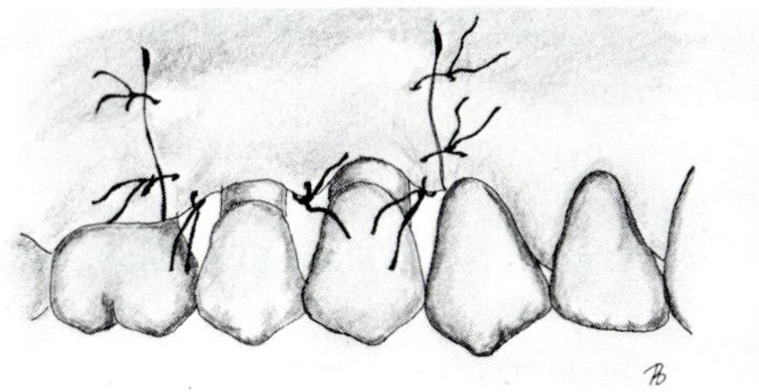

Fig. 16-23. *Original Widman flap.* The coronal ends of the buccal and lingual flaps are placed at the alveolar bone crest and secured in this position by sutures.

Flap procedures

The original Widman flap

One of the first detailed descriptions of the use of a flap procedure for pocket elimination was published in 1918 by *Leonard Widman*. In his article "The operative treatment of pyorrhea alveolaris" Widman described a mucoperiosteal flap design aimed at removing the pocket epithelium and the inflamed connective tissue, thereby facilitating optimal cleaning of the root surfaces. Sectional releasing incisions were first made to demarcate the area scheduled for surgery (Fig. 16-20). These incisons were made from the mid-buccal gingival margins of the two peripheral teeth of the treatment area and were continued several millimeters out into the alveolar mucosa. The two releasing incisions were connected by a gingival incision which followed the outline of the gingival margin and *separated the pocket epithelium and the inflamed connective tissue from the noninflamed gingiva.* Similar releasing and gingival incisions were, if needed, made on the lingual aspect of the teeth.

A mucoperiosteal flap was elevated to expose at least 2-3 mm of the marginal alveolar bone. The collar of inflamed tissue around the neck of the teeth was removed with curettes (Fig. 16-21) and the exposed root surfaces were carefully scaled. Bone recountering was recommended in order to achieve an ideal anatomical form of the underlying alveolar bone (Fig. 16-22).

Following careful debridement of the teeth in the surgical area, the buccal and lingual flaps were laid back over the alveolar bone and secured in this position with interproximal sutures (Fig. 16-23). Widman pointed out the importance of placing the soft tissue margin at the level of the alveolar bone crest, so that no pockets would remain. The surgical procedure resulted in the exposure of root surfaces. Often the interproximal areas were left without soft tissue coverage of the alveolar bone.

The main advantages of the "*original Widman flap*" procedure in comparison to the gingivectomy procedure included, according to Widman (1918), 1) less discomfort for the patient, since healing occurred by primary intention and further 2) that it was possible to reestablish a proper contour of the alveolar bone in sites with angular bony defects.

The Neumann flap

Only a few years later, *Neumann* (1920, 1926) suggested the use of a flap procedure which in some respects was different from that originally described by Widman. According to the technique suggested by Neuman, an intracrevicular incision was made through the base of the gingival pockets and the entire gingiva (and part of the alveolar mucosa) was elevated in a mucoperiosteal flap. Following its elevation, the inside of the flap was curetted to remove the pocket epithelium and the granulation tissue. The root surfaces were subsequently carefully "cleaned". Any irregularities of the alveolar bone were corrected to give the bone crest a horizontal outline. The flaps were then trimmed to allow both an optimal adaptation to the teeth and a proper coverage of the alveolar bone on both the buccal/lingual (palatal) and the interproximal sites. With regard to pocket elimination, Newmann (1926) pointed out the importance of removing the soft tissue pockets, i.e. placing the flap at the crest of the alveolar bone.

The modified flap operation

In a publication from 1931 *Kirkland* described a surgical procedure to be used in the treatment of "periodontal pus pockets". The procedure was called the "*modified flap operation*". In this procedure incisions were made intracrevicularly through the bottom of the pocket (Fig. 16-24) on both the labial and the lingual aspects of the interdental area. The incisions were extended in a mesial and distal direction. The gingiva was retracted labially and lingually to expose the diseased root surfaces (Fig. 16-25) which were carefully debrided (Fig. 16-26). Angular bony defects were curetted. Following the elimination of the pocket epithelium and granulation tissue from the inner surface of the flaps, these were *replaced* to their original position and secured with interproximal sutures (Fig. 16-27). Thus, no attempt was made to reduce the preoperative depth of the pockets.

In contrast to the "*original Widman flap*" as well as the "*Neumann flap*", the "*modified flap operation*" did not include 1) extensive sacrifice of non-inflamed tissues and 2) apical displacement of the gingival margin. Since the root surfaces were not markedly exposed thereby, the method could for esthetic reasons be useful in the anterior regions of the dentition. Another advantage of the "*modified flap operation*" was the potential for bone regeneration which, according to Kirkland (1931), in fact frequently occurred.

The main objectives of the flap procedures so far described were to 1) facilitate the de-

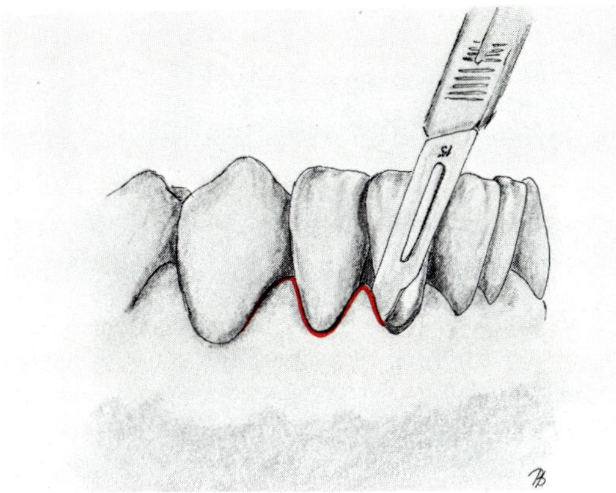

Fig. 16-24. *Modified flap operation.* Intracrevicular incision.

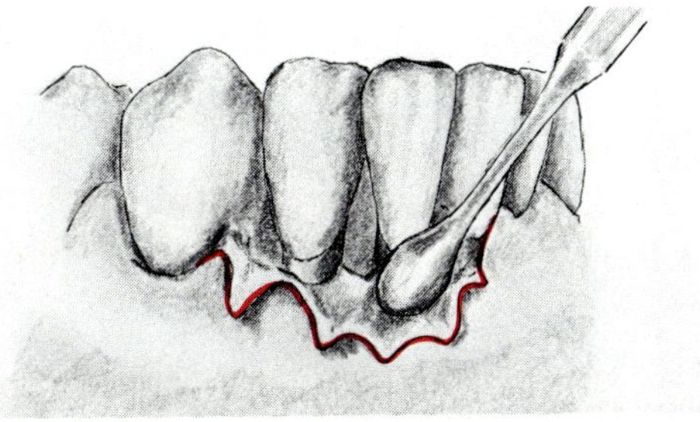

Fig. 16-25. *Modified flap operation.* The gingiva has been retracted to expose the "diseased" root surfaces.

bridement of the root surfaces as well as the removal of the pocket epithelium and the inflamed connective tissue, 2) eliminate the deepened pockets (the "*original Widman flap*" and the "*Neumann flap*") and 3) cause a minimal amount of discomfort and trauma to the patient.

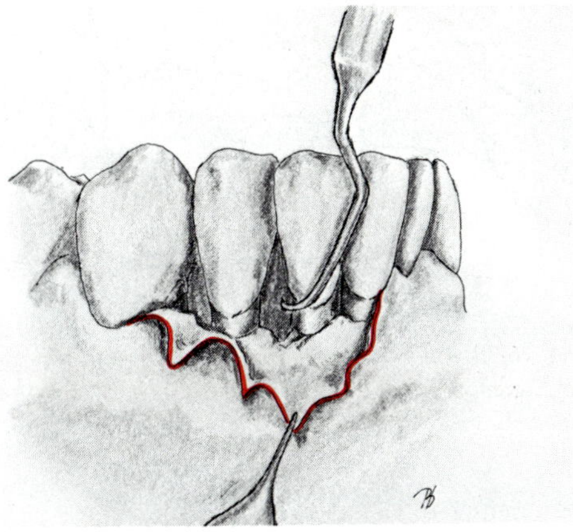

Fig. 16-26. *Modified flap operation.* The exposed root surfaces are subjected to mechanical debridement.

The apically repositioned flap

In the 1950s and 1960s new surgical techniques for the removal of soft and, when indicated, hard tissue periodontal pockets were described in the literature. The importance of maintaining "*an adequate zone of attached gingiva*" after surgery was now emphasized. One of the first authors to describe a technique for the preservation of a zone of keratinized and attached gingiva following surgery was *Nabers* (1954). The surgical technique developed by Nabers was originally denoted "repositioning of attached gingiva" and was later modified by *Ariaudo & Tyrrell* (1957). In 1962 *Friedman* proposed the term "*apically repositioned flap*" to more appropriately describe the surgical technique introduced by Nabers. Friedman emphasized the fact that, at the end of the surgical procedure, the entire complex of the soft tissues (gingiva and alveolar mucosa) rather than the gingiva alone was displaced in an apical direction. Thus, rather than excising the amount

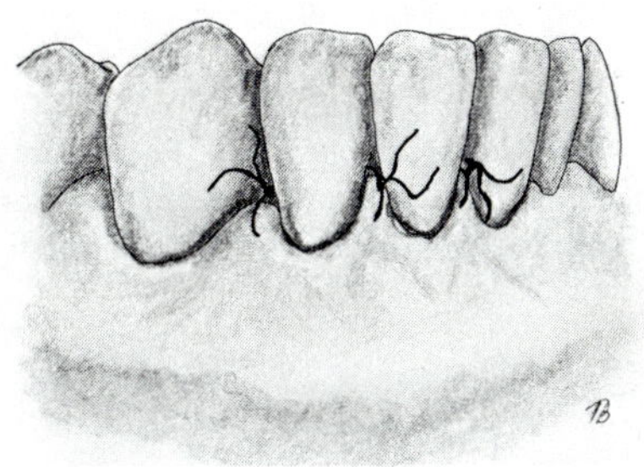

Fig. 16-27. *Modified flap operation.* The flaps are replaced to their original position and sutured.

of gingiva which would be in excess *after* osseous surgery (if performed), the whole mucogingival complex was maintained and apically repositioned. This surgical technique was used on buccal surfaces in both upper and lower jaws and on lingual surfaces in the lower jaw. According to Friedman (1962) the technique

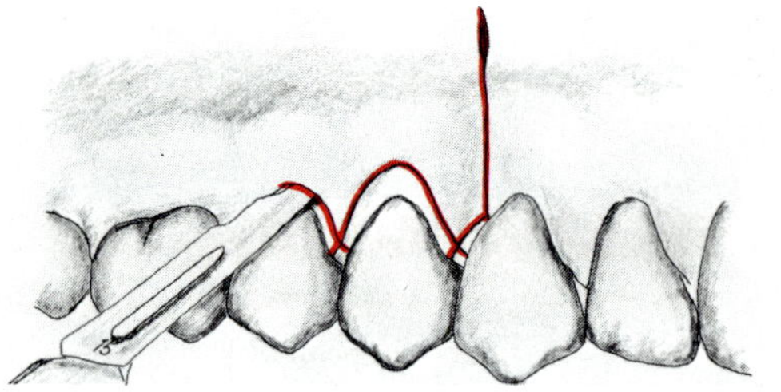

Fig. 16-28. *Apically repositioned flap*. Following a vertical releasing incision, the reverse bevel incision is made through the gingiva and the periosteum.

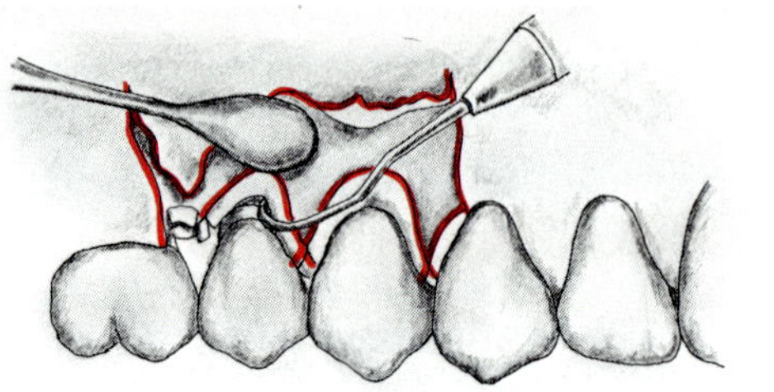

Fig. 16-29. *Apically repositioned flap*. A full thickness mucoperiosteal flap is raised and the tissue collar, including the pocket epithelium and the inflamed connective tissue, is removed with a curette.

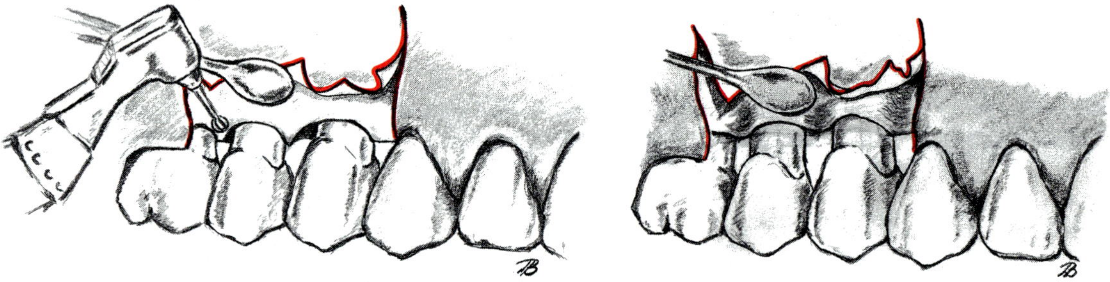

Fig. 16-30. *Apically repositioned flap*. Osseous surgery is performed with the use of a rotating bur (a) to recapture the physiologic contour of the alveolar bone (b).

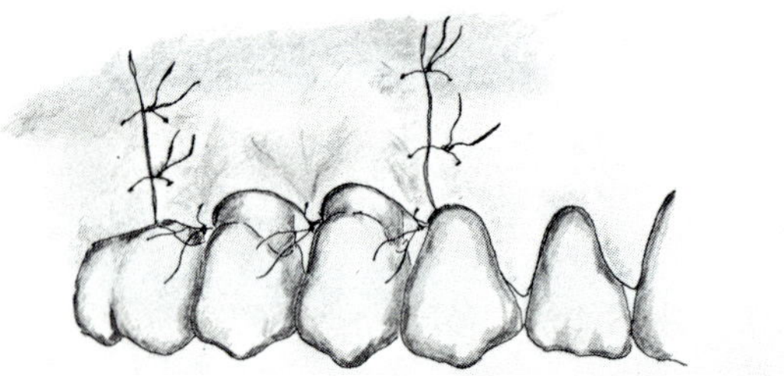

Fig. 16-31. *Apically repositioned flap*. The flaps are repositioned in an apical direction to the level of the recontoured alveolar bone crest and retained in this position by sutures.

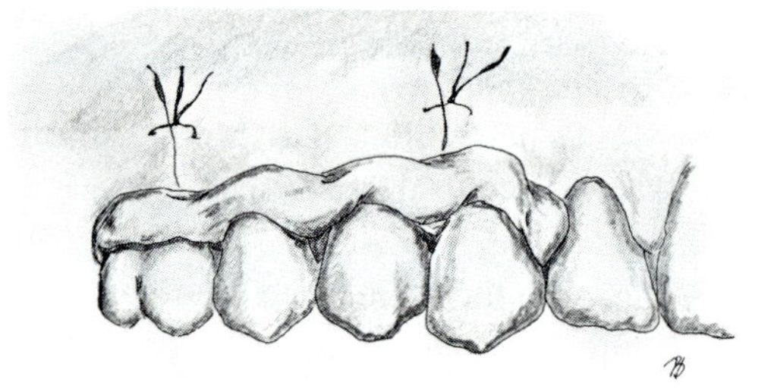

Fig. 16-32. *Apically repositioned flap*. A periodontal dressing is placed over the surgical area to ensure that the flaps remain in the correct position during healing.

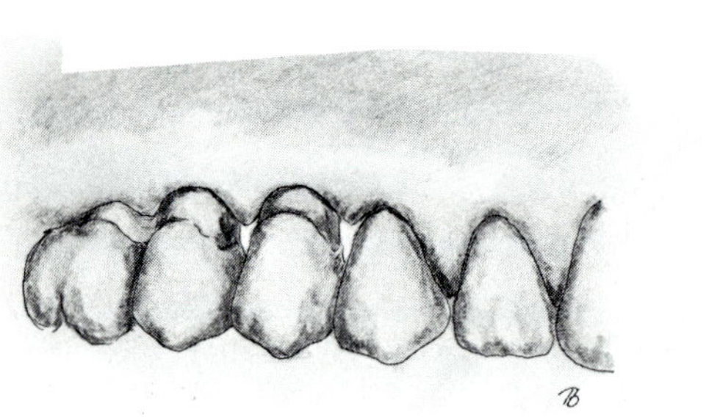

Fig. 16-33. *Apically repositioned flap*. The postoperative appearance of the surgically treated region of the dentition.

should be performed in the following way:

A reverse bevel incision is made using a scalpel with a Bard-Parker blade (No. 12B or No. 15). How far from the buccal/lingual gingival margin the incision should be made is dependent on the pocket depth as well as the thickness and the width of the gingiva (Fig. 16-28). If the gingiva preoperatively is thin and only a narrow zone of keratinized gingiva is present, the incision should be made close to the tooth. The bevelling incision should be given a scalloped outline to ensure maximal interproximal coverage of the alveolar bone, when the flap subsequently is repositioned.

Vertical releasing incisions extending out into the alveolar mucosa (i.e. past the mucogingival junction) are made at each of the end points of the reverse incision, thereby making possible the apical repositioning of the flap.

A full thickness mucoperiosteal flap including buccal/lingual gingiva and alveolar mucosa is raised by means of a mucoperiosteal elevator. The marginal collar of tissue, including pocket epithelium and granulation tissue, is removed with curettes (Fig. 16-29). The root surfaces are carefully scaled and planed.

The alveolar bone crest is recountered with the objective of recapturing the normal form of the alveolar process but at a more apical level (Fig. 16-30). The osseous surgery is performed using burs (Fig. 16-30a) and/or bone chisels.

Following careful adjustment, the buccal/lingual flap is repositioned to the level of the newly recontoured alveolar bone crest and secured in this position (Fig. 16-31). The incisional and excisional technique used means that it is not always possible to obtain proper soft tissue coverage of the denuded interproximal alveolar bone. A periodontal dressing should therefore be applied to protect the exposed bone and to retain the soft tissue at the level of the bone crest (Fig. 16-32). After healing, an "adequate" zone of keratinized gingiva is preserved and no residual pockets should remain (Fig. 16-33).

To handle periodontal pockets on the palatal aspect of the teeth, Friedman described a modification of the "apically repositioned flap", which he termed the "*bevelled flap*". Since there is no alveolar mucosa present on the palatal aspect of the teeth, it is not possible to reposition the flap in apical direction. In order to prepare the tissue of the gingival margin to properly follow the outline of the alveolar bone crest, a conventional mucoperiosteal flap is first resected (Figs. 16-34a, b). The tooth surfaces are debrided and osseous recountering is performed. The palatal flap is subsequently replaced and the gingival margin is prepared and adjusted to the alveolar bone crest by a secondary scalloped and bevelled incision (Figs. 16-35, 16-36). The flap is secured in this position with interproximal sutures (Fig. 16-37).

Among a number of suggested advantages of the "*apically repositioned flap*" procedure, the following have been emphasized:

- Minimum pocket depth postoperatively.
- If optimal soft tissue coverage of the alveolar bone is obtained, the postsurgical bone loss is minimal.
- The postoperative position of the gingival margin may be controlled and the entire mucogingival complex may be maintained.

The sacrifice of periodontal tissues by bone resection and the subsequent exposure of root surfaces (which may cause root hypersensitivity) were regarded as the main disadvantages of this technique.

The modified Widman flap

Ramfjord & Nissle (1974) described the "*modified Widman flap*" technique which is also recognized as the "*open flap curettage*" technique. It should be noted that, while the "*original Widman flap*" technique included both apical displacement of the flaps and osseous recontouring (elimination of angular bony defects) to obtain proper pocket elimination, the "*modified Widman flap*" technique is not intended to meet these objectives. Ramfjord & Nissle (1974) have described the "*modified Widman flap*" technique:

The *initial incision* (Fig. 16-38) which may be performed with a Bard-Parker knife (No 11) should be parallel to the long axis of the tooth and placed approximately 1 mm from the buccal gingival margin in order to properly separate the pocket epithelium from the flap. If the pockets on the buccal aspects of the teeth are less than 2 mm deep or if esthetic considerations are important, an intracrevicular incision may be made. Furthermore, the scalloped inci-

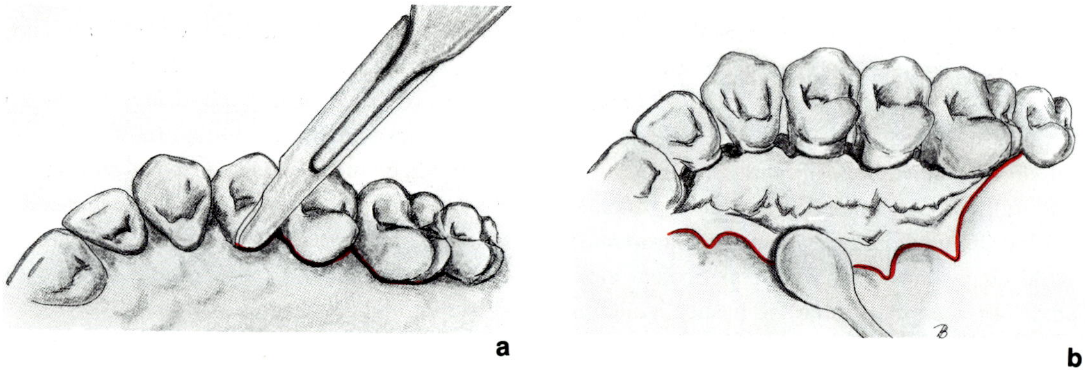

FIg. 16-34. *Bevelled flap*. A primary incision is made through the periodontal pockets (a) and a conventional mucoperiosteal flap is elevated (b).

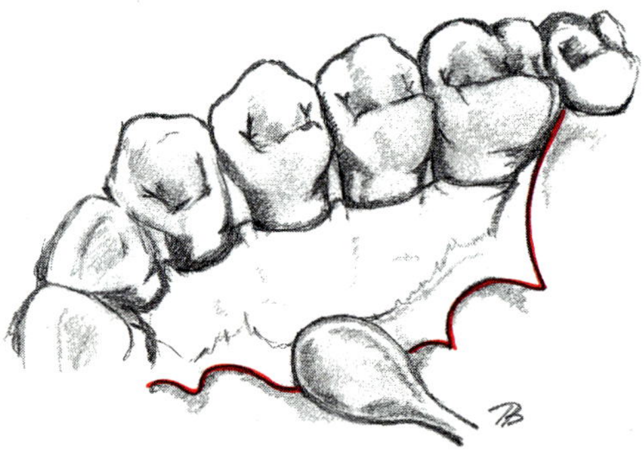

Fig. 16-35. *Bevelled flap*. Scaling, root planing and osseous recontouring have been performed in the surgical area.

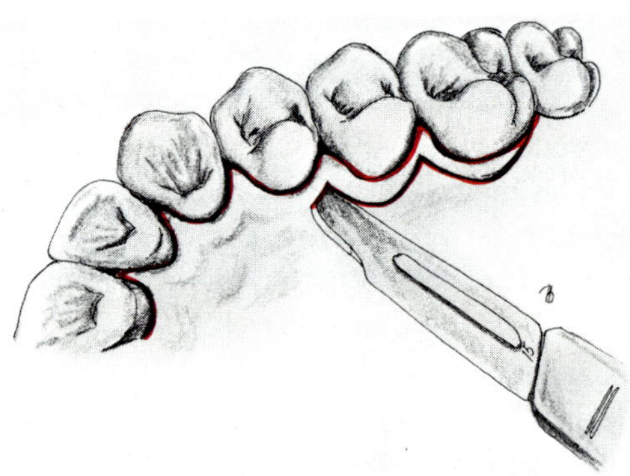

Fig. 16-36. *Bevelled flap*. The palatal flap is replaced and a secondary, scalloped, reverse bevel incision is made to adjust the length of the flap to the height of the remaining alveolar bone.

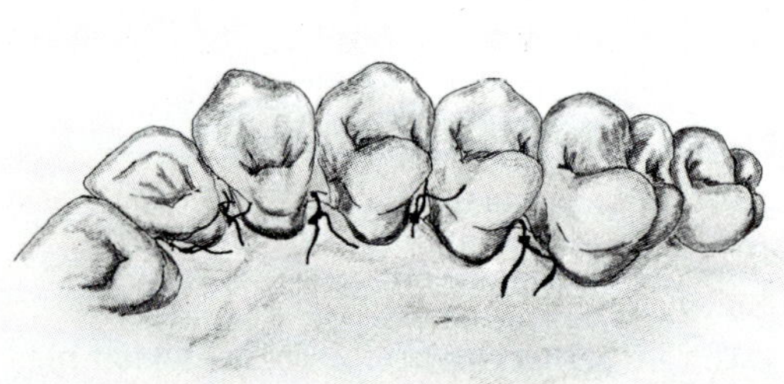

Fig. 16-37. *Bevelled flap*. The shortened flap is placed over the alveolar bone and in close contact with the root surfaces.

sion should be extended as far as possible in between the teeth, to allow maximum amounts of the interdental gingiva to be included in the flap. A similar incision technique is used on the palatal aspect. Often, however, the scalloped outline of the initial incision may be accentuated by placing the knife at a distance of 1-2 mm from the midpalatal surface of the teeth. By extending the incision as far as possible in between the teeth sufficient amounts of tissue can be included in the palatal flap to allow for proper coverage of the interproximal bone when the flap is sutured. Vertical releasing incisions are not usually required.

Buccal and palatal full thickness flaps are carefully elevated with a mucoperiosteal elevator (Fig. 16-39). The flap elevation should be limited and allow only a few millimeters of the alveolar bone crest to become exposed. To facilitate the gentle separation of the collar of pocket epithelium and granulation tissue from the root surfaces, an intracrevicular incision is

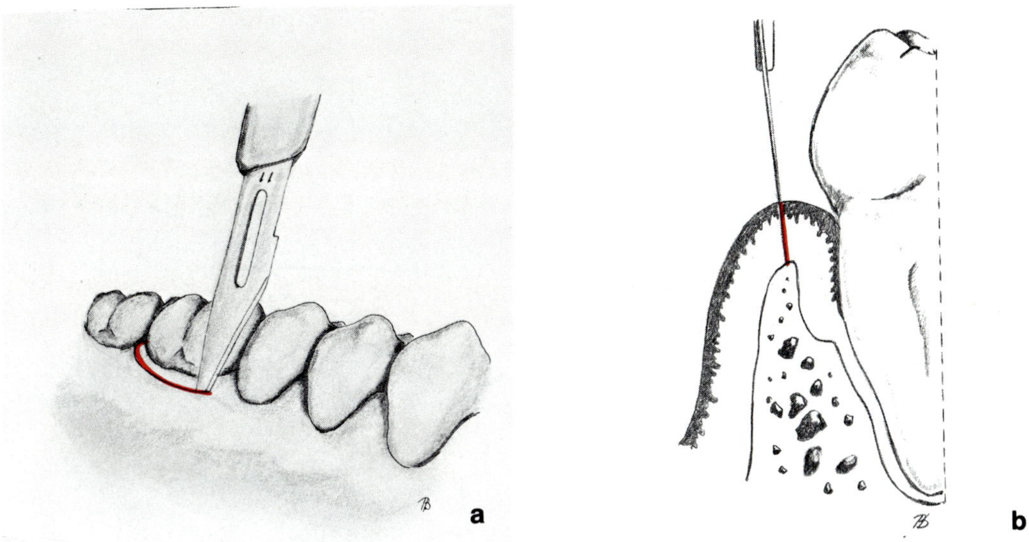

Fig. 16-38. *Modified Widman flap.* The initial incision is placed 0.5 to 1 mm from the gingival margin (a) and parallel to the long axis of the tooth (b).

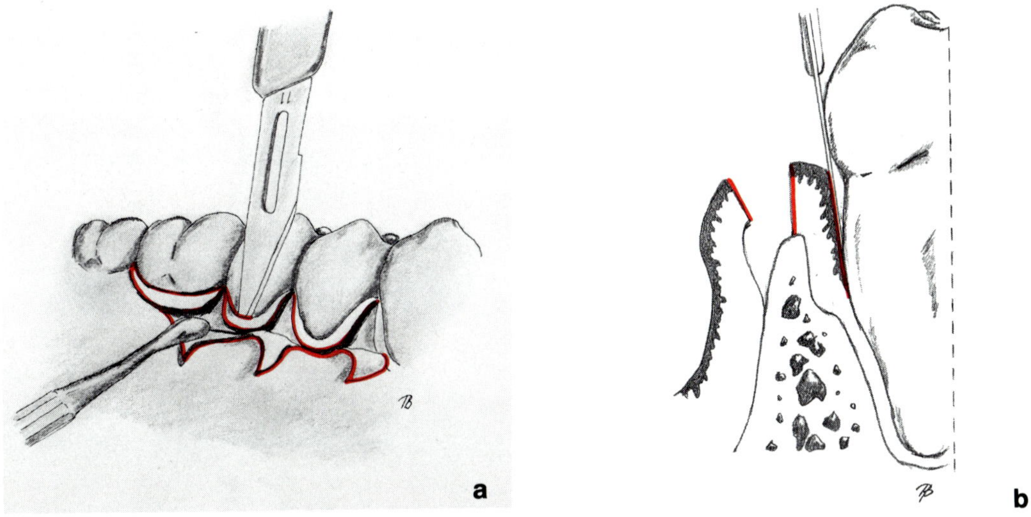

Fig. 16-39. *Modified Widman flap.* Following careful elevation of the flaps, a second intracrevicular incision (a) is made to the alveolar bone crest (b).

made around the teeth (*second incision*) to the alveolar crest.

A *third incision* (Fig. 16-40) made in a horizontal direction and in a position close to the surface of the alveolar bone crest separates the soft tissue collar of the root surfaces from the bone. The pocket epithelium and the granulation tissues are removed by means of curettes. The exposed roots are carefully scaled and planed, except for a narrow area close to the alveolar bone crest in which remnants of attachment fibers may be preserved. Angular bony defects are carefully curetted.

Following the curettage, the flaps are trimmed and adjusted to the alveolar bone to obtain complete coverage of the interproximal bone (Fig. 16-41). If this adaptation cannot be achieved by soft tissue recontouring, some

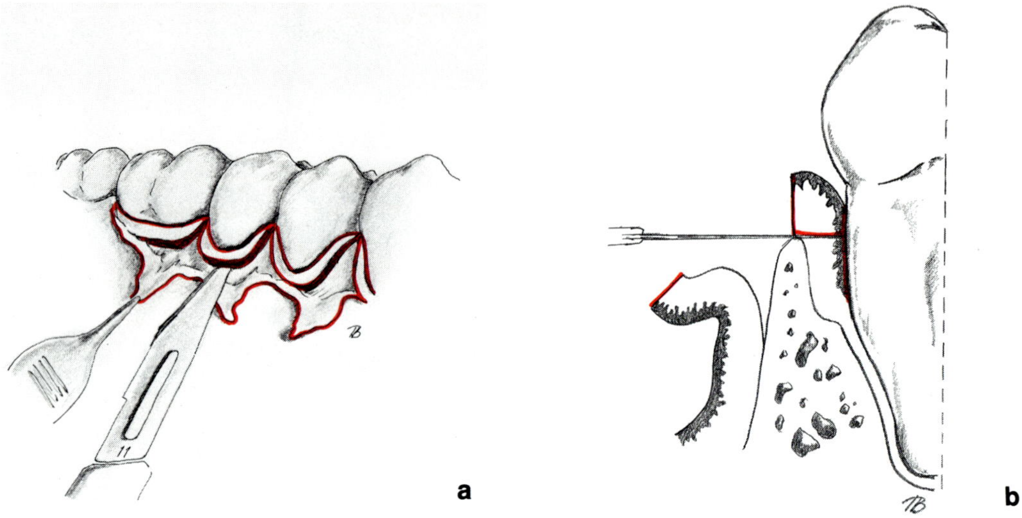

Fig. 16-40. *Modified Widman flap*. The third incision is made in a horizontal direction (a) and close to the surface of the bone crest (b), thereby separating the soft tissue collar from the root surfaces and the alveolar bone.

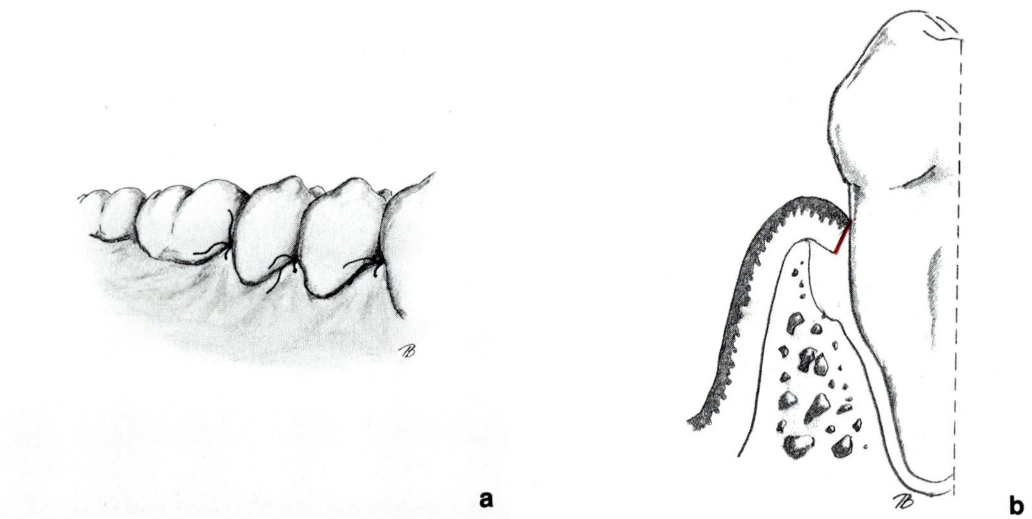

Fig. 16-41. *Modified Widman flap*. (a) Following curettage the flaps are carefully adjusted to cover the alveolar bone and sutured. (b) Complete coverage of the interproximal bone as well as a close adaptation of the flaps to the tooth surfaces should be accomplished.

bone may be removed from the outer aspects of the alveolar process in order to facilitate the all-important flap adaption. The flaps are sutured together with individual interproximal sutures. Surgical dressing may be placed over the area to ensure close adaptation of the flaps to the alveolar bone and root surfaces. The dressing, as well as the sutures, are removed after 1 week.

The main advantages of the "*modified Widman flap*" technique in comparison to other procedures previously described are 1) the possibility of obtaining a close adaptation of the soft tissues to the root surfaces and 2) the

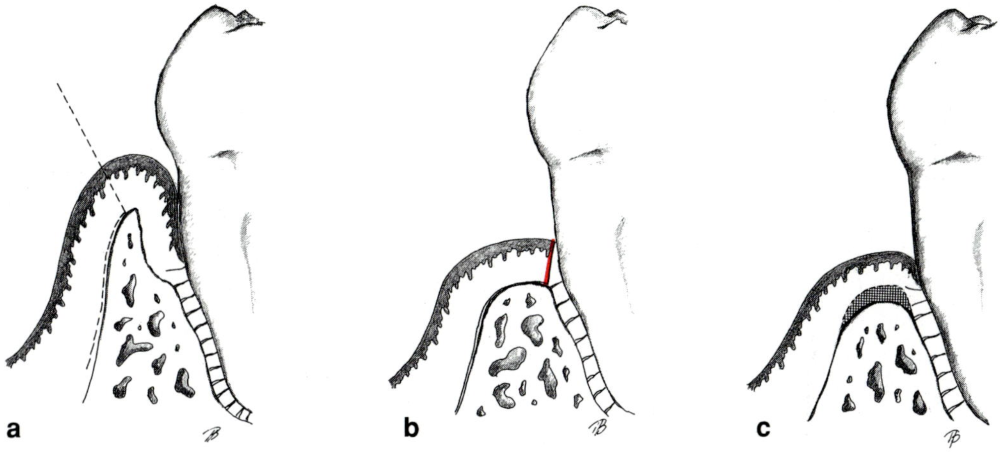

Fig. 16-42. *Apically repositioned flap*. Dimensional changes. (a) Illustrates the preoperative dimensions. The broken line indicates the site from which the mucoperiosteal flap is reflected. (b) Bone recontouring has been completed. (c) Dimensions following proper healing. Minor resorption of the marginal alveolar bone has occurred (shadowed area) as well as some loss of connective tissue attachment.

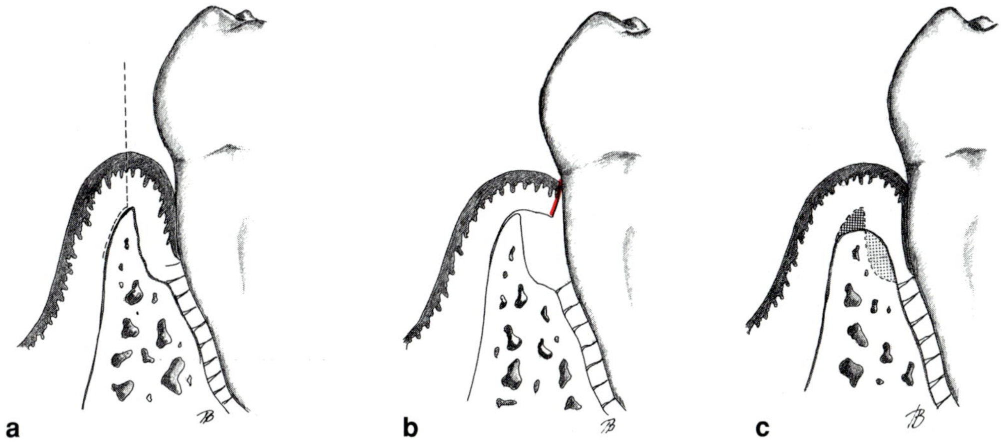

Fig. 16-43. *Modified Widman flap* - dimensional changes. (a) Illustrates the preoperative dimensions. Broken line illustrates the site from which the mucoperiosteal flap is reflected. (b) Surgery (including curettage of angular bony defects) is completed. (c) Dimensions following proper healing. Osseous repair (dotted area) as well as a small amount of crestal bone resorption (shadowed area) have occurred. Note the presence of a long junctional epithelium interposed between the regenerated bone tissue and the root surface.

minimum of trauma to which the alveolar bone and the soft connective tissues are exposed (Ramfjord & Nissle 1974). The technique also results in less exposure of the root surfaces, which from an esthetic point of view is an advantage in the treatment of anterior segments of the dentition.

Dimensional changes following flap surgery
The apically repositioned flap (Fig. 16-42): Following osseous surgery for elimination of bony defects and the establishment of "physiologic contours" and repositioning of the soft tissue flaps to the level of the alveolar bone, healing will occur primarily by first intention, especially in areas where proper soft tissue

coverage of the alveolar bone has been obtained. During the initial phase of healing, bone resorption of varying degrees almost always occurs in the crestal area of the alveolar bone (Ramfjord & Costich 1968). The extent of the reduction of the alveolar bone height resulting from this resorption is related to the thickness of the bone in each specific site (Wood et al. 1972, Karring et al. 1975).

During the phase of tissue regeneration and maturation a new dento-gingival unit will form by coronal growth of the connective tissue. This regrowth occurs in a manner similar to that which characterized healing following gingivectomy.

The "modified Widman flap" (Fig. 16-43): If a "modified Widman flap" is carried out in an area with a deep infrabony lesion, bone repair may occur within the boundaries of the lesion (Rosling et al. 1976a, Polson & Heijl 1978). However, a small amount of crestal bone resorption is also seen. The amount of bone fill obtained is dependent upon 1) the anatomy of the osseous defect (e.g. a three-walled infrabony defect often provides a better mould for bone repair than two- or one-walled defects), 2) the amount of crestal bone resorption and 3) the extent of chronic inflammation, which may occupy the area of healing. However, interposed between the regenerated bone tissue and the root surface, a long junctional epithelium is always found (Caton & Zander 1976, Caton et al. 1980). The apical cells of the newly formed junctional epithelium are found at a level on the root that closely coincides with the presurgical attachment level.

Distal Wedge procedures

In many cases the treatment of periodontal pockets on the distal surface of distal molars is complicated by the presence of bulbous tissues over the tuberosity or by a prominent retromolar pad. The most direct approach to pocket elimination in such cases in the maxillary jaw is the gingivectomy procedure. The incision is started on the distal surface of the tuberosity and carried forward to the base of the pocket of the distal surface of the molar (Fig. 16-44).

However, when only limited amounts of keratinized gingiva are present, or none at all, or if a distal angular bony defect has been diagnosed, the bulbous tissue should be reduced in size rather than being removed *in toto*. This may be accomplished by the "*distal wedge procedure*" (Robinson 1966). This technique facilitates access to the osseous defect and makes it possible to preserve sufficient amounts of keratinized gingiva and mucosa.

Technique

Buccal and lingual incisions are made in a vertical direction through the tuberosity or retromolar pad to form a triangular wedge (Fig. 16-45). The facial and lingual incisions should be extended in a mesial direction along the buccal and lingual surfaces of the distal molar to facilitate flap elevation.

The facial and lingual walls of the tuberosity or retromolar pad are deflected and the incised wedge of tissue is dissected and separated from the bone (Fig. 16-46).

The walls of the facial and lingual flaps are then reduced in thickness by undermining incisions (Fig. 16-47). Loose tags of tissue are removed and the root surfaces are scaled and planed. If necessary, the bone is recountered.

The buccal and lingual flaps are replaced over the exposed alveolar bone, and the edges trimmed to avoid overlapping wound margins. The flaps are secured in this position with interrupted sutures (Fig. 16-48). The sutures are removed after approximately 1 week.

The distal wedge procedure may be modified according to individual requirements. One such modification of the original distal wedge procedure is illustrated in Figs. 16-49 to 16-54.

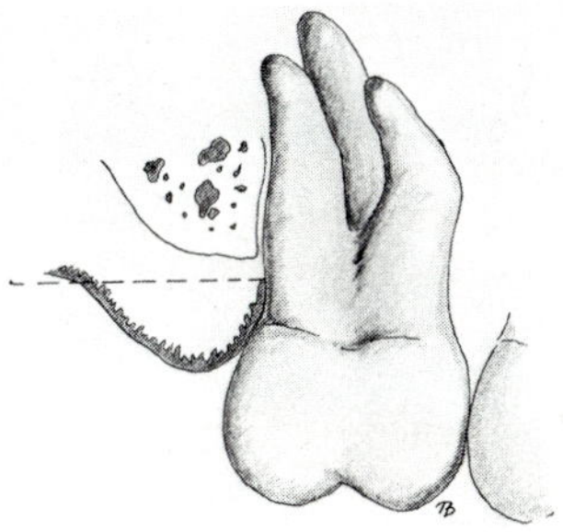

Fig. 16-44. *Distal wedge procedures.* Simple gingivectomy incision (broken line) is used to eliminate the soft tissue pocket and the fibrous tissue pad behind a second maxillary molar.

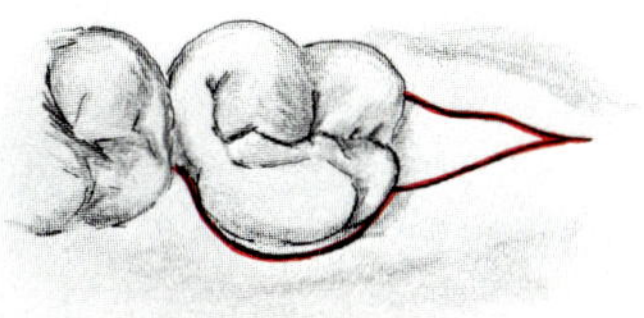

FIg. 16-45. *Distal wedge procedure.* Buccal and lingual vertical incisions are made through the retromolar pad behind a mandibular second molar.

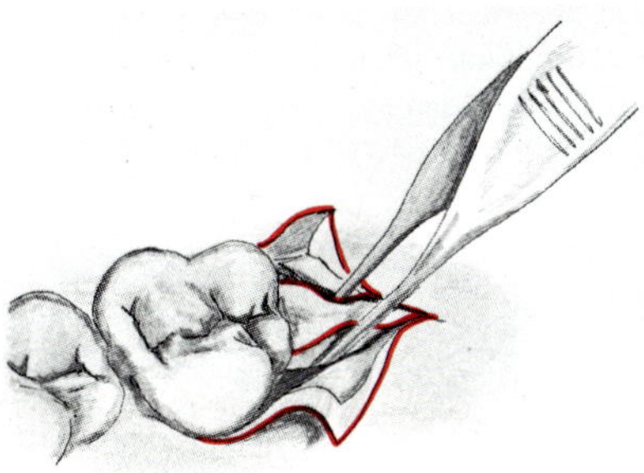

Fig. 16-46. *Distal wedge procedures.* The triangular shaped wedge of tissue, prepared by the vertical incisions, is dissected from the underlying bone and removed.

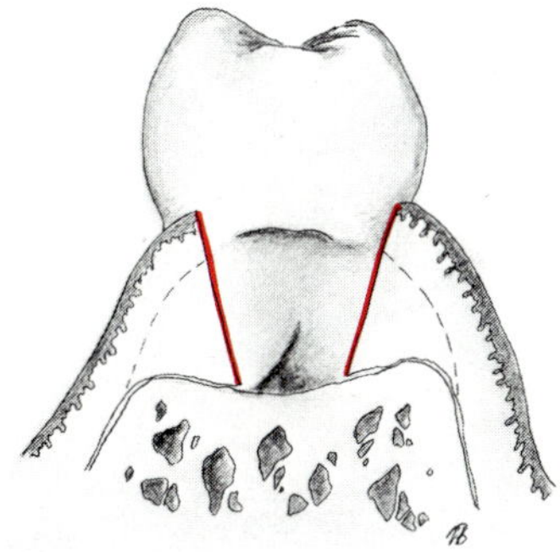

Fig. 16-47. *Distal wedge procedure.* The walls of the buccal and lingual flaps are reduced in thickness by undermining incisions (broken lines).

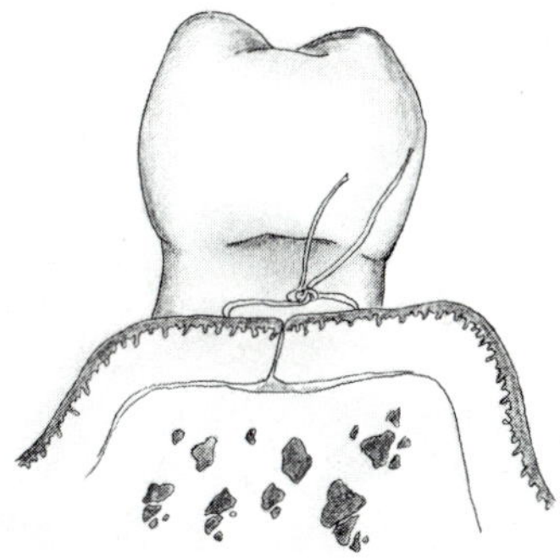

Fig. 16-48. *Distal wedge procedures.* The flaps, which have been trimmed and shortened to avoid overlapping wound margins, are sutured.

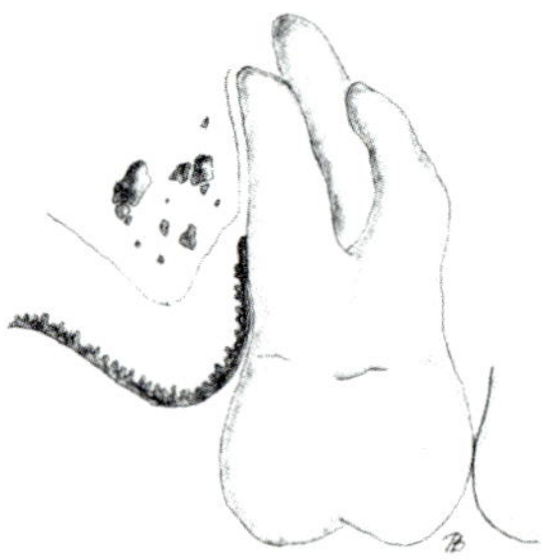

Fig. 16-49. *Distal wedge procedures.* Illustrates a deep periodontal pocket combined with an angular bony defect at the distal aspect of a second maxillary molar.

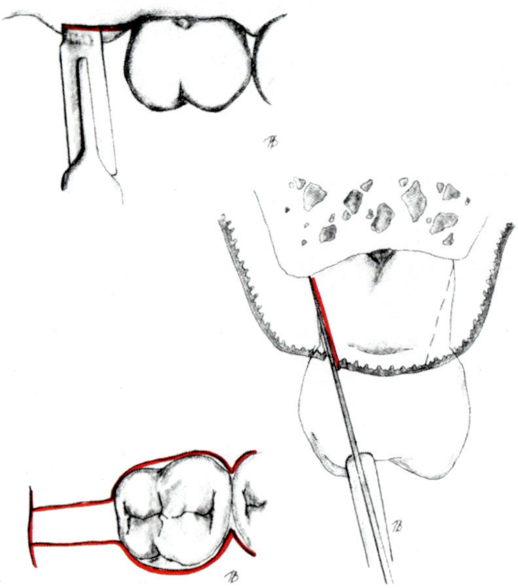

Fig. 16-50. *Distal wedge procedures.* (a, b) Two parallel reverse bevel incisions, one buccal (indicated by broken line in Fig. 16-50b) and one palatal, are made from the distal surface of the second maxillary molar to the posterior part of the tuberosity. (c) A bucco-lingual incision is then made to connect the two parallel incisions. The buccal and palatal incisions are extended in a mesial direction along the buccal and palatal surfaces of the second and first maxillary molars to facilitate flap elevation.

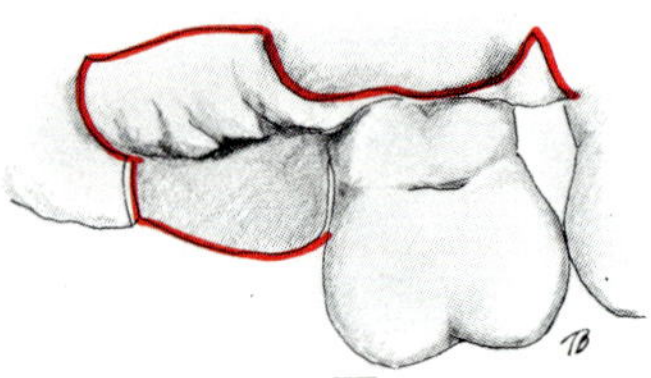

Fig. 16-51. *Distal wedge procedures.* Buccal and palatal flaps have been elevated.

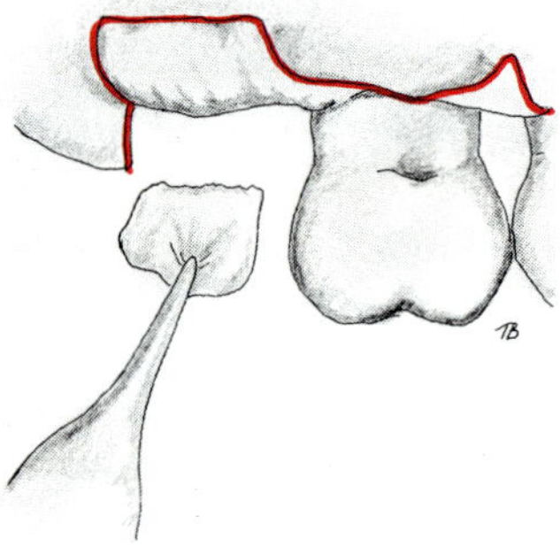

Fig. 16-52. *Distal wedge procedures.* The rectangular wedge is dissected from the underlying bone and removed.

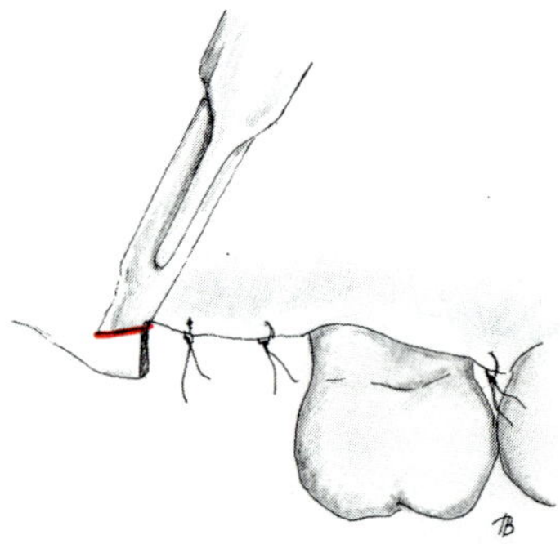

Fig. 16-53. *Distal wedge procedures.* Following bone recontouring the flaps are trimmed and shortened to avoid overlapping wound margins and sutured. The remaining fibrous tissue pad distal to the bucco-lingual incision line is "levelled" by the use of a gingivectomy incision.

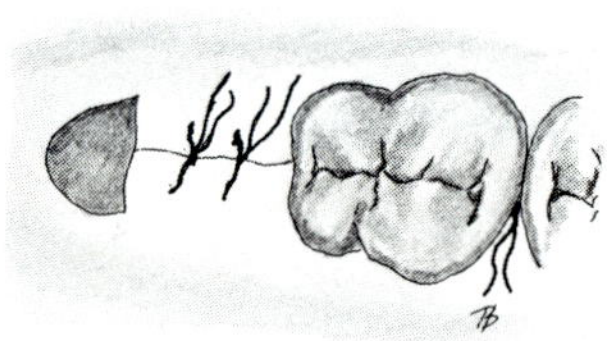

Fig. 16-54. *Distal wedge procedure.* The distal wedge procedure is completed. Note that a close soft tissue adaptation has been accomplished to the distal surface of the second maxillary molar.

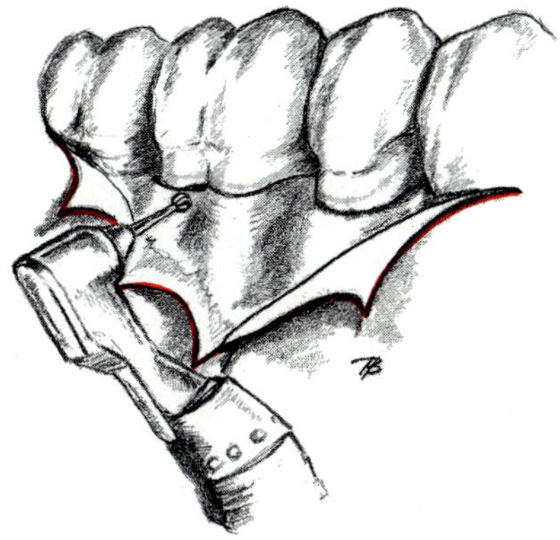

Fig. 16-55. *Osteoplasty.* Thick osseous ledges in a mandibular molar area are eliminated with the use of a round bur.

Osseous surgery

Osseous recontouring and eradication of angular bony defects and craters are excisional techniques which should be used with caution and discrimination. Sometimes deep bony defects may, for their complete elimination, require such an advanced resection of alveolar bone that the periodontal tissue support of adjacent teeth that are primarily not so seriously involved in the disease process may have to be compromised. In such cases, bone resection should be avoided.

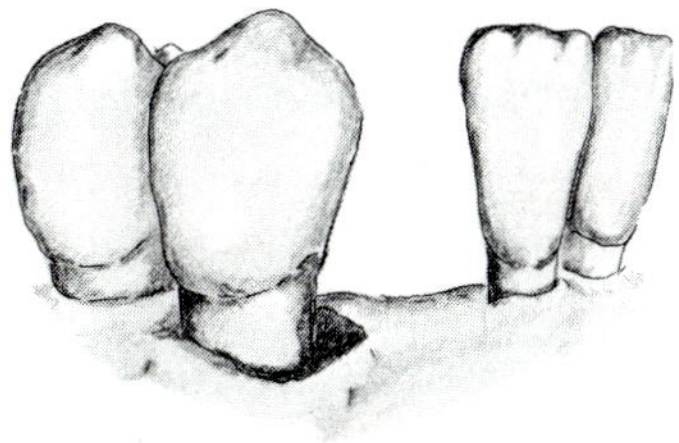

a

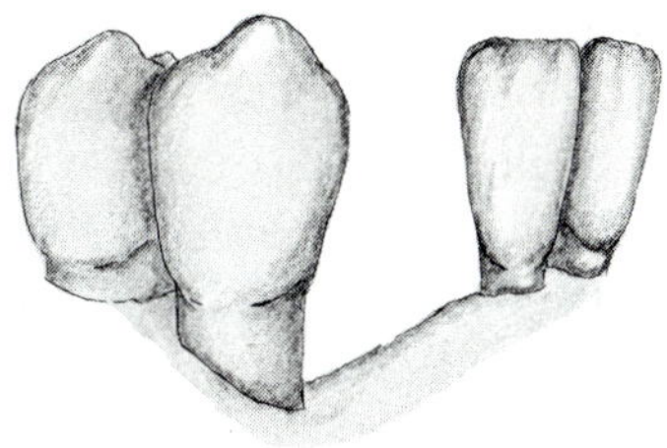

b

Fig. 16-56. *Osteoplasty.* (a) An infrabony defect is present at the mesiobuccal aspect of the mandibular right canine. (b) The osseous defect has been removed by osseous recontouring. Note that no supporting bone has been resected.

Osteoplasty

The term *osteoplasty* was introduced by Friedman in 1955. The purpose of osteoplasty is to create a physiological form of the alveolar bone *without* removing any "supporting" bone. Osteoplasty therefore is a technique analogous

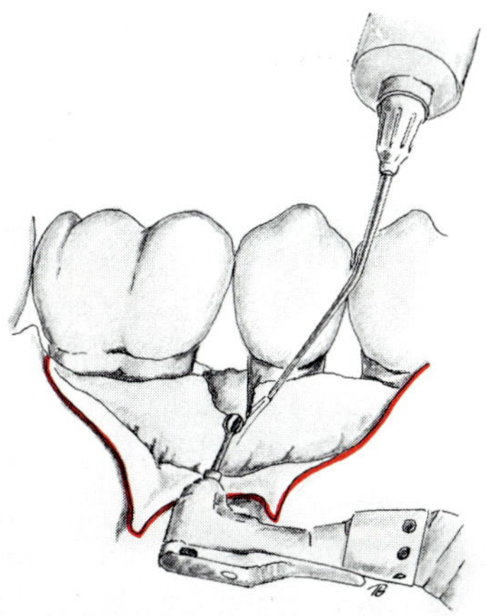

a

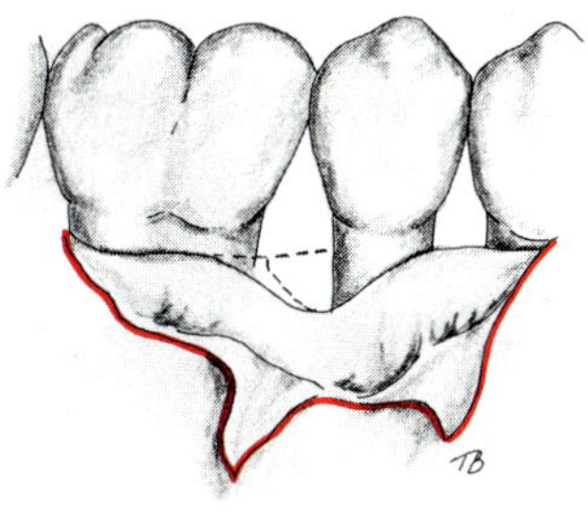

b

Fig. 16-57. *Ostectomy.* (a) An osseous defect on the distal surface of a mandibular second bicuspid has been exposed following reflection of mucoperiosteal flaps. The bone walls are reduced to the base of the defect using a rotating round bur under continuous saline irrigation. (b) The osseous recontouring procedure is completed. Note that in this illustration some supporting bone has been removed from the buccal aspect of both the second bicuspid and the first molar.

to gingivoplasty. Examples of osteoplasty are the thinning of thick osseous ledges and the establishment of a scalloped contour of the buccal (lingual and palatal) bone crest (Fig. 16-55). The levelling of interproximal craters and the elimination of bone walls of circumferential osseous defects are often referred to as "osteoplasty" since usually no resection of supporting bone is required (Figs. 16-56).

Ostectomy

Ostectomy is considered to be an important part of a surgical technique aimed at pocket elimination. However, the therapist is often faced with the dilemma of deciding whether to eliminate an angular bony defect in situations where osseous resection may compromise the periodontal tissue support of a neighboring tooth. The alternatives are 1) to maintain the area without osseous resection, 2) to compromize the amount of bone removal and accept that a certain pocket depth will remain or 3) to extract the involved tooth if the bony defect is too advanced.

After exposing the alveolar bone by the elevation of a flap, buccal and/or lingual crater walls are reduced to the base of the osseous defect using a round bur or a diamond stone under continuous saline irrigation (Fig. 16-57). Bone chisels, files and rongeurs can also be used. If bone resection has been carried out in the interdental area, the buccal and lingual/palatal bone margins may subsequently have to be recontoured to compensate for discrepancies in bone height resulting from the interdental bone resection (Fig. 16-57b). It is considered important to remove the small peaks of bone, which often remain in the area of the line angles. The objective of bone surgery is thus to establish a "physiologic" anatomy of the alveolar bone, but at a more apical level. The soft tissue flaps are recontoured and adapted to the newly created bone margin.

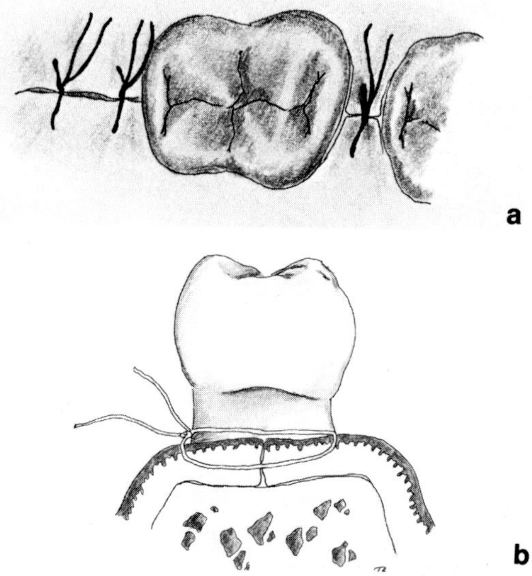

Fig. 16-58a, b. *Suturing*. Interrupted interdental suture.

Suturing

When a flap procedure has been employed it is important to ensure that, at the end of surgery, the flaps are placed in the intended position and that the flaps are properly adapted to each other and to the tooth surfaces. Preferably, full coverage of the buccal/lingual (palatal) and interdental alveolar bone should be obtained with the soft tissue flaps. If this can be achieved, healing by first intention results and the postoperative bone resorption becomes minimal. Therefore, prior to suturing, the flap margins should be trimmed to properly fit the buccal and lingual (palatal) bone margin as well as the interproximal areas; excessive soft tissue must be removed. If the amount of flap tissue present is insufficient to cover the interproximal bone, the flaps at the buccal or lingual aspects of the teeth must be recontoured and, in some cases, even coronally displaced.

Following proper trimming, the flaps are secured in the correct position by sutures. The materials most commonly used as sutures in periodontal surgery are fabricated of silk and various synthetic materials. The dimensions

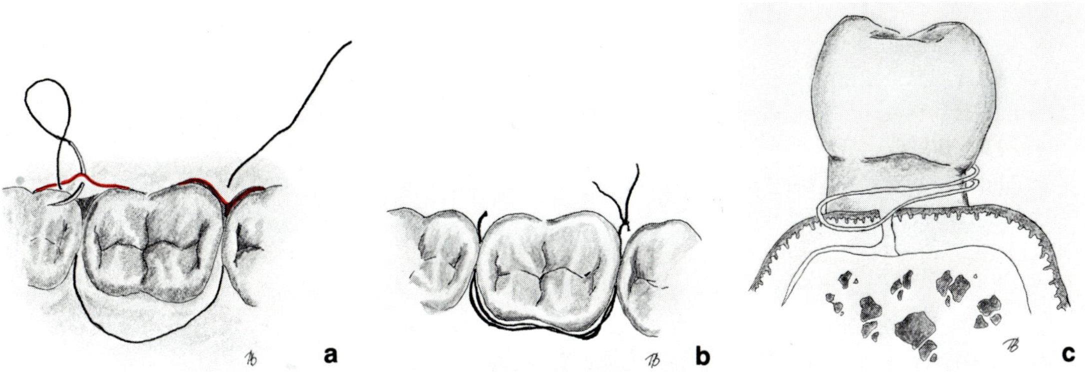

Fig. 16-59a-c. *Suturing*. Suspensory suture.

usually preferred are 3-0 or 4-0. These materials are non-resorbable and should be removed after 7 to 14 days.

Since the flap tissue following the final preparation is thin, non-traumatic needles (eyeless), either curved or straight, with a small diameter should be used. Such needles are available as rounded (noncutting) or with different cutting edges.

Technique

The three most frequently used sutures in periodontal flap surgery are 1) interrupted interdental sutures, 2) suspensory sutures and 3) continuous sutures.

The *interrupted interdental suture* (Fig. 16-58) provides a close interdental adaptation between the buccal and lingual flaps with equal tension on both units. This type of suture is therefore not recommended when the buccal and lingual flaps are repositioned at different levels. When this technique of suturing is employed, the needle is passed through the buccal flap from the external surface, across the interdental area and through the lingual flap from the internal surface, or vice versa. When closing the suture, care must be taken to avoid tearing the flap tissues.

The *suspensory suture* (Fig. 16-59) is used primarily when the surgical procedure is of

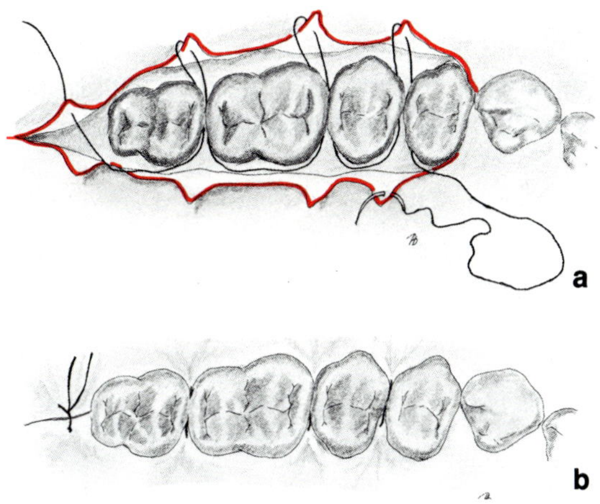

Fig. 16-60a, b. *Suturing*. Continuous suture.

limited extent and involves only the tissue of the buccal or lingual aspect of the teeth. It is also the suture of choice when the buccal and lingual flaps are repositioned at different levels. The needle is passed through the buccal flap from its external surface at the mesial side of the tooth, placed around the lingual surface of the tooth and passed through the buccal flap on the distal side of the tooth (Fig. 16-59a). The suture is brought back to the starting point via the lingual surface of the tooth and tied (Figs. 16-59a & b). If a lingual flap has been elevated as well, this is secured in the intended position using the same technique.

The *continuous suture* (Fig. 16-60) is commonly used when flaps involving several teeth are to be apically repositioned. When flaps have been elevated on both sides of the teeth, one flap at a time is secured in its correct position. The suturing procedure is started at the mesial/distal aspect of the buccal flap by passing the needle through the flap and across the interdental area. The suture is laid around the lingual surface of the tooth and returned to the buccal side through the next interdental space. The procedure is repeated tooth by tooth until the distal/mesial end of the flap is reached. Thereafter, the needle is passed through the lingual flap (Fig. 16-60a), with the suture laid around the buccal aspect of each tooth and through each interproximal space. When the suturing of the lingual flap is completed and the needle has been brought back to the first interdental area, the positions of the flaps are adjusted and secured in their proper positions by closing the suture (Fig. 16-60b). Thus, only one knot is needed.

Periodontal dressings

Periodontal dressings are mainly used 1) to protect the wound prepared during surgery, 2) to obtain and maintain a close adaptation of the mucosal flaps to the underlying bone (especially when a flap has been apically repositioned) and 3) for the comfort of the patient. In addition, periodontal dressings can, during the initial phase of healing, prevent postoperative bleeding and, if properly placed in the operated segment (especially interproximally), prevent the formation of excessive granulation tissue.

Periodontal dressings should have the following properties:

1. The dressing should be soft, but still have enough plasticity and flexibility to facilitate its placement in the operated area and to allow proper adaptation.
2. The dressing should have set within a reasonable time.
3. After setting, the dressing should have sufficient rigidity to prevent fracture and dislocation.
4. The dressing should also have a smooth surface after setting to prevent irritation to the cheeks and lips.
5. The dressing should preferably have bactericidal properties to prevent excessive plaque formation.
6. The dressing must not detrimentally interfere with healing.

It has been suggested that antibacterial agents should be incorporated in periodontal dressings to prevent bacterial growth in the wound area during healing. Results from clinical studies and *in vitro* evaluation of the antibacterial properties of various periodontal dressings, however, suggest that the antibacterial activity of most commercial dressings probably is exhausted long before the end of the 7- to 14-day period during which the dressing is frequently maintained in the operated segment (O'Neil 1975, Haugen et al. 1977).

Mouth-rinsing with antibacterial agents such as chlorhexidine does not prevent the formation of plaque *under* the dressing (Plüss et al. 1975) and should therefore not be regarded as a mean to improve or shorten the period of wound healing.

The periodontal dressings most commonly used may be divided into two groups: *eugenol containing* and *non-eugenol containing* dressings.

Eugenol dressings

These dressings have a zinc-oxide-eugenol base. The dressing is supplied as a powder and a liquid, which are mixed together. Zinc-oxide, which is used for setting material, forms when mixed with eugenol, a hardened mass. The powder also contains rosin, tannic acid, cellulose fibers and zinc acetate, while the liquid, in addition to eugenol, may contain vegetable oils, thymol and color additives. Zinc-oxide can be substituted by other similar materials such as magnesium-oxide. The setting involves both chemical and physical processes and is influenced by moisture, proportions of powder and liquid used, mixing time and temperature. The addition of a metallic salt such as zinc-acetate accelerates setting. The rosin reacts with the zinc-oxide to give the dressing better rigidity. Tannic acid has been used to improve wound healing, but its use has been prohibited in some countries because of the risk of liver damage. However, because of its suggested beneficial effects on wound healing tannic acid is still a constituent in several commercial dressings. Cellulose fibers are incorporated in order to improve the setting of the dressing material. Eugenol is weakly antiseptic and has a slight sedative effect. The vegetable oils, which are added to the liquid in order to dissolve the eugenol, will also increase the plasticity of the dressing and reduce some tissue irritation caused by the eugenol. Thymol is a weak antiseptic. Sensitivity reactions sometimes occur when zinc-oxide-eugenol dressings are used and it is usually the eugenol which provokes this kind of reaction.

Non-eugenol dressings

Since several reports have been published indicating adverse effects of eugenol and since eugenol-containing dressings have an unpleasant taste to many patients, eugenol-free dressings have been developed. Several such dressings are available, e.g. Coe-Pak® and Peripac®.

Coe-Pak®, which is frequently used in periodontal surgery, is supplied in two tubes. One tube contains oxides of various metals (mainly zinc-oxide) and lorothidol (a fungicide). The second tube contains non-ionizing carboxylic acids and chlorothymol (a bacteriostatic agent). Equal parts from both tubes are mixed together immediately prior to insertion. The setting time can be prolonged by adding a retarder. Other typical non-eugenol dressings are supplied as a powder and a liquid, which are mixed.

Cyanoacrylates have also been used as periodontal dressings with varying success. Dressings of the cyanoacrylate type are applied in a liquid directly onto the wound, or sprayed over the wound surface. Although the application of this kind of dressing is simple, its properties often do not meet clinical demands, which is why its use is rather limited at present.

It should be noted that also non-eugenol dressings may also provoke hypersensitivity reactions.

Application technique

Following gingivectomy, periodontal dressings are used primarily to protect the wound, while following flap surgery dressing is often used to keep the flaps in close contact with the underlying bone.

When bleeding from the operated tissues has ceased, the dressing material is inserted. Frequently the interproximal areas are filled with the pack material first. Thin rolls of the dressing, adjusted in length to cover the entire field of operation, are then placed against the buccal and lingual surfaces of the teeth. The rolls are pressed against the tooth surfaces and the dressing material is forced into the interproximal areas. The surface of the dressing is subsequently smoothened. The dressing should not cover more than the apical third of the tooth surfaces (Figs. 16-17, 16-32). Coe-Pak® may also be applied to the wound surfaces by means of a plastic syringe.

It is important to ensure that dressing material is never introduced between the flap and the underlying bone or root surface. To avoid such faulty placement of the pack the wound surface may occasionally be protected with, for example, tin foil prior to the insertion of the dressing. Tin foil applications are recommended in sites where an insufficient adaptation of the flap to the bone or the root has been accomplished. Furthermore, interferences of the dressing with mucogingival structures (e.g. the vestibular fold, frenula) should be carefully checked.

Concluding remarks

The objectives of surgical treatment of periodontal disease are to support the causative therapy by:

1. making subgingival root surfaces accessible for thorough scaling and root planing;
2. establishing gingival contours which facilitate the patients' home care;
3. providing for healing of periodontal lesions which preserves the maximum of supporting tissue.

Many of the technical problems experienced in periodontal surgery stem from the difficulties in assessing accurately the degree and type of breakdown that has occurred prior to surgery. Furthermore, at the time of surgery, previously undiagnosed defects may be recognized or some defects may have a more complex outline than initially anticipated. Since each of the surgical procedures described above is designed to deal with a specific situation or to meet a certain objective, it must be understood that no single standardized technique alone can be applied when periodontal surgery is undertaken in a patient. Therefore, in each surgical field, different techniques are often used and combined in such a way that the overall objectives of the surgical part of the periodontal therapy are met. As a general rule, surgical modalities of therapy which preserve or induce the formation of periodontal tissue should be preferred over those which resect or eliminate tissue.

As stated previously, postoperative plaque control is the most important variable in determining the net result of periodontal surgery. Provided proper postoperative plaque control levels are established, most surgical treatment techniques will result in conditions which favor the long-term maintenance of the periodontium. If post-operative hygiene fails, progressive loss of supporting tissue will take place regardless of surgical technique used. The relative importance of surgical therapy in the overall treatment of periodontal disease, as well as the outcome of the various techniques, is discussed in Chapter 24.

References

Ariaudo, A.A. & Tyrell, H.A. (1957) Repositioning and increasing the zone of attached gingiva. *Journal of Periodontology* **28**, 106-110.

Axelsson, P. & Lindhe, J. (1981) The significance of maintenance care in the treatment of periodontal disease. *Journal of Clinical Periodontology* **8**, 281-294.

Badersten, A., Nilveus, R. & Egelberg, J. (1981) Effect of nonsurgical periodontal therapy. I. Moderately advanced periodontitis. *Journal of Clinical Periodontology* **8**, 57-72.

Caffasse, R.G., Sweeney, P.L. & Smith, B.A. (1966) Scaling and root planing with and without periodontal flap surgery. *Journal of Clinical Periodontology* **13**, 205-210.

Caton, J., Nyman, S. & Zander, H. (1980) Histometric evaluation of periodontal surgery. II. Connective tissue attachment levels after four regenerative procedures. *Journal of Clinical Periodontology* **7**, 224-231.

Caton, J.G. & Zander, H.A. (1976) Osseous repair of an infrabony pocket without new attachment of connective tissue. *Journal of Clinical Periodontology* **3**, 54-58.

Engler, W.O., Ramfjord, S.P. & Hiniker, J.J. (1966) Healing following simple gingivectomy. A tritiated thymidine radioautographic study. I. Epithelialization. *Journal of Periodontology* **37**, 298-308.

Friedman, N. (1955) Periodontal osseous surgery: Osteoplasty and ostectomy. *Journal of Periodontology* **26**, 257-269.

Friedman, N. (1962) Mucogingival surgery. The apically repositioned flap. *Journal of Periodontology* **33**, 328-340.

Goldman, H.M. (1950) Development of physiologic gingival contours by gingivoplasty. *Oral Surgery, Oral Medicine and Oral Pathology* **3**, 879-888.

Goldman, H.M. (1951) Gingivectomy. *Oral Surgery, Oral Medicine and Oral Pathology* **4**, 1136-1157.

Grant, D.A., Stern, I.B. & Everett, F.G. (1979) *Periodontics in the tradition of Orban and Gottlieb.* 5th Ed. St. Louis: C.V. Mosby Co.

Hamp, S.E., Rosling, B. & Lindhe, J. (1975) Effect of chlorhexidine on gingival wound healing in the dog. A histometric study. *Journal of Clinical Periodontology* **2**, 143-152.

Haugen, E., Gjermo, P. & ¥rstavik, D. (1977) Some antibacterial properties of periodontal dressings. *Journal of Clinical Periodontology* **4**, 62-68.

Karring, T., Cumming, B.R., Oliver, R.C. & Löe, H. (1975) The origin of granulation tissue and its impact on postoperative results of mucogingival surgery. *Journal of Periodontology* **46**, 577-585.

Kirkland, O. (1931) The suppurative periodontal pus pocket; its treatment by the modified flap operation. *Journal of the American Dental Association* **18**, 1462-1470.

Lindhe, J., Westfelt, E., Nyman, S., Socransky, S.S., Heijl, L. & Bratthall, G. (1982) Healing following surgical/non-surgical treatment of periodontal disease. *Journal of Clinical Periodontology* **9**, 115-128.

Listgarten, M.A. (1980) Periodontal probing: What does it mean? *Journal of Clinical Periodontology* **7**, 165-176.

Nabers, C.L. (1954) Repositioning the attached gingiva. *Journal of Periodontology* **25**, 38-39.

Neuman, R. (1920) *Die Alveolar-Pyorrhöe und ihre Behandlung.*3rd Ed. Berlin: Herman Meusser.

Nyman, S., Lindhe, J. & Rosling, B. (1977) Periodontal surgery in plaque-infected dentitions. *Journal of Clinical Periodontology* **4**, 240-249.

O'Neil, T.C.A. (1975) Antibacterial properties of periodontal dressings. *Journal of Periodontology* **46**, 469-474.

Plüss, E.M., Engelberger, P.R. & Rateitschak, K.H. (1975) Effect of chlorhexidine on dental plaque formation under periodontal pack. *Journal of Clinical Periodontology* **2**, 136-142.

Polson, A.M. & Heijl, L. (1978) Osseous repair in infrabony periodontal defects. *Journal of Clinical Periodontology* **5**, 13-23.

Ramfjord, S.P. & Costich, E.R. (1968) Healing after exposure of periosteum on the alveolar process. *Journal of Periodontology* **38**, 199-207.

Ramfjord, S.P., Engler, W.O. & Hiniker, J.J. (1966) A radioautographic study of healing following simple gingivectomy. II. The connective tissue. *Journal of Periodontology* **37**, 179-189.

Ramfjord, S.P. & Nissle, R.R. (1974) The modified Widman flap. *Journal of Periodontology* **45**, 601-607.

Robicsek, S. (1884) Ueber das Wesen und Entstehen der Alveolar-Pyorrhöe und deren Behandlung. The 3rd Annual Report of the Austrian Dental Association (Reviewed in *Journal of Periodontology* **36**, 265, 1965).

Robinson, R.E. (1966) The distal wedge operation. *Periodontics* **4**, 256-264.

Rosling, B., Nyman, S. & Lindhe, J. (1976a) The effect of systemic plaque control on bone regeneration in infrabony pockets. *Journal of Clinical Periodontology* **3**, 38-53.

Rosling, B., Nyman, S., Lindhe, J. & Jern, B. (1976b) The healing potential of the periodontal tissue following different techniques of periodontal surgery in plaque-free dentitions. A 2-year clinical study. *Journal of Clinical Peridontology* **3**, 233-255.

Schluger, S. (1949) Osseous resection - a basic principle in periodontal surgery? *Oral Surgery, Oral Medicine and Oral Pathology* **2**, 316-325.

Stahl, S.S., Witkin, G.J., Cantor, M. & Brown, R. (1968) Gingival healing. II. Clinical and histologic repair sequences following gingivectomy. *Journal of Periodontology* **39**, 109-118.

Waerhaug, J. (1955) Microscopic demonstration of tissue reaction incident to removal of subgingival calculus. *Journal of Periodontology* **26**, 26-29.

Waerhaug, J. (1978) Healing of the dentoepithelial junction following subgingival plaque control. II. As observed on extracted teeth. *Journal of Periodontology* **49**, 119-134.

Widman, L. (1918) The operative treatment of pyorrhea alveolaris. A new surgical method. *Svensk Tandläkaretidskrift* (reviewed in *British Dental Journal* **1**, 293, 1920).

Wood, D.L., Hoag, P.M., Donnenfeld, O.W. & Rosenfeld, L.D. (1972) Alveolar crest reduction following full and partial thickness flaps. *Journal of Periodontology* **42**, 141-144.

Zentler, A. (1918) Suppurative gingivitis with alveolar involvement. A new surgical procedure. *Journal of the American Medical Association* **71**, 1530-1534.

CHAPTER 17

Mucogingival Surgery

Mucogingival surgery refers to "plastic surgical procedures designed to correct defects in the morphology, position and/or amount of gingiva surrounding the teeth" ("Glossary of terms" 1986). Frequently, however, the term "mucogingival surgery" is used to describe all surgical procedures which involve both the gingiva and the alveolar mucosa. Consequently, not only are techniques designed 1) to enhance the width of the attached and keratinized gingiva and 2) to correct particular soft tissue defects regarded as mucogingival procedures but 3) certain pocket elimination approaches are also included in this group of periodontal treatment modalities.

A detailed review of the large number of articles published on mucogingival surgery over the years reveals that the rationale for increasing the width of the attached and keratinized gingiva as a means to promote gingival health and to improve attachment levels is poorly supported by scientific data. Clinical impressions, case reports and anecdotal data have been used as the only reference to justify surgical intervention. Research performed during the last few years, however, has established a more proper basis for the appreciation of the role of mucogingival surgery in periodontal therapy.

Significance of the width of gingiva for the maintenance of periodontal health

For many years the presence of an "adequate" zone of keratinized and attached gingiva was considered critical for the maintenance of gingival health and for the prevention of continuous loss of connective tissue attachment (Nabers 1954, Ochsenbein 1960, Friedman & Levine 1964, Carranza & Carraro 1970, Hall 1981, Matter 1982). The concept thus prevailed that a narrow zone of gingiva was insufficient 1) to *protect* the periodontium from injury caused by friction forces encountered during mastication and 2) to *dissipate* the pull on the gingival margin created by the muscles of the adjacent alveolar mucosa (Friedman 1957, Ocsenbein 1960, Friedman & Levine 1964). Moreover, it was believed that an "inadequate" zone of gingiva would 1) *facilitate subgingival plaque formation* because of improper pocket closure resulting from the movability of the marginal tissue (Friedman 1962) and 2) *favor attachment loss and soft tissue recession* because of less tissue resistance to apical spread

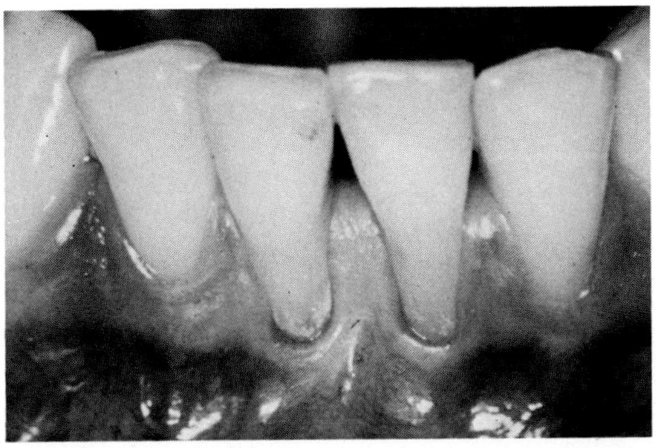

Fig. 17-1. A clinical photograph of a mandibular front tooth region. The gingiva on the buccal aspect of teeth 41 and 31 has an "inadequate" width and shows more pronounced signs of inflammation than adjacent gingival units with a wider zone of gingiva.

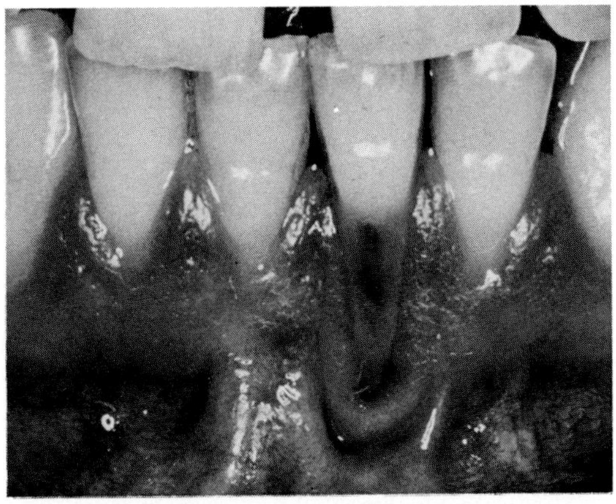

Fig. 17-2. A clinical photograph illustrating a localized gingival recession on the buccal aspect of tooth 31.

of plaque-associated gingival lesions (Stern 1976, Ruben 1979). It was also believed that a narrow gingiva and a shallow vestibular fornix might favor 1) *the accumulation of food particles during mastication* and 2) *impede proper oral hygiene measures* (Gottsegen 1954, Rosenberg 1960, Corn 1962, Carranza & Carraro 1970).

Different opinions have been expressed concerning what could be regarded as being an *adequate dimension* of the gingiva. Some authors have suggested that less than 1 mm of *attached gingiva* is sufficient (Bowers 1963), while others have claimed that the width of *keratinized gingiva* ought to exceed 3 mm (Corn 1962). A third category of authors has stated that an adequate amount of gingiva is *any width of gingiva* which 1) prevents retraction of the gingival margin during movements of the alveolar mucosa or 2) is compatible with gingival health (Friedman 1962, De Trey & Bernimoulin 1980). It has also been proposed (Maynard & Wilson 1979) that in segments of the dentition involved in restorative therapy there is a particular demand for attached gingiva. Thus, Maynard & Wilson (1979) claimed that at such sites 3 mm of *attached gingiva*, i.e. about 4-5 mm of *keratinized gingiva*, is required to maintain periodontal health.

As stated above, the opinions expressed regarding the requirement of "sufficient" width of attached and keratinized gingiva for the maintenance of the integrity of the periodontium were based on "clinical experience" rather than scientific evidence. Clinicians had the "impression" that sites with a narrow zone of gingiva (Fig. 17-1) were often inflamed while the wide zone of the gingiva found at neighboring teeth remained healthy. Moreover, it was claimed that the narrow zone of gingiva found apical to a localized soft tissue defect (Fig. 17-2) was a contributing factor in the development of the recession (for review see Hall 1981). "Support" for this clinical impression was obtained from cross-section examinations, performed in humans, showing that a correlation exists between the presence of recession defects and the width of the gingiva (e.g. Stoner & Mazdyasna 1980, Tenenbaum 1982). In this context it should be realized, however, that data derived from cross-sectional studies cannot prove or disprove a cause-effect relationship. Consequently, the data reported from such studies may also be interpreted to demonstrate that the formation of a recession defect results in a reduction of the width of the gingiva. Fig. 17-2 illustrates a lower incisor tooth region and a localized gingival recession at the buccal as-

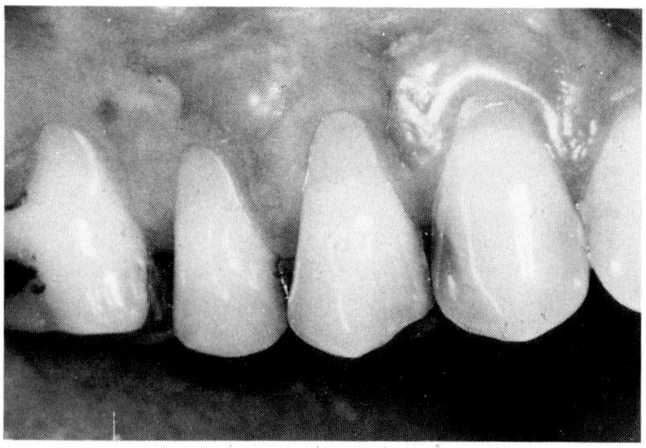

Fig. 17-3. A clinical photograph illustrating gingival recession resulting from improper toothbrushing technique. The marginal gingiva is clinically healthy and abrasion defects can be noted on the exposed roots.

pect of tooth 31. The gingiva apical to the recession defect is narrow - "insufficient" - while at neighboring teeth the gingival width appears to be "adequate". It is reasonable to assume that the gingiva at tooth 32, *before the recession defect developed*, had a width that was similar to that found at tooth 41 and tooth 31. In other words, the narrow zone of gingiva found at tooth 31 may be the result of *loss of gingival tissue during the period of recession development* rather than being the cause of the formation of the defect. If this interpretation is valid the rationale for increasing the width of the gingiva in an area *apical to the existing defect* as a means of preventing further recession may appear to be somewhat obscure.

Localized and generalized recessions of the gingival margin frequently occur in subjects with incipient as well as advanced periodontal disease (e.g. Sangnes & Gjermo 1976, Löe et al. 1978, Lindhe & Nyman 1980, Ånerud et al. 1983, Baelum et al. 1986, 1988, Miller et al. 1987, Okamoto et al. 1988). Soft tissue recessions are also often found at buccal tooth surfaces of otherwise periodontally healthy subjects (e.g. Sangnes & Gjermo 1976, Murtomaa et al. 1987) and are frequently associated with the presence of a "wedge-shaped defect in the crevicular area of one or several teeth" (Sangnes & Gjermo 1976). In subjects with periodontal disease, soft tissue recessions are frequently found also at interproximal and lingual/palatal surfaces (Miller et al. 1987, Yoneyama et al. 1988). More generalized buccal recessions seem to be more common and more advanced at single-rooted teeth than at molars (Yoneyama et al. 1988).

Localized gingival recessions are often found at malaligned teeth which have a buccally deviated position of the root with an accompanying alveolar bone dehiscence (for review see Woofter 1969, Guinard & Caffesse 1977a). Although many etiologies have been proposed for *localized gingival recessions* such as trauma from occlusion, frenal attachments, impingement of restorative margins (Gorman 1967), it is beyond dispute that 1) trauma caused by toothbrushing and 2) gingival lesions associated with plaque must be considered to be the two most important of the causative factors (Woofter 1969, Baker & Seymour 1976). Recessions resulting from improper toothbrushing techniques are often found at sites with clinically healthy gingiva and where the exposed root has a wedge-shaped defect, the surface of which is clean, smooth and polished (Fig. 17-3). Recessions occurring as a result of plaque-associated periodontal disease are found at sites (buccal and/or lingual/palatal) where the gingival tissue is thin (delicate) and where in addition the alveolar bone is thin or absent, i.e. a bone dehiscence is present. The inflammatory lesion that develops in response to subgingival plaque occupies an area of the connective tissue adjacent to the dentogingival epithelium. Measurements made by Waerhaug (1952) suggest that the distance between the periphery of microbial plaque on the tooth surface and the lateral and apical extension of the inflammatory cell infiltrate seldom exceeds 1-2 mm. Thus, if the free gingiva is voluminous the infiltrate will occupy only a small portion of the connective tissue. In a thin and delicate gingiva, however, the entire connective tissue portion may be occupied by the infiltrate. Results from a study in the rat (Baker & Seymour 1976) suggest that proliferation of epithelial cells, from the oral as well as the dento-gingival epithelium, into the thin and degraded connective tissue may bring about a subsidence of the epithelial surface which clinically becomes manifest as recession (Fig. 17-4).

One of the first studies in which attempts were made to evaluate the significance of a narrow gingival zone for the maintenance of periodontal health was carried out by Lang & Löe (1972) on dental students who had their teeth professionally cleaned once a day for 6 weeks. All buccal and lingual sites were examined for plaque, gingival conditions and width of keratinized gingiva. The results showed that gingival health was compatible with a very narrow zone of gingiva. However, despite the fact that the tooth surfaces were free from plaque, all sites with less than 2 mm of keratinized gingiva exhibited persisting clinical signs of inflammation. The authors suggested that 2 mm of *keratinized gingiva*, corresponding to 1 mm of *attached gingiva*, is adequate to maintain gingival health. Observations reported by Miyasato et al. (1977) and Grevers (1977), on the other hand, failed to support the concept that there is a need for a certain minimum width of gingiva if proper oral hygiene is maintained. In these studies it was demonstrated that it is possible to maintain clinically healthy marginal tissue even in areas with less than 1 mm of keratinized gingiva. Furthermore, when the individuals participating in the study by Miyasato et al. (1977) ceased oral hygiene for a period of 25 days, there was no difference in the development of clinical signs of gingival inflammation between areas with a minimal (≤ 1mm) and those with an appreciable (≥ 2mm) width of the gingiva.

The role of *attached gingiva* for gingival health has been studied by Wennström & Lindhe (1983a, b). Following experimentally induced periodontal tissue breakdown around premolar and molar teeth in one side of the

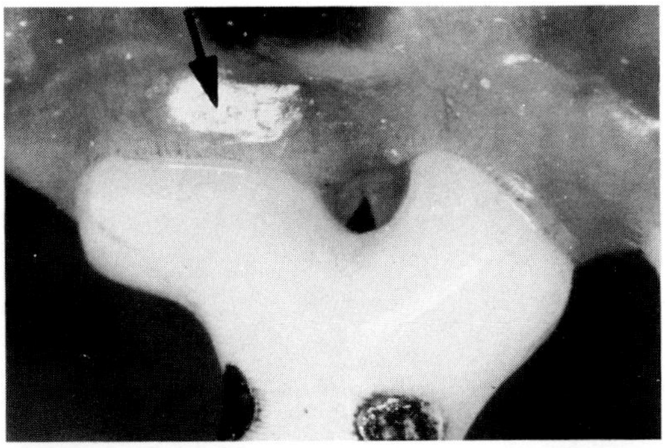

Fig. 17-4a.

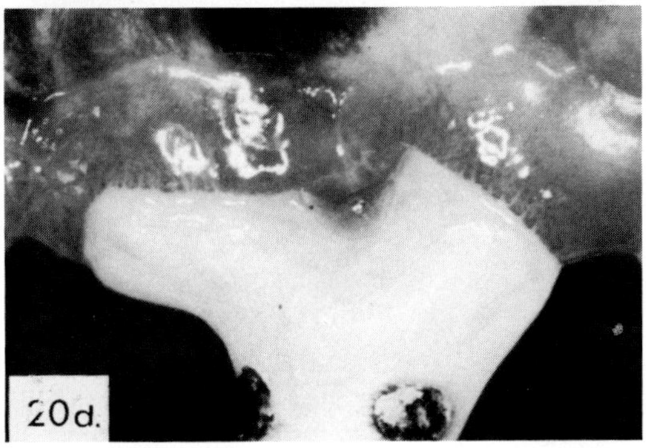

Fig. 17-4b.

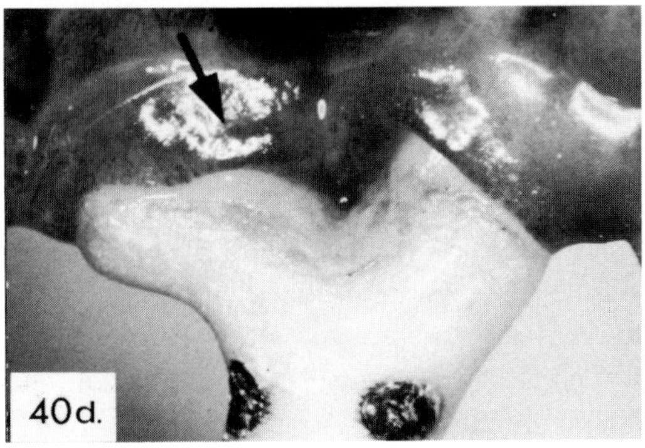

Fig. 17-4c.

Fig. 17-4a-c. Clinical photographs illustrating the development of a gingival recession as a result of plaque-induced inflammation in a beagle dog. Note the thin but healthy gingiva (arrow) at the start of the plaque accumulation period (a). Pronounced clinical signs of inflammation are seen after 20 days (b) and after 40 days of no tooth cleaning, the gingival margin has receded (c).

jaws in dogs, the resulting periodontal pockets were eliminated by a flap procedure. However, before the flaps were sutured back against the teeth, all gingival tissue was excised. Accord-

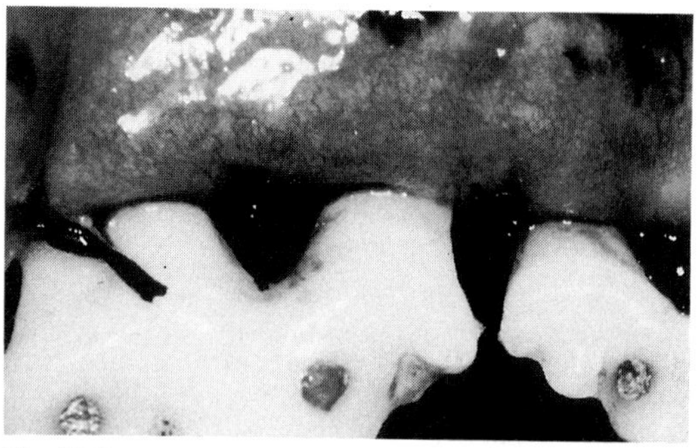

Fig. 17-5a.

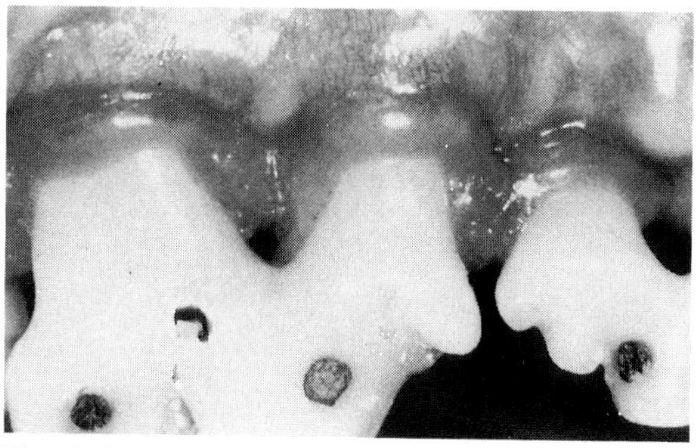

Fig. 17-5b.

Fig. 17-5a-b. All gingival tissue has been excised and the alveolar mucosa sutured to close adaptation to the roots (a). Healing consistently resulted in the reestablishment of a narrow band of keratinized gingiva even if no attached gingiva was formed (b).

ingly, the alveolar mucosa constituted the marginal tissue immediately following surgery (Fig. 17-5a). Healing consistently resulted in the reestablishment of a narrow band of keratinized gingiva (Fig. 17-5b), even if no attached gingiva was formed. A free gingival graft was subsequently placed in one of the surgically treated quadrants in order to regain a zone of attached gingiva (Fig. 17-6). In the same dogs, the teeth in one quadrant were deprived of their entire gingiva whereas one quadrant was left surgically untreated (Fig. 17-7). Hence, 4 types of dentogingival unit with different clinical characteristics were established; 1) units with recession and lack of attached gingiva, 2) units with recession and a wide zone of attached gingiva, 3) units with no recession and lack of attached gingiva, and 4)

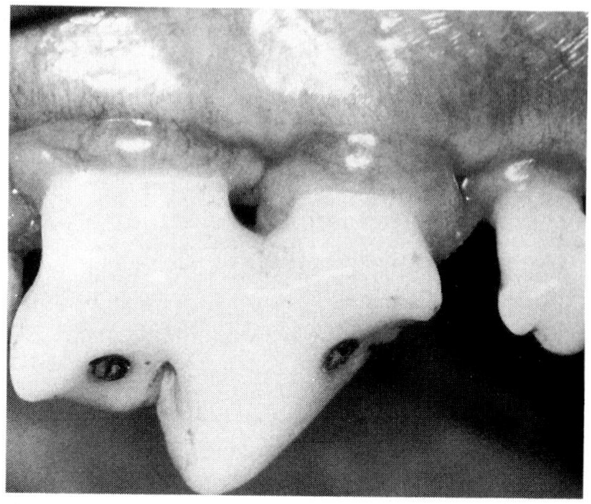

Fig. 17-6a.

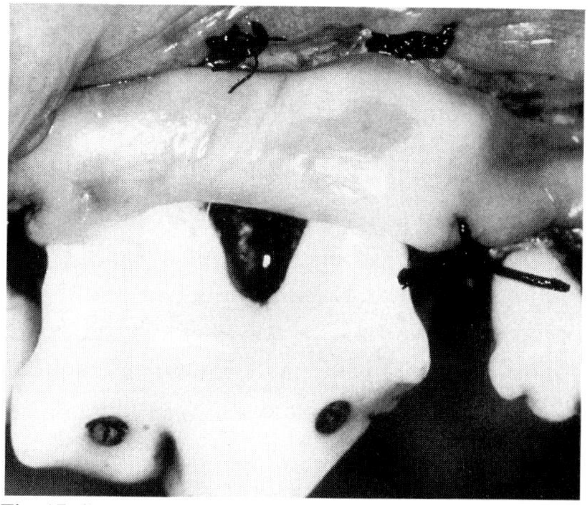

Fig. 17-6b.

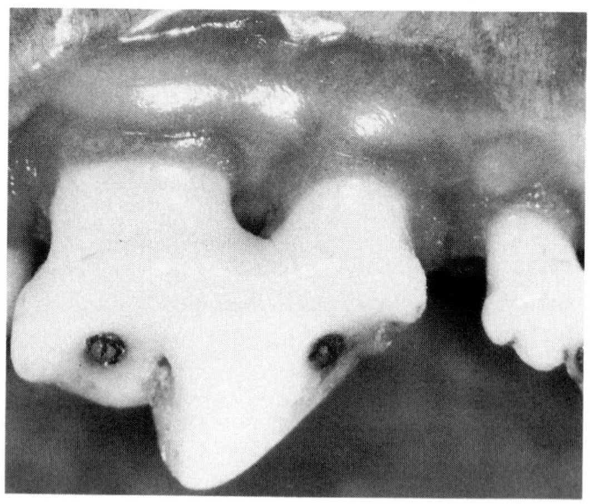

Fig. 17-6c.

Fig. 17-6a-c. A free gingival graft was placed in one of the surgically treated quadrants in order to regain a zone of attached gingiva (a-b). The healed area revealed the presence of a wide zone of attached and keratinized gingiva (c).

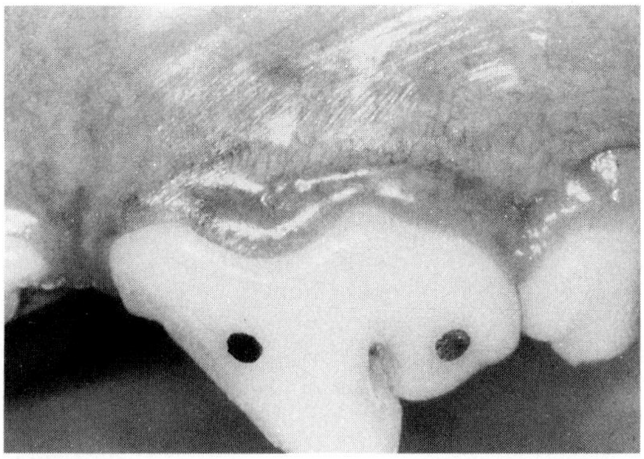

Fig. 17-7a.

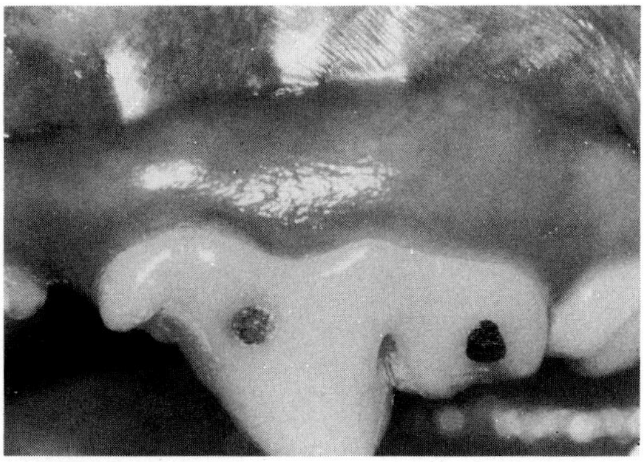

Fig. 17-7b.

Fig. 17-7a-b. Two teeth in a dog with varying dimensions of the marginal gingiva. A buccal tooth site with an unattached, narrow band of gingiva (a) and a site with a wide zone of attached and keratinized gingiva (b).

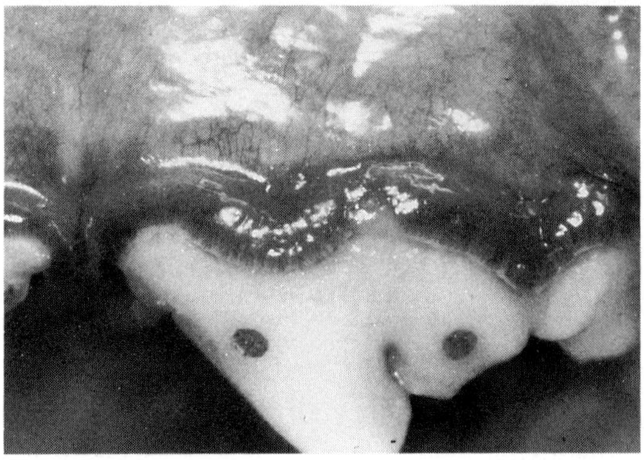

Fig. 17-8a.

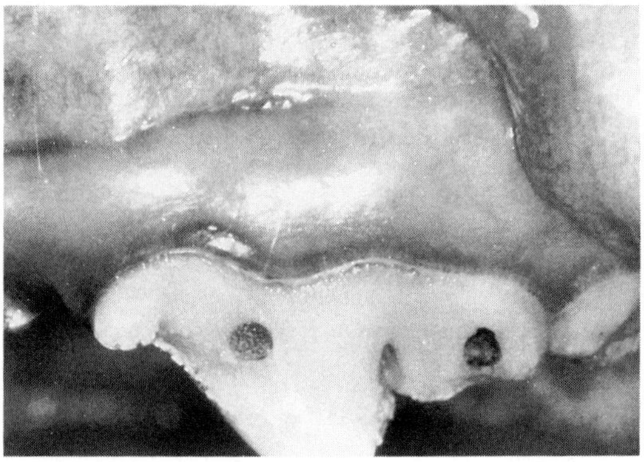

Fig. 17-8b.

Fig. 17-8a-b. The same teeth as in Fig. 17-7a,b after 40 days of plaque accumulation. The clinical signs of inflammation are more pronounced at the site with the narrow band of gingiva (a) than at the site with the wide zone of attached gingiva (b).

units with no recession and a normal wide zone of attached gingiva.

When, after the healing period, plaque was allowed to accumulate (for 40 days), clinical signs of inflammation developed which were more pronounced in tooth regions with lack of attached gingiva (Fig. 17-8a) than in areas with presence of a wide attached zone of gingiva (Fig. 17-8b). However, histologic analysis revealed that, although areas without attached gingiva exhibited more pronounced clinical signs of inflammation (redness and swelling) than areas with attached gingiva, the size of the inflammatory cell infiltrate and its extension in the apical direction (an assessment which indirectly may be used as an estimate of the apical migration of the bacterial plaque) were similar in the two categories of dentogingival units. Compared to the gingival units with a wide zone of attached gingiva, the units lacking gingiva were thinner in the buccolingual direction and their covering oral epithelium had a comparatively thinner keratin layer. This presumably made the vascular system more readily visible from the buccal aspect of the gingival units and can explain why areas with only a narrow gingival zone and lack of attached gingiva clinically appeared more inflamed than those with a wide zone of attached gingiva. Thus, the results of this study do not lend support to the view that a narrow and unattached zone of gingiva is less resistant to plaque infec-

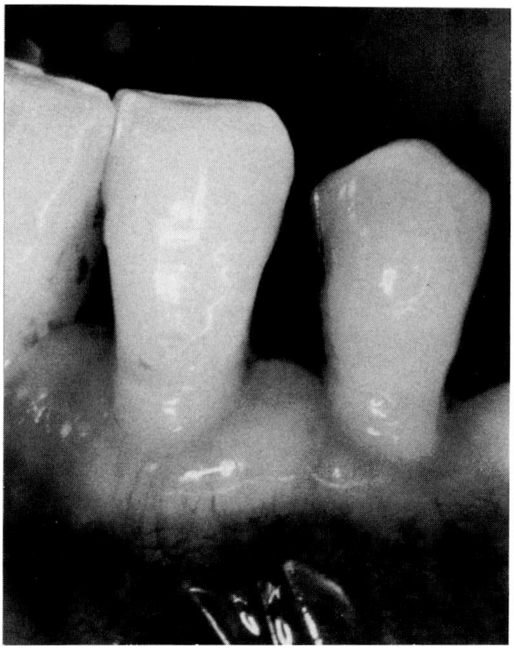

Fig. 17-9a.

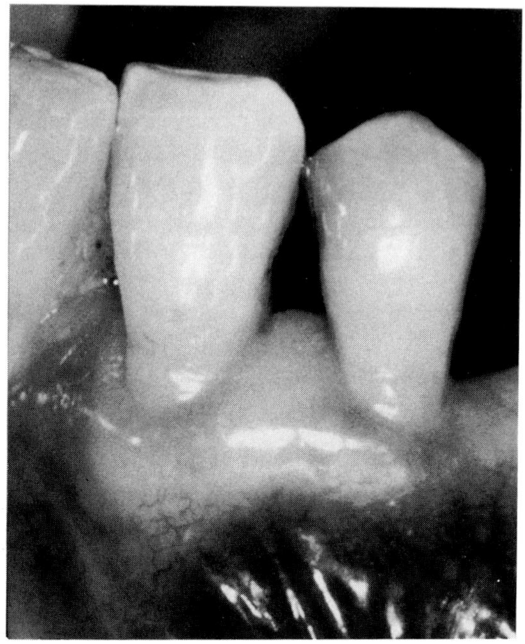

Fig. 17-9b.

Fig. 17-9a-b. Clinical photographs of a canine and a first premolar in the mandibular jaw with < 1 mm of attached gingiva 6 months after surgical treatment (a). Note the increase of the width of the gingiva at the facial aspect of the teeth and the more coronally positioned gingival margin 5 years later (b).

tion than a wide and attached gingival zone. In addition it was observed that, in the absence of microbial plaque, the gingival units were free from clinical as well as histological signs of inflammation irrespective of the presence or absence of attached gingiva or recession.

The observation made in the study by Wennström & Lindhe (1983b) that the clinical signs of gingival inflammation did not correspond with the size of the inflammatory cell infiltrate illustrates the difficulties inherent in the interpretation of data from clinical examinations made in areas with varying width of gingiva. This should be kept in mind when interpreting the data of Lang & Löe (1972) showing that clinically visible signs of inflammation, such as redness and swelling, were more frequent in areas with less than 2 mm of keratinized gingiva (i.e. approximately 1 mm of attached gingiva) than in areas with a wider zone of gingiva.

Results obtained from a number of recent longitudinal studies in patients showing areas with a minimal zone of gingiva support the conclusion that a certain quantity of gingiva is not essential for the maintenance of periodontal health and the preclusion of soft tissue recessions. Lindhe & Nyman (1980) examined the alterations of the position of the gingival margin following periodontal surgery in 43 patients with advanced periodontal breakdown. Following active treatment, all patients were recalled once every 3-6 months for maintenance care. The position of the soft tissue margin in relation to the cemento-enamel junction was assessed on the facial aspect of all teeth after initial healing and after 10-11 years of maintenance. The presence or absence of keratinized gingiva was also determined. The results showed that both in areas with and without a visible keratinized border-tissue after healing, a small coronal regrowth (=1 mm) of the soft tissue margin had occurred during the period of maintenance. In other words, no recession was observed in this group of patients maintained

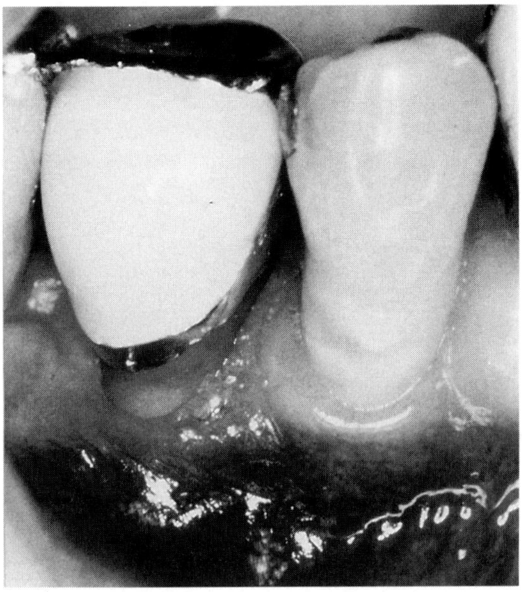

Fig. 17-10a.

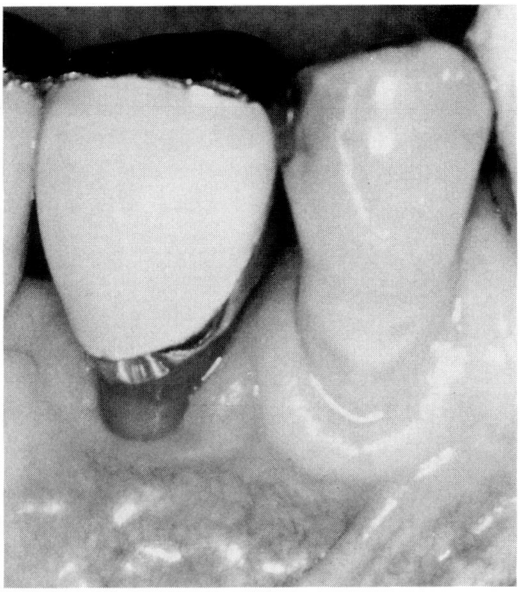

Fig. 17-10b.

Fig. 17-10a-b. A mandibular canine and first premolar tooth region showing a very narrow zone of gingiva 6 months following surgical therapy (a). No major change in the position of the soft tissue margin has occurred during a 5-year period despite the lack of attached gingiva (b).

on a careful prophylaxis program.

Dorfman et al. (1982) reported a 4-year follow-up study including 22 patients with bilateral tooth areas exhibiting gingival recession and lack of *attached gingiva.* In conjunction with scaling and root planing a free gingival graft was placed on one side while the contralateral control side was treated by scaling and root planing only. All patients were recalled for prophylaxis once every 3-6 months during a 4-year period. The data obtained from examinations of the non-grafted control areas revealed that no further recession of the soft tissue margin or loss of probing attachment had occurred despite the lack of attached gingiva. In fact, there was a slight gain of probing attachment. The authors concluded that recession sites with lack of attached gingiva will not develop further attachment loss and recession if the inflammation is controlled, a conclusion which was also valid in their 6-year report on the same patient material (Kennedy et al. 1985). The latter report also included data on 10 patients who had not participated in the maintenance phase of treatment for a period of 5 years. In these patients plaque and clinical signs of inflammation as well as some further recession were noted at the 5-year examination as compared with the data obtained after termination of active treatment. Except for the clinical signs of inflammation, which were more pronounced in non-grafted sites, no differences were observed between control sites with < 1 mm or complete lack of attached gingiva and grafted sites. These clinical observations confirm and extend the conclusion reached in the experimental study discussed above (Wennström & Lindhe 1983b) that a narrow and unattached zone of gingiva is not less resistant to plaque infection than a wide and attached gingival zone.

The lack of relationship between the width of *attached gingiva* and the development of soft tissue recession is further substantiated by results from longitudinal studies reported by Schoo & van der Velden (1985), Kisch et al.

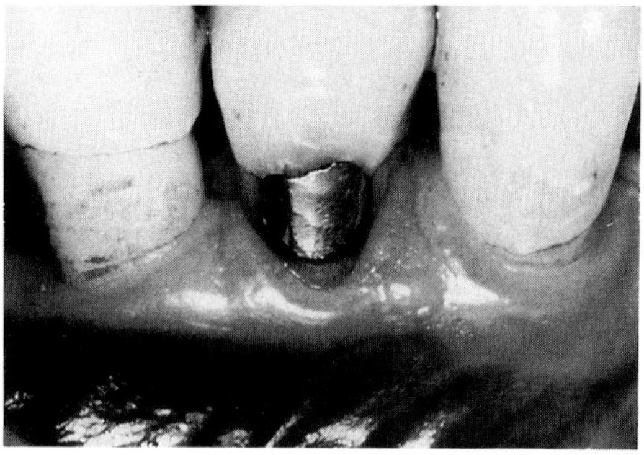

Fig. 17-11a.

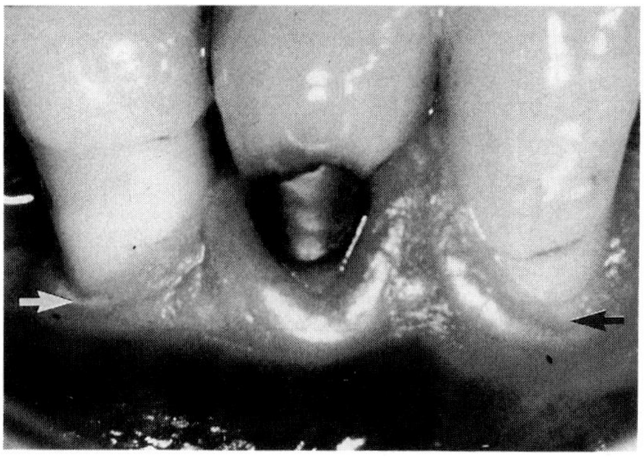

Fig. 17-11b.

Fig. 17-11a-b. Clinical photographs of the mandibular right canine-premolar tooth region in the patient showing several sites with apical displacement of the soft tissue margin during the 5 years of observation. At the initial examination the 2 premolars had < 1 mm and the canine > 1 mm of attached gingiva (a). After 5 years (b) recession and loss of gingival tissue can be seen on the buccal aspect of the canine which initially had an "adequate" width of attached gingiva (black arrow). The second premolar also showed further apical displacement of the soft tissue margin (white arrow).

(1986), Salkin et al. (1987) and Wennström (1987). The study by Wennström (1987) reports observations made at 26 buccal sites surgically deprived of all keratinized gingiva. A baseline examination carried out 6 months after treatment revealed that these sites had regained a zone of gingiva which was not attached or had a minimal (< 1 mm) portion attached to the underlying hard tissues (Figs. 17-9a and 17-10a). Adjacent teeth with > 1 mm of attached gingiva were also included in the examinations. In most sites the position of the soft tissue margin had been maintained unchanged over the 5 years (Figs. 17-9b and 17-10b). A further apical displacement of the soft tissue margin had occurred at 2 out of 26 sites with < 1 mm attached gingiva and at 3 out of 12 adjacent control sites with > 1 mm attached gingiva. Since 4 of these 5 sites were found in one patient (Fig. 17-11), and all sites were free from clinical signs of inflammation, excessive toothbrushing was considered to be the causative factor. It was also observed that the development of soft tissue recession at the control sites resulted in a decreased width of the gingiva (Fig. 17-11), an observation that supports the hypothesis that a narrow zone of gingiva apical to a localized recession is a consequence rather than a cause of the recession.

Although both anecdotal data and results from clinical research have documented that most forms of orthodontic therapy are innocuous to the periodontium (see Chapter 23), some patients obviously respond to frontal movements of incisors and lateral movements of posterior teeth by gingival recession and loss of attachment (Fig. 17-12) (Pearson 1968, Maynard & Ochsenbein 1975, Coatoam et al. 1981, Foushee et al. 1985). As discussed above, recession of the soft tissue margin is often associated with alveolar bone dehiscences. Such a "predisposing" factor is commonly found at malaligned teeth, but may also be induced by orthodontic tooth movement. It has been claimed that recession of the gingiva may occur during orthodontic therapy involving sites which have an inadequate zone of gingiva (for review see Hall 1981), and that a grafting procedure therefore should precede the initiation of orthodontic therapy in such areas (Boyd 1978, Maynard & Wilson 1980, Hall 1981).

Gingival tissue alterations occurring as a result of labial orthodontic tooth movement have been analyzed in a number of experimental studies. Batenhorst et al. (1974) and Steiner et al. (1981) used the monkey as an experimental animal and studied tissue alterations following either tipping and extrusion movements or bod-

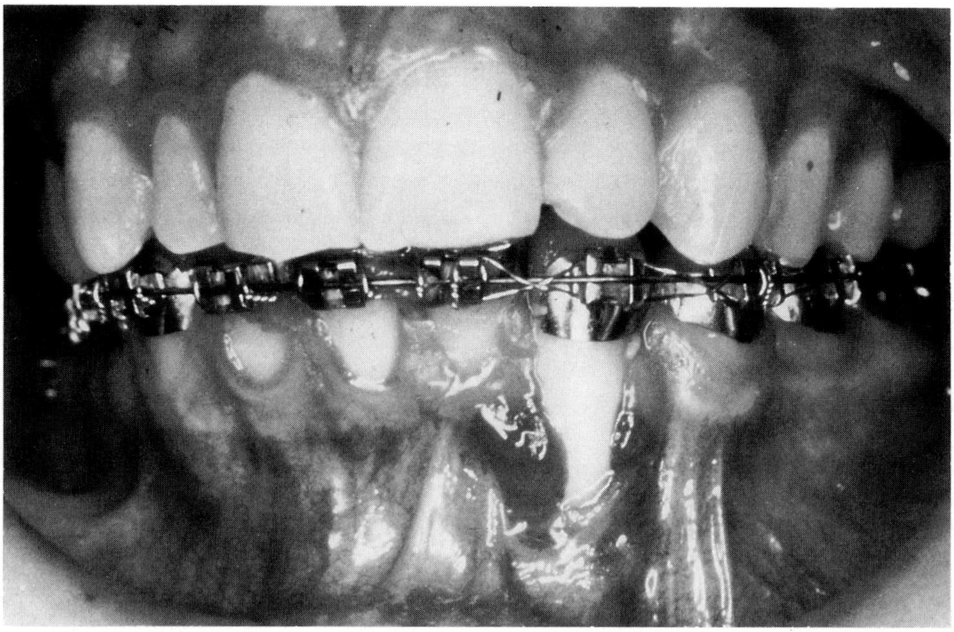

Fig. 17-12. Clinical photograph showing an advanced gingival recession on the buccal aspect of tooth 43 which developed during orthodontic treatment involving labial tooth movement of the canine.

ily movements of incisors. It was reported that such tooth movements resulted in recession of the labial gingival margin and loss of attachment. However, similar studies carried out in dogs (Karring et al. 1982, Nyman et al. 1982) or humans (Rateitschak et al. 1968) have failed to demonstrate that labial tooth movement is accompanied by gingival recession and attachment loss. This discrepancy in the response of the marginal soft tissue to orthodontic therapy in the studies referred to is difficult to conceive but may be related to differences with respect to 1) the amount of labial tooth displacement, 2) the magnitude of force applied, 3) the presence/absence of plaque and gingival inflammation in the regions subjected to tooth movement and/or 4) differences in the width of the gingiva. Steiner et al. (1981) speculated on mechanisms by which gingival tissue could be lost as a result of labial tooth movement and suggested that tension in the marginal tissue created by the forces applied to the teeth could be an important factor. If this hypothesis is valid, obviously the volume (thickness) of the gingival tissue at the pressure side rather than its apico-coronal width should determine whether or not gingival recession develops during orthodontic therapy.

Support for this hypothesis is obtained from a recently reported experimental study in monkeys (Wennström et al. 1987) in which teeth were orthodontically moved into areas with varying thickness and quality of periodontal tissues. Following extensive bodily movement of incisors in a labial direction through the alveolar bone (Fig. 17-13), most teeth showed a small apical displacement of the gingival margin but no loss of connective tissue attachment (Fig. 17-14). In other words, the apical displacement of the gingival margin was the result of a reduced height of the free gingiva (Fig. 17-15), which in turn may be related to tension - "stretching" - in the soft tissues during the facial tooth movement. At the 2 teeth which showed loss of connective tissue attachment, obvious clinical signs of inflammation were present throughout the experimental period, an observation that also was reported by Steiner et

a

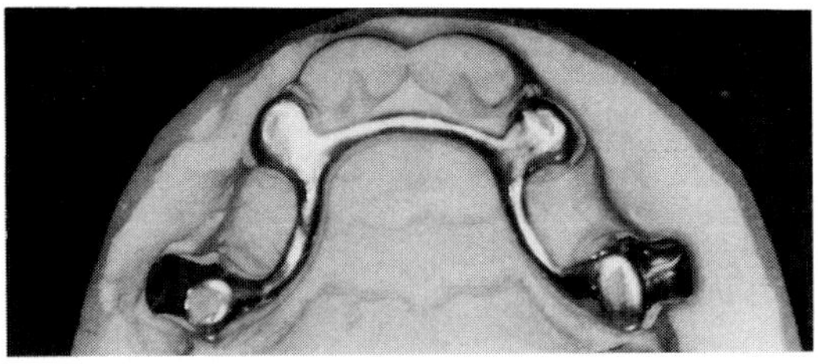

b

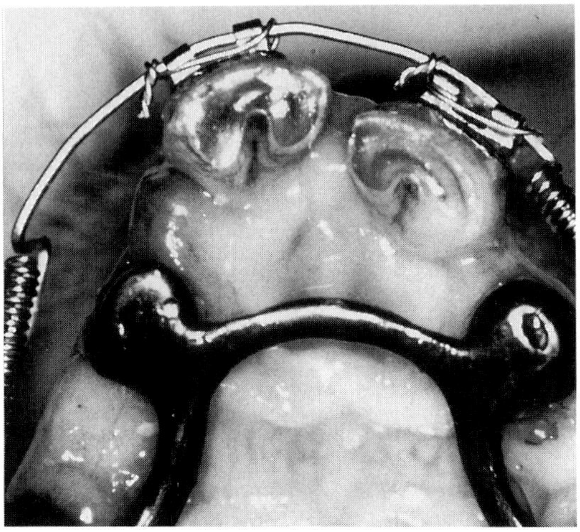

Fig. 17-13a-b. Occlusal view of the maxillary jaw in a monkey showing the position of the central incisors before (a) and after (b) the bodily movement in labial direction. The canines and the lateral incisors were joined in an individual fabricated silver splint and used as anchorage teeth.

a

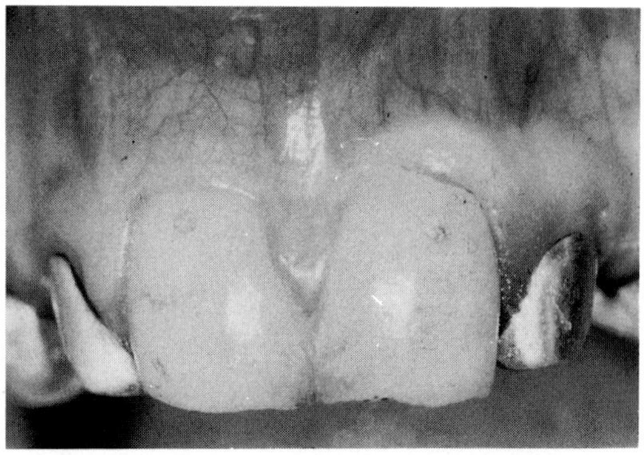

b

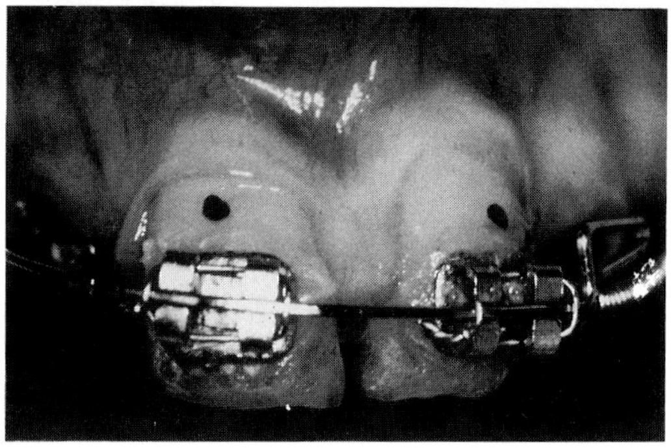

Fig. 17-14a-b. The buccal aspect of the central incisors in the same monkey as in Fig. 17-13, before (a) and after (b) the labial tooth movement. No change in the location of the gingival margin has occurred despite the pronounced labial displacement of the incisors.

al. (1981). No relationship was found between the initial apico-coronal width of keratinized and attached gingiva and the degree of apical displacement of the gingival margin during orthodontic therapy. Furthermore, there was no significant difference in terms of attachment between teeth which had been bodily moved *within the alveolar bone* into areas lined by alveolar mucosa or keratinized gingiva. Hence, the studies reported emphasize the importance of an adequate plaque control during orthodontic treatment. The clinical implication of the results is also that labial tooth movement should be preceded by careful examination of the dimensions of the tissues covering the facial aspect of the teeth to be moved. As long as the tooth can be moved within the envelope of the alveolar process, the risk of harmful side-effects in the gingival tissue is minimal, irrespective of the dimensions and quality of the soft tissues. If, however, the tooth movement is expected to result in the establishment of an alveolar bone dehiscence, the volume (thickness) of the covering soft tissue must be considered as a factor which determines whether gingival recessions will occur during and/or after the phase of active orthodontic therapy. A thin gingiva may serve as a *locus minoris resistentia* to developing soft tissue defects especially in the presence of bacterial plaque.

In conclusion, scientific data obtained from well-controlled clinical and experimental studies have unequivocally demonstrated that the apico-coronal width of gingiva and the presence or absence of an attached portion of gingiva are not of decisive importance for the maintenance of gingival health and the height of the periodontal tissues. The results of the

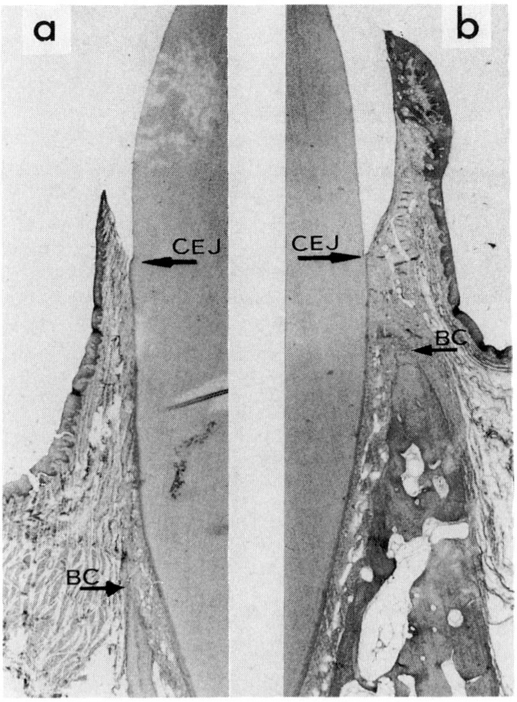

Fig. 17-15a-b. Histologic specimens showing (a) reduced alveolar bone height at an incisor bodily moved in labial direction and (b) normal alveolar bone height at a non-moved control tooth. Note the maintained level of connective tissue attachment and the reduced height of the free gingiva at the labially displaced incisor (a).

CEJ: cemento-enamel junction, BC: alveolar bone crest.

studies discussed also lend support to the concept that there are no reasons from a clinical point of view to distinguish between free and attached gingiva. As proposed by the scientific group of the World Health Organization (WHO 1978) the term *gingiva* is sufficient to describe the collagen-rich, keratinized soft tissue between the gingival margin and the mucogingival junction.

Indications for mucogingival surgery

As mentioned above, recent studies have failed to support the traditional concept that a certain width of attached and keratinized gingiva is necessary for the maintenance of periodontal health. Consequently, the presence of a narrow zone of gingiva cannot *per se* be considered as an indication for surgical intervention. However, this does not preclude that mucogingival surgery should be recommended in situations where e.g. gingival recession is creating esthetic problems and a gingival coverage of an exposed root surface is desirable. Hence, in addition to the general indications for periodontal surgery discussed in Chapter 16, the following situations may call for mucogingival therapy:

- Areas where a change of the morphology of the gingival margin would facilitate proper plaque control. This may be the case e.g. in the presence of a high frenulum attachment, a deep and narrow recession defect, and where a recession extends to the level of the vestibular fornix.
- Areas with a localized soft tissue recession which create esthetic or root sensitivity problems.
- A thin gingiva facial to a tooth which is planned for orthodontic tooth movement and where the final positioning of the tooth can be expected to result in an alveolar bone dehiscence. By increasing the thickness of the covering tissue the risk for development of soft tissue recession following orthodontic therapy may be reduced.

Modalities of surgical therapy

The treatment areas with mucogingival problems must, like all other conditions associated with destructive periodontal disease, include the removal of hard and soft bacterial deposits from the teeth and be followed by proper plaque control. In this context it should also be recalled that the two major causative factors in the development of gingival recessions are plaque-induced periodontal inflammation and trauma caused by toothbrushing. The control of these factors will in most cases prevent further progression of the recession. This means that in tooth regions with a thin covering soft tissue with or without an incipient recession, the patient must be encouraged to carry out effective but at the same time non-traumatic plaque control measures. With respect to toothbrushing technique, the Bass' method should be avoided and the patient should be instructed to use a less traumatizing technique. A soft toothbrush should be used.

The procedures included in "mucogingival surgery" are used either in combination with pocket elimination procedures or alone to correct a gingival aberration in areas without pocket formation. The earliest of these techniques are the "vestibular extension operations" which were designed mainly with the objective of extending the depth of the vestibular sulcus (Bohannan 1962a, b). In recent years, however, the use of pedicle, soft tissue grafts, free gingival grafts and subepithelial connective tissue grafts have become the most commonly used techniques in the management of mucogingival problems, because the healing results following these procedures are more predictable than those following the "vestibular extension operations".

Vestibular extension operations

The vestibular extension operations comprise a number of surgical techniques, which have been developed mainly on an empirical basis and without sufficient knowledge about the biology of the involved tissues. The treatment includes the removal of the soft tissue within an area extending from the gingival margin to a level apical to the mucogingival junction (Fig. 17-16). With the "denudation technique" all soft tissue is removed within the wound area leaving the alveolar bone completely exposed (Ochsenbein 1960, Corn 1962, Wilderman 1964).

Healing following this type of treatment often results in an increased width of the gingival zone, although in some cases only a very limited effect is observed. The exposure of alveolar bone produces severe bone resorption with permanent loss of bone height (Wilderman et al. 1961, Costich & Ramfjord 1968). In addition, the recession of marginal gingiva in the surgical area often exceeds the gain of gingiva obtained in the apical portion of the wound (Carranza & Carraro 1963, Carraro et al. 1964). Due to these complications, together with severe postoperative pain for the patient, the use of the "denudation technique" for the management of mucogingival problems can hardly be justified.

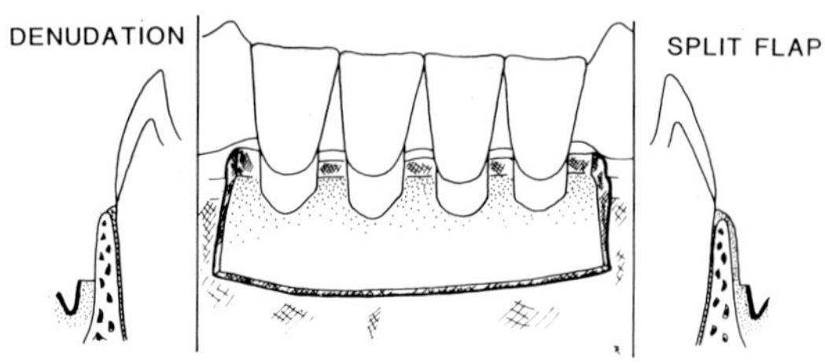

Fig. 17-16. The use of vestibular extension operations for increasing the width of the gingiva involves the production of a wound extending from the gingival margin to a level some mm apical to the mucogingival junction. With the "denudation" technique all soft tissue is removed leaving the alveolar bone exposed. With the "split flap" procedure only the superficial portion of the oral mucosa is removed leaving the bone covered with connective tissue.

With the "periosteal retention" procedure or "split flap" procedure (fig. 17-16) only the superficial portion of the oral mucosa within the wound area is removed, leaving the bone covered by periosteum (Staffileno et al. 1962, Wilderman 1963, Pfeifer 1965, Staffileno et al. 1966). Although the preservation of the periosteum implies that less severe bone resorption will occur than following the "denudation technique", loss of crestal bone height has also been observed following this type of operation unless a relatively thick layer of connective tissue is retained on the bone surface (Costich & Ramfjord 1968). If a thick layer is not secured, the periosteal connective tissue tends to undergo necrosis and the subsequent healing

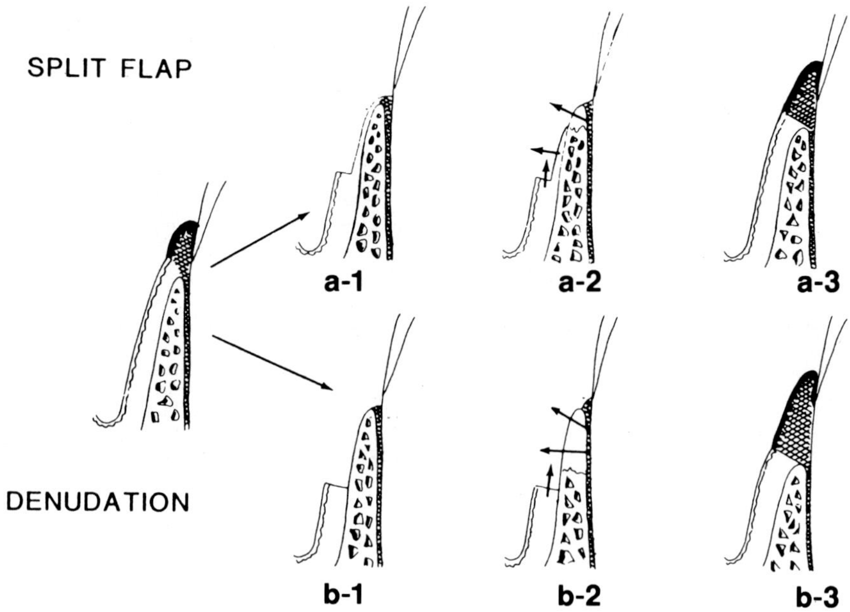

Fig. 17-17. Schematic drawing illustrating different stages of healing following the "split flap" (a) and "denudation" (b) techniques. Cells from the oral mucosa, bone and periodontal ligament (arrows) participate in granulation tissue formation. Due to the difference in the degree of bone resorption (a-2, b-2), a larger area of the coronal portion of the wound is filled with granulation tissue from the periodontal ligament following "denudation" than following the "split flap" technique. Since granulation tissue from the periodontal ligament possesses the ability to induce a keratinized epitelium, "denudation" usually results in a wider zone of keratinized gingiva than is the case following the "split flap" technique (a-3, b-3).

will closely resemble that following the "denudation technique" described above.

Other vestibular extension operations or mucogingival procedures which have been used for increasing the width of the gingival zone may in fact be considered as modifications of the "denudation" and "split flap" techniques or combinations of these procedures. The apically repositioned flap procedure (Friedman 1962), for instance, involves the elevation of soft tissue flaps and their displacement during suturing in an apical position, often leaving 3-5 mm of alveolar bone denuded in the coronal part of the surgical area. This involves the same risk for extensive bone resorption as the "denudation technique". It has been reported that a predictable post-surgical result with respect to increase of the width of the gingiva may be obtained following the "apically repositioned flap" (Friedman 1962), while other studies have indicated that the presurgical width is retained or becomes only slightly increased (Donnenfeld et al. 1964, Carranza & Carraro 1970).

The use of vestibular extension operations for increasing the width of the gingival zone was based on the assumption that it is the frictional forces encountered during mastication which determine the presence of a keratinized gingiva adjacent to the teeth (Orban 1957, Pfeifer 1963). Therefore, it was believed that by the displacement of muscle attachments and the extension of vestibular depth, the regenerating tissue in the surgical area would be sub-

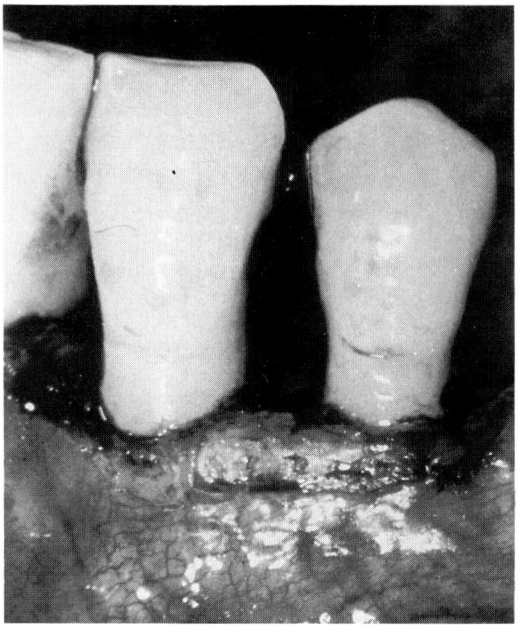

Fig. 17-18a.

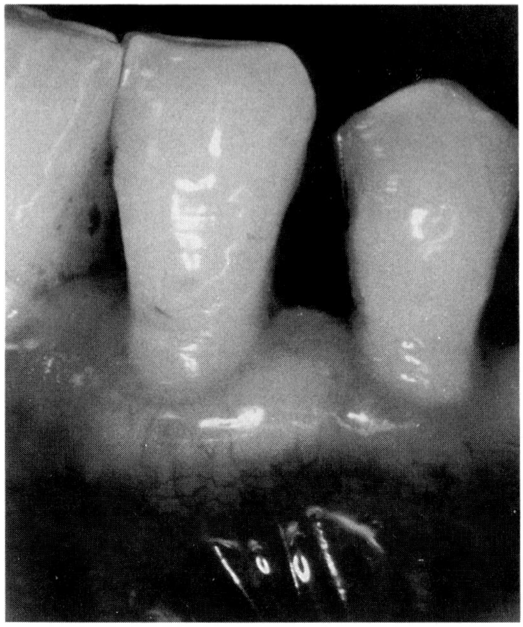

Fig. 17-18b.

Fig. 17-18a-b. Clinical photographs of the buccal aspect of a canine and a premolar following the removal of the entire zone of gingiva by a gingivectomy procedure (a). The healing results 9 months after surgery (b) shows the regain of a certain zone of keratinized gingiva.

jected to physical impacts and adapt to the same functional requirements as those met by "normal" keratinized gingiva (Ivancie 1957, Bradley et al. 1959, Pfeifer 1963). Later studies, however, have shown that the characteristic features of the gingiva are determined by some inherent factors in the tissue rather than being the result of functional adaptation and that the differentation (keratinization) of the gingival epithelium is controlled by morphogenetic stimuli from the underlying connective tissue (see Chapter 1).

Healing

Since the specificity of the gingiva is determined by some inherent factor in the tissues, the postoperative results of vestibular extension procedures depend on the degree to which the various tissues contribute to the formation of granulation tissue in the wound area (Karring et al. 1975a,b). Following the "denudation" or "split flap technique", the wound area is filled with granulation tissue derived from the periodontal ligament, the tissue of the bone marrow spaces, the retained periosteal connective tissue, and the surrounding gingiva and alveolar mucosa (Fig. 17-17). The degree of bone resorption induced by the surgical trauma influences the relative amount of granulation tissue which grows into the wound from these various tissue sources. The resorption of crestal bone exposes varying amounts of the periodontal ligament tissue in the marginal area, allowing granulation tissue from the periodontal ligament to fill out the coronal portion of the wound. The greater the bone loss, the greater the portion of the wound which becomes filled with granulation tissue from the periodontal ligament. This particular tissue possesses the ability to induce keratinization of the gingival epithelium. This means that the widening of the keratinized gingiva following "denudation" and "split flap" operations is achieved at the expense of a reduced bone height. The "denu-

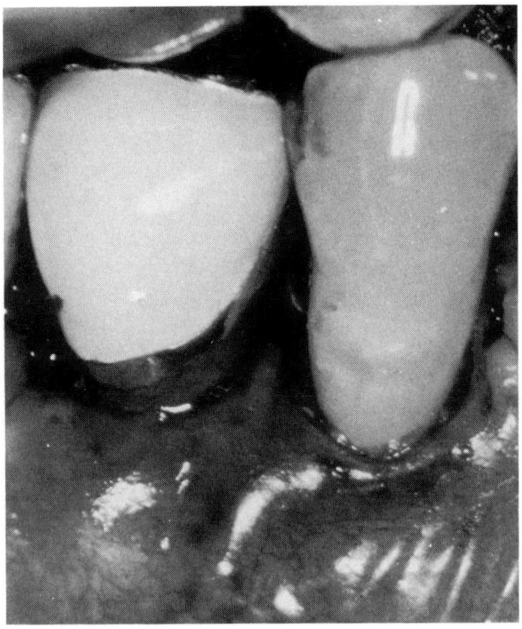

Fig. 17-19a.

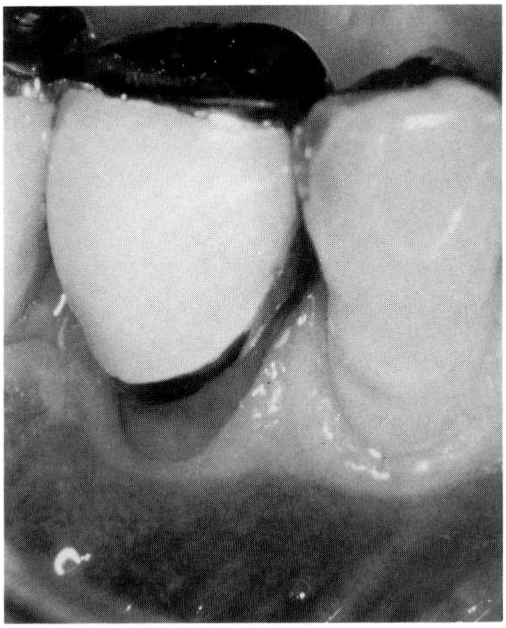

Fig. 17-19b.

Fig. 17-19a-b. Clinical photographs of a tooth region subjected to excision of the entire zone of gingiva by a flap procedure. The alveolar mucosa has been coronally displaced to achieve complete coverage of the surgically exposed alveolar bone (a). Healing has resulted in the reformation of a narrow zone of keratinized gingiva on the buccal aspect of the teeth; 9 months post-surgery (b).

dation technique" results usually in more bone loss than the "split flap technique". Therefore, a greater amount of granulation tissue with the ability to induce a keratinized gingival epithelium develops in the marginal area following the "denudation technique" than following the "split flap technique". This is in accordance with the clinical observation that the "denudation technique" usually is superior to the "split flap technique" in increasing the width of keratinized gingiva (Bohannan 1962a, b).

It is concluded that the success or failure in extending the width of keratinized gingiva by the "denudation" or "split flap" techniques rests with the origin of granulation tissue which is related to the extent of bone loss induced by the surgical trauma. This in turn means that the result with respect to increasing the gingival width by methods involving periosteal exposure or denudation of the alveolar bone is unpredictable. The use of such methods is therefore not justified in periodontal therapy. The procedures discussed represent examples on how lack of knowledge about basic biological principles may lead to the development of inappropriate therapeutic methods.

In the clinical study by Wennström (1983), periodontal pockets were eliminated by the use of a "gingivectomy" or a "flap" procedure, both of which involved the complete removal of the keratinized gingiva. In the "gingivectomy" procedure the wounded area was left to heal by second intention, while in the "flap" procedure the alveolar mucosa was repositioned to achieve complete coverage of the surgically exposed bone (Figs. 17-18a and 19a). Irrespective of the surgical technique used, healing resulted in the reformation of keratinized gingiva, the width of which, however, was greater following the "gingivectomy" procedure than following the "flap" procedure (Figs. 17-18b and 19b). The gingiva was

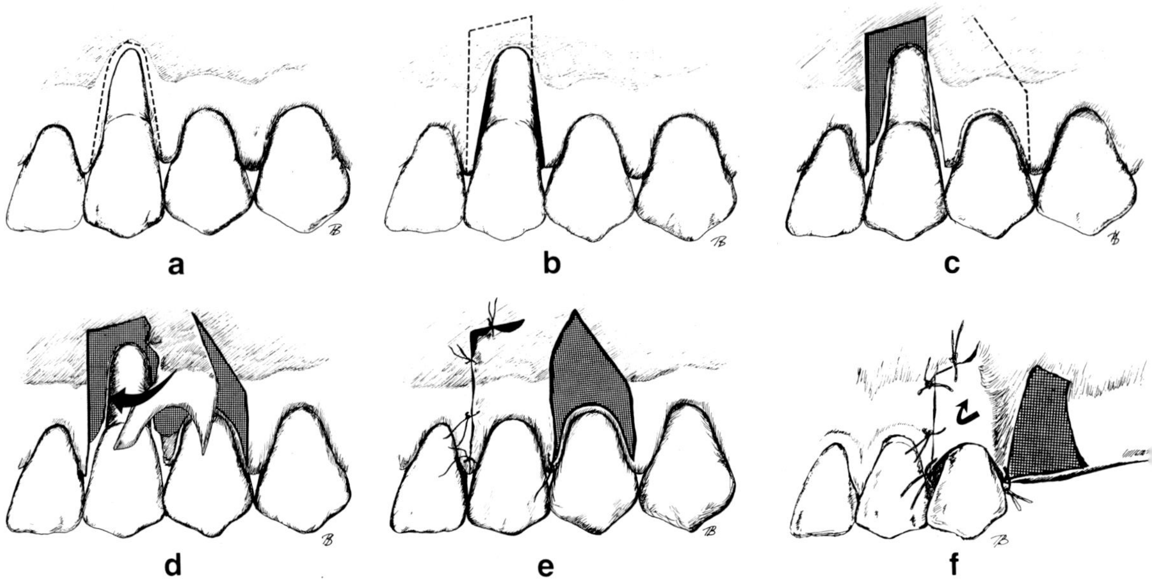

Fig. 17-20a-f. Schematic drawings illustrating the surgical technique for utilizing pedicle grafts to cover localized gingival recessions. Fig. 17-20e illustrates a laterally repositioned flap, and Fig. 17-20f a rotated flap.

formed because granulation tissue from the periodontal ligament with capacity to induce a keratinized epithelium had proliferated coronally along the root surface. This granulation tissue formation was obviously favored by a more pronounced bone resorption during the healing following the "gingivectomy" procedure.

Transplantation of gingiva and palatal mucosa

Studies have shown that gingival and palatal soft tissues maintain their original characteristics after transplantation to areas of the alveolar mucosa (see Chapter 1). Thus, in contrast to vestibular extension operations, the use of transplants offers the potential to predict the postsurgical result. For that reason, transplants have become commonly used in the treatment of mucogingival problems in recent years (Haggerty 1966, Nabers 1966, Sullivan & Atkins 1968a, b, Hawley & Staffileno 1970, Edel 1974, Matter 1982, Raetzke 1985). The type of transplants used can be divided into 1) pedicle grafts, which after placement at the recipient site maintain their connection with the donor site and 2) free grafts which are completely deprived of their connection with the donor area.

Pedicle grafts (sliding flaps; lateral, coronal)
Laterally repositioned flaps were introduced in periodontal therapy to cover areas with localized gingival recession and to gain keratinized or attached gingiva (Grupe & Warren 1956). This technique involves the reflection of a full thickness flap in a donor area adjacent to the defect and the subsequent displacement of this flap to cover the exposed root surface. More recent modifications of this technique (Staffileno 1964, Pfeifer & Heller 1971) utilize a split thickness flap in order to prevent recession of the gingiva at the donor site. A modification of the sliding procedure is the double papilla flap (Cohen & Ross 1968).

The laterally repositioned flap procedure is initiated with the preparation of the recipient site (Fig. 17-20). A reverse bevel incision is made all along the gingival margin of the defect (Fig. 17-20a). After removal of the dissected pocket epithelium, the exposed root surface is thoroughly curetted. At a distance of approximately 3 mm from the wound edge which delineates the defect at the side opposite the donor site, a superficial incision is made extending from the gingival margin to a level approximately 3 mm apical to the defect (Fig. 17-20b). Another superficial incision is then placed horizontally from this incision to the opposite wound edge (Fig. 17-20b). The epithelium and the outer portion of the connective tissue within the area delineated by these incisions and the wound edges is removed by sharp dissection (Fig. 17-20c). In this way a 3-mm wide recipient bed is created at the one side of the defect, and apically to the defect.

After preparation of the recipient site, a tissue flap to cover the recession is dissected in the adjacent donor area. The preparation of this flap is initiated by a vertical superficial incision placed parallel to the wound edge of the adjacent donor site and at a distance which exceeds the width of the recipient bed by approximately 3 mm (Fig. 17-20c). This incision is extended apically to the apical level of the recipient bed and is terminated within the alveolar mucosa with an oblique releasing incision directed towards the gingival recession. An incision connecting the vertical incision and the incision previously made around the gingival recession is placed along the gingival margin of the donor site (Fig. 17-20c). A split thickness flap is then prepared by sharp dissection within the area delineated by these incisions so that a thin layer of connective tissue is covering the bone in the donor area when the flap is laterally displaced over the denuded root surface and sutured (Figs. 17-20d and 20e). It is important that the oblique releasing incision is made so far apically that the tissue flap can be placed on the recipient bed without being subjected to tearing forces when adjacent soft tissues are moved.

In sites where the gingival recession is deep, the width of gingiva in the adjacent donor area is often insufficient for preparation of a flap which can cover the entire defect with keratinized tissue. This implies that by laterally repositioning the flap, only the coronal part of the defect would be covered by keratinized gingiva while the remaining apical part becomes covered by alveolar mucosa. If the gingival tissue necrotizes during healing, this may result in a gingival recession with no keratinized gingiva apical to the defect. In order to avoid this complication it is often appropriate to place the laterally repositioned flap in such a way that it covers only the most apical portion of the defect. However, the prepared tissue flap can also be rotated about 90° when sutured at the recipient bed (Fig. 17-20f). In this way the entire defect becomes covered by keratinized gingiva. Obviously, this rotation of the tissue flap must be prepared during the operation since the width of the tissue flap in that case must be equal to the vertical extension of the defect (Pennel et al. 1965).

After suturing, pressure must be applied against the flap for 2-3 minutes in order to secure a good adaptation to the underlying recipient bed. Before the placement of periodontal dressing a piece of dry foil is placed over the flap in order to provide a sliding film between the dressing and the graft. This prevents tearing forces from being transferred to the graft by movements of the periodontal dressing. The periodontal dressing and the sutures can be removed after 1 week.

Healing

Following the surgical treatment the laterally repositioned flap is in close contact with the underlying recipient bed and is only separated from the recipient tissue by a thin fibrin layer. In the areas surrounding the defect, where the recipient bed consists of bone covered by connective tissue, the pattern of healing is similar to that observed following a traditional flap

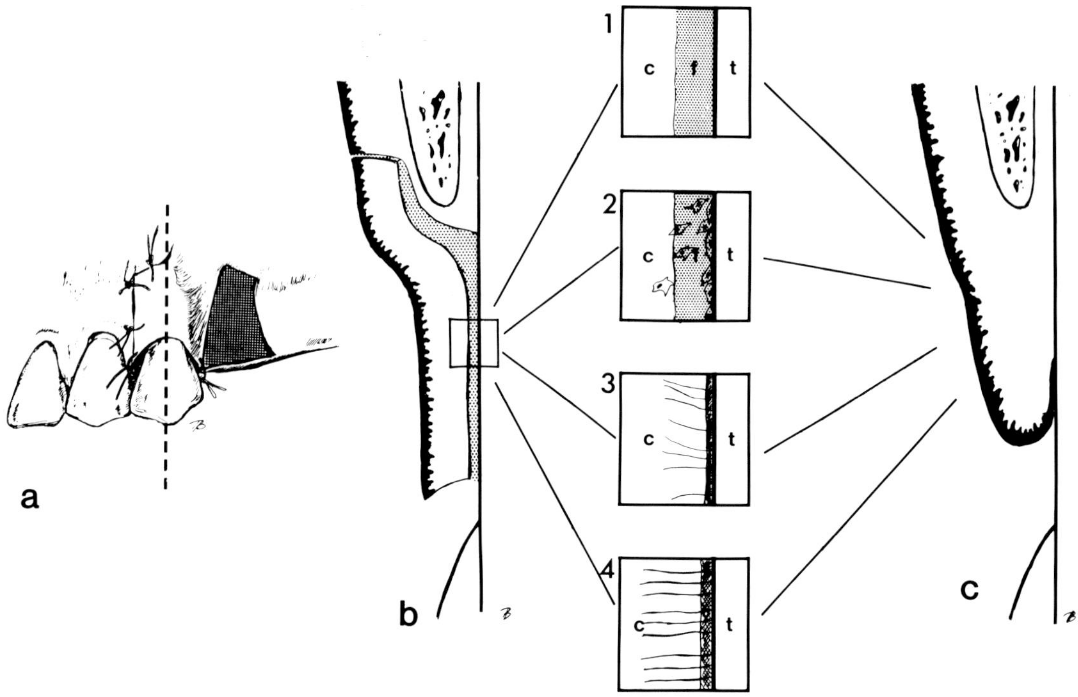

Fig. 17-21a-c. Schematic drawing illustrating healing following treatment of a localized gingival recession with a pedicle graft (a). Fig. 17-21b shows a cross-section through the area immediately after operation. Fig. 17-21c shows the area after healing. The framed areas (1-4) illustrate the 4 stages into which the healing process can be divided.

c: connective tissue, f: fibrin layer, t: tooth.

operation. Cells and blood vessels from the recipient bed as well as from the graft invade the fibrin layer, which gradually becomes replaced by connective tissue. Already after 1 week a fibrous reunion is established between the graft and the underlying tissue.

Healing in the area where the graft is in contact with the denuded root surface has been studied by Wilderman & Wentz (1965) in dogs. According to these authors the healing process can be divided into four different stages (Fig. 17-21).

1. *The adaptation stage (from 0 to 4 days)*
The laterally repositioned flap is separated from the exposed root surface by a thin fibrin layer. The epithelium covering the transplanted tissue flap starts to proliferate and reaches contact with the tooth surface at the coronal edge of the flap after a few days.

2. *The proliferation stage (from 4 to 21 days)*
In the early phase of this stage the fibrin layer between the root surface and the flap is invaded by connective tissue proliferating from the subsurface of the flap. In contrast to areas where healing occurs between two connective tissue surfaces, growth of connective tissue into the fibrin layer can only take place from one surface. After 6-10 days a layer of fibroblasts is seen in apposition to the root surface. These cells are believed to differentiate into cementoblasts at a later stage of healing. At the end of the proliferation stage, thin collagen fibers are formed adjacent to the root surface, but fibrous union between the connective tissue and the root has not been observed. From the coronal edge of the wound, epithelium is proliferating apically along the root surface. According to Wilderman & Wentz (1965), the apical proliferation of epithelium may stop within the coro-

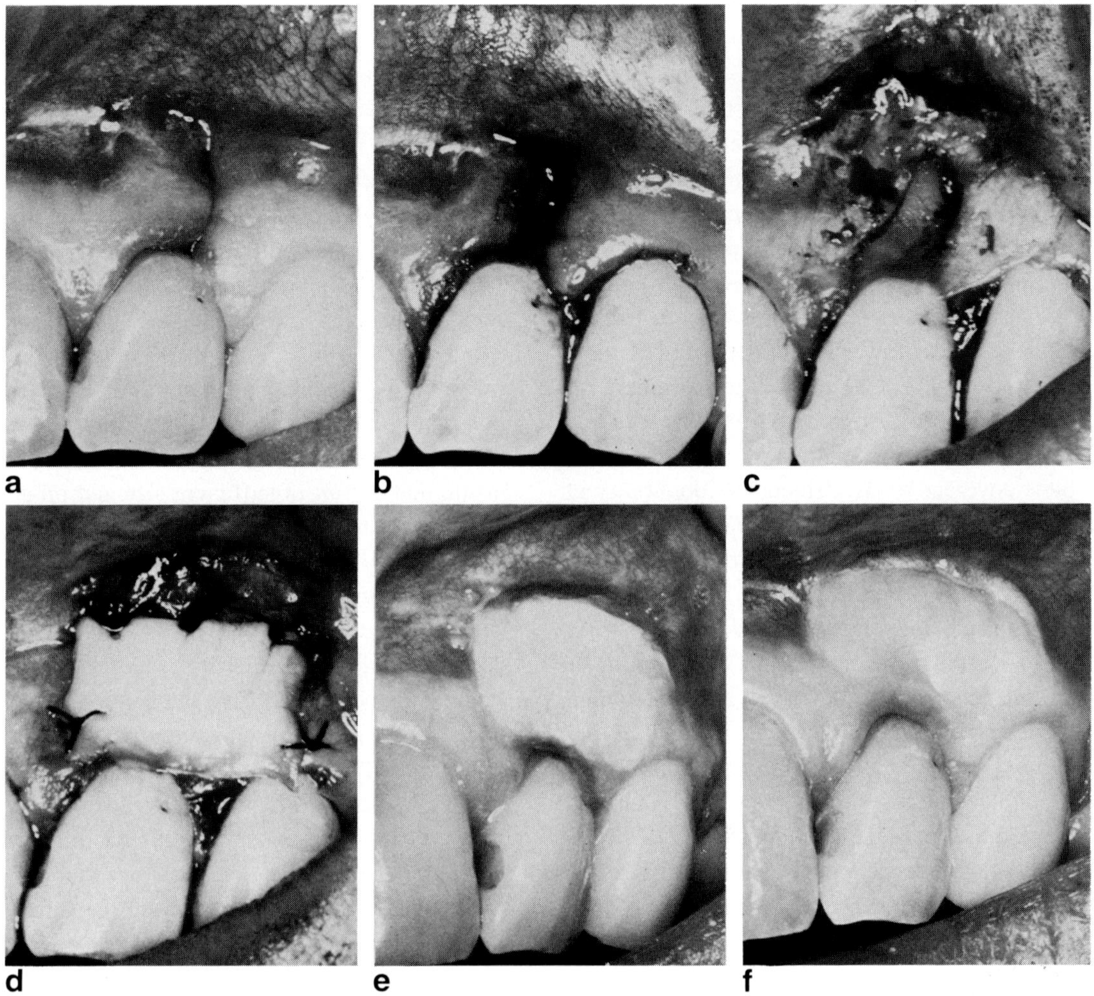

Fig. 17-22a-f. Clinical photographs of a maxillary front tooth region illustrating a narrow gingival recession on the labial aspect of tooth 21 (a). This recession was treated with a free gingival graft. The pocket epithelium all around the defect was removed (b). A recipient bed was then prepared (c). The transplant dissected from the palate was placed in the recipient site and secured by sutures (d). (e) shows the area 14 days and (f) 3 months after treatment.

nal half of the defect, although further downgrowth of epithelium was also frequently observed. Wilderman & Wentz (1965) concluded that it is not the establishment of a fibrous union between the tooth and the flap which arrests the apical migration of the epithelium along the root surface.

3. *The attachment stage (from 27 to 28 days)*
During this stage of healing, thin collagen fibers become inserted in a layer of new cementum formed at the root surface in the apical portion of the recession.

4. *The maturation stage*
This last stage of healing is characterized by continuous formation of collagen fibers. After 2-3 months bundles of collagen fibers are inserting into the cementum layer on the curetted root surface in the apical portion of the recession. This observation is in accordance with results presented by Gottlow et al. (1986). These

authors found that the newly formed cementum was consistently in continuity with the original cementum in the apical, non-instrumented portion of the roots, indicating that the newly formed attachment was produced by cells originating from the periodontal ligament.

Although there are several publications describing the use of laterally repositioned flaps for the treatment of gingival recession, only a few studies have presented well-documented clinical results following this type of therapy (McFull 1968, Sugarman 1969, Guinard & Caffesse 1977b). Apparently it is only in a few cases that this type of therapy results in complete coverage of the defect. The possibility of achieving a new connective tissue attachment in the apical portion of the defect seems to be considerably better in narrow gingival recessions than in wider ones most probably because the periodontal ligament at the lateral parts of the defect serve as a source of granulation tissue from which a new attachment can develop (Gottlow et al. 1986). Even if a new connective tissue attachment most likely fails to form in the entire depth of the defect, the treatment procedure evidently rarely results in the formation of a deep periodontal pocket.

Free grafts

Free grafts of gingiva or palatal mucosa and subepithelial connective tissue grafts are utilized to increase the zone of gingiva at the buccal or lingual aspect of a single tooth or groups of teeth. In addition, free grafts of gingiva or palatal mucosa are used to cover gingival recessions when these are relatively narrow and there is no acceptable donor tissue present in adjacent areas. A two-stage procedure, which involves the placement of a free gingival graft and coronally repositioning after healing, has been reported by Bernimoulin et al. (1975) to be the most effective treatment approach to soft tissue recessions.

The principles of utilizing free mucosal grafts were outlined by Sullivan & Atkins (1968a, b). Like the treatment with pedicle grafts, the surgical procedure is initiated with the preparation of the recipient site. A reverse bevel incision is placed at the gingival margin all around the recession (Fig. 17-22a) in order to remove the pocket epithelium (Fig. 17-22b). After thorough planing of the root surface, a 3- to 4-mm wide recipient bed is prepared around the defect by removing the epithelium, the outer portion of the connective tissue, and muscle fibers (Fig. 17-22c). The free mucosal graft may be obtained from any area having a sufficient quantity of masticatory mucosa (e.g. attached gingiva or palatal mucosa). In order to ensure that a graft of sufficient size and proper contour is removed from the donor area, it is often appropriate to place a tin foil template over the recipient site. This template is transferred to the donor site where it is outlined by a shallow incision. A graft with a thickness of 2-3 mm is then dissected from the donor area and placed at the previously prepared recipient bed (Fig. 17-22d). It is advocated to place the sutures in the graft before it is cut completely free from the donor area since this may facilitate its transfer to the recipient site. In order to immobilize the graft at the recipient site the sutures must be placed in the periosteum or the adjacent attached gingiva (Fig. 17-22d). After suturing, pressure is exerted against the graft for 2-3 minutes in order to eliminate blood and exudate between the graft and the recipient bed. Before the placement of periodontal dressing a piece of dry foil is placed over the flap. The sutures and periodontal dressing can be removed after 1 to 2 weeks. A 2-week-old graft from the palate is shown in Fig. 17-22e immediately after removal of the periodontal dressing. Fig. 17-22f shows the same transplant 3 months after treatment.

Healing

Healing of free gingival grafts placed entirely on a connective tissue recipient bed has been studied in monkeys by Oliver, Löe & Karring

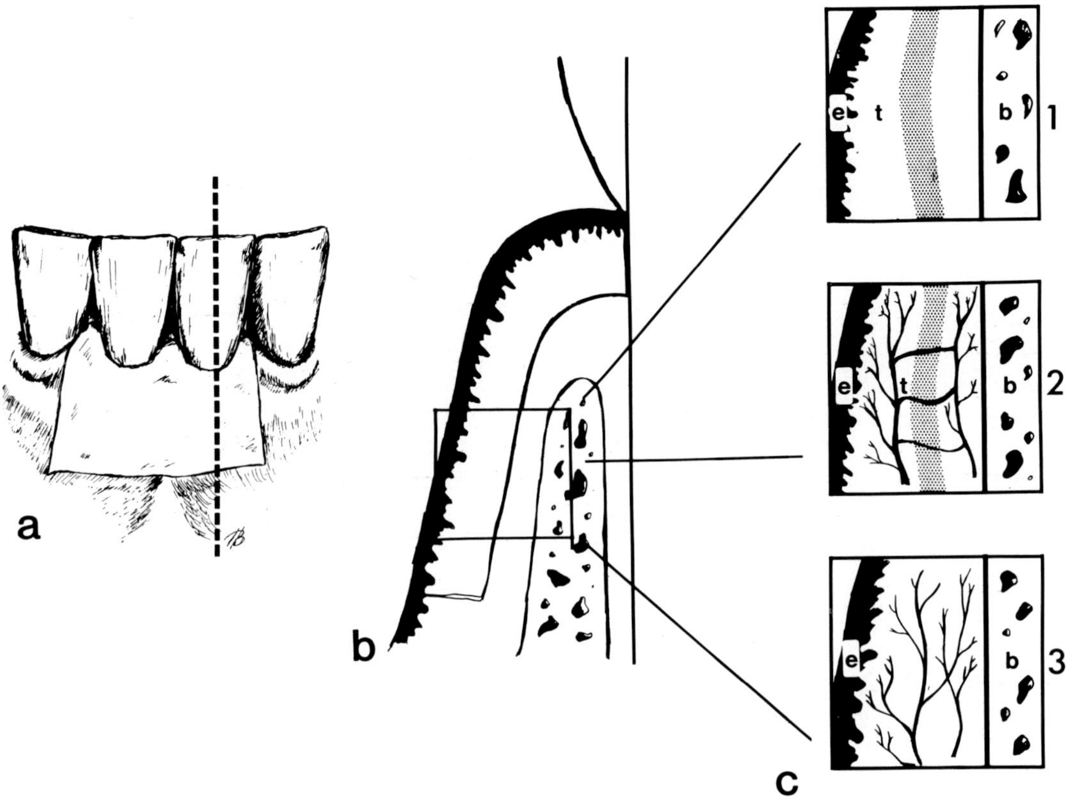

Fig. 17-23a-b. Schematic drawings illustrating healing of a free gingival graft placed entirely on a connective tissue recipient bed (a). A cross-section through the area is shown in (b). The framed areas (1-3) illustrates the 3 phases into which the healing process can be divided.

e: epithelium, t: transplant, b: bone.

(1986). According to these authors healing can be divided into the following three phases (Fig. 17-23).

1. *The initial phase (from 0 to 3 days)*
During these first days of healing a thin layer of exudate is present between the graft and the recipient bed. During this period the grafted tissue survives with an avascular "plasmatic circulation" from the recipient bed. Therefore, it is essential for the survival of the graft that a close contact is established to the underlying recipient bed at the time of operation. A thick layer of exudate or a blood clot may hamper the "plasmatic circulation" and result in the rejection of the graft. The epithelium of the free graft degenerates early in the initial healing phase, and subsequently it becomes desquamated. In placing a graft over a recession, part of the recipient bed will be the avascular root surface. Since the graft is dependent on the nature of its bed for diffusion of plasma and subsequent revascularization, the utilization of free grafts in the treatment of gingival recessions involves a great risk of failure. The area of the graft over the avascular root surface must receive nutrients from the connective tissue bed that surrounds the recession. Thus, the amount of tissue that can be maintained over the root surface is limited by the size of the avascular area. Therefore, it is mainly relatively narrow gingival recessions that can be treated successfully with a free gingival graft.

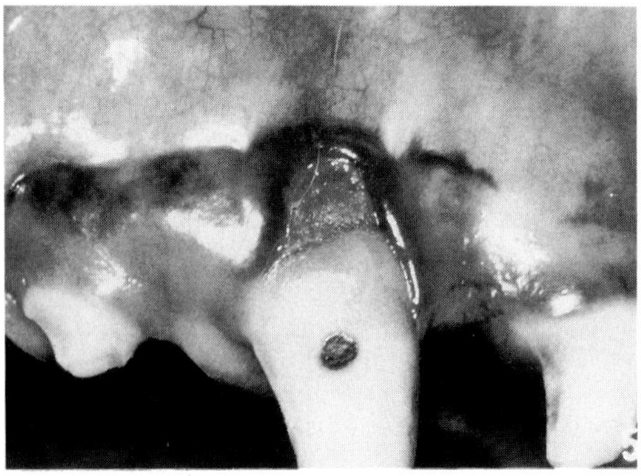

Fig. 17-24a.

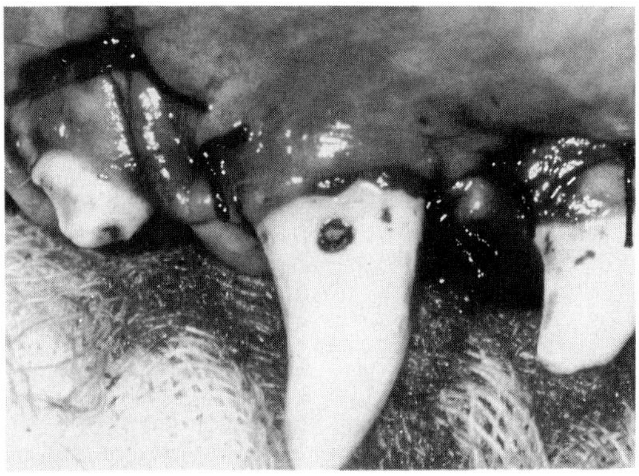

Fig. 17-24b.

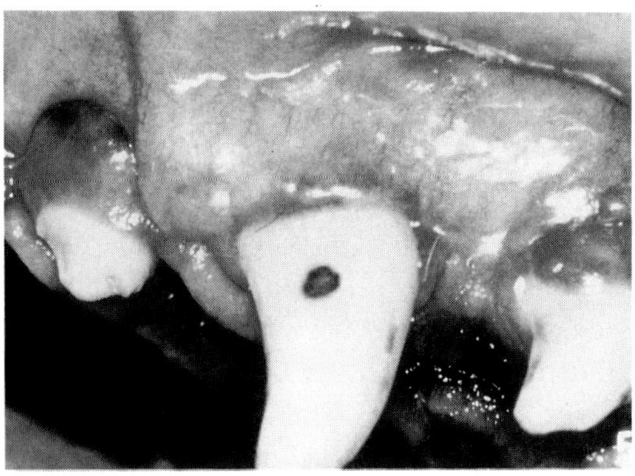

Fig. 17-24c.

Fig. 17-24a-c. Clinical photographs illustrating the treatment of an experimentally induced localized gingival recession in a dog with a coronally displaced flap. Presurgical appearance of the localized gingival recession (a). The site following flap closure of the defect (b) and following 3 months of healing (c).

2. *Revascularization phase (from 2 to 11 days)*
After 4 to 5 days of healing, anastomoses are established between the blood vessels of the recipient bed and those in the grafted tissue. Thus, the circulation of blood is reestablished in the pre-existing blood vessels of the graft. The subsequent time period is characterized by capillary proliferation, which gradually results in a dense network of blood vessels in the graft. At the same time a fibrous union is established between the graft and the underlying connective tissue bed. The re-epithelialization of the graft occurs mainly by proliferation of epithelium from the adjacent tissues. If a free graft is placed over the denuded root surface, apical migration of epithelium along the root surface may take place at this stage of healing.

3. *Tissue maturation phase (from 11 to 42 days)*
During this period the number of blood vessels in the transplant becomes gradually reduced, and after approximately 14 days the vascular system of the graft appears normal. Also, the epithelium gradually matures with the formation of a keratin layer during this stage of healing.

The establishment and maintenance of a "plasmatic circulation" between the recipient bed and the graft during the initial phase of healing is critical for the result of this kind of therapy. Differences between grafts or portions of grafts in their ability to survive transplantation is most likely to be due to variations in the establishment of an adequate plasmatic diffusion. Therefore, in order to ensure ideal conditions for healing, blood between the graft and the recipient site must be removed by exerting pressure against the graft following suturing.

The effect of grafting procedures

Although successful treatment of gingival recessions by pedicle grafts or free grafts has been reported in a number of publications (for review see Matter 1982), it is still an open question as to what extent this type of treatment results in the establishment of a new connective tissue attachment to the denuded root surface or if a long junctional epithelium facing the root surface is established.

In a study in dogs, Björn (1961) demonstrated that a new connective tissue attachment could be obtained to the denuded root surface in experimentally produced gingival recessions when infection and migrating epithelial cells were prevented from interfering with healing. Root resorption, however, was also observed.

In a study by Nyman et al. (1980), roots deprived of their periodontal ligament tissue and cementum layer were implanted in the jaws of monkeys and dogs in such a way that half their circumference was embedded into bone while the remaining portion was covered by gingival connective tissue. In this model system, healing never resulted in new attachment formation, but in a passive adaptation of the gingival connective tissue to the root surface. In several specimens, considerable resorption had affected the root portions facing the gingival connective tissue. The results of this study were interpreted to indicate that gingival tissue cells lack the ability to form a new connective tissue attachment (see Chapter 18). This finding is of particular interest when considering the rationale for the treatment of gingival recessions by free or pedicle gingival grafts. Since in these surgical procedures gingival connective tissue is placed in contact with a denuded root surface, root resorption should be expected to occur. The reason why it is not a common complication following this type of treatment can be explained by two possible events. Either cells from the periodontal ligament form a fibrous attachment to the root surface, or epithelial cells proliferate apically to form a root protective barrier (long junctional epithelium) towards the gingival connective tissue (see Chapter 18).

Histological studies on whether it is the one or the other type of attachment that results following treatment of gingival recessions are few. Wilderman & Wentz (1965) evaluated the dimensional changes of the gingival tissues that occurred following a pedicle flap procedure. Retraction of the gingival margin in this study amounted to 50% of the initially covered portion of the defect, while a new connective tissue attachment of around 2 mm and an epithelial attachment of the same height had formed in the soft tissue covered portion of the defect.

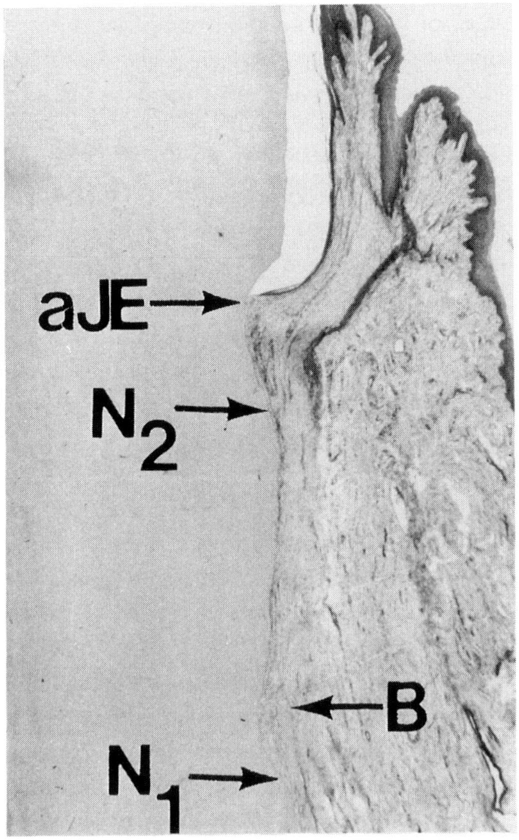

Fig. 17-25. Microphotograph of the healing following a coronally displaced flap in the dog as illustrated in Fig. 17-24. A new connective tissue attachment is formed and extends coronally from the apical border of the notch prepared at the surgically created bone crest (N_1) to the apical termination of the epithelium (aJE) located within the notch indicating the presurgical level of the gingival margin (N_2). B: alveolar bone crest.

In a recent study, Gottlow et al. (1986) examined the result of healing following treatment of localized gingival recessions with coronally placed flaps in dogs (Fig. 17-24). The histological analysis after 3 months of healing disclosed that, on average, 20% of the apicocoronal length of the original defect had been exposed due to recession, 40% was covered by epithelium and 40% demonstrated new connective tissue attachment (Fig. 17-25). However, it was also observed that in 5 out of 16 roots treated, resorption had occurred in the root area between the most apical portion of the dentogingival epithelium and the newly formed cementum. Determining factors for the type of healing result were the size and the shape of the defect. Obviously, the periodontal ligament tissue in both the apical and lateral parts of the defect may serve as a source of granulation tissue from which a new attachment can develop. This means that the chance for a narrow defect to heal with complete new attachment and proper soft tissue coverage is greater than for a wider defect. Furthermore, coronal placement of the flap and the elongation of the distance which the epithelial cells have to cover enhances the chance for new attachment, but also increases the risk for root resorption. Such root resorption occurs when granulation tissue originating from the connective tissue of the gingiva and alveolar mucosa reaches contact with the root surface before it is protected by epithelium or newly formed cementum.

Dorfman et al. (1980) examined the necessity for and effectiveness of the free gingival grafting procedure in maintaining periodontal attachment. Ninety-two patients with bilateral facial tooth surfaces exhibiting inadequate keratinized gingiva (i.e. less than 2 mm) had a free gingival graft placed on one side, while the contralateral side served as the untreated control. Prior to and after surgery the patients were subjected to scaling and root planing and instruction in oral hygiene measures. Not surprisingly, the investigators found a significant increase (approximately 4 mm) in the width of keratinized and attached gingiva at the grafted sites. This increased width of gingiva was maintained for a 2-year follow-up period. The attachment level was also maintained throughout this time period. In the control sites the width of keratinized gingiva was less than 2 mm and did not vary significantly during the 2 years of observation. However, also in the non-grafted areas the attachment level was maintained unchanged. Thus, a narrow zone of gingiva apparently has the same resistance to continuous attachment loss as a wider zone of gingiva. Subsequent 4 and 6 years follow-up reports of this patient material (Dorfman et al. 1982, Kennedy et al. 1985) confirmed the 2-year follow-up findings.

Hangorsky & Bissada (1980), who evaluated the long-term clinical effect of free gingival grafts on the periodontal condition in 34 patients, also failed to observe any difference between grafted and non-grafted sites after 1 to 8 years with regard to gingival health and pocket depth. They concluded that "while the free gingival graft is an effective means to widen the zone of the attached and keratinized gingiva, there is no indication that this increase bears a direct influence upon periodontal health". This result is an agreement with the findings of De Trey & Bernimoulin (1980), who examined the effect of free gingival grafts in 12 patients with less than 1 mm of attached gingiva on homologous contralateral pairs of mandibular teeth. In this study no significant differences were found in gingival health when test and control sites were compared longitudinally.

In summary, on the basis of our present knowledge it can be concluded that no scientific data lend support to the traditional concept that a narrow zone of gingiva or localized gingival recessions need further treatment than the control of plaque in order to maintain the height of the periodontal tissues.

References

Ånerud, K.E., Robertson, P.B., Löe, H., Ånerud, Å., Boysen, H. & Patters, M.R. (1983) Periodontal disease in three young adult populations. *Journal of Periodontal Research* **18**, 655-668.

Baelum, V., Fejerskov, O. & Karring T. (1986) Oral hygiene, gingivitis and periodontal breakdown in adult Tanzanians. *Journal of Periodontal Research* **21**, 221-232.

Baelum, V., Fejerskov, O. & Manji, F. (1988) Periodontal diseases in adult Kenyans. *Journal of Clinical Periodontology* **15**, 445-452.

Baker, D.L. & Seymour, G.J. (1976) The possible pathogenesis of gingival recession. A histological study of induced recession in the rat. *Journal of Clinical Periodontology* **3**, 208-219.

Batenhorst, K.F., Bowers, G.M. & Williams, J.E. (1974) Tissue changes resulting from facial tipping and extrusion of incisors in monkeys. *Journal of Periodontology* **45**, 660-668.

Bernimoulin, J.P., Lüscher, B. & Mühlemann, H.R. (1975) Coronally repositioned periodontal flap. Clinical evaluation after one year. *Journal of Clinical Periodontology* **2**, 1-13.

Björn, H. (1961) Experimental studies on reattachment. *Dental Practitioner and Dental Records* **11**, 351-354.

Bohannan, H.M. (1962a) Studies in the alteration of vestibular depth. I. Complete denudation. *Journal of Periodontology* **33**, 120-128.

Bohannan, H.M. (1962b) Studies in the alteration of vestibular depth. II. Periosteum retention. *Journal of Periodontology* **33**, 354-359.

Bowers, G.M. (1963) A study of the width of attached gingiva. *Journal of Periodontology* **34**, 201-209.

Boyd, R.L. (1978) Mucogingival considerations and their relationship to orthodontics. *Journal of Periodontology* **49**, 67-76.

Bradley, R.E., Grant, J.C. & Ivancie, G.P. (1959) Histologic evaluation of mucogingival surgery. *Oral Surgery* **12**, 1184-1199.

Carranza, F.A. & Carraro, J.J. (1963) Effect of removal of periosteum on post-operative results of mucogingival surgery. *Journal of Periodontology* **34**, 223-226.

Carranza, F.A. & Carraro, J.J. (1970) Mucogingival techniques in periodontal surgery. *Journal of Periodontology* **41**, 294-299.

Carraro, J.J., Carranza, F.A., Albano, E.A. & Joly, G.G. (1964) Effect of bone denudation in mucogingival surgery in humans. *Journal of Periodontology* **35**, 463-466.

Coatoam, G.W., Behrents, R.G & Bissada, N.F. (1981) The width of keratinized gingiva during orthodontic treatment: its significance and impact on periodontal status. *Journal of Periodontology* **52**, 307-313.

Cohen, D. & Ross, S. (1968) The double papillae flap in periodontal therapy. *Journal of Periodontology* **39**, 65-70.

Corn, H. (1962) Periosteal separation - its clinical significance. *Journal of Periodontology* **33**, 140-152.

Costich, E.R. & Ramfjord, S.F. (1968) Healing after partial denudation of the alveolar process. *Journal of Periodontology* **39**, 5-12.

De Trey, E. & Bernimoulin, J. (1980) Influence of free gingival grafts on the health of the marginal gingiva. *Journal of Clinical Periodontology* **7**, 381-393.

Donnenfeld, O.W., Marks, R.M. & Glickman, I. (1964) The apically repositioned flap - a clinical study. *Journal of Periodontology* **35**, 381-387.

Dorfman, H.S., Kennedy, J.E. & Bird, W.C. (1980) Longitudinal evaluation of free autogenous gingival grafts. *Journal of Clinical Periodontology* **7**, 316-324.

Dorfman, H.S., Kennedy, J.E. & Bird, W.C. (1982) Longitudinal evaluation of free gingival grafts. A four-year report. *Journal of Periodontology* **53**, 349-352.

Edel, A. (1974) Clinical evaluation of free connective tissue grafts used to increase the width of keratinized gingiva. *Journal of Clinical Periodontology* **1**, 185-196.

Foushee, D.G., Moriarty, J.D. & Simpson, D.M. (1985) Effects of mandibular orthognatic treatment on mucogingival tissue. *Journal of Periodontology* **56**, 727-733.

Friedman, N. (1957) Mucogingival surgery. *Texas Dental Journal* **75**, 358-362.

Friedman, N. (1962) Mucogingival surgery: The apically repositioned flap. *Journal of Periodontology* **33**, 328-340.

Friedman, N. & Levine, H.L. (1964) Mucogingival surgery: Current status. *Journal of Periodontology* **35**, 5-21.

"Glossary of terms" (1986) *Journal of periodontology* **57**, Supplement.

Gorman, W.J. (1967) Prevalence and etiology of gingival recession. *Journal of Periodontology* **38**, 316-322.

Gottlow, J., Nyman, S., Karring, T. & Lindhe, J. (1986) Treatment of localized gingival recessions with coronally displaced flaps and citric acid. A experimental study in the dog. *Journal of Clinical Periodontology* **13**, 57-63.

Gottsegen. R. (1954) Frenulum position and vestibular depth in relation to gingival health. *Oral Surgery* **7**, 1069-1078.

Grevers, A. (1977) Width of attached gingiva and vestibular depth in relation to gingival health. Thesis. University of Amsterdam.

Grupe, J. & Warren, R. (1956) Repair of gingival defects by a sliding flap operation. *Journal of Periodontology* **27**, 290-295.

Guinard, E.A. & Caffesse, R.G. (1977a) Localized gingival recessions. II. Treatment. *The Journal of the Western Society of Periodontology* **25**, 10-21.

Guinard, E.A & Caffesse, R.G. (1977b) Treatment of localized gingival recessions. I. Lateral sliding flap. *Journal of Periodontology* **49**, 351-356.

Haggerty, P.C. (1966) The use of a free gingival graft to create a healthy environment for full crown preparation. *Periodontics* **4**, 329-331.

Hall, W.B. (1981) The current status of mucogingival problems and their therapy. *Journal of Periodontology* **52**, 569-575.

Hangorsky, U. & Bissada, N.B. (1980) Clinical assessment of free gingival graft effectiveness on maintenance of periodontal health. *Journal of Periodontology* **51**, 274-278.

Hawley, C.E. & Staffileno, H. (1979) Clinical evaluation of free gingival grafts in periodontal surgery. *Journal of Periodontology* **41**, 105-112.

Ivancie, G.P. (1957) Experimental and histological investigation of gingival regeneration in vestibular surgery. *Journal of Periodontology* **28**, 259-263.

Karring, T., Cumming, B.R., Oliver, R.C. & Löe, H. (1975a) The origin of granulation tissue and its impact on postoperative results of mucogingival surgery. *Journal of Periodontology* **46**, 577-585.

Karring, T., Lang, N.P. & Löe, H. (1975b) The role of gingival connective tissue in determining epithelial differentiation. *Journal of Periodontal Research* **10**, 1-11.

Kennedy, J.E., Bird, W.C., Palcanis, K.G. & Dorfman, H.S. (1985) A longitudinal evaluation of varying widths of attached gingiva. *Journal of Clinical Periodontology* **12**, 667-675.

Kisch, J., Badersten, A. & Egelberg, J. (1986) Longitudinal observation of "unattached", mobile gingival areas. *Journal of Clinical Periodontology* **13**, 131-134.

Lang, N.P. & Löe, H. (1972) The relationship between the width of keratinized gingiva and gingival health. *Journal of Periodontology* **43**, 623-627.

Lindhe, J. & Nyman, S. (1980) Alterations of the position of the marginal soft tissue following periodontal surgery. *Journal of Clinical Periodontology* **7**, 525-530.

Löe, H., Ånerud, A., Boysen, H. & Smith, M. (1978) The natural history of periodontal disease in man. The rate of periodontal destruction before 40 years of age. *Journal of Periodontology* **49**, 607-620.

Matter, J. (1982) Free gingival grafts for the treatment of gingival recession. A review of some techniques. *Journal of Clinical Periodontology* **9**, 103-114.

Maynard, J.G. & Ochsenbein, D. (1975) Mucogingival problems, prevalence and therapy in children. *Journal of Periodontology* **46**, 543-552.

Maynard, J.G. & Wilson, R.D. (1979) Physologic dimensions of the periodontium significant to the restorative dentist. *Journal of Periodontology* **50**, 170-174.

Maynard, J.G. & Wilson, R.D. (1980) Diagnosis and management of mucogingival problems in children. *The Dental Clinics of North America* **24**, 683-703.

McFull, W.T. (1968) The laterally repositioned flap - criteria for success. *Periodontics* **5**, 89-92.

Miller, A.J., Brunelle, J.A., Carlos, J.P., Brown, L.J. & Löe, H. (1987) Oral health of United States adults. NIH Publication No. 87-2868, National Institute of Dental Research, Bethesda, Maryland.

Miyasato, M., Crigger, M. & Egelberg, J. (1977) Gingival condition in areas of minimal and appreciable width of keratinized gingiva. *Journal of Clinical Periodontology.* **4**, 200-209.

Murtomaa, H., Meurman, J.H., Rytömaa, I. & Turtola, L. (1987) Periodontal status in university students. *Journal of Clinical Periodontology* **14**, 462-465.

Nabers, C.L. (1954) Repositioning the attached gingiva. *Journal of Periodontology* **25**, 38-39.

Nabers, C.L. (1966) Free gingival grafts. *Periodontics* **4**, 243-245.

Nyman, S., Karring, T. & Bergenholtz, G. (1982) Bone regeneration in alveolar bone dehiscences produced by jiggling forces. *Journal of Periodontal Research* **17**, 316-322.

Nyman, S., Karring, T., Lindhe, J. & Plantén, S. (1980) Healing following implantation of periodontitis-affected roots into gingival connective tissue. *Journal of Clinical Periodontology* **7**, 394-401.

Ochsenbein, C. (1960) Newer concept of mucogingival surgery. *Journal of Periodontology* **31**, 175-185.

Okamoto, H., Yoneyama, T., Lindhe, J., Haffajee, A.D. & Socransky, S.S. (1988) Methods of evaluating priodontal disease data in epidemiological research. *Journal of Clinical Periodontology* **15**, 430-439.

Oliver, R.G., Löe, H. & Karring, T. (1968) Microscopic evaluation of the healing and re-vascularization of free gingival grafts. *Journal of Periodontal Research* **3**, 84-95.

Orban, B.J. (1957) *Oral Histology and Embryology.* 4th ed., pp. 221-264. St. Louis: C.V. Mosby Company.

Pearson, L.E. (1968) Gingival height of lower central incisors orthodontically treated and untreated. *Angle Orthodontist* **38**, 337-339.

Pennel, B.M., Higgison, J.D., Towner, T.D., King, K.O., Fritz, B.D. & Salder, J.F. (1965) Oblique rotated flap. *Journal of Periodontology* **36**, 305-309.

Pfeifer, J.S. (1963) The growth of gingival tissue over denuded bone. *Journal of Periodontology* **34**, 10-16.

Pfeifer, J.S. (1965) The reaction of alveolar bone to flap procedures in man. *Periodontics* **3**, 135-140.

Pfeifer, J. & Heller, R. (1971) Histologic evaluation of full and partial thickness lateral repositioned flaps. A pilot study. *Journal of Periodontology* **42**, 331-333.

Raetzke, P.B. (1985) Covering localized areas of root exposure employing the "envelope" technique. *Journal of Periodontology* **56**, 397-402.

Rateitschak, K.H., Herzog-Specht, F. & Hotz, R. (1968) Reaktion und Regeneration des Parodonts auf Behandlung mit festsitzenden Apparaten und abnehmbaren Platten. *Fortschritte der Kieferorthopädie* **29**, 415-435.

Rosenberg, N.M. (1960) Vestibular alterations in periodontics. *Journal of Periodontology* **31**, 231-237.

Ruben, M.P. (1979) A biological rationale for gingival reconstruction by grafting procedures. *Quintessence International* **10**, 47-55.

Salkin, L.M., Freedman, A.L., Stein, M.D. & Bassiouny, M.A. (1987) A longitudinal study of untreated mucogingival defects. *Journal of Periodontology* **58**, 164-166.

Sangnes, G. & Gjermo, P. (1976) Prevalence of oral soft and hard tissue lesions related to mechanical tooth cleaning procedures. *Community Dentistry and Oral Epidemiology* **4**, 77-83.

Schoo, W.H. & van der Velden, U. (1985) Marginal soft tissue recessions with and without attached gingiva. *Journal of Periodontal Research* **20**, 209-211.

Staffileno, H. (1964) Management of gingival recession and root exposure problems associated with periodontal disease. *Dental Clinics of North America*, March, 111-120.

Staffileno, H., Levy, S. & Gargiulo, A. (1966) Histologic study of cellular mobilization and repair following a periosteal retention operation via split thickness mucogingival surgery. *Journal of Periodontology* **37**, 117-131.

Staffileno, H., Wentz, F. & Orban, B. (1962) Histologic study of healing of split thickness flap surgery in dogs. *Journal of Periodontology* **33**, 56-69.

Steiner, G.G., Pearson, J.K. & Ainamo, J. (1981) Changes of the marginal periodontium as a result of labial tooth movement in monkeys. *Journal of Periodontology* **52**, 314-320.

Stern, J.B. (1976) Oral mucous membrane. In: *Orban's oral histology and embryology*. ed. Bhaskar, S.N., Chapter 8, St. Louis: C.V. Mosby.

Stoner, J. & Mazdyasna, S. (1980) Gingival recession in the lower incisor region of 15-year-old subjects. *Journal of Periodontology* **51**, 74-76.

Sugarman, E.F. (1969) A clinical and histological study of the attachment of grafted tissue to bone and teeth. *Journal of Periodontology* **40**, 381-387.

Sullivan, H.C. & Atkins, J.H. (1968a) Free autogenous gingival grafts. I. Principles of successful grafting. *Periodontics* **6**, 121-129.

Sullivan, H.C. & Atkins, J.H. (1968b) Free autogenous gingival grafts. III. Utilization of grafts in the treatment of gingival recession. *Periodontics* **6**, 152-160.

Tenenbaum, H. (1982) A clinical study comparing the width of attached gingiva and the prevalence of gingival recessions. *Journal of Clinical Periodontology* **9**, 86-92.

Waerhaug, J. (1952) The gingival pocket. Anatomy, pathology, deepening and elimination. *Odontologisk Tidskrift* **60**, Supplement.

Wennström, J.L. (1983) Regeneration of gingiva following surgical excision. A clinical study. *Journal of Clinical Periodontology* **10**, 287-297.

Wennström, J.L. (1987) Lack of association between width of attached gingiva and development of gingival recessions. A 5-year longitudinal study. *Journal of Clinical Periodontology* **14**, 181-184.

Wennström. J.L. & Lindhe, J. (1983a) The role of attached gingiva for maintenance of periodontal health. Healing following excisional and grafting procedures in dogs. *Journal of Clinical Periodontology* **10**, 206-221.

Wennström. J.L. & Lindhe, J. (1983b) Plaque-induced gingival inflammation in the absence of attached gingiva in dogs. *Journal of Clinical Periodontology* **10**, 266-276.

Wennström, J.L., Lindhe, J., Sinclair, F. & Thilander, B. (1987) Some periodontal tissue reactions to orthodontic tooth movement in monkeys. *Journal of Clinical Periodontology* **14**, 121-129.

Wilderman, M.N. (1963) Repair after a periosteal retention procedure. *Journal of Periodontology* **34**, 484-503.

Wilderman, M.N. (1964) Exposure of bone in periodontal surgery. *Dental Clinics of North America*, March, 23-26.

Wilderman, M.N. & Wentz, F.M. (1965) Repair of a dentogingival defect with a pedicle flap. *Journal of Periodontology* **36**, 218-231.

Wilderman, M.N., Wentz, F.M. & Orban, B.J. (1961) Histogenesis of repair after mucogingival surgery. *Journal of Periodontology* **31**, 283-299.

Woofter, C. (1969) The prevalence and etiology of gingival recessions. *Periodontal Abstracts* **17**, 45-49.

World Health Organization (WHO 1978) Epidemiology, etiology and prevention of periodontal disease. *Technical Report Series* No. 621.

Yoneyama, T., Okamoto, H., Lindhe, J. Socransky, S.S. & Haffajee, A.D. (1988) Probing depth, attachment loss and gingival recession. Findings from a clinical examination in Ushiku, Japan. *Journal of Clinical Periodontology* **15**, 581-591.

CHAPTER 18

Reattachment - New Attachment

Definition

The ultimate goal of periodontal therapy entails not only the arrest of progressive periodontal disease but also the restitution of those parts of the supporting apparatus which have been destroyed, i.e. *restitutio ad integrum*.

Reattachment is a term used to describe the reunion of connective tissue with a root surface on which viable periodontal ligament tissue is present. Since, however, the aim of so-called regenerative procedures involves *de novo* formation of connective tissue attachment to root surfaces which have lost such attachment, the term *New Attachment* should be preferred. In other words, *New Attachment* signifies the formation of new cementum with inserting collagen fibers in an area where the root has been deprived of its connective tissue attachment.

New attachment procedures

Root planing and soft-tissue curettage

A variety of surgical techniques have been developed and tested for their potential to restore the periodontal tissues lost in destructive periodontal disease. The first methods used in attempts to obtain new attachment included scaling and root planing in conjunction with soft-tissue curettage, i.e. mechanical removal of the "diseased" root cementum and the pocket epithelium. Studies in humans (e.g. Younger 1899, McCall 1926, Beube 1947, 1952, Orban 1948, Waerhaug 1952, Schaffer & Zander 1953, Carranza 1954, 1960) and animals (e.g. Beube 1947, Ramfjord 1951, Kon et al. 1969), showed that this type of periodontal therapy frequently resulted not only in the establishment of gingival health but also in a reduction of the initially recorded pocket depth. This decrease in the depth of the periodontal pocket was suggested to be the result partly of shrinkage of the initially inflamed gingiva but partly also the effect of the formation of a new connective tissue attachment in the apical part of the pocket.

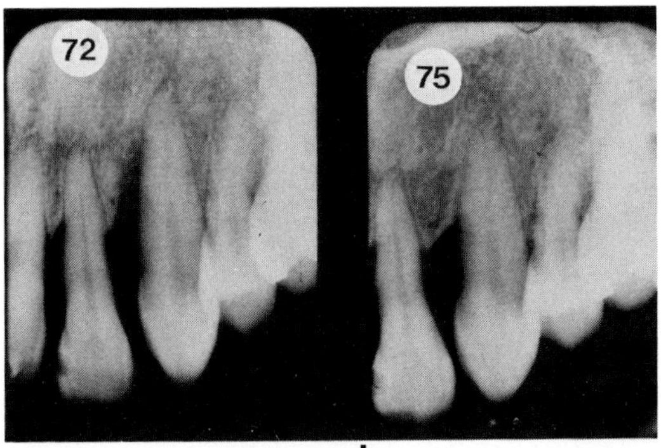

a b

Figs. 18-1a,b. An angular bony defect at the mesial aspect of tooth 23 was in 1972 (a) treated by scaling and root planing in conjunction with a modified Widman flap procedure. Three years after therapy bone repair ("bone fill") had occurred in this site (b).

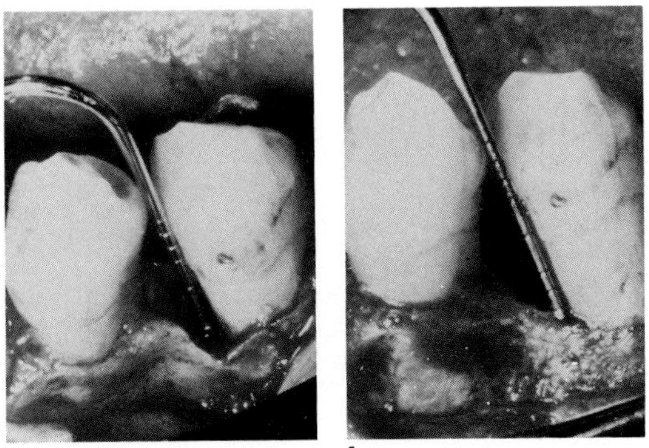

a b

Figs. 18-2a,b. Photographs showing healing of an angular bony defect. The defect at the time of surgery (left) and at reentry after 3 months of healing (right). (From Polson & Heijl 1978).

Flap procedures

Since the 1950s most new attachment attempts, in particular in the treatment of angular osseous defects (i.e. infrabony pockets), have besides root planing included the elevation of flaps (e.g. Prichard 1957a,b, Patur & Glickman 1962, Wade 1962, 1966, Ellegaard & Löe 1971, Yukna et al. 1976). After elevation of a soft-tissue flap (split-thickness or full-thickness flap) the granulation tissue in the osseous defect is removed and the root surface is carefully scaled and planed. In order to enhance regeneration of bone, small perforations are often made with a bur at several sites of the bony walls. The flap is then sutured to accomplish coverage of the alveolar bone.

Many clinical investigators claimed that new attachment resulted following this type of treatment. Patur & Glickman (1962) reported that bone regeneration and new attachment occurred in 2- and 3-wall infrabony pockets but not in l-wall pockets. Ellegaard & Löe (1971) presented results from a study comprising 191 lesions in 24 patients with periodontal disease which indicated that after 2-3 years of healing *complete regeneration* had occurred in around 70% of the 3-wall defects, in 40% of the combined 2- and 3-wall and in 45% of the 2-wall defects. In a study by Rosling et al. (1976) 124 angular bony defects in 12 patients were treated by means of the modified Widman flap procedure (Ramfjord & Nissle 1974). Reexamination performed 2 years after therapy demonstrated that all osseous defects, irrespective of their initial classification as 2- or 3-wall defects, were refilled with bone. The authors suggested that this bone fill was indicative of the formation also of new connective tissue attachment and ascribed the successful healing mainly to the optimal standard of oral hygiene which was maintained in all patients during healing. (Radiographs illustrating the healing of an infrabony pocket from this study are shown in Fig. 18-1). A similar clinical study with almost identical results (Fig. 18-2) was presented by Polson & Heijl (1978) who concluded: "It appears that infrabony periodontal defects may predictably remodel throughout their circumferential extent after *surgical debridement and establishment of optimal plaque control*".

Grafting procedures

In a number of clinical trials and animal experiments the flap approach has been combined with the insertion of different kinds of implant materials into the curetted bony defects in order to improve healing (e.g. Yuktanandana 1959, Nabers & O'Leary 1965, 1967, Robinson 1969, Schallhorn et al. 1970, Rosenberg 1971, Dragoo & Sullivan 1973a,b, Hiatt & Schallhorn 1973, Froum et al. 1975a,b, 1976, Ellegaard et al. 1976, Hiatt et al. 1978, Dragoo 1981, Bowers et al. 1985). The various implant materials which have been used so far can be grouped into 4 categories (Gara & Adams 1981):

1. *Autograft:* a graft transferred from one position to another within the same individual:
   a) cortical bone (osseous coagulum)
   b) cancellous bone and marrow obtained either from intra-oral or extra-oral donor sites
   c) combination of cortical and cancellous bone (bone blend).

2. *Allograft:* a graft transferred between genetically dissimilar members of the same species:
   a) viable cancellous bone and marrow
   b) sterilized cancellous bone and marrow
   c) freeze-dried bone

3. *Heterograft or xenograft:* a graft taken from a donor of another species.

4. Grafts of *bone substitutes* and *synthetic materials.*

The literature suggests that autografts in the form of cancellous bone and hemopoietic marrow establish the most favorable conditions for new attachment during healing after periodontal therapy (Schallhorn 1977, Dragoo 1981). Hiatt et al. (1978) reported that in 66 out of 79 grafted areas new cementum was formed and moved coronally on the root surface, while in only 7 out of 21 non-grafted cases new cementum was formed. The use of bone and marrow as either autografts or allografts, however, appeared to involve certain risks such as root resorption and ankylosis with the use of fresh material, additional surgical insult to the patient with autografts and possible antigenicity with allografts. Because of such undesired side effects with autografts and allografts, bone substitutes and synthetic materials have been introduced (Alderman 1969, Levin et al. 1974, Bump et al. 1975, Strub et al. 1979) and reports have been published claiming that, following the use of such materials, healing occurs with the formation of new attachment (for review see Bowers et al. 1982).

A critical analysis of the literature reveals, however, that the methods used to induce new attachment are by no means predictable. The inconsistency in the results obtained may be illustrated by the findings of Waerhaug (1952), Schaffer & Zander (1953), Carranza (1954) and Ellegaard & Löe (1971). Waerhaug reported that coronal gain of attachment occurred following subgingival curettage in *only 4 out of 32 treated teeth*, while Schaffer & Zander (1953) observed new connective tissue attachment in 5 teeth out of 8. Carranza (1954) claimed to have obtained new attachment in *41 out of 103 infrabony pockets* following root planing and curettage. Ellegaard & Löe (1971), who used a flap approach, claimed that complete regeneration had occurred in *70% of 3-wall pockets*, in *40% of 2- or combined 2- and 3- wall bony defects*, and that failure resulted in *20-40% of all defects treated.* Also, the effect of grafting procedures in reconstructive therapy shows considerable variation. For extensive review on methods used in new attachment therapy and the result reported, the reader is referred to papers by Gara & Adams (1981) and Wirthlin (1981).

Errors inherent in the assessment of new attachment

Clinical methods

In recent years criticism has been directed toward the methods which have been used to assess new attachment formation following therapy. This is particularly the case when the result of treatment has been evaluated by clinical means only, i.e. *attachment level* measurements, *radiographic* analysis and *reentry* operations. The reliability of such clinical methods to determine gain of new attachment is open to criticism.

Periodontal probing

Findings by Listgarten et al. (1976), Armitage et al. (1977), van der Velden & de Vries (1978) and others have demonstrated the inability of periodontal probing to determine accurately the coronal level of the connective tissue attachment. It has been pointed out that improvement of attachment levels following periodontal treatment assessed by probing does not necessarily demonstrate the formation of a new connective tissue attachment to the root surface. Rather, improved clinical attachment levels merely describe the resolution of the inflammatory process within the gingiva without an accompanying "true" gain of attachment, i.e. a connective tissue attachment formed in an area coronal to the level of this attachment before treatment. In other words, *the resolution of the inflammatory lesion in the gingiva will increase the resistance of the tissue to probing.* This change will in a probing depth measurement be registered as an improved attachment level (for a detailed discussion on errors inherent in clinical probing of periodontal pockets see Chapter 12).

Radiographic analysis; reentry operations

Regeneration of bone tissue, which frequently occurs within angular bony defects following so-called reconstructive therapy, has been documented by *measurements made in radiographs* obtained in a standardized and reproducible manner and/or in conjunction with reentry operations. Analysis of radiographs obtained of an angular bony defect before and after therapy and inspection of the treated area during a reentry operation can certainly provide evidence of new bone formation. Such "bone fill", however, does not document formation of new root cementum and a new periodontal ligament. In fact, it was demonstrated by Caton & Zander (1976), Moskow et al. (1979) and others that bone regeneration in infrabony pockets can occur opposite a junctional epithelium interposed between the newly formed bone and the curetted root surface. This means that methods such as radiographic analysis and measurements made at reentry operations are unreliable for the identification of formation of new cementum and new periodontal ligament tissue.

Histological methods

In several studies healing has been analyzed in histological sections of block biopsies obtained after various forms of therapy. In such experiments the location of the attachment level prior to therapy has often been assessed by clinical probing. Since it is not possible, however, by clinical means (see above) to identify properly the coronal level of the connective tissue attachment, not even such combined clinical and histological methods are ideal for studying the formation of new connective tissue attachment.

A discriminating animal model

Many efforts have been made to develop research models in which the coronal level of the

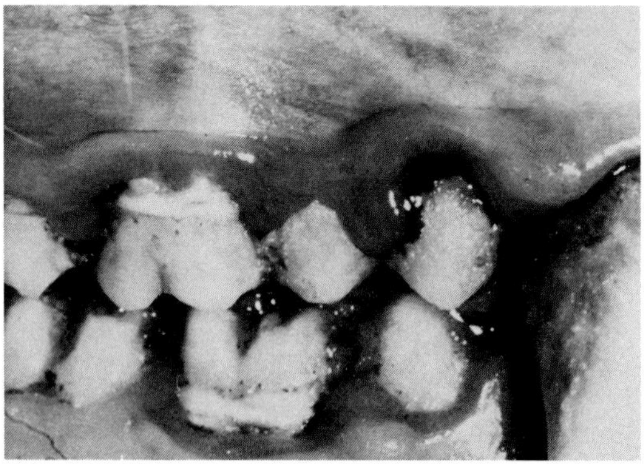

Fig. 18-3. Periodontal tissue breakdown was produced by the placement of orthodontic elastics around the neck of the teeth and by allowing plaque accumulation. Note the recession and the swelling of the marginal gingiva. (From Caton & Zander 1975).

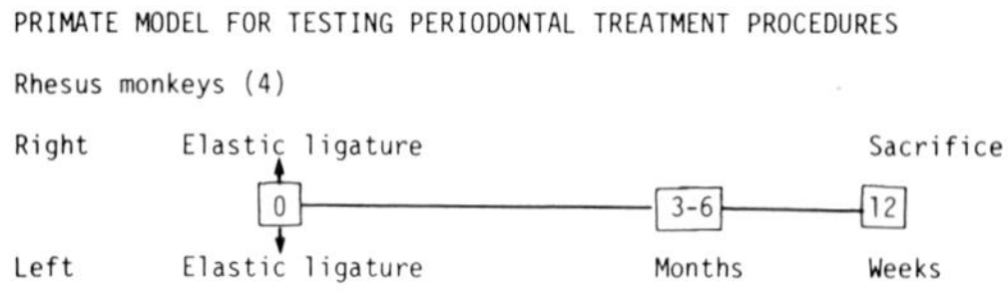

	Right	Left	
CEJ-JE	2.47 mm	2.53 mm	N.S.
CEJ-CR	2.57 mm	2.59 mm	N.S.
CEJ-AAD	3.01 mm	2.97 mm	N.S.

Fig. 18-4. Diagram describing the outline of the experiment by Caton & Kowalsky (1976). Elastic ligatures (orthodontics elastics) were placed around the teeth on Day 0 and were removed 3-6 months later. The animals were sacrificed 12 weeks after removal of the elastics. Measurements made in histological sections revealed that pockets of almost identical depth and morphology had been produced around contralateral teeth.

connective tissue attachment on the root surface both *before* and *after* treatment can be properly assessed. A reliable animal model was described (Caton & Zander 1975, Caton & Kowalski 1976), by means of which periodontal lesions of almost identical depth and morphology could be produced around contralateral teeth in the monkey. The periodontal lesions were produced by placing and retaining orthodontic elastics of identical size and elasticity around contralateral teeth for the same period of time and allowing plaque accumulation (Figs. 18-3 and 18-4). The periodontal lesions, often accompanied by angular bony defects, were treated in one side of the jaw. Healing was studied using the contralateral lesions as untreated controls. Hence, in histological sections, differences in the connective tissue attachment levels between treated test sites and untreated control sites could be assessed.

Regenerative potential of the periodontal structures

How this model has been used to study the potential of the peridontal tissues to form new attachment will be described below. But first some elementary principles must be outlined regarding wound healing in the periodontium. In 1976, Melcher in a review paper postulated that the cells which repopulate the root surface after surgery determine the nature (quality) of the attachment that will form. This is illustrated in Figs. 18-5a,b. After a reverse bevel incision and removal of the granulation tissue, the curetted root surface may be repopulated by 4 different types of cells: epithelial cells, cells originating from the gingival connective tissue, cells originating from the bone tissue, and cells originating from the periodontal ligament.

If the cells from the epithelium proliferate apically to its presurgical level, an epithelial attachment (long junctional epithelium) will result. (Fig. 18-6). The contact between the root surface and this junctional epithelium is maintained by cuticular structures and hemidesmosomes.

If cells originating from the *gingival connective tissue* migrate into contact with the root surface, it has been assumed that some kind of connective tissue adhesion or attachment between the soft and hard tissues may be established (Fig. 18-7). But do cells originating from the connective tissue of the gingiva have a potential to form a new fibrous attachment?

If cells originating from *bone tissue* are migrating into contact with the curetted root surface, root resorption and ankylosis can occur (Fig. 18-8). The question remains, however, if bone cells have the potential to stimulate the formation of cementum and periodontal ligament fibers.

Ideal conditions for healing may develop in situations where cells originating from the *periodontal ligament* proliferate to cover the previously diseased root surface (Fig. 18-9). Such cells have, according to Melcher (1976), the capacity to form cementum and periodontal ligament fibers. But is it possible to obtain colonization of such cells on a root surface which has been 1) exposed to a periodontal pocket and 2) instrumented during scaling and root planing?

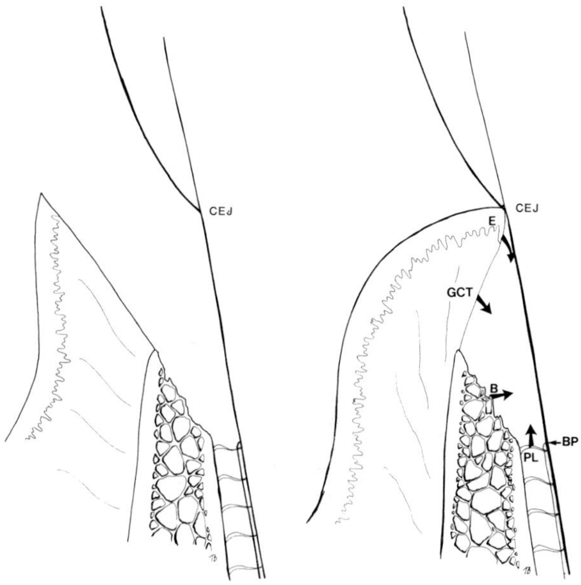

Figs. 18-5a,b. Schematic drawings illustrating the wound after flap elevation and removal of plaque, calculus, pocket epithelium and infiltrated portions of connective tissue (a). The cells which repopulate the wound determine the quality of the attachment (b); epithelial cells (E), gingival connective tissue cells (GCT), bone cells (B), periodontal ligament cells (PL). BP = preoperative bottom of the pocket.

Epithelium

The monkey model (Caton & Zander 1975, Caton & Kowalski 1976) was used by Caton and co-workers (1980) to study the healing of

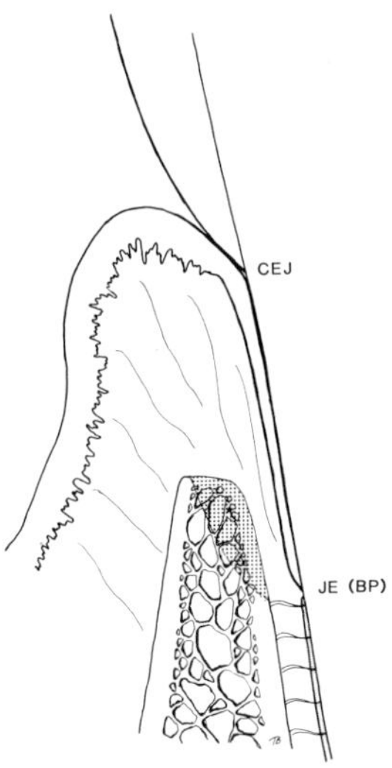

Fig. 18-6. Epithelial attachment - long junctional epithelium - which has formed during healing. JE = apical extent of the junctional epithelium. BP = preoperative level of the pocket epithelium. Shadowed area = bone repair.

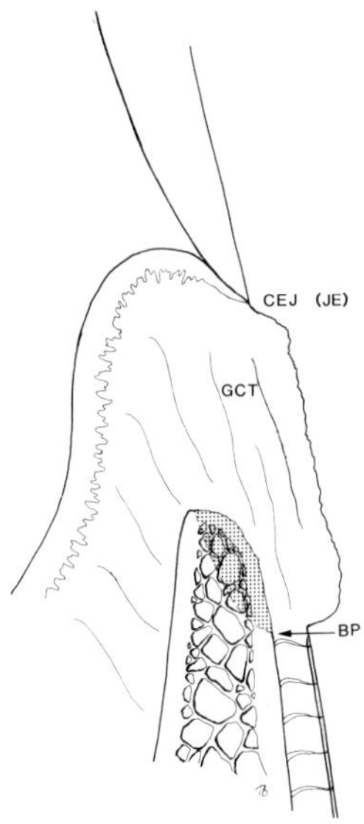

Fig. 18-7. If cells from the gingival connective tissue (GCT) repopulate the root surface, tbe attachment occurs in the form of connective tissue adhesion. In addition, root resorption may occur. Shadowed area = bone repair.

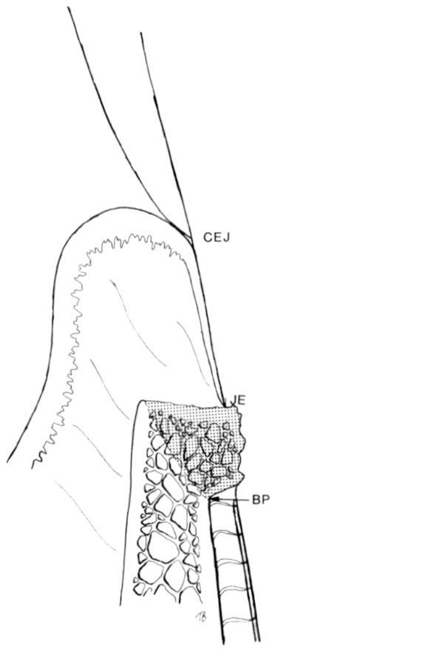

Fig. 18-8. If bone cells migrate into contact with the scaled root surface, root resorption and ankylosis occur. JE = apical extent of the junctional epithelium. BP = preoperative level of the pocket epithelium.

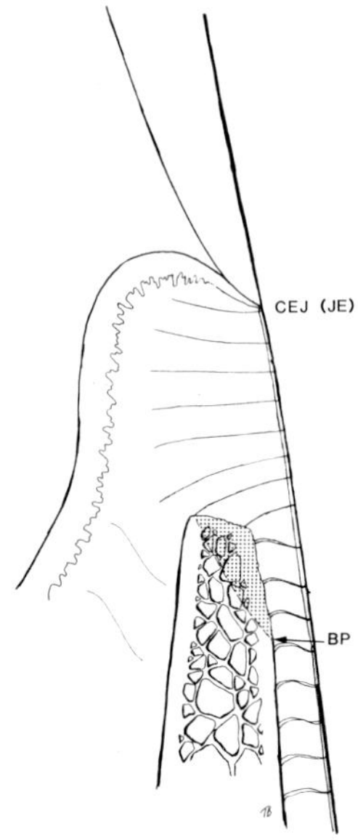

Fig. 18-9. Ideal conditions for healing may develop if cells from the periodontal ligament proliferate to cover the denuded root surface.

the periodontal structures after different modalities of periodontal therapy. The lesions in the test sites were subjected to 1) periodic *root planing and soft tissue curettage*, 2) root planing in combination with the *modified Widman flap* operation without osseous surgery, 3) root planing in combination with the *modified Widman flap* operation without osseous surgery but with *implantation into the defects of previously frozen autogenous, red marrow and cancellous bone*, and 4) root planing in combination with the *modified Widman flap* operation without osseous surgery but with *implantation of a bone substitute*, beta tricalcium phosphate.

Histometric measurements made in sections from block biopsies demonstrated that healing following all 4 treatment procedures resulted in the reformation of a long junctional epithelium facing the instrumented root surfaces. The apical cells of the junctional epithelium were consistently located at or close to their presurgical level in all teeth treated (Figs. 18-10,a,b), i.e. at the same level as in the untreated control lesions. This development of a long junctional epithelium occurred at sites with suprabony as well as at sites with infrabony pockets. The findings by Caton & Nyman (1980) and Caton et al. (1980) were confirmed by Yukna (1976), Nyman et al. (1981) and others in similar experiments.

The results of the studies referred to should not, however, be interpreted to mean that formation of a new connective tissue attachment is impossible. They only demonstrate that new attachment formation is inhibited by the apically migrating dentogingival epithelium. During periodontal wound healing the proliferating epithelial cells reach the presurgical level of the pocket epithelium about 1 week following surgery (Moskow 1964, Kon et al. 1969, Proye & Polson 1982, Karring et al. 1983). This rapid proliferation of the epithelium prevents the gingival connective tissue from establishing a close contact with the root surface. *An early contact between the gingival connective tissue and the root has been regarded as the prime prerequisite for the formation of a new attachment* (Björn 1961, Björn et al. 1965, Hiatt et al.

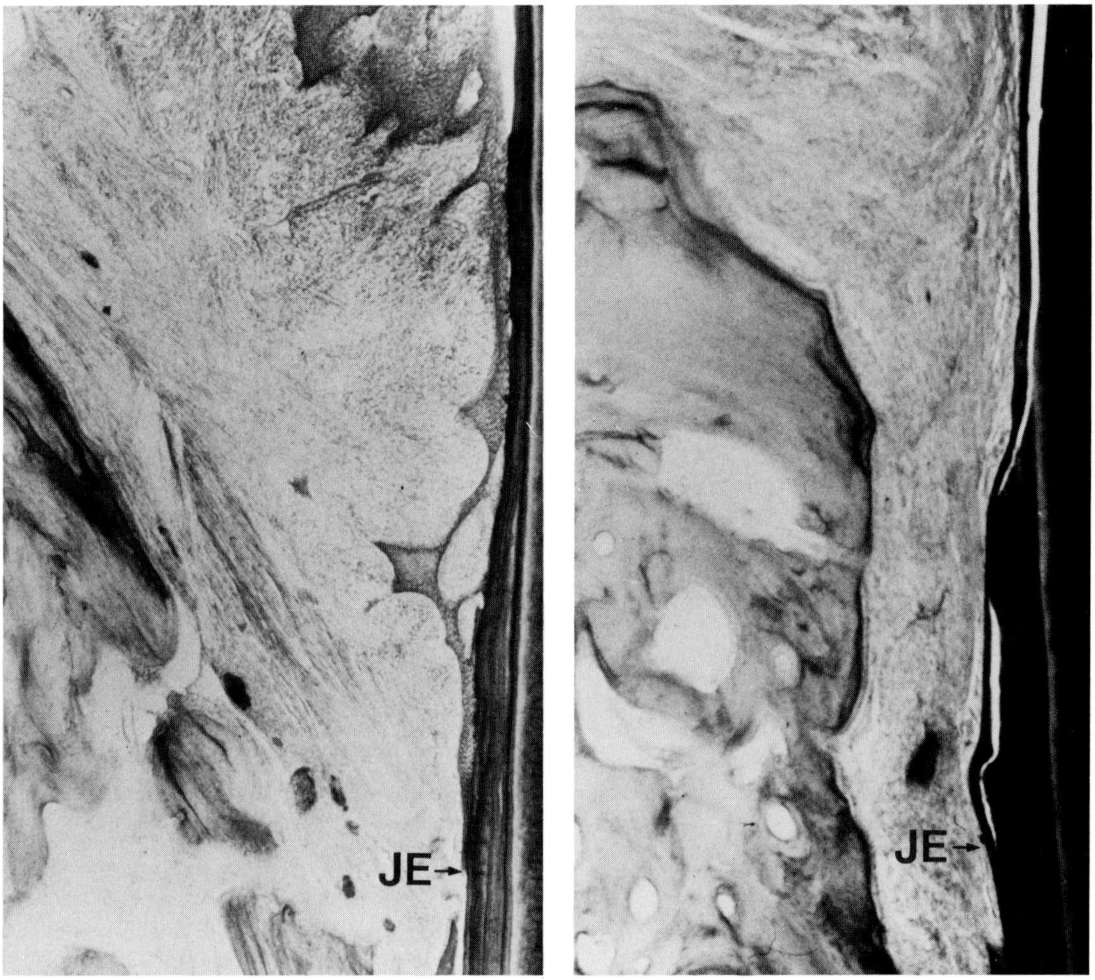

a b

Figs. 18-10a,b. Microphotographs illustrating an infrabony pocket before (a) and after (b) treatment. Note that "bone fill" has occurred but also that the epithelium has migrated apically to the same level as its apical extension before treatment. JE = apical extent of the junctional epithelium. (From Caton & Nyman 1980).

1968). Björn (1961) also claimed that complete new attachment with reorganization of root cementum, periodontal membrane and alveolar bone would be obtained following periodontal therapy, provided the epithelium could be excluded from the healing wound and proper contact between the gingival connective tissue and the root surface was established.

Gingival connective tissue and alveolar bone

In order to evaluate whether the exclusion of the epithelium during healing would in fact result in new attachment, the following experiment was carried out (Nyman et al. 1980): Periodontal tissue breakdown was produced around certain teeth (experimental teeth) in monkeys and dogs using the method described by Caton & Zander (1975). When the destruction of the supporting tissues had progressed to

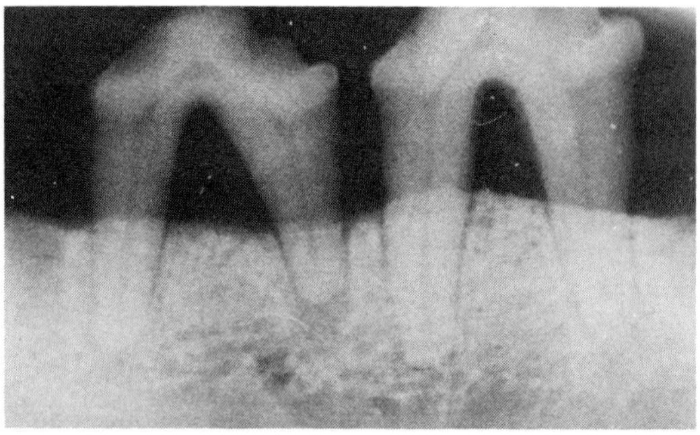

Fig. 18-11. Radiograph of mandibular dog premolars showing destruction of the alveolar bone to approximately half the length of the roots.

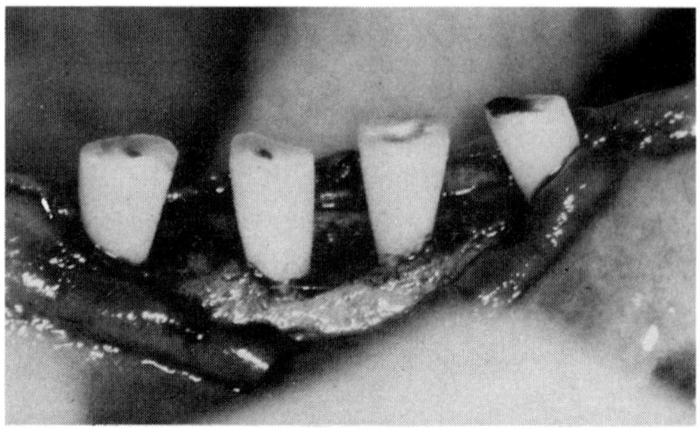

Fig. 18-12. Photograph of experimental roots following separation. Scaling and root planing of the coronal, diseased portions of the separated roots have been carried out.

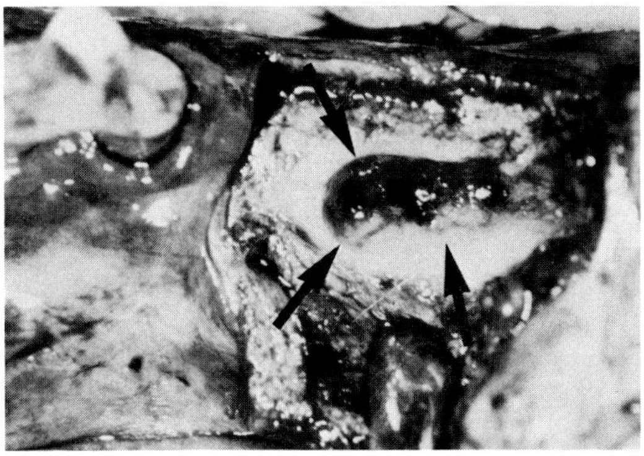

Fig. 18-13. Photograph showing location and size of one groove (arrows) prepared in the buccal surface of the jaw bone. The experimental roots were extracted and placed in such grooves.

approximately half the length of the roots (Fig. 18-11), the plaque-collecting ligatures were removed. Other teeth in the dentition were extracted to provide space (recipient sites) for subsequent implantation of the diseased roots of the experimental teeth (see below).

Following removal of the ligatures the crowns of the experimental teeth were resected. Full-thickness flaps were raised at the facial and lingual/palatal aspects of the teeth, and the denuded (diseased) parts of the root surfaces were thoroughly scaled and planed (Fig. 18-12). Notches were prepared in the roots at the level of the marginal bone crest.

At each recipient site a full-thickness flap was prepared. Grooves, corresponding in size to the roots to be implanted, were prepared in the buccal surface of the jaw bone (Fig. 18-13). The roots of the experimental teeth were extracted and placed in the grooves in the alveolar bone. The flaps were repositioned and sutured to complete coverage of the implanted root and the surrounding bone. With this experimental design, the epithelium was prevented from migrating into the wound. Each implanted root was embedded to half its circumference into bone, and the remaining part was covered by the gingival connective tissue of the flap (Fig. 18-14).

After 3 months of healing, the implanted roots with surrounding tissue were excised and subjected to histological examination. The analysis revealed the following: in the apical portion of the roots, where a viable periodontal ligament tissue was preserved, both on the side facing gingival connective tissue and on the side facing bone, there was a fiber reunion between the root surface and the surrounding tissue (Fig. 18-15). In other words, reattachment was the result of healing. In the coronal, "diseased" portion of the roots (i.e. in areas of the roots which had previously been pathologically exposed) there were no signs of regeneration. In the particular zone of the "diseased" root which faced the gingival connective tissue, collagen fibers were seen with an orientation parallel to the root surface (Fig. 18-15). These fibers were in no instance attached to the implanted roots and *de novo* formation of root

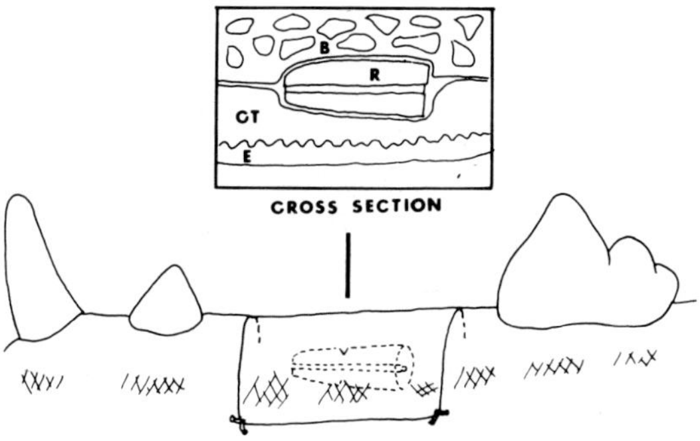

Fig. 18-14. Schematic drawing illustrating the position of a transplanted experimental root. The root (R) is embedded to half its circumference into bone tissue (B). The remaining part is covered by a tissue flap containing gingival connective tissue (CT) and epithelium (E).

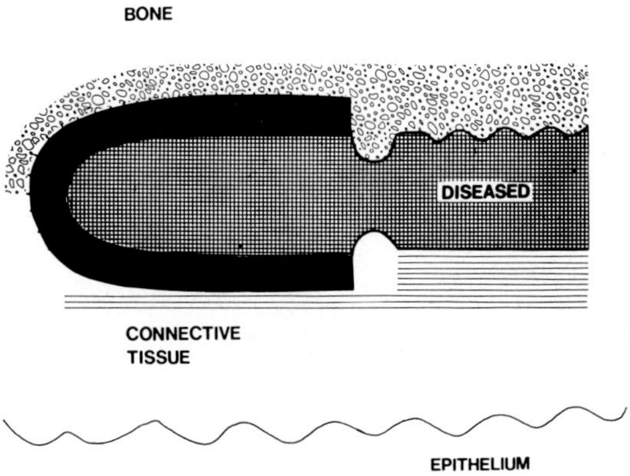

Fig. 18-15. Schematic drawing illustrating the result of healing following root transplantation. In the apical, "non-diseased" portion of the root, a fibrous reunion (reattachment) between the root surface and surrounding tissue was established (black areas). In the coronal, "diseased" root portion new attachment failed to occur.

cementum was never observed. In addition, large resorption lacunae containing multinucleated cells were found along the root surface. In the zone, where the previously "diseased" root surface was facing bone tissue, healing had consistently resulted in extensive root resorption and ankylosis (Fig. 18-15).

This experiment demonstrated that formation of a new attachment is not promoted by the mere exclusion of the epithelium from the healing wound. When in a periodontal wound granulation tissue, derived from the gingival connective tissue or from the bone, reaches contact with the root surface, a process of root resorption is initiated. The experiment thus revealed that *granulation tissue originating from bone or gingival connective tissue lacks the ability to establish a new connective tissue attachment.*

The fact that granulation tissue derived from gingival connective tissue produced root resorption and that granulation tissue derived from bone produced resorption and ankylosis concurs with results reported from several studies on reimplantation and transplantation of teeth (Löe & Waerhaug 1961, Andreasen & Hjörting-Hansen 1966, Karring et al. 1980, 1983, Andreasen 1981, Andreasen & Kristerson 1981, Nyman et al. 1985). On the basis of these findings, it may seem surprising that root resorption is not a common complication following traditional flap surgery, especially when the soft-tissue flap is repositioned with its connective tissue in close contact with the curetted root surface. It may also seem surprising that ankylosis is a rare complication following treatment of infrabony pockets. In fact, since the alveolar bone surrounding the bony defect constitutes a source of granulation tissue during healing, resorption and ankylosis might well be expected to occur on root surfaces located adjacent to surgically treated infrabony defects. The reason why such complications only occasionally take place is evidently the ability of the epithelial cells to proliferate rapidly to the presurgical location of the pocket epithelium. Hereby, the newly formed epithelial lining acts as a barrier which effectively protects the root from granulation tissue from the alveolar bone and the gingiva. This conclusion is further supported by the results presented by Björn et al. (1965) who treated 11 periodontally diseased teeth in 7 human volunteers, using a technique which prevented apical migration of the dentogingival epithelium. They reported that root resorption was indeed a common complication

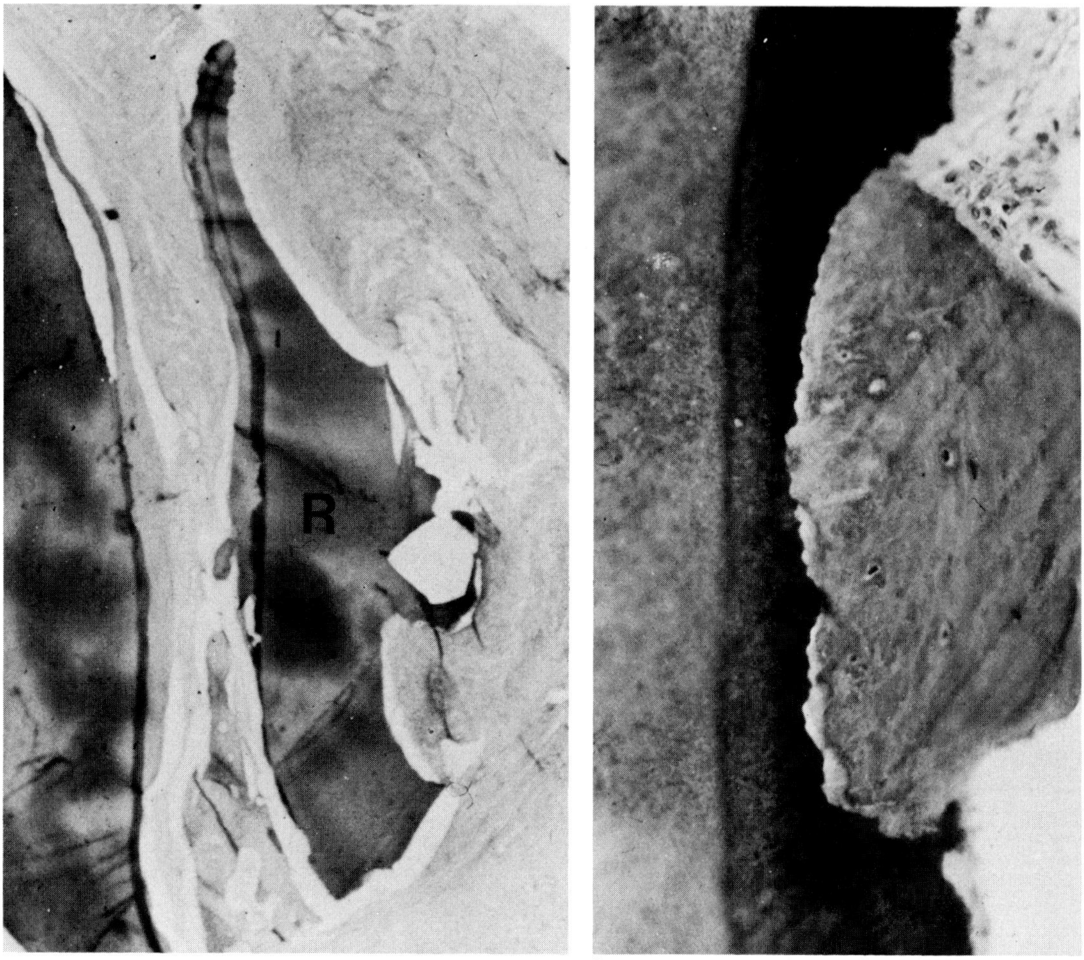

a b

Figs. 18-16a,b. Extensive root resorption (a) and root resorption in conjunction with ankylosis (b) following treatment of advanced periodontal disease in humans using a surgical technique which prevented apical migration of the dentogingival epithelium during healing. R = remaining part of the root. (From Björn et al. 1965)

following this type of therapy (Figs. 18-16a,b).

From the above description it is obvious that attempts aiming at preventing apical downgrowth of the epithelium in order to allow new attachment to form may instead result in root resorption.

In this context, a study in the monkey by Karring et al. (1983) should be briefly described. Roots which to half the root length had been exposed to periodontal disease were, following treatment, implanted into bone and gingival connective tissue in a manner similar to that described above (Nyman et al. 1980). After varying time intervals the roots were exposed by a secondary incision through the covering mucosa. The epithelium was thereby enabled to migrate into the wound. If this incision was made within 2 weeks after root implantation, the epithelium migrated into the wound and covered the previously diseased part of the root which showed no signs of resorption or ankylosis (Fig. 18-17). With increasing intervals between implantation of the roots and the secondary incision, the migrating epithelium covered the root surface to a diminishing degree and signs of root resorption and ankylosis

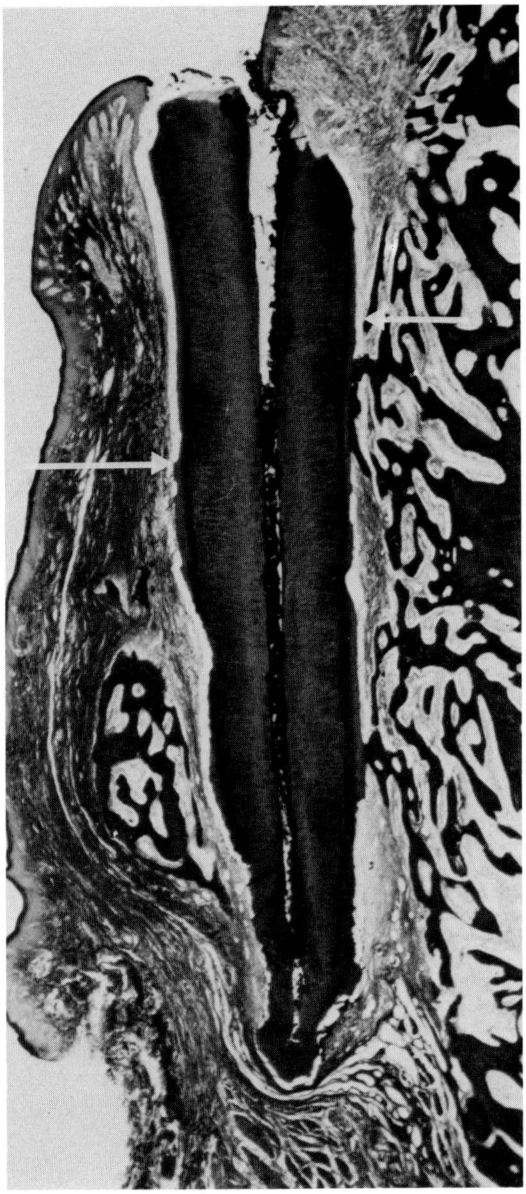

Fig. 18-17. Microphotograph of a transplanted root. The surgical procedure prevented during a 2-week period the epithelium from migrating into the wound. The epithelium has migrated along the coronal, previously periodontitis involved root surfaces down to a level indicated by the arrows. In the areas covered by epithelium there are no signs of resorption. Apical to this level the root surfaces are characterized by resorption.

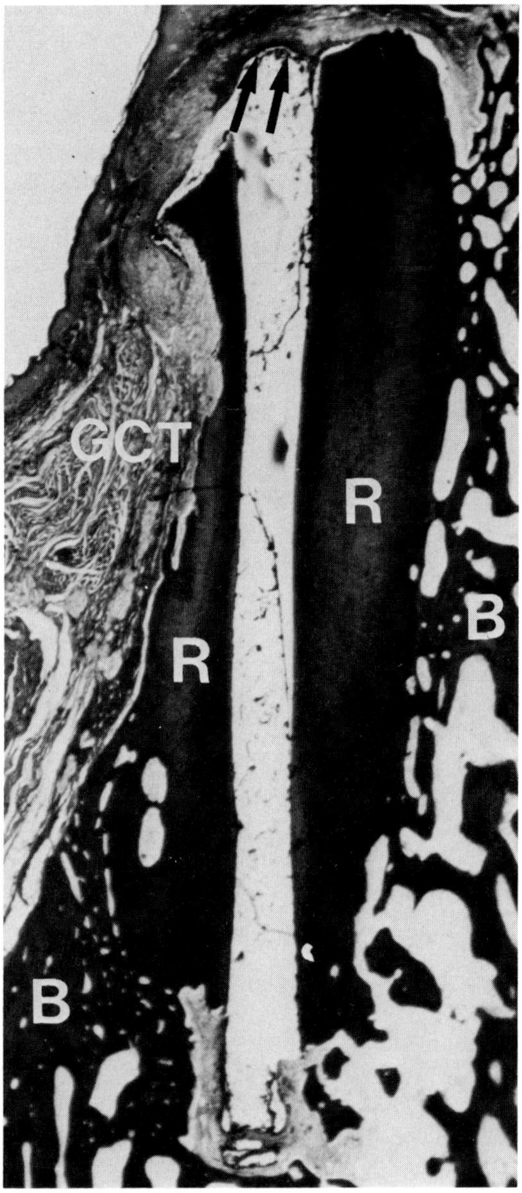

Fig. 18-18. Microphotograph of an implanted root. After 8 weeks of healing the epithelium was allowed to proliferate in apical direction. The epithelium (arrows) covers only part of the coronal, cut-root surface. Extensive root resorption is seen on the surface facing the gingival connective tissue (GCT). Resorption and ankylosis characterized the surface facing the bone tissue. R = root, B = bone.

became more pronounced (Fig. 18-18). Taken together with the data reported previously, these findings demonstrated that *the migrating epithelium functions as a protective barrier towards root resorption and ankylosis during healing following periodontal therapy.*

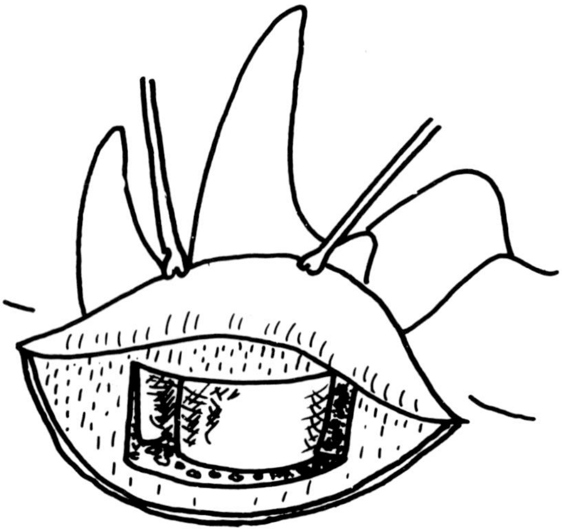

Fig. 18-19. Schematic drawing illustrating the surgical procedure used in the study by Nyman et al. (1982a).

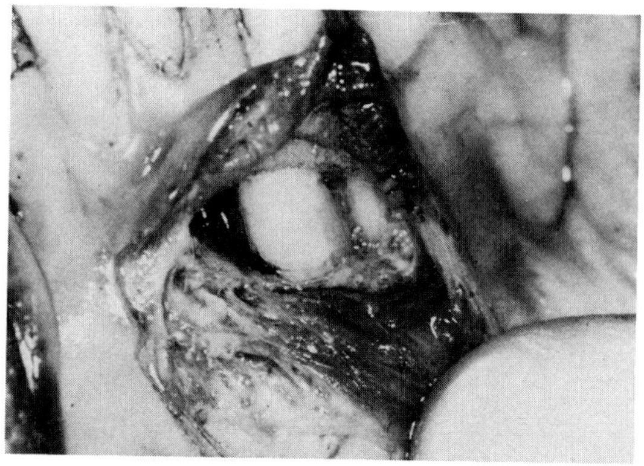

Fig. 18-20. Photograph showing the wound with the denuded part of the root. The cementum layer of this part of the root was removed.

This fact is, of course, of particular interest with respect to the use of bone transplants in the treatment of infrabony pockets (for review see Gara & Adams 1981). The rationale behind such treatment is the concept that bone regeneration in an angular bony defect may favor the formation of new cementum and new connective tissue attachment. The results of the studies discussed above, as well as of other investigators (e.g. Melcher 1969, 1970, Atrizadeh et al. 1971, Line et al. 1974, Boyko et al. 1981), demonstrating that granulation tissue derived from bone induces root resorption and ankylosis, however, seem to invalidate the use of bone grafts in periodontal surgery. In fact, when viable bone cells are transferred with fresh iliac bone-marrow grafts into infrabony periodontal defects, replacement resorption identified by root resorption and ankylosis often occurs (Schallhorn et al. 1970, Seibert 1970, Sullivan et al. 1971, Burnette 1972, Schallhorn 1972, Dragoo & Sullivan 1973a,b, Dragoo 1981).

Periodontal ligament

An important observation made in studies on the regenerative potential of the periodontal tissues is that deposition of new cementum with inserting collagen fibers occasionally occurs during healing in the most apical part of periodontal wounds (Skillen & Lundqvist 1937, Linghorne & O'Connell 1950, Morris 1953, Listgarten 1972, Frank et al. 1974, Caton & Nyman 1980, Cole et al. 1980, Karring et al. 1980, Nyman et al. 1981). This formation of new cementum may be indicative of a potential for coronal migration (along the root surface) of cells from the remaining periodontal ligament which have the capacity to form a new attachment. Result from animal experiments by e.g. Melcher (1970), Line et al. (1974) (for review see Melcher 1976) have provided support for the hypothesis that cells derived from the periodontal ligament possess an ability to produce new cementum.

In order to learn if periodontal ligament cells do indeed have this ability, a research model was developed (Nyman et al. 1982a) by which not only the dentogingival epithelium was prevented from interfering with the wound, but by which also granulation tissue, derived from the gingiva, was inhibited from reaching contact with the root surface during healing. At the

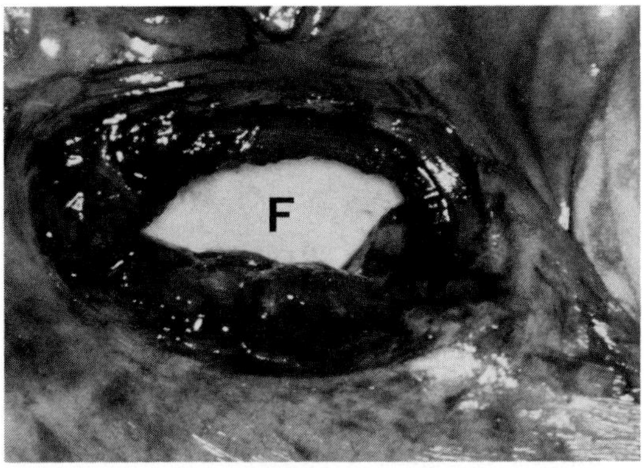

Fig. 18-21. The fenestration of the alveolar bone was covered by a membrane (F) over which the tissue flap was subsequently positioned.

buccal aspect of canine teeth in monkeys a U-shaped incision was made through the oral mucosa (Fig. 18-19). A mucoperiosteal flap was raised on the coronal side of the incision to expose the buccal alveolar bone. Within an area extending from a level approximately 3mm coronal to the apex to a level 2 mm apical to the marginal bone crest, the buccal and approximal alveolar bone was resected and the root surface thoroughly planed to remove all cementum (Fig. 18-20). By preserving the most marginal portion of the periodontium, wound healing was allowed to occur *without interference from an apically migrating dentogingival epithelium.* In order to *prevent the gingival connective tissue from reaching* contact with the root surface, a membrane (Millipore®; Millipore Corporation) was placed to cover the fenestration in the alveolar bone (Fig. 18-21). The flap was repositioned to the facial surface of the membrane and sutured.

The histological analysis of block sections representing 3 months of healing disclosed that new formation of attachment had occurred, including newly formed cementum with inserting collagen fibers and also supporting alveolar bone (Fig. 18-22). This finding demonstrates that periodontal ligament cells have a considerable potential for regeneration. However, this ability of the periodontal ligament cells evidently may manifest itself only if the epithelium and the gingival connective tissue are prevented from occupying the wound area adjacent to the root.

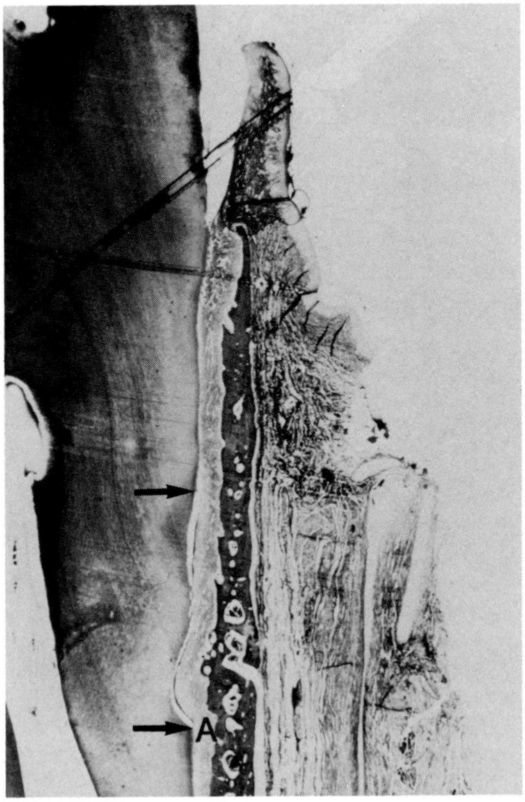

Fig. 18-22. Microphotograph of a histological specimen demonstrating new cementum (between arrows) and regenerated bone along the curetted root surface. A split has occurred between the dentine and the new cementum layer during histological preparation. A = the apical notch prepared in the root surface.

In the study described, new attachment was obtained on root surfaces which were indeed deprived of their periodontal ligament and cementum but, on the other hand, had not been exposed to plaque or to a periodontal pocket. In order to test the hypothesis that new cementum with inserting principal fibers also could be formed on a previously diseased root surface provided cells from the periodontal ligament were enabled to repopulate this portion of the root, the following experiment was performed (Nyman et al. 1982b):

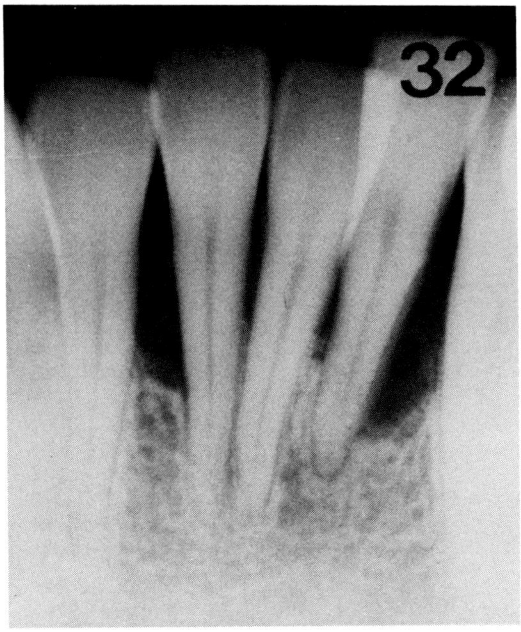

Fig. 18-23. A radiograph demonstrating advanced bone loss in the mandibular incisor part of the dentition of a patient with longstanding periodontal disease.

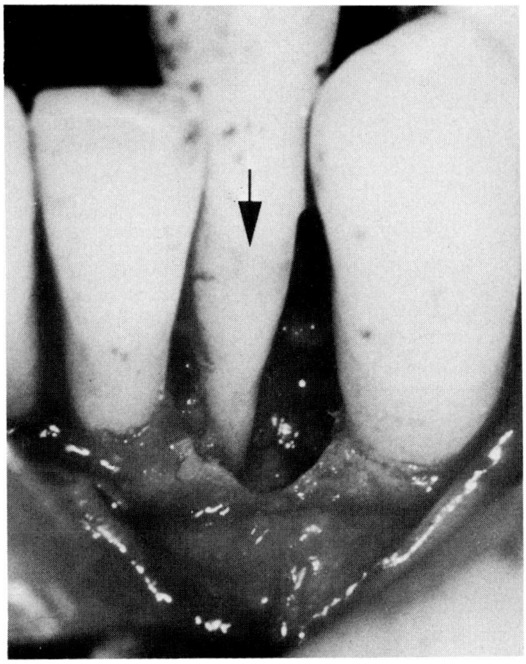

Fig. 18-24. The degree of loss of periodontal tissue in the area of tooth 32 is illustrated after flap elevation. The location of the cemento-enamel junction is identified by the arrow. Note the angular bony defect at the buccal and distal aspects of the tooth.

A male patient (47 years of age) suffered from advanced periodontal disease of a generalized character. A mandibular incisor with deep pockets of long standing and scheduled for extraction was treated using a flap technique. A radiograph of this tooth obtained immediately before treatment is shown in Fig. 18-23. The attachment level at the buccal surface of this tooth was found to be located 11mm apical to the cemento-enamel junction (CEJ). Following elevation of soft tissue flaps (Fig. 18-24), a notch was prepared in the buccal root surface at the level of the alveolar bone crest. The distance between CEJ and this notch was 9mm. An angular bony defect, 2 mm deep, was found to be present apical to the notch. Following removal of all granulation tissue and careful scaling and root planing (to the bottom of the angular defect), a membrane was adjusted to cover the buccal and approximal tooth surfaces from a level around 2 mm coronal to CEJ to a level 1mm apical to the bone crest (Figs. 18-25a-c).

The membrane was placed in position and adapted to the enamel surface by means of a resin. The buccal flap was then repositioned to the facial surface of the membrane and secured to the lingual flap by interdental sutures. The location of the membrane in relation to the tooth and the surrounding periodontal tissues is illustrated in Fig. 18-25c. With this design of the wound, the membrane prevented the gingival connective tissue from contacting the facial and proximal parts of the root. The proliferating oral epithelium was thus during healing guided along the outer surface of the membrane rather than along the root surface. The result of treatment after 3 months of healing is shown in Fig. 18-26. The histological section illustrates that the epithelium had proliferated along the facial surface of the membrane. New cementum with inserting collagen fibers was observed on the facial root surface extending in coronal direction from the apical level of the previous angular bony defect via the notch area to a level 5mm coronal to the apical border of the notch. Figs. 18-26a-d show the newly formed connective tissue attachment at different levels coronal to the notch.

From the findings of this experiment it was concluded that new attachment can in fact be established on a previously diseased root surface. Hence, the concept that the periodontitis-affected root surface is a major preventive factor for new attachment seems to be invalid. A subsequent study (Gottlow et al. 1984) was designed in order to evaluate the predictability of new attachment formation on previously plaque-exposed root surfaces using the method of guiding the periodontal ligament cells (PDL-cells) into the wound (Guided tissue regeneration). This study was carried out in the monkey. A soft-tissue flap was raised at the buccal aspect of the experimental teeth. 50-70% of the buccal alveolar bone, between the mesio-buccal and disto-buccal line angels of the root, was removed. Before flap repositioning the coronal portion of the flap was excised so that its cut margin coincided with the reduced bone crest. Hereby the coronal portion of the roots was left open to plaque accumulation.

After 6 months of experimentation, a notch was prepared in the buccal root surface at the level of the gingival margin. This was done in order to demarcate the coronal, denuded and plaque-exposed root portion. A soft-tissue flap was again raised at the buccal aspect of the experimental teeth (Fig. 18-27a). The root surface coronal to the notch was thoroughly scaled. The crowns of the teeth were then resected (Fig. 18-27b) and the flaps sutured to the lingual wound edge to accomplish complete coverage of the roots. However, before suturing of the flaps, a teflon membrane was placed over the denuded root surfaces on one side of the jaw (test roots) in order to prevent granulation tissue from the soft tissue flap from reaching contact with the roots (Fig. 18-27c). No membrane was placed over the contralateral roots (control roots).

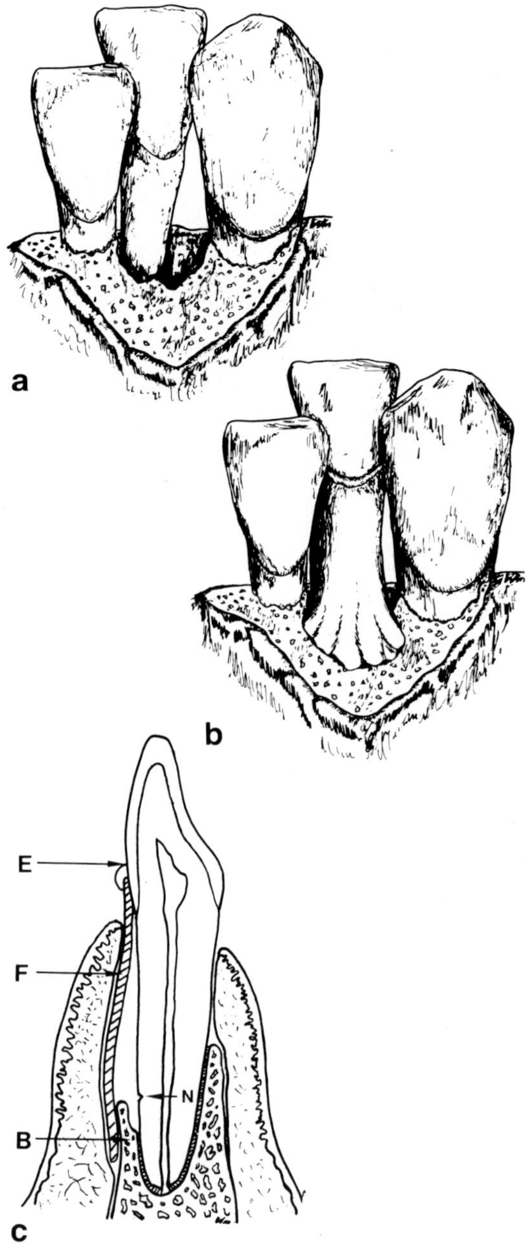

Figs. 18-25a-c. Schematic drawings illustrating the root and bone architecture before (a) and after (b) the placement of the membrane (F). Fig. 18-25c demonstrates that the membrane (F) covers an area extending from the enamel surface (E) to the aleolar bone (B). A notch (N) was prepared in the root surface at the level of the alveolar bone crest.

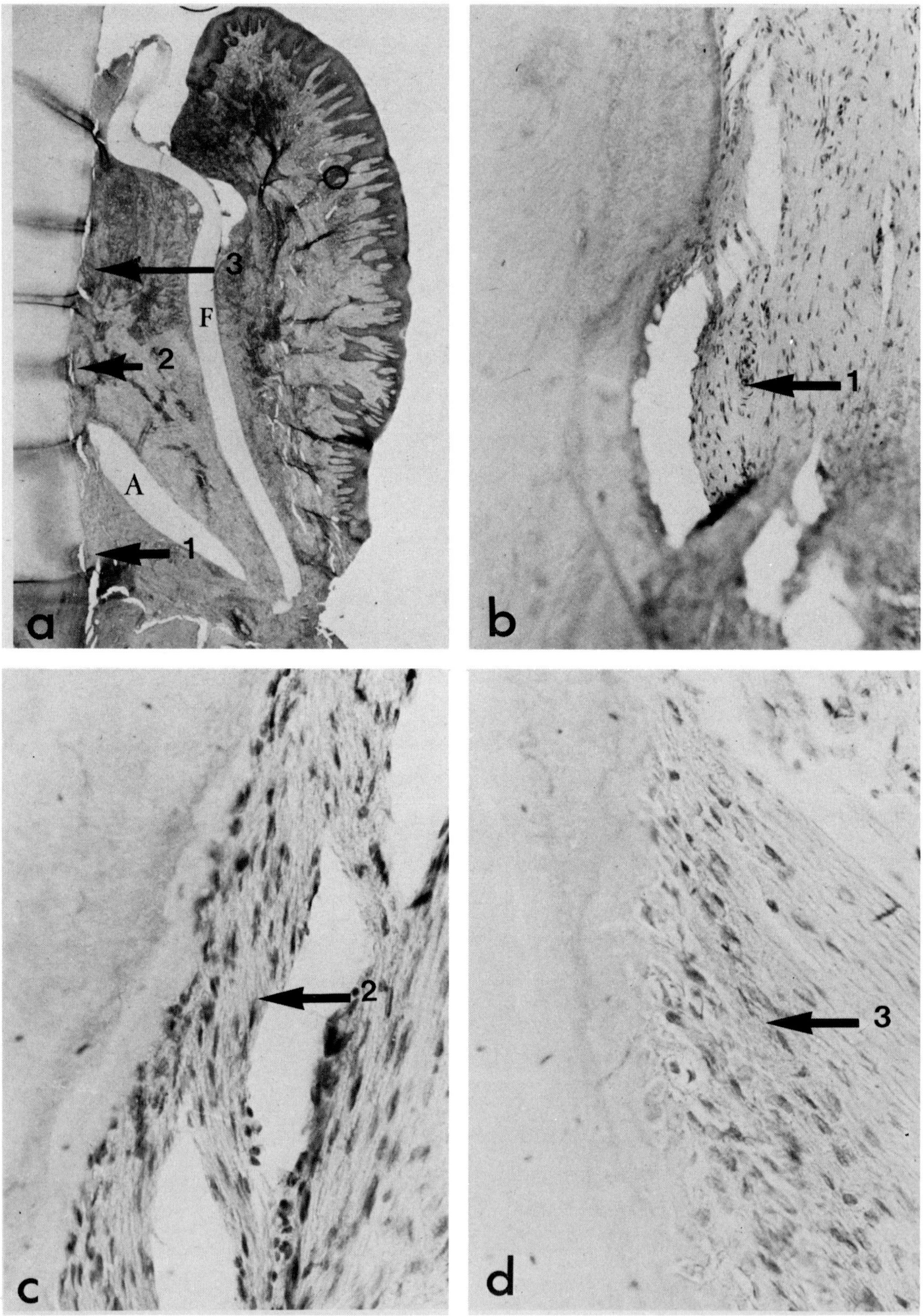

Figs. 18-26a-d. The upper left microphotogram (a) illustrates the location of the membrane (F) in relation to the gingiva and the root surface. Arrow 1 denotes the notch area. Arrows 2 and 3 denote previously exposed root areas coronal to the notch with newly formed cementum and inserting principal fibers. A = artifact. Figs. 18-26b-d = magnifications of the 3 different areas of arrows 1, 2 and 3.

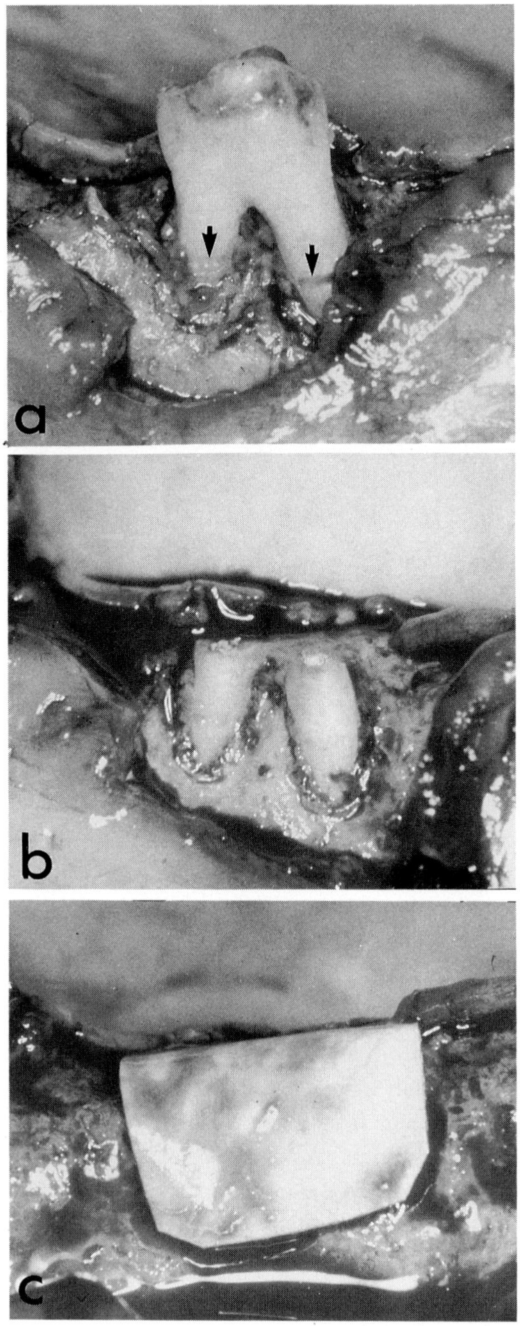

Figs. 18-27a-c. Illustration of the experimental procedure. After 6 months of plaque accumulation on surgically exposed test and control roots, a soft tissue flap was raised. Notches (arrows) were prepared in the roots at the apical border of the plaque-exposed portion of the root surface (a). After root instrumentation, the crown of the tooth was resected (b). Prior to flap replacement, a membrane was placed to cover the denuded surfaces of the test roots (c).

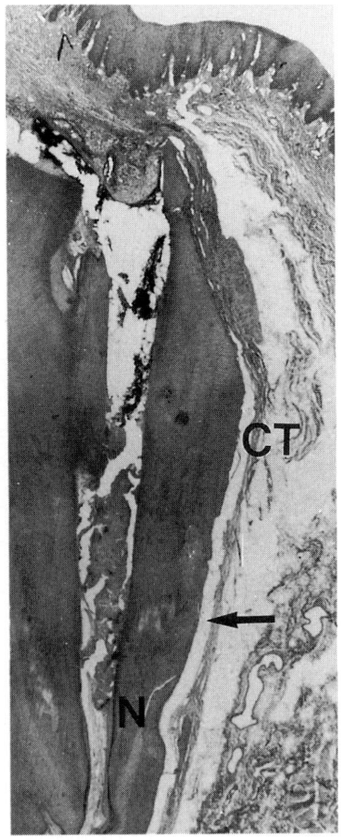

Fig. 18-28. Microphotograph of a control root. New cementum is formed on the root surface within the notch area and extends a small distance (arrow) coronally to the notch (N). The root surface coronal to the newly formed cementum is covered by a non-attached connective tissue (CT).

The material available for histological examination comprised 9 test roots and 6 control roots. New cementum with inserting collagen fibers was observed on the curetted surfaces of all test roots and on 5 of the 6 control roots. In specimens with new fibrous attachment, the newly formed cementum was always in continuity with the cementum of the apical part of the roots. Furthermore, the newly formed cementum was thicker in the apical than in the coronal portions. In the control roots (Fig. 18-28), the length of the newly formed fibrous attachment varied between 0 and 2.5 mm, while in the test roots (Fig. 18-29) the range was 0.9 to 6.8 mm. In 4 of the 9 test roots, new cementum covered the entire length of the root por-

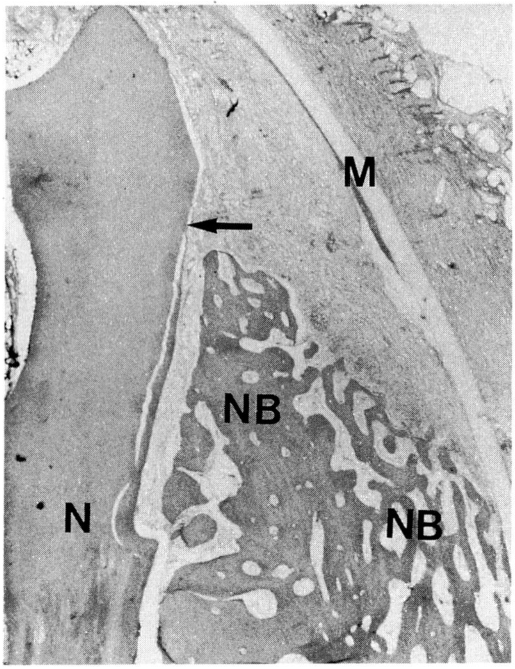

Fig. 18-29. Microphotograph of a test root. Newly formed cementum extends from the apical border of the notch (N) to a level exceeding half the length of the previously exposed portion of the root (arrow). Significant regrowth of bone has occurred in the coronal as well as in the buccal direction. NB = new bone; M = membrane.

tion coronal to the notch and, in 3 of these 4 roots, even part of the coronal cut surface (Fig. 18-30a-c). Only 3 of 9 test roots exhibited a new fibrous attachment which covered less than 60% of the length of the previously exposed root surface, while only 1 control root exhibited a new attachment which exceeded 60% of corresponding root portion (Table 18-1). In all control specimens, the surface coronal to the newly formed cementum was characterized by the presence of multinucleated cells and resorption cavities. In one control specimen, virtually half the root had become resorbed (Fig. 18-31). However, areas without sign of root resorption were also observed. The root surface in such areas was covered by a non-attached connective tissue with collagen fibers running parallel to the surface (Fig. 18-28).

Table 18-1

Frequency distribution describing the varying length (as a percentage of the total length of the exposed root surface) of new attachment in test and control roots

	Test (n=9)	Control (n=6)
100%	4	0
80-99%	2	0
60-79%	0	1
40-59%	1	1
20-39%	2	2
0-19%	0	2

Coronal regrowth of alveolar bone had occurred to a varying extent adjacent to 7 of the 9 test roots and 2 of the 6 control roots. No relationship was found between the amount of new cementum formation and the degree of bone regrowth, a finding which concurred with observations by Bogle et al. (1983) and Lindhe et al. (1984). The most important information derived from this study was, however, that the gingival connective tissue evidently lacks the ability to form a new attachment and that the prevention of the gingival tissues (i.e. both the gingival connective tissue and the epithelium) from interfering with healing facilitates new attachment formation by giving preference to the periodontal ligament cells to repopulate the wound area adjacent to the root.

The findings from the studies described above prompted the initiation of a clinical trial, the objective of which was to assess if new attachment would predictably form also in human teeth when treatment is based on the principle of guided tissue regeneration.

In this study (Gottlow et al. 1986), 12 periodontally involved teeth in 10 patients were used. The comprehensive treatment plan for the patients called for extraction of 5 of the 12 teeth. Four of these 5 teeth were treated with the guided tissue regeneration (GTR) tech-

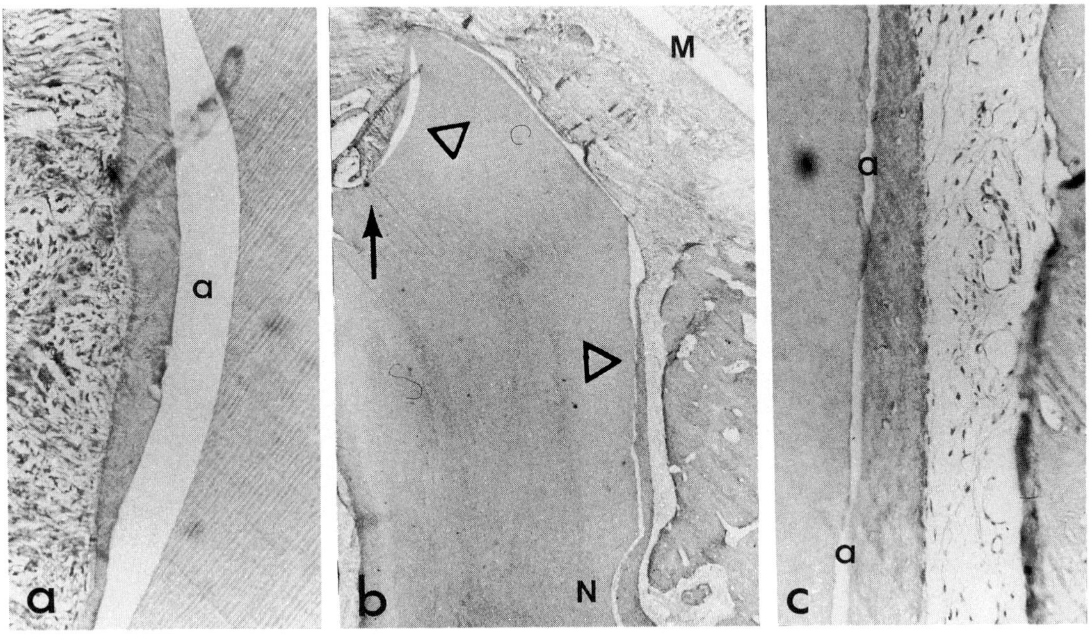

Figs. 18-30a-c. Microphotographs of a test root. New cementum covers the entire length of the buccal root surface coronal to the notch (N in b) and also part of the coronal cut surface (to the arrow in b). Higher magnifications (a and c) of the areas at the upper and lower triangles in b show that collagen fibers are inserted into the newly formed cellular cementum. a = artifact; M = membrane.

nique. One of the 5 teeth was surgically treated without placement of membrane. Following healing these 5 teeth were extracted and subjected to histological examination.

The remaining 7 teeth were treated with the GTR method and retained. The result of healing in these teeth was evaluated using clinical parameters, i.e. probing attachment level (PAL), probing bone level (PB), radiographic analysis and clinical inspection during reentry operation.

Following incision through the bottom of the pockets, full-thickness flaps were raised at the buccal and lingual aspects of the teeth. Epithelium and granulation tissue on the inner surface of the flap were removed. The root surfaces were scaled and planed. In 11 teeth, a teflon membrane (Goretex® W.L. Gore and Ass. Inc., Flagstaff, Arizona, USA) was adjusted to cover the root surfaces from a level around 5 mm api-

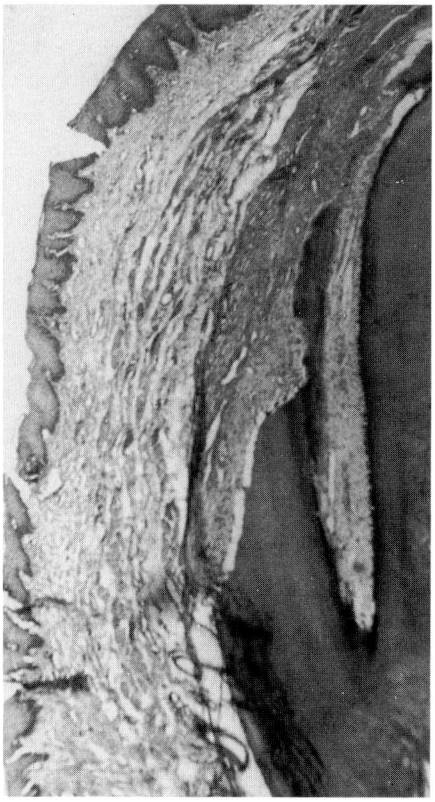

Fig. 18-31. Microphotograph of a control root exhibiting extensive resorption.

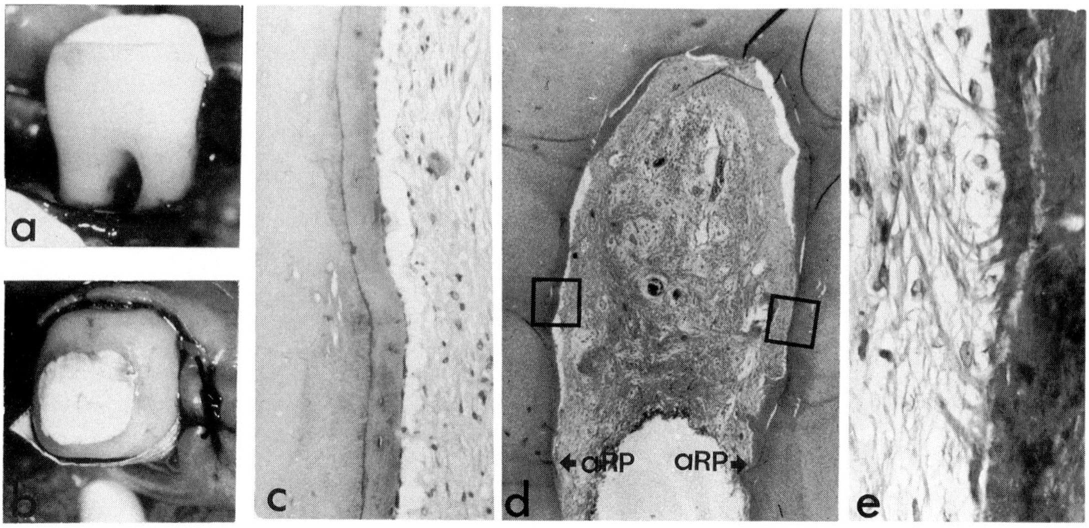

Figs. 18-32a-e. Case 1. Male, 54 years of age. The clinical status of the lingual furcation area of tooth 47 after flap elevation is shown in (a). The membrane was placed to cover the lingual root surfaces and the entrance to the interradicular area and the flap was repositioned and secured with sutures (b). Mesio-distal sections from the lingual portion of the furcation, obtained after 3 months of healing, showed that the entire circumference of this area was covered by newly formed cementum (d). The delineated areas in (d) are shown in higher magnification in (c) and (e). Healing had resulted in complete closure of the furcation defect.

cal to the bone crest to a level approaching the CEJ. The membrane was retained in this position and the mucoperiosteal flaps were placed on the outer surface of the membrane and secured with interdental sutures in such a way that the coronal border of the membrane was consistently located around 1-2 mm above the flap margin. This wound preparation was designed to prevent the oral epithelium and the gingival connective tissue from reaching contact with the root.

After 3 months of healing, the 5 teeth which had been scheduled for extraction were removed together with surrounding periodontal tissues. The biopsies were subjected to routine histological preparation. The amount of new attachment, i.e. the linear distance from the apical extension of root-planed surface (aRP) to the coronal level of newly formed cementum with inserting collagen fibers (C), was assessed in 5 sections obtained from the central portion of each experimental root.

In the group of 7 teeth which were retained, a second surgical procedure was carried out after 3 months of healing for the removal of the membranes. The level of the alveolar bone crest and the apical extension of angular defects were determined by probing. After another 3-month period of healing, a final examination was made including measurements of the probing attachment level (PAL). The result of treament is exemplified by the following two cases, one documented histologically and the other with the use of clinical parameters.

Case presentation

Case 1

Male, 54 years of age (Figs. 18-32a-e). The clinical status of the lingual furcation area of tooth 47 after flap elevation is shown in (a). The membrane was placed to cover the lingual root surfaces and the entrance to the interradicular area and the flap was repositioned and secured with sutures (b). Mesio-distal sections from the lingual portion of the furcation, obtained after 3 months of healing, showed that the entire circumference of this area was

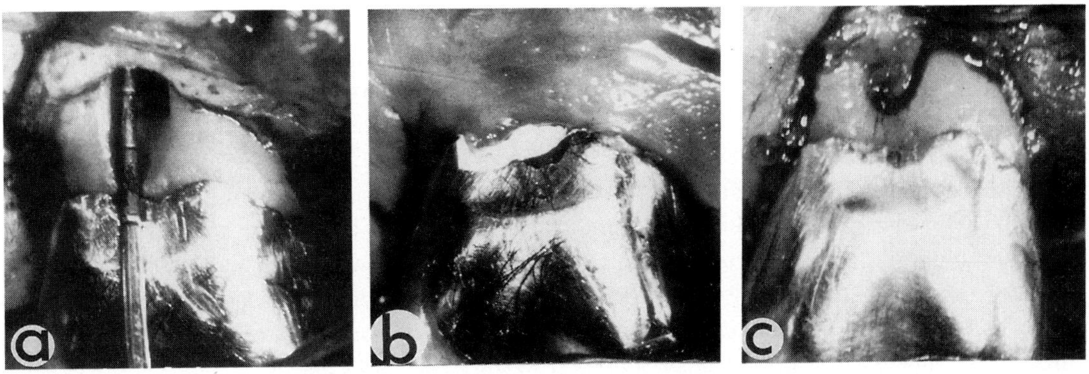

Figs. 18-33a-c. Case 2. Male, 62 years of age. Tooth 16 exhibited loss of periodontal tissues at the buccal aspect of the tooth and, in addition, a deep buccal furcation involvement associated with an angular bony defect within the furcation area (a). Following the placement of a membrane to cover the buccal surfaces and the entrance to the furcation, the flap was repositioned and sutured (b). At the time of removal of the membrane, the furcation defect was found to be completely closed by newly formed alveolar bone (c). The tooth did not show any signs of ankylosis by percussion or mobility tests.

covered by newly formed cementum (d). The delineated areas in (d) are shown in higher magnification in (c) and (e). Healing had resulted in complete closure of the furcation defect.

Case 2

Male, 62 years of age (Figs. 18-33a-c). Tooth 16 exhibited loss of periodontal tissues at the buccal aspect of the tooth and, in addition, a deep buccal furcation involvement associated with an angular bony defect within the furcation area (a). Following the placement of a membrane to cover the buccal surfaces and the entrance to the furcation, the flap was repositioned and sutured (b). At the time of removal of the membrane, the furcation defect was found to be completely closed by newly formed alveolar bone (c). The tooth did not show any signs of ankylosis by percussion or mobility tests.

In this context it should be mentioned that no sign of new attachment was found in the histological sections obtained from the tooth which was surgically treated without placement of membrane.

The result of this study suggests that a regenerative surgical therapy, based on the principle of guided tissue regeneration, predictably results in new connective tissue attachment. The amount of fibrous attachment formed in this clinical trial, however, varied considerably from one tooth to the other. In some teeth, treatment resulted in a complete new attachment, while in other sites only a few mm of new cementum were formed. Several factors are responsible for this variability. One factor is the degree of gingival recession that occurs during healing. The more the gingiva recedes, the shorter becomes the root surface portion that is available for PDL-cell repopulation. Another factor that may influence the degree of new attachment formation is the morphology of the periodontal defect. In the situation of a "horizontal"-type defect circumscribing the root, new attachment is entirely dependent on a coronal upgrowth of PDL-tissue from remaining periodontium in the apical part of the root. In angular defects and in furcation involvements of partial character, PDL-cells may migrate into the wound area not only from the apical part of the defect but also from its lateral borders. This may enhance the potential for new attachment formation.

As described above, the membrane used was consistently placed with its apical portion on the outer surface of the remaining alveolar bone even in the case of angular defects. Such placement of the membrane allows in fact not only periodontal ligament tissue but also bone tissue with a potential to produce root resorption to invade the wound area adjacent to the root. However, no signs or symptoms of ankylosis were found in any of the treated teeth as evaluated histologically in the extracted teeth and by percussion and mobility tests in the retained teeth. This must mean that the periodontal ligament tissue had established contact with the root surface before granulation tissue originating from the bone reached the tooth.

Recently a clinical trial was reported in which the regenerative potential of the periodontal tissues was assessed in Degree II furcation defects at mandibular molars using a surgical treatment technique based on the principles of guided tissue regeneration (Pontoriero et al. 1988). The patient sample included 21 subjects. The patients had periodontal lesions in the right and left molar regions including advanced periodontal tissue destruction within the interradicular area. The furcation-involved molars were in each patient randomly assigned to either a test or a control treatment procedure. The test procedure included the elevation of mucoperiosteal flaps at the buccal and lingual aspect of the alveolar process. The inner surface of each flap was carefully curetted to remove epithelium and granulation tissue. The root surfaces were scaled and planed. A teflon membrane was adjusted to cover the entrance of the furcation area and the adjacent root surfaces as well as a portion of the alveolar bone apical to the crest. The flaps were repositioned and placed on the outer surface of the membrane and secured with interdental sutures. A second surgical procedure was performed after a healing period of 1-2 months to remove the membrane. A procedure identical to the one used at the test teeth was performed at the control tooth regions with the exception of the placement of the teflon membrane. The findings from the investigation demonstrated that treatment of Degree II furcation defects at mandibular molars using a technique in compliance with the principles of guided tissue regeneration at most sites resulted in the disappearance of the anatomical defect. More than 90% of the sites treated with the membrane technique showed complete resolution of the furcation problem. Conventional therapy reached the same treatment goal in less than 20% of the cases treated.

Conclusion

The results of this series of experiments have clearly demonstrated that a method of treatment aimed at restitution of the attachment apparatus must be based on the principle of guided tissue regeneration, i.e. guiding those particular cells into the periodontal wound which have the biological ability to regenerate the connective tissue attachment.

Citric acid: an adjunct for new attachment formation ?

Studies on repair of surgical wounds in animals have led to the use of citric acid as a means of promoting new attachment (Register & Burdick 1976, Ririe et al. 1980). Following removal of the root cementum from the periodontitis affected part of the root, citric acid at pH 1 is applied to the dentin surface for 3 min. The surperficial zone of the root dentin hereby becomes demineralized, which leads to denudation of the collagen fibrils of the dentin matrix. A connective tissue attachment will, according to Ririe et al. (1980), be established by "interdigitation of new and old collagen fibrils at the tooth-gingiva interface". Citric acid conditioning has demonstrated some remarkable success in periodontal defects in dogs (Crigger et al. 1978, Nilveus 1978) and also enabled the demonstration of new attachment in humans (Cole et al. 1980). However, other studies indicate only a limited regeneration following acid conditioning (Cole et al. 1981, Renvert & Egelberg 1981).

References

Alderman, N. (1969) Sterile plaster of Paris as an implant in the infrabony environment: A preliminary study. *Journal of Periodontology* **40**, 11-13.

Andreasen, J.O. (1981) Periodontal healing after replantation and autotransplantation of permanent incisors. *International Journal of Oral Surgery* **60**, 54-61.

Andreasen, J.O. & Hjörting-Hansen, E. (1966) Replantation of teeth. II. Histological study of 22 replanted anterior teeth in humans. *Acta Odontologica Scandinavica* **24**, 290-306.

Andreasen, J.O. & Kristerson, L. (1981) The effect of limited drying or removal of the periodontal ligament. Periodontal healing after replantation of mature permanent incisors in monkeys. *Acta Odontologica Scandinavica* **1**, 1-13.

Armitage, G.C., Svanberg, G.K. & Löe, H. (1977) Microscopic evaluation of clinical measurements of connective tissue attachment levels. *Journal of Clinical Periodontology* **4**, 173-190.

Atrizadeh, F., Kennedy, J. & Zander, H. (1971) Ankylosis of teeth following thermal injury. *Journal of Periodontal Research* **6**, 157-159.

Beube, F.E. (1947) A study of reattachment of the supporting structures of the teeth. *Journal of Periodontology* **18**, 55-66.

Beube, F.E. (1952) A radiographic and histologic study on reattachment. *Journal of Periodontology* **23**, 158-164.

Björn, H. (1961) Experimental studies on reattachment. *Dental Practitioner and Dental Reconstruction* **11**, 351-354.

Björn, H. Hollender, L. & Lindhe, J. (1965) Tissue regeneration in patients with periodontal disease. *Odontologisk Revy* **16**, 317-326.

Bogle, G., Garrett, S., Crigger, M. & Egelberg, J. (1983) New connective tissue attachment in beagles with advanced natural periodontitis. *Journal of Periodontal Research* **18**, 220-228.

Bowers, G.M., Schallhorn, R.G. & Mellonig, J.T., (1982) Histologic evaluation of new attachment in human intrabony defects. *Journal of Periodontology* **53**, 509-514.

Bowers, G.M., Granet, M., Steven, M., Emerson, J., Corio, R., Mellonig, J., Lewis, S.B., Peltzman, B., Romberg, E. & Risom, L. (1985) Histologic evaluation of new attachment in humans. A preliminary report. *Journal of Periodontology* **56**, 381-396.

Boyko, G.A., Melcher, A.H. & Brunette, D.M. (1981) Formation of new periodontal ligament by periodontal ligament cells implanted in vivo after culture in vitro. A preliminary study of transplanted roots in the dog. *Journal of Periodontal Research* **16**, 73-88.

Bump, R.L., Salimeno, T., Hooker, S.P. & Wilkinson, E.G. (1975) The use of woven ceramic fabric as a periodontal allograft. *Journal of Periodontology* **46**, 453-458.

Burnette, E.W. (1972) Fate of an iliac crest graft. *Journal of Periodontology* **43**, 88-90.

Carranza, F.A. (1954) A technique for reattachment. *Journal of Periodontology* **25**, 272-277.

Carranza, F.A. (1960) A technique for treating infrabony pockets so as to obtain reattachment. *Dental Clinics of North America*, March, 75-83.

Caton, J.G. & Kowalski, C.J. (1976) Primate model for testing periodontal treatment procedures. II. Production of contralaterally similar lesions. *Journal of Periodontology* **47**, 506-510.

Caton, J. & Nyman, S. (1980) Histometric evaluation of periodontal surgery. I. The modified Widman flap procedure. *Journal of Clinical Periodontology* **7**, 212-223.

Caton, J., Nyman, S. & Zander, H. (1980) Histometric evaluation of periodontal surgery. II. Connective tissue attachment levels after four regenerative procedures. *Journal of Clinical Periodontology* **7**, 224-231.

Caton, J.G. & Zander, H.A. (1975) Primate model for testing periodontal treatment procedures. I. Histologic investigation of localized periodontal pockets produced by orthodontics elastics. *Journal of Periodontology* **46**, 71-77.

Caton, J. & Zander, H.A. (1976) Osseous repair of an infrabony pocket without new attachment of connective tissue. *Journal of Clinical Periodontology* **3**, 54-58.

Cole, R.T., Crigger, M., Bogle, G., Egelberg, J. & Selvig, K.A. (1980) Connective tissue regeneration to periodontally diseased teeth. A histologic study. *Journal of Periodontal Research* **15**, 1-9.

Cole, R.T., Nilvéus, R., Ainamo, J., Bogle, G., Crigger, M. & Egelberg, J. (1981) Pilot clinical studies on the effect of topical citric acid application on healing after replaced periodontal flap surgery. *Journal of Periodontal Research* **16**, 117-122.

Crigger, M., Bogle, G., Nilvéus, R., Egelberg, J. & Selvig, K.A. (1978) The effect of topical citric acid application on the healing of experimental furcation defects in dogs. *Journal of Periodontal Reserach* **13**, 538-549.

Dragoo, M.R. (1981) *Regeneration of the Periodontal Attachment in Humans*. Philadelphia: Lea & Febiger.

Dragoo, M.R. & Sullivan, H.C. (1973a) A clinical and histological evaluation of autogenous iliac bone grafts in humans. I. Wound healing 2 to 8 months. *Journal of Periodontology* **44**, 599-613.

Dragoo, M.R. & Sullivan, H.C. (1973b) A clinical and histologic evaluation of autogenous iliac bone grafts in humans. II. External root resorption. *Journal of Periodontology* **44**, 614-625.

Ellegaard, B. & Löe, H. (1971) New attachment of periodontal tissue after treatment of infrabony lesions. *Journal of Periodontology* **42**, 648-652.

Ellegaard, B., Nielsen, I.M. &.Karring, T. (1976) Composite jaw and iliac cancellous bone grafts in intrabony defects in monkeys. *Journal of Periodontal Research* **11**, 299-310.

Frank, R., Fiore-Donno, G., Cimasoni, G. & Matter, J. (1974) Ultrastructural study of epithelial and connective gingival reattachment in man. *Journal of Periodontology* **45**, 226-235.

Froum, S.J., Ortiz, M., Witkin, R.T. Thaler, R., Scopp, I.W. & Stahl, S.S. (1976) Osseous autografts. III. Comparison of osseous coagulum-bone blend implant with open curettage. *Journal of Periodontology* **47**, 287-294.

Froum, S.J., Thaler, R., Scopp, I. W. & Stahl, S.S. (1975a) Osseous autografts. I. Clinical responses to bone blend or hip marrow grafts. *Journal of Periodontology* **46**, 515-521.

Froum, S.J., Thaler, R., Scopp, I.W. & Stahl, S. S. (1975b) Osseous autografts. II. Histological responses to osseous coagulum-bone blend grafts. *Journal of Periodontology* **46**, 656-661.

Gara, G.G. & Adams, D.E. (1981) Implant therapy in human intrabony pockets: A review of the literature. *Journal of the Western Society of Periodontology, Periodontal Abstracts* **2**.

Gottlow, J., Nyman, S., Karring, T. & Lindhe, J. (1984) New attachment formation as the result of controlled tissue regeneration. *Journal of Clinical Periodontology* **11**, 494-503.

Gottlow, J., Nyman, S., Lindhe, J., Karring, T. & Wennstrom, J. (1986) New attachment formation in the human periodontium by guided tissue regeneration. *Journal of Clinical Periodontology* **13**, 604-616.

Hiatt, W.H. & Schallhorn, R.G. (1973) Intraoral transplants of cancellous bone and marrow in periodontal lesions. *Journal of Periodontology* **44**, 194-208.

Hiatt, W.H., Schallhorn, R.G. & Aaronian, A.J. (1978) The induction of new bone and cementum formation. IV. Microscopic examination of the periodontium following human bone and marrow allograft, autograft and non-graft periodontal regenerative procedures. *Journal of Periodontology* **49**. 495-512.

Hiatt, W.H., Stallard, R.E., Butler, E.D. & Badgett, B. (1968) Repair following mucoperiosteal flap surgery with full gingival retention. *Journal of Periodontology* **39**, 11-16.

Karring, T., Nyman, S. & Lindhe, J. (1980) Healing following implantation of periodontitis affected roots into bone tissue. *Journal of Clinical Periodontology* **7**, 96-105.

Karring, T., Nyman, S., Lindhe, J. & Sirirat, M. (1984) Potentials for root resorption during periodontal healing. *Journal of Clinical Periodontology* **11**, 41-52.

Kon, S., Novaes, A.B., Ruben, M.P. & Goldman, H.M. (1969) Visualization of microvascularization of the healing periodontal wound II. Curettage. *Journal of Periodontology* **40**, 96-105.

Levin, M.P., Getter, L. Adrian, J. & Cutright, D.E. (1974) Healing of periodontal defects with ceramic implants. *Journal of Clinical Periodontology* **1**, 197-205.

Lindhe, J., Nyman, S. & Karring, T. (1984) Connective tissue attachment as related to presence or absence of alveolar bone. *Journal of Clinical Periodontology* **11**, 33-40.

Line, S.E., Polson, A.M. & Zander, H.A. (1974) Relationship between periodontal injury, selective cell repopulation and ankylosis. *Journal of Periodontology* **45**, 725-730.

Linghorne, W.J. & O'Connell, D.C. (1950) Studies in the regeneration and attachment of supporting structures of the teeth. I. Soft tissue reattachment. *Journal of Dental Research* **29**, 419.

Listgarten, M.A. (1972) Electron microscopic study of the junction between surgically denuded root surfaces and regenerated periodontal tissues. *Journal of Periodontal Research* **7**, 68-90.

Listgarten, M.A., Moa, R. & Robinson, P.J. (1976) Periodontal probing and the relationship of the probe to the periodontal tissues. *Journal of Periodontology* **47**, 511-513.

Löe, H. & Waerhaug, J. (1961) Experimental replantation of teeth in dogs and monkeys. *Archieves of Oral Biology* **3**, 176-184.

McCall, J.O. (1926) An improved method of inducing reattachment of the gingival tissue in periodontoclasia. *Dental Items of Interest* **48**, 342-358.

Melcher, A.H. (1969) Healing of wounds in the periodontium. In: *Biology of the Periodontium*. ed. Melcher, A.H. & Bowen, W.H., pp. 497-529.

London: Academic Press.

Melcher, A.H. (1970) Repair of wounds in the periodontium of the rat. Influence of periodontal ligament on osteogenesis. *Archives of Oral Biology* **15**, 1183-1204.

Melcher, A.H. (1976) On the repair potential of periodontal tissues. *Journal of Periodontology* **47**, 256-260.

Morris, M.L.(1953) The reattachment of human periodontal tissues following surgical detachment: A clinical and histological study. *Journal of Periodontology* **24**, 220.

Moskow, B.S. (1964) The response of the gingival sulcus to instrumentation: A histological investigation. *Journal of Periodontology* **35**, 112-126.

Moskow, B.S., Karsh, F. & Stein, S.D. (1979) Histological assessment of autogeneous bone graft. A case report and critical evaluation. *Journal of Periodontology* **6**, 291-300.

Nabers,.C.L. & O'Leary, T.J. (1965) Autogenous bone transplant in the treatment of osseous defects. *Journal of Periodontology* **36**, 5-14.

Nabers, C.L. & O'Leary, T.J. (1967) Autogenous bone grafts: case report. *Periodontics* **5**, 251-253.

Nilvéus, R. (1978) Treatment of periododontal furcation pockets. *Experimental studies in dogs.* Thesis, Malmö, Sweden.

Nyman, S., Gottlow, J., Karring, T. & Lindhe, J. (1982a) The regenerative potential of the periodontal ligament. An experimental study in the monkey. *Journal of Clinical Periodontology* **9**, 157-265.

Nyman, S., Houston, F., Sarhed, G., Lindhe, J. & Karring, T. (1985) Healing following reimplantation of teeth subjected to root planing and citric acid treatment. *Journal of Clinical Periodontology* **12**, 294-305.

Nyman, S., Karring T., Lindhe, J. & Planten, S. (1980) Healing following implantation of periodontitis-affected roots into gingival connective tissue. *Journal of Clinical Periodontology* **7**, 394-401.

Nyman, S., Lindhe, J. & Karring, T. (1981) Healing following surgical treatment and root demineralization in monkeys with periodontal disease. *Journal of Clinical Periodontology* **8**, 249-258.

Nyman, S., Lindhe, J., Karring, T. & Rylander, H. (1982b) New attachment following surgical treatment of human periodontal disease. *Journal of Clinical Periodontology* **9**, 290-296.

Orban, B. (1948) Pocket elimination or reattachment? *New York Dental Journal* **14**, 227-232.

Patur, B. & Glickman, I. (1962) Clinical and roentgenographic evaluation of the post-treatment healing of infrabony pockets. *Journal of Periodontology* **33**, 164-171.

Polson, A.M. & Heijl, L. (1978) Osseous repair in infra-bony defects. *Journal of Clinical Periodontology* **5**, 13-23.

Pontoriero, R., Lindhe, J., Nyman, S., Karring, T., Rosenberg, E. and Sanavi, F. (1988) Guided tissue regeneration in degree II furcation involved mandibular molars. A clinical study. *Journal of Clinical Periodontology* **15**, 247-254.

Prichard, J. (1957a) Regeneration of bone following periodontal therapy. *Oral Surgery* **10**, 247-252.

Prichard, J. (1957b) The infrabony technique as a predictable procedure. *Journal of Periodontology* **28**, 202-216.

Proye, M. & Polson, A.M. (1982) Effect of root surface alterations on periodontal healing. I. Surgical denudation. *Journal of Clinical Periodontology* **9**, 428-440.

Ramfjord, S.P. (1951) Experimental periodontal reattachment in Rhesus monkeys. *Journal of Periodontology* **22**, 67-77.

Ramfjord, S.P. & Nissle, R.R. (1974) The modified Widman flap. *Journal of Periodontology* **45**, 601-607.

Register, A.A. & Burdick, F.A. (1976) Accelerated reattachment with cementogenesis to dentin, demineralized in situ. II. Defect repair. *Journal of Periodontology* **47**, 497-505.

Renvert, S. & Egelberg, J. (1981) Healing after treatment of periodontal intraosseous defects. II. Effect of citric acid conditioning of the root surface. *Journal of Clinical Periodontology* **8**, 459-473.

Ririe, C.M., Crigger, M. & Selvig, K.A. (1980) Healing of periodontal connective tissue following surgical wounding and application of citric acid in dogs. *Journal of Clinical Periodontology* **15**, 314-327.

Robinson, R.E. (1969) Osseous coagulum for bone induction. *Journal of Periodontology* **40**, 503-510.

Rosenberg, M.M. (1971) Free osseous tissue autografts as a predictable procedure. *Journal of Periodontology* **42**, 195-209.

Rosling, B., Nyman, S. & Lindhe, J. (1976) The effect of systematic plaque control on bone regeneration in infrabony pockets. *Journal of Clinical Periodontology* **3**, 38-53.

Schaffer, E.M. & Zander, H.A. (1953) Histological evidence of reattachment of periodontal pockets. *Parodontologie* **7**, 101-107.

Schallhorn, R.G. (1972) Postoperative problems associated with iliac transplants. *Journal of Periodontology* **43**, 3.

Schallhorn, R.G. (1977) Present status of osseous grafting procedures. *Journal of Periodontology* **48**, 570-576.

Schallhorn, R.G., Hiatt, W.H. & Boyce, W. (I970) Iliac transplants in periodontal therapy. *Journal of Periodontology* **41**, 566-580.

Seibert, J.S. (1970) Reconstructive periodontal surgery: Case report. *Journal of Periodontology* **41**, I13-117.

Skillen, W.G. & Lundquist, G.R. (1937) An experimental study of periodontal membrane re-attachment in healthy and pathologic tissues. *Journal of the American Dental Association* **24**, 175-185.

Strub, J.R., Gaberthuel, T.W. & Firestone, A.R. (1979) Comparison of tricalcium phosphate and frozen allogenic bone implants in man. *Journal of Periodontology* **50**. 624-629.

Sullivan, H.C., Vito, A.A., Meltzer, A.M. & Rabinowitz, J.L. (1971) A histological evaluation of the use of hemopoietic marrow in intrabony periodontal defects. Program and abstract of papers. *International Association of Dental Research*: meeting.

van der Velden, U. & de Vries, J.H. (1978) Introduction of a new periodontal probe: the pressure probe. *Journal of Clinical Periodontology* **5**, 188-197.

Wade, A.B. (1962) An assessment of the flap operation. *Dental Practitioner and Dental Record* **13**, 11-20.

Wade, A.B. (1966) The flap operation. *Journal of Periodontology* **37**, 95-99.

Waerhaug, J. (1952) The gingival pocket. *Odontologisk Tidsskrift*. **60**, Supplement 1.

Waerhaug, J. (1978) Healing of the dento-epithelial junction following subgingival plaque control. I. As observed in human biopsy material. *Journal of Periodontology* **49**, 1-8.

Wirthlin, M.R. (1981) The current status of new attachment therapy. *Journal of Periodontology* **52**, 529-544.

Younger, W.J. (1899) Pyorrhea alveolaris from a bacteriological standpoint with a report of some investigations and remarks on the treatment. *International Dental Journal* **20**, 413-423.

Yukna, R.A. (1976) A clinical and histologic study of healing following the excisional new attachment procedure in rhesus monkeys. *Journal of Periodontology* **47**, 701-709.

Yukna, R.A., Bowers, G.M. Lawrence, J.J. & Fedi, P.F. (1976) A clinical study of healing in humans following the excisional new attachment procedure. *Journal of Periodontology* **47**, 696-700.

Yuktanandana, I. (1959) Bone graft in the treatment of intrabony periodontal pockets in dogs. A histological investigation. *Journal of Periodontology* **30**, 17-26.

CHAPTER 19

Esthetics and Periodontal Therapy

Pocket elimination procedures

Biotypes of periodontal tissues

Gingivectomy and flap procedures are frequently employed in the treatment of periodontal disease in order to 1) gain access for proper root debridement and 2) eliminate or reduce the depth of pathological periodontal pockets. The undesired but often unavoidable side-effects of this type of treatment include 1) additional loss of attachment and bone as well as 2) recession of the marginal soft tissue. The long clinical crowns, the irregular contour of the gingival margin and the loss of papillary tissue often have an adverse influence on *dental-facial esthetics*.

In order to be able to properly evaluate what effect pocket elimination therapy may have on the position of the gingival margin, the configuration of interdental papillae and the alveolar bone at individual teeth and tooth surfaces, *and the esthetic result that will be attained*, the clinician must develop a sense of *tissue appreciation*. In other words he/she must not only be familiar with results from clinical studies describing overall dimensional changes which occur in the periodontal tissues following therapy (for review see Chapter 24) but must also learn *how to read tissue*.

A range exists in types and forms (*biotypes*) of periodontal tissues. The THICK-FLAT and the THIN, HIGHLY-SCALLOPED biotypes are found at either end of the spectrum. Different biotypes of periodontal tissues have a tendency to respond differently to inflammation and surgical injury. Thus, while a THIN gingiva often moves away from a source of irritation and recedes following periodontal therapy (see Chapter 18), a THICK gingiva frequently dis-

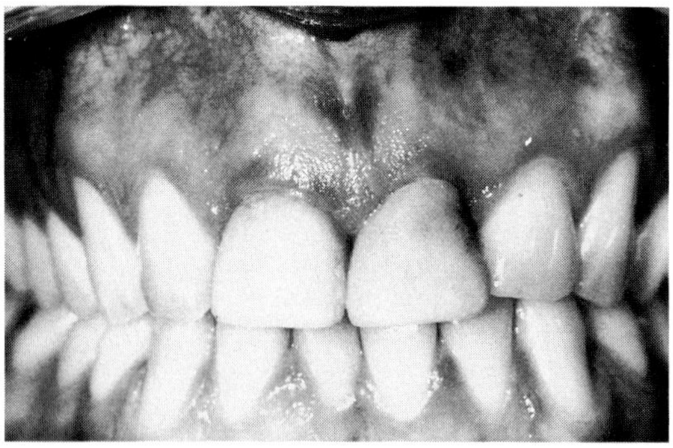

Fig. 19-1a.

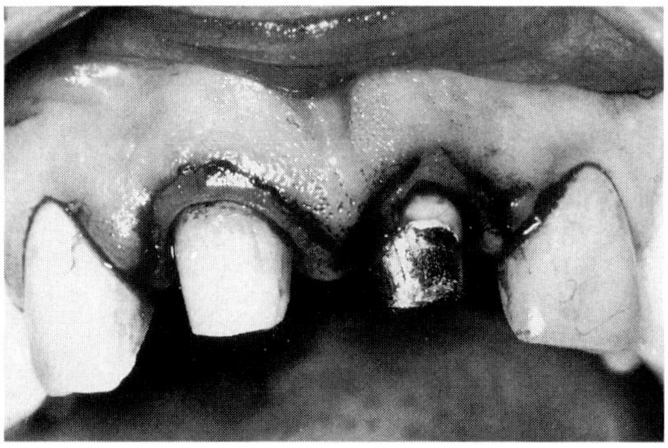

Fig. 19-1b.

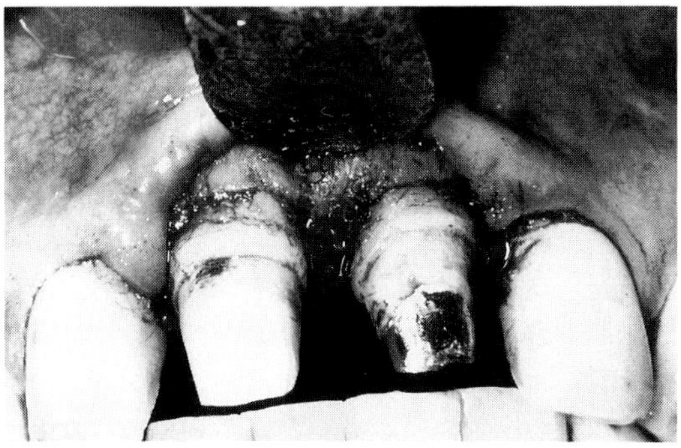

Fig. 19-1c.

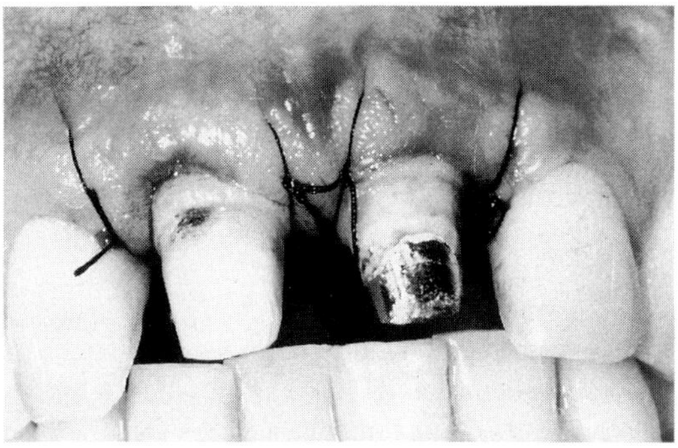

Fig. 19-1d.

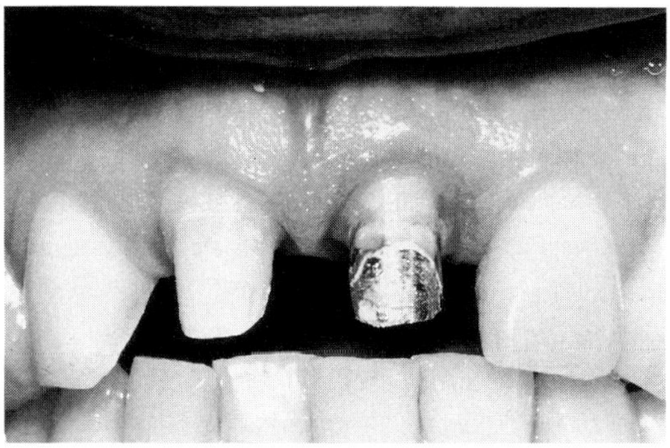

Fig. 19-1e.

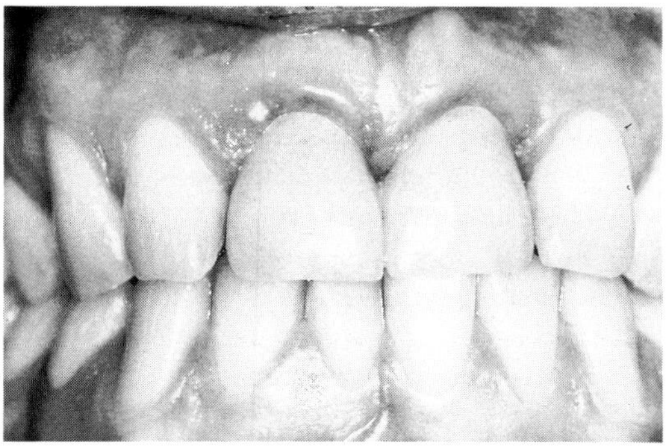

Fig. 19-1f.

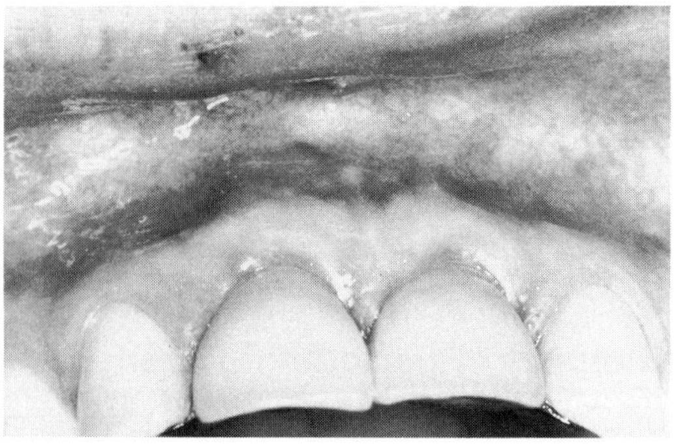

Fig. 19-1g.

Fig. 19-1. (a) *Crown lengthening* was required to gain access to the submarginal area of the crowns of the central incisors. The patient in this illustration had a thick periodontium. The finish line of the provisional crowns was improperly prepared. (b) An internally beveled submarginal path of incision was used to 1) thin the tissue, 2) apically position the gingival margins, 3) gain access to the bone margins. (c) The attached gingiva was reflected to expose the margins of the bone and the improperly prepared finish lines. Note that the gingiva was not reflected apical to the mucogingival junction. (d) The *thinned* and shortened labial and palatal flaps were replaced and stabilized with interrupted silk sutures. (e) 10 weeks post-treatment. The crowns were reprepared and final impressions were taken. The gingival tissues were thin at this stage. (f) 18 months post-treatment. The gingival tissues had healed to their normal, *thicker* biotype and a rolled, red gingival margin had formed. (g) Incisal view. Note the flat contours of the crowns in the cervical area.

plays a hyperplastic response to irritation and tends to revert to its original form and dimension during repair following treatment.

In order to avoid unnecessary recession and tooth exposure, the treatment of a patient with a THIN periodontium should be planned on a tooth-by-tooth basis. If such a patient is treated by a uniform procedure, e.g., gingivectomy, flap or subgingival root planing, a combination of overtreatment and undertreatment may result. Undertreatment will occur in areas with deep pockets by denying the clinician proper access for root debridement, while overtreatment will result in areas of shallow pockets by exposing such sites to unnecessary attachment loss and recession.

The treatment of a patient with a THICK periodontium must also be planned with caution. To improve dental-facial esthetics, attempts may be made to surgically recontour the gingiva and the alveolar bone of a THICK biotype into a THIN, HIGHLY-SCALLOPED periodontium. If such a patient is carefully documented before and after treatment, a marked change in tissue topography will usually be observed during the first few months after the completion of active therapy. The thick periodontium may, indeed, have been converted to resemble a periodontium of the thin biotype. With the passage of time, however, the characteristics of the thick biotype gradually return. This process of remodelling is most often completed within a 12- to 24-month period after surgery (Fig. 19-1).

There are three different general case categories that have to be considered with respect to the effect of pocket elimination procedures on overall esthetics:

- Patients who *will not* be exposed to extensive restorative therapy after periodontal therapy;
- Patients *who will be* restored after periodontal therapy;
- Patients who *already have been* restored.

The method of periodontal treatment to be selected should, in all three categories of patients, ideally be determined not only after proper assessment of *degree of disease progression* (probing depth, attachment loss, bone loss; extent and shape of deformities in the bone) in various parts of the dentition and *biotype of periodontium*, but also with respect to:

- Location of the lip line - low and high smile lines; even or uneven exposure of the teeth and gingivae;
- Location of the gingival margins - located at or coronal to the cemento-enamel junction, or being receded;
- Form and shape of the interdental papillae - normal, narrow, wide, blunted, cratered or missing.

Goldstein (1984), Tjan et al. (1984) and Abrams (1987) emphasized the importance of a proper lip line examination for the esthetically concerned periodontal patient. The lips limit the amount of teeth and mucosal tissues that are displayed. The form of the lips, the location of the relaxed smile line and the high smile line should be recorded in this kind of patient with the same attention that is given to probing depths, attachment levels, bone levels, restorations and carious lesions. The form of the lips and the position of the lips during speech and smiling cannot be easily changed, but the dentist may, if necessary, modify/control the form of the teeth and interdental papillae as well as the position of the gingival margin. In other words, it is possible by a combination of periodontal and prosthetic treatment measures to improve dental-facial esthetics in this category of patient.

Patient who will not be exposed to extensive restorative therapy

Periodontal therapy in a patient with deep (> 5 mm) pockets may result in considerable dimensional alterations of the periodontium (Chapter 24). If the pattern of attachment and bone loss in the anterior segments of the dentition is of an even character, the generalized recession of the periodontium that follows treatment may resemble a normal architectural form but at a more apical level. If, however, the pattern of tissue destruction is uneven and varies greatly from tooth to tooth or between teeth on either side of the midline, treatment unfortunately often results in an uneven pattern of periodontal tissue recession. The asymmetry that follows may severely compromise dental-facial esthetics. In the planning of the treatment of such a patient the clinician has to make some difficult decisions, e.g.: Should all of the deep pockets be eliminated or should a compromise be made and some pockets be retained? Should moderate or large amounts of alveolar bone be resected in an attempt to produce even and symmetrical contours in the profile of the crest of the alveolar bone?

Patients who will be restored

The various factors that govern the post-treatment location and topography of the gingival margins and the interdental papillae in the non-restored case are also relevant in patients who are scheduled for additional restorative therapy. There are, however, some additional problems to consider in such cases. Patients who have undergone pocket elimination therapy may complain about 1) the dark triangles that occur in the interdental areas 2) the uneven outline of the gingival margin and 3) the display of root structure. Such esthetic problems may be overcome by restorative treatment measures. Thus, the location and symmetry of the gingival margins can be levelled and blended into harmonious balance by intentionally reducing the height of the periodontal tissues. The facial-proximal contours of restorations and the location of the interproximal contact areas can be adjusted to hide many of the soft and hard tissue defects that may be present. In other words, the prosthesis may restore the *illusion* of a healthy dentition.

With respect to the planning of restorative therapy after the completion of periodontal treatment, the following guidelines may be considered:

- In the THIN, HIGHLY-SCALLOPED periodontal biotype the gingival tissues undergo an immediate phase of recession that appears to stabilize after 2 months following surgery. In some patients, however, there may be a secondary phase of recession that continues for another 2-4 months. In such cases it is therefore prudent to postpone the completion of definitive prosthetic therapy until about 6 months after active periodontal therapy.
- The THICK periodontal biotype following treatment has a tendency to slowly revert to its original form. If the tissues of a thick periodontium are thinned during periodontal surgery, they may retain the morphology of a thin biotype during the first few months after treatment. Within 6-12 months, however, the tissues tend to regain their original form; the thin gingival margins return to the more rounded and bulky form that characterize this biotype (Fig. 19-1). In such a case, therefore, the definitive phase of restorative treatment should not be completed until 12-24 months after the end of periodontal therapy.

Patients who have already been restored

Since pocket elimination therapy results in gingival recession and the exposure of root structure, there is a risk that this type of treatment in a patient with fixed bridgework may expose crown margins that were initially placed within the confines of the gingival sulcus. Clinicians must carefully weigh the advantages of pocket elimination therapy against the esthetic problems that may ensue by the exposure of restorative crown margins. It is important that patients of this kind fully understand that dimensional changes will occur as a result of pocket elimination therapy, and that the clinician does not undertake such treatment until informed consent has been obtained from the patient.

Surgical management of interdental papillae

The papillae derive their shape and size from the proximal surfaces of adjacent teeth, the interdental bone surface, the outline of the cemento-enamel junctions and the amount of space that exists between adjacent teeth. If the papillae properly fill the interproximal spaces, they impart an appearance of periodontal health. Conversely, if the size and/or shape of the interdental papillae are compromised, the periodontium may appear diseased. Thus the papillae play an important role in dental-facial esthetics.

Loss of papillary tissue may also cause many patients to have problems with phonation. Since an effective air seal cannot be established between the lips and the tongue, droplets of saliva may be expelled during speaking. In addition, food particles may be trapped in the open interproximal spaces.

The damaged interdental papillae are difficult or impossible to repair or regenerate. It is important, therefore, that during surgery special attention is paid to the interdental tissues. Whenever possible, an incision technique should be used which makes it possible to preserve normal papillary form. Improperly planned or carelessly executed surgical therapy causes much of the disfigurement that is observed post-surgically in the interproximal regions of the dentition.

The alveolar crest acts as a scaffolding to support the overlying veneer of gingival tissue. Thus, the topography of the bone crest has a direct influence on the post-treatment shape of the interdental papillae. If the bone crest has receded but retained its normal shape, normal papillary form can be regained following surgical therapy and proper healing. If, on the other hand, angular bony defects or craters are present in the interdental region, treatment without bone recontouring will most likely result in less than normal papillary form.

The following technical aspects should be considered to ensure that *optimal* esthetics are attained in the papillary areas upon final healing and maturation of the surgical site:

- surgical techniques used to release papillae
- surgical techniques used to reflect papillae
- surgical techniques used to stabilize papillae

Surgical techniques used to release papillae

If the gingival tissues are THIN, and a narrow zone of attached gingiva is present at the buccal or lingual surfaces, an incision should preferably be made in the pockets and be directed parallel to the long axis of the teeth. If the gingival tissues are THICK, and a wide zone of attached gingiva is present, the incision should start at the crest of the gingival margin or at an appropriate apical (lateral) distance from this level. Also this internal bevel incision should be made parallel to the long axis of the teeth and be carried to the bone crest (Fig. 19-2).

Once the decision has been made as to how thick or thin the papillae should be dissected, the manner in which the scalpel blade is directed around the teeth while making the horizontal entrance incision becomes important (Fig. 19-2). It is in these first critical stages of the surgical procedure that most of the errors are made. The three most common errors are:

– *creating short or narrow papillae*

The path of incision is not sufficiently scalloped (made too flat or linear) or the scalpel is not carried deeply enough into the interproximal area. The papillae are thereby transsected and a critical amount of connective tissue is lost. To avoid this problem the papillae must be viewed in three dimensions. The pretreatment

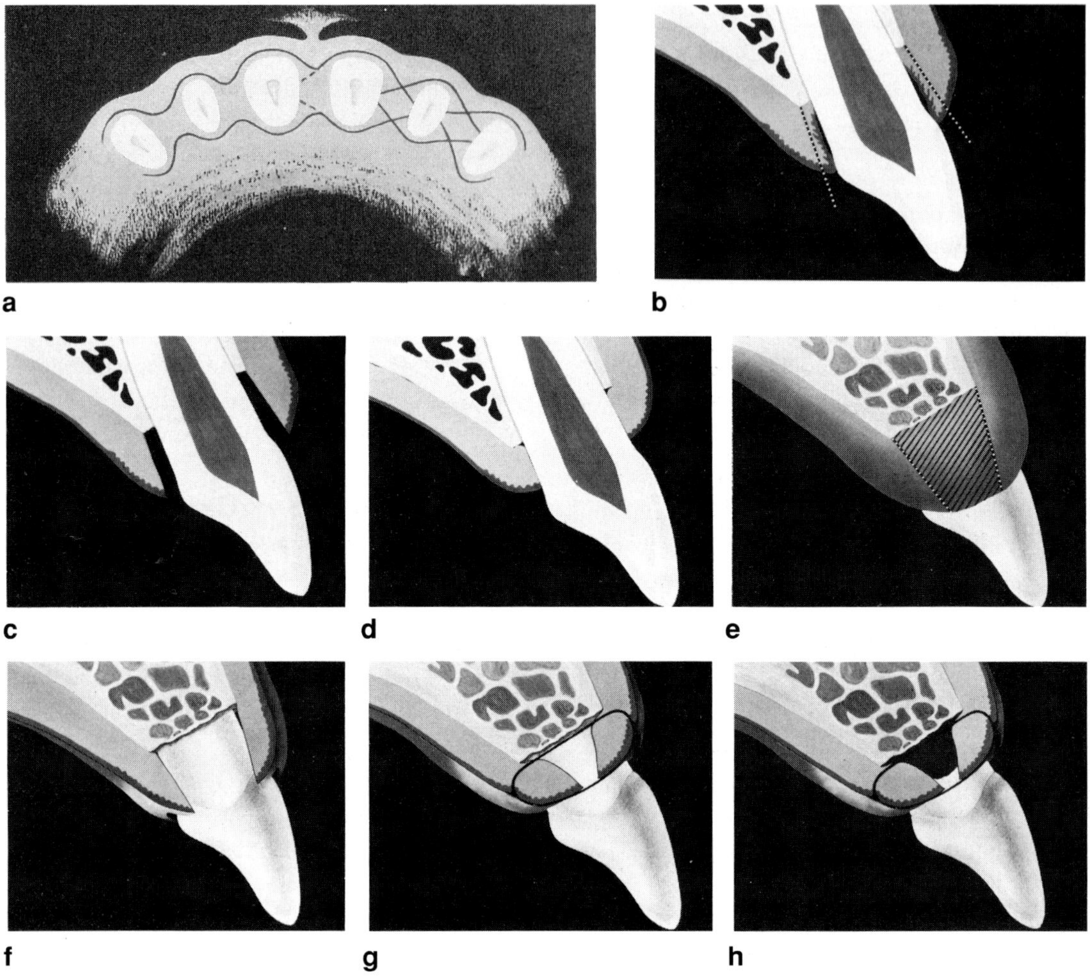

Fig. 19-2. Surgical design used to create flaps for periodontal procedures. The schematic drawing illustrates problems that are created by bone loss in the interproximal areas. (a) Incisal view showing the horizontal crestal incision made as a continuous incision on the left side, and as an interrupted series of arcs on the right side of the midline. (b) On the labial and lingual surfaces of the teeth, the scalpel blade was directed towards the crestal bone (dotted line) to (i) create an internally beveled flap, and (ii) thin the flaps. (c) The pocket lining and inflamed connective tissue adjacent to the the pocket were removed. (d) Properly placed sutures positioned the flaps tightly against the labial and lingual surfaces of the teeth. (e) The drawing depicts moderate to advanced bone loss in the interproximal areas and the amount of tissue (cross-hatched lines) that was removed in creating the flaps. (f) When root debridement was completed, the papillary segments of the flaps collapsed into the defects. (g) The angular edges of the interproximal ledges should reduced to permit adaptation of the buccal and lingual segments of the papillae. If the edges of the flaps are not brought tightly together, a soft tissue crater will form. (h) A blood clot is shown filling the space remaining in the interproximal areas of the flap. The clot will contract upon wound healing and be replaced by granulation tissue.

volume of each papilla must be assessed and the incisions performed in such a way that the desired volume of connective tissue is retained.

– *creating bulbous papillae*

If a flap is intended to be *replaced to its former position* it is important to retain as much as possible of the connective tissue of the papillae. If too much of the connective tissue is removed the papillae will shrink during healing and fail to properly fill the interproximal spaces.

If a flap is intended to be *apically positioned*, on the other hand, a substantial amount of connective tissue of the papillae must be excised. If too much connective tissue is retained, the papillary segments of the flap will have a triangular shape (bucco-lingually) with the apex of the triangle facing the bone surface. The thin and flat non-papillary sections of the flap, but not the V-shaped undersurface of the papillae, will adapt closely to the surface of the alveolar bone. *Bulbous papillae will result.* To avoid the formation of bulbous papillae the entire undersurface of the flap - the papillary as well as the non-papillary - must be made as smooth and flat as possible.

The retained papillae procedure: As stated above, the surgical removal of connective tissue from the interdental papillae results in shrinkage of the interdental tissues during healing and the establishment of open interdental spaces. The risk of creating an esthetically unacceptable soft tissue defect in the interdental area increases if the embrasure space is large in the anterior segments of the dentition. Areas with diastemata constitute a particular problem in this respect. In such areas the interdental papillae are usually broad, rounded and smooth. If the incision separates the papilla into one facial and one lingual segment, healing frequently results in the establishment of a depression at the tip of the interdental tissue unit. Evian et al. (1985) recommended the use of the *retained papilla procedure* to preserve the integrity of the papillae at sites with diastemata. The papillae are incised at the lingual side of the dental arch and are subsequently retained in the facial segment of the flap (Fig. 19-3). Sufficient space must exist between the teeth to properly maneuver the lingual segments of the papillae through the interproximal areas. Care must be exercised when the papillae are reflected to the facial surface. If unduly traumatized, large portions of the papillary tissue may be lost during healing. Lingually anchored sutures are used to return the papillae to their original position and to join them with the lingual segment of the flap.

– *creating improperly shaped papillae*
This error usually occurs if *direct vision* is used when the horizontal incision is prepared; from the distal to the anterior area of the dentition. In this situation the scalpel is frequently carried too far mesially towards the distal line angle of each tooth as the blade passes from the buccal, or the lingual, surface through the interproximal area. The location of the peak of the papillae is thereby moved from the center of the interproximal space towards the distal surface. This error can be avoided by viewing the surgical area through *mirrored vision*.

Surgical techniques used to reflect papillae
Before the flap is reflected it is important to ascertain that the connective tissue of the gingiva and the papillae has been properly incised. The dense connective tissue of the gingiva has great tensile strength, and it takes only a few unsevered collagen fibers to make it difficult to retract the incised tissue. If difficulty is encountered the surgeon may choose to employ additional pressure on the elevator. This should, however, be avoided because the excess force may create unnecessary tissue damage with concomitant loss of tissue volume.

Surgical techniques used to stabilize papillae
The technique(s) to be used to close the surgical wound and to stabilize the soft tissues must be determined *before* the surgical procedure is initiated. If the suturing technique is not properly planned, the operator may find that the most advantageous method of suture placement cannot be utilized, because the required tissue or anchorage units were removed in earlier stages of the surgical procedure. The most common errors encountered in stabilizing the papillary area of a flap and moving the papillae to the intended post-treatment location are:

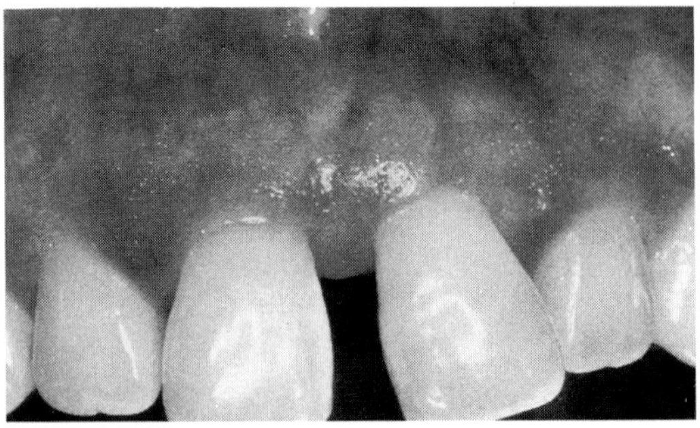

Fig. 19-3a.

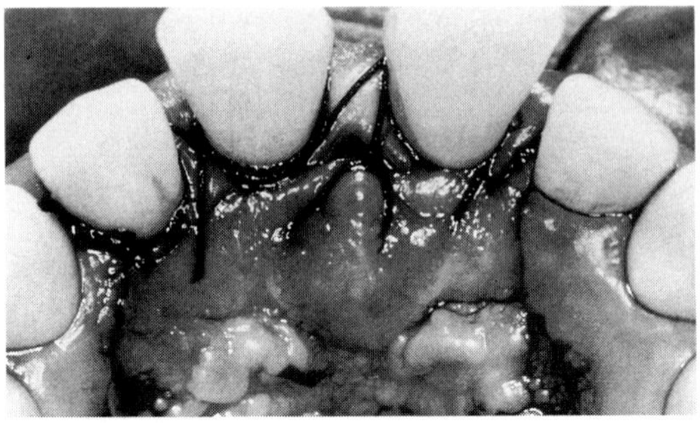

Fig. 19-3b.

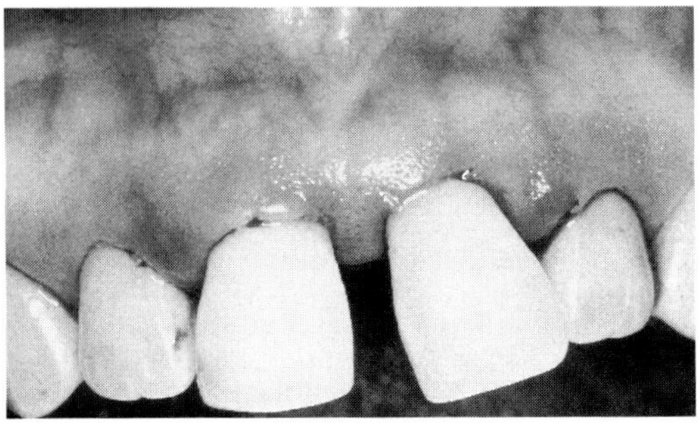

Fig. 19-3c.

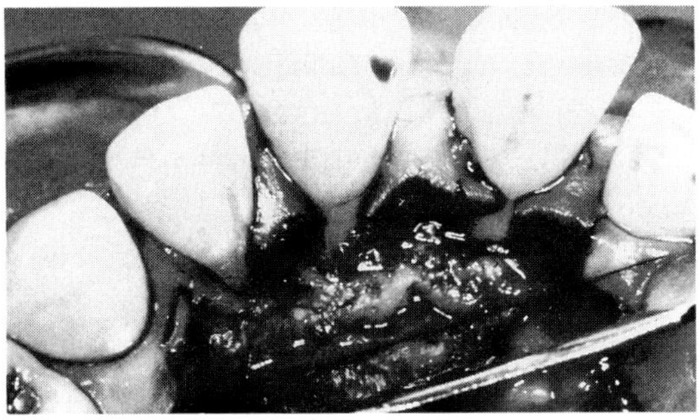

Fig. 19-3d.

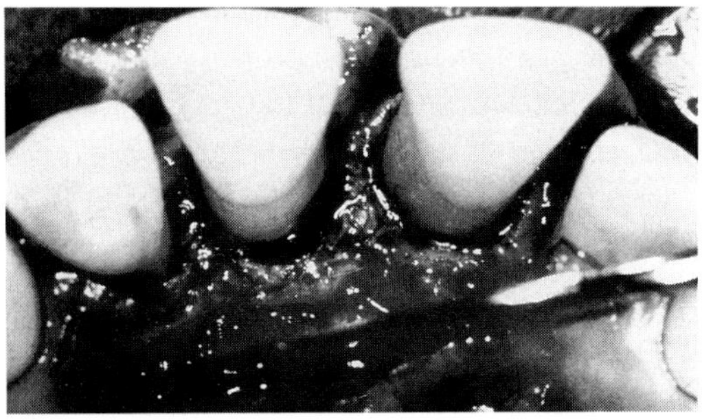

Fig. 19-3e.

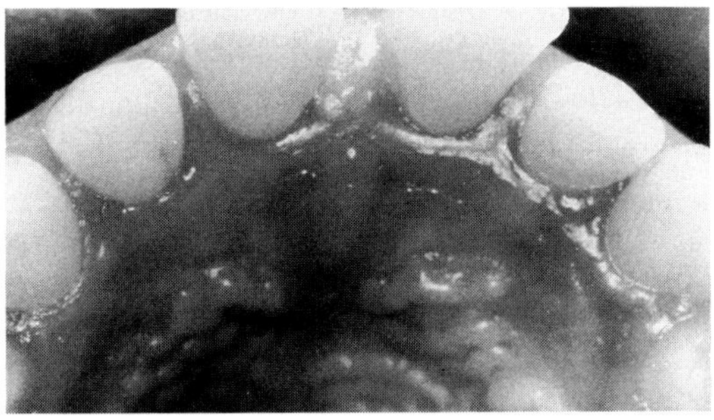

Fig. 19-3f.

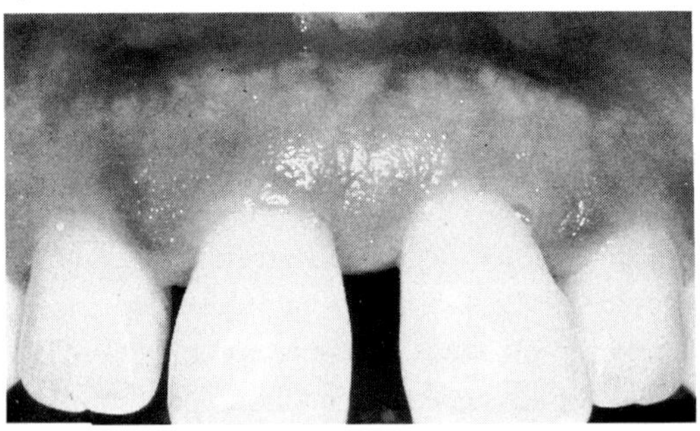

Fig. 19-3g.

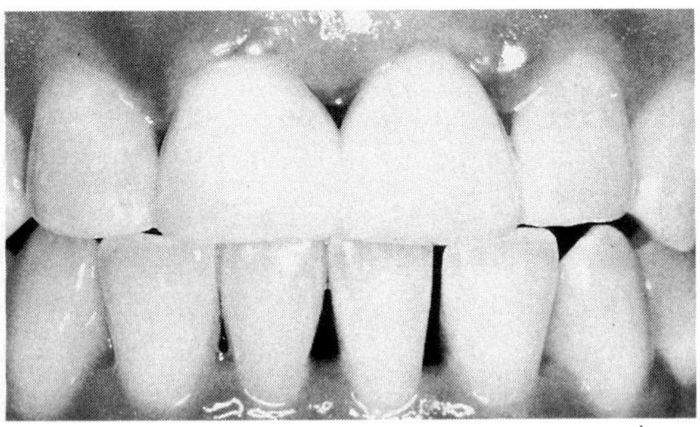

Fig. 19-3h.

Fig. 19-3. *Retained papillae procedure.* (a-b) Labial and lingual pretreatment views. (c) Labial and interproximal incisions were made in the pocket to maintain the papillae in the labial segment of the flap. (d) The horizontal releasing incision for the lingual segment of the flap was started in the lingual pocket or laterally to it. Note the retention of the papillae in the labial segment of the flap. (e) Access was provided for root debridement and treatment of the infrabony pockets. (f) The flaps were returned to their former position and the papillae were sutured to the lingual flap. (g) 2 weeks postsurgery, the tissue contours were preserved. (h) Minor tooth movement was used to align the central incisors. The teeth were reshaped by selective grinding and bonded to close the diastema. (Courtesy of Dr. R. Pontoriero).

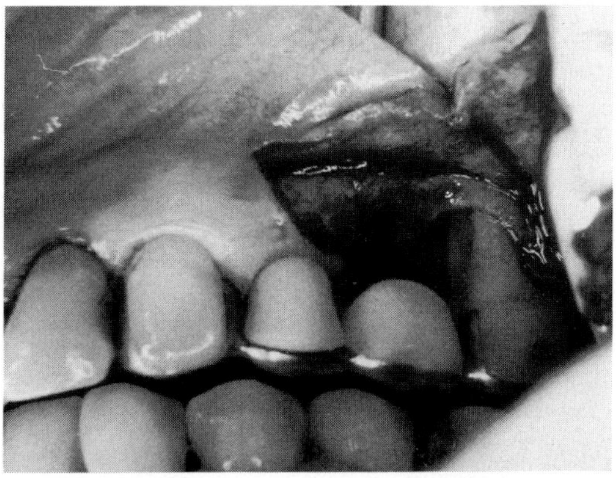

Fig. 19-4a.

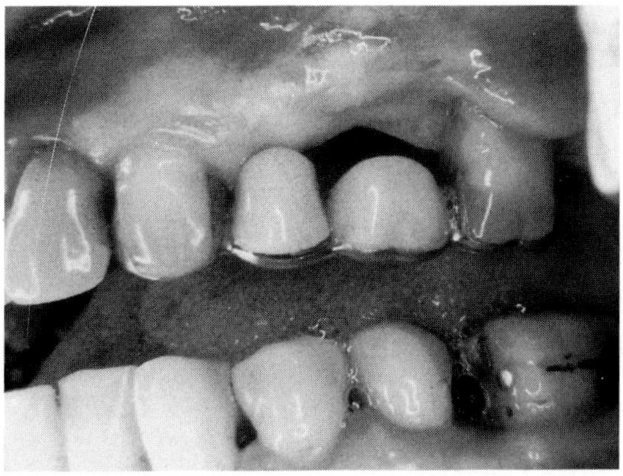

Fig. 19-4b.

Fig. 19-4. (a) A horizontal midline incision was made along the crest of the ridge to release the gingival tissue under the pontics in order to gain access to the infrabony pocket on the proximal surface of the molar. Bone recontouring was accomplished to eliminate the osseous defect. When the flaps were made thinner prior to flap closure, the thick connective tissue that formerly existed over the ridge and under the pontics was discarded. (b) Post-treatment view showing the large space under the pontic teeth that the pocket elimination procedure created.

– *apico-coronal placement error*

The flaps are positioned too far coronally or apically from their intended location.

– *mesio-distal placement error*

The flaps are displaced mesially or distally, thereby preventing the papillae from residing in the center of the interproximal spaces.

– *failure to adapt and unite the facial and lingual segments*

This results in the establishment of an interdental col or even in the formation of one facial and one lingual tip of the papilla. In such a case the papillae will not properly reside under the contact area.

– *traumatizing the papillae*

This may occur if a large suture needle is used or if repeated passes are made with the needle through the papillary tissue. Tissue necrosis may also result if the papillae are sutured too tightly, thereby constricting the blood supply to the tissue unit.

– *tissue displacement caused by the periodontal dressing*

This error results from improper mixing and placement of the dressing. If the dressing is mixed to a stiff consistency and is pressed with excessive force against the teeth and the periodontal tissues, the flaps may be displaced. Soft, slow-setting dressings may also cause flap displacement. A soft dressing has a tendency to flow and may therefore be forced under the flap by lip or tongue pressure.

Papillae in advanced periodontal disease

In cases with advanced periodontal disease the interdental septae are often markedly resorbed and deep interdental bony defects or craters have formed. If a periodontal flap procedure is performed in a segment of the dentition where deep angular bony defects and infrabony pockets are present, the interproximal areas of the flap will usually collapse into the hard tissue defects. This inability of the interdental tissues to form proper papillae is unrelated to flap design, surgical skill, papillae positioning or suturing (Fig. 19-2). Marked postoperative recession in such a case is inevitable. This is one of the unfortunate consequences of treating patients with advanced breakdown of the periodontal tissue. There are presently no techniques available that can be used to predictably restore severely truncated papillae.

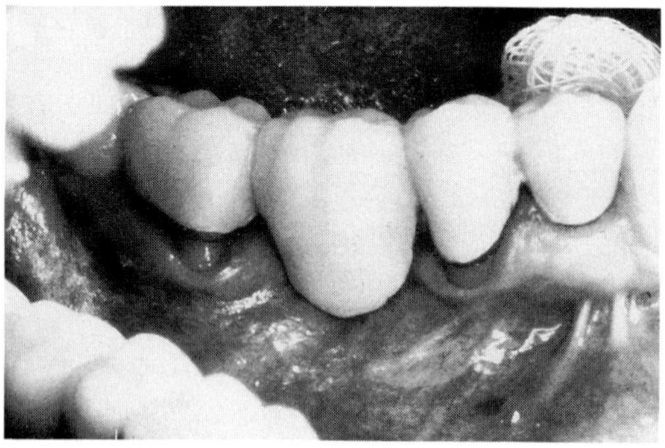

Fig. 19-5a.

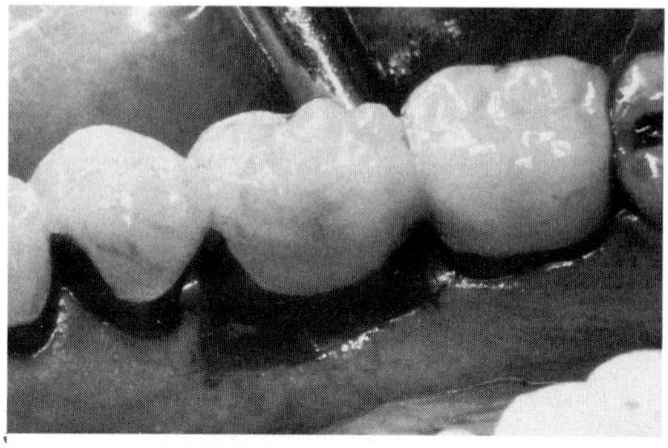

Fig. 19-5b.

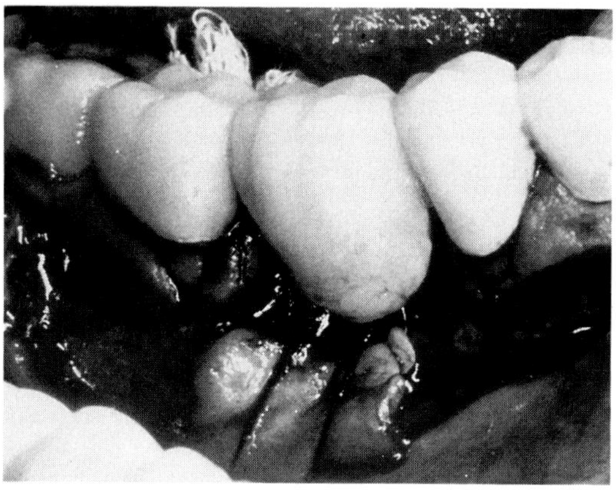

Fig. 19-5c.

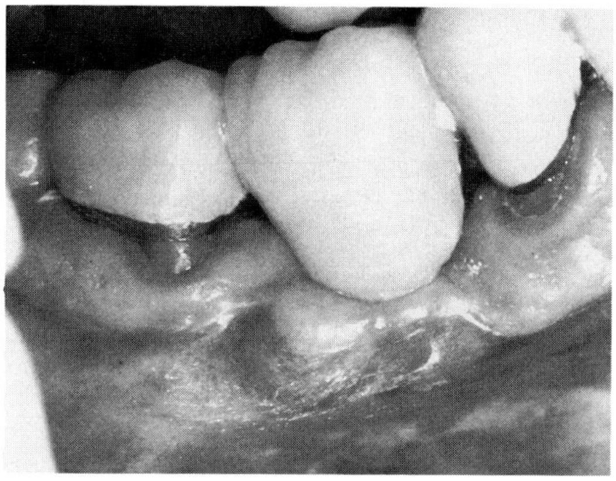

Fig. 19-5d.

Fig. 19-5. (a) Pretreatment view of a prosthesis that was constructed with a "*modified ridge lap pontic*". (b) The horizontal releasing incision was made on the lingual side of the ridge to conserve all of the gingiva that was present under the pontic. (c) The path of dissection was made from the lingual to the buccal surface of the ridge and followed the contour of the bone. This permitted the flap to be pushed to the buccal side of the ridge. The gingiva in the coronal area of the flap was apically positioned and stabilized by sutures on the buccal side of the ridge. (d) One year post-treatment. The buccal vestibule was deepened and attached gingiva now exists under the pontic. (Courtesy of Dr. H. Corn).

Surgical management of pontic areas

Pocket elimination therapy involving the periodontal tissues at abutment teeth and pontic areas often results in the establishment of ridge defects which may jeopardize both function and dental-facial esthetics (Fig. 19-4). In patients with fixed bridgework it is therefore frequently necessary to accept a compromise with respect to pocket reduction. This is especially the case in the anterior region, where the establishment of a ridge defect may be entirely unacceptable. If a fixed bridge has an acceptable design, every effort should be made during periodontal therapy to retain the periodontal tissue volume in the pontic area. In the patient shown in Fig. 19-4, the pontics fit properly against the ridge prior to periodontal surgery. The patient regarded the bridge as being esthetically acceptable and the treatment plan did not include provisions for remaking the bridge. The probing depth at the interproximal surfaces of the abutment teeth ranged from 5 to 7 mm. The objective of periodontal surgery was to gain access for root debridement. The pocket elimination therapy performed certainly accomplished the objective set for the procedure,

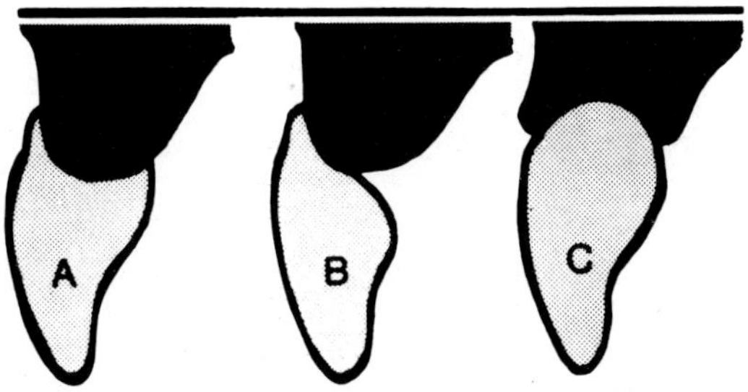

Fig. 19-6. Pontic designs. (A) *Total ridge lap pontic.* (B) *Modified ridge lap pontic.* (C) *Ovate pontic* (From Garber D. & Rosenberg, E. (1981) "The edentulous ridge in fixed prosthodontics". Compendiun of Continuing Education in Dentistry).

but a large ridge defect was created in the pontic area. A large black space was noticeable when the patient smiled.

The creation of ridge defects can often be prevented by employing a technique such as the *retained papillae procedure* (Evian et al. 1985) described above. Instead of making a mesial-distal midline incision along the edentulous span of the ridge, the entrance incision is made well to the palatal/lingual side of the pontic region. The gingival tissues under the pontic section are dissected from the bone surface and included in the buccal flap. Bone recontouring, if performed, should be limited to the palatal/lingual alveolar bone. The palatal/lingual flap, but not the buccal flap, is apically positioned. Hereby, the soft tissues which formerly filled the space between the pontic teeth and the ridge can be returned to their original location. The use of the "pull through" component of the *retained papillae procedure* illustrated in Fig. 19-5 makes it possible to avoid many of the esthetic and functional problems that arose in the patient illustrated in Fig. 19-4.

Ridge lap designed pontics (Fig. 19-6) are often difficult to work around. Access to the tissue-facing surface (tissue surface) of the pontic may be entirely blocked from both the buccal and the lingual surfaces by the pontic extensions. In order to preserve the soft tissue located under the pontic and to gain access for the "pull through" procedure it is often necessary to remove the lingual extension of the pontic.

If the treatment plan includes the construction of a new bridge, pocket elimination procedures can be performed with less concern for creating ridge defects. After surgery, the clinical crowns of the abutment teeth are longer and therefore the pontics can also be made longer and still harmonize with the abutment teeth. In this particular situation, it is the treatment of the proximal surfaces of the abutment teeth adjacent to the pontic segment that is critical for dental-facial esthetics. Every attempt must be made to retain the papillae in these regions. If the interdental papillae at the abutment teeth are shortened or eliminated as the ridge is flattened, an open space - a dark triangle - is created between the pontic and the abutment section. As discussed previously, the presence of dark triangles often compromises dental-facial esthetics.

Crown lengthening procedures

To overcome problems with a "gummy" smile

In most patients, the lower edge of the upper lip assumes a "gull-wing" profile which limits the amount of gum tissue that is exposed. Patients who have a high lip line and "short front teeth" expose a broad zone of gingival tissue and often express concern about their "gummy" smile. Different techniques can be used to reduce the amount of gingiva which is exposed, and to alter the shape and forms of the anterior teeth. The following factors must be considered:

- Location of the gingival margin in relation to the cemento-enamel junction and the bone crest;

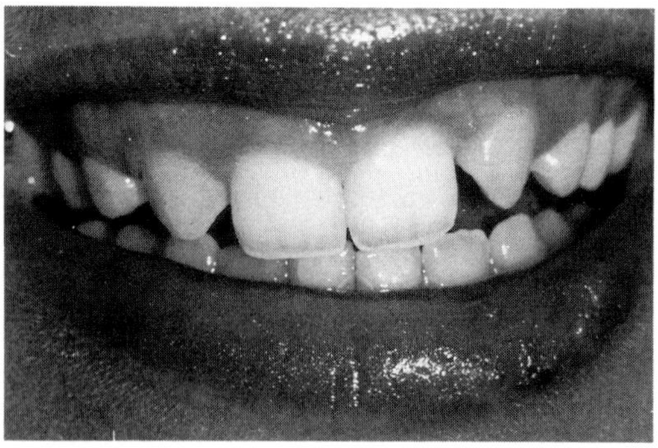

Fig. 19-7a.

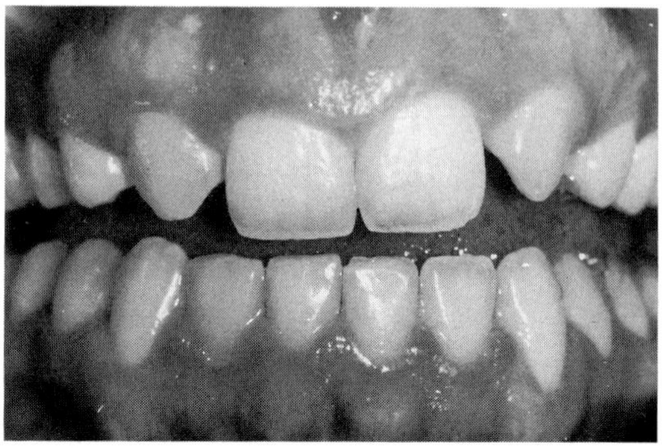

Fig. 19-7b.

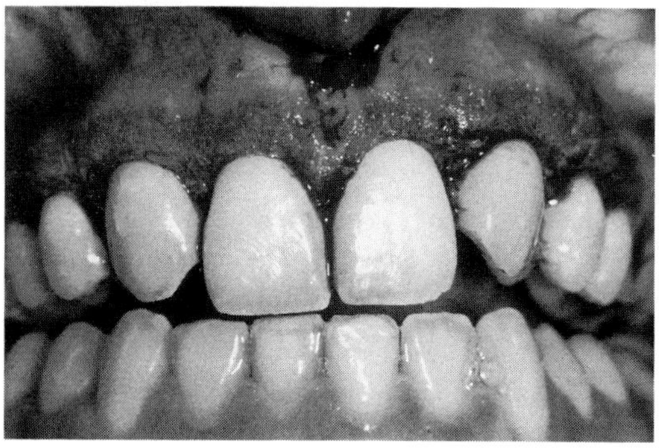

Fig. 19-7c.

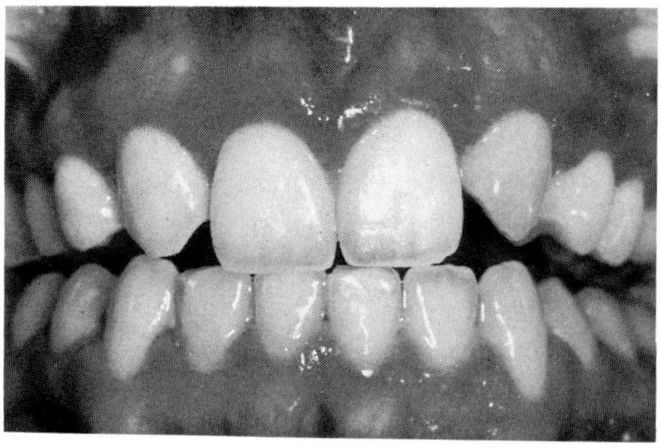

Fig. 19-7d.

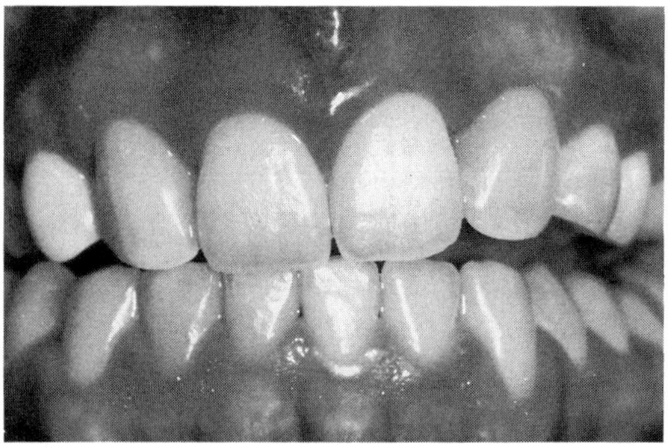

Fig. 19-7e.

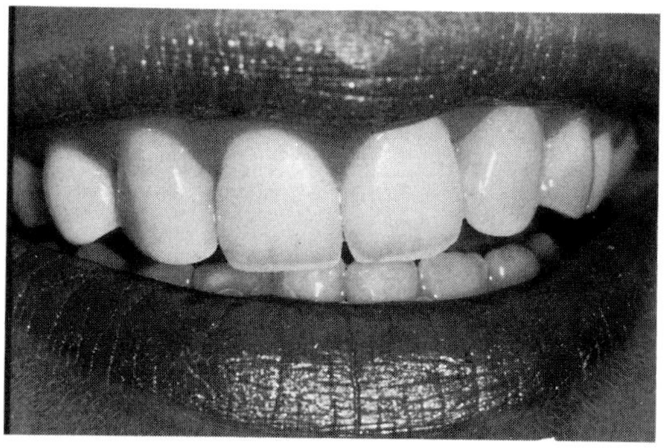

Fig. 19-7f.

Fig. 19-7. *Crown lengthening procedure.* (a-b) Pretreatment views. The lateral incisiors were congenitally missing and orthodontic treatment had been accomplished to move the posterior teeth anteriorly. The canine teeth in the position of the lateral incisors added to the esthetic disharmony. (c) A gingivectomy was performed to expose the anatomical crowns of the teeth. (d) One month postsurgery. At this appointment the canine and first premolar teeth were reshaped and bonded. (e) Tooth form and proportional balance was improved by bonding. (f) At completion of therapy. Compare with Fig. 19-7a.

– Crown-root-alveolar bone relationships;
– Size and shape of the upper lip;
– Location of the lip line during speech and during a broad, relaxed smile.

In the normal young adult the healthy gingival margin resides about 1 mm coronal to the cemento-enamel junction. Some patients who complain about their "small front teeth", however, have a free gingiva that is more than 1

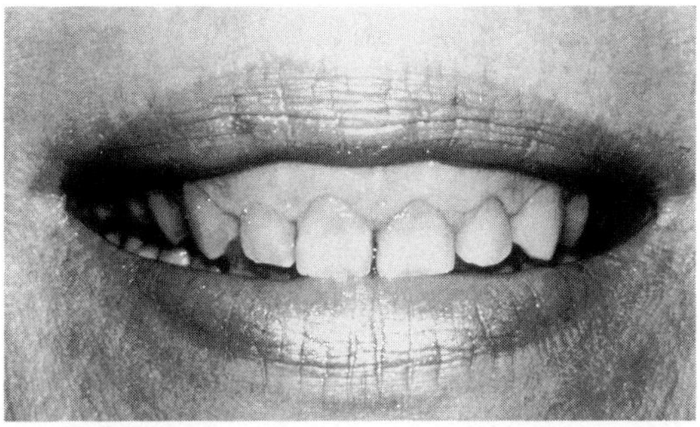

Fig. 19-8a.

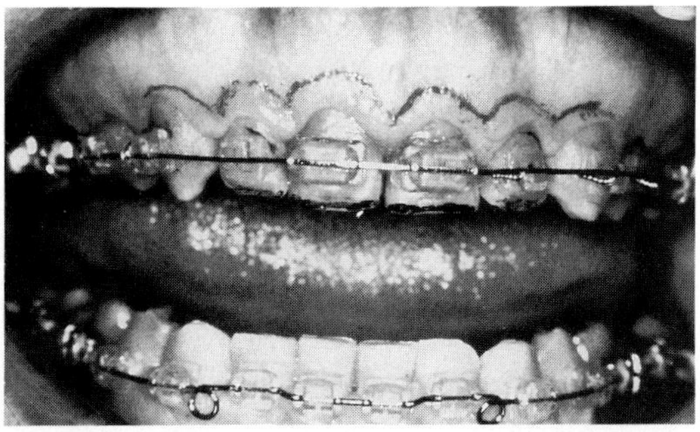

Fig. 19-8b.

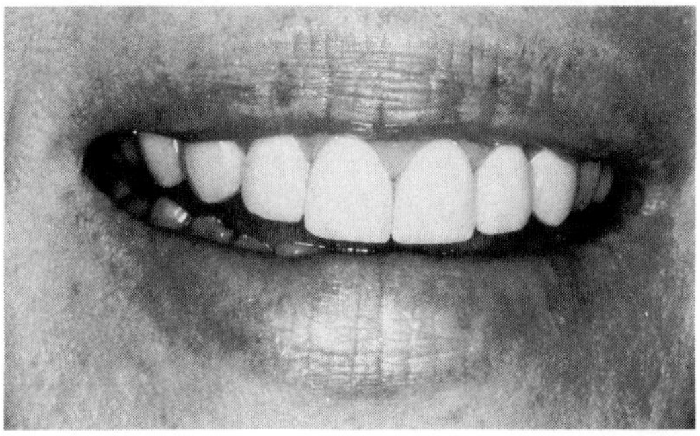

Fig. 19-8c.

Fig. 19-8. *Crown lengthening* by surgical and prosthetic procedures. (a) Pretreatment view. The patient displayed "short front teeth" and a broad exposure of gum tissue. (b) The patient had an unusually wide zone of attached gingiva. The *gingival margins* were positioned apically by making an internally beveled flap with a submarginal entrance incision as outlined in red ink. The crest of the bone was reduced in height. (c) After the tissues had matured following surgery, individual crowns were prepared for each of the anterior teeth. Crown lengthening was achieved and the patient no longer exposed a broad expanse of gum tissue. (Courtesy of Dr. D. Garber).

mm high. In other words the *clinical crown* is shorter than the *anatomical crown*. If, in such a patient, the periodontium is of the THIN biotype, full exposure of the *anatomical crown* can be accomplished by a gingivectomy procedure (Fig. 19-7). If the periodontium is of the THICK biotype, an apically positioned flap procedure should be preferred. This will, if necessary, allow for minor osseous recontouring.

More extensive bone recontouring is required to solve esthetic problems found in patients who do indeed have short *anatomical crowns* in the anterior segment of the dentition. In this category of patients prosthetic measures must be used after resective periodontal therapy to increase the apico-coronal dimension of the crowns. Patients who are candidates for this kind of resective therapy can be divided into two categories (Garber 1987):

- Subjects who have *normal* occlusal relationships and incisal guidance. In this category the incisal line of the front teeth must remain unaltered but the clinical crowns can be made longer by surgically exposing root structure and by locating the cervical margins of the restorations apical to the cemento-enamel junction (Fig. 19-8).

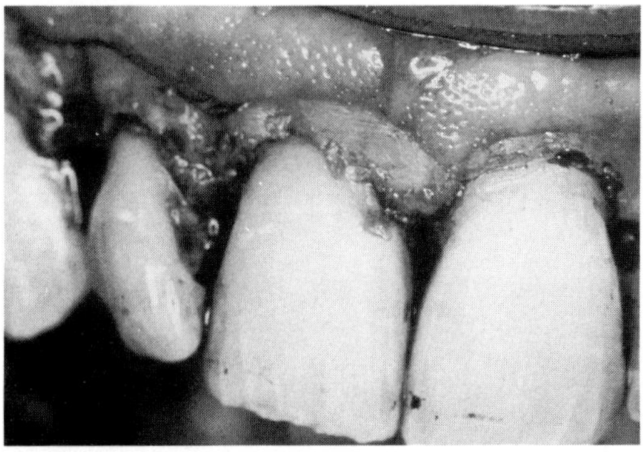

Fig. 19-9. *Crown lengthening* by apically positioned flaps and prosthetic procedure to overcome problems of a "gummy" smile. This patient had a deep overbite and the incisors could be shortened by 2mm without interfering with the incisal guidance. The gingival tissues were apically positioned and the alveolar crest was reduced sufficiently to attain the degree of crown lengthening desired. (Courtesy of Dr. D. Garber).

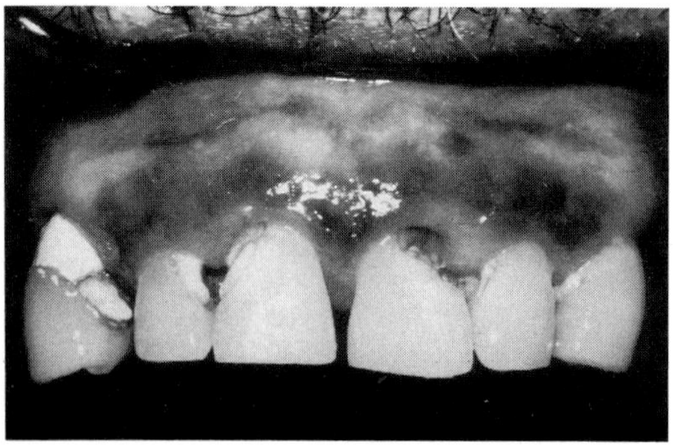

Fig. 19-10a.

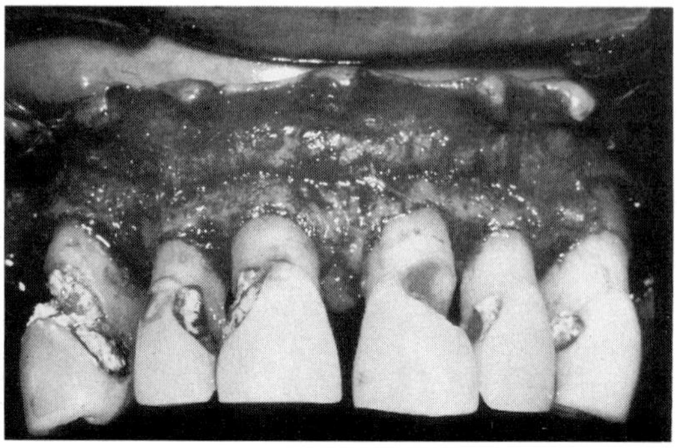

Fig. 19-10b.

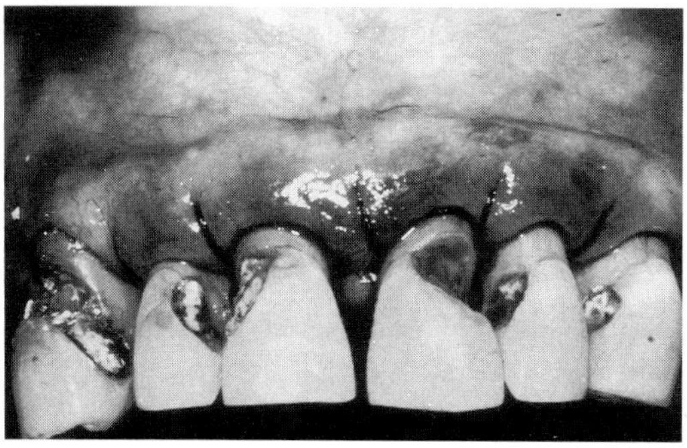

Fig. 19-10c.

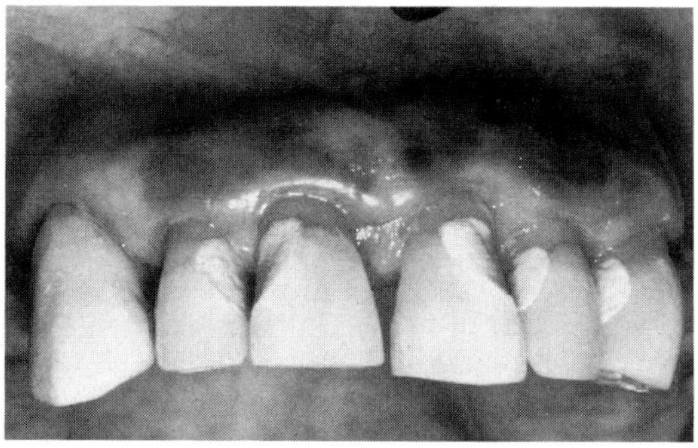

Fig. 19-10d.

Fig. 19-10. (a-c) The subgingival location of the carious lesions required the exposure of sound tooth structure. Apically positioned flaps and osseous resection procedures were used to expose sound tooth structure and recreate normal gingival form at a more apical level. (d) 4 months postsurgery. Gingival symmetry and dental-facial esthetics were maintained (Courtesy Dr. F. Celenza Jr.).

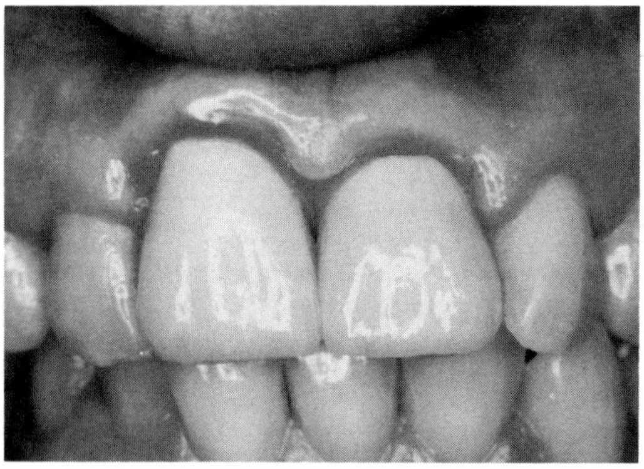

Fig. 19-11. A deformity which interfered with dental-facial esthetics was created at the right central incisor by using a surgical crown lengthening procedure at one single tooth to expose sound tooth structure.

- Subjects who have *abnormal* occlusal relationships with excessive interocclusal space in the posterior dentition when the anterior teeth are in edge-to-edge contact. In this category of patients the length of the maxillary front teeth can be reduced without inducing posterior occlusal interferences. In addition, the marginal gingiva can be resected or relocated to an apical position before crown restorations are made (Fig. 19-9).

It should be realized that patients who have teeth with short tapering roots are not proper candidates for this type of treatment. In such patients the amount of periodontium available is often insufficient for the necessary bone resective measures.

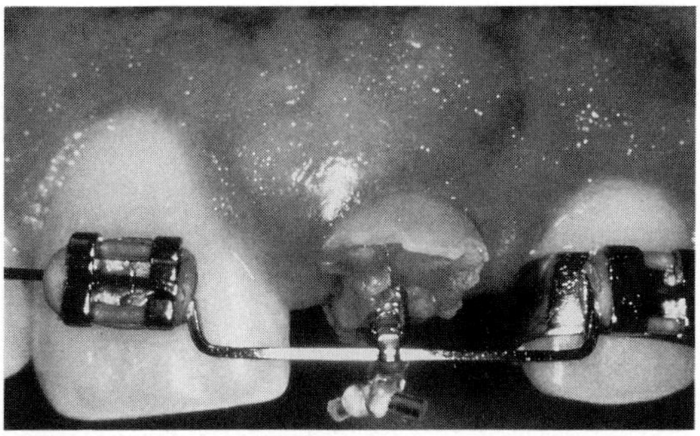

Fig. 19-12a.

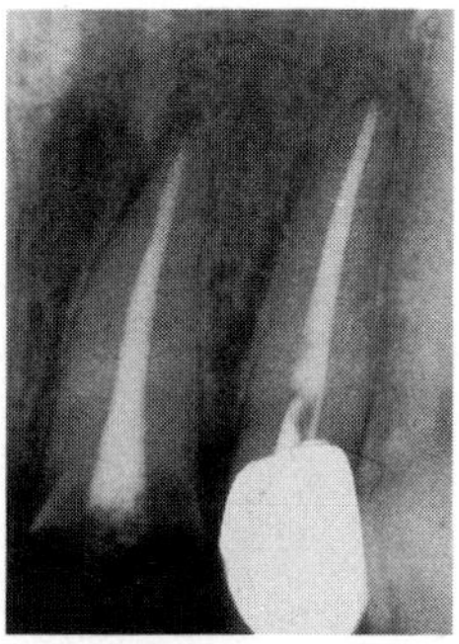

Fig. 19-12b.

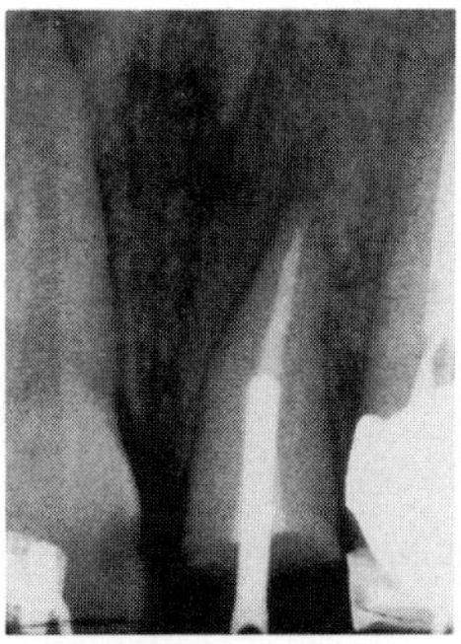

Fig. 19-12c.

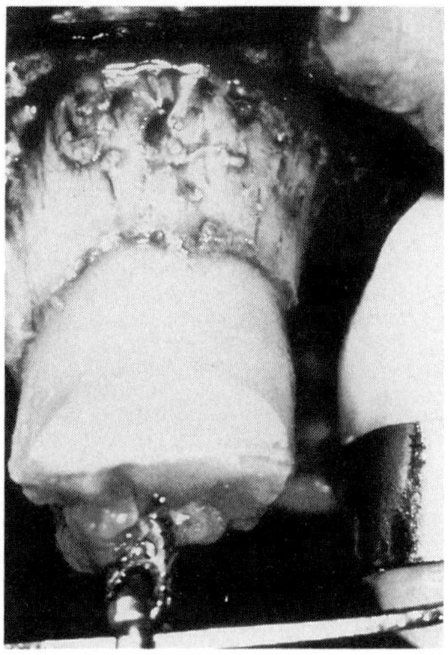

Fig. 19-12d.

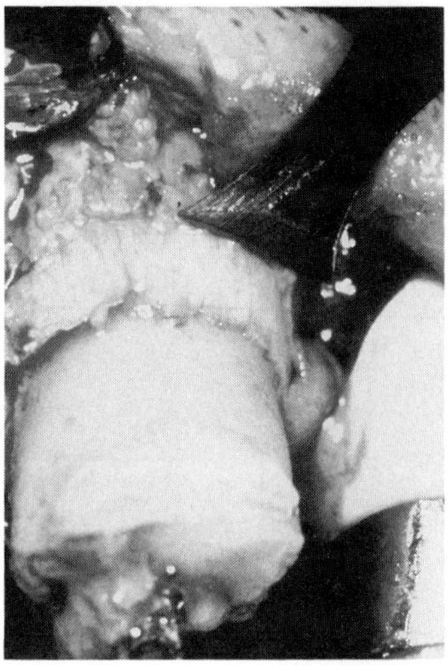

Fig. 19-12e.

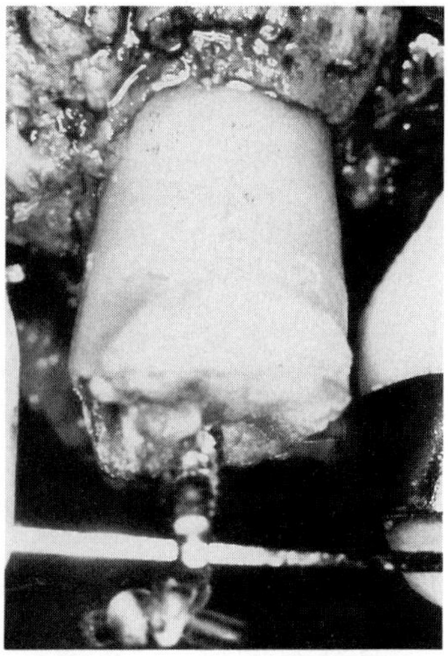

Fig. 19-12f.

Fig. 19-12. *Slow tooth eruption* in conjunction with apically positioned flap and bone resection procedures. (a) The crown of the left central incisor was fractured above the gingival margin. (b) Pretreatment radiograph. Note the form of the interdental septae. (c) Radiograph taken after 6 weeks of slow tooth eruption. Note how the alveolar bone followed the root coronally, creating a "positive" angular crest. (d-f) An access flap (that was later apically positioned) was created to remove bone and recontour the marginal bone to its former shape and level. (g) The attachment levels were not altered on the adjacent teeth.

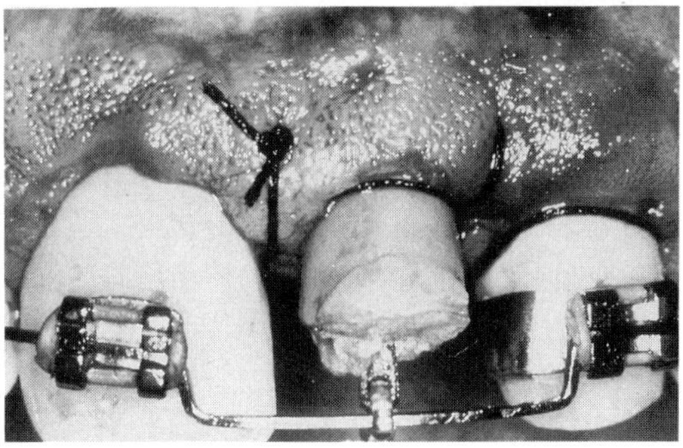

Fig. 19-12g.

To expose sound tooth structure

Crown lengthening procedures may be required to solve different problems such as:

- subgingival location of carious lesions
- subgingival location of fracture lines
- inaccessibility of subgingival margins of failing restorations
- inaccessibility of subgingivally prepared tooth structure for proper impressions

The techniques used to accomplish crown leng-

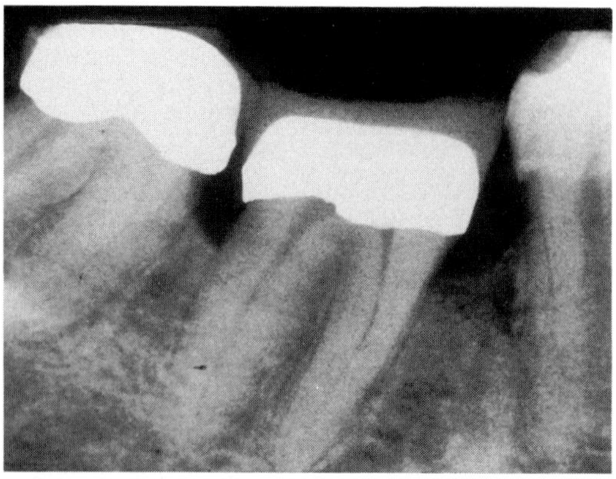

Fig. 19-13a.

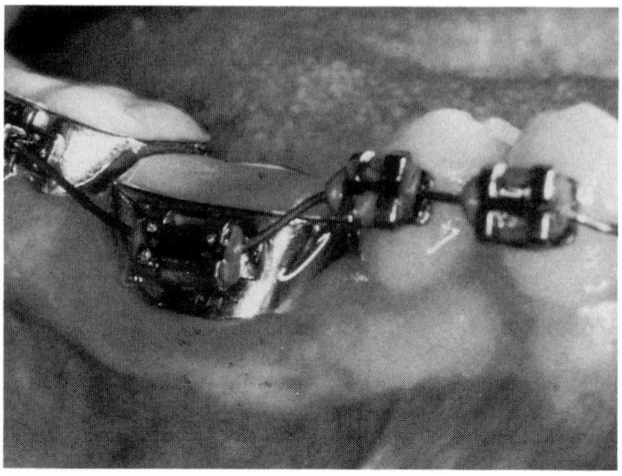

Fig. 19-13b.

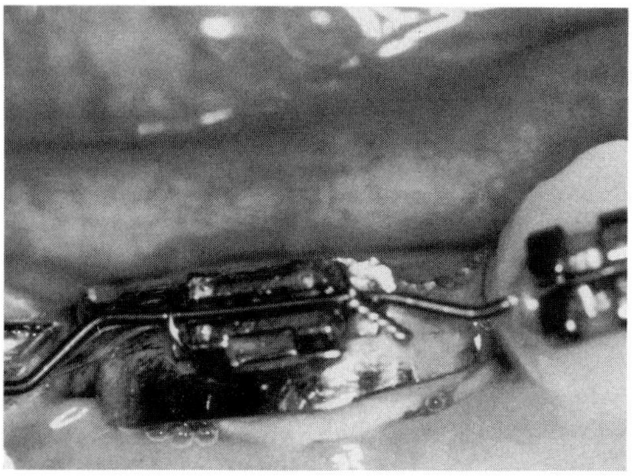

Fig. 19-13c.

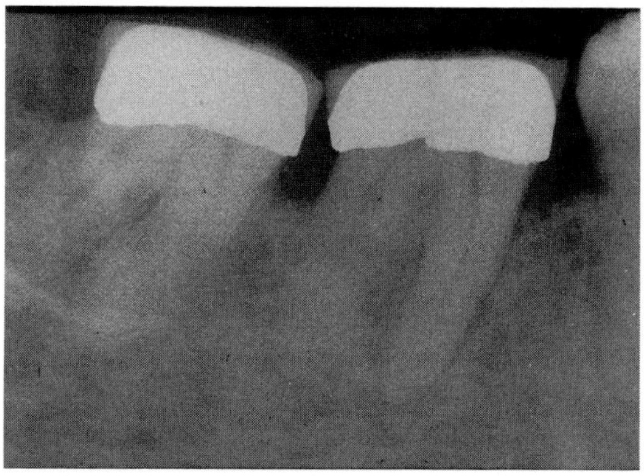

Fig. 19-13d.

Fig. 19-13. *Slow tooth eruption* procedure used to level cementoenamel junctions and angular bone crests. (a) Pretreatment radiograph. (b) A nitol wire was used to erupt the molar. (c) The crown was shortened over a period of 4 months by selective grinding. (d) Radiograph taken 8 months after the start of treatment. The angular bone defects were eliminated.

thening include 1) apically positioned flap procedure including bone resection, 2) slow eruption of teeth, 3) rapid eruption of teeth.

Apically positioned flap with bone recontouring

The apically positioned flap technique with bone recontouring (resection) is frequently used to expose sound tooth structure. As a general rule, at least 4 mm of sound tooth structure must be exposed between the most apical extension of a fracture line or a carious lesion and the bone crest. During healing the supracrestal soft tissues will proliferate to cover 2-3 mm of the root, thereby leaving only 1-2 mm of supragingivally located sound tooth structure. When this technique is used for crown lengthening it must be realized that gingival tissues have an inherent tendency to bridge abrupt changes in the contour of the bone crest. Thus, in order to retain the gingival margin at its new and more apical position, bone recontouring (resection) must be performed not only at the problem tooth but also at the adjacent teeth. Substantial amounts of attachment may consequently have to be sacrificed when crown lengthening is accomplished with an apically positioned flap technique. It is also important to remember that, for esthetic reasons, symmetry of tooth length must be maintained between the right and left side of the dental arch. This may, in some situations,

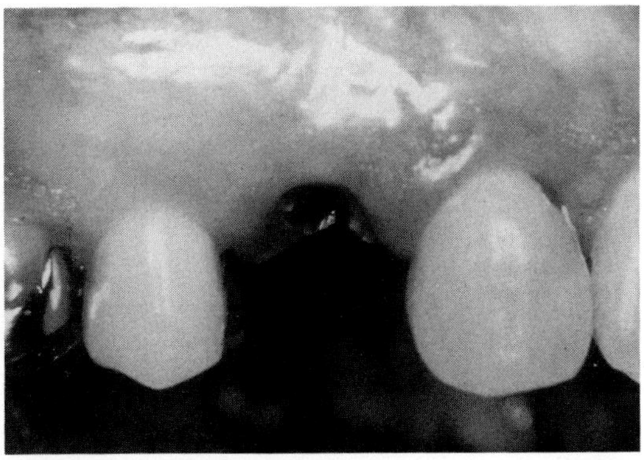

Fig. 19-14a.

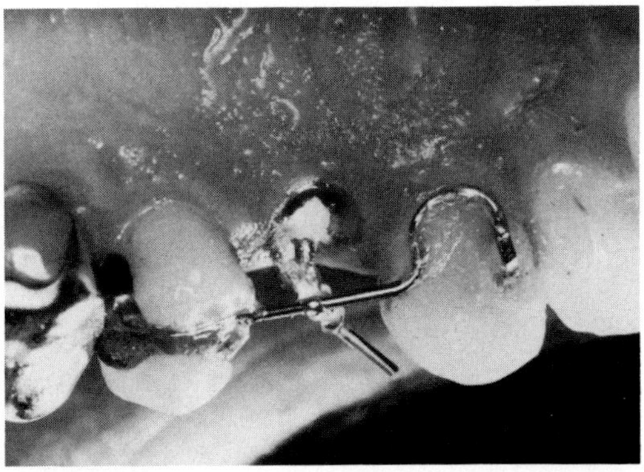

Fig. 19-14b.

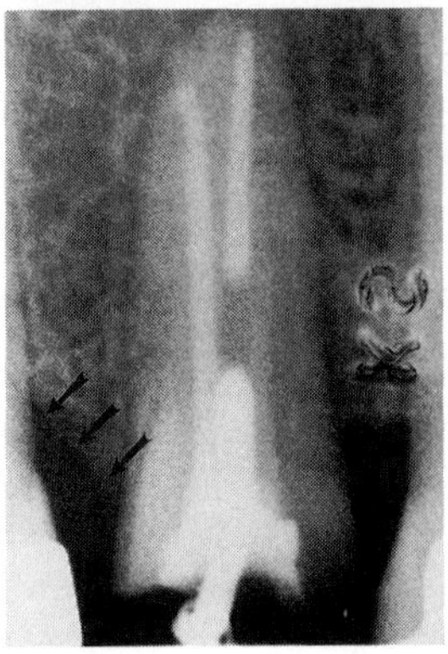

Fig. 19-14c.

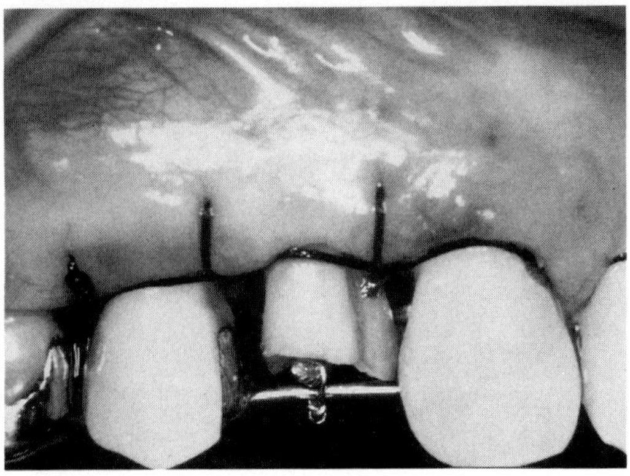

Fig. 19-14d.

Fig. 19-14. *Rapid tooth eruption procedure* in conjunction with fiberotomy procedure. (a) Buccal view, the fracture on the first premolar extended subgingivally. (b) Palatal view as eruption was initiated. Sulcular fiber resection was performed at the mesial half of the tooth to the level of the bone crest. The distal half remained as a control surface. The fiber resection was repeated once a week during the 3-week eruption phase. The tooth was stabilized for 6 weeks, and at that time a full-thickness flap was raised. (c) The bone crest had a "positive" angulation at the distal surface and remained unchanged at the mesial surface. (d) Ample crown lengthening was obtained and the gingival margins healed to their former shape and location.

call for the involvement of even more teeth in the surgical procedure.

Indication: crown lengthening of multiple teeth in a quadrant or sextant of the dentition (Fig. 19-10).

Contraindication: crown lengthening of single teeth, especially in the anterior regions (Fig. 19-11).

Technique: the apically positioned flap technique and methods used for bone recontouring are presented in Chapter 14.

Slow eruption of teeth

Orthodontic tooth movement can be used to erupt teeth in adults (Reitan 1967, Heithersay 1973, Ingber 1974, 1976, Simon et al. 1978, Lythgoe et al. 1980, Antrium 1981, Potashnick et al. 1982, Guilford et al. 1984). If moderate eruptive forces are used, the entire attachment apparatus will move in unison with the tooth. The tooth must be extruded a distance equal to or slightly longer than the portion of sound tooth structure that will be exposed in the subsequent surgical treatment. After the tooth has reached the intended position and been stabi-

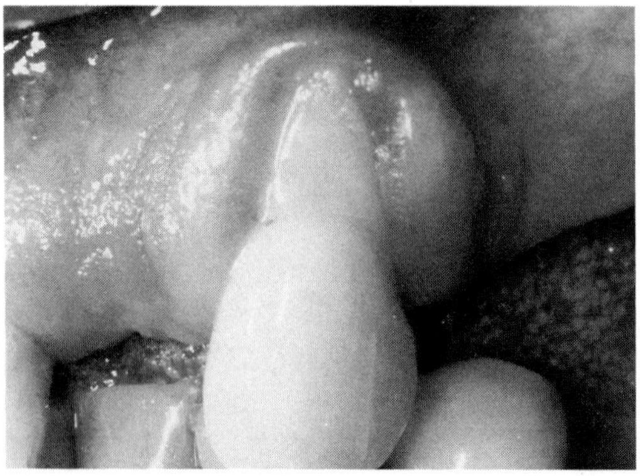

Fig. 19-15a.

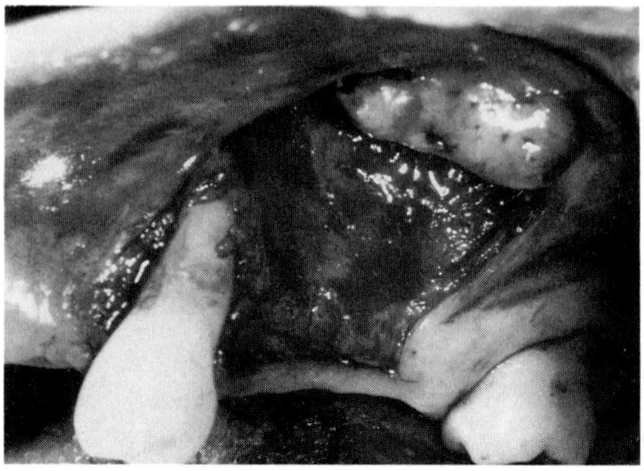

Fig. 19-15b.

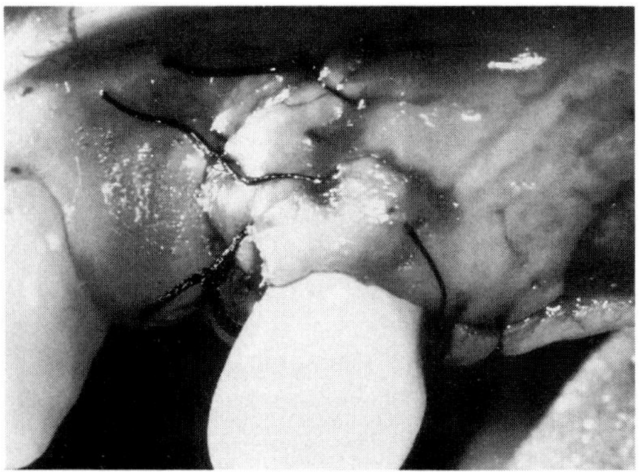

Fig. 19-15c.

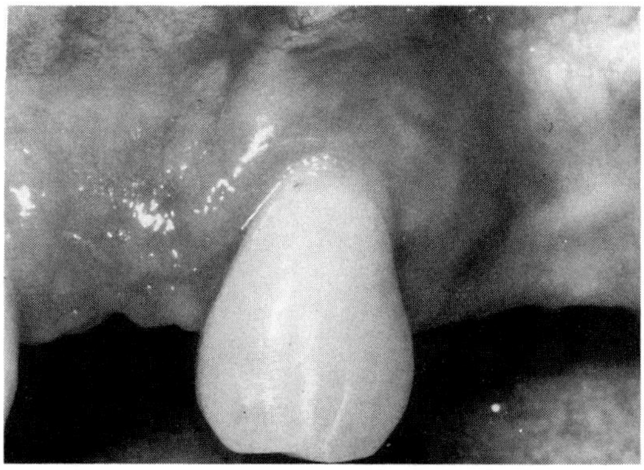

Fig. 19-15d.

Fig. 19-15. (a) Advanced, localized gingival recession at the buccal surface of the maxillary left canine. (b) A partial-thickness pedicle flap was raised. (c) The flap was stabilized with sutures and retracting muscle pull was eliminated by undermining dissection. (d) 4 months postsurgery.

lized, a full thickness flap is elevated and bone recontouring is performed to expose sound root structure at the problem tooth. It is important that the bone and soft tissue levels at adjacent teeth remain unchanged (Fig. 19-12).

Indication: crown lengthening at sites where removal of attachment and bone from adjacent teeth must be avoided. The slow eruption technique can also be used as a means of reducing pocket depths at sites with angular bony defects (Brown 1973, Ingber 1974, 1976). The angular bony defect at the problem tooth can be reduced while the attachment level at the adjacent tooth surface remains unchanged (Fig. 19-13).

Contraindication: The slow eruption technique requires the use of fixed orthodontic appliances. Thus, in patients who have only a few teeth remaining, an alternative approach for crown lengthening has to be selected.

Technique: Orthodontic brackets are banded to the teeth adjacent to the problem tooth and are combined with an arch wire. Another type of mechanical system can be utilized by placing a heavy gauge bar in grooves prepared in the adjacent teeth and over the problem tooth. If sufficient crown structure remains on the problem tooth a bracket can be bonded to its cervical portion. A power elastic is tied from the bracket to the arch wire (or the bar) which pulls the

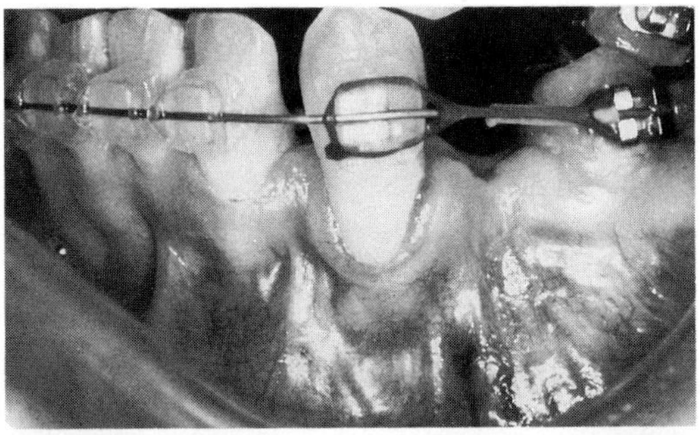

Fig. 19-16a.

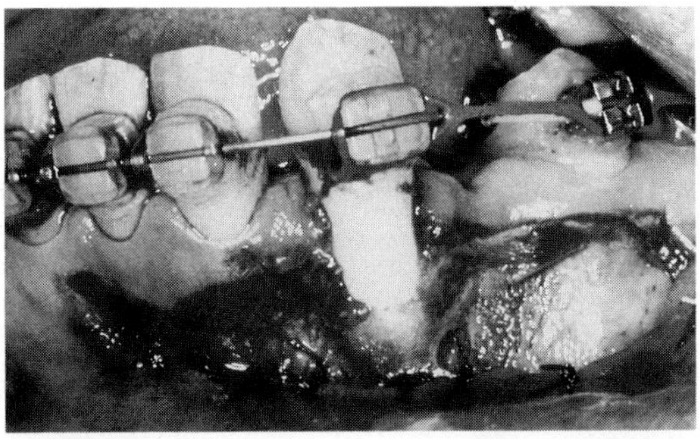

Fig. 19-16b.

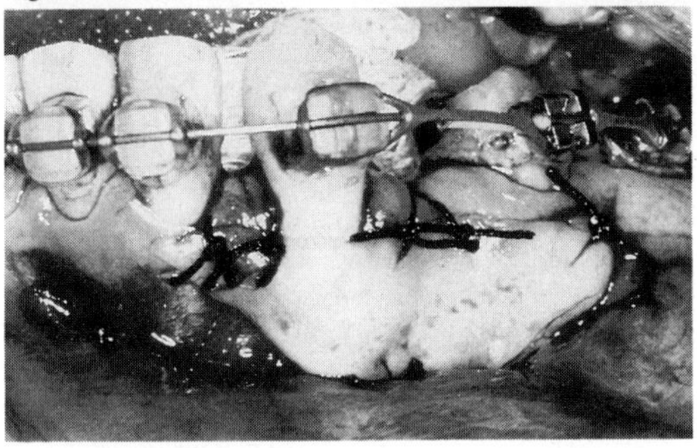

Fig. 19-16c.

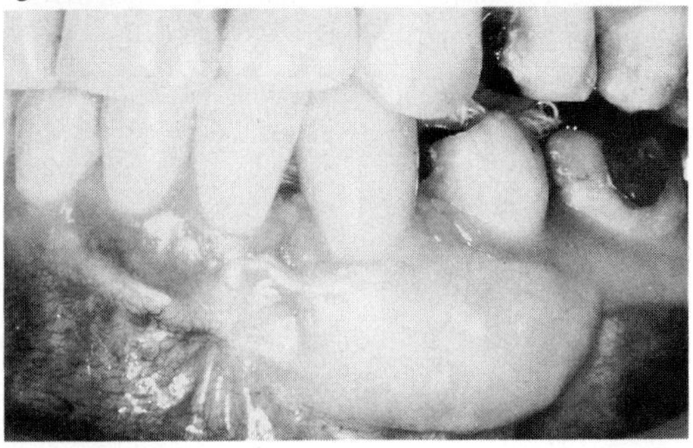

Fig. 19-16d.

Fig. 19-16. (a) A deep-wide area of recession was present on the buccal surface of the mandibular left canine. (b) The recipient site was prepared with a marginal dissection to receive a thick, free gingival graft. (c) The graft was positioned over the root in an attempt to gain root coverage in addition to augmenting the zone of attached gingiva. (d) One year postsurgery. (Courtesy of Dr. H. Corn).

tooth coronally. If most of the crown structure is lost, root canal therapy is required. A post placed in the root canal is fitted with a power elastic which is also joined with the arch wire. The direction of the tooth movement must be carefully checked to ensure that the problem tooth is not tilted or moved towards the adjacent tooth surfaces (Fig. 19-12).

Rapid eruption of teeth

In the rapid tooth eruption procedure the problem tooth is moved coronally and out of its socket. The crestal bone and the gingival margin are retained at their pretreatment locations. The tooth-gingiva interface at adjacent teeth is unaltered. In this technique more force is used than in the slow eruption procedure. In addition, *fiberotomy* must be performed at 7- to 10-day intervals to sever the supracrestal connective tissue fibers. In Fig. 19-14, *fiberotomy* had been performed only at the mesial half of the root. Radiographs obtained after 9 weeks demonstrate that crestal bone migration has occurred at the distal but not at the mesial surface of the problem tooth (Pontoriero et al. 1987).

Indication: crown lengthening at sites where it is important to maintain the location of the gingival margin at adjacent teeth unchanged.

Contraindication: the rapid tooth eruption technique should not be employed at teeth associated with angular bone defects. In such cases the slow eruption technique should be preferred.

Technique: Similar to the technique described under the slow eruption procedure, but heavier forces are used to pull the problem tooth out of

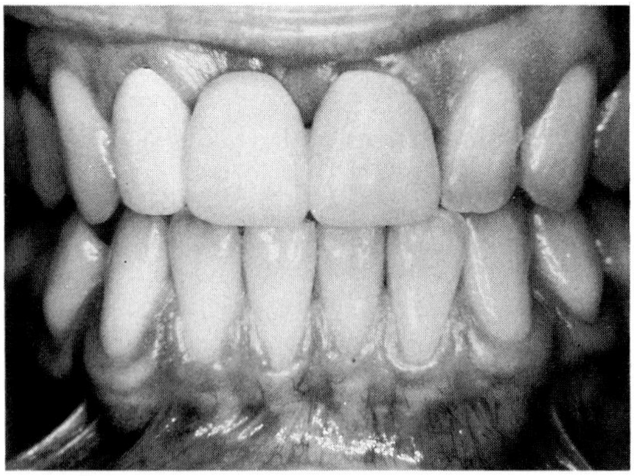

Fig. 19-17a.

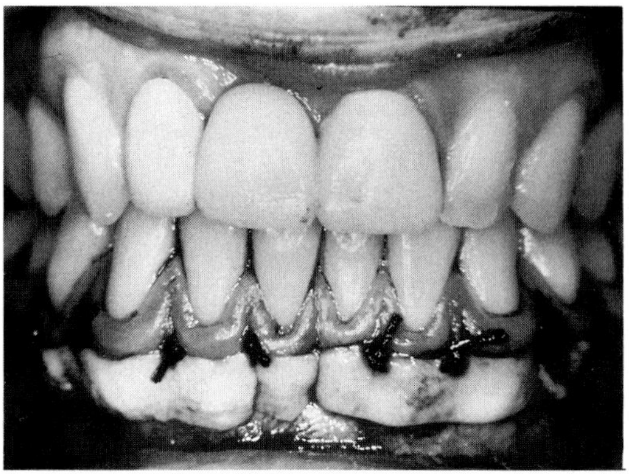

Fig. 19-17b.

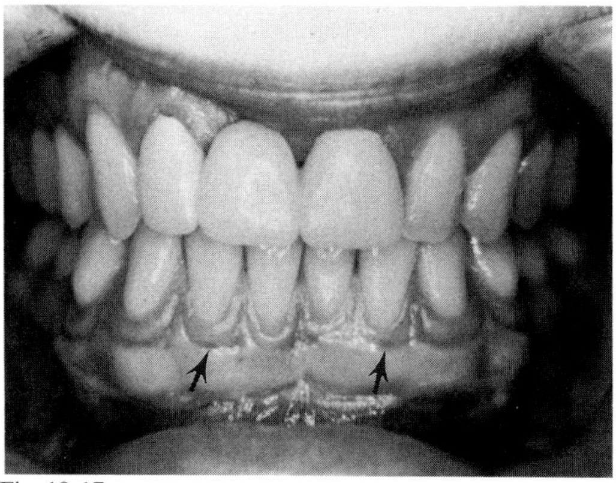

Fig. 19-17c.

Fig. 19-17. (a) Pretreatment view. A minimal zone of attached gingiva existed on the labial surfaces of the mandibular incisors. (b) A submarginal path of incision, perpendicular to the tissue surface, was started at the mucogingival junction to prepare the recipient site. The coronal edges of the grafts (2 sections) were trimmed to a square surface to form a *buttjoint* with the remaining gingiva. (c) One year postsurgery. This illustration shows the red line that formed between the graft and the marginal gingiva.

its socket and *fiberotomy* must be performed once every 7-10 days.

Reconstructive procedures

Reconstruction of gingiva at sites with recession

Pedicle graft or *free grafts of masticatory mucosa* are used to reconstruct gingiva over exposed root surfaces (Grupe & Warren 1956, Nabers 1966, Mlinek et al. 1973, Livingstone 1975, Ruben et al. 1976, Corn 1980, Corn & Marks 1983A, 1983B, Miller 1982, Holbrook & Ochsenbein 1982, Miller 1987).

Pedicle grafts

The pedicle graft procedures are probably the most predictable of all procedures described to obtain proper root coverage. A functional blood supply is maintained through the pedicle of the flap (Fig. 19-15) and, when healed, the graft provides a proper match with the color and texture characteristics of the adjacent gingiva.

The amount of gingiva than can be transposed to cover a recipient site is dependent on the thickness and surface area of the gingiva present at adjacent teeth. Thus, if the recession defect is wide and deep, and the gingiva at adjacent teeth is moderate with respect to thickness and width, the pedicle graft procedure may not provide enough donor tissue. The pedicle graft procedure should also be avoided at sites where the gingiva and alveolar bone of the donor sites are thin. Findings reported by Sullivan et al. (1971 a,b) and Caffesse et al. (1978) demonstrate that severe recessions may in such situations occur at the donor sites.

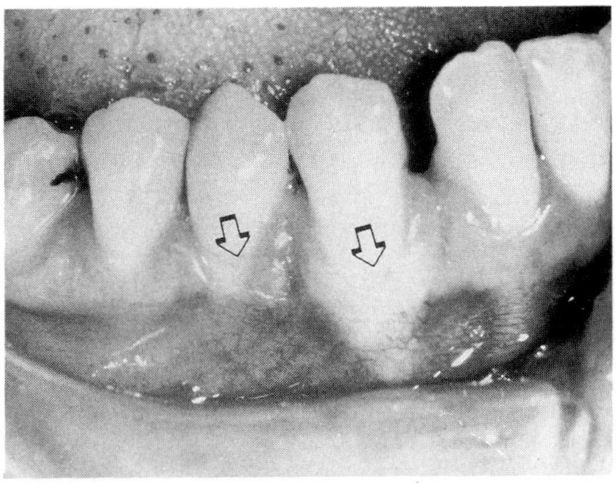

Fig. 19-18a.

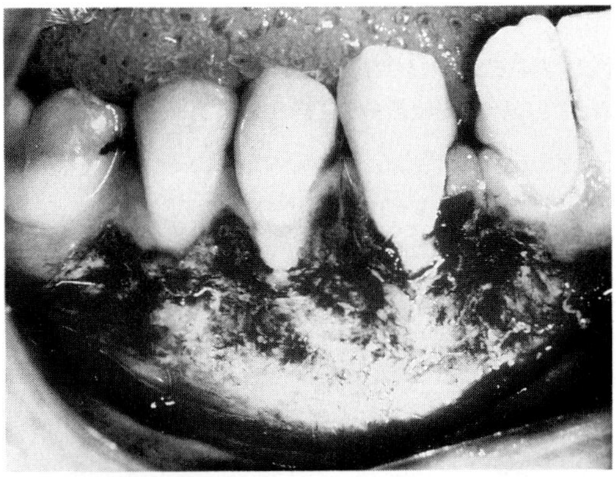

Fig. 19-18b.

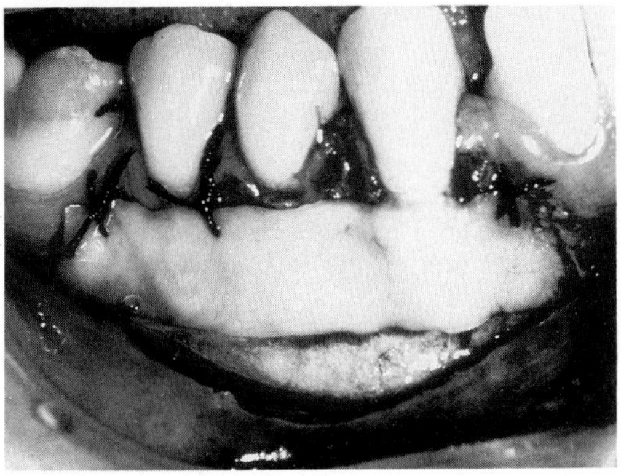

Fig. 19-18c.

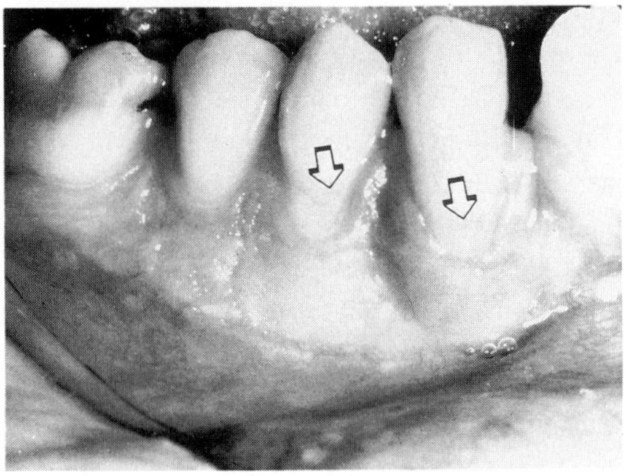

Fig. 19-18d.

Fig. 19-18. (a) Pretreatment view. (b) A marginal path of incision that started in the gingival sulcus was employed to prepare the recipient site. The labial surfaces of the papillae were deepithelialized by using a gingivoplasty diamond point in a high-speed turbine handpiece. (c) 9 months post-treatment. The surface texture and contour of the graft blended smoothly into the surface of the gingiva. Note the amount of recession that was produced by removing the gingival sulcus and failing to cover this area of the teeth with the graft. (Courtesy of Dr. S. Soehren).

Free grafts of masticatory mucosa

The free graft procedure used to cover exposed root surfaces is technically demanding (Miller 1987). A thick graft must be used and the recipient site must be prepared to ensure rapid revascularization of the graft (Fig. 19-16). The free graft procedure is often used as a two-stage operation (Harvey 1965, 1970, Restrepo 1973, Bernimoulin et al. 1975, Maynard 1977, Guinard & Caffesse 1978, Matter 1979). A free graft of the required dimensions is first placed apical to the recession defect in a conventionally prepared recipient site. In a second stage pedicle graft procedure, performed 6-8 weeks later, the grafted gingiva is shifted coronally to cover the exposed root surface.

Advantages: With the use of the free graft procedure a large volume of donor tissue can be obtained. The donor tissue is frequently harvested from edentulous areas of the mouth.

Disadvantages: Delay in the revascularization of the graft often results in partial or complete necrosis. The healed recipient site may appear blanched and fail to match the color of the adjacent gingival tissue.

Augmentation of a narrow zone of gingiva

Free grafts of masticatory mucosa (free gingival grafts) are used to augment zones of narrow gingiva. For details regarding indications for grafting and the biological principles of healing, see Chapter 18. Free gingival grafts are normally harvested from the palate and at the recipient sites are positioned and stabilized over an exposed bed of richly vascularized connective tissue. Grafting of masticatory mucosa may in some situations give rise to esthetical problems. The grafted tissue frequently becomes lighter in color and appears more blanched than the unoperated gingiva. Thus, patients who have naturally occurring heavy pigmentation within their gingivae are in many situations poor candidates for this kind of therapy. If pink palatal tissue is grafted into a zone of darker gingiva a marked color disharmony will be the result. If for some reason it is regarded as necessary to augment the gingiva in such a patient, the graft should, for esthetic reasons, be extended from second premolar to second premolar. This will ensure uniformity of gingival color on both sides of the midline.

Placement of graft margins: The recipient site for the graft can be prepared in two different ways. The horizontal incision used to dissect the alveolar mucosa from the recipient site can be started either at *the mucogingival junction* or in *the gingival sulcus*. If the incision is started in the gingival sulcus the entire gingiva must be removed from the recipient site. This is referred to as *marginal preparation*. If the incision is started at the mucogingival junction, the marginal gingiva is left intact and the technique is denoted *submarginal preparation*.

The incision at the submarginal preparation site can be made either perpendicular to the tissue or with a bevelled outline. If a perpendicular incision is used, the margins of the graft should be trimmed to form a square edge. Hereby a butt-joint is established between the graft and the recipient tissue. During healing, free gingival grafts shrink and lose about 15-25 % of their surface area and consequently contract along both the apico-coronal and the mesio-distal axes. This frequently causes the butt-joint to open and granulation tissue from the recipient site tissue (alveolar mucosa) fills the void. After healing, a red line of alveolar mucosa will separate the marginal gingiva and the pale grafted tissue (Fig. 19-17). This may compromise esthetics in patients who have a high lip line. To overcome this problem, the bevelled incision technique may be preferred for the submarginal preparation. The bevelled edge of the graft is fitted against the bevelled gingiva of the recipient site and an overlapping joint is established (Soehren et al. 1973). The graft must overlap the recipient area by a distance large enough to compensate for the shrinkage that will occur during healing. This preparation technique usually provides an esthetically acceptable gingiva (Fig. 19-18). But if the graft fails to heal properly, gingival recession may occur.

The edentulous ridge and ridge augmentation

The normal ridge

A partially or completely edentulous ridge may have retained the general shape of the alveolar process. Such a ridge is traditionally referred to as a *normal ridge*. Even though this *normal ridge* has retained the bucco-lingual and apico-coronal dimensions of the alveolar process, it is *not* normal in many other respects; the eminences that existed in the bone over the roots are no longer present, and the interdental papillae are missing.

The smooth contours of the *normal ridge* create problems for the restorative dentist. In a fixed bridge the pontics 1) frequently give the impression that they rest on the top of the ridge rather than emerge from within an alveolar pro-

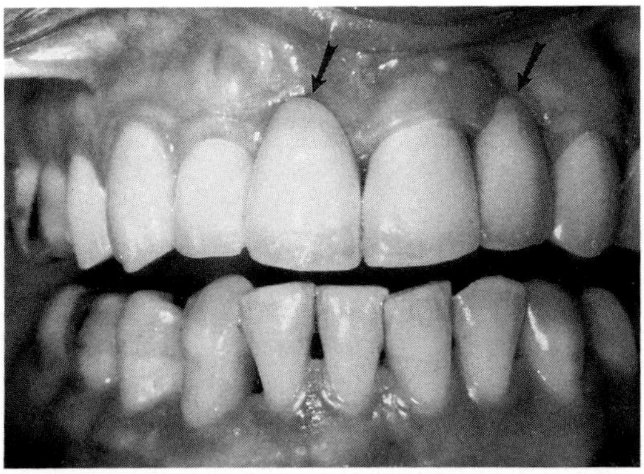

Fig. 19-19. *Blended pontics.* The facial contour in the cervical one-third of the pontics replacing the right central and left lateral incisor was "blended" in a gradual arc to contact the concavity in the residual ridge. The pontics are longer than the contralateral abutment teeth.

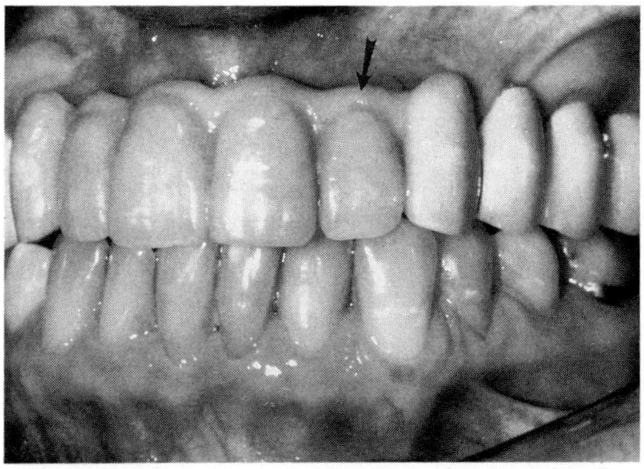

Fig. 19-20. *Pontics with a flange.* In order to keept the pontics in the 5-tooth span (right lateral incisor to left canine) from appearing too long, a flange of pink acrylic was added to hide the deformity in the ridge. (Courtesey of Dr. L. Abrams).

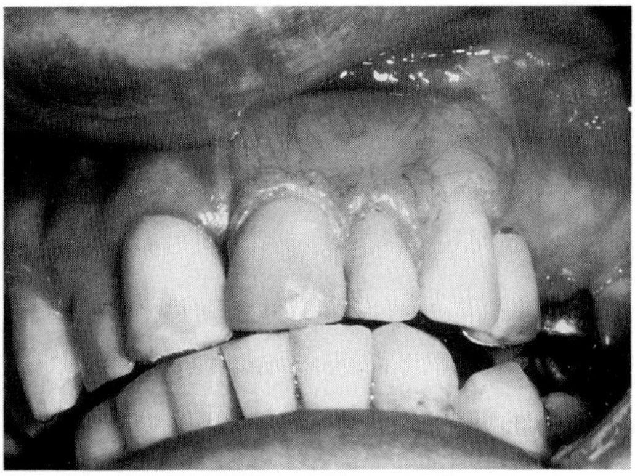

Fig. 19-21a.

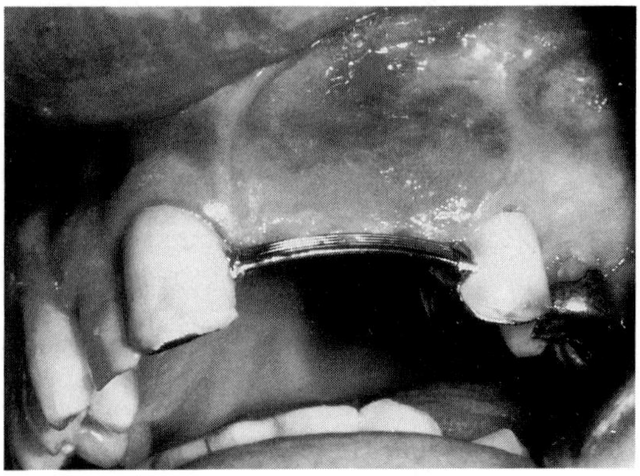

Fig. 19-21b.

Fig. 19-21. *Andrew's bridge system.* (a) A 3-tooth unit with an acrylic flange in position over the supporting bar. (b) The clip-retained removable section was removed to show the abutment crowns and the supporting bar section of the prosthesis.

cess, 2) lack a root eminence, 3) lack marginal gingivae and interdental papillae. Dark triangles, which almost always interfere with dental-facial esthetics, are present in the embrasure area between the pontics and between the abutment and the pontics. In other words, also in the presence of a *normal ridge* it may be difficult or impossible to produce a fixed prosthesis which truly restores the esthetics and function of the natural dentition.

The deformed ridge

A *deformed ridge* may result from, e.g., clefts from birth defects, trauma, tumors, tooth extractions, advanced periodontal disease, abscess formations etc. The deformity that exists in the ridge is directly related to the volume of root structure and associated bone that is missing or has been destroyed.

Classification: Ridge defects can be divided into three classes according to Seibert (1983a):

Class I: Loss of tissue in bucco-lingual direction, normal height in apico-coronal direction.

Class II: Loss of tissue in apico-coronal direction, normal width in bucco-lingual direction.

Class III: A combination of Class I and Class II, i.e. loss of both height and width.

A number of different surgical implant and graft procedures have been developed in attempts to reconstruct the partially edentulous ridge and ridge defects (Meltzer 1979, Abrams 1980a, Seibert 1980, 1983a, Langer & Calagna 1980, 1982, Garber & Rosenberg 1981, Kaldahl et al. 1982, McHenry et al. 1982, Rosenberg et al. 1984, Allen et al. 1985, Miller 1986, Seibert & Cohen 1987). Some of these procedures will be described below.

Prosthetic treatment of ridge defects

Prosthetic means are most frequently used to restore dental-facial esthetics and function in patients with ridge defects. In a fixed bridge the pontic teeth are modified and extended to reach the surface of the defect. This extension, however, frequently makes the pontics markedly longer than the adjacent teeth and, if used in the front tooth regions, such a prosthetic solution to a ridge defect may severely interfere with dental-facial esthetics.

In a fixed bridge the cervical portion of the pontic is usually curved lingually to bring the prosthetic unit in contact with the *normal ridge* (blended pontic; Abrams 1980a, Fig. 19-19). For esthetic reasons (differences in height between neighboring teeth), it is difficult to use blended pontics in patients with advanced *ridge defects*. In such situations a flange of pink stained plastic can be added to the apical portion of the pontic. Such a flange will give the illusion of gingival tissue and may fill the space between the pontic and the deformed ridge (Fig. 19-20). Another device frequently employed in the treatment of patients with large ridge defects is Andrew's Bridge System (Fig. 19-21). The bridge system consists of a fixed retainer and a rectangular bar system, which employs a clip-retained removable pontic and a flange section.

Various types of precision attachments have also been devised for multiple pontic spans at ridge defects. Such attachments are used in both fixed and removable prosthetic appliances. The addition of a flange of simulated gum tissue may improve the esthetic value of the prosthesis and may also control airflow and improve phonation.

While the flange type of a prosthesis may be the only practical solution for certain types of large volume ridge defects, a variety of plastic surgical procedures have been described which can be used to predictably and successfully augment ridge defects of moderate dimensions.

Surgical treatment of ridge defects

Presurgical treatment planning

A provisional bridge must be made prior to surgery. The soft tissue at the surgically treated recipient site for a graft or implant will undergo considerable swelling during the early phase of healing. The tissues will conform to the tissue-facing surfaces (tissue surfaces) of the bridge. The prosthesis is thus used to help in preparing the surface of the augmented ridge to the desired form. The location and shape of the interproximal embrasure areas in the provisional bridge will determine where the papillae of the ridge will be located.

Presurgical-preprosthetical treatment planning and joint consultations involving the surgeon and the restorative dentist are required for an optimal result. The following factors should be determined prior to the initiation of therapy:

- The volume of tissue required to eliminate the ridge deformity
- The type of graft or implant to be used
- The location of donor sites for grafts
- The number and timing of various treatment procedures
- The design of the provisional bridge
- The design of a surgical stent
- Possible problems with tissue discolorations (Fig. 19-22) and tissue color matching

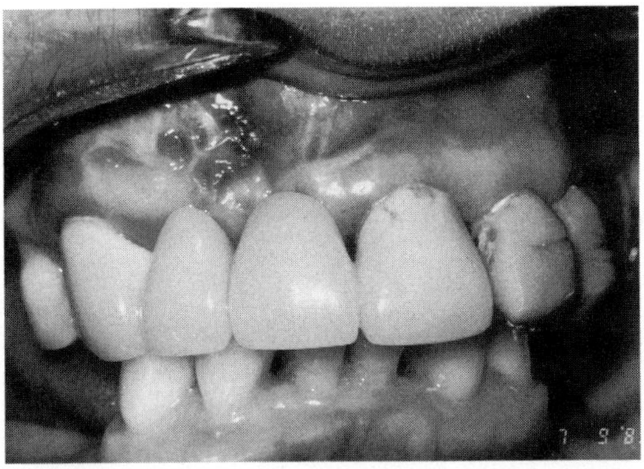

Fig. 19-22a.

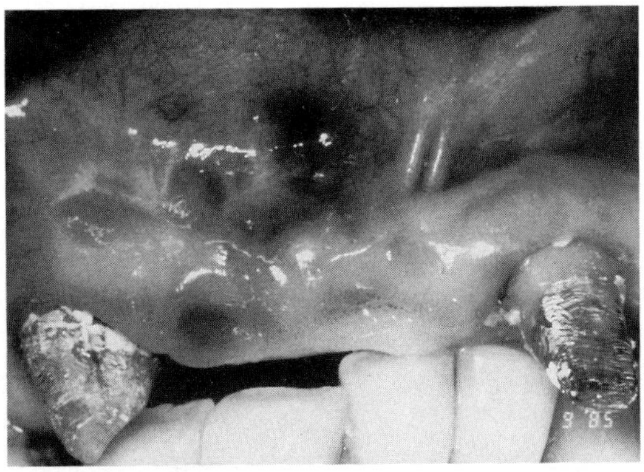

Fig. 19-22b.

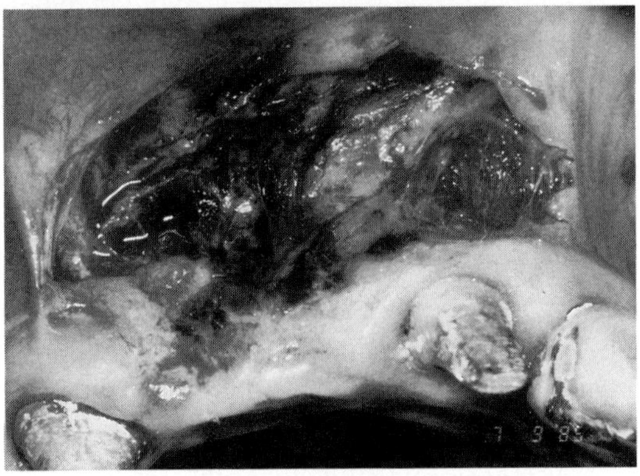

Fig. 19-22c.

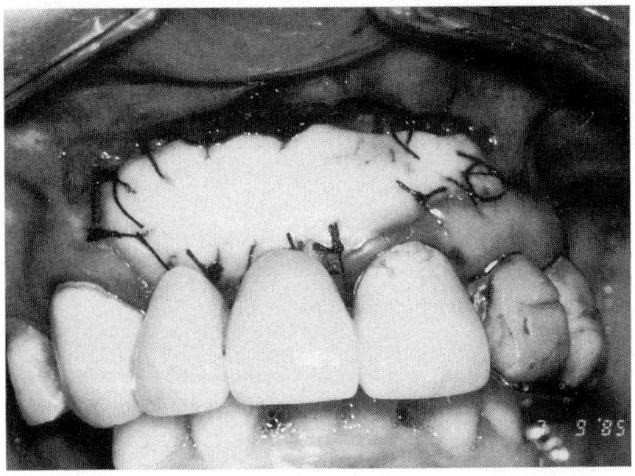

Fig. 19-22d.

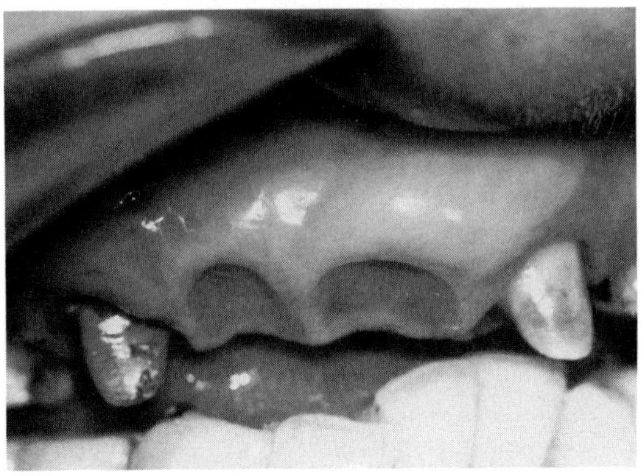

Fig. 19-22e.

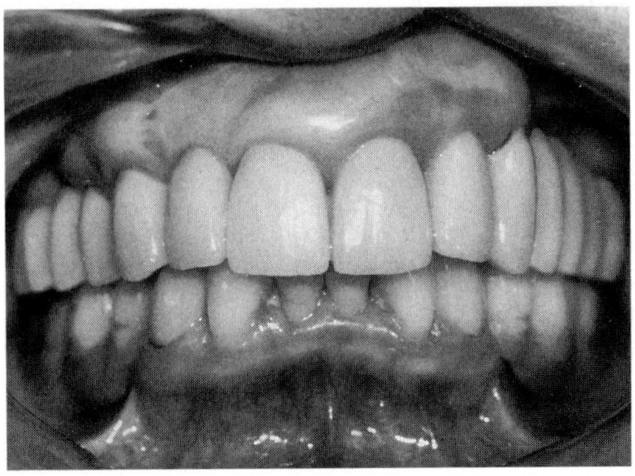

Fig. 19-22f.

Fig. 19-22. *Class I ridge deformity* with an amalgam tattoo. (a) Pretreatment view with a failing fixed prosthesis in position. (b) Pretreatment view with the fixed prosthesis removed. (c) Recipient site prepared to receive a free graft from the palate; to augment the ridge and to mask the stained tissues. (d) The graft in place. (e) A gingivoplasty procedure was used to create the ovate receptacle sites in the healed ridge. This view shows the form of the ridge 20 months after surgery. (f) The final prosthesis placed in provisional cementation. Note that, at 20 months after surgery, the amalgam tattoo had not returned.

The Roll procedure

Surgical concept: The Roll procedure (Abrams 1980b) involves the preparation of a de-epithelialized connective tissue pedicle graft which is

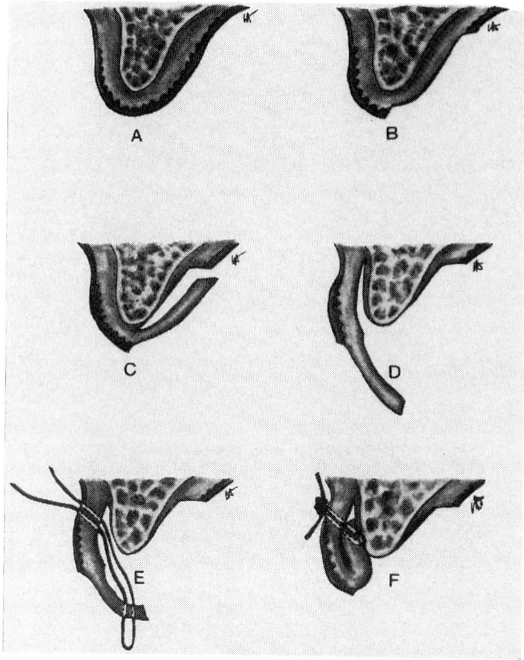

Fig. 19-23. Sequence of steps in the *pedicle graft (Roll) procedure.* (A) Cross section of the residual edentulous ridge prior to treatment. (B) The removal of the epithelium. (C) The elevation of the pedicle. (D) The pouch was created. (E) Sutures were placed at the mucogingival junction to catch the tip of the pedicle flap and pull it into place in the pouch. (F) The flap was secured. A convexity in the ridge was created. (Courtesy Dr. L. Abrams).

subsequently placed in a subepithelial pouch (Fig. 19-23). This procedure is used in the treatment of small to moderate Class I ridge defects. The technique enables the surgeon to augment tissue apically and labially to the cervical area of a pontic and to give the recipient site the appearance of a normal tooth-gingiva interface. A bucco-lingual ridge concavity can be converted into a ridge convexity resembling the eminence produced by the roots of the adjacent teeth (Fig. 19-24).

Technique: A rectangular shaped pedicle of connective tissue is prepared on the palatal side of the defect. The length of the pedicle must match the amount of apico-coronal augmentation that is planned. This, in turn, is related to the amount of root eminence that exists on either side of the defect. If a 2 or 3 tooth pontic space is treated with the Roll technique, 2 or 3 separate pedicles are raised. Each of these pedicles will form a new "root-cervical margin".

The epithelium on the palatal surface of the donor site is first removed. A maximum of *supraperiosteal* connective tissue is raised from the palate using sharp dissection. The void that is produced at the donor site will gradually fill in with granulation tissue. Caution must be exercised in dissecting the pedicle flap so that tissue perforation is avoided, when the plane of dissection approaches the facial (labial) surface (Figs. 19-23, 19-24). A pouch or tunnel is made in the *supraperiosteal* connective tissue at the facial (labial) surface of the ridge. In order to preserve as much connective tissue and blood supply as possible at the recipient site, the dissection must be made as close as possible to the periosteum of the facial bone.

The pedicle is tucked into the pouch as a try-in procedure. Adjustment of the pedicle size should now be made. Once the pedicle fits as desired it is made ready for the stabilizing suture. The suturing scheme is illustrated in Fig. 19-23. The suture must be positioned close to the muco-buccal fold. This enables the surgeon to pull the pedicle to the apical portion of the pouch. The suture should not be tightly tied, since it only serves as a positioning and stabilizing device. The use of a resorbable suture material is recommended.

Adjustment of pontic contours

Measures used to adapt the tissue surface of the pontic to the contour of the surgically treated ridge are common to all ridge augmentation procedures in patients with fixed bridgework. A *light pressure* must be maintained between the pedicle graft or the implant surface and the tissue surface of the pontics. The postoperative swelling, as discussed above, will cause the tissue to conform to the shape of the pontic.

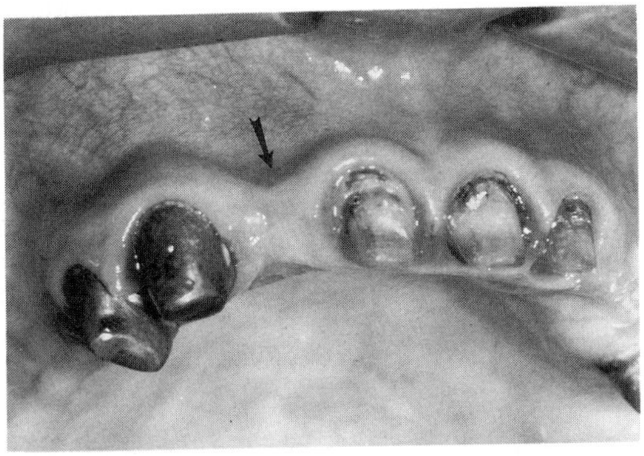

Fig. 19-24a.

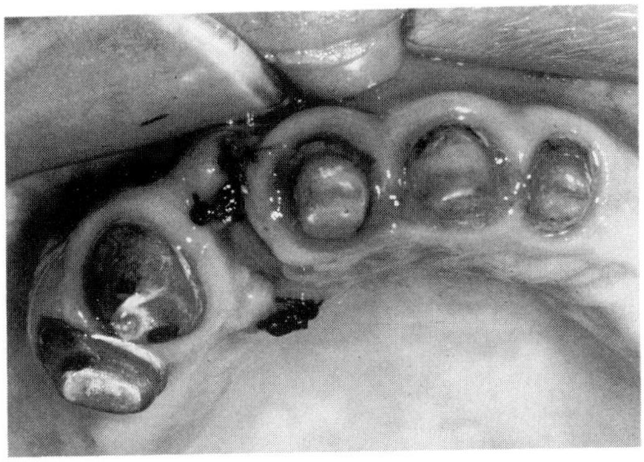

Fig. 19-24b.

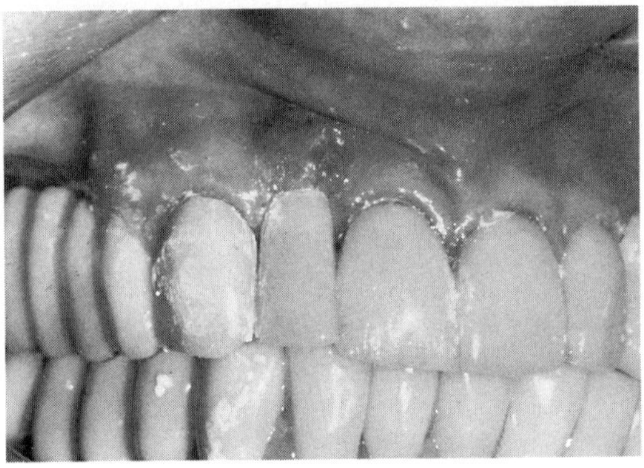

Fig. 19-24c.

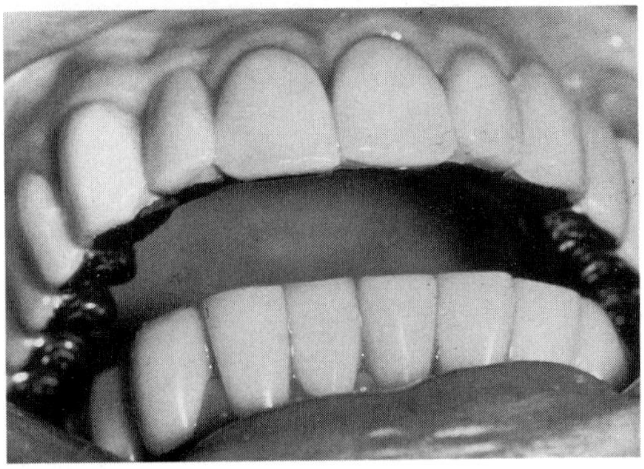

Fig. 19-24d.

Fig. 19-24. (a) Pretreatment view of a *class I ridge defect* in the area of the right lateral incisor. Note the marked concavity in the ridge. (b) This view shows the surgical site 1 week after surgery and prior to the removal of the sutures. (c) The tissue surface of the pontic was relined with autopolymerizing resin. (d) Final prosthesis in place. Note the illusion of a root eminence and a free gingival margin apical to the lateral incisor pontic tooth. (Courtesy of Dr. L. Abrams).

This enables the clinician to shape the soft tissue into a form that is intended for the augmented site. Autopolymerizing resin is added to the tissue surface of the pontics and is allowed to cure until the resin reaches a dough-like state. The bridge is then seated and pressed into the grafted site. When the resin has set to a firm consistency, the bridge is removed and placed in hot water to complete the process of polymerization (Fig. 19-24). The tissue surface of the pontics and the embrasure areas are then carved to the shape that is intended for the definitive bridge. The surface of the pontic is polished and the bridge put in place using an appropriate temporary cement.

Postoperative care

A periodontal dressing is placed over the donor site. No dressing should be placed over the facial (labial) surface of the implanted or grafted area where swelling will occur. *No steps should be taken to avoid swelling.* The dressing at the donor site should be changed at weekly intervals and maintained until wound healing has progressed to a point where the tissue is no longer tender to touch.

A "dead" space has been created in the connective tissue of the pouch and has been intentionally sealed off. It is likely that, during surgery, bacteria from the oral cavity are introduced in the pouch. For this reason an appro-

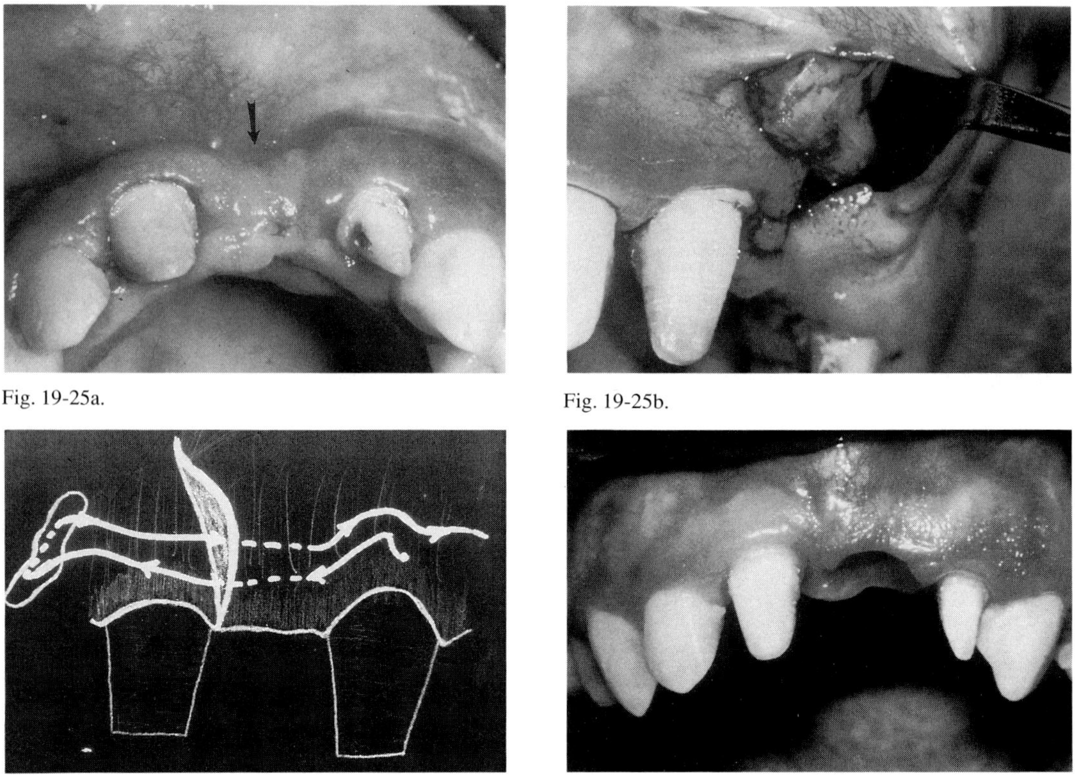

Fig. 19-25a.

Fig. 19-25b.

Fig. 19-25c.

Fig. 19-25d.

Fig. 19-25. (a) Pretreatment view of a *class I ridge defect.* (b) A lateral pouch procedure was used to augment the ridge with connective tissue obtained from the second molar-tuberosity area. (c) Diagram of the method of suturing used to pull the connective tissue into the desired place within the pouch. (d) At 2 months postsurgery, a gingivoplasty procedure was used to accentuate the receptacle site for an ovate pontic. (Courtesy of Dr. D. Garber).

priate prophylactic antibiotic regimen is warranted.

Pouch procedures for free grafts and implants

Surgical concept: Three different varieties of pouch preparation techniques have been designed for free grafts of connective tissue, or implants of bone or bone substitutes. The techniques vary only with respect to *direction of entrance incision* and *plane of dissection* (Langer & Calagna 1980, 1982, Garber & Rosenberg 1981, Kaldahl et al. 1982, Seibert 1983a, Rosenberg et al. 1984, Allen et al. 1985, Miller 1986). The subepithelial pouch is created in the same manner as described for the Roll procedure. A free graft of connective tissue, autogenous bone chips, allograft bone material or bone substitutes (e.g. hydroxylapatite) is placed in the pouch and molded to create the desired contour of the ridge. The entrance incision is closed with sutures.

The *entrance incision* and the *plane of dissection* are made in the following way:

– *coronal-apically:* the horizontal incision is made on the palatal or lingual side of the defect and the plane of dissection carried in an apical direction
– *apical-coronally:* the horizontal entrance incision is made high in the vestibule near the muco-buccal fold and the plane of dissection is carried coronally to the crest of the ridge
– *laterally:* one or two vertical entrance inci-

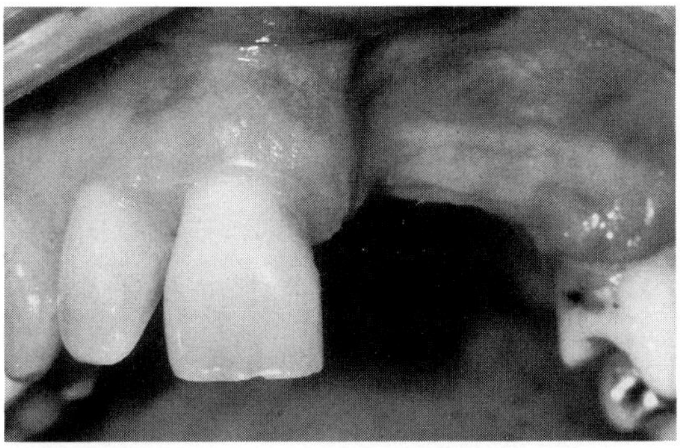

Fig. 19-26a.

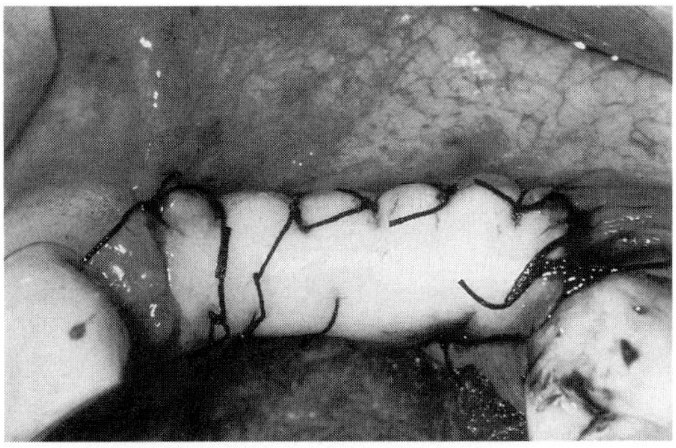

Fig. 19-26b.

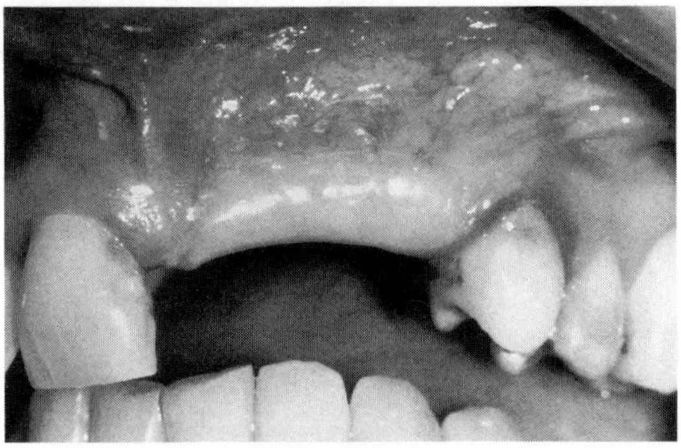

Fig. 19-26c.

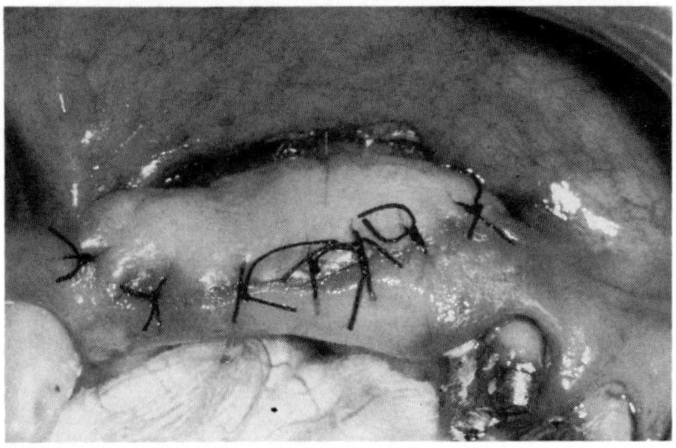

Fig. 19-26d.

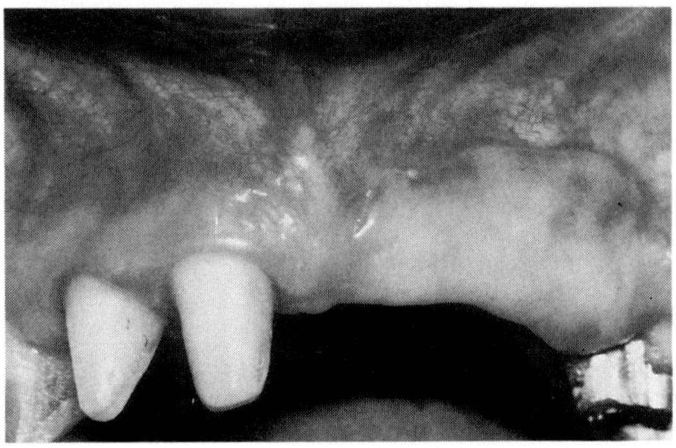

Fig. 19-26e.

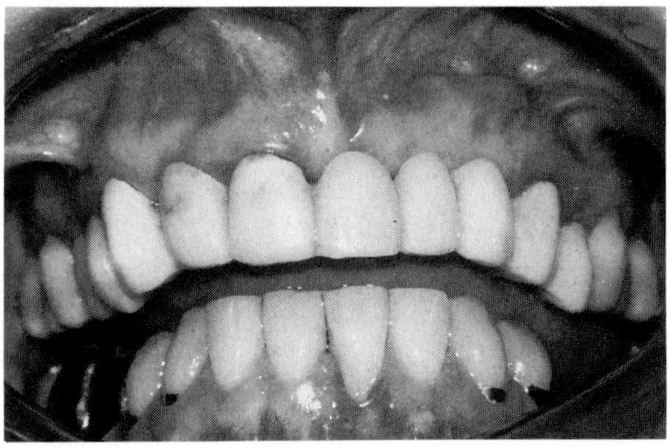

Fig. 19-26f.

Fig. 19-26. (a) Pretreatment view of an extensive *class III ridge defect*. The patient has used a removable prosthesis for many years and wished to have a fixed prosthesis made. (b) First-stage of the soft tissue reconstruction. A large, thick onlay graft was sutured into position. (c) 2 months postsurgery. The onlay graft produced gain in ridge height. A second procedure was performed to augment the ridge further in a buccolingual dimension. (d) A veneer type of free graft was used to gain augmentation in buccolingual direction. (e) Appearance of the reconstructed ridge 2 months after the final grafting procedure. Compare the contour of the healed augmented ridge with that shown in Fig. 19-26A. (f) Provisional prosthesis in place.

sions are started from either side of the defect (Fig. 19-25). The plane of dissection is made laterally across the span of the deformity.

Indication: The techniques are used to correct small, moderate and large size Class I defects. Patients with large volume defects may have thin palatal tissues which are insufficient to se-

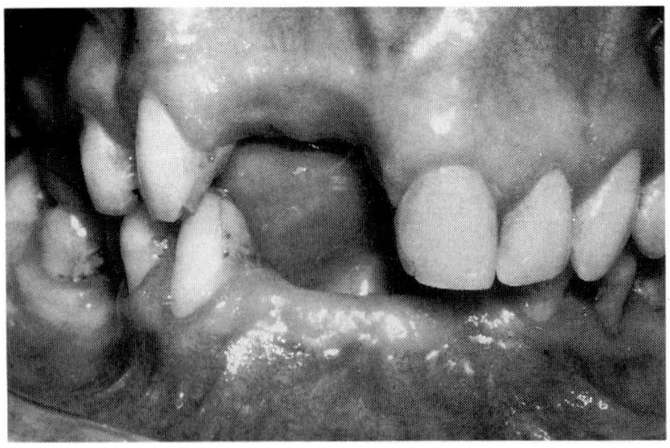

Fig. 19-27a.

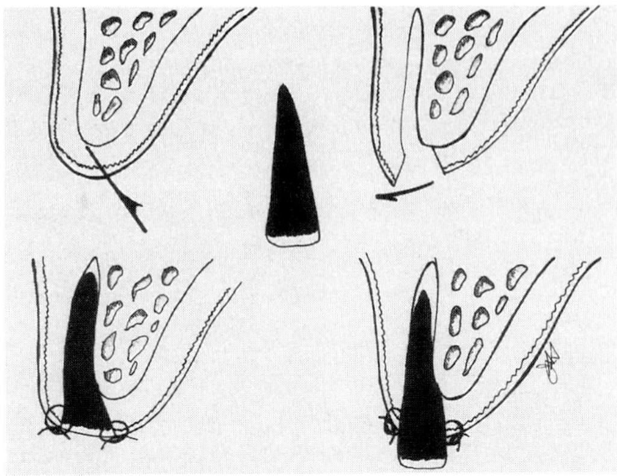

Fig. 19-27b.

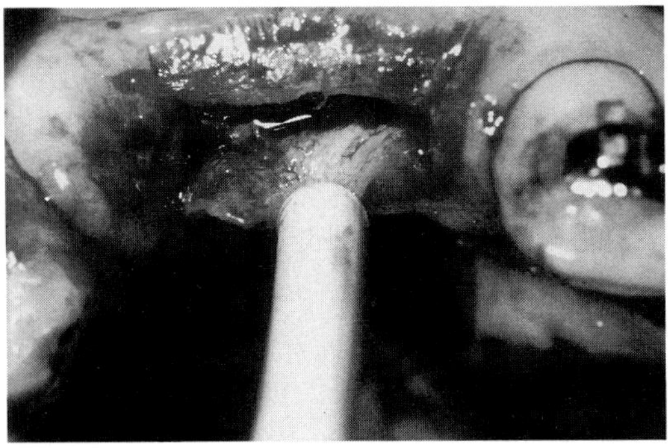

Fig. 19-27c.

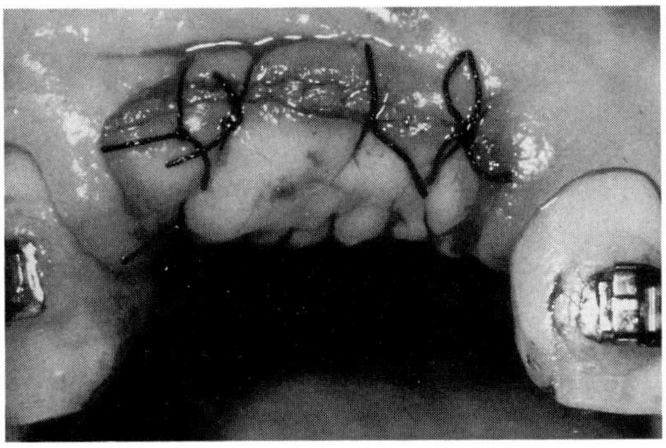

Fig. 19-27d.

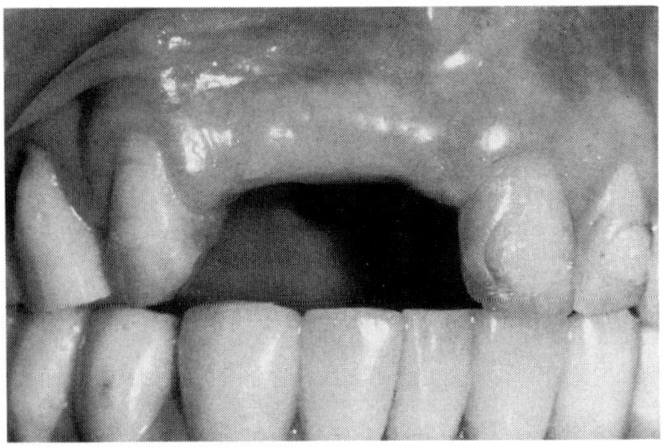

Fig. 19-27e.

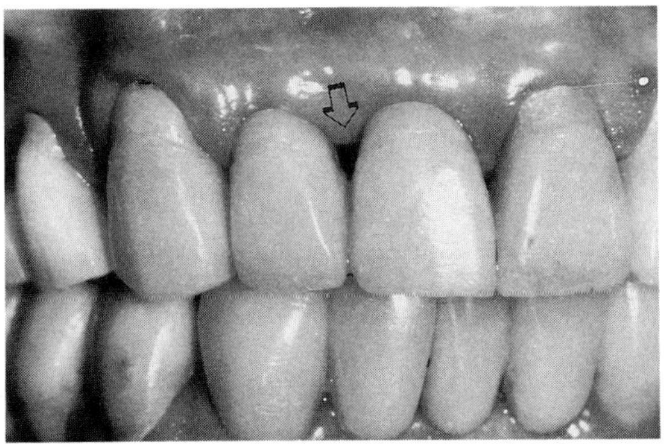

Fig. 19-27f.

Fig. 19-27. *Wedge procedure* in conjunction with second-stage onlay graft. (a) Pretreatment view. The patient had a large class III ridge defect. (b) Sequence of steps in the wedge procedure. A wedge-shaped section of connective tissue with its epithelium was removed from the palate and was inserted between the elevated pouch-like flap and the ridge. (c) The pouch was prepared to receive the wedge (inlay-onlay) graft. (d) The graft was sutured into position. (e-f) 2 months postsurgery. Note the amount of ridge height that was obtained. A second-stage procedure was performed to gain more ridge height and to fill

cure the volume of donor tissue to fill the deformity. Bone grafts or bone substitutes can in such cases aid in restoring ridge contour.

Technique: The pouch is first prepared. If a graft of connective tissue is used to augment the ridge, the plane of dissection should be made above the periosteum. If bone or bone substitutes are used, the periosteum must be raised and the implant material inserted between the periosteum and the bone surface.

,The mesio-distal entrance incision for the

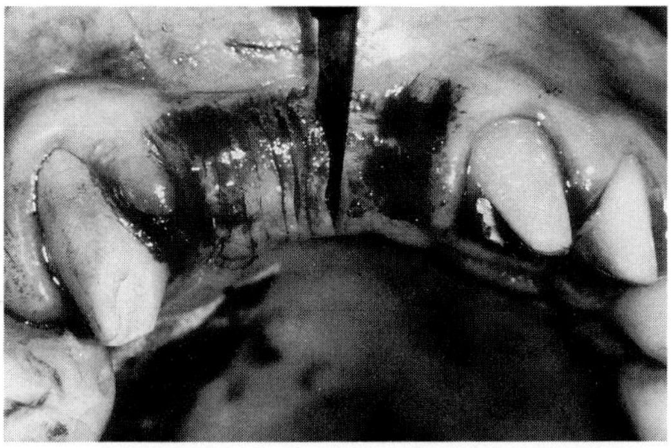

Fig. 19-27g.

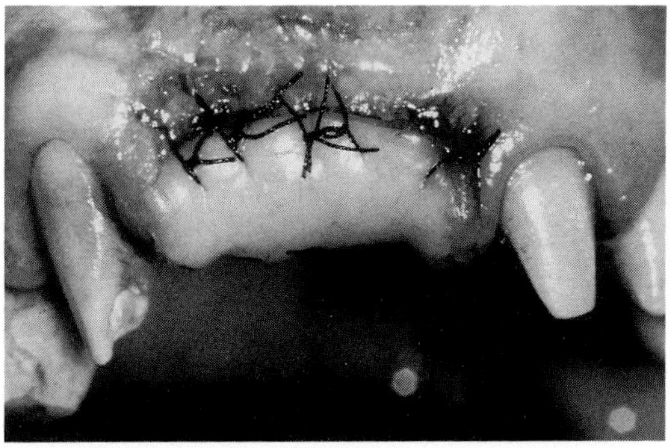

Fig. 19-27h.

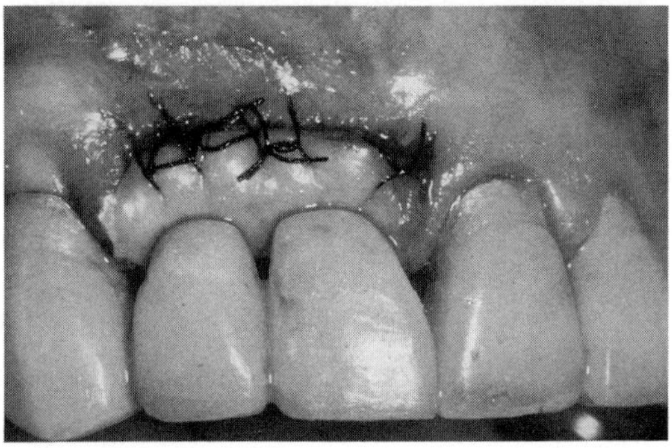

Fig. 19-27i.

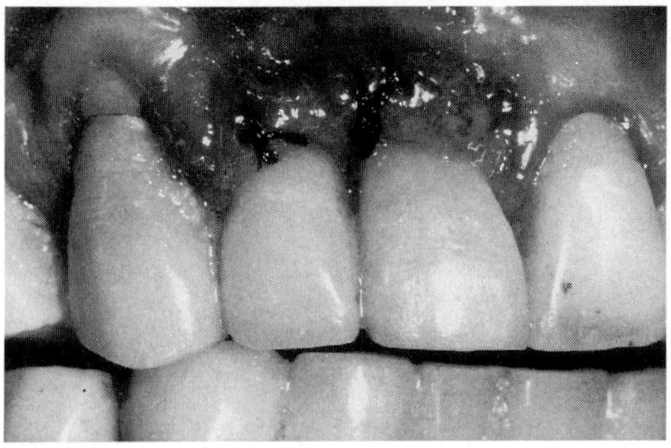

Fig. 19-27j.

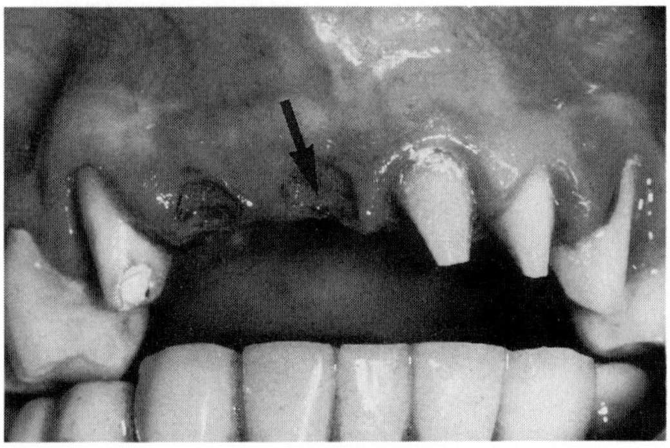

Fig. 19-27k.

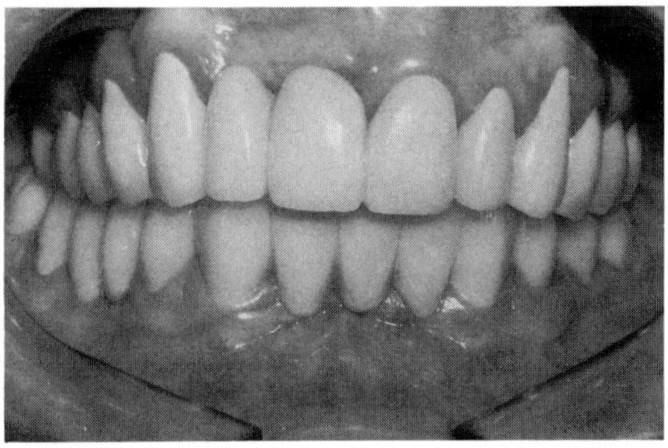

Fig. 19-27l.

in the "dark triangles" between the teeth. (g) 2 months after the first surgical procedure, the ridge was de-epithelialized and cuts were made into the connective tissue prior to placing the second-stage onlay graft into position. (h) The onlay graft was sutured into position. (i) The pontics were adjusted and brought into light contact with the graft. (j) Marked swelling occurred within the graft at 14 days postsurgery. (k) 2 months following the second surgical procedure, a gingivoplasty was performed to deepen the pontic receptacle sites for the ovate pontics. (l) Post-treatment view 1 year after the final surgical procedure.

pouch should be made with a long bevel and must be started well to the palatal (lingual) side of the defect (Fig. 19-27). After the pouch has been filled with graft or implant material, the facial tissue will be stretched. The long bevel of the entrance incision permits the palatal edge of the flap to slide towards the facial surface without opening a gap at the incision line. Sometimes vertical releasing incisions have to be made lateral to the border of the defect. The palatal entrance incision as well as the releasing incisions are closed with sutures.

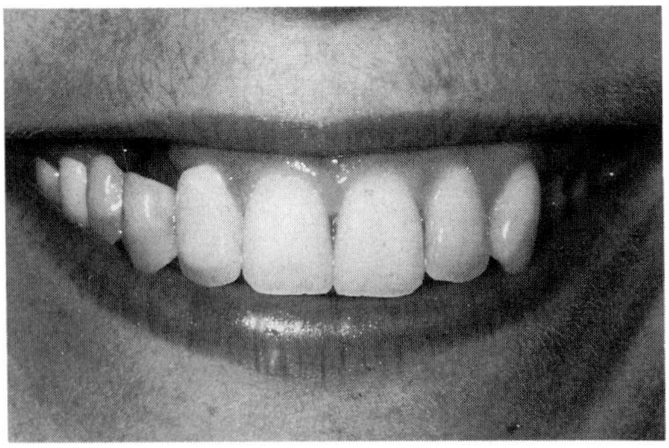

Fig. 19-28a.

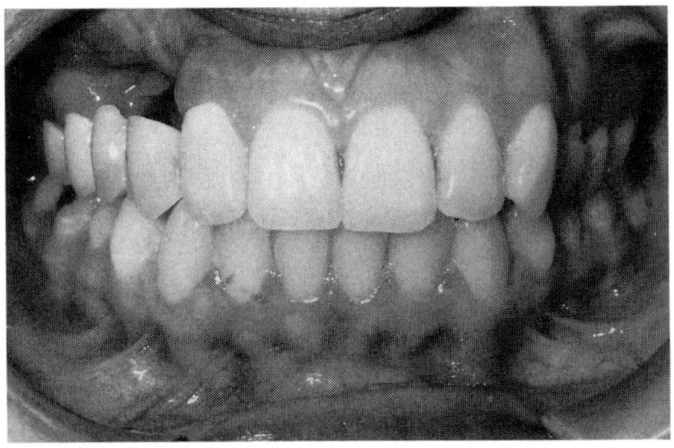

Fig. 19-28b.

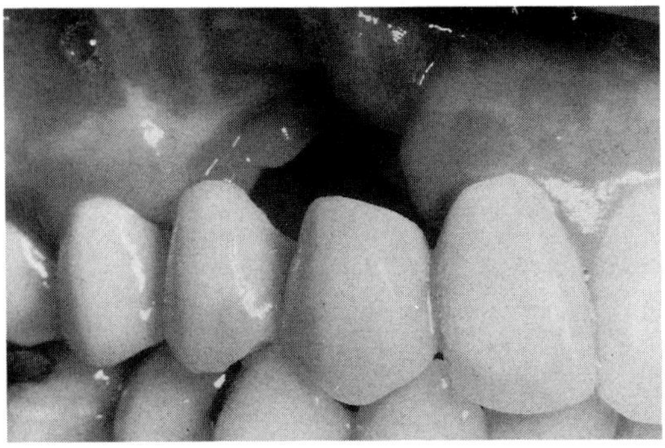

Fig. 19-28c.

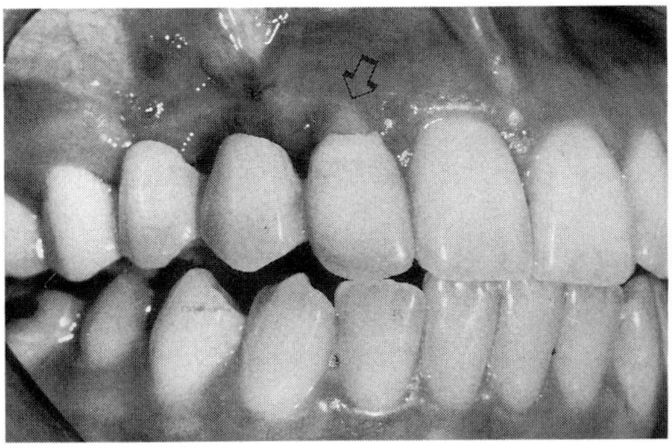

Fig. 19-28d.

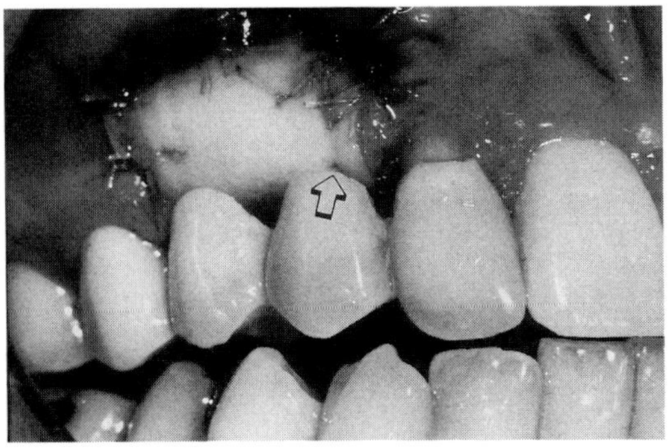

Fig. 19-28e.

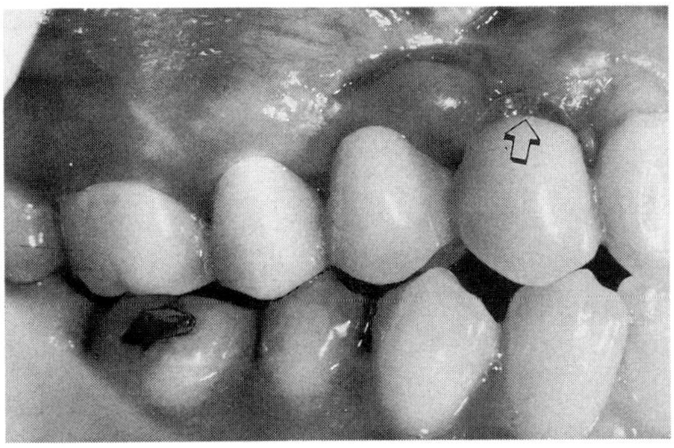

Fig. 19-28f.

Wedge and inlay procedures

Surgical concept: The labial surface of a pouch is first elevated, in a facial direction, the distance required to eliminate the ridge defect. A wedge shaped graft is placed in the pouch to maintain the facial surface of the pouch in the intended position. If augmentation is required not only in the bucco-lingual but also in the apico-coronal direction, a portion of the wedge must be positioned above the surface of the tissue surrounding the recipient site. Thereby a certain amount of the grafted connective tissue will be exposed to the oral cavity.

Indications: Wedge-inlay procedures are used to correct Class I as well as small and moderate Class II defects.

Technique: A pouch is made in the manner previously described, or a proper full or split thickness flap may be prepared at the facial

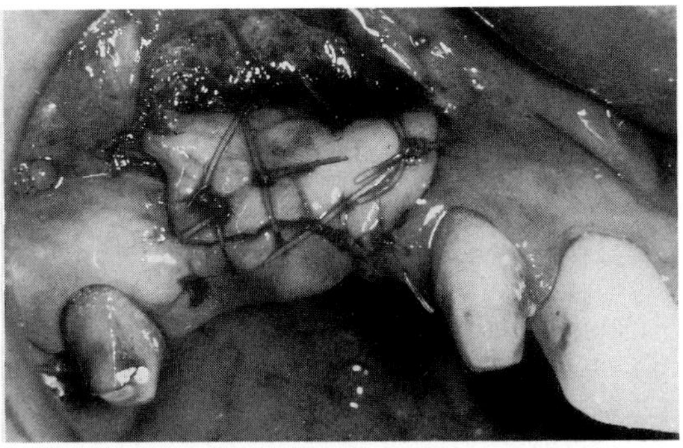

Fig. 19-28g.

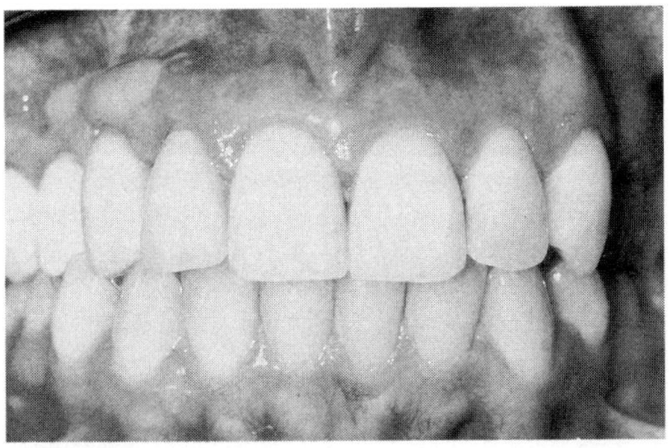

Fig. 19-28h.

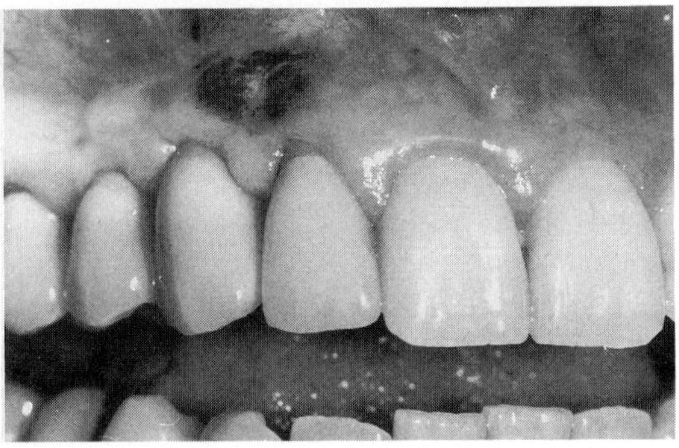

Fig. 19-28i.

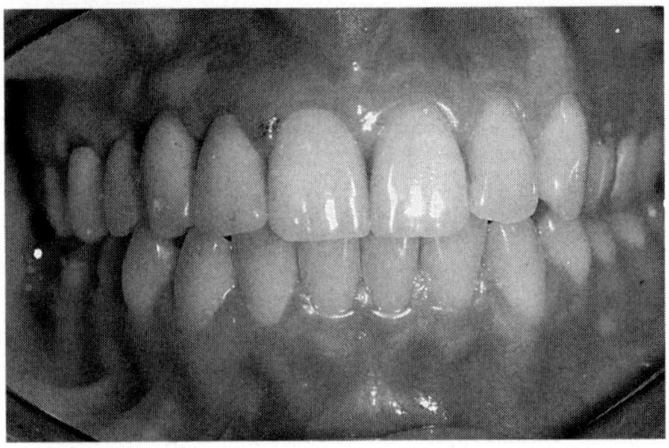

Fig. 19-28j.

Fig. 19-28. (a-c) Pretreatment views. The right first premolar and canine teeth were avulsed in a car accident. (d) An iliac bone graft consisting of 3 cc of hemopoietic marrow was placed via a tunnel procedure into the space of the deformity in the maxilla. At 3 months postsurgery, some amount of ridge augmentation was obtained by the first surgical procedure. The labial flap made for the tunnel procedure produced the recession that can be seen on the lateral incisor. (e) A second-stage onlay graft was performed at 3 months to gain additional ridge height. (f) This view shows the additional ridge augmentation that was achieved. Clear acrylic was added to the tissue facing surface of the canine pontic to bring it into contact with the ridge. (g) 3 months later, another onlay graft procedure was performed to (1) eliminate the scar in the area of the vestibular fornix and (2) create the illusion of a root eminence above the canine pontic. (h-i) These views show the final prosthesis in place and the overall amount of ridge augmentation that was obtained. Note that the pontic teeth have the same length as the teeth on the contralateral side of the arch. A gingivoplasty was performed at this visit to eliminate the "crease" in the tissue mesial to the "canine eminence". (j) This view shows the topography of the augmented ridge 17 months after the last onlay graft procedure. Restoration by Dr. Abraham Ingber.

surface of the defect area (Fig. 19-27). The provisional bridge is placed in position to serve as a reference when estimates are made regarding the amount of tissue that has to be grafted to fill the defect. A periodontal probe may be used to measure the length, width and depth of the void of the pouch. A suitable donor site is selected - in the palate, the tuberosity area, or in an edentulous area - and a free graft of epithelium-connective tissue is excised. *Selection of donor site, surgical care and wound healing will be discussed in a subsequent section of this chapter.*

The donor tissue is transferred to the recipient site and placed in position. If gain in ridge height is not intended, the epithelial surface of the graft is placed flush with the surrounding epithelium. The graft is sutured along its entire circumference to the tissues of the recipient site.

The provisional bridge is once again placed in position and the pontics are trimmed and ad-

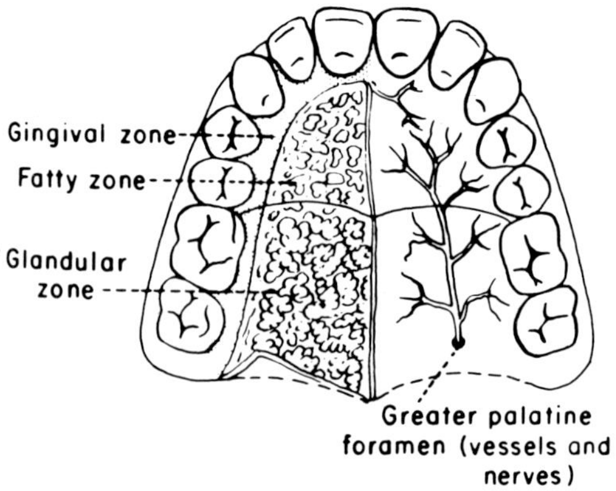

Fig. 19-29. Basic anatomical - histological zones of the palate. Note the normal location of the greater palatine foramen.

justed as discussed above. No dressing is used to cover the recipient site.

If gain also in ridge height is intended a certain portion of the graft has to be kept above the surface of the surrounding tissue (Fig. 19-27). Granulation tissue formed during healing will eventually make the border between the graft and the adjacent tissue smooth and properly epithelialized. The swelling which occurs postoperatively will, as discussed above, assist in sculpting the contour of the ridge.

Onlay graft procedures

Surgical concept: The onlay procedure was designed to augment ridge defects in the apico-coronal plane, i.e. to gain ridge height (Seibert 1980, 1983a). Onlay grafts are full thickness free gingivial grafts which, following placement, receive their nutrition from the deepithelialized connective tissue of the recipient site. The amount of apico-coronal augmentation that can be obtained is related to the initial thickness of the graft, the events of the wound healing process and the amount of graft tissue that survives (Figs. 19-26, 19-27, 19-28). The grafting procedure can be repeated at 2-month intervals to gradually increase the ridge height.

Indications: Onlay-graft procedures are used in the treatment of large Class II and III defects. They are not well suited in areas where the blood supply at the recipient site has been compromised by scar tissue formation from previous wound healing.

Technique: An attempt must be made to retain as much as possible of the lamina propria of the recipient site. The anesthetic solution should be placed high in the vestibular fornix and in the palate, thus keeping vasoconstriction in the recipient site to a minimum. A scalpel blade is used to remove the epithelium. The scalpel is moved with short, sawlike strokes across the recipient site at a level approximately 1 mm below the outer surface of the epithelium. The *least amount of connective tissue* possible should be excised. The margins of the recipient site can be prepared with either a butt-joint or a beveled margin. The prepared recipient site should be covered with a surgical gauze moistened with isotonic saline while the donor tissue is dissected.

A series of parallel cuts (striations) may be made deep into the exposed lamina propria of the recipient site to sever large blood vessels (Fig. 19-27). The striations are made 1 mm apart and perpendicular to the surface of the ridge. It is believed that this tissue injury stimulates blood vessels to heal with extensive capillary loop formations which protrude into the graft. A hematoma-like reaction occurs, the graft tissues swell and adapt to the surface contours of the temporary bridge. The swelling phenomenon is illustrated in Fig. 19-27. It should be emphasized that striations of this kind must only be made in areas of the recipient site which are supported by bone.

During healing most of the connective tissue of the graft appears to survive while the original epithelial surface is lost. It is sometimes observed that the volume of the graft has increased during healing. The reason for this addition of tissue volume is presently unknown.

Selection of donor site

Wedge procedures, inlay-onlay procedures and onlay graft procedures require large amounts of donor tissue. The palatal vault region of premolars and first molars, midway between the gingival margin and the midline raphae is, as a general rule, the only area in the maxilla that contains the necessary volume of tissue required to augment large size ridge defects. During the presurgical planning phase the tissue of the palate should be probed with a 30-gauge syringe needle to ensure that an acceptable volume of tissue can be obtained at the time of surgery.

The major palatine artery emerges from the palatine foramen located adjacent to the distal surface of the maxillary second molar, midway between the gingival margin and the midline raphae (Fig. 19-29). The artery passes in an anterior direction close to the surface of the palatal bone. It is important therefore that the second and third molar regions are *not used* as donor sites for large volume grafts.

Planning the graft preparation

A periodontal probe can be used to measure the length and width of donor tissue required for the recipient site. As a rule the graft should be made a few mm wider and longer than the dimensions required at the recipient site. The dimensions of the graft are outlined on the palate with the use of a scalpel and light bleeding is provoked to define the surface borders. In order to avoid interference with the palatine artery, the borders of the graft must be planned in such a way that its thinner portions are located high in the palatal vault or in the first molar area. The thicker portions should be harvested from the premolar areas. If during graft preparation the palatine artery or one of its major branches is severed, a deep suture must be passed around the segment of the artery that remains anterior to the foramen. Bleeding will hereby be arrested.

Dissection of donor tissue

The base of the graft should be V- or U-shaped to match the shape of the defect in the ridge. The different planes of incision prepared in the palate must therefore converge towards an area under the center or towards one edge of the donor site. It is comparatively easy, with the use of a scalpel, to dissect in an antero-posterior or from an area high in the palate in a lateral direction towards the teeth. It is, however, difficult to dissect in an anterior direction from the distal edge of the donor site. There are a variety of blade holders available which permit the scalpel blade to be positioned at different angles to the holder and which enable the surgeon to cut with a back-action.

When the donor tissue has been removed, it must at all times be stored in pieces of surgical gauze moistened with isotonic saline.

Treatment of the donor site

Since it difficult to anchor and maintain a periodontal dressing at the donor site in the palatal vault, an acrylic stent should be fabricated prior to surgery. The stent should be made with wrought wire clasps on each side to add retention and to aid the patient in removing and inserting the device.

The donor site must be inspected carefully for signs of arterial bleeding. If any small-vessel bleeding is observed, a circumferential suture must be placed around the vessel distal to the bleeding point. Immediately thereafter, the void at the donor site should be packed with a suitable hemostatic agent and the edges of the wound be brought closer together with sutures. The stent is then put in position.

It usually requires 20-30 minutes to suture the graft in position and to adjust the provisional bridge. This time is almost always sufficient to allow for proper hemorrhage control at the donor site and to avoid problems with postoperative bleeding. The patient is instructed to leave the stent in position for 2-3 days before proper plaque control measures can be initiated.

Wound healing in the donor site

Granulation tissue will gradually fill the donor site. Initial healing is usually complete within 2-3 weeks after the removal of a 4- to 5-mm thick graft. Patients should wear the surgical stent for about 2 weeks to protect the healing wound. After the 3rd day of wound healing, the stent can be removed for oral hygiene measures. The palate returns to its presurgical contour after about 3 months.

Try-in and stabilization of graft

The graft is transferred with tissue forceps to the recipient site for a try-in. The graft is trimmed to the proper shape and adjusted to fit the connective tissue surface of the prepared ridge, whereupon it is returned for temporary storage. Final preparations are made for suturing. *It is at this stage that striations are made in the connective tissue of the recipient site.* For orientation purposes a *tacking* suture is placed in two corners along one border of the onlay graft. A series of interrupted sutures is placed along this border. The dental assistant should stabilize the onlay graft against the surface of the recipient site, while the surgeon completes the placement of sutures along the borders of the graft (Figs. 19-26, 19-27, 19-28). The sutures should not be placed too close to the borders of the recipient tissue and the graft.

Wound healing in the recipient site

Considerable postoperative swelling often occurs during the 1st week after pouch, wedge, inlay-onlay and onlay augmentation procedures. The epithelium of the graft will slough during the 1st week of healing. The epithelial cells, together with fibrin, form a *white film* on the surface of the graft. Patients must be informed that 1) it is normal for the augmented area to pass through a *white stage* of 4- to 7-days duration, 2) they should rinse 2-4 times per day with an antimicrobial mouthwash during this period but 3) refrain from mechanical cleaning measures until a new epithelial covering has formed over the graft.

Epithelium will not cover the grafted tissue until a functional capillary circulation has been reestablished. During the 2nd and 3rd week after surgery, therefore, the graft will pass through its *red stage*.

The grafted tissue assumes a normal color as epithelialization is completed and the epithelium thickens via stratification. The graft gradually reverts to its original volume - or remains slightly larger - as the swelling subsides. Tissue form is usually stable after 2 months, but some shrinkage may occur between the 2nd and 4th months after surgery. Final restorative measures should not be initiated until after 4-6 months.

Refinement of pontic contours

When the tissues of the augmented ridge have adapted to their final shape, minor adjustments may be made at the tissue surface of the pontics as well as in the soft tissue ridge. The adjustments are made to shape and refine the *emergence profile* of the pontics from the edentulous ridge. Hereby an illusion is created that the pontic teeth are contained within the corpus of the ridge rather than resting on its surface.

The tissue surfaces of *ridge lap pontics* are rebased with autopolymerizing resin to 1) obtain proper contact with the ridge and 2) refine the shape of the cervical area. If *ovate pontics* are used, *gingivoplasty* is often performed to deepen the indentations or the *receptacle socket sites*, which were initially shaped as the soft tissues healed against the pontics of the provisional bridge (Garber & Rosenberg 1981). *Gingivoplasty* is often performed with the use of *tissue sculpting diamond stones* fitted in an ultraspeed handpiece (Figs. 19-22, 19-25, 19-27). The tissue surface of the *ovate pontics* are immediately thereafter rebased with resin.

This final tissue sculpting procedure is minor

but aids greatly in defining the shape of the papillae and creating the illusion of the presence of a cuff of *free gingiva* at the pontic/ridge interface.

References

Abrams, L. (1980a) Augmentation of the deformed residual edentulous ridge for fixed prosthesis. *The Compendium of Continuing Education in General Dentistry* **1**(3), 205-214.

Abrams, L. (1980b) Pontic classification. Personal communication.

Abrams, L. (1987) Preventing esthetic failures in clinical practice. Presentation, D. Walter Cohen Periodontal Symposium, University of Pennsylvania, Philadelphia.

Allen, E.P., Gainza, C.S., Farthing, G.G., et al. (1985) Improved technique for localized ridge augmentation. *Journal of Periodontology* **56**, 195.

Antrim, D.D. (1981) Vertical extrusion of endodontically treated teeth. *U.S. Navy Medicine* **72**(9), 23-28.

Bernimoulin, J.P., Luscher, B. & Muhlemann, H.R. (1975) Coronally repositioned periodontal flap. *Journal of Clinical Peridontology* **2**, 1.

Brown, S.I. (1973) The effect of orthodontic therapy on certain types of periodontal defects. I. - Clinical findings. *Journal of Periodontology* **44**, 742-756.

Corn, H. (1980) Reconstructive mucogingival surgery, in Goldman, H.M., Cohen, D.W. (eds): *Periodontal Therapy*, 6th edn. St. Louis: the C.V. Mosby Co., pp. 914-922.

Corn, H. & Marks, M. (1983a) Gingival grafting for deep-wide recession - A status report. Part I. Rationale, Case selection, and root preparation. *The Compendium of Continuing Education in General Dentistry* **IV** (No. 1), 53-66.

Corn, H. & Marks, M. (1983b) Gingival grafting for deep-wide recession - A status report. Part II. Surgical Procedures. *The Compendium of Continuing Education in General Dentistry* **IV** (No. 2), 167-182.

Evian, C., Corn, H. & Rosenberg, E. (1985) Retained interdental papilla procedure for maintaining anterior esthetics. *The Compendium of Continuing Education in General Dentistry* **IV** (No. 1), 58-65.

Garber, D.A. (1987) *Periodontal esthetics problem solving - unique problems require unique solutions*. Presentation, D. Walter Cohen Periodontal Symposium, University of Pennsylvania, Philadeplhia.

Garber, D.A. & Rosenberg, E.S. (1981) The edentulous ridge in fixed prosthodontics. *The Compendium of Continuing Education in General Dentistry* **2**, 212-224.

Goldstein, R.E. (1984) *Change Your Smile*. Chicago: Qiuntessence Publishing Company.

Grupe, H.E. & Warren, R.F. (1956) Repair of gingival defects by a sliding flap operation. *Journal of Periodontology* **27**, 290.

Guilford, H.J., Gruble, T.A. & Pence, D.L. (1984) Vertical extrusion: A standardize technique. *The Compendium of Continuing Education in General Dentistry* **V** (No. 7): 562-568.

Guinard, E.A. & Caffesse, R.G. (1978) Treatment of localised gingival recessions. Part III. Comparison of results obtained with lateral sliding and coronally repositioned flaps. *Journal of Periodontology* **49**, 457.

Harvey, P.M. (1956) Management of advanced periodontitis. I. Preliminary report of a method of surgical reconstruction. *New Zealand Dental Journal* **61**, 180.

Harvey, P.M. (1970) Surgical reconstruction of the gingiva. II Procedures. *New Zealand Dental Journal* **66**, 42.

Heithersay, G.S. (1973) Combined endodontic-orthodontic treatment of transverse root fractures in the region of the alveolar crest. *Oral Surgery* **36**, 404-415.

Holbrook, T. & Ochsenbein, C. (1982) Root Coverage. Presented to Continuing Education Program, University of Pensylvania School of Dental Medicine, Philadelphia, May 20.

Ingber, J.S. (1974) Forced eruption: Part I. A method of treating isolated one and two wall infrabony osseous defects - Rationale and case report. *Journal of Periodontology* **45**, 199-206.

Ingber, J.S. (1976) Forced eruption: Part II. A method of treating non-restorable teeth - periodontal and restorative considerations. *Journal of Periodontology* **47**, 203-216.

Kaldahl, W.B., Tussing, G.J., Went, F.M., et al. (1982) Achieving an esthetic appearance with a fixed prosthesis by submucosal grafts. *Journal of the American Dental Association* **104**, 449-452.

Langer, B. & Calagna, L. (1980) The subepithelial connective tissue graft. *Journal of Prosthetic Dentistry* **44**, 363-367.

Langer, B. & Calagna, L. (1982) The subepithelial connective tissue graft: A new approach to the enhancement of anterior cosmetics. *International*

Journal of Periodontics and Restorative Dentistry **2**, 22-23.

Livingston, H.L. (1975) Total coverage of multiple and adjacent denuded root surfaces with a free gingival autograph - A case report. *Journal of Periodontology* **46**, 209-220.

Lythgoe, J.R., Torabinejad, M. & Simon, J.H.S. (1980) Extrusion techniques for the general dentist. *General Dentistry* **28**, 42.

Matter, J. (1979) Free gingival graft and coronally repositioned flap. *Journal of Clinical Periodontology* **6**, 437.

Maynard, J.G. Jr. (1977) Coronal positioning of a previously placed autogenous gingival graft. *Journal of Periodontology* **48**, 151.

McHenry, K., Smutko, G. & McMullen, J.A. (1982) Restructuring the topography of the mandibular ridge with gingival autographs. *Journal of the American Dental Association* **104**, 478.

Meltzer, J.A. (1979) Edentulous area tissue graft correction of an esthetic defect. A case report. *Journal of Periodontology* **50**, 320-322.

Miller, P.D. Jr. (1982) Root coverage using a free soft tissue autograph following citric acid application, Part I: Technique. *International Journal of Periodontology and Restorative Dentistry* **1**, 65-70.

Miller, P.D. Jr. (1986) Ridge augmentation under existing fixed prosthesis: Simplified technique. *Journal of Periodontology* **57**, 742.

Miller, P.D. Jr. (1987) Root coverage with the free gingival graft - Factors associated with incomplete coverage. *Journal of Periodontology* **58**, 674-681.

Mlinek, A., Smukler, H. & Buchner, A. (1973) The use of free gingival grafts for the coverage of denuded roots. *Journal of Periodontology* **44**, 248.

Nabers, J.M. (1966) Free gingival grafts. *Periodontics* **4**, 243.

Pontoriero, R., Celenza, F., Jr., Ricci, G. & Carnevale, M. (1987) Rapid extrusion with fiber resection: A combined orthodontic-periodontic treatment modality. *The International Journal of Periodontics & Restorative Dentistry* **5**, 30-43.

Potashnick, S.R. & Rosenberg, E.S. (1982) Forced eruption: Principles in periodontics and restorative dentistry. *Journal of Prosthetic Dentistry* **48**(2), 141-148.

Reitan, K. (1967) Clinical and histologic observations on tooth movement during and after orthodontic treatment. *American Journal of Orthodontics* **53**, 721-745.

Restrepo, O.J. (1973) Coronally repositioned flap - report of four cases. *Journal of Periodontology* **44**, 564.

Rosenberg, E.S., Garber, D.A. & Evian, C.I. (1980) Tooth lengthening procedures. *The Compendium of Continuing Education in General Dentistry* **I** (No. 3): 161-173.

Rosenberg, S., Greenberg, J. & Cucharale, N. (1984) Use of ceramic material for augmentation of the partially edentulous ridge: A case report. *The Compendium of Continuing Education in General Dentistry* **V**, 279-284.

Ruben, M.P., Goldman, H.M. & Janson, W.A. (1976) Biological considerations fundamental to successful employment of laterally repositioned pedicle flaps and free autogenous gingival grafts in periodontal therapy, in Stahl, S.S. (ed): *Periodontal Surgery - Biologic Basis and Technique*. Springfield, IL: Charles C. Thomas, pp. 235-282.

Seibert, J.S. (1980) Soft tissue grafts in periodontics, in Robinson, P.J., Guernsey, L.H. (eds): *Clinical Transplantation in Dental Specialities*. St. Louis: C.V. Mosby Co., pp. 107-145.

Seibert, J.S. (1983a) Reconstruction of deformed, partially edentulous ridges, using full thickness onlay grafts: I. Technique and wound healing. *The Compendium of Continuing Education in General Dentistry* **4**(5), 437-453.

Seibert, J.S. (1983b) Reconstruction of deformed, partially edentulous ridges, using full thickness onlay grafts: II. Prosthetic/periodontal interrelationships. *The Compendium of Continuing Education in General Dentistry* **4**(6), 549-562.

Seibert, J.S. & Cohen, D.W. (1987) Periodontal considerations in preparation for fixed and removable prosthodontics, in Full Mouth Reconstruction: Fixed Removable. *Dental Clinics of North America* (July) **31**, 529-555.

Simon, J.H.S., Kelly, W.H., Gordon, D.G. & Ericksen, G.W. (1978) Extrusion of endodontically treated teeth. *Journal of the American Dental Association* **97**, 17-23.

Soehren, S.E., Allen, A.L., Cutright, D.E. & Seibert, J.S. (1973) Clinical and histologic studies of donor tissues utilized for free grafts of masticatory mucosa. *Journal of Periodontology* **44**, 727.

Sullivan, H.C., Carmen, D. & Dinner, D. (1971a) Histologic evaluation of the laterally positioned flap. Abstract no. 467, I.A.D.R. Program and Abstract of Papers, p. 169.

Sullivan, H.C., Dinner, D. & Carman, D. (1971b) Clinical evaluation of the laterally positioned flap. Abstract no. 466, I.A.D.R. Program and Abstract of Papers, p. 169.

Tjan, A.H., Miller, G.D. & The, H.G. (1984) Some esthetic factors in a smile. *Journal of Prosthetic Dentistry* **51**, 24-28.

CHAPTER 20

Treatment of Furcation-Involved Teeth

Objectives

Studies on humans and laboratory animals have documented the decisive role played by the bacterial plaque in the etiology of gingivitis and destructive periodontal disease. Consequently, therapeutic measures aimed at eliminating gingival inflammation and arresting progression of periodontal tissue breakdown must include the careful removal of the microbial deposits from the tooth surfaces and the establishment of a home-care program which prevents recurrence of gross amounts of plaque and calculus (for reviews see Hamp 1973, Rosling 1976, Badersten 1984, Westfelt 1984).

Treatment of advanced forms of periodontal disease frequently includes surgical procedures. The objectives of these procedures are (see also Chapter 13):

1. to obtain visibility and access to the root surfaces for proper professional debridement
2. to eliminate the pathologically deepened pockets
3. to establish a morphology in the dento-gingival region which facilitates proper, self-performed tooth cleaning.

The third of these objectives is particularly valid in the treatment of periodontal disease around multirooted teeth when the destruction of the supporting tissues has involved the furcation areas. The elimination of pathologically deepened pockets and the establishment of a morphology in the furcation areas which facilitates self-performed plaque control measures require elaborate therapeutic techniques, since progressive loss of attachment and bone resorption in such sites proceed not only in the apical direction along the root surfaces but also in the horizontal direction in between the roots.

Anatomical characteristics

The anatomy of the roots and the topography of the alveolar bone in the furcation areas of multirooted teeth in a periodontal patient can

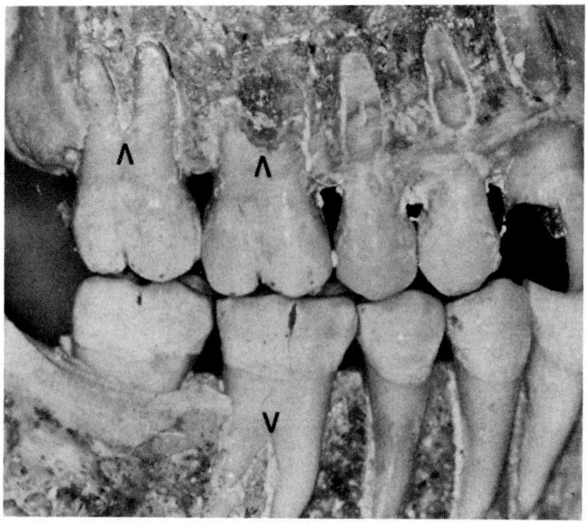

Fig. 20-1a. Autopsy showing the right maxillary and mandibular tooth areas after removal of the buccal cortical bone. The buccal entrance of the furca of three molars is marked with arrows.

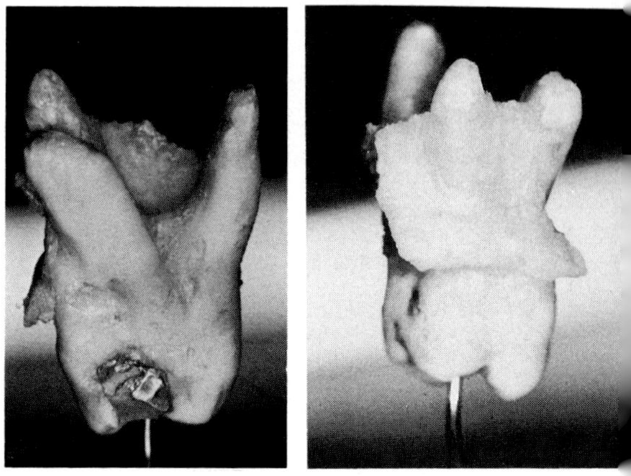

Figs. 20-1b,c. Photographs demonstrating a maxillary first molar with buccally angulated buccal roots (b). The thin bone plate covering the buccal roots can be seen in (c).

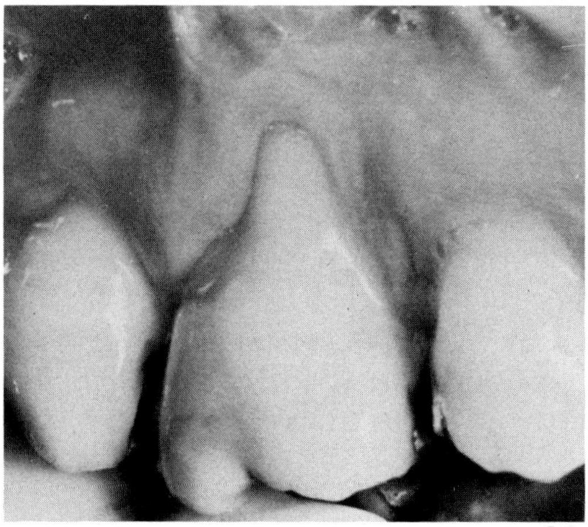

Fig. 20-1d. Dehischence in combination with gingival recession at the mesiobuccal root of a maxillary first molar.

be best examined if a mucoperiosteal flap is elevated. Since a surgical approach for diagnostic purposes is only occasionally adopted, detailed knowledge regarding the anatomy of the root system of different teeth as well as the natural progress of periodontal disease in such sites is a fundamental prerequisite for the proper interpretation of data obtained by clinical probing and radiographic examination.

General information regarding the anatomy of the furcation areas of multirooted teeth may be gained from *autopsy material*. If the buccal bone plates are removed from an autopsy preparation the buccal furcas are exposed (arrows; Fig. 20-1a) as well as the location of the furcas in relation to the cementoenamel junctions. The position and spread of the roots of the maxillary molars often give rise to a large area of interradicular supporting bone (Fig. 20-1b). A thin buccal bone plate is sometimes associated with the presence of fenestrations (Fig. 20-1c) and/or dehiscences in combination with gingival recessions (Fig. 20-1d).

The position and anatomy of the various roots of maxillary and mandibular posterior teeth can also be illustrated in cross-sections of the jaws. Figs. 20-2a and b are schematic drawings from such cross sections prepared at a distance of a few mm apical to the cementoenamel junction.

In Fig. 20-2a the roots of the *maxillary* second premolar (P2) and the maxillary molars (M1, M2 and M3) are identified as well as the buccal and palatal bone plates. From this drawing it becomes obvious that the mesiobuccal roots of the first and second molars are comparatively wide in the buccopalatal direction, while the distobuccal roots are of considerably smaller dimension. The palatal roots are often wider in the mesiodistal than in the buccopala-

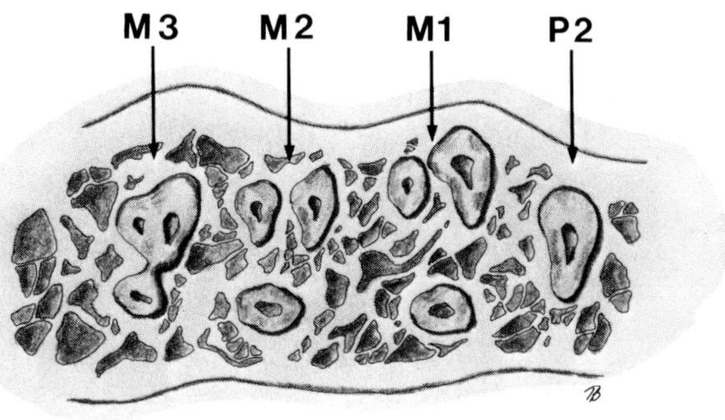

Fig. 20-2a.

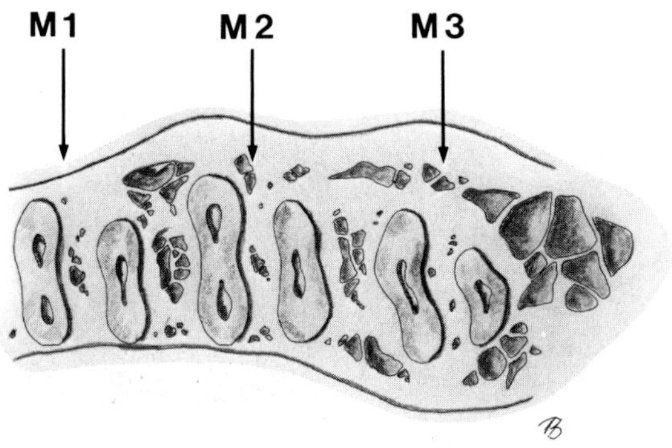

Fig. 20-2b.

Figs. 20-2a,b. Schematic illustrations depicting some important anatomical characteristics of the maxillary (a) and the mandibular (b) molar areas in a cross-sectional view a few millimeters apical to the furcas of the molars. Observe the position of the roots in relation to the facial cortical bone plates.

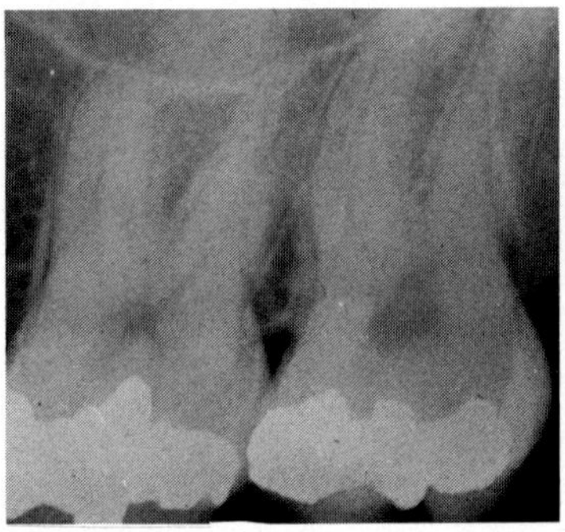

Fig. 20-3a.

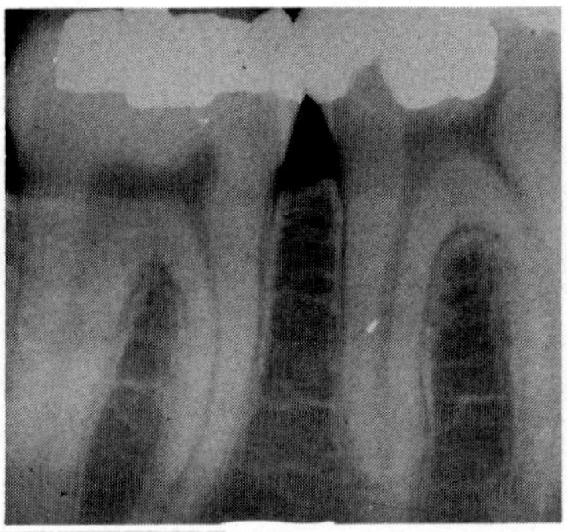

Fig. 20-3b.

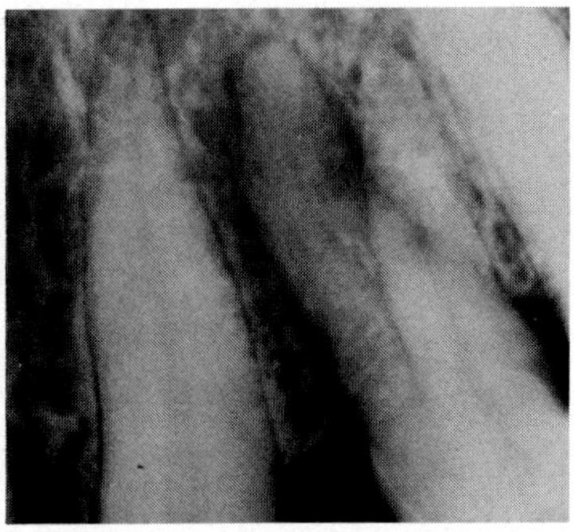

Fig. 20-3c.

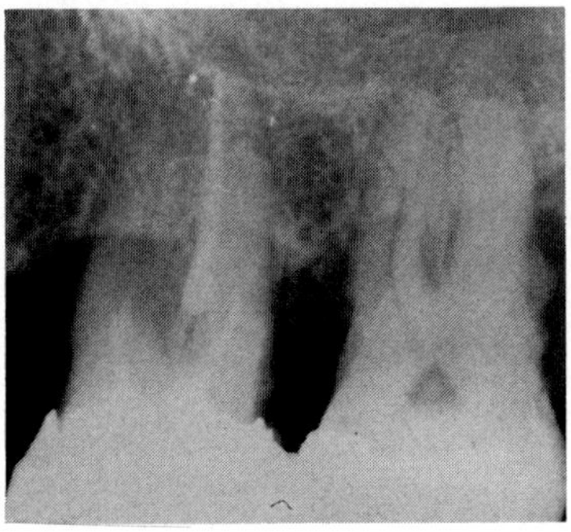

Fig. 20-3d.

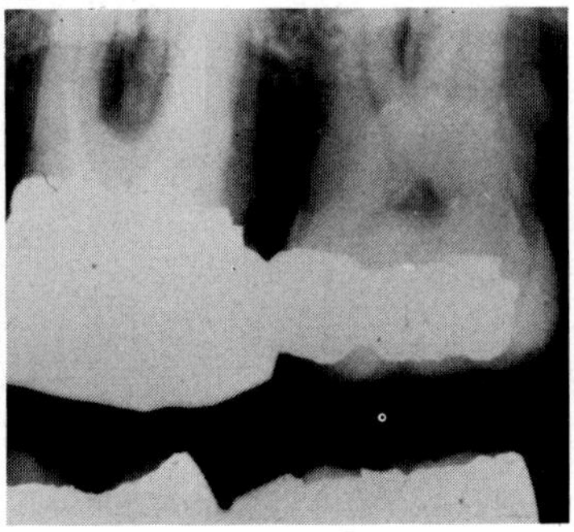

Fig. 20-3e.

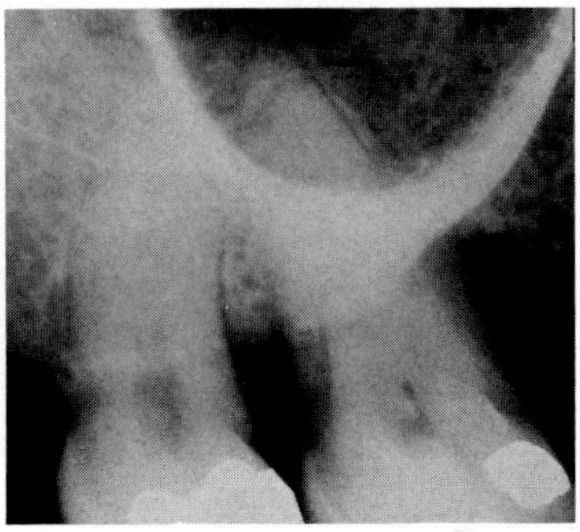

Fig. 20-3f.

Figs. 20-3a-f. Radiographs of furcation areas in health (a,b) and disease (c-f). Note the difficulties in diagnosing the presence of furcation involvements due to superimposition of surrounding hard tissues.

tal direction. The oval-shaped mesiobuccal roots often have marked invaginations while the distobuccal roots generally have a more rounded outline and less frequently exhibit distinct invaginations.

In Fig. 20-2b the roots of the *mandibular* molars can be identified. Note the differences in the anatomy between the mesial and distal roots. The mesial roots are normally wider in the buccolingual direction than the distal roots

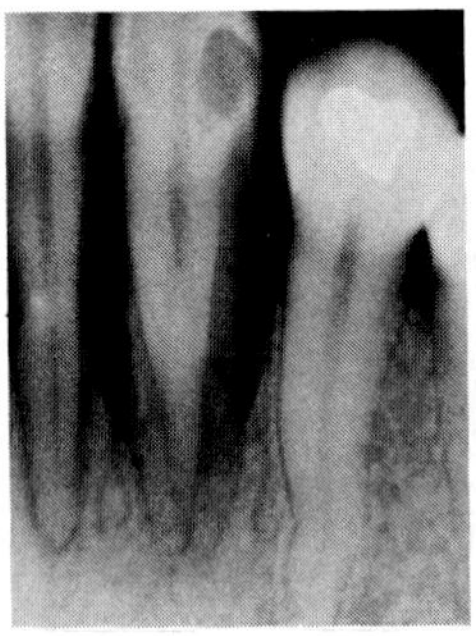

Fig. 20-4a.

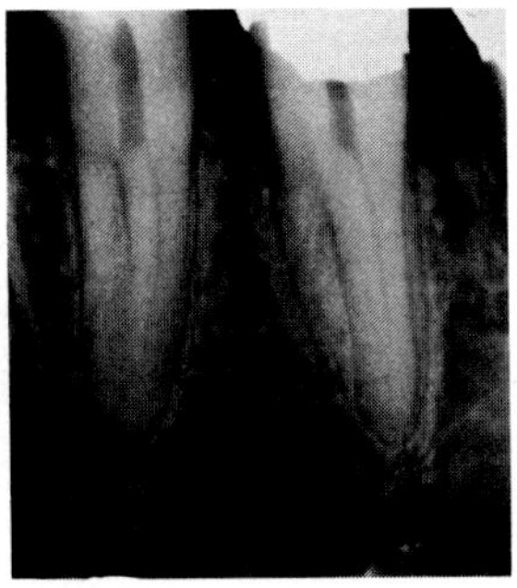

Fig. 20-4b.

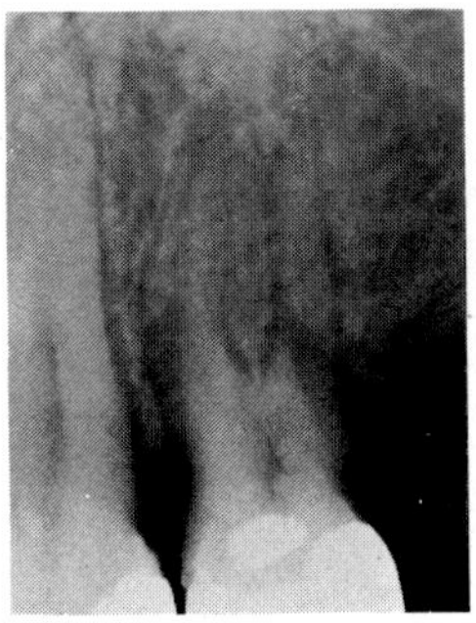

Fig. 20-4c.

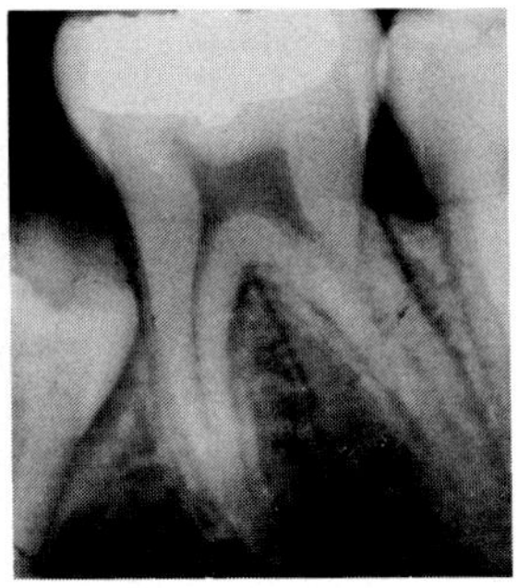

Fig. 20-4d.

Figs. 20-4a-d. Anatomical variations exemplified by 2-rooted mandibular canine (a) and premolars (b), 3-rooted maxillary first premolar (c) and 4-rooted mandibular molar (d).

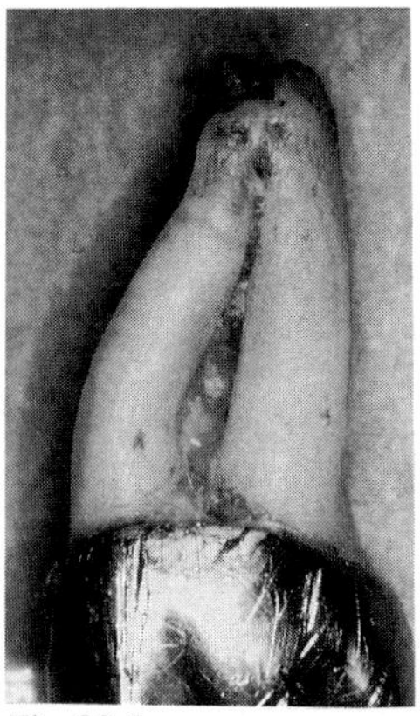

Fig. 20-5a.

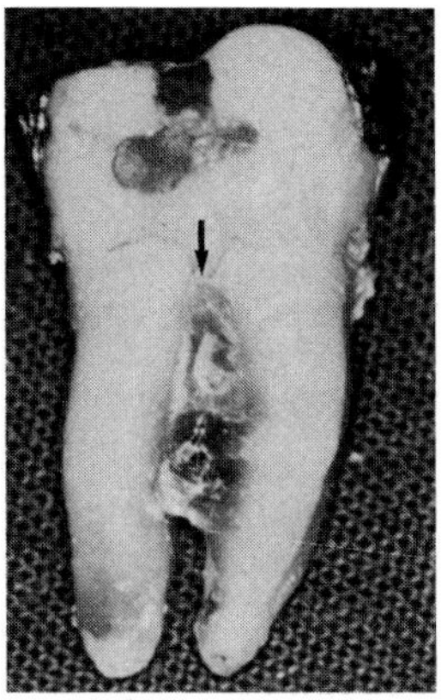

Fig. 20-5b.

Figs. 20-5a,b. Morphological variations illustrated by (a) fusion between the roots of a maxillary second molar, and (b) cervical enamel projection into the furca entrance of a mandibular first molar (arrow).

and they have frequently more pronounced root furrows or invaginations. It should also be observed that the buccal bone plate is thinner adjacent to the roots of the first molars than at the second and, in particular, the third molars.

The use of *radiographs* to identify the structures in the furcation areas is generally of limited value. Hence, in maxillary molars (Fig. 20-3a) frequently only the buccal furca can be properly identified and in mandibular molars (Fig. 20-3b) the images of the buccal and lingual furcas cannot always be distinguished since tooth and bone structures often become superimposed over the furcation areas. It should be noted that the furcation area of the maxillary premolars may be best identified in a radiograph obtained by directing the central beam towards the canine (Fig. 20-3c). The information obtained from radiographs is improved if the radiographic examination includes pictures obtained both by parallelling periapical and bite-wing techniques (Figs. 20-3d,e). Fig. 20-3f illustrates a second maxillary molar in which the furcation area is obscured by superimposed hard-tissue structures.

The fact that furcas may be present in teeth which normally have only one root should also be taken into consideration. Thus, 2-rooted incisors or canines (Fig. 20-4a) and mandibular premolars (Fig. 20-4b) may exist. Occasionally, 3-rooted maxillary premolars (Fig. 20-4c) and 4-rooted mandibular molars (Fig. 20-4d) can be found.

Other morphological variations to consider in the diagnosis and treatment of furcation-involved teeth are "fusions" between divergent roots (Fig. 20-5a), cervical enamel projections or enamel pearls in the furcation areas (arrow; Fig. 20-5b), and the presence of accessory pulp canals which communicate with the furcation area, etc.

Rationale for diagnosis

Treatment of periodontal disease around a multirooted tooth should not be initiated until

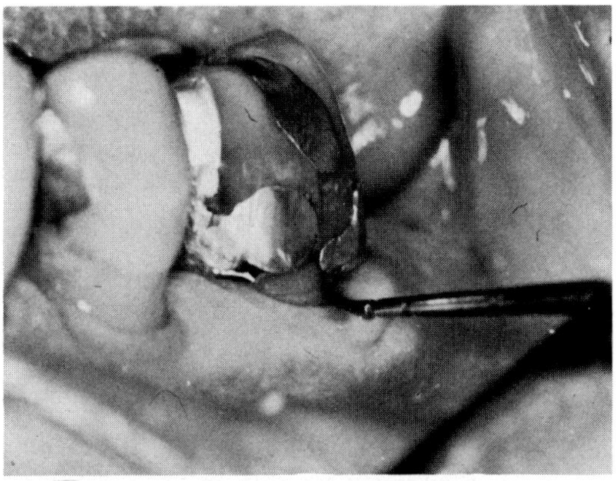

Fig. 20-6a.

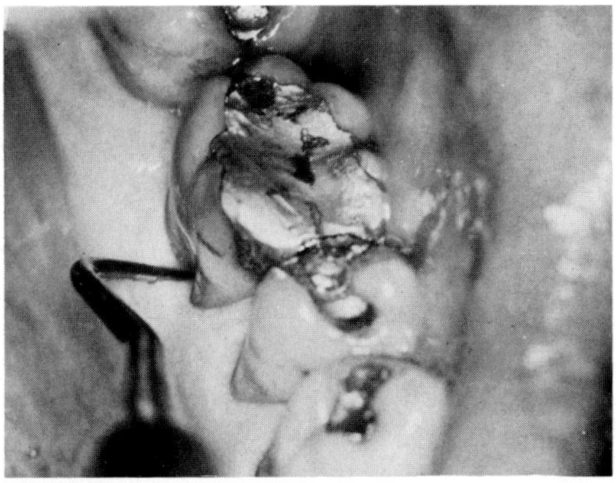

Fig. 20-6b.

Figs. 20-6a,b. A periodontal probe inserted into the furcation areas of a mandibular first molar demonstrating (a) a buccal *Degree 1* and (b) a lingual *Degree 2*-involvement.

the tooth has been examined for the presence of a furcation involvement. Such an examination should comprise both *clinical probing* and *radiographic analysis*. Graduated curved periodontal probes, explorers or small curettes should be used for the clinical examination. Sometimes the vitality of the affected tooth must be tested in order to differentiate between a plaque-associated lesion and a lesion of pulpal origin in the furcation area (see Chapter 9).

Furcation involvements may be *classified* into three degrees, depending on the extension of the destruction in the horizontal direction within the interradicular area:

Degree 1 (initial) -denotes horizontal loss of periodontal tissue support not exceeding 1/3 of the width of the tooth.

Degree 2 (partial) -denotes horizontal loss of periodontal tissue support exceeding 1/3 of the width of the tooth but not encompassing the total width of the furcation area.

Degree 3 (total) -denotes horizontal "through-and-through" destruction of the periodontal tissues in the furcation area.

The buccal furca of the maxillary molars and the buccal (Fig. 20-6a) and lingual (Fig. 20-6b) furcas of the mandibular molars are normally accessible for examination by clinical probing.

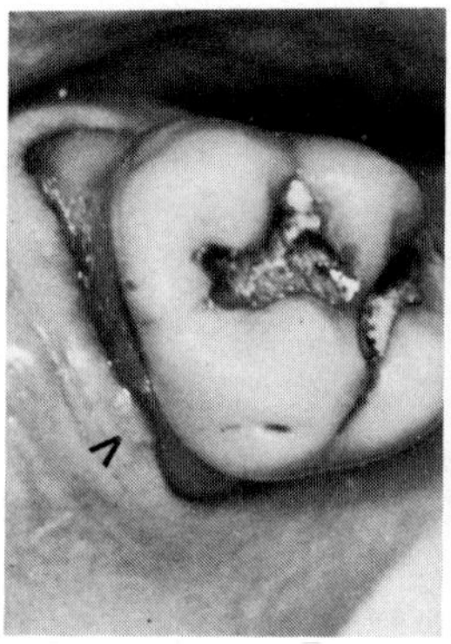

Fig. 20-7a.

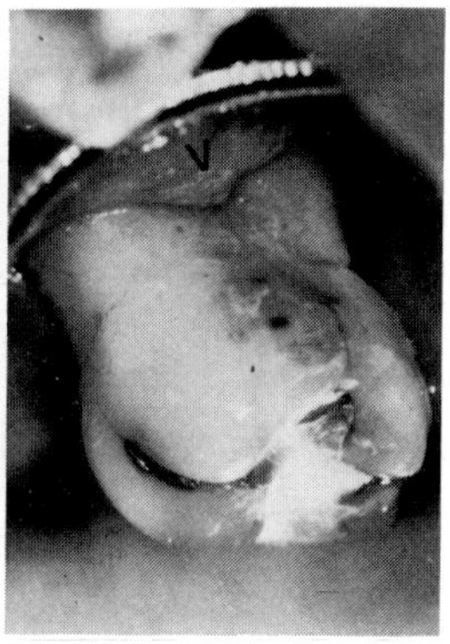

Fig. 20-7b.

Figs. 20-7a,b. Photographs showing the entrances (marked with arrows) of the proximal furcas of maxillary molars. The mesial furca is located palatally (a) while the distal furca is centred to the mid-portion of the tooth (b).

The clinical examination or furcas on the approximal tooth surfaces may be more difficult when neighboring teeth are present, especially if the contact area between the teeth is large. This is particularly the case in maxillary molars. As a rule, however, the furca in the mesial surface of a maxillary molar should be probed from the palatal aspect of the tooth (Fig. 20-7a) while the furca in the distal surface is probed

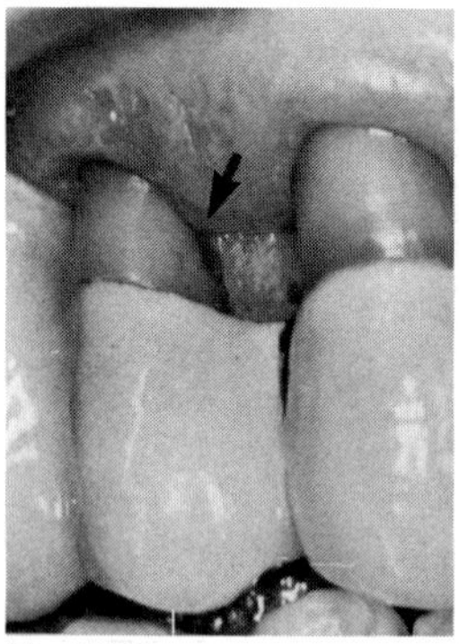

Fig. 20-8a.

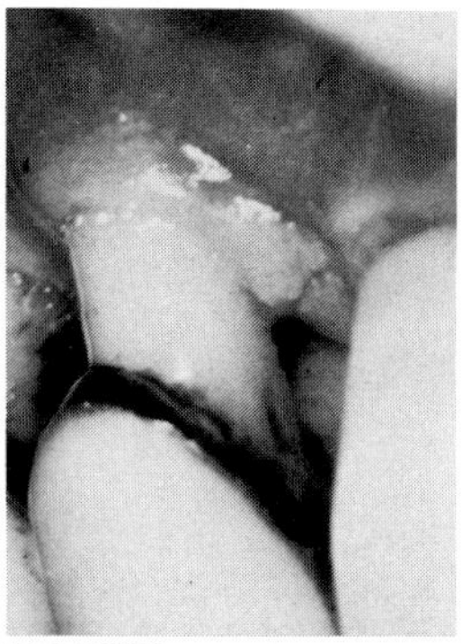

Fig. 20-8b.

Figs. 20-8a,b. Photographs of maxillary first premolars with different root anatomy, one with a mesial root furrow (arrow in a) and the other with an open *Degree 2*-involvement close to the cementoenamel junction (b).

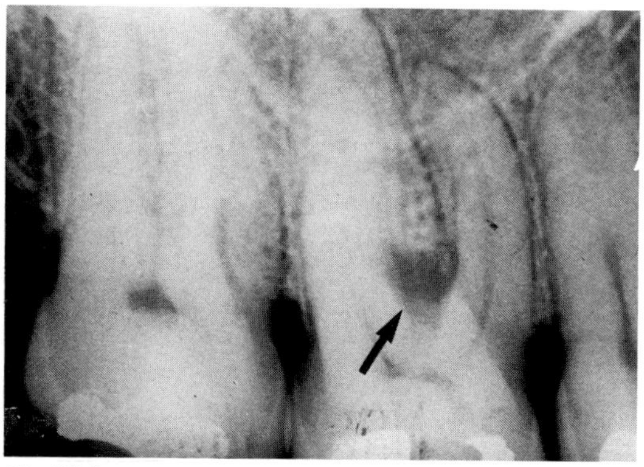

Fig. 20-9a.

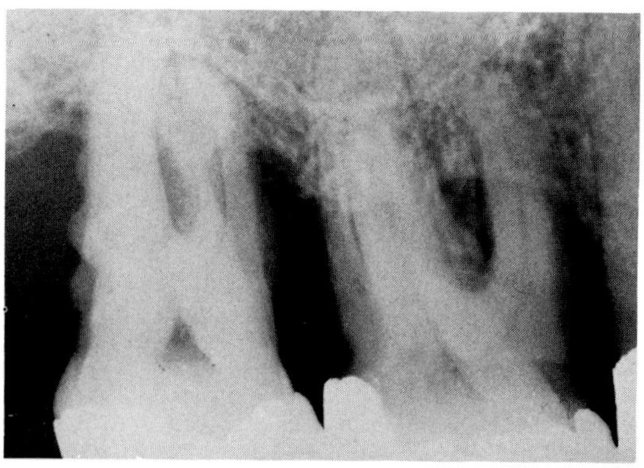

Fig. 20-9b.

Figs. 20-9a,b. Radiographic analysis as an aid to diagnosis of buccal furcation involvement of a maxillary first molar (a). The level of the interproximal bone crest, as seen in the radiograph (b) indicates severe molar furcation involvements.

from either the buccal or the palatal aspect (Fig. 20-7b).

Premolars - in particular the first maxillary premolars - often have a varying root anatomy. In addition, the roots harbor irregularities such as longitudinal furrows, invaginations (arrow; Fig. 20-8a) or true furcas (Fig. 20-8b) which may open up at different levels from the cementoenamel junction. The clinical examination of maxillary premolars is often difficult due to limited access for probing. It may not always be possible to identify the presence and the degree of furcation involvement in such teeth until a flap is raised in an explorative (surgical) procedure in the area.

In addition to *clinical probing*, a *radiographic analysis* should be made as a supplementary examination of possible furcation involvements. The information obtained should be related to findings from the clinical examination. Fig. 20-9a (arrow) shows a radiolucency in the buccal furcation area of a maxillary first molar which corresponds to an involvement of *Degree 2* as assessed by clinical probing. No further involvements could be diagnosed in the molar region, either by probing or by the radiographic analysis.

In cases of advanced destruction of the supporting apparatus in the molars (Fig. 20-9b), the occurrence of furcation involvements at the mesial and distal aspects of the teeth may be anticipated when the image of the interdental alveolar bone crest in the radiograph is located apical to the "normal" level of the furcas. In the two molars (17 and 16), illustrated in Fig. 20-9b, there were *Degree 3* involvements from the buccal, mesial and distal aspects of the teeth. This diagnosis was confirmed by probing the furcas by means of a curved probe.

In this context, it should be observed that even extensive loss of alveolar bone in the interradicular area of maxillary molars is often not disclosed in the radiograph due to the superimposition of remaining bone structures and of the palatal root (arrows; Figs. 20-10a,b).

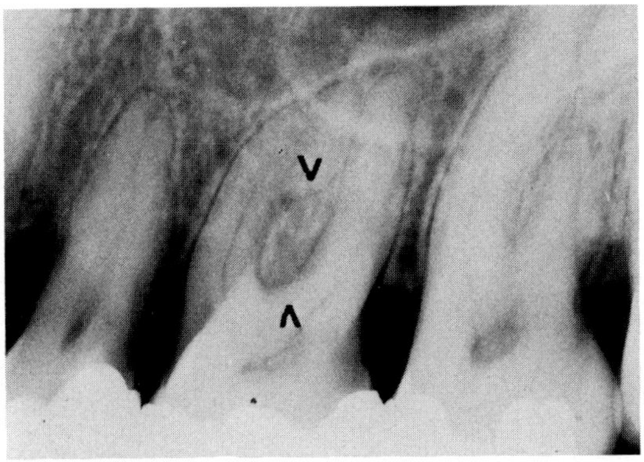

Fig. 20-10a.

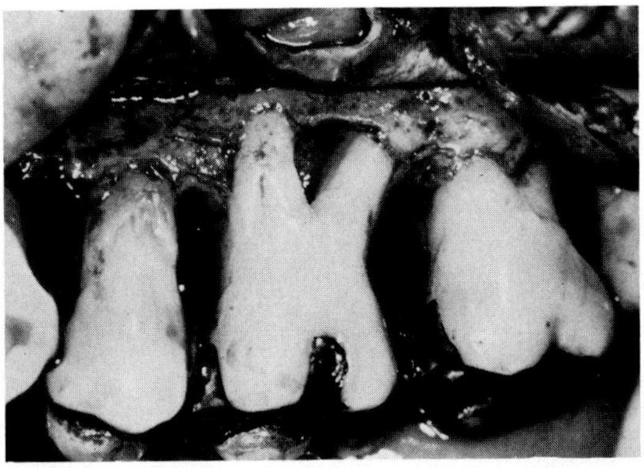

Fig. 20-10b.

Figs. 20-10a,b. Radiograph indicating buccal furcation involvement in a maxillary first molar (a). The clinical appearance after flap elevation reveals the extent of the destruction (b).

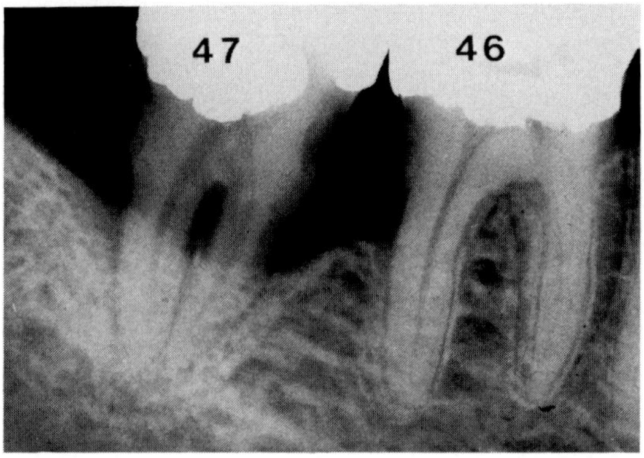

Fig. 20-11a.

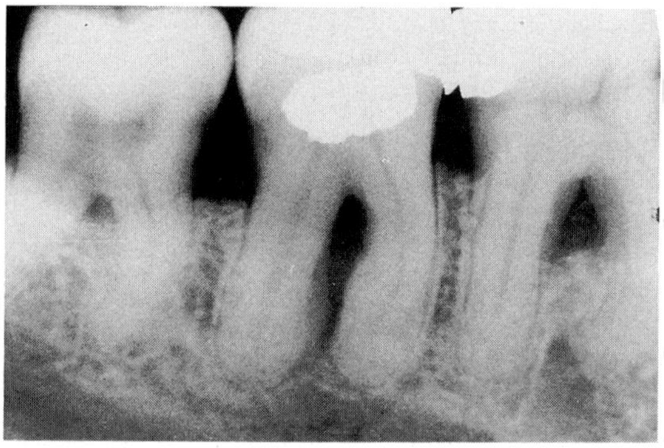

Fig. 20-11b.

Figs. 20-11a,b. Radiographs showing different degrees of furcation involvements in mandibular molars (see text).

Different degrees of furcation involvements in mandibular molars are illustrated in Figs. 20-11a,b. In Fig. 20-11a a through-and-through furcation involvement in tooth 47 can be distinguished in the radiograph. This diagnosis was verified by the clinical examination, which revealed pathologically deepened pockets (8 mm at the buccal and lingual aspects of the tooth), furcation involvement of *Degree 3* and a tooth mobility of *Degree 2*. On the other hand, it was not possible from the radiograph to detect the *Degree 1* involvements which were probed from both the buccal and lingual aspect of tooth 46. In this radiograph, persisting inter-radicular alveolar bone in the mid-portion of the furcation area obscured these initial furcation involvements.

In the teeth seen in Fig. 20-11b, the clinical assessments of furcation involvements gave the following result: tooth 48 *Degree 1* (from the lingual aspect), tooth 47 *Degree 3* and tooth 46 *Degree 2* (from the buccal aspect). The *Degree 1* involvement in the lingual surface of tooth 48 is clearly visible in this radiographic projection, as is the *Degree 3* involvement in tooth 47. The *Degree 2* involvement at the buccal aspect of tooth 46 is reproduced in a characteristic way. By thorough analysis of the radiograph, the trabecular structure of bone tissue can be detected within the radiolucent zone of

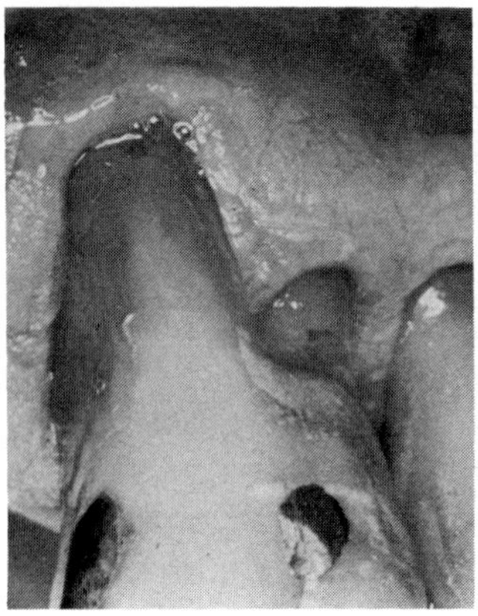

Fig. 20-12a.

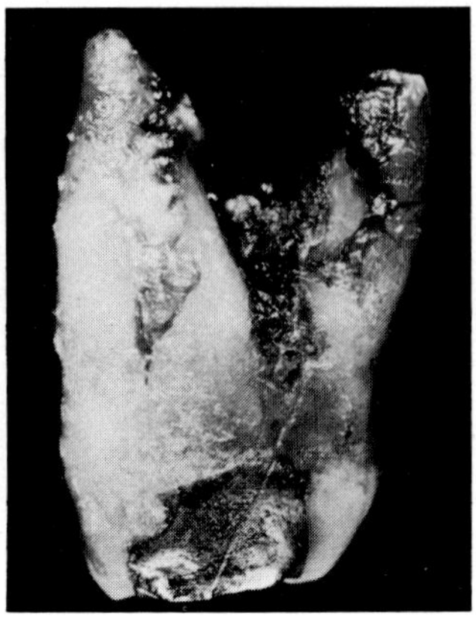

Fig. 20-12b.

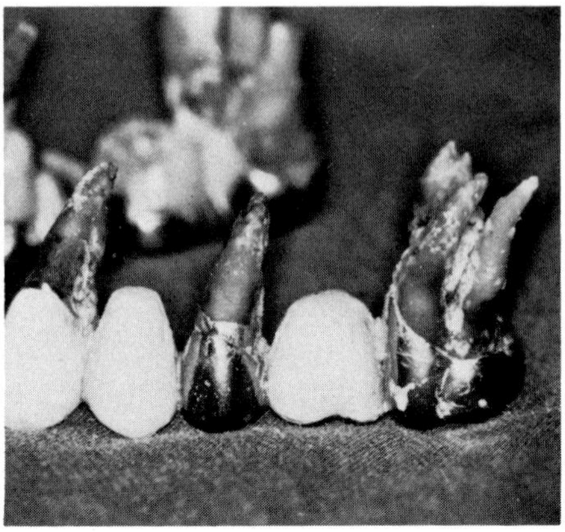

Fig. 20-12c.

Figs. 20-12a-c. Photographs illustrating success (a) and failure (b) of scaling and root planing of furcation-involved maxillary molars. The loss of a cross-arch bridge may be the end result of extended accumulation of plaque and calculus (c).

the interradicular area; the alveolar bone at the lingual aspect of the tooth is normal in height - no lingual furcation involvement was recorded - and, in the radiograph, this bone mass is projected over the buccally located lesion in the furcation area.

Rationale for therapy

Since the distance between the cementoenamel junction and the furcas of multirooted teeth - particularly first molars - often is comparatively short, furcation involvements may already develop at initial or moderate stages of breakdown of the attachment apparatus. Proper diagnosis and treatment of periodontal disease at an early stage, i.e. before the furcas have become involved in the destructive process, are therefore important in order to prevent such complications. In cases where furcation involvements have developed, different therapeutic alternatives are available, alternatives which often relate to the different degrees of involvement:

Degree of involvement	Therapy
Degree 1	Scaling and root planing Furcation plasty
Degree 2	Furcation plasty Tunnel preparation Root resection Tooth extraction
Degree 3	Tunnel preparation Root resection Tooth extraction

Scaling and root planing

The removal of hard and soft bacterial deposits from the tooth and root surfaces is the only procedure in the treatment of most furcation involvements of *Degree 1*. The successful result of this simple treatment is illustrated in Fig. 20-12a. It should be borne in mind that healing must result in a morphology in the furcation area which is optimal for self-performed plaque control. If this is not fulfilled, plaque and calculus will again accumulate in the critical area and recurrence of the progressive destruction may occur (Figs. 20-12b,c). If proper condi-

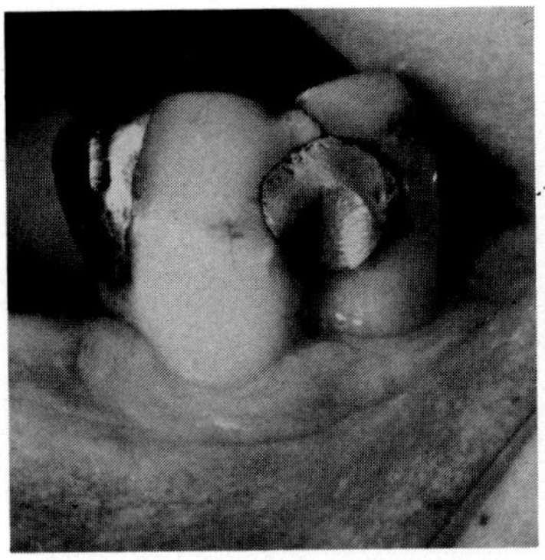

Fig. 20-13a.

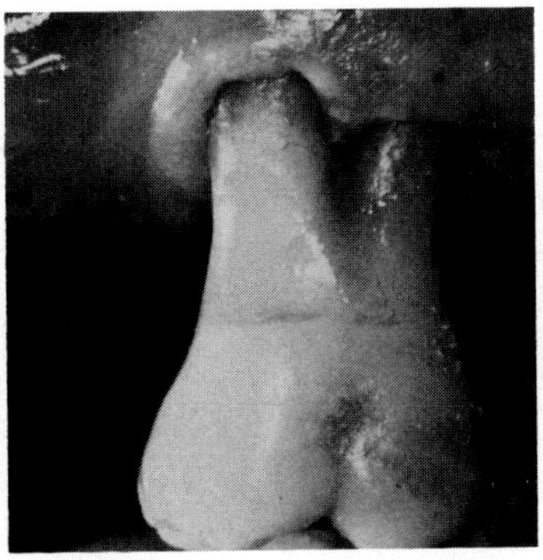

Fig. 20-13b.

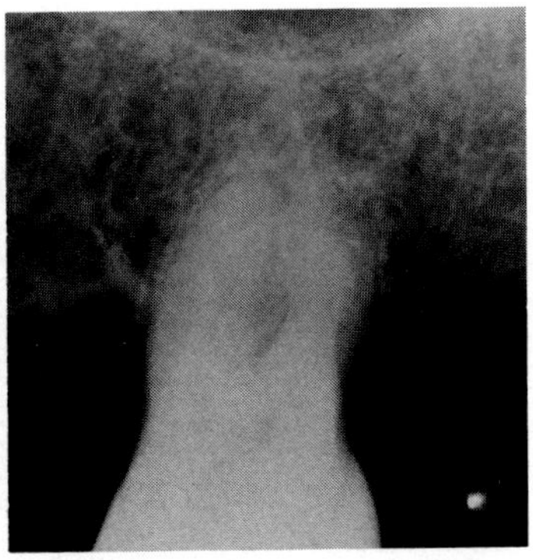

Fig. 20-13c.

Figs. 20-13a-c. Furcation plasty carried out as odontoplasty at the buccal aspect of a mandibular molar (a) and a maxillary molar (b). The radiographic appearance of the maxillary molar after treatment is shown in (c).

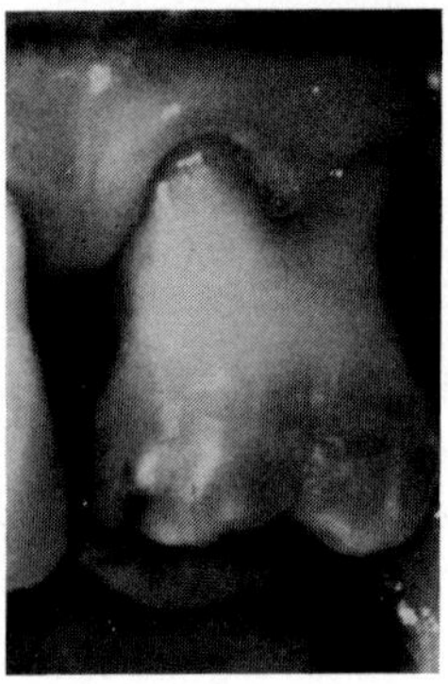

Fig. 20-14a.

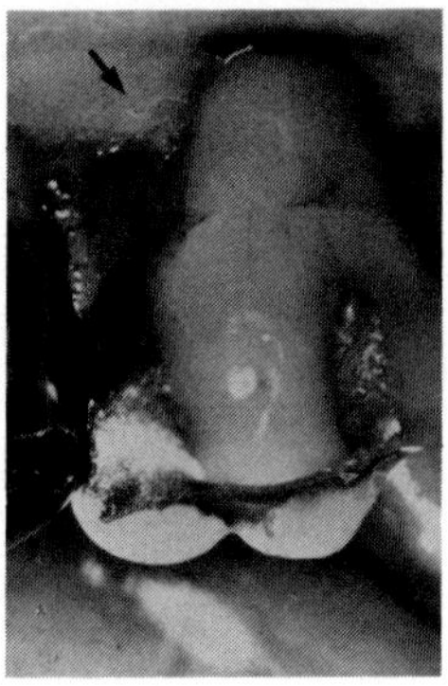

Fig. 20-14b.

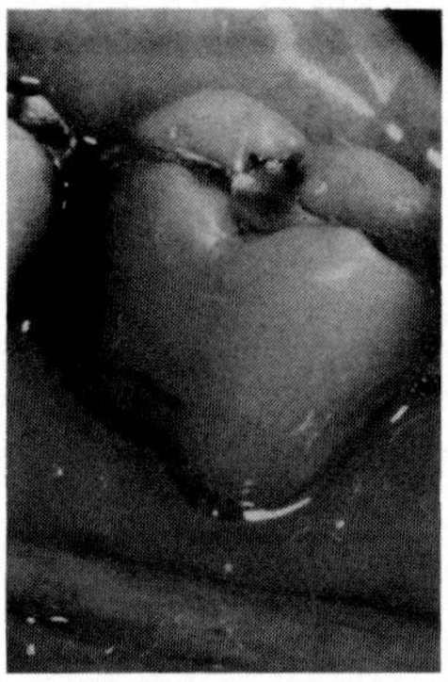

Fig. 20-14c.

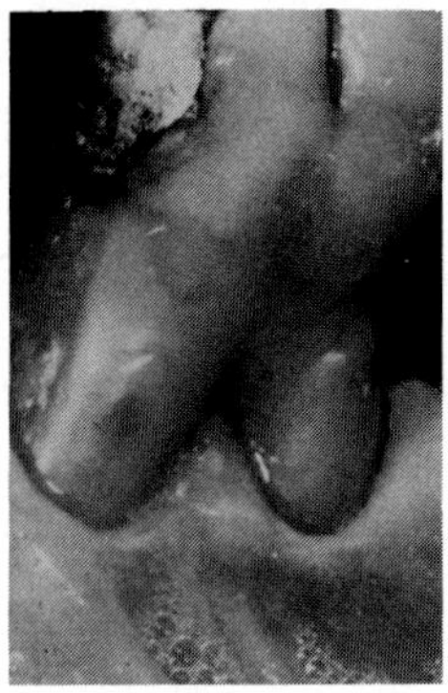

Fig. 20-14d.

Figs. 20-14a-d. Photographs showing the result of furcation plasty in four molars; buccally and mesially at maxillary molars (a,b) and buccally and lingually at mandibular molars (c,d) at different levels of supporting tissues.

tions for plaque control measures cannot be established by scaling and root planing alone, other therapeutic methods must be used.

Furcation plasty

This includes the following procedures:

- reflection of a mucoperiosteal flap to obtain proper access to the interradicular area,
- removal of soft and hard bacterial deposits and inflammatory soft tissue from the furcation area,
- odontoplasty, i.e. removal of tooth substance in the furcation area in order to widen a narrow entrance of the furca and to reduce the horizontal depth of the involvement,
- osteoplasty, i.e. recontouring of bony defects in the furcation area, if indicated,
- repositioning and suturing of the flap.

Furcation plasty is a therapeutic measure preferably used in the treatment of advanced *Degree 1* and initial *Degree 2* involvements. Owing to limitations of access and difficulty in securing optimal plaque control, such recontouring encounters difficulties in the areas of proximally located furcas, i.e. in maxillary molars and premolars, when neighboring teeth have approximal contacts. The result of this

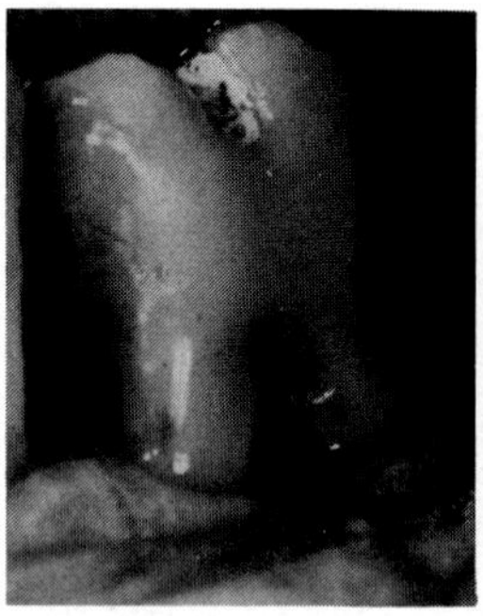

Fig. 20-15a.

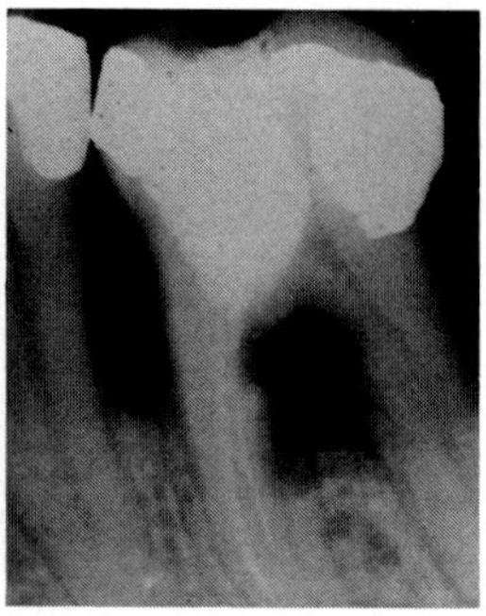

Fig. 20-15b.

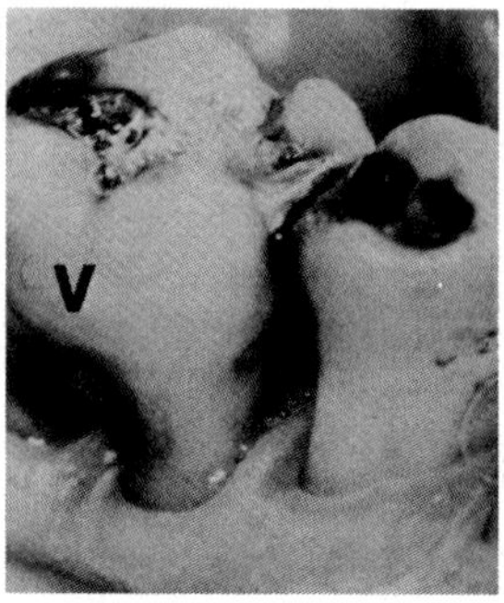

Fig. 20-15c.

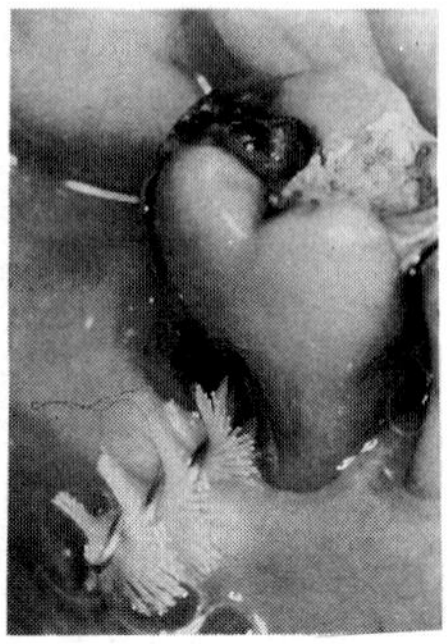

Fig. 20-15d.

Figs. 20-15a-d. Tunnel preparation of a *Degree 3* - involved mandibular first molar (a). A radiograph (b) and photographs (c,d) obtained 7 years after treatment reveal a pronounced carious lesion at the entrance of the lingual furca despite the accessibility to the areas with oral hygiene aids (d).

type of treatment is exemplified in Figs. 20-13a-c and 20-14a-d. The treatment should result in the establishment of a soft-tissue papilla which covers the entrance to the interradicular periodontal tissues. It should again be emphasized that the purpose of the procedure is - besides the removal of plaque and calculus - to establish a condition in the dentogingival region which facilitates self-performed plaque control.

In this context, however, there is reason to *warn against* too extensive recontouring of the tooth by grinding since this procedure may result in hypersensitivity problems, be detrimental to a vital pulp and also increase the risk of root surface caries. In addition, osteoplasty should be performed with caution so that no additional, unintended, loss of periodontium occurs at the site of operation.

Tunnel preparation

This implies surgical exposure of the entire furcation area. Following elevation of mucoperiosteal flaps at the buccal and lingual aspects of the affected tooth, the root surfaces are scaled and planed and an irregular alveolar bone crest recontoured, if necessary. The flaps are repositioned to the interradicular alveolar bone crest and secured in this position by interdental and interradicular sutures. Surgical packs may be applied to prevent excessive granulation tissue forming in the tunnel space during healing. For technical reasons the mandibular molars are most suited for this mode of therapy. Fig. 20-15a illustrates the clinical appearance of a mandibular first molar following tunnel preparation. It should be stressed that there is a pronounced risk of carious lesions developing in the denuded root surfaces within and adjacent to such tunnels (Figs. 20-15b,c) if the self-performed plaque control is not maintained on a very high level. Consequently, the method should be used with caution and restricted to situations where there is space enough between roots to permit interradicular cleansing by means of an interproximal toothbrush. Despite this, caries may develop (Fig. 20-15d).

Root resection

This is the procedure of choice in cases of deep *Degree 2* and *Degree 3* involvements and includes the removal of one or more roots from a multirooted tooth. The risk of leaving "overhangs" of tooth substance behind during tooth hemisection and root resection (Fig. 20-16) is an incitement to carry out these procedures after flap elevation, which makes proper inspection of the surgically cut dentine surface possible. A radiograph should also be obtained of the area immediately after surgery to verify that such "overhangs" do not persist.

As a rule, endodontic treatment of the root to be retained following tooth hemisection and root resection should be performed prior to surgery. Information on the result of the endodontic measures will hereby be obtained before extraction of root(s), which may possibly be maintained as an alternative. In multirooted teeth with advanced destruction of the supporting tissues it may not always be possible to decide until surgery which root or roots it is possible or most favorable to preserve. As an alternative to permanent filling of all root canals with gutta-percha before surgery, pulpectomy can be performed and the canals filled with calcium hydroxide. Each of the openings to the root canals is sealed with zinc oxide eugenol cement. Root separation and resection can thus be carried out without risk of bacterial contamination of the root canals. Permanent filling of the root(s) is in such cases performed after surgery.

In the selection of root(s) to be retained following root separation, the following factors should be considered:

- the amount of supporting tissue remaining around the various roots,
- the stability of the individual roots,
- the root and root canal anatomy with respect to endodontic and restorative treament procedures,
- the periodontal condition,
- the position of the various roots in the alveolar process in relation to adjacent and opposing teeth.

In a case where, for example, the furcation of a first mandibular molar is involved to an extent which calls for root resection, it is usually easy to decide which root is preferable to maintain from the periodontal aspect. If the amount of remaining periodontium around the 2 roots is similar, it is often preferable from the endodontic point of view to maintain the distal root. This root has generally only one, wide, root canal and is therefore easily accessible for endodontic treatment. However, the extraction and loss of the mesial portion of the tooth often requires prosthetic replacement by means of a bridge construction. Figs. 20-17a-d demonstrate a case where the two mandibular molars on one side of the jaw were furcation-involved (*Degree 3*). The loss of alveolar bone had progressed to, on average, the same level around all 4 roots (Fig. 20-17a). The distal roots were exposed to endodontic therapy (Fig. 20-17b), tooth hemisection including extraction of the mesial roots was performed (Fig. 20-17c) and, following healing (Fig. 20-17d), the mesial portions of the molars were replaced by a fixed bridge, extending from the distal root of the second molar to the second premolar. On the other hand, provided the mesial root of a mandibular molar has a root canal anatomy which allows for proper root filling and insertion of a proper post, this root can be preserved and used as abutment for a single crown. Extensive bridge therapy can hereby be avoided. Such a treatment is exemplified in Figs. 20-18a,b.

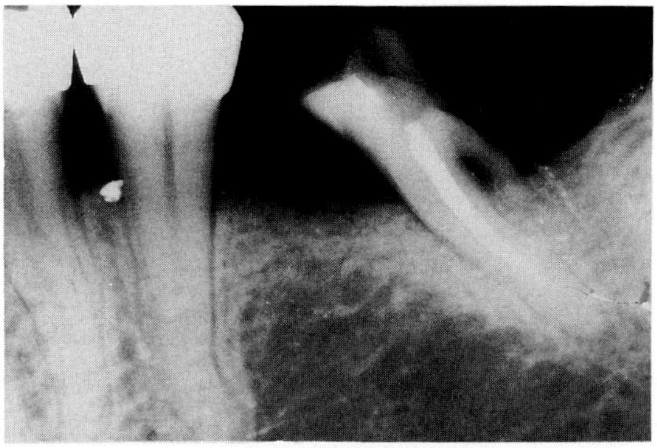

Figs. 20-16. Radiograph of a mandibular second molar subjected to hemisection. "Overhang" is left behind as a consequence of oblique sectioning distal to the furca.

Difficult problems arise when root resection is performed in maxillary molars. Since these teeth often have 3 roots, 1 or 2 roots can be preserved after separation. In spite of careful

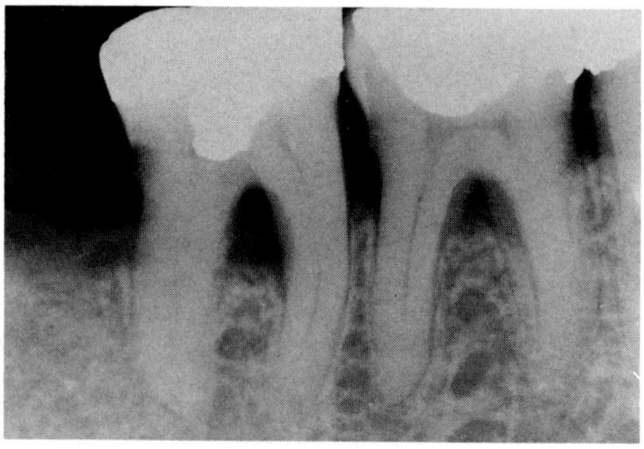

Fig. 20-17a.

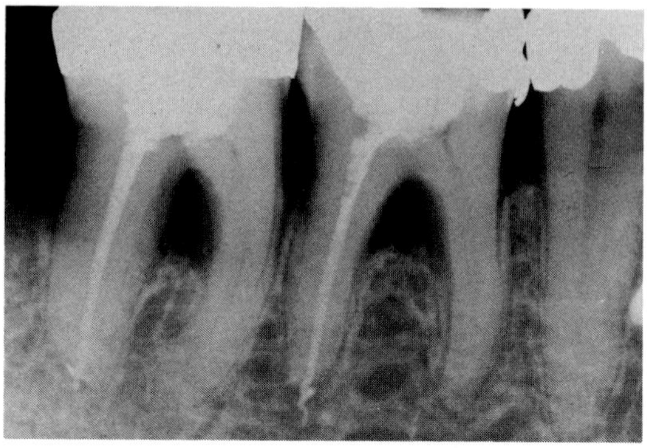

Fig. 20-17b.

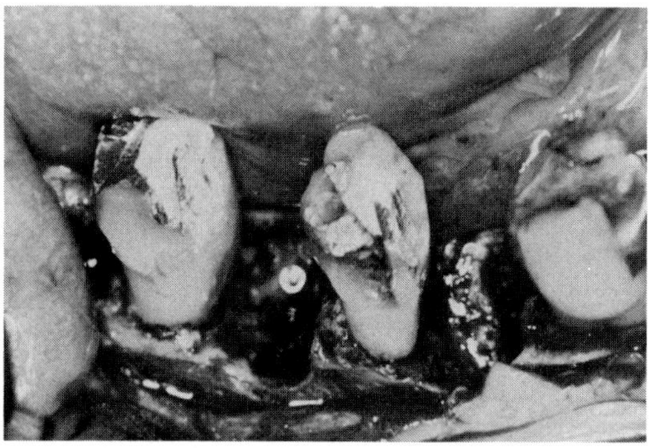

Fig. 20-17c.

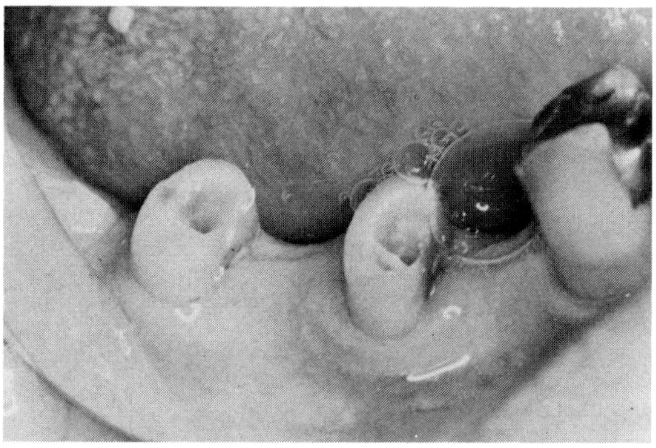

Fig. 20-17d.

Figs. 20-17a-d. The sequential stages of root resection of two mandibular molars. Both teeth were *Degree 3*-involved (a), endodontically treated (b), root resected and the mesial roots extracted (c). After complete healing, the distal roots were prepared for abutments for a fixed bridge (d).

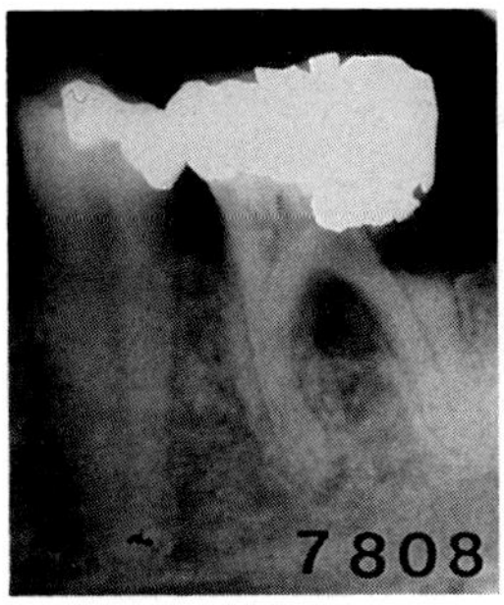

Fig. 20-18a.

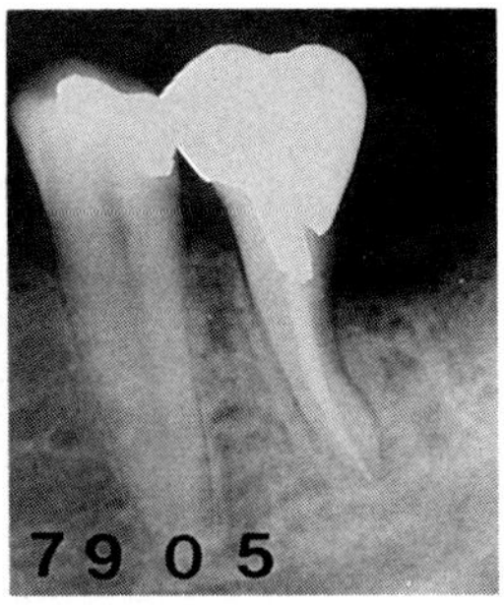

Fig. 20-18b.

Figs. 20-18a,b. Radiographs showing the use of the mesial root of a mandibular first molar as an abutment for a single crown restoration after hemisection.

clinical and radiographic examination it is often impossible to properly evaluate the extension of the furcation defect until a flap procedure makes direct inspection possible. In cases of advanced periodontal disease around maxillary molars it is often necessary to separate all 3 roots from each other to obtain access to the interradicular area for assessment of the height of the remaining bone at, for example, the buccal surface of the palatal root and the palatal surfaces of the buccal roots.

The series of photographs presented in Figs. 20-19a-c demonstrates root resection in a maxillary first molar. Fig. 20-19a illustrates how the roots are separated from each other using a fissure bur. In Fig. 20-19b the alveolar bone crest at the buccal surface of the palatal root is indicated by the tip of the probe after extraction of the 2 buccal roots. Subsequent to the root resection therapy on tooth 26, the two neighboring teeth (25, 27) which could not be treated were extracted and a 3-unit bridge was

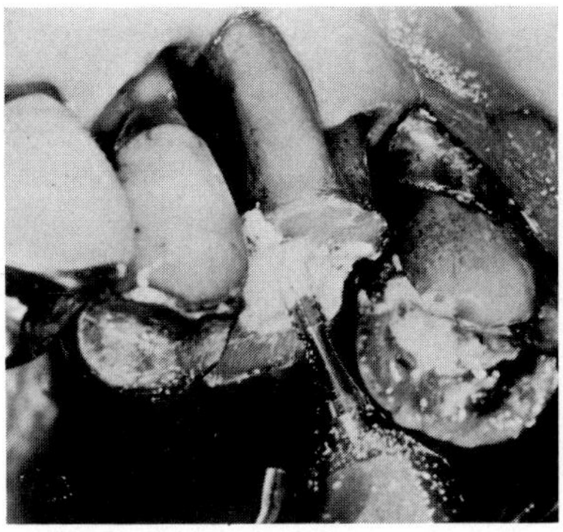

Fig. 20-19a.

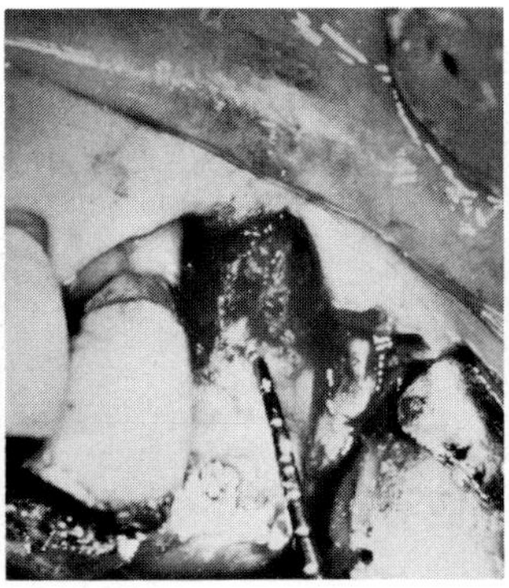

Fig. 20-19b.

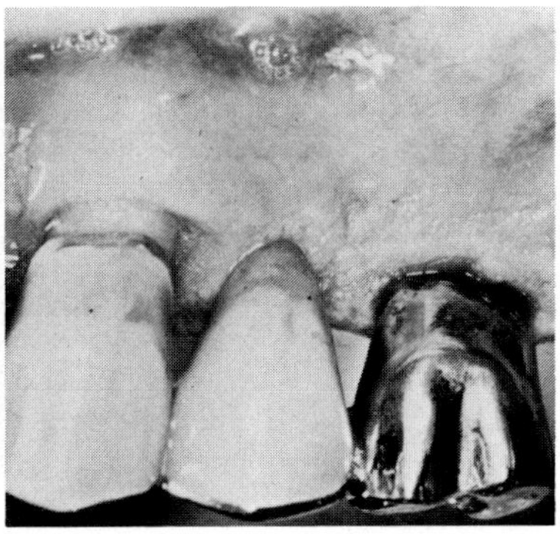

Fig. 20-19c.

Figs. 20-19a-c. The sequential stages of root resection of a maxillary first molar and extraction of the second premolar and the second molar. After endodontic treatment of the first molar, the roots were separated through the furcation area (a) and the buccal roots extracted (b) making it possible to use the palatal root as an abutment for a 3-unit bridge (c).

inserted (Fig. 20-19c) with the extension 24 ^{25} 26 (palatal root).

When a maxillary molar exhibits furcation involvement from the buccal aspect only, or when the buccal furca and one of the proximal furcas are periodontally involved, (e.g. the buccal and the distal furcas), the tooth may be treated as illustrated in Figs. 20-20a,b. The mesiobuccal and palatal roots were root filled (Fig. 20-20a) and the distobuccal root was resected (Fig. 20-20b). Such a root resection can often be performed without the removal of excessive amounts of tissue from the crown of the tooth, i.e. there may be no need for the placement of an artificial crown following surgery.

A similar treatment of a molar with a *Degree 2* involvement in the mesial surface is illustrated in Figs. 20-21a-d. No involvements were present at the distal and buccal aspects of the tooth. The radiographic analysis (Fig. 20-21a) and the findings during surgery (Fig. 20-21b) disclosed bone loss at the mesial surface to apex of the mesiobuccal root. Figs. 20-21c and d present the result of the treatment, i.e. extraction of this root, after 6 months of healing.

Resection of the palatal root might be an unusual way to solve a furcation problem. However, in a situation where the buccal furca is intact but the presence of a mesial and/or a distal furcation involvement is combined with advanced loss of attachment around the palatal root, the removal of this root and the maintenance of the buccal portion of the tooth including the 2 buccal roots may be the procedure of choice. In the case presented in Fig. 20-22a, the second premolar and the second molar were extracted. The root canals of the first premolar and the buccal roots of the first molar were filled. Root resection was carried out in the first molar, including extraction of the palatal root. Following healing (Fig. 20-22b) a fixed bridge with the extension 16 ^{15} 14 was inserted (Fig. 20-22c).

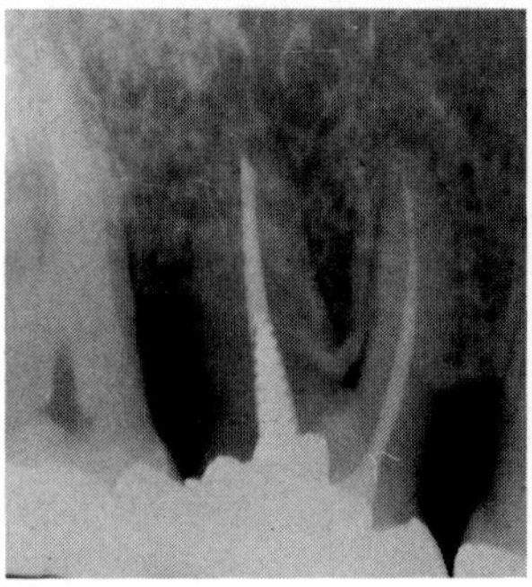

Fig. 20-20a.

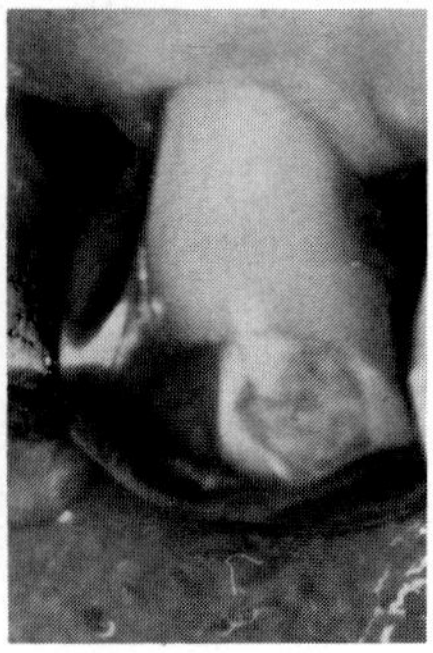

Fig. 20-20b.

Figs. 20-20a,b. Resection and extraction of the distobuccal root of a maxillary first molar. Radiograph (a) and photograph of the tooth with restored crown (b).

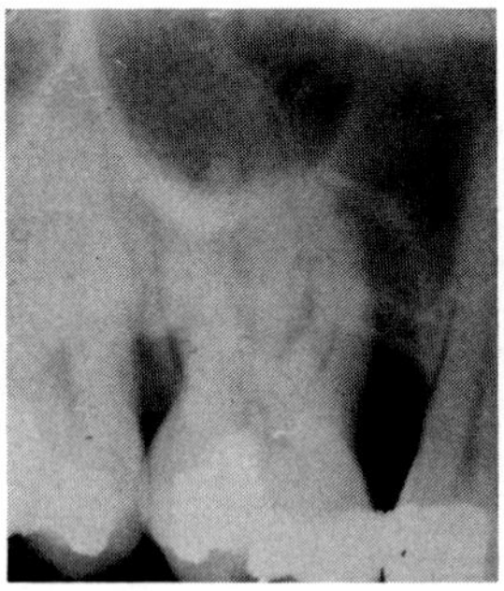
Fig. 20-21a.

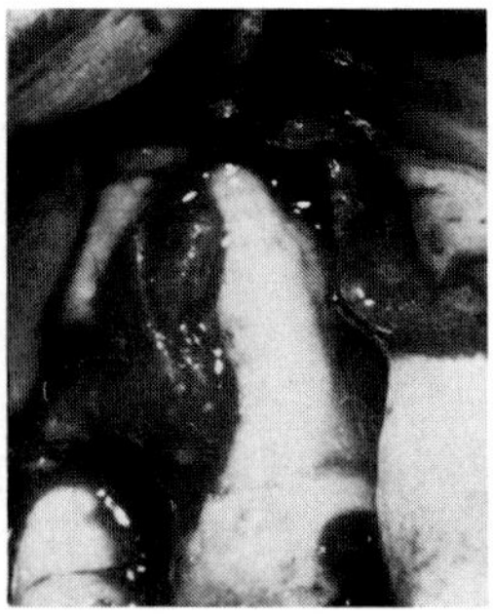
Fig. 20-21b.

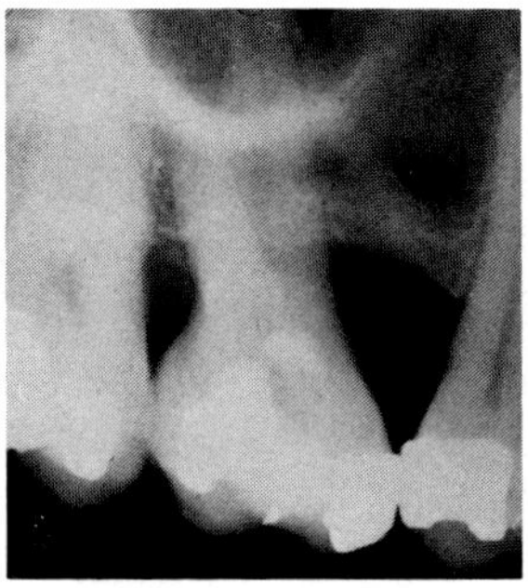
Fig. 20-21c.

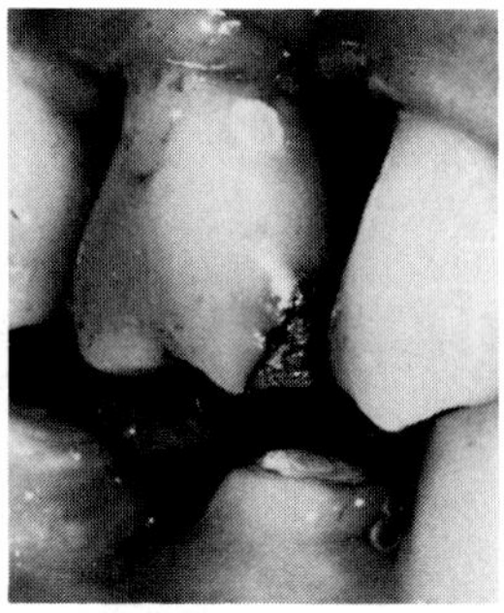
Fig. 20-21d.

Figs. 20-21a-d. Resection of the mesiobuccal root of a maxillary first molar. Radiograph and photograph before (a,b) and after (c,d) the resection.

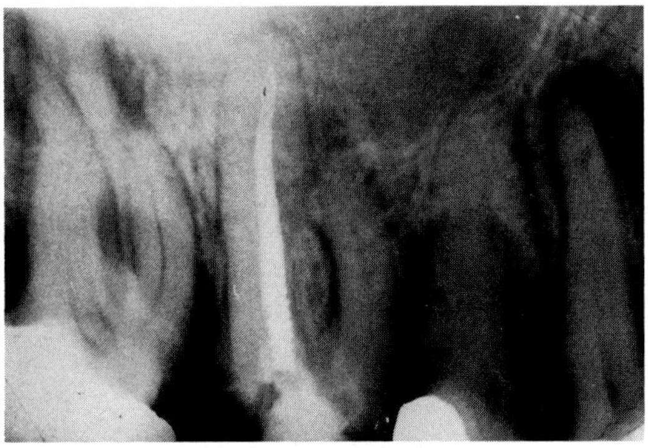
Fig. 20-22a.

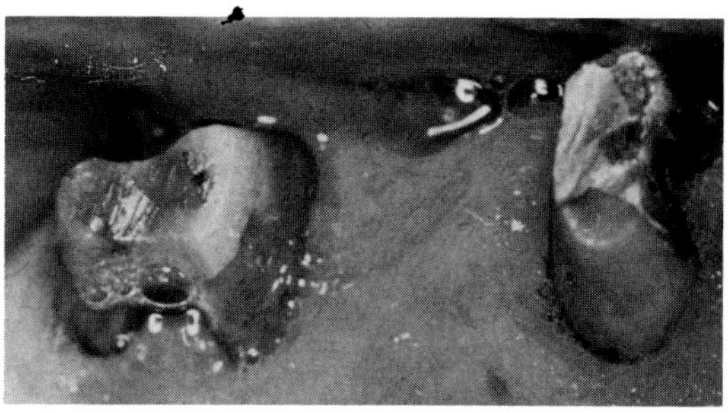
Fig. 20-22b.

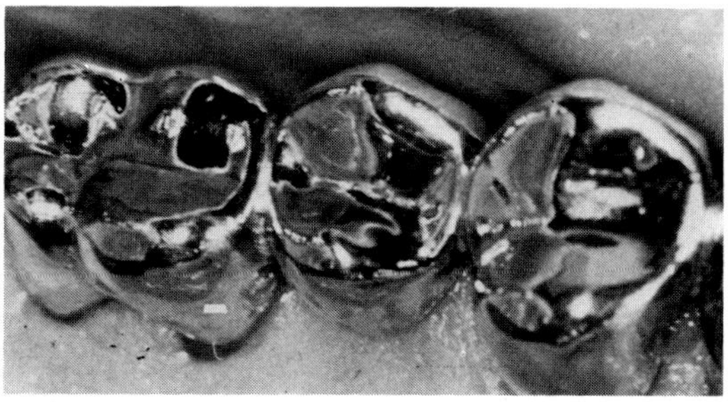
Fig. 20-22c.

Figs. 20-22a-c. Radiograph (a) showing pulpal and periodontal pathology around maxillary molars and premolars. The second molar and the second premolar were extracted and the first molar and first premolar endodontically treated. After root resection and extraction of the palatal root of the first molar (b), the 2 buccal roots were maintained as distal abutment for a 3-unit bridge (c).

Root resection of maxillary first premolars is possible only in rare instances due to the anatomy of the tooth. The furca is often located at such an apical level that the maintenance of 1 root serves no meaningful purpose. In most cases, therefore, a furcation involvement of *Degree 3* in a maxillary first premolar calls for tooth extraction (Figs. 20-23a,b).

In the selection of roots that can or should be retained in a case with multiple furcation involvements in the maxillary molars, the position of the various roots in the jaw in relation to neighboring teeth must be considered. The buccal roots, provided they can be subjected to proper endodontic treatment, may be preferred to a palatal root. For example, if the maxillary second premolar is present (see Fig. 20-24a), one or several of the buccal roots of the molars - later to be used as distal abutments in a cross-arch bridge - should be preserved because of their more favorable position in the dental arch in relation to the premolar in comparison with

Figs. 20-23a,b. Radiograph and photograph (after extraction and dyeing of the remaining periodontal ligaments) of a maxillary first premolar demonstrating the apically located furca.

the palatal roots. In this particular example, the mesiobuccal root of the second molar was preserved and used as the distal abutment tooth. Fig. 20-24b demonstrates another case before bridge insertion. Here the mesiobuccal root of each of the first molars was used as distal abutments in a cross-arch bridge.

Another example of the problems involved in the selection of roots to be retained in a

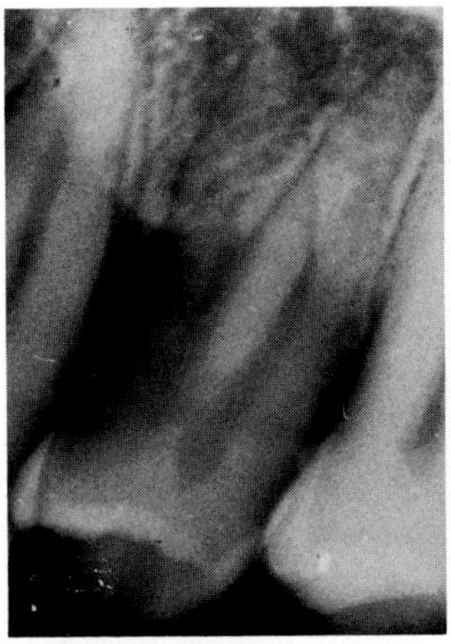

Fig. 20-23a.

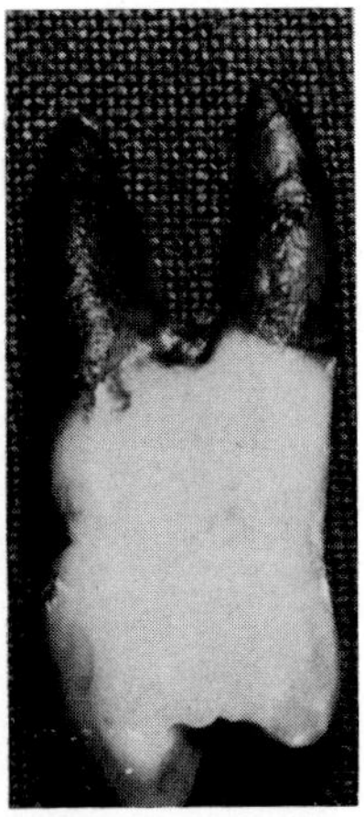

Fig. 20-23b.

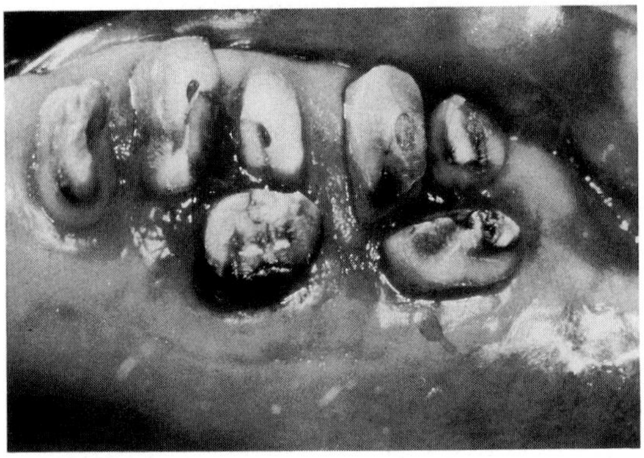

Fig. 20-24a.

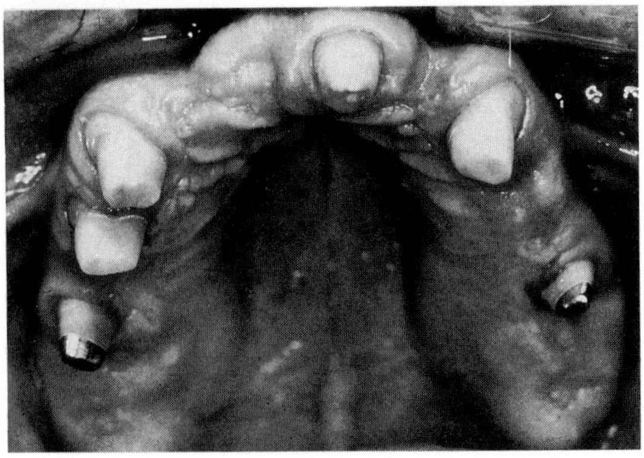

Fig. 20-24b.

Figs. 20-24a,b. Photographs after total root sectioning showing the root anatomy of maxillary molars and their position in the dental arch. The mesiobuccal roots are wide in the buccopalatal dimension (a), and frequently favorably located in the arch to serve as abutments for subsequent bridgework (b).

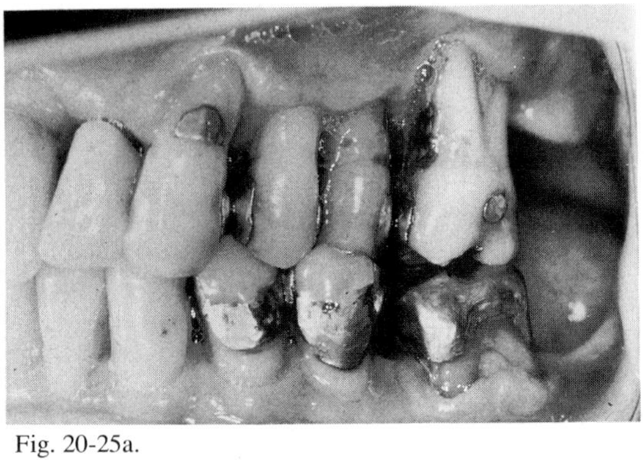

Fig. 20-25a.

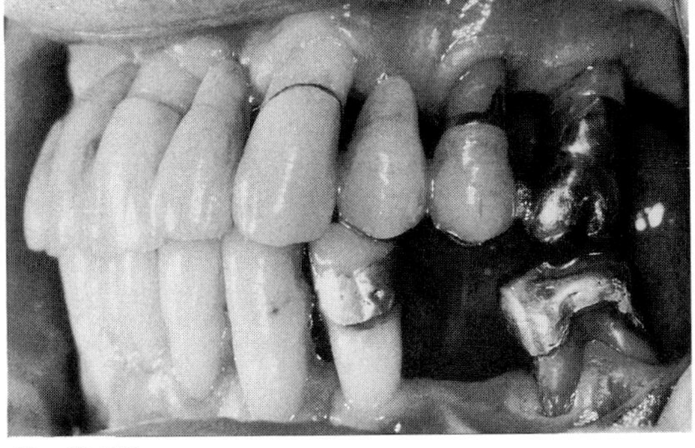

Fig. 20-25b.

Figs. 20-25a,b. Photographs (a,b) demonstrating the use of the palatal root of a maxillary molar as bridge abutment.

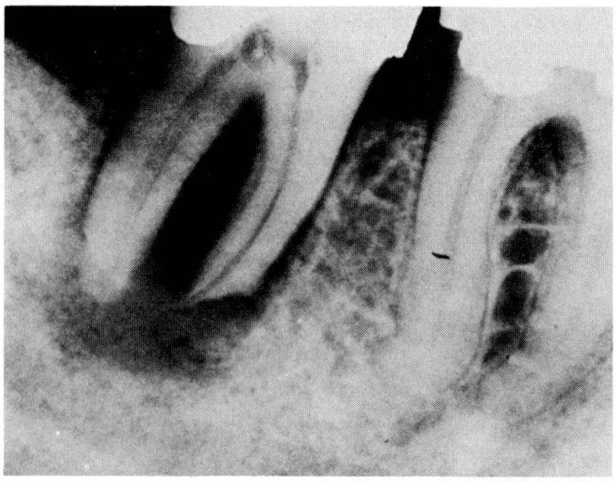

Fig. 20-26a.

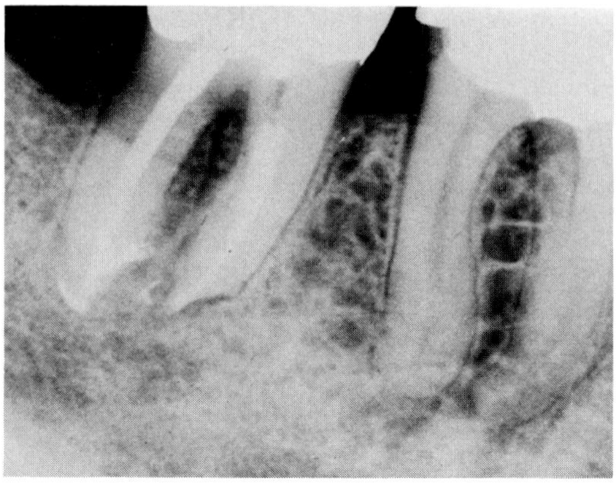

Fig. 20-26b.

Figs. 20-26a,b. Radiographs demonstrating severe destruction of interradicular bone including periapical lesions and resorptions in both roots of a mandibular second molar (a). Rapid bone healing occurred after endodontic treatment (b).

given case is illustrated in Figs. 20-25a,b. The palatal root was the only root of the maxillary first molar that could be preserved. Following resection of the buccal roots, the palatal root was found to have a high mobility. Due to the fact that the second premolar was palatally displaced in the jaw (cross-bite position; see Fig. 20-25a) and thus located in the same plane as the retained molar root, a splint with proper design could be placed (Fig. 20-25b).

Finally, it should be pointed out that all forms of periodontal surgery, including root resection, result in exposed root dentine surfaces which may be susceptible to carious lesions. Fluorides should routinely be applied topically to such surfaces after completion of surgery.

Tooth extraction

The extraction of a periodontally involved 2- or multirooted tooth will of course predictably eliminate the disease in this particular area. This therapy is indicated when the destruction of the periodontium has progressed to such a level that no root can be preserved. Extraction may also be performed when the maintenance of the affected tooth will not improve the overall treatment or when treatment of the furcation-involved tooth will not result in conditions which can be properly maintained by self-performed plaque control measures.

In the diagnosis and treatment of furcation-involved teeth it should be realized that loss of alveolar bone within the interradicular area - besides being caused by periodontal disease - may also be the effect of infection derived from a necrotic pulp. Such a situation is illustrated in Fig. 20-26a. Examination of the affected molar disclosed a nonvital pulp. The tooth was endodontically treated and complete healing of the bony lesion occurred within a few months (Fig. 20-26b). For detailed discussion on interrelationships between periodontics and endodontics, see Chapter 9.

Prognosis

A 5-year follow-up study of the results of treatment of 175 furcation-involved 2- and multirooted teeth was presented by Hamp et al. 1975 (Table 20-1). The teeth included had been treated in accordance with the principles described in this chapter. Out of the 175 teeth, 32 had been treated by scaling and root planing alone. Scaling and root planing in conjunction with furcation plasty, including odonto- and/or

Table 20-1

Frequency and distribution of various procedures in furcation-involved teeth (from Hamp et al. 1975)

Therapy \ Teeth	36/46	37/47	16/26	17/27	18/28	14/24	Other premolars	Total
Scaling/root planing	8	4	12	6	2	-	-	32
Furcation plasty	12	15	14	8	-	-	-	49
Tunnel preparation	6	-	-	-	-	1	-	7
Root resection	30	14	28	11	-	3	1	87
Total	56	33	54	25	2	4	1	175

osteoplasty, had been carried out in 49 teeth: 87 furcation-involved teeth had been subjected to root resection while a tunnel had been prepared in 7 teeth only. Following the active treatment phase, all patients were enrolled in a maintenance-care program including recall appointments once every 3-6 months. At each recall appointment the patients were instructed in oral hygiene measures, and scaling, root planing and polishing of the teeth were performed. *Presence of plaque* and *gingival conditions* at the furcation areas of all teeth were assessed immediately before active treatment and once a year postoperatively using the Plaque and Gingival Index systems described by Löe & Silness (1963) and Silness & Löe (1964). The mean PlI scores for all types of therapeutic procedures at the final examination varied between 0.2 and 0.3. The corresponding GI scores were 0.2-0.4.

Pocket depth measurements at the final control revealed that only 16 out of the 175 teeth subjected to furcation treatment had a probing pocket depth exceeding 3 mm. The distribution of these pockets in relation to the different therapeutic procedures is given in Table 20-2.

Table 20-2

Probing pocket depths in the furcation areas at the final examination (from Hamp et al 1975)

Therapy	≤ 3mm	4-6 mm	> 6 mm	Total
Scaling/ root planing, Furcation plasty	77	4	-	81
Tunnel preparation	4	3	-	7
Root resection	78	7	2	87
Total	159	14	2	175

During the observation period (5 years) carious lesions were detected on 12 treated tooth surfaces which had been subjected to scaling, root planing and furcation plasty (3 surfaces), root resection (5 surfaces) and tunnel preparation (4 surfaces).

It should be stressed that different modalities of periodontal surgery, including the various procedures for treatment of furcation involvements described above, constitute only part of the overall teatment of periodontal disease in a given case. The factor which determines success or failure in the long perspective following surgery is the degree of plaque control that can be obtained and maintained (Hamp et al. 1975, Lindhe & Nyman 1975, 1984, Rosling 1976). Successful treatment requires that all tooth surfaces are properly cleaned during the active phase of treatment and that patients are thereafter enrolled in a profesionally supervised maintenance program including measures which prevent recurrence of the disease (Nyman et al. 1975, Axelsson & Lindhe 1981, Ravald & Hamp 1981, Westfelt et al. 1983, Ravald et al. 1986, Bühler 1988).

Regeneration of furca defects

During the last few years, encouraging results have emerged from extensive research based on the Guided Tissue Regeneration approach (Nyman et al. 1982a,b, Gottlow et al. 1984, 1986, Isidor et al. 1986). The possibility of periodontal tissue regeneration is of particular importance in the treatment of furcation-involved teeth, enabling a more conservative therapeutic approach to be adopted. Recent reports (Pontoriero et al. 1987, 1988) have demonstrated that GTR therapy brings a high rate of success and predictability in the treatment of *Degree 2* furcation involvements of mandibular molars. There is therefore reason to presume that Guided Tissue Regeneration is a potentially superior mode of treatment of furcation-involved teeth. For detailed discussion on new attachment, see Chapter 18.

For further reading on the management of teeth with furcation involvements the reader is referred to publications by Bergenholtz (1972), Klavan (1975), Hirschfeld & Wasserman (1978), Ross & Thompson (1978), Waerhaug (1980), Langer et al. (1981), Newell (1981), Erpenstein (1983), Green (1986), Martin et al. (1986) and Svärdström & Wennström (1988).

References

Axelsson, P. & Lindhe, J. (1981) The significance of maintenance care in the treatment of periodontal disease. *Journal of Clinical Periodontology* **8**, 281-294.

Badersten, A. (1984) Nonsurgical periodontal therapy. *Thesis*. University of Lund, Malmö, Sweden.

Bergenholtz, A. (1972) Radectomy of multirooted teeth. *Journal of the American Dental Association* **85**, 870-875.

Bühler, H. (1988) Evaluation of root-resected teeth. Results after 10 years. *Journal of Periodontology* **59**, 805-810.

Erpenstein, H. (1983) A 3-year study of hemisectioned molars. *Journal of Clinical Periodontology* **10**, 1-10.

Gottlow, J., Nyman, S., Karring, T. & Lindhe, J. (1984) New attachment formation as the result of controlled tissue regeneration. *Journal of Clinical Periodontology* **11**, 494-503.

Gottlow, J., Nyman, S., Lindhe, J., Karring, T. & Wennström, J. (1986) New attachment formation in the human periodontium by guided tissue regeneration. *Journal of Clinical Periodontology* **13**, 604-616.

Green, E.N. (1986) Hemisection and root amputation. *Journal of American Dental Association* **112**, 511-518.

Hamp, S.-E. (1973) On the development and prevention of periodontal disease in the Beagle dog. *Thesis*. University of Göteborg, Göteborg, Sweden.

Hamp, S.-E., Nyman, S. & Lindhe, J. (1975) Periodontal treatment of multirooted teeth. Results after 5 years. *Journal of Clinical Periodontology* **2**, 126-135.

Hirshfeld, L. & Wasserman, B. (1978) A long-term survey of tooth loss in 600 treated periodontal patients. *Journal of Periodontology* **49**, 225-237.

Isidor, F., Karring, T., Nyman, S. & Lindhe, J, (1986) The significance of coronal growth of periodontal ligament tissue for new attachment formation. *Journal of Clinical Periodontology* **13**, 145-150.

Klavan, B. (1975) Clinical observations following

root amputation in maxillary molar teeth. *Journal of Periodontology* **46**, 1-5.

Langer, B., Stein, S.D. & Wagenberg, B. (1981) An evaluation of root resections. A ten-year study. *Journal of Periodontology* **52**, 719-722.

Lindhe, J. & Nyman, S. (1975) The effect of plaque control and surgical pocket elimination on the establishment and maintenance of peridontal health. A longitudinal study of periodontal therapy in cases of advanced disease. *Journal of Clinical Periodontology* **2**, 67-79.

Lindhe, J. & Nyman, S. (1984) Long-term maintenance of patients treated for advanced periodontal disease. *Journal of Clinical Periodontology* **11**, 504-514.

Löe, H. & Silness, J. (1963) Periodontal disease in pregnancy. I. Prevalence and severity. *Acta Odontologica Scandinavica* **21**, 533-551.

Martin, M., Gantes, B., Garret, S. & Egelberg, J. (1988) Treatment of periodontal furcation defects (1). Review of the literature and description of a regenerative surgical technique. *Journal of Clinical Periodontology* **15**, 227-231.

Newell, D.H. (1981) Current status of the management of teeth with furcation invasions. *Journal of Periodontology* **52**, 559-568.

Nyman, S., Rosling, B. & Lindhe, J. (1975) Effect of professional tooth cleaning on healing after periodontal surgery. *Journal of Clinical Periodontology* **2**, 80-86.

Nyman, S., Gottlow, J., Karring, T. & Lindhe, J. (1982a) The regenerative potential of the periodontal ligament. An experimental study in the monkey. *Journal of Clinical Periodontology* **9**, 257-265.

Nyman, S., Lindhe, J., Karring, T. & Rylander, H. (1982b) New attachment following surgical treatment of human periodontal disease. *Journal of Clinical Periodontology* **9**, 290-296.

Pontoriero, R., Nyman, S. & Lindhe, J. (1987) Guided tissue regeneration in the treatment of furcation defects in man. *Journal of Clinical Periodontology* **14**, 618-620.

Pontoriero, R., Lindhe, J., Nyman, S., Karring, T., Rosenberg, E. & Sanavi, F. (1988) Guided tissue regeneration in degree II furcation-involved mandibular molars. A clinical study. *Journal of Clinical Periodontology* **15**, 247-254.

Ravald, N. & Hamp, S.-E. (1981) Prediction of root surface caries in patients treated for advanced periodontal disease. *Journal of Clinical Periodontology* **8**, 400-414.

Ravald, N., Hamp, S.-E. & Birkhed, D. (1986) Long-term evaluation of root surface caries in periodontally treated patients. *Journal of Clinical Periodontology* **13**, 758-767.

Rosling, B. (1976) Plaque control. A determining factor in the treatment of periodontal disease. *Thesis*. University of Göteborg, Göteborg, Sweden.

Ross, I.F. & Thompson, R.H. (1978) A long-term study of root retention in the treatment of maxillary molars with furcation involvement. *Journal of Periodontology* **49**, 238-244.

Silness, J. & Löe, H. (1964) Periodontal disease in pregnancy. II. Correlation between oral hygiene and periodontal condition. *Acta Odontologica Scandinavica* **22**, 121-135.

Svärdström, G. & Wennström, J.L. (1988) Furcation topography of the maxillary and mandibular first molars. *Journal of Clinical Periodontology* **15**, 271-275.

Waerhaug, J. (1980) The furcation problem. Etiology, pathogenesis, diagnosis, therapy and prognosis. *Journal of Clinical Periodontology* **7**, 73-95.

Westfelt, E. (1984) Effect of periodontal therapy. *Thesis*. University of Göteborg, Göteborg, Sweden.

Westfelt, E., Nyman, S., Socransky, S. & Lindhe, J. (1983) Significance of frequency of professional tooth cleaning for healing following periodontal surgery. *Journal of Clinical Periodontology* **10**, 148-156.

CHAPTER 21

Occlusal Therapy

Clinical symptoms of trauma from occlusion

Angular bony defect

It has been claimed that *angular bony defects* and *increased tooth mobility* are important symptoms of trauma from occlusion (Glickman 1965, 1967). The validity of this suggestion has, however, been questioned (see Chapter 8). Angular bony defects have been found at teeth affected by *trauma from occlusion* as well as at teeth with normal occlusal function (Waerhaug 1979). *This means that the presence of angular bony defects cannot* per se *be regarded as an exclusive symptom of trauma from occlusion.*

Increased tooth mobility

Increased tooth mobility, determined clinically, is expressed in terms of amplitude of displacement of the crown of the tooth. Increased tooth mobility can, indeed, be observed in conjunction with *trauma from occlusion.* It may, however, also be the result of a reduction of the height of the alveolar bone with or without an accompanying angular bony defect caused by plaque-associated periodontal disease (see Chapter 8). Increased tooth mobility resulting from occlusal interferences may further indicate that the periodontal structures have become adapted to an altered functional demand, i.e. a widened periodontal ligament with a normal tissue composition has become the end result of a previous phase of progressive tooth mobility (see Chapter 8) associated with trauma from occlusion.

Progressive (increasing) tooth mobility

In Chapter 8, it was concluded that the diagnosis trauma from occlusion should be used

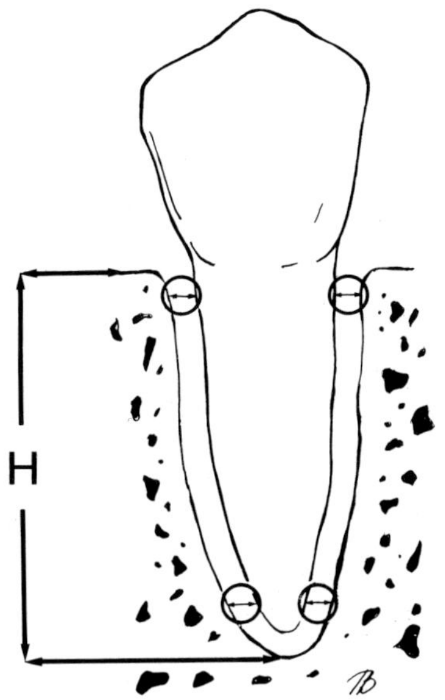

Fig. 21-1. The mobility of a tooth in horizontal direction is dependent on the height of the alveolar bone (H), the width of the periodontal ligament (encirled arrows) and the shape and number of roots.

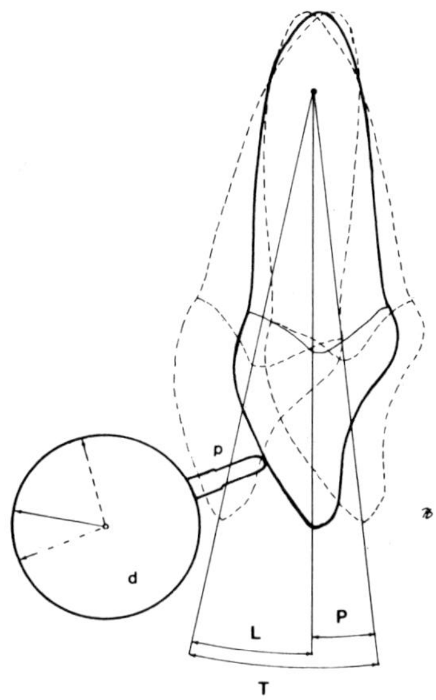

Fig. 21-2. Tooth mobility measurements by means of the Periodontometer. d: dial indicator, p: pointer. L: labial excursion of the crown, P: palatal excursion of the crown, T = L+P: total excursion of the crown.

solely in situations where a progressive mobility could be observed. Progressive tooth mobility can be identified only through a series of repeated tooth mobility measurements carried out over a period of several days or weeks.

Tooth mobility crown excursion/root displacement

Initial and secondary tooth mobility

A tooth which is surrounded by a normal periodontium may be moved (displaced) in horizontal and vertical directions and may in addition be forced to perform limited rotational movements. Clinically, tooth mobility is usually assessed by exposing the crown of the tooth to a certain force and determining the distance the crown can be displaced in buccal and/or lingual direction. The mobility (= movability) of a tooth in a horizontal direction is closely dependent on the height of the surrounding supporting bone, the width of the periodontal ligament as well as the shape and number of roots present (Fig. 21-1).

The mechanism of tooth mobility was studied in detail by Mühlemann (1954, 1960) who described a standardized method for measuring even minor tooth displacements. By means of the "Periodontometer" a small force (~100 pounds) is applied to the crown of a tooth (Fig. 21-2). The crown starts to tip in the direction of the force. The resistance of the tooth-supporting structures against displacement of the root is low in the initial phase of force application and the crown is moved only 5/100-10/100 mm. This movement of the tooth was called *"initial" tooth mobility-ITM"* by Mühlemann (1954) and is the result of an *intraalveolar* displacement of the root (Fig. 21-3). In the pressure zone (see Chapter 8) there is a 10% reduction in the width of the periodontal ligament

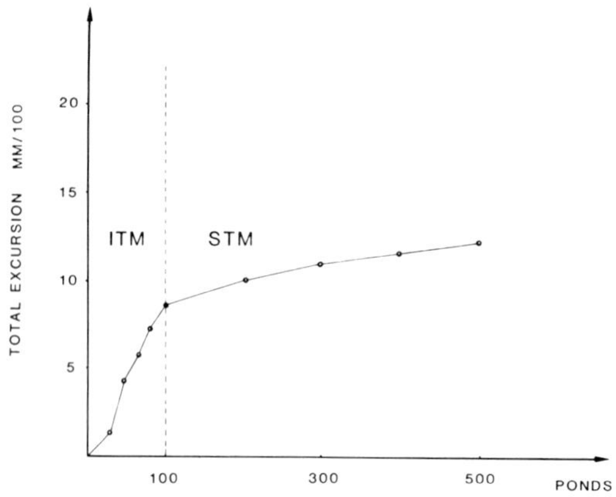

Fig. 21-3. Initial tooth mobility (ITM) means the excursion of the crown of a tooth when a force of 100 ponds is applied to the crown. Secondary tooth mobility (STM) means the excursion of the crown of the tooth when a force of 500 ponds is applied.

and in the tension zone there is a corresponding increase. Mühlemann & Zander (1954) stated that "there are good reasons to assume that the initial displacement of the root *(initial-TM)* corresponds to a reorientation of the periodontal membrane fibers into a position of functional readiness towards tensile strength". The magnitude of the *"initial-TM"* varies from individual to individual, from tooth to tooth, and is mainly dependent on the structure and organization of the periodontal ligament. The *"initial-TM"* value of ankylosed teeth is therefore zero.

When a larger force (~ 500 pounds) is applied to the crown, the fiber bundles on the tension side can not offer sufficient resistance to further root displacement. The additional displacement of the crown that is observed in *"secondary tooth mobility-secondary-TM"* (Fig. 21-3) is allowed by distortion and compression of the periodontium in the pressure side. According to Mühlemann (1960) the magnitude of *"secondary-TM"*, i.e. the excursion of the crown of the tooth when a force of 500 pounds is applied, 1) varies between different types of teeth (e.g. incisors 10-12/100 mm, canines 5-9/100 mm, premolars 8-10/100 mm and molars 4-8/100 mm), 2) is larger in children than in adults, 3) is larger in females than males and increases during e.g. pregnancy. Furthermore, tooth mobility seems to vary during the course of the day; the lowest value is found in the evening and the largest in the morning.

Clinical assessment of tooth mobility (Physiologic and pathologic tooth mobility)

If, in the traditional clinical measurement of tooth mobility, a comparatively large force is placed on the crown of a tooth surrounded by a normal periodontium, the tooth will tip within its alveolus until a closer contact has been established between the root and the marginal (or apical) bone tissue. The magnitude of this tipping movement, which is normally assessed using the tip of the crown as a reference point, is referred to as the *"physiologic"* tooth mobility. The term *"physiologic"* implies that *"pathologic"* tooth mobility may also occur.

What then is "pathologic" tooth mobility?

1. If a similar force is applied to a tooth which is surrounded by a periodontal ligament with an increased width, the excursion of the crown in horizontal direction will become increased; the clinical measurement consequently demonstrates that the tooth has an increased mobility. Should this increased mobility be regarded as *"pathologic"*?
2. An increased tooth mobility, i.e. an increased displacement of the crown of the tooth after force application can also be found in situations where the height of the alveolar bone has been reduced but the remaining periodontal ligament has a normal width. At sites where this type of bone loss is extensive the degree of tooth mobility (i.e. excursion of the crown) may be pronounced. Should this increased tooth mobility be regarded as "pathologic"? Fig. 21-

4b illustrates a tooth which is surrounded by alveolar bone of reduced height. The width of the remaining periodontal ligament, however, is within normal limits. A horizontally directed force applied to the crown of the tooth will in this case result in a larger excursion of the crown than if a similar force is applied to a tooth with normal height of the alveolar bone and normal width of the periodontal ligament (Fig. 21-4a.). There are reasons to suggest that the *so-called increased mobility* measured in the case of Fig. 21-4b is, indeed, *"physiologic"*. The validity of this statement can easily be demonstrated if the displacement of the 2 teeth is assessed not from the crown but from a point on the root at the level of the bone crest. If a horizontal force is directed to the teeth as indicated in Figs. 21-4a,b the reference points (*) on the root surfaces will be displaced a similar distance in both instances. *Obviously it is not the length of the excursive movement of the crown that is important from a biologic point of view, but the displacement of the root within its remaining periodontal ligament.*

In plaque-associated periodontal disease bone loss is a prominent feature. Another so-called classical symptom of periodontitis is "increased tooth mobility". It is important to realize, however, that in many situations with even or horizontal bone loss, the increased crown displacement (tooth mobility) which is assessed in clinical measurements should, according to the above discussion, also be regarded as physiologic; the movement of the root within the space of its remaining "normal" periodontal ligament is normal.

3. Increased crown displacement (tooth mobility) may also be detected in a clinical measurement where a "horizontal" force is applied to teeth with angular bony defects and/or increased width of the periodontal ligament. If this mobility is not gradually increasing - from one observation time to the next - the root is surrounded by a periodontal ligament of increased width but normal composition. Also this mobility should be considered as *"physiologic"* since the movement is a function of the height of the alveolar bone and the width of the periodontal ligament.

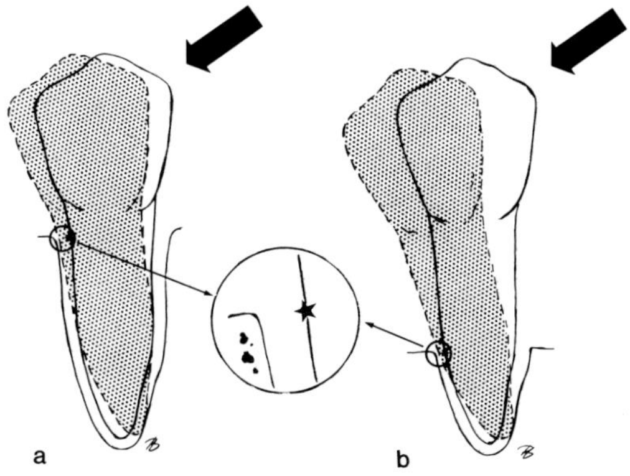

Figs. 21-4a, b. (a) illustrates the normal "physiologic" mobility of a tooth with normal height of the alveolar bone and normal width of the periodontal ligament but reduced height of the alveolar bone. It should be observed that the distance of the horizontal displacement of the reference point (*) on the roots is the same in the two situations.

4. Only *progressively increasing tooth mobility* which occurs during trauma from occlusion and which is characterized by active bone resorption (see Chapter 8) and which indicates the presence of inflammatory alterations within the periodontal ligament tissue, may be considered *"pathologic"* .

Treatment of increased tooth mobility

A number of situations will be described below which may call for treatment aimed at reducing an increased tooth mobility .

Situation I

Increased mobility of a tooth with increased

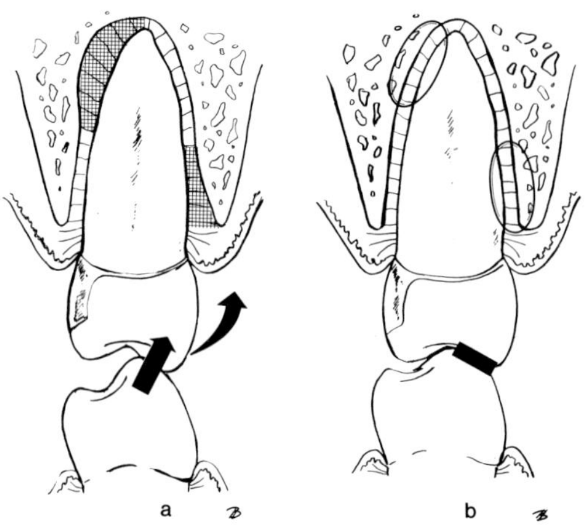

Figs. 21-5a, b. (a) illustrates the contact relationship between a mandibular and a maxillary premolar in occlusion. The maxillary premolar is fitted with an artificial restoration with an improperly designed occlusal surface. Occlusion results in horizontally-directed forces which may produce an undue stress concentration within the encircled areas of the periodontium of the maxillary tooth. Resorption of the alveolar bone occurs in these areas. A widening of the periodontal ligament can be detected as well as increased mobility of the tooth. Following adjustment of the occlusion the horizontal forces are reduced. This results in bone apposition and a normalization of the tooth mobility (b).

width of the periodontal ligament but normal height of the alveolar bone

If a tooth (for instance a maxillary premolar) is fitted with an improper filling or crown restoration, occlusal interferences develop and the surrounding periodontal tissues become the seat of inflammatory reactions, i.e. trauma from occlusion (Fig. 21-5). If the restoration is so designed that the crown of the tooth in occlusion is subjected to undue forces directed in a buccal direction, bone resorption phenomena develop in the buccal-marginal and lingual-apical pressure zones with a resulting increase of the width of the periodontal ligament in these zones. The tooth becomes hypermobile or moves away from the "traumatizing" position. Since such traumatizing forces in teeth with normal periodontium or overt gingivitis cannot result in pocket formation or loss of connective tissue attachment, the resulting increased mobility of the tooth should be regarded as a physiologic adaptation of the periodontal tissues to the altered functional demands. A proper correction of the anatomy of the occlusal surface of such a tooth, i.e. occlusal adjustment, will normalize the relationship between the antagonizing teeth in occlusion, thereby eliminating the excessive forces. As a result apposition of bone will occur in the zones previously exposed to resorption, the width of the periodontal ligament will become normalized and the tooth stabilized, i.e. it reassumes its normal mobility (Fig. 21-5). In other words, resorption of alveolar bone which is caused by trauma from occlusion is a reversible process which can be treated by the elimination of occlusal interferences.

The capacity for bone regeneration after resorption following trauma from occlusion has been documented in a number of animal experiments (Waerhaug & Randers-Hansen 1966, Polson et al. 1976a, Karring et al. 1982, Nyman et al. 1982). In such experiments, the induced bone resorption not only involved the bone within the alveolus but also the alveolar bone crest. When the traumatizing forces were removed, bone tissue was deposited not only in the walls of the alveolus, thereby normalizing the width of the periodontal ligament, but also on the bone crest area whereby the height of the alveolar bone was normalized (Fig. 21-6; Polson et al. 1976a). In the presence of an untreated, plaque-associated lesion in the soft tissue, however, substantial bone regrowth did not always occur (Fig. 21-7; Polson et al. 1976b) .

Situation II

Increased mobility of a tooth with increased width of the periodontal ligament and reduced height of the alveolar bone

When a dentition has been properly treated for plaque-associated periodontal disease, gingival health is established in areas of the dentition

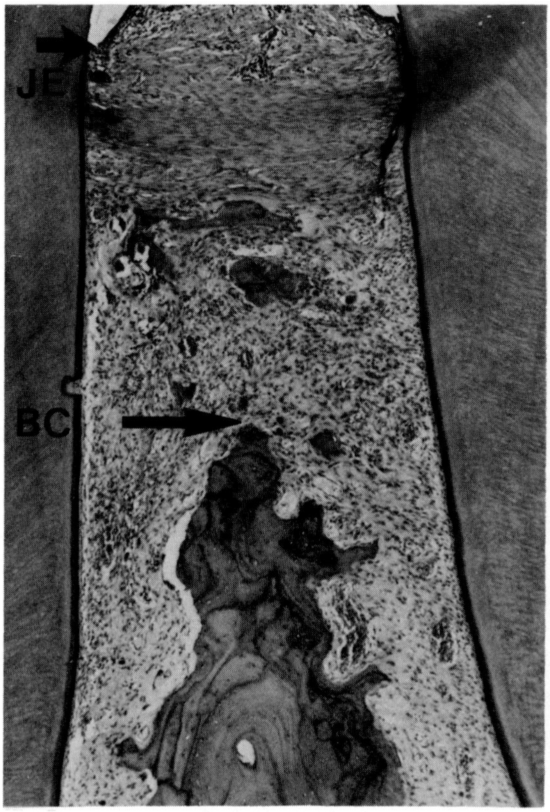

Fig. 21-6a.

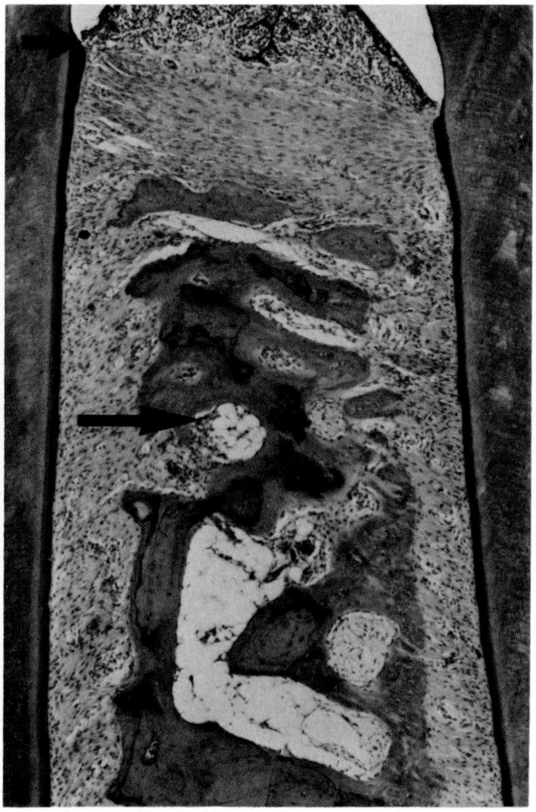

Fig. 21-6b.

Figs. 21-6a, b. Photomicrograph illustrating the interdental area between 2 mandibular premolars in the monkey. In (a) the 2 premolars are exposed to jiggling forces. Note the reduction of alveolar bone in the area and the location of the bone crest (arrow;BC). Ten weeks after the elimination of the jiggling forces (b) a considerable regeneration of bone has occurred. Note the increase of the height of the interdental bone and the normalization of the width of the periodontal ligaments. The apical end of the junctional epithelium (JE) is located at the cementoenamel junction. (Courtesy of Dr. Polson; from Polson et al. 1976a.)

where teeth are surrounded by periodontal structures of reduced height. If a tooth with a reduced periodontal tissue support is exposed to excessive horizontal forces (trauma from occlusion), inflammatory reactions develop in the pressure zones of the periodontal ligament with

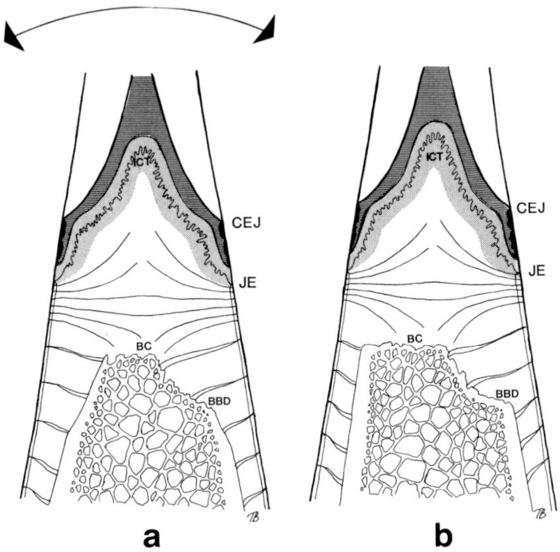

Figs. 21-7a, b. In the presence of an existing marginal inflammation, alveolar bone, lost by jiggling trauma (a), will not always regenerate following elimination of the traumatic forces (b). ICT: infiltrated connective tissue; CEJ: cementoenamel junction; JE: apical end of junctional epithelium; BC: alveolar bone crest; BBD: bottom of angular bony defect (From Polson et al. 1976b).

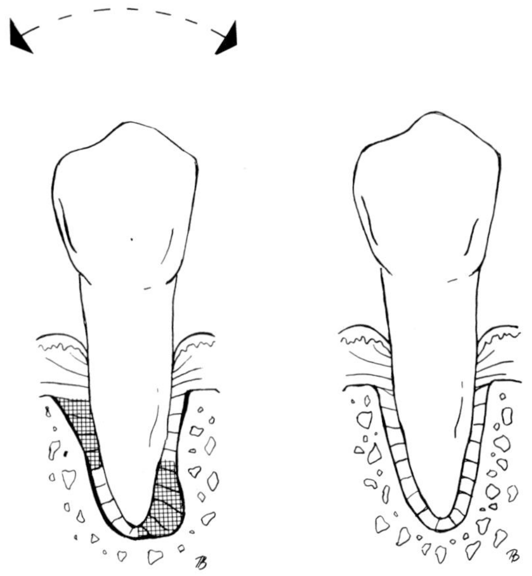

Figs. 21-8a, b. If a tooth with reduced periodontal tissue support (a) has been exposed to excessive horizontal forces a widened periodontal ligament space (encircled areas) and increased mobility (arrow) results. Following reduction or elimination of such forces bone apposition will occur and the tooth will become stabilized (b).

accompanying bone resorption. These alterations are similar to those which occur around a tooth with normal height of the supporting structures; the alveolar bone is resorbed, the width of the periodontal ligament is increased in the pressure/tension zones and the tooth becomes hypermobile (Fig. 21-8a). If the excessive forces are reduced or eliminated by occlusal adjustment, bone apposition to the "pre-trauma" level will occur, the periodontal ligament will regain its normal width and the tooth will become stabilized (Fig. 21-8b).

Conclusion: Situations I and II

Occlusal adjustment is an effective therapy against increased tooth mobility when such mobility is caused by an *increased width* of the periodontal ligament.

Situation III

Increased mobility of a tooth with reduced height of the alveolar bone and normal width of the periodontal ligament

The increased tooth mobility which is the result of a reduction in height of the alveolar bone without a concomitant increase in width of the periodontal membrane cannot be reduced or eliminated by occlusal adjustment since, in teeth with normal width of the periodontal ligament, no further bone apposition on the walls of the alveoli can occur. If such an increased tooth mobility does not interfere with the patient's chewing function or comfort no treatment is required. If the patient experiences the tooth mobility as disturbing, however, the mobility can in this situation be reduced only by splinting, i.e. by joining the mobile tooth/teeth together with other teeth in the jaw into a fixed unit-a SPLINT.

A SPLINT is according to the Glossary of Periodontic Terms (American Academy of Periodontology 1986) "an appliance designed to stabilize mobile teeth". A splint can be fabricated in the form of joined composite fillings, fixed bridges, removable partial prostheses, etc.

Example: Case A, 64-year-old male

The periodontal condition of this patient is illustrated by the probing depth, furcation involvement and tooth mobility data as well as the radiographs from the initial examination in Fig. 21-9. Periodontal disease has progressed to a level where, around the maxillary teeth, only the apical third or less of the roots are invested in supporting alveolar bone. The following discussion is related to the treatment of the maxillary dentition:

In the treatment planning of this case it was decided that the first premolars (teeth 14 and 24) had to be extracted due to advanced periodontal disease and furcation involvement of Degree 3. For the same reasons teeth 17 and 27 were scheduled for extraction. Also 16 and 26

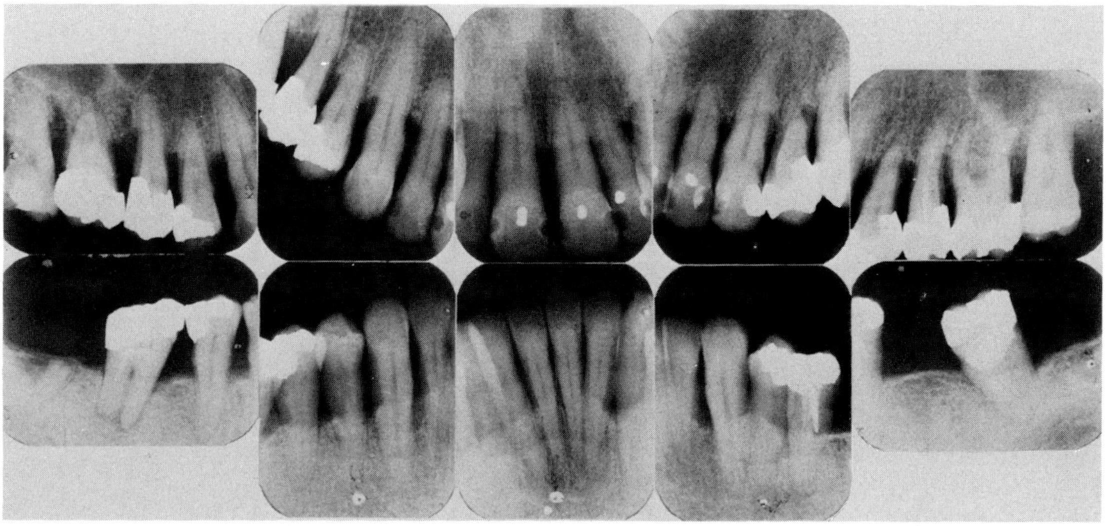

Fig. 21-9. Case A, 64-year-old male. Periodontal status and radiographs prior to therapy.

were found to have advanced loss of periodontal tissue support in combination with deep furcation involvements. The most likely *definitive* treatment should include periodontal and adjunctive therapy in the following parts of the dentition: 15 and 25, and 13, 12, 11, 21, 22, 23. For functional and esthetic reasons, obviously 14 and 24 had to be replaced. The question now arose as to whether these 2 premolars should be replaced by 2 separate unilateral bridges, using 13, 15 and 23, 25 as abutment teeth, or if the increased mobility of these teeth and also of the anterior teeth (12, 11, 21, 22; Fig. 21-9) called for a bridge of cross-arch design with the extension 15-25 to obtain a splinting effect. If 14 and 24 are replaced by 2 unilateral bridges, each one of these 3-unit bridges will exhibit the same degree of mobility in buccolingual direction as the individual abutment teeth (degree 2: Fig. 21-9), since a unilateral straight bridge will not have a stabilizing effect on the abutment teeth in this force direction.

From the radiographs it can be seen that the increased mobility observed in the maxillary teeth of this patient is associated mainly with reduced height of the alveolar bone and not with increased width of the periodontal liga-

Periodontal chart

Tooth	Pocket depth M	B	D	L	Furcation involvement	Tooth mobility
~~18~~						
17	6	6	8	8	b2, m2, d1	
16	6	6	8	8	m1, d2	2
15	8	4	6	7		2
14	7	4	7	4	3	2
13	8	4	8	4		2
12	8	4	8	4		2
11	6	4	7	4		1
21	6	4	6	4		1
22	6	5	7			2
23	6		6	4		2
24	7		8		3	2
25	6	8	8	4		2
26	8		6		b2, m2, d2	
27	6	6	10	8	b2, d2	1
~~28~~						
~~48~~						
~~47~~						
46	8	6	6	7	b1, l2	
45	6		7	4		1
44	6		6	4		
43	7	7	6	4		
42	4		4	4		1
41	6	4				1
31	6					1
32	4		6	4		1
33	6		6	6		2
34	4		7	4		
35	7		4	6		2
~~36~~						
37	8	5	6	4	b2, l1	3
~~38~~						

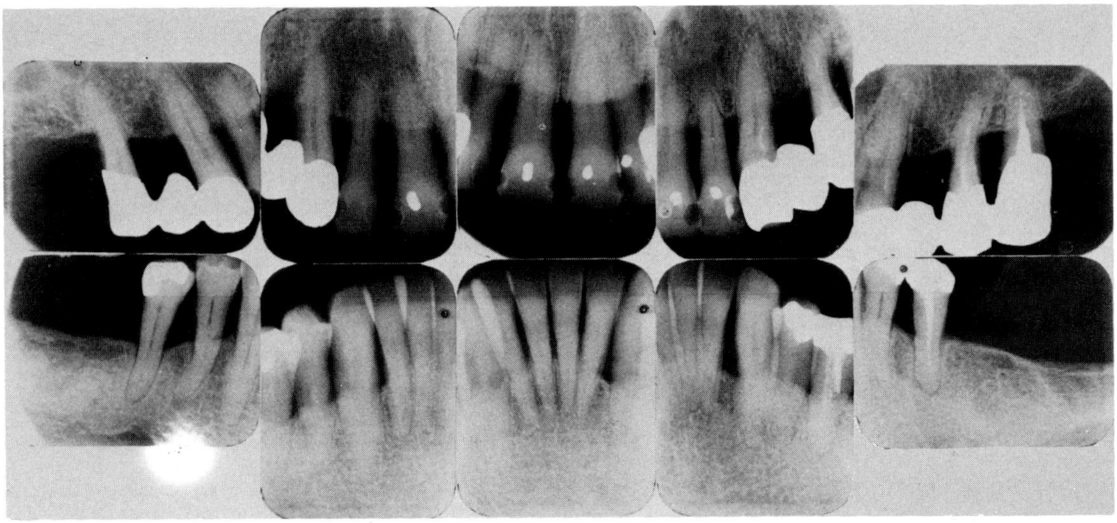

Fig. 21-10. Case A. Radiographs obtained 10 years after periodontal therapy and installation of 2 unilateral bridges in the maxilla.

ments. This means that the mobility of the individual teeth should be regarded as normal or "physiologic" for teeth with such a reduced height of the supporting tissues. This in turn implies that the increased tooth mobility in the present case does not call for treatment unless it interferes with the chewing comfort or jeopardizes the position of the front teeth. This particular patient had not recognized any functional problems related to the increased mobility of his maxillary teeth. Consequently there, was no reason to install a cross-arch bridge in order to splint the teeth, i.e. to reduce tooth mobility.

Following proper treatment of the plaque-associated periodontal lesions, 2 separate provisional bridges of unilateral design were produced (15, 14, 13; 23, 24, 25, 26 palatal root). The provisional acrylic bridges were used for 6 months during which the occlusion, the mobility of the 2 bridges and the position of the front teeth were all carefully monitored. When, after 6 months, no change of position of the lateral and central incisors had occurred and no increase of the mobility of the 2 provisional bridges had been noted, the definitive restorative therapy was performed.

Fig. 21-10 presents radiographs obtained 10 years after initial therapy. The position of the front teeth and the mobility of the incisors and the 2 bridges have not changed during the course of the maintenance period. There has been no further loss of periodontal tissue support during the 10 years of observation, no further spread of the front teeth and no widening of the periodontal ligaments around the individual teeth, including the abutment teeth for the bridgework.

Conclusion: Situation III

Increased tooth mobility (or bridge mobility) as a result of reduced height of the alveolar bone can be accepted and splinting avoided, provided the occlusion is stable (no further migration or further increasing mobility of individual teeth), and provided the degree of mobility existing does not disturb the patient's chewing ability or comfort. Consequently: splinting is indicated when the mobility of a tooth or a group of teeth is so increased that chewing ability and/or comfort are disturbed.

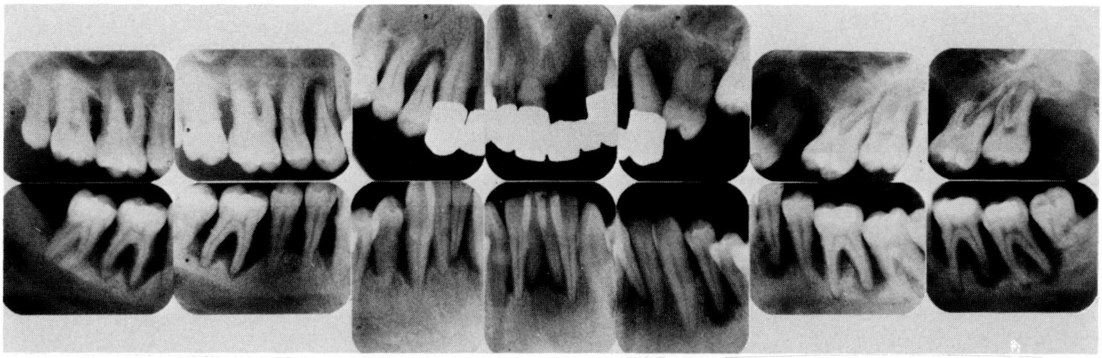

Fig. 21-11. Case B, 26-year-old male. Radiographs illustrating the periodontal conditions prior to therapy.

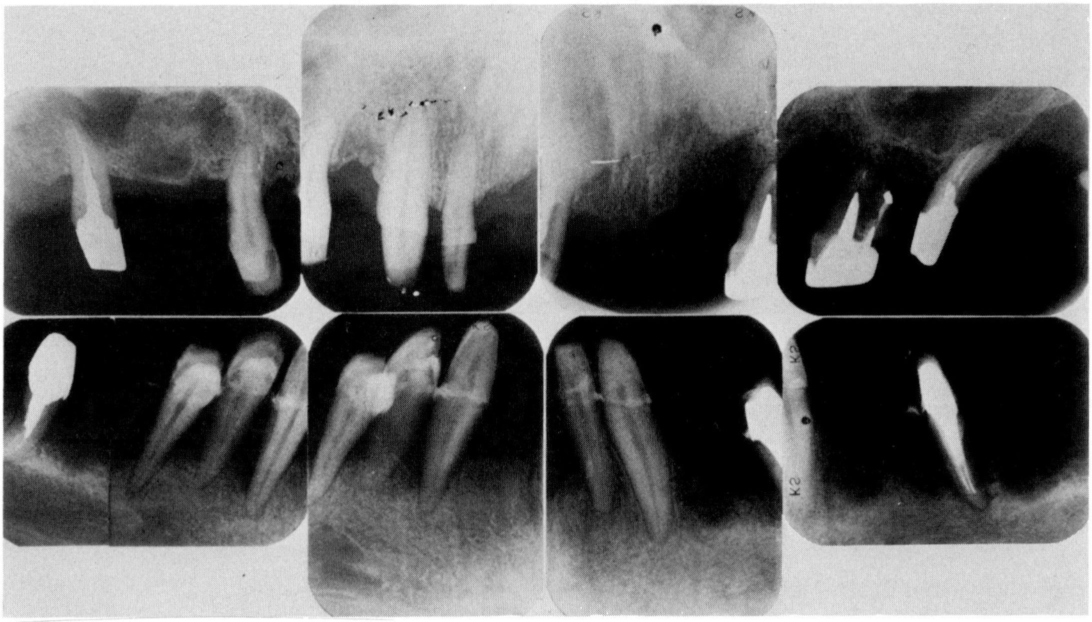

Fig. 21-12. Case B. Radiographs obtained after periodontal treatment and preparation of the abutment teeth for 2 fixed splints.

Situation IV

Progressive (increasing) mobility of a tooth (teeth) as a result of gradually increasing width of the periodontal ligament in teeth with a reduced height of the alveolar bone

Often in cases of advanced periodontal disease the tissue destruction may have reached a level where extraction of one or several teeth cannot be avoided. Teeth which in such a dentition are still available for periodontal treatment may, after therapy, exhibit such a high degree of mobility - or even signs of progressively increasing mobility - that there is an obvious risk that the forces elicited during function may mechanically disrupt the remaining periodontal ligament components and cause extraction of the teeth. Only by means of a splint will it be possible to maintain such teeth. In such cases a fixed splint has 2 objectives: namely 1) to stabilize hypermobile teeth and 2) to replace missing teeth.

Example: Case B, 26-year-old male

Fig. 21-11 Presents radiographs taken prior to therapy and Fig. 21-12 those obtained after

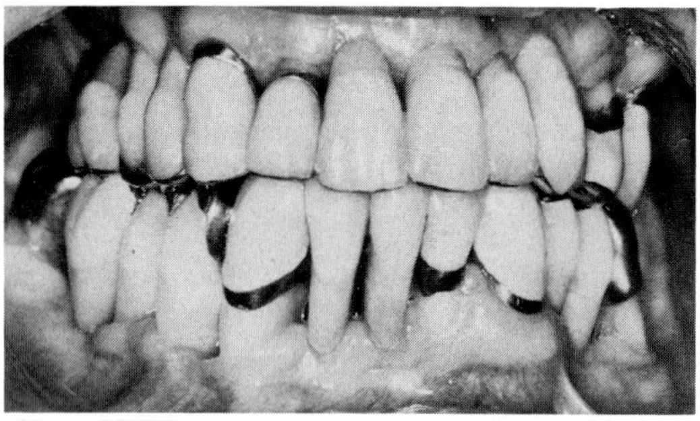

Fig. 21-13a.

Fig. 21-13a-c. Case B. Clinical status 9 years after therapy.

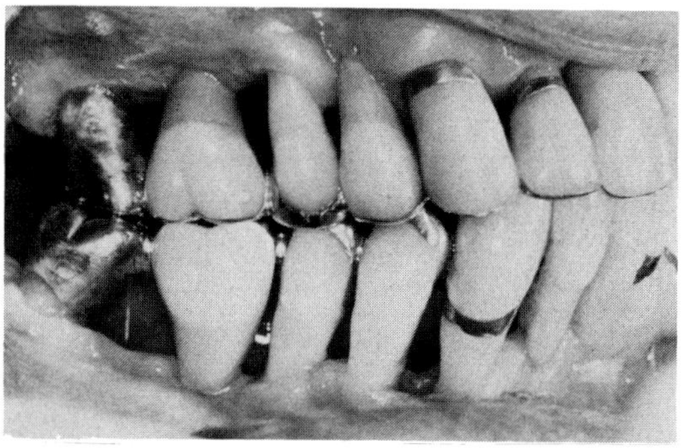

Fig. 21-13b.

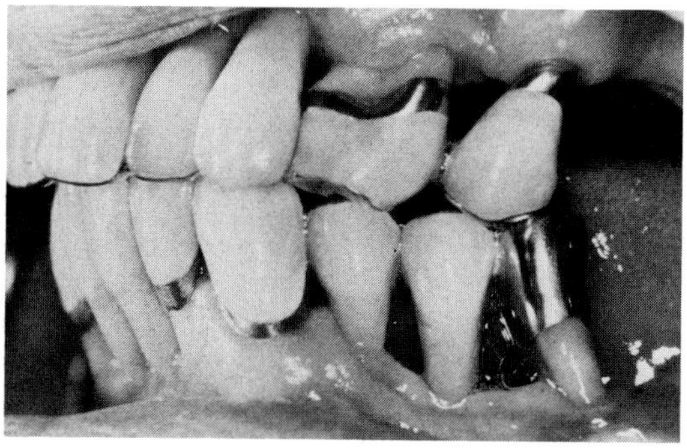

Fig. 21-13c.

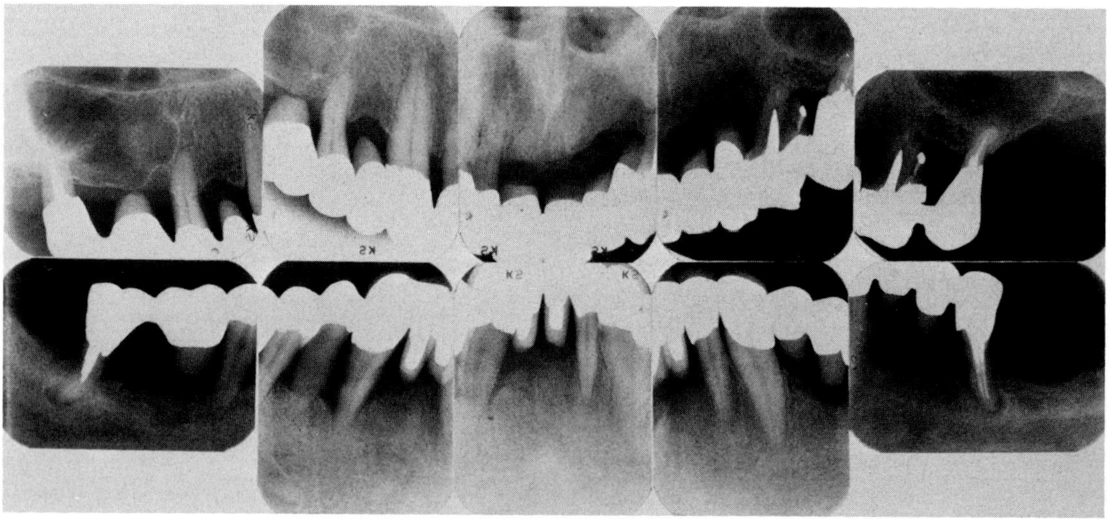

Fig. 21-14. Case B. Radiographs obtained 10 years after therapy.

periodontal treatment and preparation of the remaining teeth as abutments for 2 fixed splints. All teeth except 13,12 and 33 have lost around 75% or more of the alveolar bone and widened periodontal ligaments are a frequent finding. The 4 distal abutments for the 2 splints are root-separated molars, the maintained roots being the following: the palatal root of 17, the mesio-buccal root of 26 and the mesial roots of 36 and 47. It should be observed that tooth 24

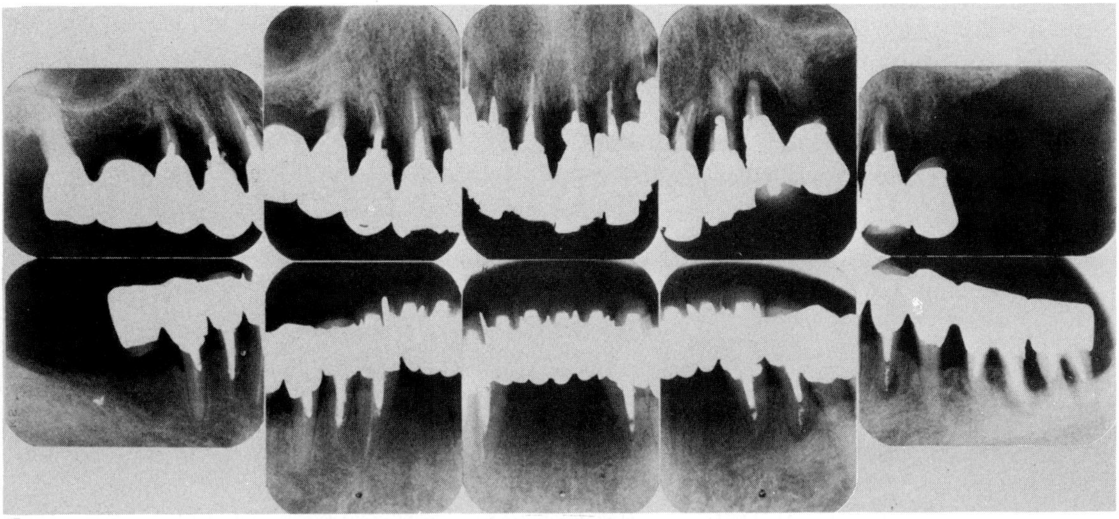

Fig. 21-15. Case C, 52-year-old female. Radiographs obtained at the initial examination.

is root-separated and the palatal root maintained with only minute amounts of periodontium left. Immediately prior to insertion of the 2 splints all teeth except 13, 12 and 33 displayed a mobility varying between Degrees 1 and 3. From the radiographs in Fig. 21-12 it can be noted that there is an obvious risk of extraction of a number of teeth such as 24, 26, 47, 45, 44, 43 and 36, if the patient is allowed to bite with a normal chewing force without the splints in position.

Despite the high degree of mobility of the individual teeth, the splints were, after insertion, entirely stable and have maintained their stability during a maintenance period of more than 12 years. Figs. 21-13a,b,c describe the clinical status and Fig. 21-14 presents the radiographs obtained 10 years after therapy. From these radiographs it can be observed (compare with Fig. 21-12) that during the maintenance period there has been no further loss of alveolar bone or widening of the various periodontal ligament spaces.

Conclusion: Situation IV

Splinting is indicated when the periodontal support is so reduced that the mobility of the teeth is progressively increasing, i.e. when a tooth or a group of teeth during function are exposed to extraction forces.

Situation V

Increased bridge mobility despite splinting

In patient with advanced periodontal disease it can often be observed that the destruction of the periodontium has progressed to varying levels around different teeth and tooth surfaces in the dentition. Following proper treatment of the plaque-associated lesions, often including multiple extractions, the remaining teeth may not only display an extreme reduction of the supporting tissues concomitantly with increased or progressive tooth mobility, but they may also be distributed in the jaw in such a way as to make it difficult, or impossible, to obtain a proper splinting effect even by means of a cross-arch bridge. The entire bridge/splint may exhibit mobility in frontal and or lateral directions.

It was stated above (Situation III) that a certain mobility of a tooth or a bridge of unilateral design can be accepted provided this mobility does not interfere with the patient's chewing

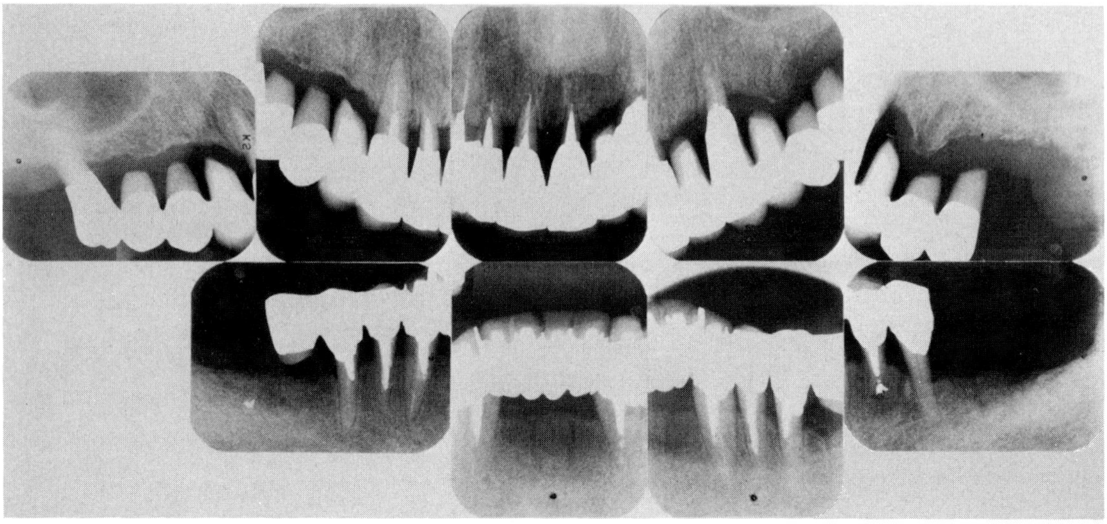

Fig. 21-16. Case C. Radiographs obtained 5 years after therapy.

ability or comfort. This is also valid for a cross-arch bridge/splint. From a biologic point of view there is no difference between increased tooth mobility on the one hand and increased bridge mobility on the other. However, neither progressive tooth mobility nor progressive bridge mobility can be accepted. In cases of extremely advanced periodontal disease a cross-arch splint with an increased mobility may be regarded as an acceptable result of rehabilitation. The maintenance of status quo of the bridge/splint mobility and the prevention of tipping or orthodontic displacement of the total splint, however, requires particular attention regarding the design of the occlusion. Below, a case is reported which may serve as an interesting illustration of this particular clinical problem.

Example: Case C, 52-year-old female

Fig. 21-15 shows radiographs obtained at the initial examination. A 12-unit maxillary bridge was installed 10-15 years prior to the present examination using 18, 15, 14, 13, 12, 11, 21, 22, 23 and 24 as abutments. After a detailed clinical examination it was obvious that 15, 14, 22 and 24 could not be maintained because of severe symptoms of caries and periodontal disease. The remaining teeth were subjected to periodontal therapy and maintained as abutments for a new bridge/splint in the maxilla extending from tooth 18 to the region of 26, i.e. a cross-arch splint was installled which carried 3 cantilever units namely 24, 25 and 26. The mobility of the individual abutment teeth immediately prior to insertion of the splint was the following: Degree 1 (tooth 18), Degree 0 (tooth 13), Degree 2 (teeth 12 and 11), Degree 3 (tooth 21) and Degree 2 (tooth 23).

Radiographs obtained 5 years after therapy are shown in Fig. 21-16. The bridge/splint had a mobility of Degree 1 immediately after its insertion and this mobility was unchanged 5 years later. The radiographs demonstrate that no further widening of the periodontal ligament has occurred around the individual teeth during the maintenance period.

When a cross-arch bridge/splint exhibits increased mobility the center (fulcrum) of the movement must be identified. In order to prevent further increase of the mobility and/or to prevent displacement of the bridge it is essential to design the occlusion in such a way that the bridge/ splint, when in contact with the teeth of the opposing jaw, is subjected to a balanced load, i.e. equal force on each side of the fulcrum. If this can be achieved the force to which the bridge is exposed in occlusion can be used to retain the fixed prosthesis in proper balance (further increase of the mobility being thereby prevented).

Balanced loading of a mobile bridge/splint has to be established not only in the intercuspal position (IP) and centric occlusion (CP) but also in frontal and lateral excursive movements of the mandible, if the bridge shows mobility or a tendency for tipping in the direction of such movements. In other words, a force which tends to displace the bridge in a certain direction has to be counteracted by the introduction of a balancing force on the opposite side of the fulcrum of the movement. If, for instance, a cross-arch splint in the maxilla exhibits mobility in frontal direction in conjunction with protrusive movements of the mandible, the load applied to the bridge in the frontal region has to be counterbalanced by a load in the distal portions of the splint; this means that there must be a simultaneous and equal contact relationship between the occluding teeth in both the frontal and the posterior regions of the splint. If the splint is mobile in a lateral direction, the force acting on the working side of the jaw must be counteracted by a force established by the introduction of balancing contacts in the non-working side of the jaw. The principle for establishing stability of a mobile cross-arch splint is consequently the same as that used to obtain stability in a complete denture. In situations where distal abutment teeth are missing in a cross-arch bridge/splint with increased mobility, balance and functional stability may be obtained by means of cantilever units. It is important in this context to point out that balancing contacts on the nonworking side should not be introduced in a bridge/splint in which no increased mobility can be observed.

The maxillary splint in the patient described in Figs. 21-13 to 21-16 exhibited increased mobility in frontal direction. Considering the small amount of periodontal support left around the anterior teeth, it is obvious that there would have been a risk of frontal displacement of the total bridge, had the bridge terminated at the last abutment tooth (23) on the left side of the jaw. The installation of cantilever units in the 24 and 25 region prevented such a displacement of the bridge/splint by the introduction of a force counteracting against frontally directed forces during protrusive movements of the mandible (Fig. 21-17). In addition, the cantilever units provide bilateral contact relationship towards the mandibular teeth in the intercuspal position, i.e. bilateral stability of the bridge.

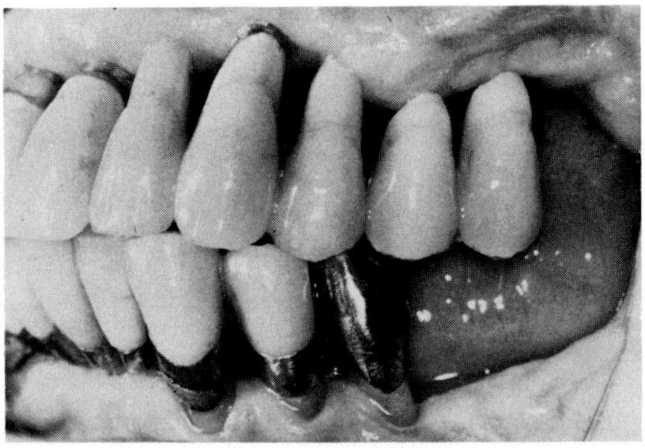

Fig. 21-17. Case C. The cantilever section including teeth 24, 25 and 26.

In cases similar to the one described above, cantilever units can thus be used to prevent increasing mobility or displacement of a bridge/splint. It should, however, be pointed out that the insertion of cantilever units increases the risk of failures of a technical and biophysical character (fracture of the metal frame, fracture of abutment teeth, loss of retention, etc). For details regarding the technical aspects of fixed bridgework in patients with advanced periodontal disease, see Chapter 22.

In cases of severely advanced periodontal disease it is often impossible to anticipate in the planning phase whether a bridge/splint after insertion will show signs of instability and increasing (Progressive) mobility. In such cases a provisional splint should always be inserted. Any alterations of the mobility of the bridge/splint can be observed over a prolonged period of time and the occlusion continuously adjusted until, after 4-6 months, it is known whether stability (i.e. no further increase of the mobility) can be achieved. The design of the occlusion of the provisional acrylic bridge is then reproduced in the permanent bridge construction. If, on the other hand stability cannot be obtained, the rehabilitation of the case cannot be achieved with a fixed splint. The alternative treatment then is a complete denture.

Conclusion: Situation V

An increased mobility of a cross-arch bridge/ splint can be accepted provided the mobility does not disturb chewing ability or comfort and the mobility of the splint is not progressively increasing.

References

Glickman, I. (1965) Clinical significance of trauma from occlusion. *Journal of the American Dental Association* **70**, 607-618.

Glickman, I. (1967) Occlusion and periodontium. *Journal of Dental Research* **46**, Supplement, 53

Glossary of Periodontic Terms (1986) *Journal of Periodontology*. Supplement.

Karring, T., Nyman, S., Thilander, B. & Magnusson, I. (1982) Boneregeneration in orthodontically produced alveolar bone dehiscenes. *Journal of Periodontal Research* **17**, 309-315.

Muhlemann, H.R. (1954) Tooth mobility. The measuring method. Initial and secondary tooth mobility. *Journal of Periodontology* **25**, 22-29.

Muhlemann, H.R. (1960) Ten years of tooth mobility measurements. *Journal of Periodontology* **31**, 110-122.

Muhlemann, H.R. & Zander, H.A. (1954) Tooth mobility, III. The mechanism of tooth mobility. *Journal of Periodontology* **25** 128.

Nyman, S., Karring, T., Bergenholtz, G. (1982) Bone regeneration in alveolar bone dehiscences produced by jiggling forces. *Journal of Periodontal Research* **17**, 316-322.

Polson, A.M., Meitner, S.W. & Zander, H.A. (1976a) Trauma and progression of marginal periodontitis in squirrel monkeys. III Adaptation of interproximal alveolar bone to repetitive injury. *Journal of Periodontal Research* **11**, 279-289.

Polson, A.M., Meitner, S.W. & Zander, H.A. (1976b) Trauma and progression of marginal periodontitis in squirrel monkeys. IV. Reversibility of bone loss due to trauma alone and trauma superimposed upon periodontitis. *Journal of Periodontal Research* **11**, 290-298.

Waerhaug, J. (1979) The infrabony pocket and its relationship to trauma from occlusion and subgingival plaque. *Journal of Periodontology* **50**, 355-365

Waerhaug, J. & Randers-Hansen, E. (1966) Periodontal changes incident to prolonged occlusal overload in monkeys. *Acta Odontologica Scandinavica* **24**, 91-105.

CHAPTER 22

Technical and Biophysical Aspects of Crown and Bridge Therapy

Often in cases of advanced periodontal disease the destruction of the supporting tissues, in one or more parts of the dentition, has progressed to a level which calls for extraction of several teeth (Fig. 22-1). Following treatment of such cases only a few teeth may remain, teeth which not only have a minimum of periodontal tissue support left, but which also frequently show signs of markedly increased mobility. In such cases there is an obvious need for prosthetic treatment in order to 1) restore lost function, 2) improve esthetics and 3) stabilize mobile teeth. The principles of periodontal treatment and the biological rationale for splinting in the treatment of periodontitis are discussed in Chapters 13, 14 and 21.

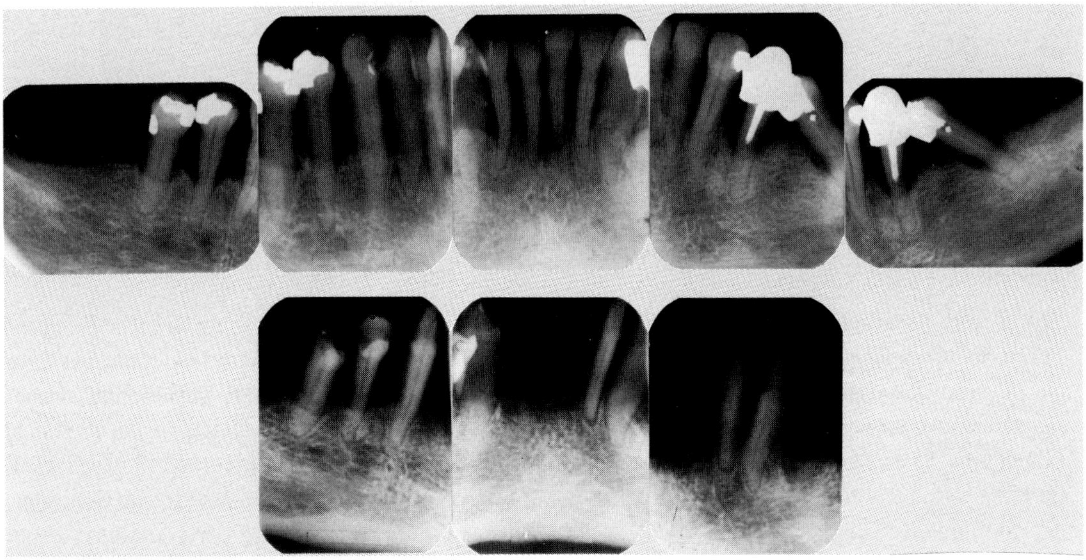

Fig. 22-1. Radiographs illustrating periodontal conditions before (top) and after (bottom) treatment of advanced periodontal disease. The remaining teeth have reduced periodontal tissue support.

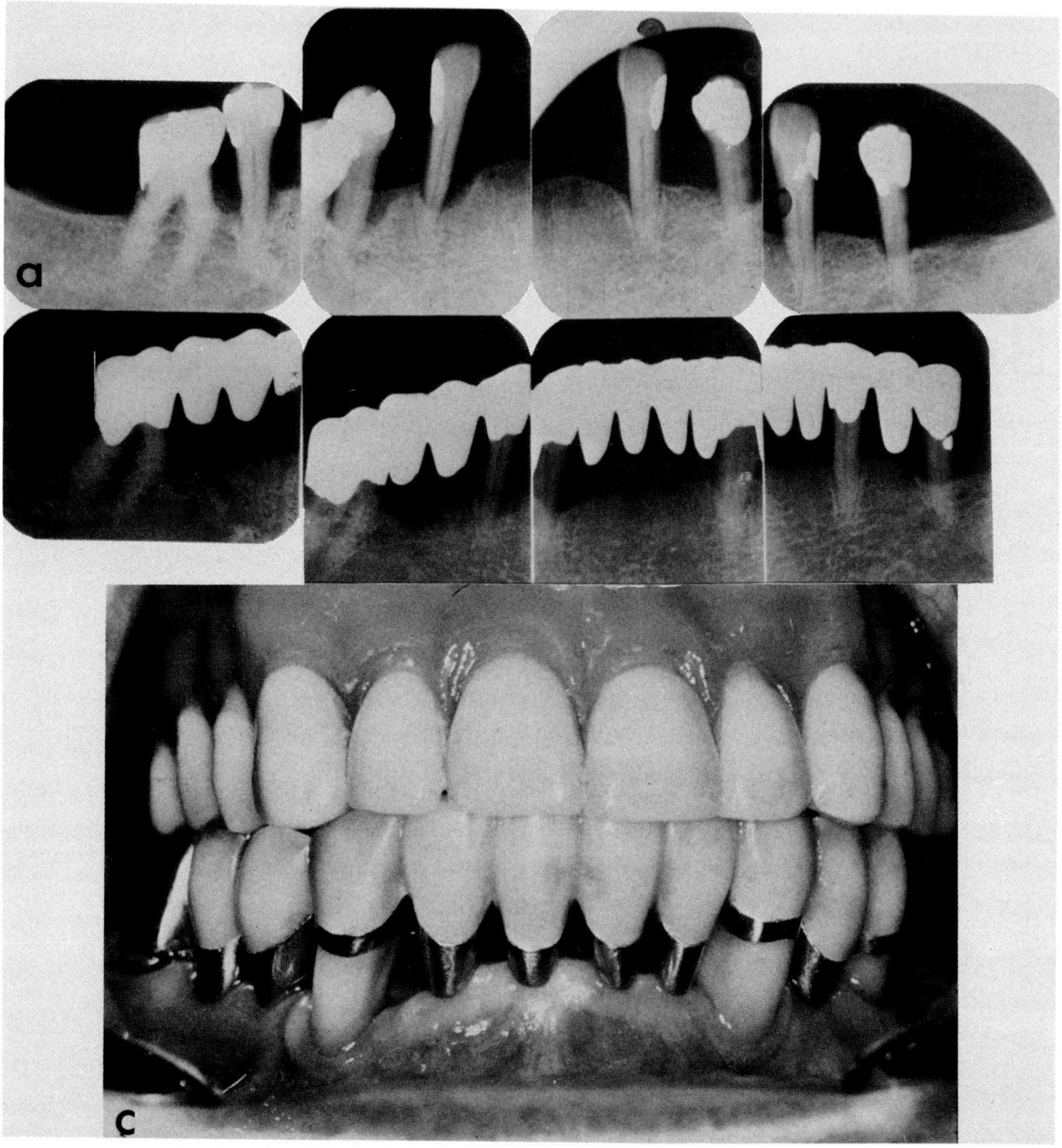

Figs. 22-2a, b, c. Radiographs of a patient with advanced loss of the periodontal tissues (a) before and (b) after combined periodontal and prosthetic treatment. The clinical status 5 years after treatment is shown in (c).

As a rule, in patients with pronounced loss of periodontal support, fixed bridges are preferable to removable partial dentures (Fig. 22-2). In contrast to removable partial dentures, fixed bridges provide a degree of rigidity and a more favorable force distribution to the remaining periodontium (see Chapter 21).

Recently published long-term results of combined periodontal and prosthetic treatment have shown that the limiting criteria for fixed bridgework in patients with few abutment teeth and reduced, but healthy, periodontal tissues around these teeth are related to the technical and biophysical factors involved in the fabrication of the bridges rather than to the biological capacity of the remaining periodontium to support the bridges successfully (Nyman & Lindhe 1979, Nyman & Ericsson 1982, Randow et al.

1986). The results showed in fact that it was possible in such patients to prevent recurrence of gingivitis of clinical importance and to arrest further progression of periodontal tissue breakdown by proper periodontal treatment and the institution of a carefully designed postoperative plaque control program. No abutment teeth were lost in these patients as the result of recurrence of periodontal disease during the observation period of more than 10 years. However, technical failures did occur. These failures were caused 1) by loss of retention of retainers, 2) fracture of metal components and 3) fracture of abutment teeth. A further analysis revealed that the fundamental principles regarding design and construction of bridgework had often been overlooked in the unsuccessful prostheses. These principles will be discussed in detail in this chapter.

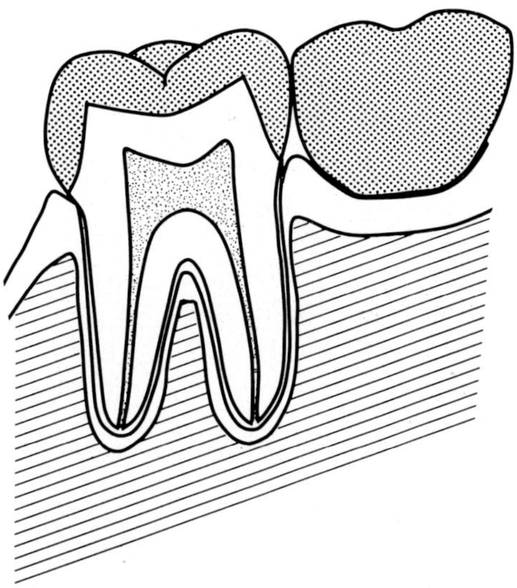

Fig. 22-3. A bridge construction includes not only the metal component and the veneer material of the prosthesis but also the cementing agent, the abutment teeth, the periodontal ligaments and the supporting alveolar bone.

General principles

The basic principles for constructing fixed bridges for patients with few available abutments and reduced periodontal tissue support do not differ from those for patients with many available abutments. The clinical and technical difficulties are, however, more pronounced. Some technical and biophysical factors are discussed here, factors which *per se* have universal applicability in all bridge treatment, but which are of utmost importance when restoring peridontally weak dentitions with fixed bridgework.

It should be emphasized first that the term "bridge" or "bridge construction" is not restricted to the metal component and the veneer material (Fig. 22-3), but refers also to the cementing agent, abutment teeth, the periodontal ligaments and the supporting alveolar bone.

In any object (e.g. a bridge construction) exposed to loading, transferred forces will create stress (~ force/surface area) which in turn causes strain (Fig. 22-4). It is a fundamental requirement of a bridge construction that in none of the components (i.e. the metal frame, the veneer material, the cementing agent, the abutment teeth, the periodontal ligaments and the alveolar bone) must strain reach such levels during function that permanent deformation or fractures occur. In this context it should be recognized that the different components of a bridge construction have different physical properties. The periodontal ligament and, to a

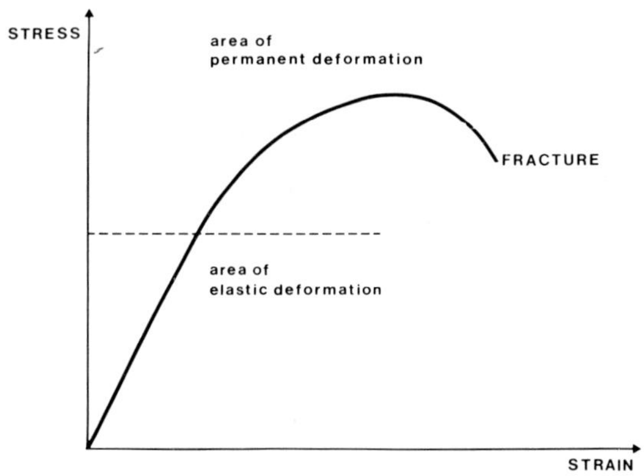

Fig. 22-4. In any object exposed to loading, the created stress will cause strain in the form of elastic/plastic deformation or fracture.

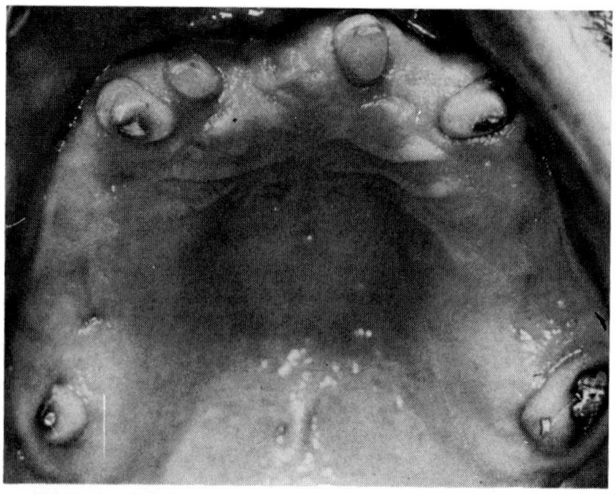

Figs. 22-5, 22-6. The magnitudes of loading forces, the proper dimensions of the prosthesis and the threshold values for permanent deformation of the various components of a prosthetic appliance depend on the individual design and extension of the prosthesis and on the distribution of the abutments.

⇐ Fig. 22-5.

Fig. 22-6. ⇓

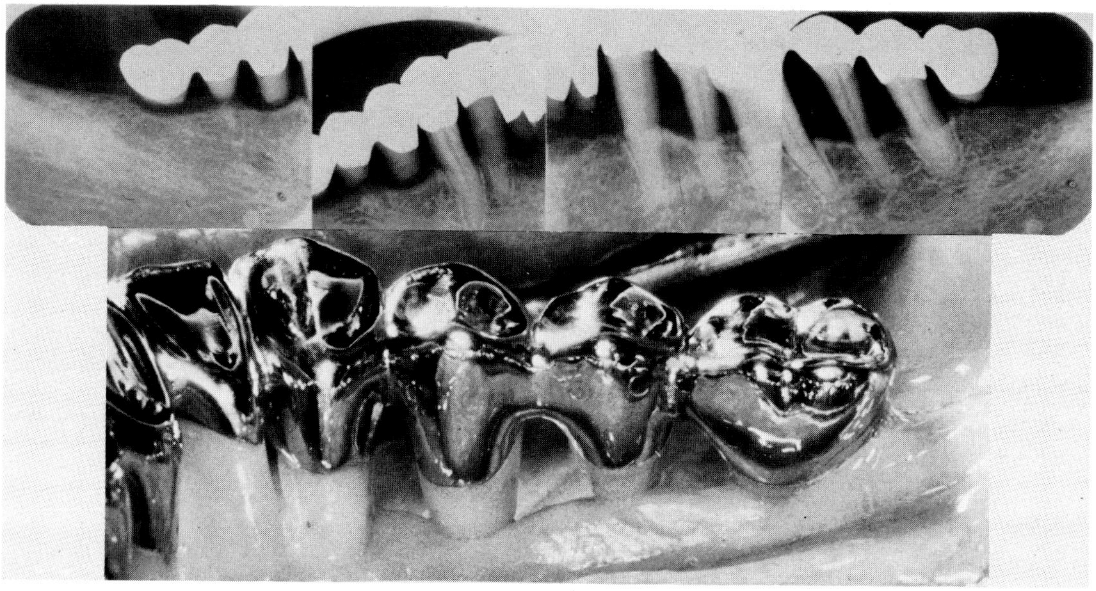

certain degree the alveolar bone, are elastic tissues with good ability to withstand and distribute forces, thereby reducing the risk of adverse stress concentration. On the other hand, dental alloys, ceramics and cementing agents are materials which can withstand only limited amounts of strain without exhibiting permanent deformation or fracture.

To prevent failures of a technical and biophysical nature in fixed bridgework it is mandatory to locate and define the dimension and shape of each component of a bridge (abutments, cementing agents, retainers, pontics, solderings, etc.) in such a way that not even maximum stress will result in unfavorable strain in any part of the construction. Few available abutments, unfavorably distributed in relation to the extent of the bridge, make it difficult to avoid permanent deformation or fracture. It should be understood, however, that within a bridge construction there are the mechanoreceptors of the periodontal ligaments and the alveolar bone, which possess a controlling effect on the load induced by the masticatory muscles (Hannam 1976). This, in turn, implies that all other bridge components must be located and designed in such a way that they do not exhibit permanent deformation before the mechanoreceptors are activated. The function of the mechanoreceptors is also stress-depend-

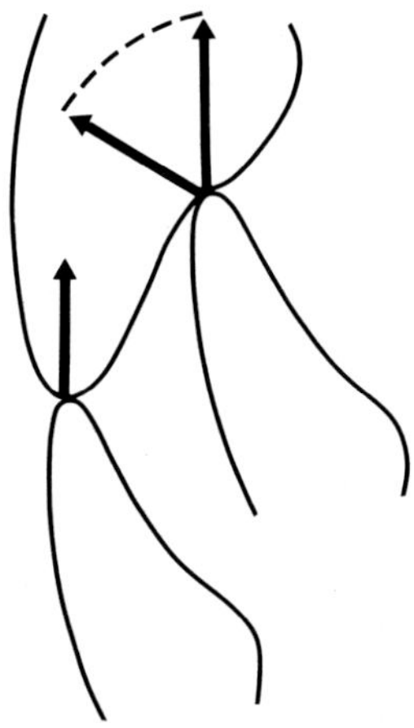

Fig. 22-7. In dentitions with deep vertical overlap the horizontal forces elicited during function are higher than in dentitions with shallow horizontal overlap.

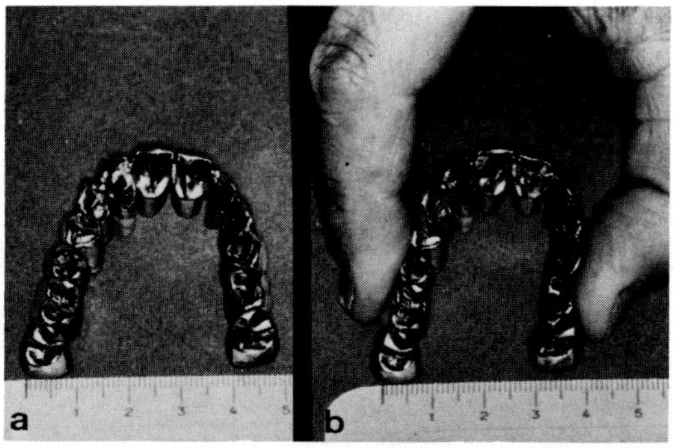

Fig. 22-8. A 13-unit bridge which, evidently, has insufficient rigidity for lateral loading.

ent and there is experimental support for the hypothesis that the threshold level of the mechanoreceptor function is lower in teeth with reduced periodontal tissue support than in teeth with normal height of the supporting apparatus (Lundgren et al. 1975) and lower in vital teeth (Randow & Glantz 1986). This is an advantage when a fixed bridge is made for a patient with vital teeth with reduced periodontal tissue support since it facilitates the possibilities to give the various components of the bridge sufficient dimensions. Consequently, what can be accomplished in extensive fixed bridges for periodontally involved patients does not apply directly to "normal" patients (Randow et al. 1986). It is also important to realize that the threshold level for the mechanoreceptor function is not definite but can be changed, e.g. through adaption (Öwall & Möller 1974, Goldberg 1976). Therefore, the gap between the threshold for receptor function and permanent deformation of the other bridge components (prosthetic materials, abutment teeth etc.) should be kept wide. In other words, all other physical components (i.e. prosthetic materials, abutment teeth, etc.) must be capable of withstanding more load than the periodontal tissues.

Depending on the individual design, extension and distribution of abutment teeth, for each bridgework no formula exists for the relationship between the magnitude of loading forces, the dimensions of the prosthesis and the threshold values for permanent deformation of the various bridge components (Figs. 22-5, 22-6). When relevant model systems are used, it can be demonstrated that deformation can be kept within tolerable limits by reducing the length of pontic segments, particularly cantilever segments, and by giving all components sufficient height in all directions of loading which occur during function (Timoshenko & Goodier 1970).

When, as a consequence of a reduced number of available abutment teeth, long pontic spans cannot be avoided or when cantilever must be used to obtain stability of a mobile bridge (see Chapter 21), the increased stress produced by the pontics must be compensated for by a sufficient increase of the height of the prosthesis in the directions of loading (Lindhe & Nyman 1977). Also in this respect the periodontally involved patient offers advantages over the "normal " patient. Resorption of alveolar bone provides abutment teeth with long clinical crowns and a wide distance between the alveolar crest of edentulous areas and the occlusal surfaces of opposing teeth.

To secure a proper design for bridge construction, all functional loading directions must

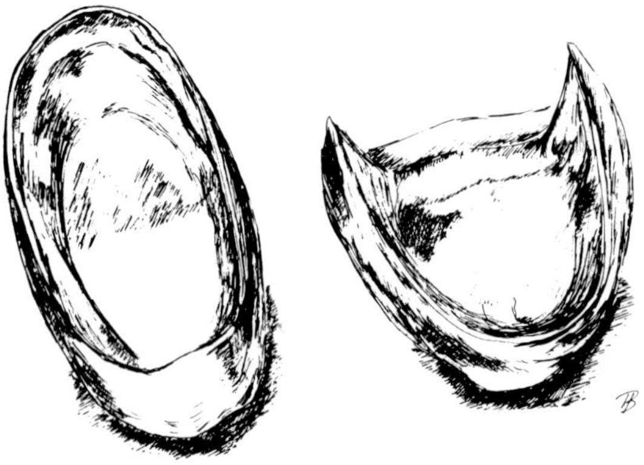

Fig. 22-9. A complete crown has a higher degree of rigidity than a partial crown.

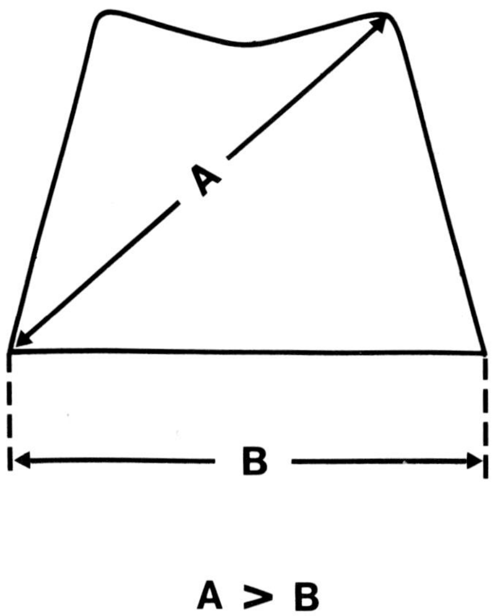

Fig. 22-10. A complete crown obtains "self retention" to the prepared tooth if the length of the diagonal of the prepared portion of the tooth (A) exceeds the diameter of its base (B).

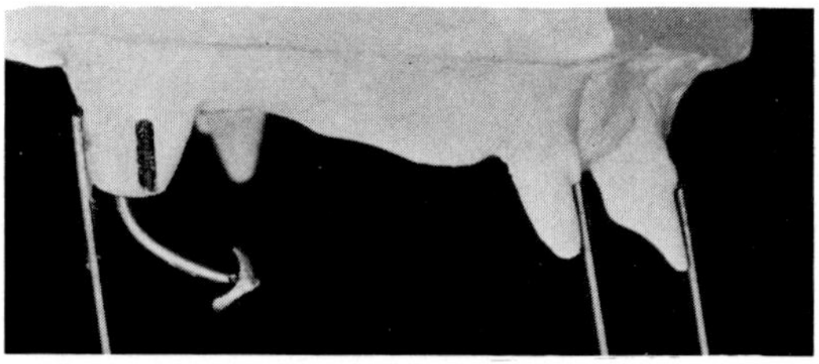

Fig. 22-11. Model of a case in which abutment teeth have been prepared for a maxillary fixed prosthesis. Protrusive contact movements will produce occlusoanteriorly directed forces on the distal abutment.

be carefully analyzed. For example in a dentition with a deep vertical overlap (Fig. 22-7), the horizontal forces acting on the maxillary teeth during function are large. The horizontal dimensions of the prosthesis must receive special attention to secure rigidity. If rigidity is not obtained in such a case, sooner or later fracture will occur in one or the other of the bridge components (Randow et al. 1986) (Fig. 22-8).

Selection of retainer crowns

Partial crowns such as inlays, pin-ledges and 3/4 crowns often give good esthetic results particularly when the buccal tooth surfaces are intact. It is well known, however, that the rigidity of an intact tube, such as a complete crown, is much higher than that of a tube with a longitudinal opening (Timoshenko & Goodier 1970). This means that, in comparison to a complete crown, a partial veneer crown has less resistance to deformation. Therefore, complete crowns are preferable as retainers in dentitions with few abutments related to the extension of the bridge (Fig. 22-9).

Preparation design

A fundamental demand, when preparing a tooth for a complete crown, is to ensure "self retention" against horizontally directed forces; that is, strength of the cement film must not be the sole retentive factor. This demand is met by preparing the abutment teeth with maximum height and minimum taper (Fig. 22-10). *The length of any diagonal of the prepared tooth must exceed the diameter of its base* (for discussion see Hegdahl & Silness 1977).

Fig. 22-11 illustrates a maxilla in which a bridge with a cross-arch design is to be inserted. Assuming that "normal" horizontal and vertical overlaps exist, protrusive movements will produce a force in occlusoanterior direction (arrow, Fig. 22-11) operating on the distal abutment. A dislodging effect of such a force can be prevented if the distal surface of the molar is prepared parallel to the mesial and distal surfaces of the canine and the labial and lingual surfaces of the incisor. In addition, the direction of insertion should have a distal angulation in relation to the direction of the dislocating force. To further improve the retention, boxes or grooves which are parallel to the distal surface of the molar can be prepared in the *buccal* (and/or the *lingual*) surfaces.

If a molar abutment tooth has tilted mesially it may no longer be possible, with slice preparation, to obtain parallelism between its distal surface and the opposite surfaces of the front teeth (Fig. 22-12). If this is the case, the distal surface of the molar can often be made parallel to the labial surfaces of anterior teeth by a shoulder preparation. To secure proper retention against laterally dislocating forces, the buccal and lingual surfaces of premolars and molars on each side of the jaw must be parallel to each other and to the proximal surfaces of anterior teeth, if present (Fig. 22-13). If boxes or grooves are added to increase retention they should be prepared on the *proximal* surfaces of posterior teeth.

Pins parallel to the path of insertion and/or horizontal pins can improve retention of cast restorations. Pins can also be used in abutments where the diameter of the base of the preparation is longer than the diagonals. However, pin retention should only be used in a tooth with thick dentine (Fig. 22-14); otherwise, there is an obvious risk of dentine fracture with subsequent loss of retention.

Following periodontal treatment, the remaining teeth may exhibit different degrees of mobility. When these teeth are used as abutments, the most stable tooth (arrow, Fig. 22-15) will act as the fulcrum for rotational and dislocating movements. The establishment of proper retention for this retainer is of critical importance. Therefore, maximum height of the clinical

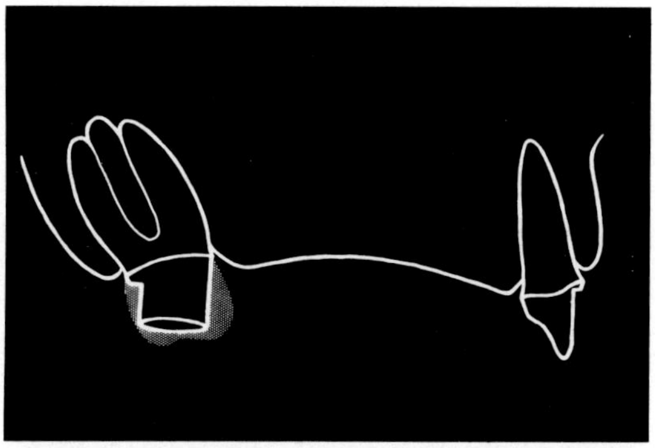

Fig. 22-12. Schematic drawing of a case with a mesially tilted molar abutment. When preparing this tooth the distal surface can be made parallel to the labial surface of the canine by a shoulder preparation.

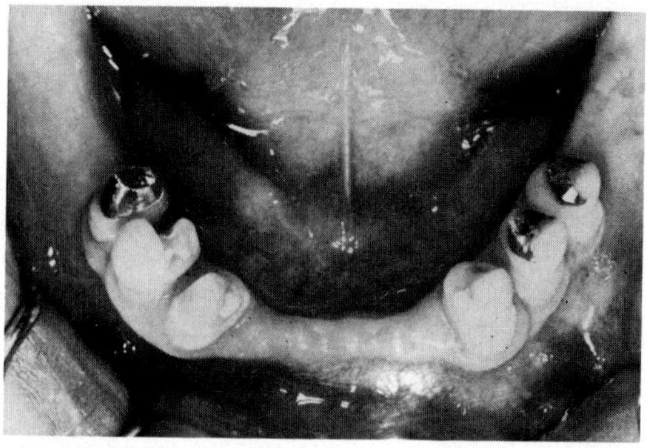

Fig. 22-13. Preparations for a fixed mandibular prosthesis demonstrating how proper retention against dislocating forces in lateral excursion has been secured by preparing the buccal and lingual surfaces of the teeth on each side of the jaw parallel to one another.

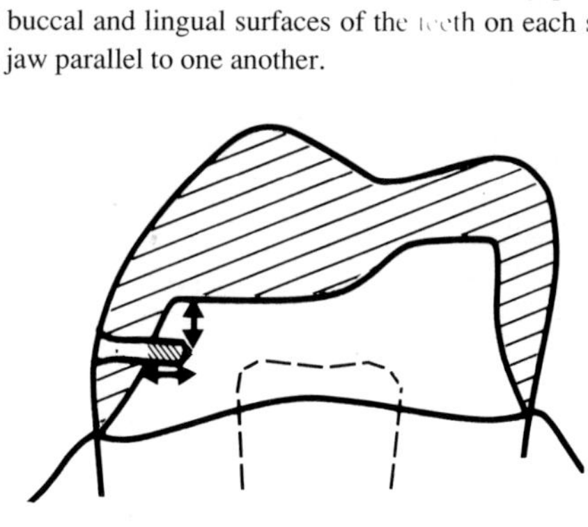

Fig. 22-14. Horizontal pins may be inserted into the preparation to improve retention. Note that the pin is surrounded by a comparatively thick layer of dentine.

crown should be used when the tooth is prepared. In addition, boxes or grooves may be

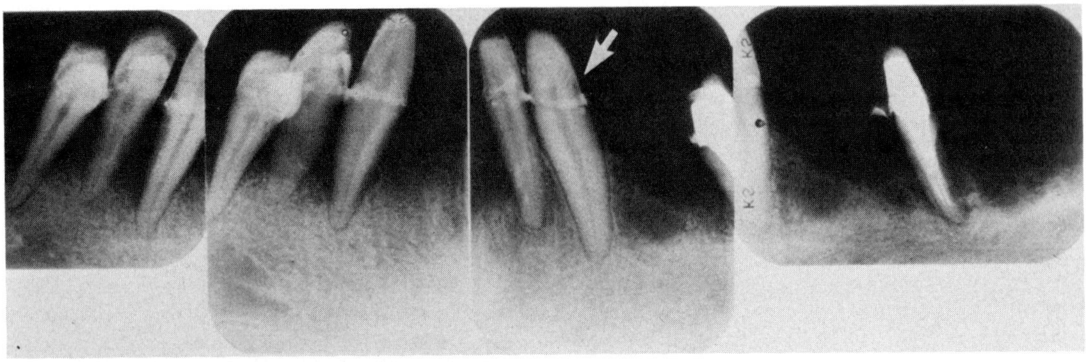

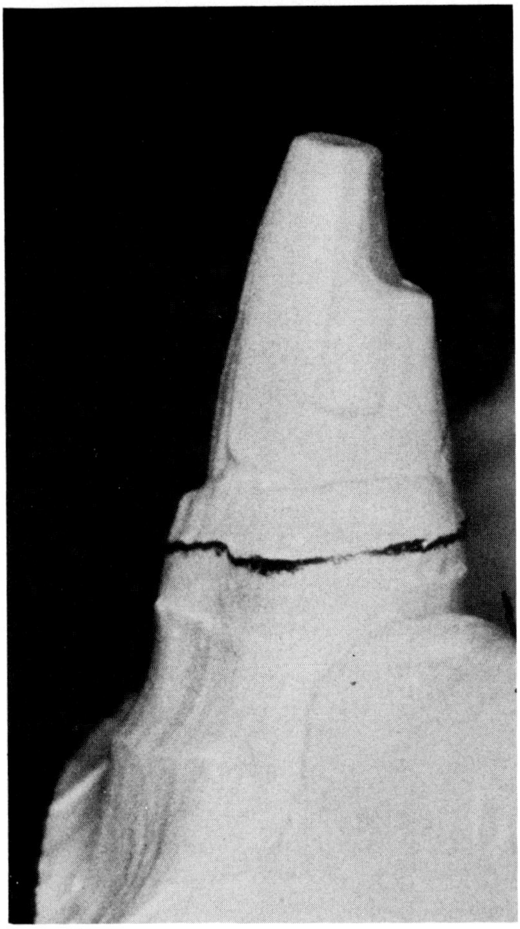

⇐ Fig. 22-16. Fig. 22-15. ⇑

Figs. 22-15, 22-16. Radiogram of a mandibular dentition with retainers exhibiting different degrees of mobility. The most stable retainer (arrow, Fig. 22-15) will act as a fulcrum for dislocating movements. On this retainer optimal retention was established during preparation by using 1) maximum height of the clinical crown and 2) including vertical grooves (Fig. 22-16).

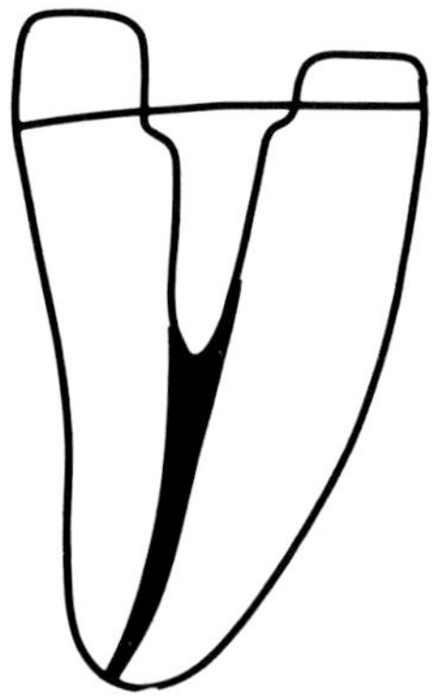

Fig. 22-17. Preparation for insertion of a dowel. The root canal and circumferential bevel are prepared with low angles of convergence.

prepared to further improve retention (Fig. 22-16).

The same demands on parallelism that apply to the design of core preparations must also be met when preparing root canals for insertion of dowels (Fig. 22-17). The root canal and the circumferential bevel should be prepared with as low an angle of convergence as possible.

In summary: if the preparations are given low

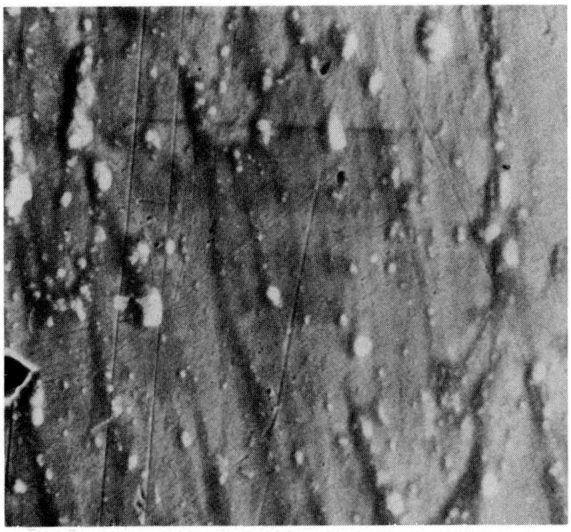

Fig. 22-18. Scanning electron micrograph (X 2500) showing the dentine surface of a prepared tooth coated with foreign material which must be removed before cementation of the crown.

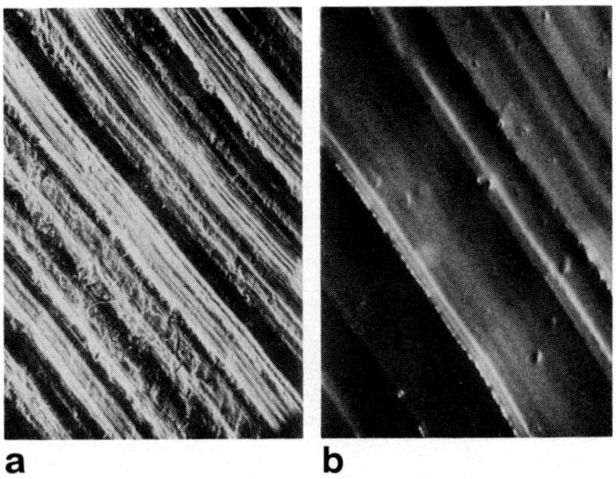

Figs. 22-19a, b. Prepared dentine surface before (a) and after (b) application of a liner. The liner fills the irregularities in the dentine surface.

angles of convergence (<20°), the strength of cement films is generally sufficient to prevent loss of retention resulting from forces acting in the opposite direction to the direction of the path of insertion of the bridge. The strength of the cement is not sufficient, however, to withstand horizontally directed forces if the preparations and the retainers do not have sufficient height and correct dimensions.

Surface treatment of prepared teeth

The surfaces of prepared teeth may be coated with various materials such as dentine chips, impression material, temporary cement, absorbed salivary components, microorganisms and food debris (Fig. 22-18). In order to achieve optimum retention, all such materials must be removed before cementation. Otherwise the necessary close contact between the cement film and the prepared tooth surface will not be obtained. For the maintenance of the microstructure and the quality of the prepared surface, the removal of the foreign materials should be managed with methods and cleaning agents which are non-destructive to the dentine. Effective cleaners such as strong acids and bases should therefore be avoided. Studies by Brännström et al. (1982) indicate that surface active cleaning agents are more effective than the commonly used combination of 3% hydrogen peroxide solution and ethanol. However, considering the wide range of the physical and chemical properties of the various foreign materials, the most effective cleansing procedure includes separate application of 1) an oxidizing agent such as a weak hydrogen peroxide solution, 2) a solvent such as ethanol and 3) a surfactant cleanser. Following the application of each of these cleansers, the tooth should be rinsed with water to remove loosened material and to prevent the different agents from inhibiting the cleansing effect of the others.

It has been claimed that liners should be applied to prepared dentine before cementation of a crown to protect the pulp. Such treatment drastically reduces the retention of dental cements (Glantz et al. 1978), since the liners fill the irregularities in the dentine (Fig. 22-19) where the cement gains retention.

If the remaining dentine is so thin that the

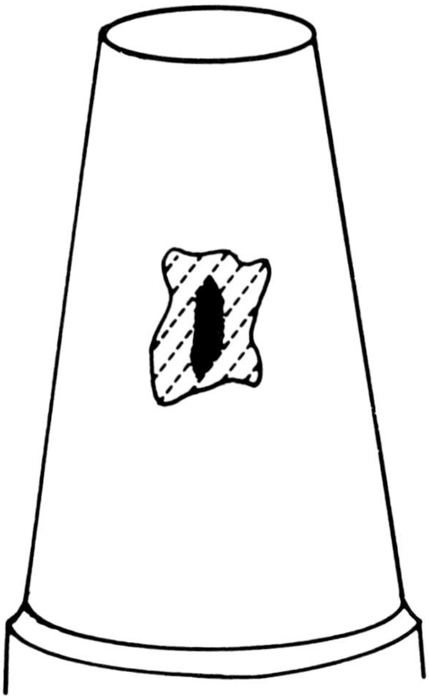

Fig. 22-20. Liner applied to protect the pulp in an area where the covering dentine is thin. Note that the liner covers only the critical area.

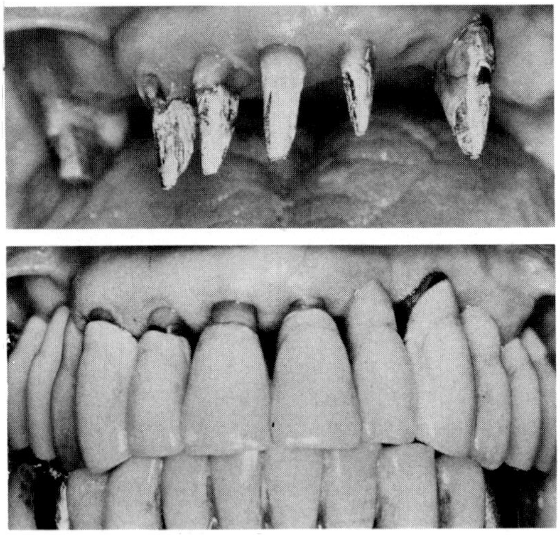

Fig. 22-22. Patient with long clinical crowns (top) and a shallow overlap (bottom). This facilitates proper dimensioning of the metal frame.

pulp must be protected, the liner should only cover the critical area (Fig. 22-20) and not the entire surface of the preparation. Since liners

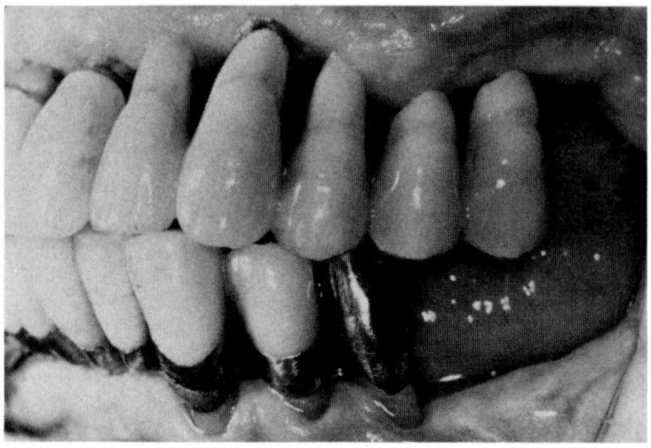

Fig. 22-21. Cantilever pontics used for the stabilization of a mobile bridge.

have chemical and mechanical properties inferior to those of cements, they must not be applied at or close to crown margins. Low viscous liners are preferred since the retentive capacity of the cement film will decrease with increased viscosity of the liner (Glantz et al. 1978).

During cleansing and cementation procedures it is of primary importance to prevent saliva from reaching the prepared tooth surfaces. Even after momentary contact with saliva a thin organic film is adsorbed to the surface, thereby obstructing the direct contact between cement and tooth (Baier & Glantz 1978).

Specific aspects of strength

Fracture of bridgework

Fracture of the metal frame can be prevented by giving the frame adequate dimensions. Cantilever pontics may be used to achieve the balanced loading necessary to obtain stability of a mobile bridge (see Chapter 21). Such a prosthesis (Fig. 22-21) should have increased thickness of the metal frame in the loading directions to compensate for the increased stress produced by the cantilever segment (Nyman et al. 1975). Such compensating increase can, however, only be made in patients with long

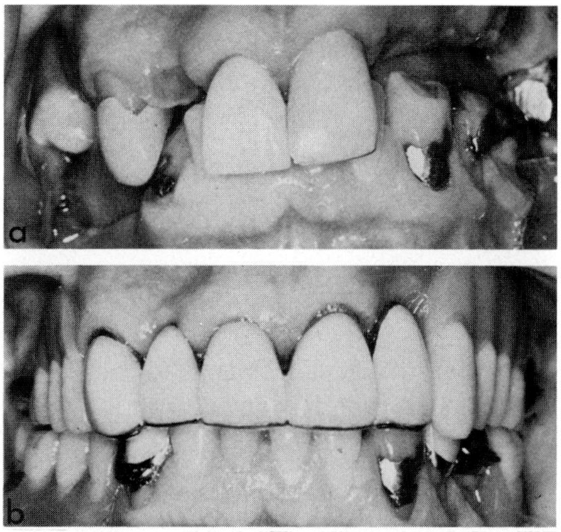

Figs. 22-23a, b. Patient with short clinical crowns and a deep overbite (a). In such cases removable restorations or combinations of fixed and removable restorations (b) should be favored at the prosthetic rehabilitation.

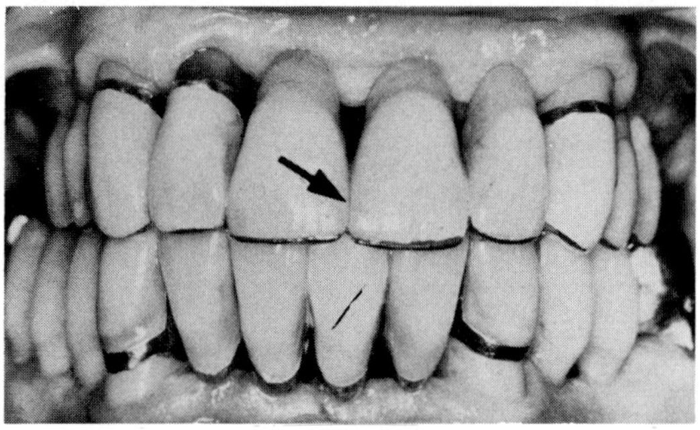

Fig. 22-25. A 10-unit maxillary bridge with 3 retainers (teeth 13, 12 and 23). This bridge has only 1 soldered joint (arrow).

clinical crowns and a shallow vertical overlap (Fig. 22-22). This implies that cantilever segments should be avoided where the space is not available, such as in patients with short clinical crowns or with deep overbite (Fig. 22-23a). In such individuals, prosthetic treatment with removable restorations or combinations of fixed and removable restorations should be favored (Fig. 22-23b).

Soldered joints are common sites for fractures (Fig. 22-24). The reason is generally poor design and occasionally inferior physical properties in the areas of such joints (Bergman

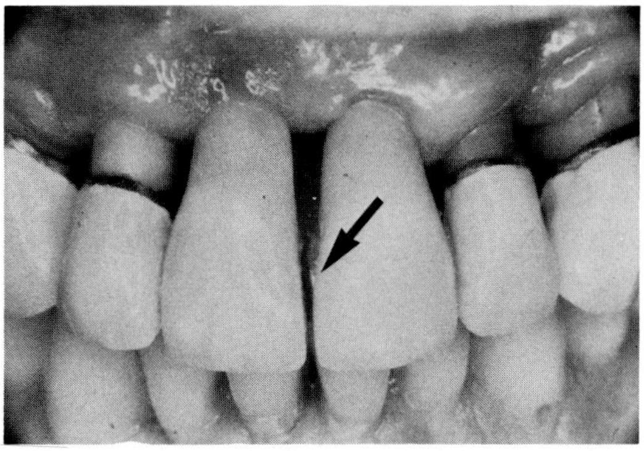

Fig. 22-24. Maxillary bridge showing a fracture of a soldered joint (arrow).

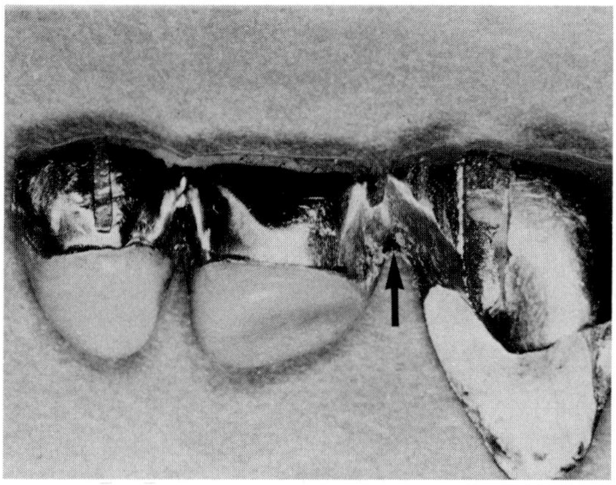

Fig. 22-26.

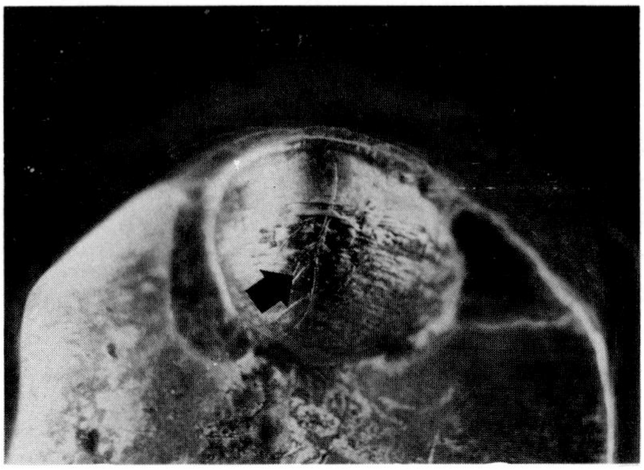

Fig. 22-27.

Figs. 22-26, 22-27. Corrosion products on soldered joints (arrow) (Fig. 22-26), and the occlusal surface of a complete crown (cast in gold alloy) which for 7 years has been located in contact with a denture frame of a partial removable denture (cast in Co/Cr-alloy) (Fig. 22-27).

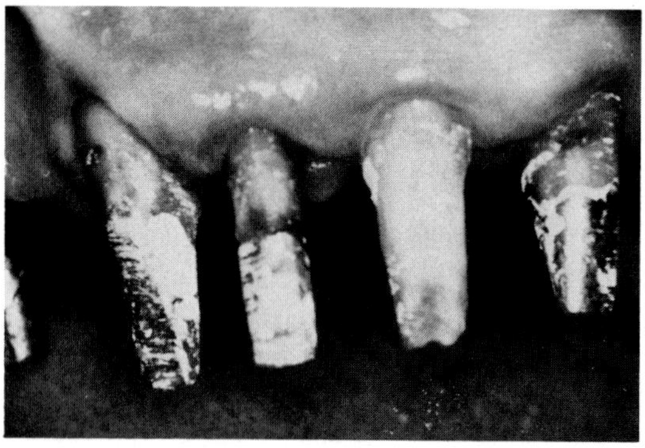

Fig. 22-28. Preparations with large surface areas for maximum cement contact and retention.

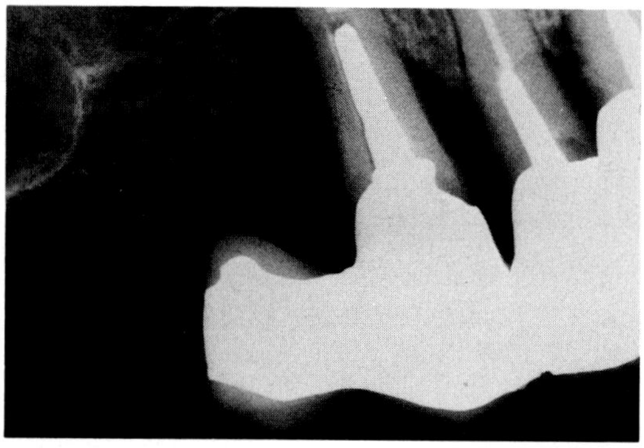

Fig. 22-29. Radiograph showing a cantilever bridge with root fracture in the terminal abutment at the tip of the dowel. Note the bony defect.

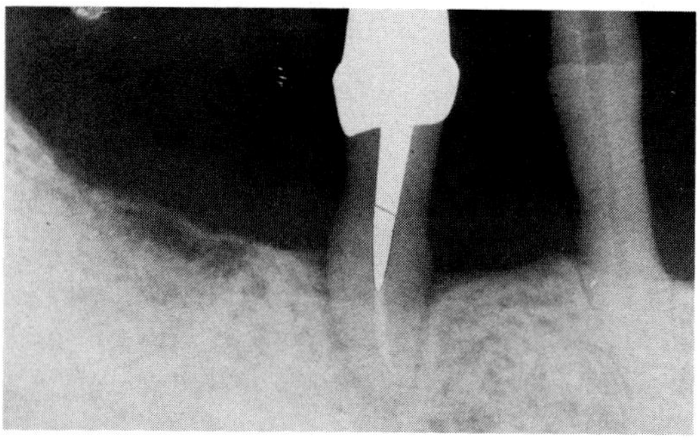

a

Fig. 22-30a. Radiograph and clinical picture of root filled abutment teeth with proper dowel.

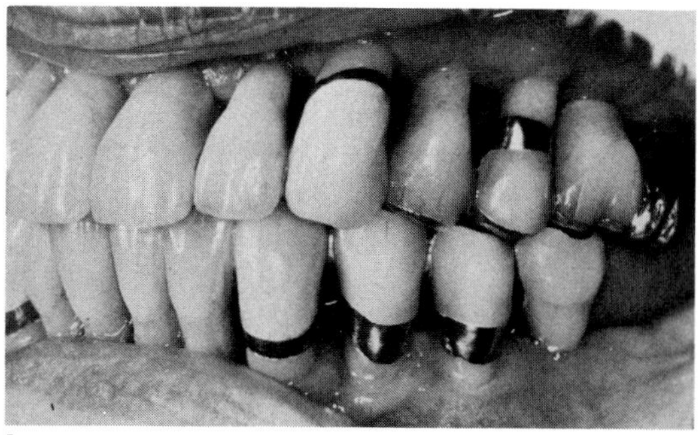

b

Fig. 22-30b. Radiograph and clinical picture of root filled abutment teeth with metal copings.

1976). Solderings should therefore be avoided by casting as many bridge units as possible in one. Soldered joints should not be located in areas subjected to high strain. Examples of such areas are the mesial and distal surfaces of retainers next to cantilever pontics (Glantz et al. 1984). In the maxillary bridge extending from second premolar to second premolar (Fig. 22-25) there are only 3 abutments (right lateral incisor, canine and left canine). The frame was cast in 2 segments and there is only 1 soldered joint which is located between the central incisors.

The metal frame of all bridges consists of one or several metal alloys. When different metals or alloys are present in the same biological environment, interactions that lower their individual properties occur between the materials. Corrosion is the most common reaction and it appears as soon as different metals or alloys are in contact with each other (Figs. 22-26, 22-27). Noble metal alloys should be used whenever possible and the types of alloys to be used in 1 patient should be as few as possible, ideally only 1.

Fracture of luting cement

As already discussed, fracture of the luting agent results in loss of retention of the retainer. In this context it should be stressed that the larger the area of the cement film, the higher is its total retentive capacity (Fig. 22-28). This fact further strengthens the importance of using the maximum length and maximum surface area of the clinical crown for retention, particularly in bridges with few abutments.

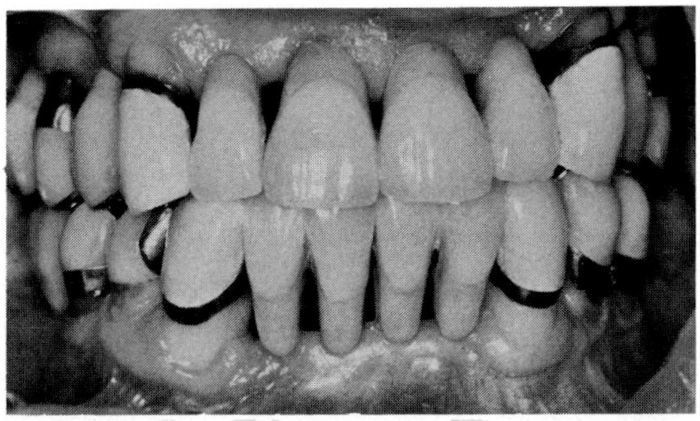

Fig. 22-31. Clinical picture of extensive fixed bridges designed to facilitate proper oral hygiene.

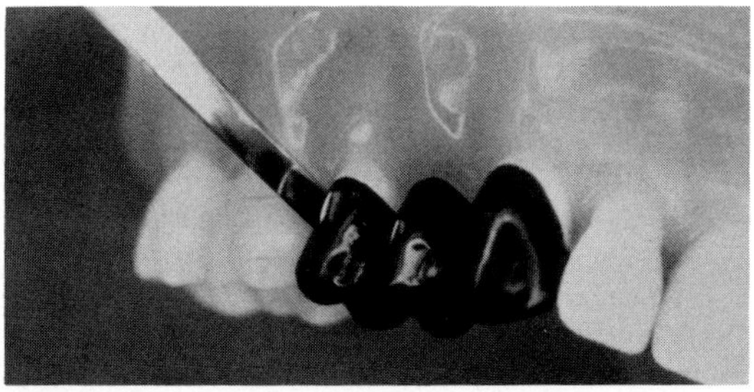

a

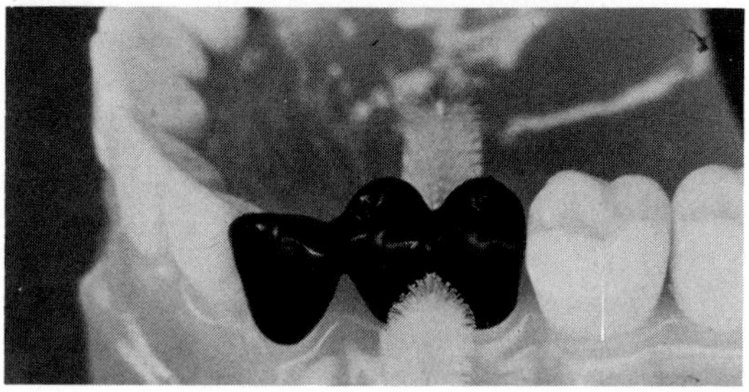

b

Figs. 22-32a,b. Toothpicks and interdental toothbrushes should be used during waxing of brdiges (in this case two 3-unit bridges) to ensure a proper outline of the interdental area.

Fracture of abutment teeth

Fracture of abutment teeth has been reported to occur more frequently in root filled (Fig. 22-29) than in vital teeth (Randow et al. 1986) and primarily in teeth containing root dowels and serving as terminal abutments for cantilever bridges. To minimize the risk of such fractures the root canal should not be so widened as to undermine the dentine walls (Fig. 22-30a). Furthermore a metal coping should circumscribe the cervix to the tooth (Fig. 22-30b). Using standard model systems, it can be demonstrated that the strength of a root filled tooth with a dowel and a metal coping is about 10 times that of a corresponding root without a coping. The wider the coping, the higher is its retentive capacity.

In addition to these technical and biophysical aspects on fixed bridges in patients with reduced periodontal tissue support, it should be emphasized that all complete crowns, used as retainers and pontics, should be designed to facilitate proper oral hygiene (Fig. 22-31). The margins of the complete crowns should be placed in a supragingival position whenever possible and the buccal and lingual surfaces must not be overcontoured.

In addition, the width of the embrasures should be matched to the size of the particular interdental cleaning device (Fig. 22-32a, b) recommended to the patient.

References

Baier, R.E. & Glantz, P.-O. (1978) Characterization of oral *in vivo* films formed on different types of solid surfaces. *Acta Odontologica Scandinavica* **36**, 289-301.

Bergman, M. (1976) Chemical and thermodynamic studies of dental gold alloys with special reference to homogenization, electrical corrosion and cluster formation. Thesis. University of Umeå, Sweden.

Brännström, M., Glantz, P.-O. & Nordenvall, K.-J. (1982) Cavity cleaners and etchants. In *Biocompatibility of Dental Materials*, vol. II, ed. Smith, D.C. & Williams, D.F. Boca Raton, FL, U.S.A.: CRC Press.

Glantz, P.-O., Gwinnett, A.J. & Jendresen, M.D. (1978) Effects of cavity varnish on surface morphology and retention. *Journal of Dental Research* **57**, Special Issue A, 126.

Glantz, P.-O., Nyman, S., Strandman, E. & Randow, K. (1984) On functional strain in fixed mandibular reconstructions II, an in vivo study, *Acta Odontologica Scandinavica*, **42**, 269-276.

Goldberg, L.J. (1976) Changes in the excitability of elevator and depressor motoneurons produced by stimulation of intra-oral nerves. In *Mastication*, ed. Anderson, D.J. & Matthews, B. Bristol, U.K.: John Wright & Sons Ltd.

Hannam, A.G. (1976) Periodontal mechanoreceptors. In *Mastication*, ed. Anderson, D.J. & Matthews, B. Bristol, U.K.: John Wright & Sons Ltd.

Hegdahl, T. & Silness, J. (1977) Preparation areas resisting displacement of artificial crowns. *Journal of Oral Rehabilitation* **4**, 201-207.

Lindhe, J. & Nyman, S. (1977) The role of occlusion in periodontal disease and the biological rationale for splinting in treatment of periodontitis. *Oral Sciences Reviews* **10**, 11-43.

Lundgren, D., Nyman, S., Heijl, L. & Carlsson, G.E. (1975) Functional analysis of fixed bridges on abutment teeth with reduced periodontal support. *Journal of Oral Rehabilitation* **2**, 105-116.

Nyman, S. & Ericsson, I. (1982) The capacity of reduced periodontal tissues to support fixed bridgework. *Journal of Clinical Periodontology* **9**, 409-414.

Nyman, S., Lindhe, J. & Lundgren, D. (1975) The role of occlusion for the stability of fixed bridges in patients with reduced periodontal support. *Journal of Clinical Periodontology* **2**, 53-66.

Nyman, S. & Lindhe, J. (1979) A longitudinal study of combined periodontal and prosthetic treatment of patients with advanced periodontal disease. *Journal of Periodontology* **50**, 163-169.

Randow, K. & Glantz, P.-O. (1986) On cantilever loading of vital and non-vital teeth. *Acta Odontologica Scandinavica* **44**, 271-277.

Randow, K., Glantz, P.-O. & Zöger, B. (1986) Technical failures and some related clinical complications in extensive fixed prosthodontis, *Acta Odontologica Scandinavia* **44**, 241-255.

Timoshenko, S.P. & Goodier, J.N. (1970) *Theory of Elasticity*. 3rd ed. New York: McGraw-Hill Book Company.

Öwall, B. & Möller, E. (1974) Oral tactile sensibility during biting and chewing. *Odontologisk Revy* **25**, 327-346.

CHAPTER 23

Orthodontic Tooth Movement in Periodontal Therapy

The continuous migration of teeth is a physiological process caused by alterations in the periodontal tissues initiated by such forces as occlusal and approximal attrition. Loss of teeth and/or periodontal tissues affects physiological tooth migration and can result in malocclusion or malalignment of teeth, changes which can be aggravated by occlusal trauma and/or oral habits, such as tongue thrust and nail biting. Pathological tooth migration can involve a single tooth or a group of teeth, and result in 1) the development of medial diastema or general spacing of the teeth, particularly in the anterior segments of the dentition; 2) in spacing of the teeth combined with proclination of upper incisors; 3) in rotated and tipped bicuspids and molars with collapse of the posterior occlusion and the development of reduced height of the bite. All these symptoms are common in individuals with advanced periodontal disease. Thus, the overall treatment plan for a patient with advanced periodontal disease often involves orthodontic realignment of the teeth to reestablish satisfactory 1) occlusion, 2) esthetic conditions and 3) chewing comfort.

In many cases the orthodontic treatment can be accomplished by comparatively simple measures. All tooth movements, however, must be preceded by a comprehensive orthodontic analysis and treatment planning. Without such an analysis even so-called "minor tooth movements" may produce more problems than they solve.

There are no standardized methods to follow in orthodontic treatment of adult individuals. The biomechanical principles used in orthodontics must be adapted to the individual anatomy of the areas in the dentition where tooth movement is planned. Radiographic examination should be performed at predetermined intervals during the course of orthodontic treatment to ensure early disclosure, and to counteract undesired iatrogenic side effects.

Factors to be considered in orthodontic therapy

Basic differences

It should be remembered that orthodontic treatment in patients with advanced periodontal disease is performed not in children or adolescents, but in adult individuals. Since growth in such patients is completed, it is not possible by orthodontic measures to influence *zones of growth* and, therefore, treatment in the adult individual is restricted to different types of tooth *alignment*. This limitation of the possibility for orthodontic therapy in an adult patient is important to recognize. The following example may illustrate the difficulty discussed.

A deep bite is frequently found in patients with advanced forms of periodontal disease. This deep bite or reduced height of the bite is often the result of loss of molar support for the occlusion and may be rehabilitated by means of a bite plane in order to increase the height of the bite. However, if the deep bite is of genuine character and is combined with postnormal malocclusion or occurs in individuals with neutral occlusion with low anterior facial height, an increase of vertical dimension is indeed a doubtful procedure, owing to the risk of development of muscular dysfunction and/or temporomandibular joint (TMJ) problems. Treatment, including intrusion of the incisors in such cases, involves a great risk for root resorption and is, therefore, an orthodontic measure hardly ever indicated in adult patients with periodontal disease.

Patient problems

It is far more difficult for an adult individual to adapt to an orthodontic appliance than for a child. Phonetic adjustment to a removable appliance, for instance, generally requires more time in an adult. In the initial phase of treatment, the patient often has difficulty in fitting the active elements (i.e. springs, elastics) into place, with the risk that the appliance may only be used sporadically. As a consequence, the induced orthodontic treatment fails. A fixed appliance is usually better tolerated by adult patients. However, a fixed appliance may for esthetic reasons be difficult to accept by such a patient, even if plastic or ceramic brackets are used. The adult patient must thus be very thoroughly prepared for the consequences and implications of orthodontic treatment, and it should not be initiated unless the patient is in full physical and mental health. As a rule, however, patients with advanced periodontal disease are strongly motivated for orthodontic treatment and will normally cooperate excellently.

Periodontal tissue response

Mesial migration of teeth is dependent on osteoclastic and osteoblastic activity in the periodontium. These are physiological processes that throughout life permit a constant remodelling of bone. With increasing age, however, cellular activity decreases and the tissue becomes richer in collagen. Age *per se* is not a contraindication to orthodontic treatment. But in the elderly the tissue response to orthodontic forces, including both cell mobilization and conversion of collagen fibers, is considerably slower than in children and teenagers. This means that in adults hyalin zones are formed more easily on the pressure side of the orthodontically treated tooth. Such zones may at least temporarily prevent the tooth from moving in the intended direction.

Biomechanical considerations are of the utmost importance in adult orthodontics. *The orthodontic force* applied must be *light*. Light forces will result in the desired tooth movement and prevent tissue damage. If the force is strong enough to exceed the capillary blood pressure in the periodontal ligament, local ischemia occurs, followed by degenerative changes in the ligament tissue, a hyalinization. No osteoclasts can differentiate in this tissue, i.e. tooth movement cannot occur until the hyalinized zones are eliminated through the undermining resorption from the marrow spaces and adjacent areas of the unaffected alveolar bone. Tissue elements invade from the adjacent viable tissue and reorganization of the posthyalinized area will then occur. Provided there is no invasion of inflammatory elements from the gingival structures, all the changes described above are reversible (see also Chapter 8).

The force applied in the adult patient should preferably be of the *interrupted* type. While the *continuous* force acts for longer periods of time, the *interrupted* force is of comparatively short duration (up to a few weeks). As the magnitude of the force rapidly decreases, the tissue will become properly reorganised before the active elements are reactivated. Thus, if a hyalinized zone is formed in this type of treatment it will be rapidly eliminated. There is also less risk for root resorption and pulpal damage when *interrupted* forces are used.

In the initial stage of orthodontic treatment in adults, an *interrupted* force of 20-30 g is recommended. Later on, the force may be increased (up to 30-50 g in tipping and 50-80 g in bodily movements, corresponding to a distance of movement of 0.5-1 mm per month), depending on the degree of marginal bone loss and the amount of remaining alveolar bone. Clinically, a proper orthodontic force is distinguished by the fact that the treated teeth are tender for not more than 1 or 2 days after reactivation.

Root filled or traumatized teeth which have a normal radiographic appearance may be moved orthodontically provided *light interrupted* forces are used. The selection of proper *anchorage* for the orthodontic tooth movement may present major problems in adult orthodontics, especially in partially edentulous patients and in individuals with reduced amounts of alveolar bone. Transversal palatal bars are recommended for stabilizing molars and/or premolars.

The retention period

From observations made in children subjected to orthodontic therapy, Reitan (1959) pointed out that the Sharpey's fibers of the newly formed bundle bone, as well as the principal fibers of the periodontal ligament, will undergo rearrangement even after a retention period of several months. The supraalveolar and transseptal fibers, on the other hand, change very slowly. In order to achieve proper rearrangement of the tissue structures involved in orthodontic therapy and to prevent relapse, the teeth must therefore be retained for a varying period of time.

In adults the retention period is generally long, owing to decreased ability of the periodontal tissue to react to mechanical stimuli. Risk for relapse always exists as long as the tissue reorganization is still in progress. Thus, permanent retainers must often be applied after completion of active orthodontic therapy. It is important to discuss also the duration of the retention period with the patient *before* the orthodontic treatment is initiated.

In orthodontic treatment of children and teenagers it is sometimes recommended to "over-adjust" the orthodontically moved teeth to compensate for relapse. It is difficult, however, to predict the degree of over-correction needed to counteract relapse. In adult orthodontics such over-corrections are not advisable, especially not in dentitions with reduced periodontal tissue support. The retention after the

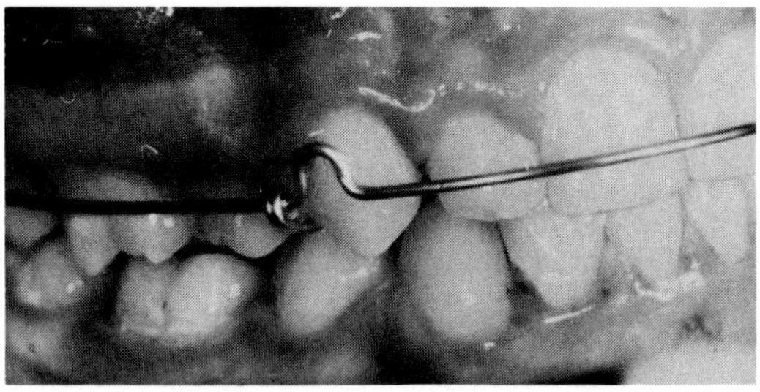

a

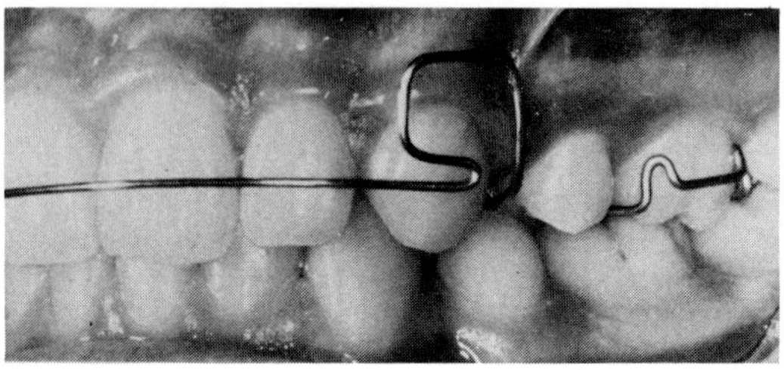

b

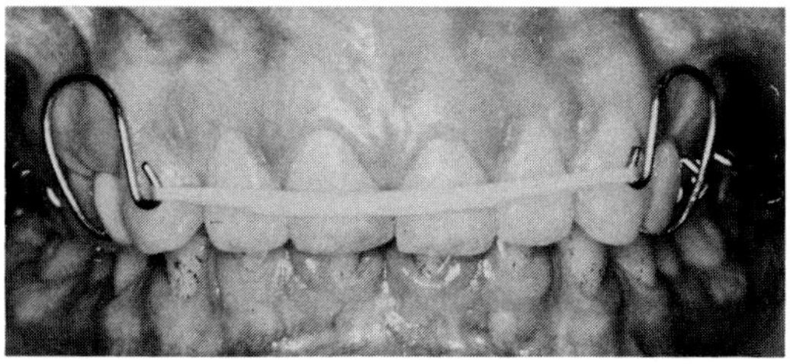

c

Figs. 23-1a-c. Different kinds of removable retainers. a) Hawley plate. b) Plate with Adams clasps and a modification of the labial arch for retaining the cuspids. c) The labial arch is replaced by an elastic (in this case 3/8" light) for esthetic reasons.

active orthodontic movement can be activated with removable or fixed appliances. Different types of removable retainers have been described (Fig. 23-1). A proper retainer should keep each orthodontically treated tooth in the acquired position. The appliance should be designed to be as inconspicuous as possible, yet be strong enough to achieve its objective during the entire period of use. It should also be easy for the patient to clean. Temporary or semi-permanent fixed retainers are often preferred to the removable varieties (Fig. 23-2). The retainer has to be properly designed to facilitate self-performed tooth cleaning. When removable retainers are used, the dentist is often too dependent on the cooperation of the patient. In well documented experiments, Reitan (1967) showed that most relapse following orthodontic tooth movement occurred during the first 5 h after the appliance had been removed. As already mentioned, removable appliances often cause the patient speech problems and inconvenience during chewing. It is therefore understandable that patients often use their removable retainers only in the evening and at night. This, however, results in a daily repeated minor relapse of the tooth movement. This "jiggling" results in alternate bone deposition and resorption and in a further prolongation of the retention period.

Iatrogenic effects associated with orthodontic treatment

Orthodontic treatment may cause injuries to the teeth and periodontium but in most instances this damage is reversible and regeneration or repair of the tooth structures and periodontal tissues occurs. In some cases, however, the changes may get out of control, resulting in irreparable damage. In order to prevent such damage a proper basic knowledge is required of biomechanical principles as well as tissue reactions in orthodontic treatment. Radiography should be performed at regular intervals to disclose any iatrogenic effects during the orthodontic treatment.

Root resorption

This can hardly be avoided during orthodontic tooth movement. The majority of the resorption lacunae which develop are small and insignificant. They generally appear at the border of the hyalinized zone within the marginal and middle thirds of the root and are soon repaired by apposition of cellular cementum. In con-

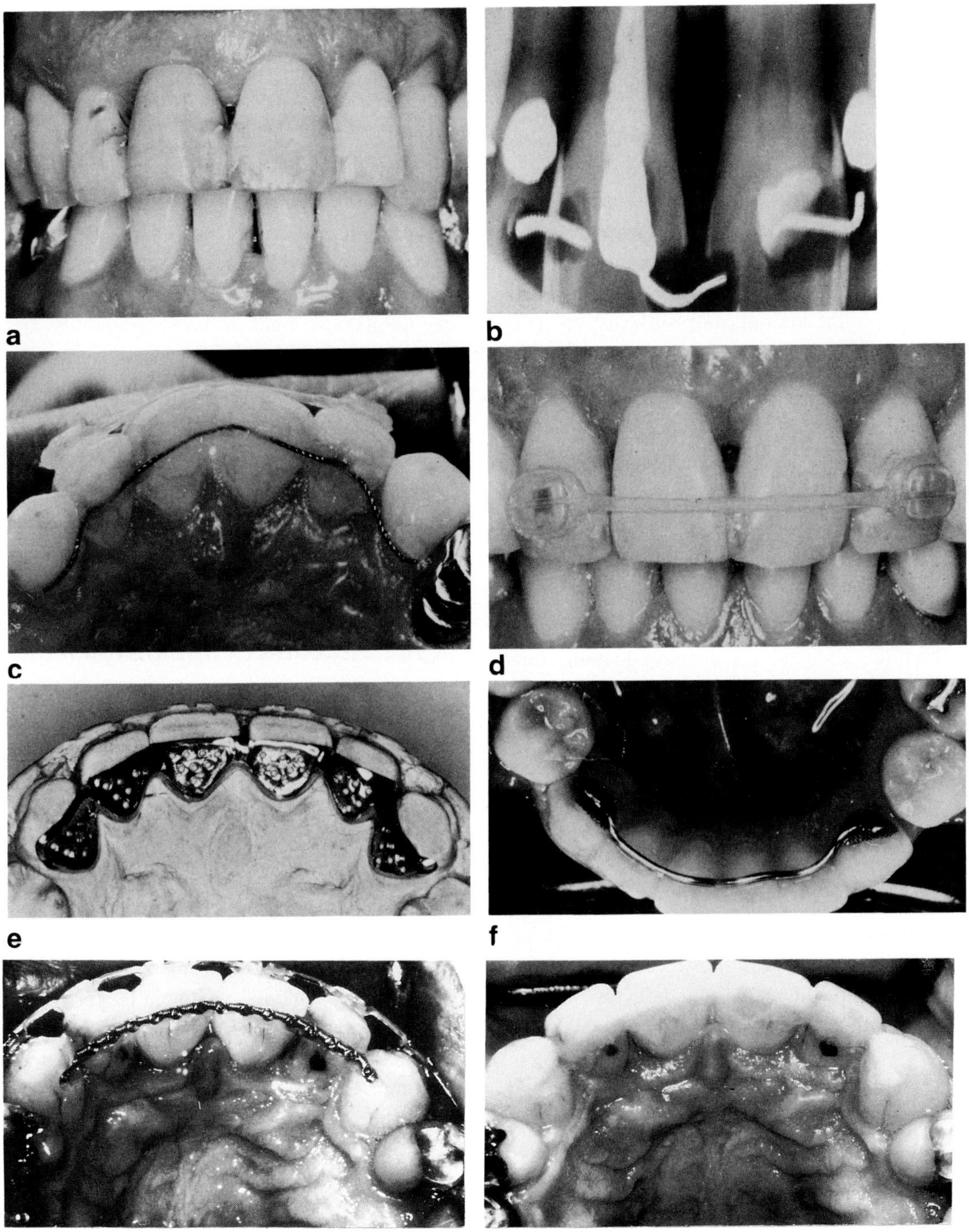

Figs. 23-2a-h. Different kinds of temporary and semipermanent fixed retainers. a, b) Interapproximate bonding with intradental pins in the composite fillings. c, d) Bonded lingual retainer in the upper jaw (Wildcat .0175). The retention is strengthened bucally for 1 month with an Alastic K2. e) Bonded gold skeleton. f) Bonded lingual retainer in the lower jaw (blue Elgiloy .019) strengthened with nets at the cuspids. g, h) Bonded lingual retainer set into an enamel groove.

trast, apical root resorption is an irreversible injury, resulting in a permanent shortening of the root. An unfavorable change in the crown-to-root ratio is thereby established. This is particularly alarming in dentitions with marginal bone loss, in which the extraalveolar leverage is already increased. In experimental studies of orthodontically displaced premolars, less resorption was found to occur with tipping than with bodily tooth movements and less resorption occurred on the mesial root surfaces of teeth moved mesially into extraction sites than on the distal surfaces. Clinical studies have shown that root resorptions predominantly occur in incisors and that the risk for root resorption is increased in situations where 1) large orthodontic forces are used, 2) prolonged continuous bodily movements and 3) intrusive movements are performed.

It should be remembered that there is also a risk for root resorption in the anchorage teeth, which are often subject to heavy loading. Further, it should be kept in mind that in patients with periodontal disease the resistance of the anchorage unit may be reduced, not only by loss of alveolar bone but also, in many dentitions, by loss of proper anchorage teeth.

Loss of alveolar bone

The possible association between malocclusion and periodontal disease has received much attention in the literature but little support has been found for such an association. Conversely, it has been claimed that orthodontic treatment may have adverse effects on the gingival and periodontal tissues which may hasten or promote periodontal tissue breakdown later in life.

Dentitions with normal height of the attachment apparatus

A number of experiments have demonstrated that in animals with either normal gingiva or overt gingivitis, orthodontic forces cause no damage to the supraalveolar connective tissue and orthodontic treatment will therefore not result in periodontal tissue breakdown and pocket formation.

Some clinical studies, however, report that in children and young adults orthodontic treatment can in fact aggravate a preexisting plaque induced gingival lesion and cause some loss of alveolar bone and periodontal attachment. Recent follow-up studies stressing the importance of the use of light orthodontic forces and proper self performed oral hygiene during the treatment period have reported insignificant or only slight marginal bone loss in orthodontically treated children and teenagers. Compared to subjects who had never received orthodontic therapy, no difference in the general prevalence of periodontal disease was observed.

Dentitions with reduced height of the attachment apparatus

Surprisingly little has been published about adult orthodontics in patients with periodontal disease, and the effect of orthodontic treatment in these patients has been controversial. Thus, some 10 years ago we raised the following questions: Is it possible to move teeth which have reduced amounts of periodontal tissue support? Will the orthodontic movement cause an aggravation of the periodontal lesions and further promote loss of attachment and bone? Should the orthodontic treatment be performed before or after the cause related or the corrective phase of periodontal therapy? How and for how long should the teeth be stabilized subsequent to orthodontic treatment in patients with reduced amounts of periodontium?

Experiments in beagle dogs

Results were obtained which provided some basic answers to the above questions (Ericsson et al 1977, 1978, Ericsson & Thilander 1978, 1980). In these experiments it was demonstrated that 1) in the absence of plaque, orthodontic forces and tooth movements failed to induce gingivitis. In the presence of plaque, similar forces caused angular bone defects, and with tipping and intruding movements the forces were capable of converting an overt gingival lesion into a lesion associated with attachment loss. The experiments also demonstrated that 2) orthodontic forces, kept within biological limits, failed to cause gingival inflammation in tooth regions where the periodontal tissue support was markedly reduced but *non*inflammatory, and that 3) the most important factor in initiation, progression and recurrence of periodontal disease in dogs was the microbial plaque present within the gingival pocket.

In discussing the prevention of posttreatment orthodontic relapse, the difference in reaction between the supraalveolar and the periodontal ligament fibers has been pointed out. It has also been shown in man, in the monkey and in the dog, that fibrotomy of the supraalveolar fibers reduces the degree of relapse after orthodontic derotation of teeth. This suggests that periodontal surgery in dentitions with reduced periodontal tissue support should preferably be performed after completion of active orthodontic therapy in order to minimize the risk for and degree of relapse. In the beagle dog experiments described above it was demonstrated, however, that 4) no significant difference existed regarding the tendency for relapse between teeth treated with periodontal surgery before or after orthodontic tipping movements.

Treatment planning

Recently it was suggested that orthodontic therapy, e.g. extrusion, intrusion, tipping, lateral movements of teeth, may result in new attachment formation. Since the biological mechanisms by which such new attachment can occur are not fully understood, there are reasons to recommend that the clinician exercise caution when utilizing orthodontic forces for the purpose of obtaining new attachment.

From our experiments in the beagle dog, it was concluded that:

1. individual teeth can be moved by means of light orthodontic forces in markedly reduced, but healthy, periodontal tissue
2. the connective tissue which regenerated after orthodontic tipping movements was incapable of preventing relapse.

The findings from the experimental studies have been tested in the clinic. Thus, the effect of orthodontic treatment of patients with advanced periodontal disease has been followed in comprehensive long-term follow-up examinations. Based on experience thus gained from clinical and experimental studies, the following treatment protocol may be suggested for patients with a reduced but otherwise healthy periodontium.

Initial planning

Proper *records* (including casts, photographs, intraoral radiographs) and a thorough *clinical examination* (including Plaque Index, Gingival Index, probing depth and clinical attachment level) are required for the *treatment planning*, in which the following aspects are included: the aim of therapy; the feasibility and means of achieving the aims listed; the periodontal status after cause related and corrective therapy phases; the esthetic and functional improvements required; the expected stability of the dentition; the long-term prognosis.

In simple cases the treatment planning can be performed by the general practitioner, but in more complicated and advanced cases consultation with the orthodontist and the periodontist is necessary. The treatment plan, with its advantages and disadvantages, must be explained in detail to the patient, after which treatment can start.

Treatment of periodontal disease

This includes the elimination of plaque and retention factors for plaque as well as the establishment of a morphology in the dentogingival region which facilitates proper self performed tooth cleaning. Deepened gingival pockets are eliminated and the root surfaces properly debrided before the orthodontic treatment is initiated.

Orthodontic treatment

Light forces of the *interrupted continuous* type are used. The forces are kept within biological limits, and frequent follow-up visits are scheduled for radiographic and clinical assessment of the periodontal status.

The orthodontic appliance has to be properly designed. It must provide stable anchorage without causing tissue irritation from bands, wires, loops, coils and elastics used in fixed appliances or from clasps and springs used in removable appliances. Furthermore, the appliance must be fashioned so as to permit proper self performed plaque control measures.

At each follow-up visit for reactivation (usually every 3-4 weeks) all bands must be checked since loosened bands may stimulate the accumulation of plaque and promote caries. For esthetic reasons bonded plastic or ceramic brackets are frequently used in adult orthodontics. Excess of bonding material close to the gingival margin promotes plaque accumulation and will rapidly cause gingival inflammation. Loss of bonding material, on the other hand, will result in leakage and risk for demineralization on the buccal tooth surfaces. When elastics are used, the patient must be thoroughly instructed in how they should be applied. There is a risk that elastics may become dislodged into the gingival pocket and cause an inflammatory reaction with additional loss of attachment and bone. It is therefore important to probe the pockets of the anchorage and orthodontically moved teeth at each visit to discover foreign material. In order to facilitate the tooth movements, occlusal adjustment is recommended in appropriate situations during the phase of orthodontic therapy.

In orthodontic treatment the following factors must be considered: 1) a suitable orthodontic appliance must be chosen; 2) proper anchorage teeth must be selected; 3) light and interrupted forces should be used; 4) thorough clinical and/or radiographic assessments must be made at each follow-up visit; 5) the occlusion should be adjusted if indicated; 6) the oral hygiene technique must be checked; 7) proper records must be prepared (see under Initial planning) to enable a proper evaluation of the result of the orthodontic treatment.

Final occlusal adjustment and surgical pocket elimination

After the orthodontic treatment, final adjustment of the occlusion is performed to ensure good functional stability. If necessary, additional surgical pocket elimination is also carried out.

Retention

The phase of *retention* is initiated. Appliances of temporary, semipermanent or permanent types are inserted. During this phase assessments must be made regarding esthetics and functional stability of the treatment result. The oral hygiene must be checked and proper recordings and thorough clinical examinations performed (see Initial planning) to facilitate the evaluation of the final result.

Posttreatment controls

These have to be undertaken to evaluate objectively also the long-term effects of the treatment.

Case presentations

On the following pages are some examples of planned treatment performed according to the principles described above.

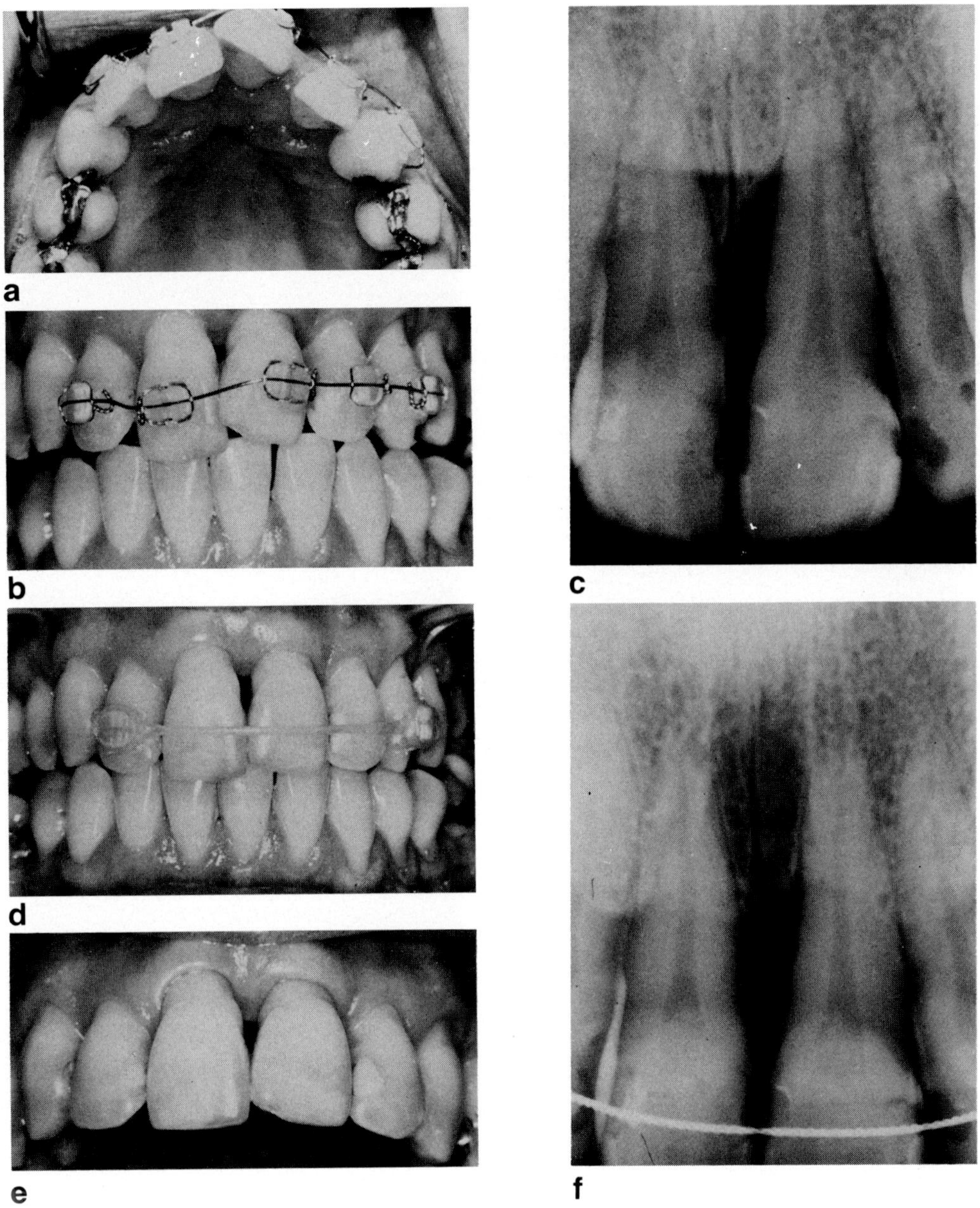

Fig. 23-3a-f.

Case No. 1

A 45-year-old woman (Figs. 23-3a-f) had to be treated orthodontically because of tooth migration and rotation of the left central incisor (a, b, c). The periodontal conditions had been treated by a periodontist and the level of plaque control was excellent. The incisor was derotated with a sectional light arch wire (.016 green Elgiloy). Three months later retention was performed by means of a bonded lingual retainer (.0175 Wildcat) together with a temporary buccal elastic retainer for 6 weeks (Alastic K2) (d). Posttreatment control 5 years later (e, f). Note the improvement of the vertical bony pocket mesially to the left central incisor.

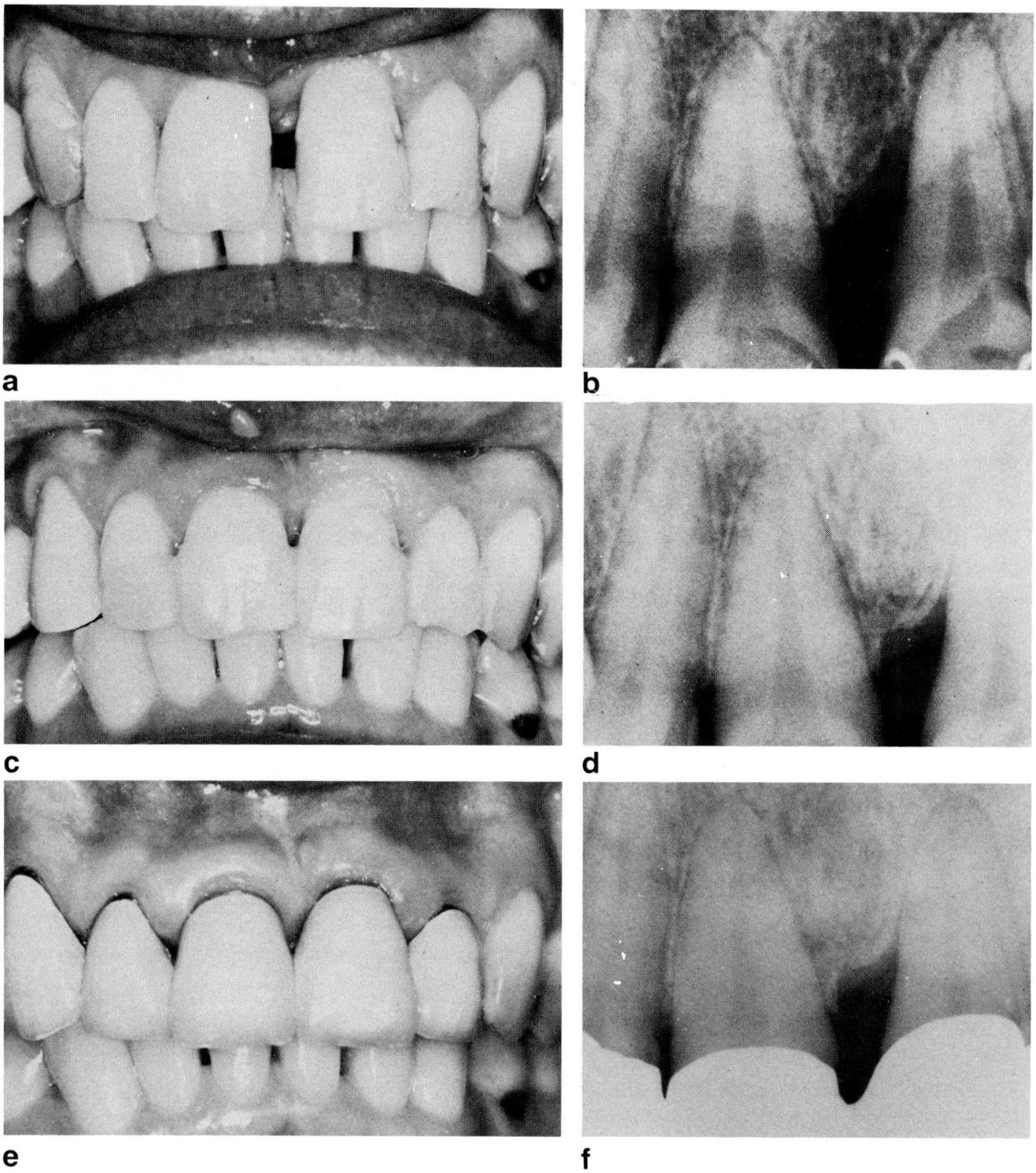

Fig. 23-4a-f.

Case No. 2

A 40-year-old woman (Figs. 23-4a-f) had been treated for periodontal disease. The spaces in the upper incisor segment (a, b) were orthodontically closed by means of a light arch wire (.016 green Elgiloy). Four months later semipermanent retention was performed with intradental anchorage pins by refilling the approximal cavities (c, d). Posttreatment control 5 years later with a permanent bridge as retention (e, f). Note the improvement of the vertical bony defect mesially to the left central incisor.

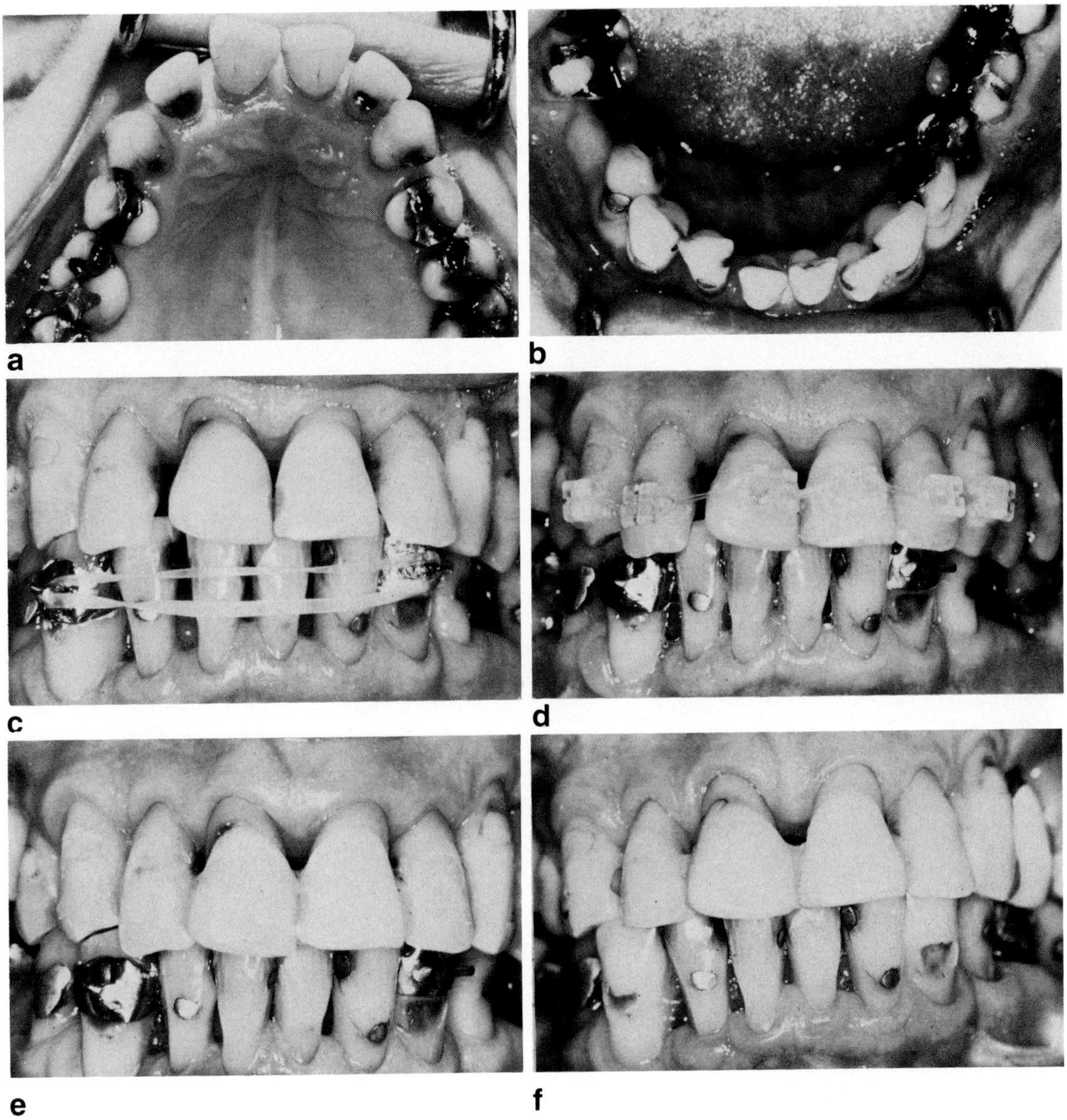

Fig. 23-5a-f.

Case No. 3

A 49-year-old woman (Figs. 23-5a-j) had to be treated orthodontically because of tooth migration in the upper and lower frontal segments (a, b, g, h). She had been treated for periodontal disease. Her plaque control was excellent. The incisor spaces were comparatively small and evenly distributed and were closed by means of 3/8" light latex ligatures in the lower jaw and an Alastic chain in the upper jaw (c, d). After 2 months of treatment, the teeth were retained by interproximal bonding and bonded lingual retainers in both jaws (e). Special care was taken to allow space for cleaning the teeth and for plaque control. Posttreatment control 5 years later (f, i, j).

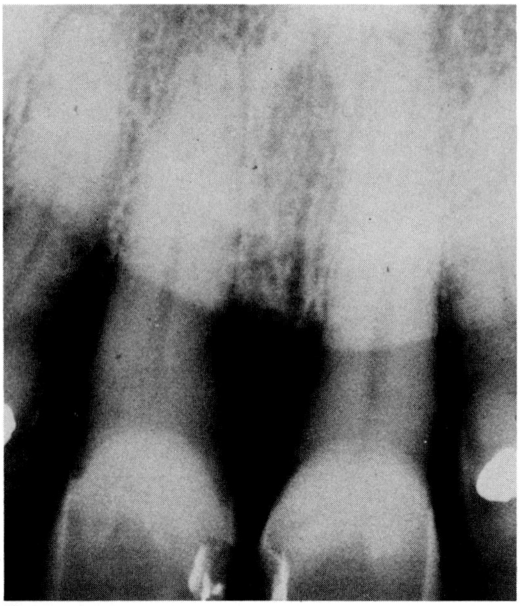
g

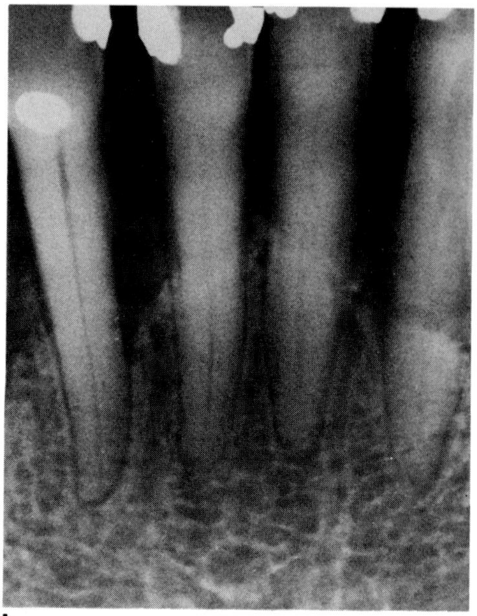
h

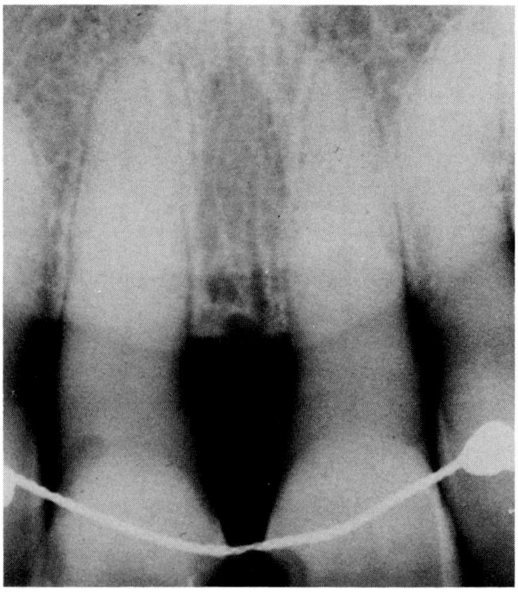
i

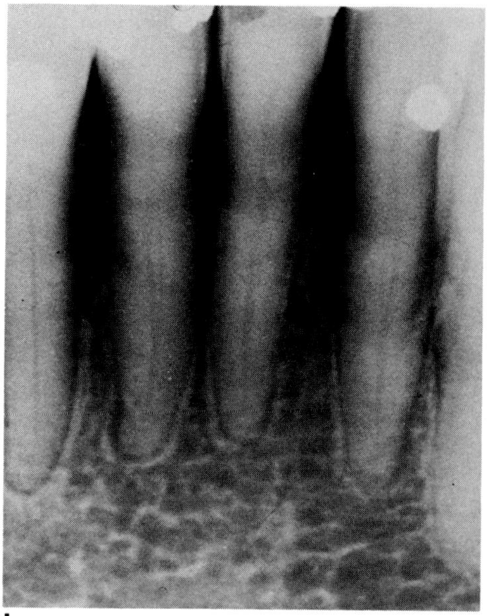
j

Fig. 23-5g-j.

Case No. 4

A 42-year-old man (Figs. 23-6a-f) had been treated for periodontal disease. The bucally tipped and elongated left upper incisor had to be orthodontically realigned (a, b). The incisor was repositioned in the arch by very light forces (c, d). Six months later retention was performed with a bonded lingual retainer (.032 spiral twisted wire, strengthened with a net) (e). Note the improvement of the bone structure around the realigned incisor (f).

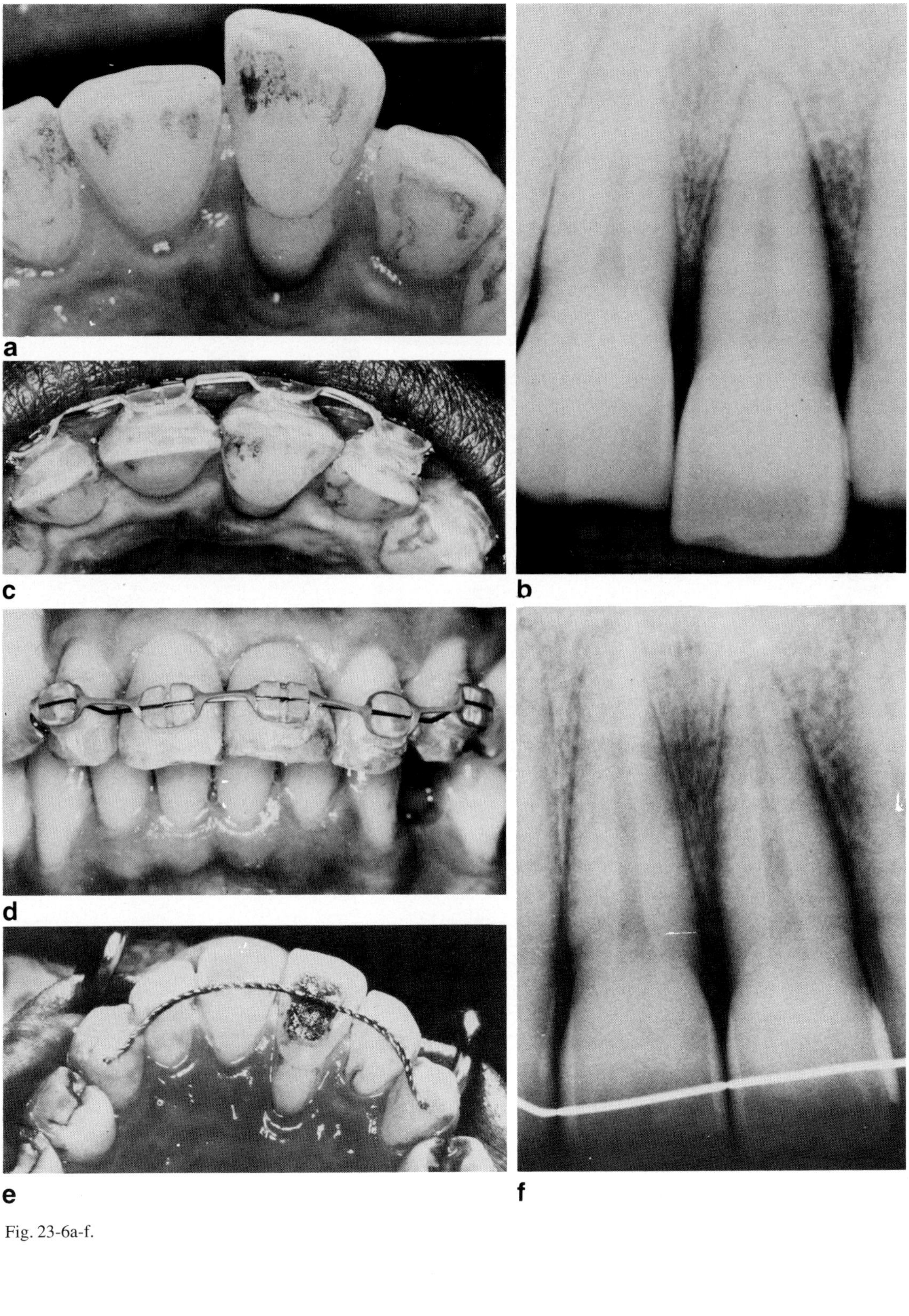

Fig. 23-6a-f.

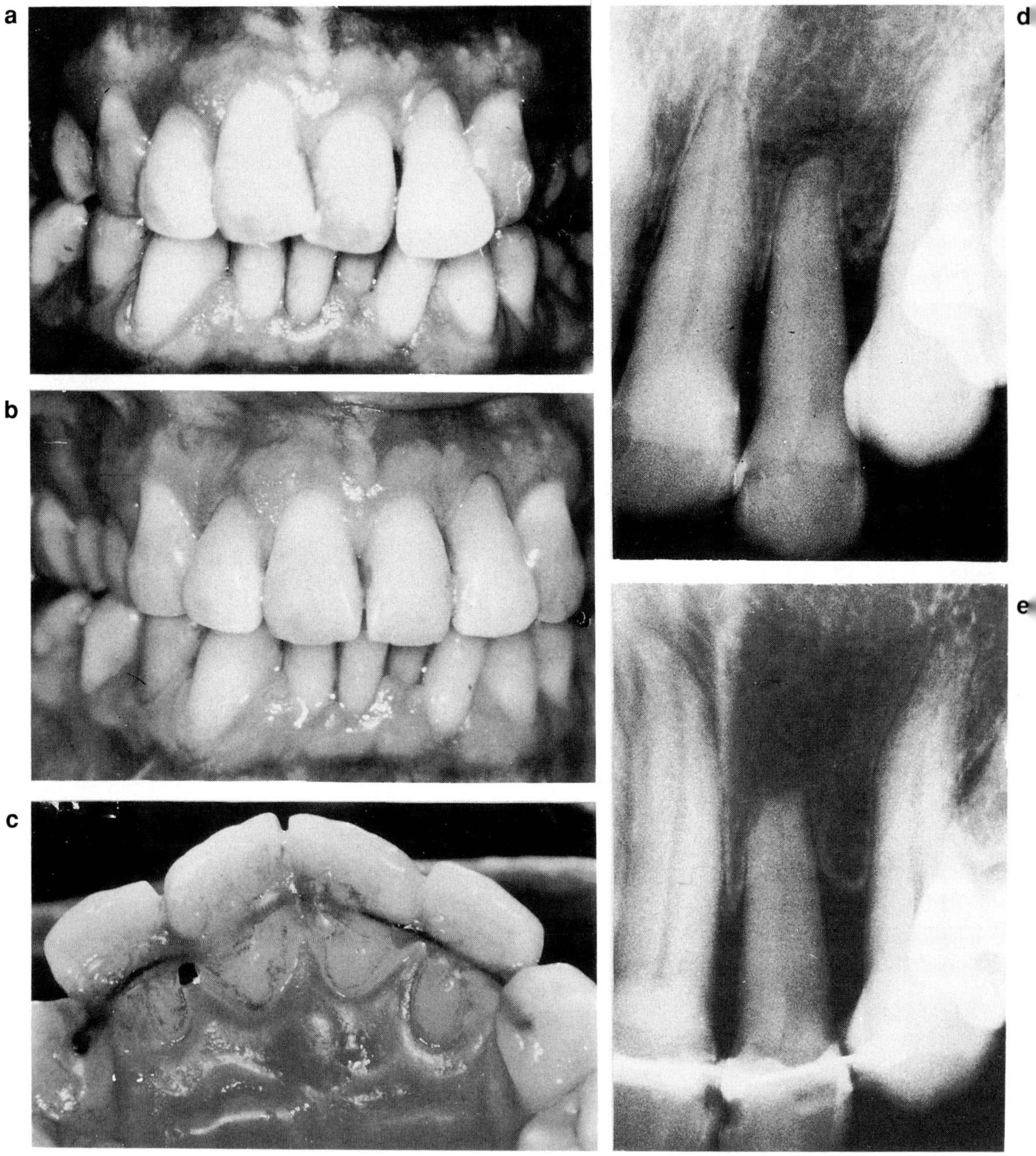

Fig. 23-7a-e.

Case No. 5

A 55-year-old woman had been treated for periodontal disease (Fig. 23-7a, d). The upper incisors had to be orthodontically realigned. The left lateral incisor was intruded by very light forces. Seven months later retention was accomplished with a bonded lingual retainer (.032 spiral twisted wire) placed in an enamel groove (b, c, e). The positive effect of the intrusive tooth movement on the marginal bone was in part compromized by the apical root resorption.

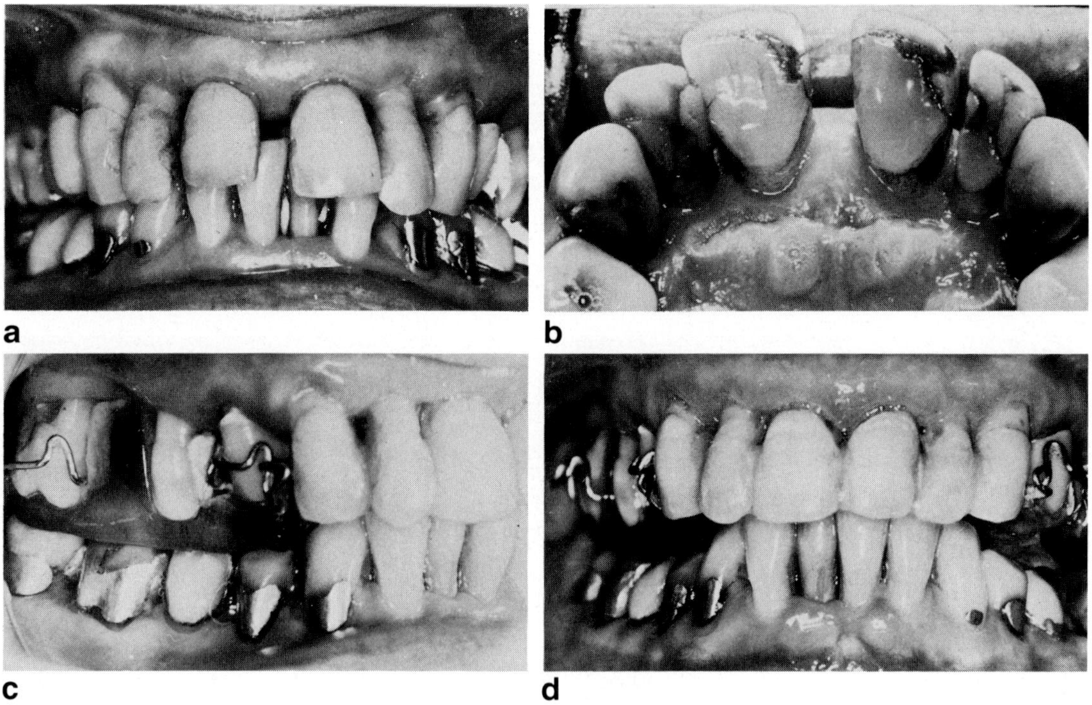

Fig. 23-8a-d.

Case No. 6

A 52-year-old woman (Figs. 23-8a-d) was referred by a general practitioner for excessive overbite and tooth migration in the maxillary frontal segment (a, b). The patient suffered from chronic fissures at the corners of the mouth and discomfort and periodic tenderness of the temporomandibular joint and of the masseter and temporal muscles. The patient tolerated a bite plane well, and the muscle and joint symptoms resolved. Periodontal treatment was carried out and the diastemas in the upper jaw were then closed by means of a fixed appliance. Retention with interproximal bonding and a lingual retainer was inserted after 4 months (c, d). A bite plane was used in the upper jaw until a fixed bridge could be inserted to obtain proper stability of the vertical dimension of the dentition.

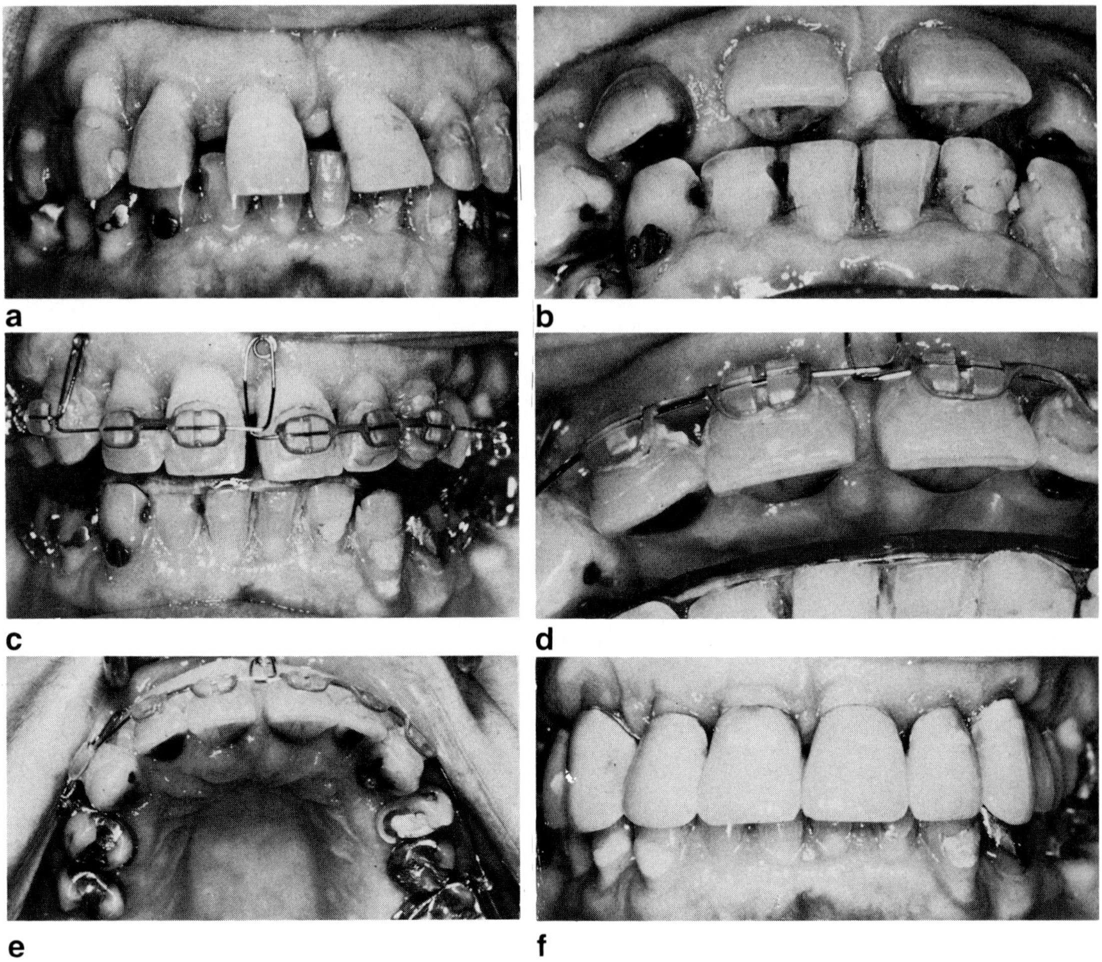

Fig. 23-9a-f.

Case No. 7

A 39-year-old woman (Figs. 23-9a-f) was referred by a general practitioner for excessive overbite and tooth migration in the maxillary frontal segment (a, b). An occlusal splint was placed in the lower jaw to raise the bite. The patient tolerated this splint therapy well, periodontal treatment was carried out, after which the diastemas in the upper jaw were closed by means of a fixed appliance (.016 green Elgiloy with contraction loops) (c, d, e). The final result, 4 years after orthodontic treatment and after construction of the crown prosthesis (f).

Case No. 8

A 50-year-old man had been treated for periodontal disease (Fig. 23-10a, b). He showed signs of tooth migration in the upper frontal segment in combination with excessive overjet. The diastemas were closed by means of a fixed appliance with contraction loops (c, d) and edge-wires (.016 x .016) with elastic chains (e, f). Note the transversal palatal bar (d, f) used to obtain proper anchorage of the molars. The retention was performed 12 months later (g, h) with a bonded lingual retainer placed in an enamel groove (see Fig. 23-2g, h).

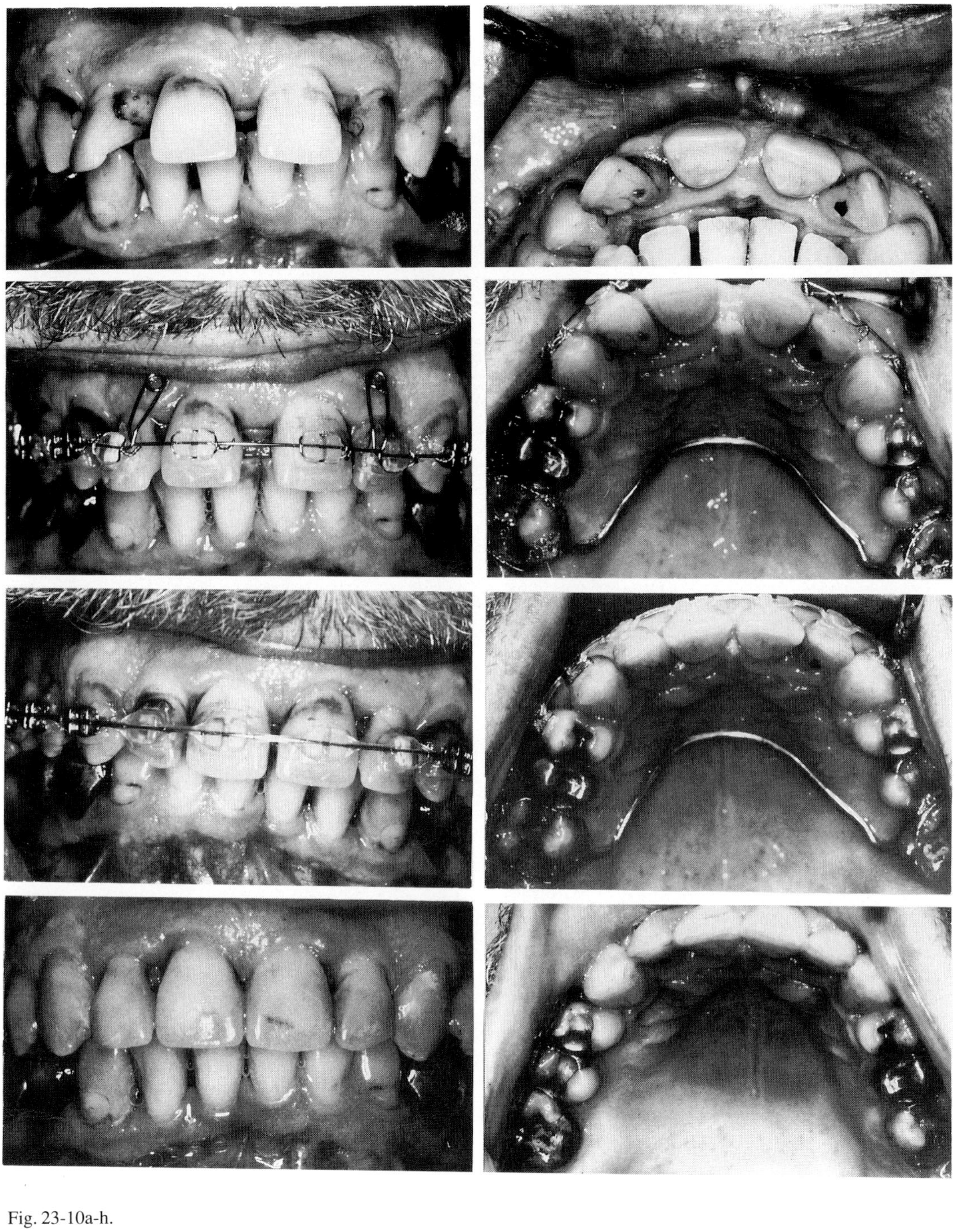

Fig. 23-10a-h.

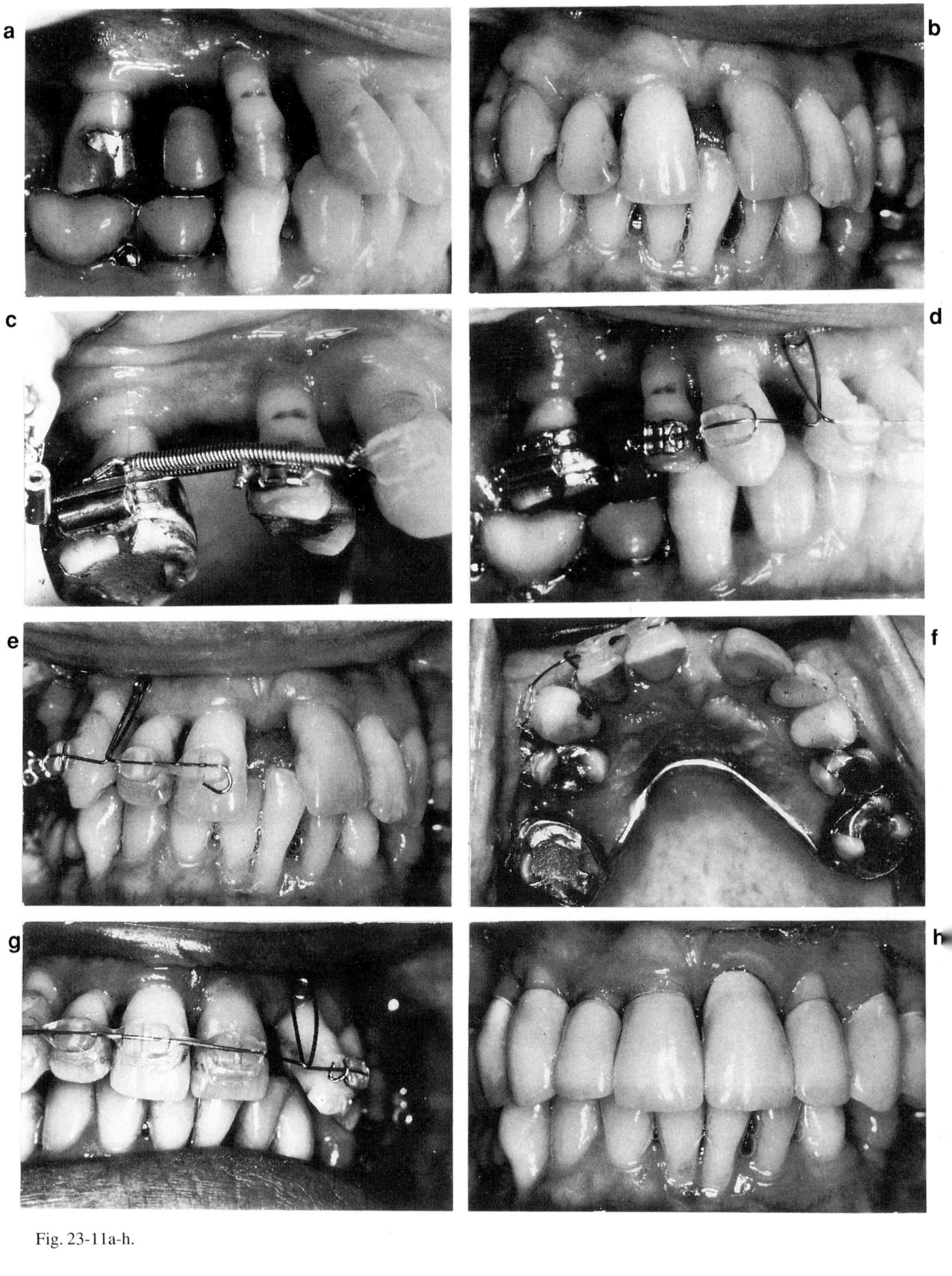

Fig. 23-11a-h.

Case No. 9

A 37-year-old woman had been treated for periodontal disease (Fig. 23-11a, b). Orthodontic treatment was performed because of generalized tooth migration in the maxilla. The right second premolar was extracted. The right first premolar was distalized and retained, after which the canine was distalized using an open coil (c). The frontal diastemas were then closed by fixed appliances with contraction loops (d-g). A transversal palatal bar was used for proper anchorage of the bifurcated molars. The final result with a fixed bridge for proper retention (h) 1 year after the end of orthodontic treatment is shown in (h).

Case No. 10

A 51-year-old woman (Figs. 23-12a-f) was referred to the Dental School for full mouth rehabilitation (a). It was agreed that after endodontic treatment in the frontal segment of the lower jaw and periodontal treatment in both jaws the patient should have orthodontic treatment of the anterior cross-bite. The treatment was carried out with a removable appliance which also raised the bite (b, c, d). The clasps were free from occlusal acrylic to permit proper anchorage. The small helical springs and the double, looped spring were reactivated only 1 mm every 3rd week. The cross-bite was eliminated after 5 1/2 months of treatment (e). After treatment, the periodontal conditions in the frontal segments were good. Note the alignment of the gingival margins. The final result after construction of a crown prosthesis (f).

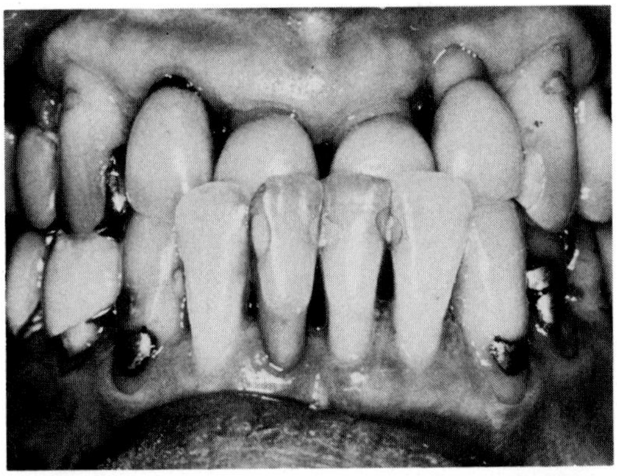

a

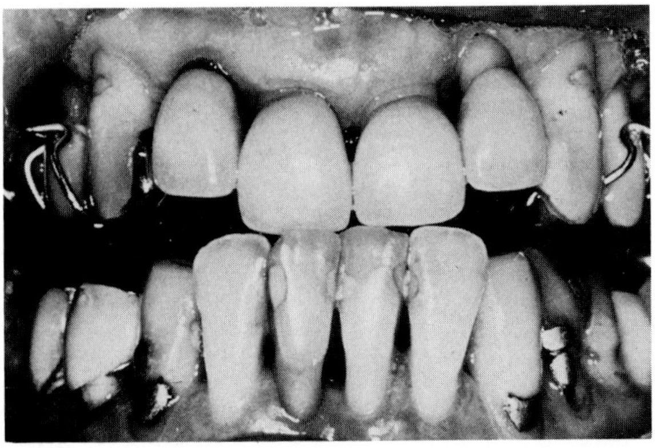

b

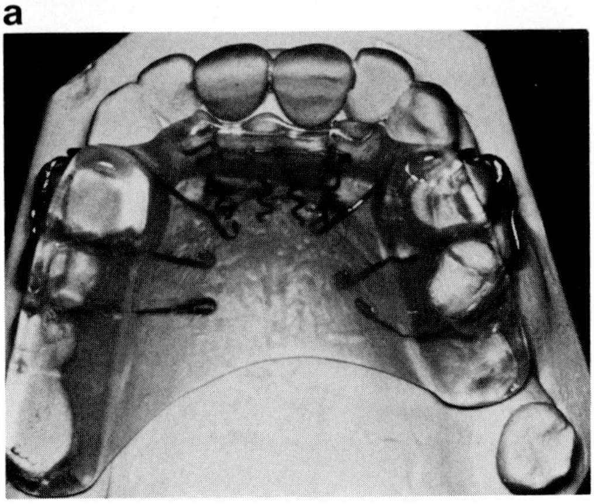

c

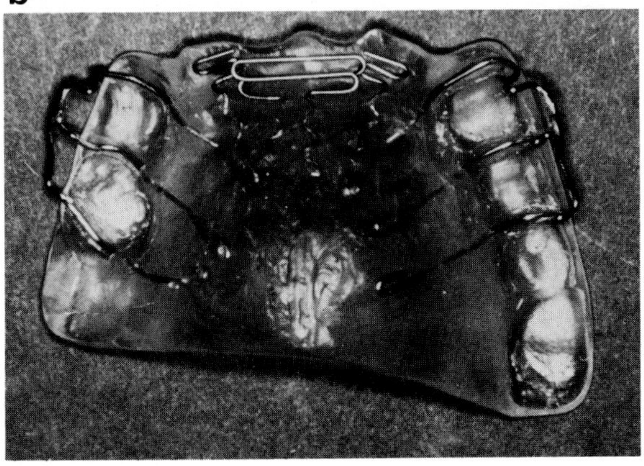

d

Fig. 23-12a-d.

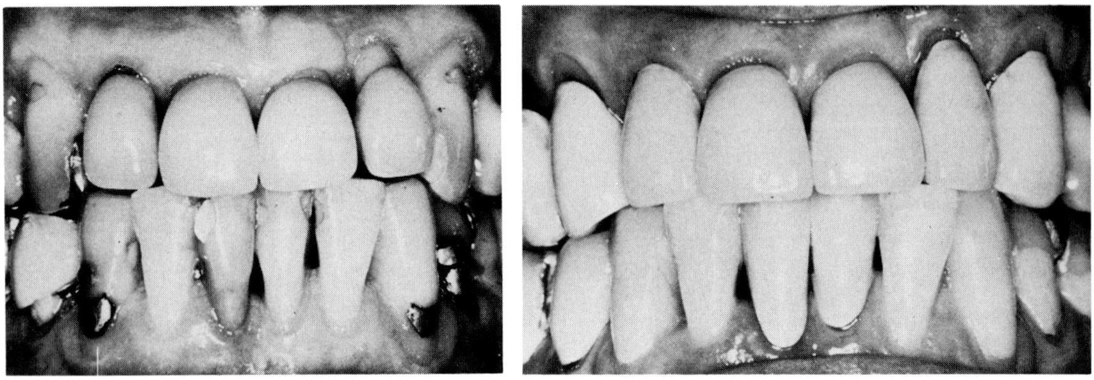

e f

Fig. 23-12e-f.

Case No. 11

A 30-year-old woman (Figs. 23-13a-j) had been treated for juvenile periodontitis (a, b). Orthodontic alignment of the teeth was undertaken preparatory to prosthetic reconstruction (c, d). Orthodontic treatment with coiled springs lasted 4 months, after which a bridge was constructed (e, f). Radiographs at the beginning and end of the periodontal treatment (g, h) and at the end of the orthodontic treatment as well as 1 year later (i, j).

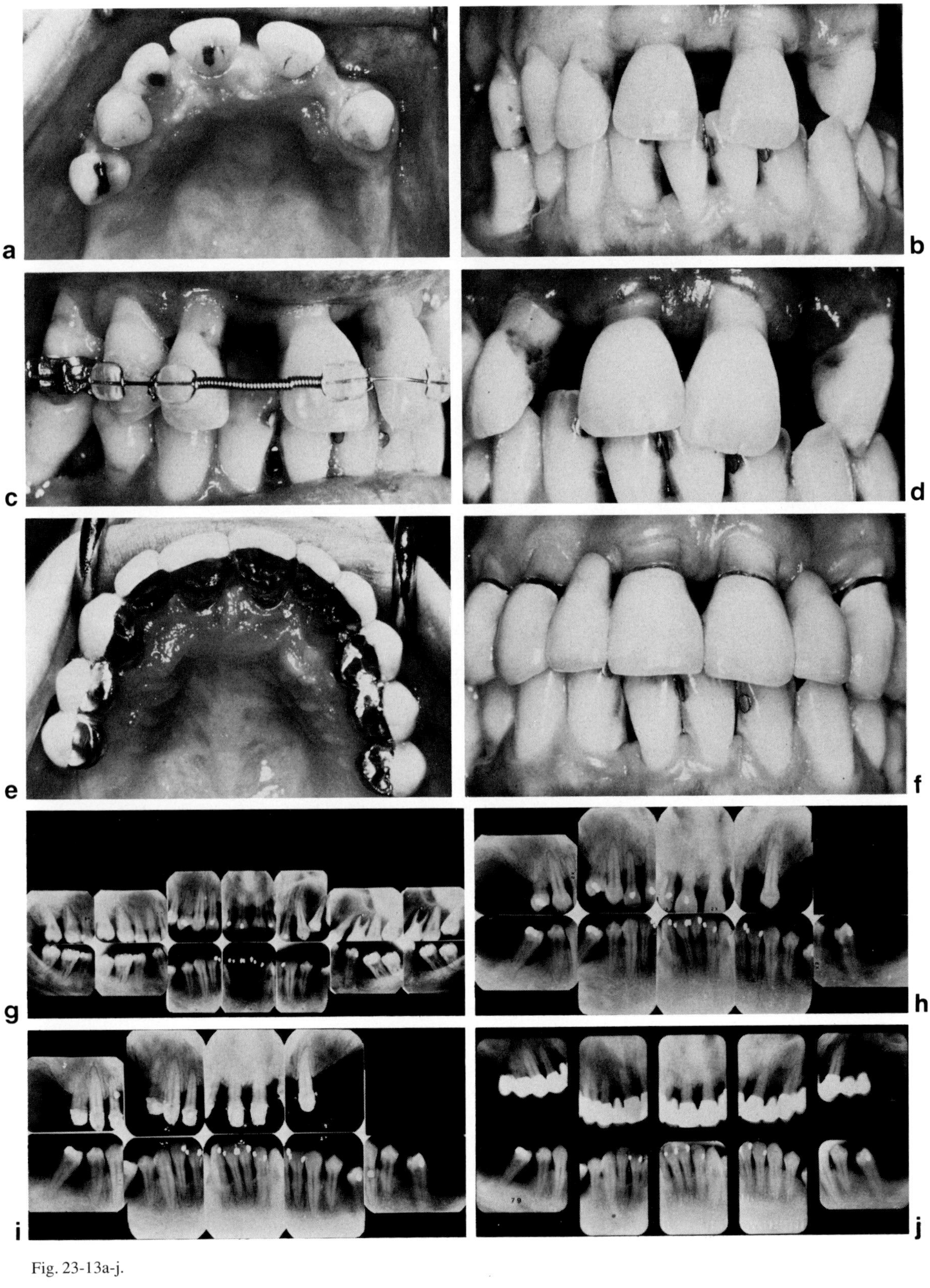

Fig. 23-13a-j.

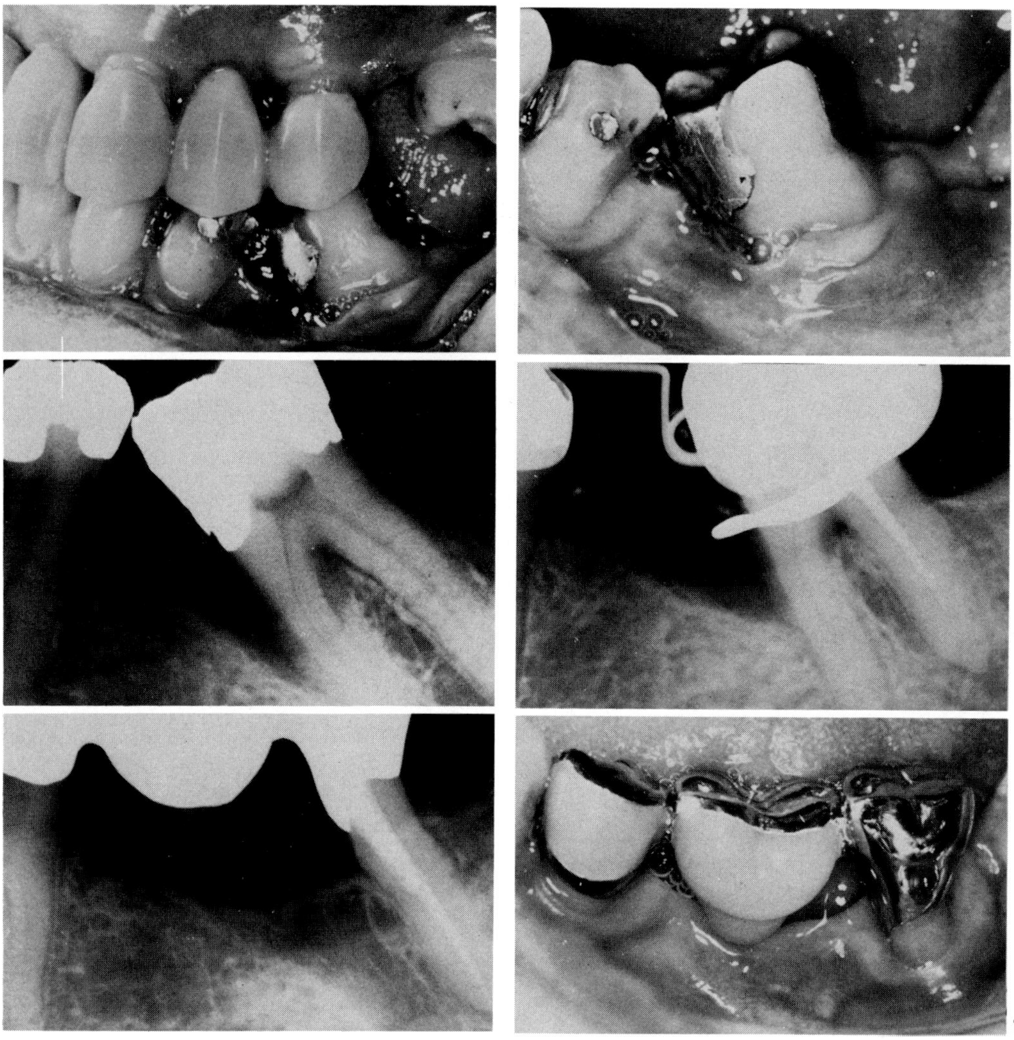

a b c d e f

Fig. 23-14a-f.

Case No. 12

A 45-year-old woman (Figs. 23-14a-f) was referred by a periodontist for treatment of a mesially tipped left mandibular second molar with a pronounced bony pocket and involvement of the bifurcation (a, b, c). It was considered important to preserve the distal root as abutment for a bridge prosthesis. After periodontal surgery, the tooth was tipped distally with an uprighting spring (.014 Australian) and this was followed by bone regeneration (d). After 7 months of treatment, the distal root was treated endodontically, the tooth was separated, the mesial root was extracted and the bridge prosthesis was constructed (e, f).

Case No. 13

A 49-year-old man had been treated for periodontal disease. The bucally tipped upper incisors had to be orthodontically realigned (Fig. 23-15a-d). Fixed appliance and a transversal palatal bar were used for proper anchorage. Retention was performed with a bonded lingual retainer. The left lower molars showed involve-

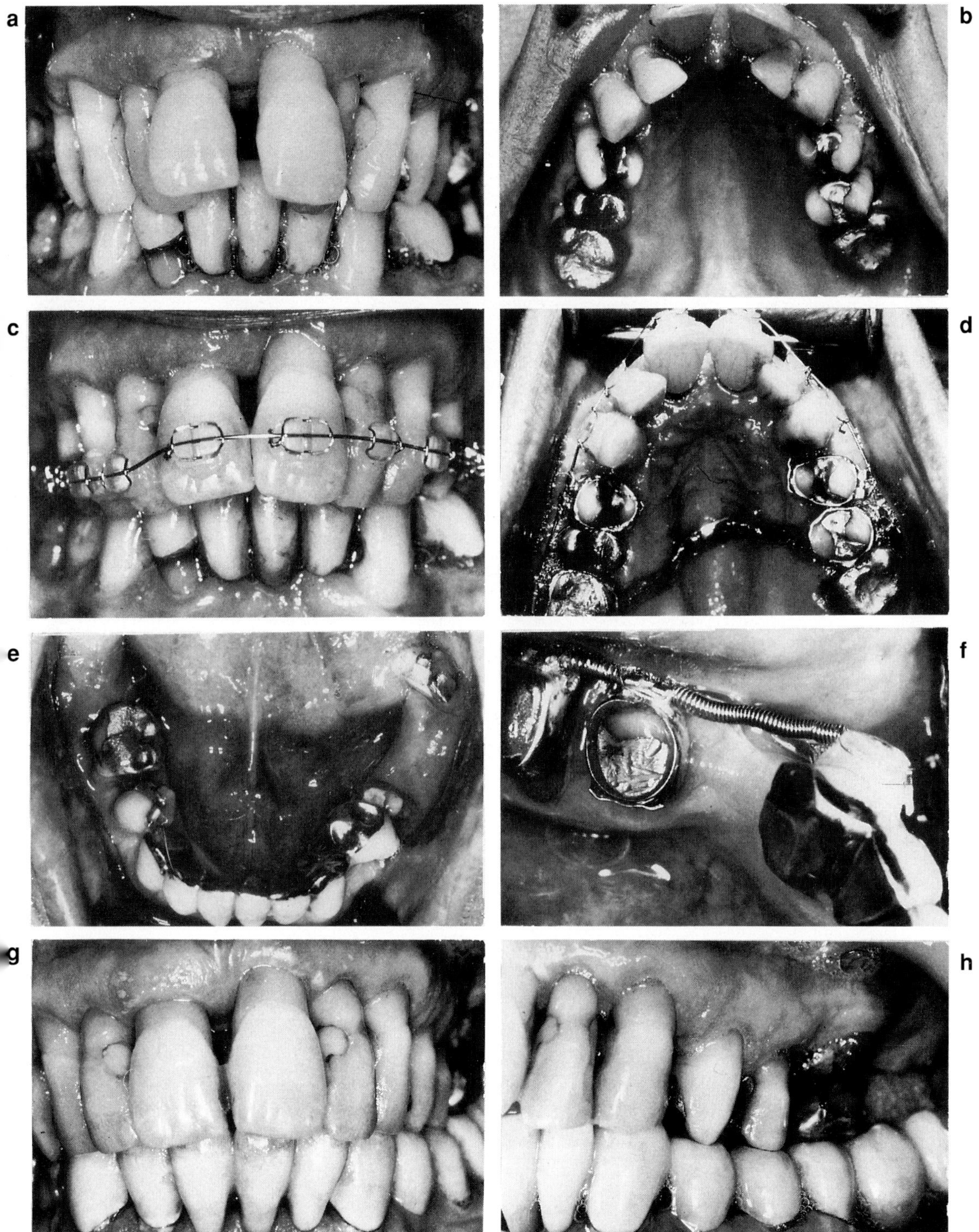

Fig. 23-15a-h.

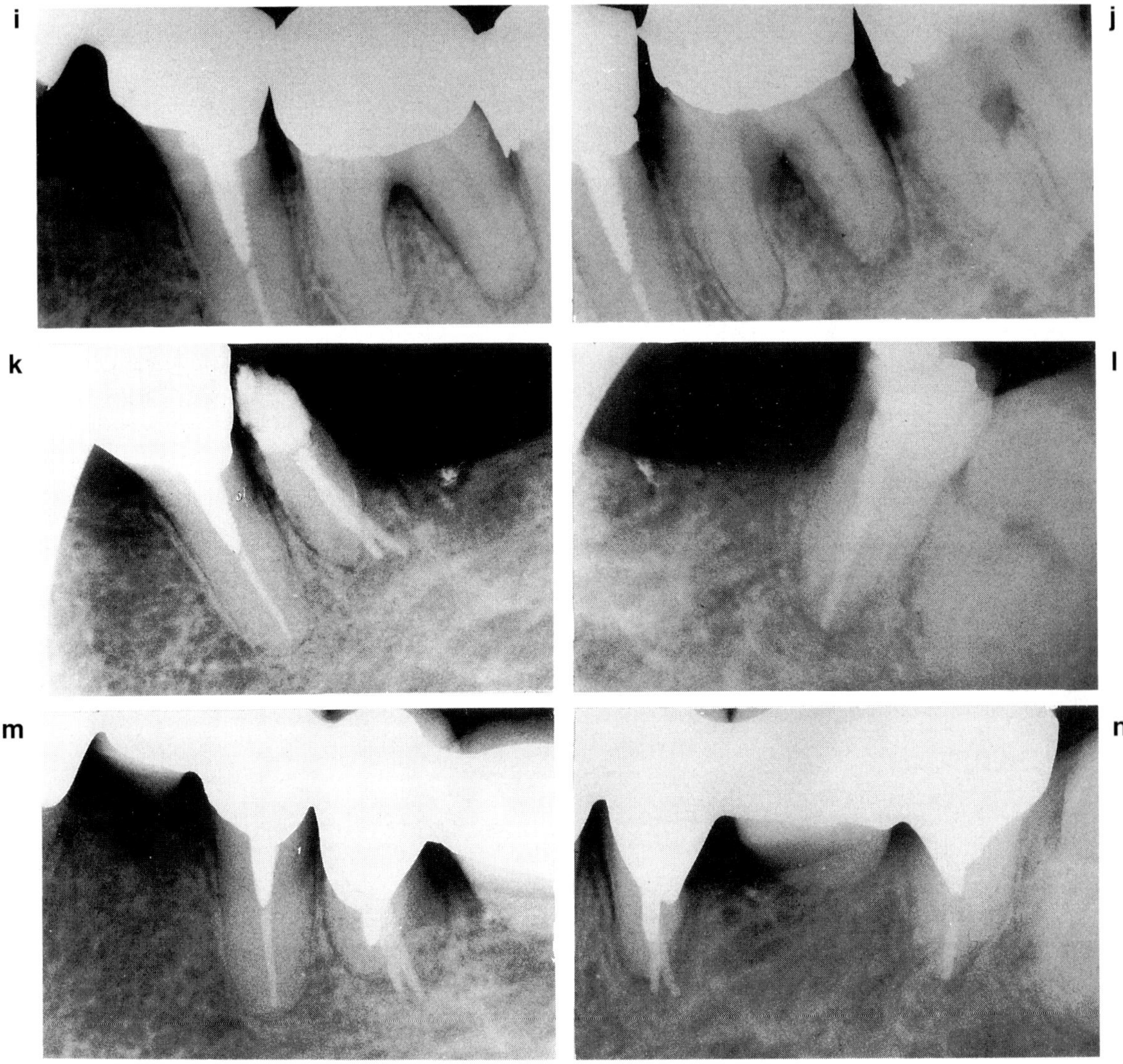

Fig. 23-15i-n.

ment of the bifurcation area (i, j). They were rootfilled, separated and the mesial root of the first molar and the distal root of the second molar were maintained (k, l, e). The tipped second premolar was separated from the fixed bridge and the crown was removed. The mesial root of the first molar was moved distally about 7 mm. This was followed by distalizing of the second premolar (j) using a coil. After an orthodontic treatment period of 8 months, fixed bridges were constructed in the left lower jaw. The final result, 2 years after treatment, is shown in (g,h).

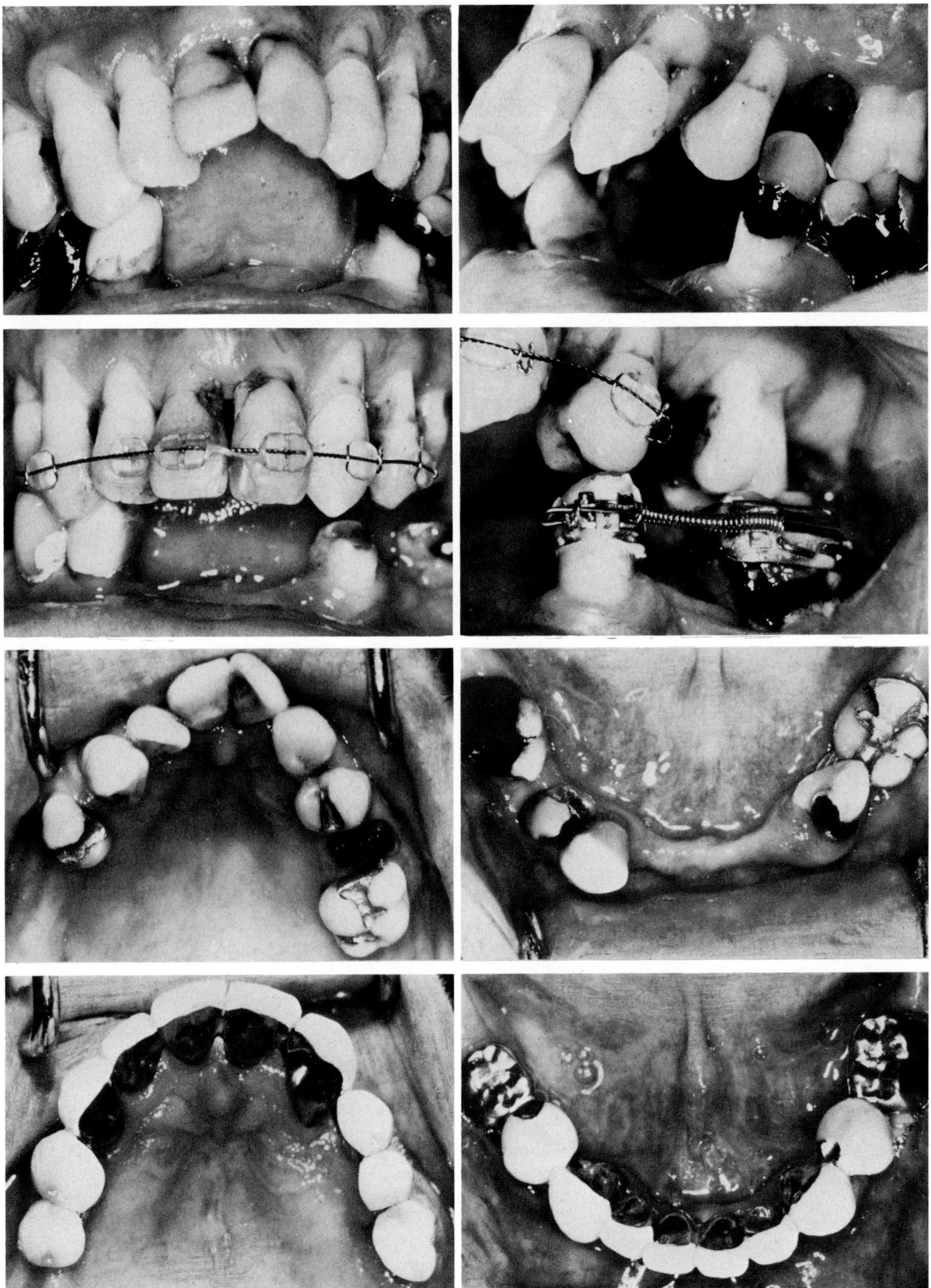

Fig. 23-16a-h.

Case No. 14
A 42-year-old man (Figs. 23-16a-h) was referred by a general practitioner for crowding and tipped mandibular teeth following tooth extractions (a, b, e, f). The intention was to use the few lower teeth as abutments for a fixed bridge. Periodontal treatment was carried out. The lower teeth were forced upright (d) with a coiled spring and the upper teeth were aligned (.016 green Elgiloy) (c). After 8 months of orthodontic treatment, bridges were constructed in both jaws (g, h).

References

Ahterton, J.D. (1970) Gingival response to orthodontic treatment. *American Journal of Orthodontics* **58**, 179-186.

Alstad, S. & Zachrisson, B. (1979) Longitudinal study of periodontal condition associated with orthodontic treatment in adolescents. *American Journal of Orthodontics* **76**, 277-286.

Baer, P.N. & Cocarro, P.J. (1964) Gingival enlargement coincident with orthodontic treatment. *Journal of Periodontology* **34**, 436-439.

Chasens, A.I. (1972) Indications and contraindications for adult tooth movement. *Dental Clinics of North America* **16**, 423-437.

Eliasson, L-Å., Hugosson, A., Kurol, J. & Siwe, H. (1982) The effects of orthodontic treatment on periodontal tissues in patients with reduced periodontal support. *European Journal of Orthodontics* **4**, 1-9.

Ericsson, I. & Thilander, B. (1978) Orthodontic forces and recurrence of periodontal disease. *American Journal of Orthodontics* **74**, 41-50.

Ericsson, I. & Thilander, B. (1980) Orthodontic relapse in dentitions with reduced periodontal support. An experimental study in dogs. *European Journal of Orthodontics* **2**, 51-57.

Ericsson, I., Thilander, B. & Lindhe, J. (1978) Periodontal conditions after orthodontic tooth movement in the dog. *Angle Orthodontist* **48**, 210-218.

Ericsson, I., Thilander, b., Lindhe, J. & Okamoto, H. (1977) The effect of orthodontic tilting movements on the periodontal tissues if infected and non-infected dentitions in dogs. *Journal of Clinical Periodontology* **4**, 278-293.

Follin, M., Ericsson, I. & Thilander, B. (1986) Occurrence and distribution of root resorption in orthodontically moved premolars in dogs. *The Angle Orthodontist* **56**, 164-175.

Glickman, I. (1972) *Clinical Periodontology*. 4th ed., Ch. 56. Philadelphia: W.B. Saunders Co.

Goldman, H.M. & Cohen, D.W. (1973) *Periodontal Therapy*. 5th ed., Ch. 23. St. Louis: C.V. Mosby Co.

Goldson, L. & Henrikson, C.O. (1975) Root resorption during Begg treatment. A longitudinal roentgenologic study. *American Journal of Orthodontics* **68**, 55-66.

Hollender, L., Rönnerman, A. & Thilander, B. (1980) Root resorption, marginal bone support and clinical crown length in orthodontically treated patients. *European Journal of Orthodontics* **2**, 197-205.

Iyer, V.S. (1962) Reaction of gingiva to orthodontic force - A clinical study. *Journal of Periodontology* **33**, 26-28.

Kloehn, J.S. & Pfeifer, J.S. (1974) The effect of orthodontic treatment on the periodontium. *Angle Orthodontist* **44**, 127-134.

Kvam, E. (1972) Scanning electron microscopy of tissue changes on the pressure surface of human premolars following tooth movement. *Scandinavian Journal of Dental Research* **80**, 357-368.

Linge, B. & Linge, L. (1980) Apikale Wurzelresorptionen der oberen Frontzähne. Eine longitudinelle, röntgenologische Untersuchung in einer kieferorthopädischen Praxis. *Fortschritte Kieferorthopädie* **41**, 276-288.

Melsen, B. (1986) Tissue reaction following application of extrusive and intrusive forces to teeth in adult monkeys. *American Journal of Orthodontics* **89**, 469-475.

Morse, P.H. (1971) Resorption of upper incisors following orthodontic treatment. *Dental Practitioner* **22**, 21-35.

Pearson, L.E. (1968) Gingival heights of lower central incisors orthodontically treated and untreated. *Angle Orthodontist* **38**, 337-339.

Polson, A., Caton, J., Polson, A.P., Nyman, S., Novak, J. & Reed, B. (1984) Periodontal response after tooth movement into infrabony defects. *Journal of Periodontology* **55**, 197-202.

Pritchard, J.F. (1975) The effect of bicuspid extraction orthodontics on the periodontium. *Journal of Periodontology* **46**, 534-542.

Reitan, K. (1959) Tissue rearrangement during retention of orthodontically rotated teeth. *Angle Orthodontist* **20**, 106-113.

Reitan, K. (1967) Clinial and histologic observations on tooth movement during and after orthodontic treatment. *American Journal of Orthodontics* **53**, 721-745.

Reitan, K. (1969) Principles of retention and avoidance of post-treatment relapse. *American Journal of Orthodontics* **55**, 776-790.

Reitan, K. (1975) Biomechanical principles and reactions. In *Current Orthodontic Concepts and Techniques*, ed. Graber & Swain, 2nd ed., Ch. 2. Philadelphia: W.B. Saunders Co.

Rönnerman, A., Thilander, B. & Heyden, G. (1980) Gingival tissue reactions to orthodontic closure of extraction sites. Histologic and histochemical studies. *American Journal of Orthodontics* **77**, 620-625.

Rygh, P. (1973) Ultrastructural changes in pressure zones of human periodontium incident to orthodontic tooth movement. *Acta Odontologica Scandinavica* **31**, 109-122.

Rygh, P. (1974) Elimination of hyalinized periodontal tissues associated with orthodontic tooth movement. *Scandinavian Journal of Dental Research* **82**, 57-73.

Sadowsky, C. & BeGole, E. (1981) Long-term effects of orthodontic treatment on periodontal health. *American Journal of Orthodontics* **80**, 156-172.

Schlossberg, A. (1975) *Adult Tooth Movement in General Dentistry*. Philadelphia: W.B. Saunders Co.

Sjölien, T. & Zachrisson, B. (1973) Periodontal bone support and tooth length in orthodontically treated and untreated persons. *American Journal of Orthodontics* **64**, 28-37.

Struteville, O.H. (1937) Injuries caused by orthodontic appliances and methods of preventing these injuries. *Journal of the American Dental Association* **24**, 1494-1507.

Thilander, B. (1979a) Ortodontisk behandling i adult ålder. *Tandläkartidningen* **71**, 1036-1046.

Thilander, B. (1979b) Indications for orthodontic treatment in adults. *European Journal of Orthodontics* **1**, 227-241.

Thilander, B. (1982) Orthodontic treatment in dentitions with reduced periodontal support. *Revue Belge de Médecine Dentaire* **37**, 119-125.

Thilander, B. (1986) The role of the orthodontist in the multidisciplinary approach to periodontal therapy. *International Dental Journal* **36**, 12-17.

Thilander, B. & Lennartsson, B. (1988) Vuxen ortodonti. Behandlingsbehov och åtgärder. *INVEST-ODONT AB Bjuv.*

Thilander, B., Nyman, S., Karing, T. & Magnusson, I. (1983) Bone regeneration in alveolar bone dehiscences related to orthodontic tooth movements. *European Journal of Orthodontics* **5**, 105-114.

Trosello, V.K. & Gianelly; A.A. (1979) Orthodontic treatment and periodontal status. *Journal of Periodontology* **50**, 665-671.

Wennström, J., Lindhe, J., Sinclair, F. & Thilander, B. (1987) Some periodontal tissue reactions to orthodontic tooth movement in monkeys. *Journal of Clinical Peridontology* **14**, 121-129.

Zachrisson, B. & Alnaes, L. (1973) Periodontal condition in orthodontically treated and untreated individuals. I. Loss of attachment, gingival pocket depth and clinical crown height. *Angle Orthodontist* **43**, 402-411.

Zachrisson, B. & Alnaes, L. (1974) Periodontal condition in orthodontically treated and untreated individuals. II. Alveolar bone loss: Radiographic findings. *Angle Orthodontist* **44**, 48-55.

CHAPTER 24

An Overview of the Effect of Periodontal Therapy

Objectives and means of therapy

The overall objectives of dental therapy for an adult patient may include measures to: 1) obtain relief from pain, 2) arrest dental diseases, and 3) satisfy the patient's demands regarding a) esthetics, b) chewing comfort.

Treatment plan

Objectives	**Means**
I. Eliminate inflammation II. Maintain/regain periodontal tissue support III. Maintain/regain stability of remaining teeth	I+II. Reduce/eliminate infections 1. Plaque control measures 2. Scaling and root planing 3. Periodontal surgery A) access for proper debridement B) establish conditions which favor regain of supporting tissue III. Occlusal adjustment - splinting

Fig. 24-1. Different objectives and procedures available for the treatment of a patient with periodontal disease.

Often a patient who suffers from periodontal disease also shows signs of a number of other dental and oral disorders such as caries (primary or recurrent), pulpal disease, mucous membrane disease, temporomandibular joint dysfunction, etc. In this chapter only procedures which are used in the treatment of periodontal disease will be discussed (Fig. 24-1). It should be understood, however, that the proper overall therapy for patients with periodontal disease includes also the detailed diagnosis and treatment of all other dental and oral disorders present.

Plaque control measures to eliminate gingival inflammation

The efficiency of oral hygiene measures to eliminate infection in deep periodontal pockets has been studied in humans by Tagge et al. (1975), Listgarten et al. (1978), Badersten et al. (1984), and others.

Tagge et al. (1975) treated 2 supra-bony pockets in each of 22 individuals with periodontal disease in two different ways. Three sites (A,B and C) were first examined regarding gingivitis, probing depth and clinical attachment level. Following this examination, one site (A) was excised and sectioned for histological examination. Site B was subjected to careful scaling and root planing while site C received no professional therapy. The patients were instructed to use meticulous oral hygiene measures for 2 months, following which sites B and C were reexamined. After a clinical examination the soft tissue of the 2 sites was excised and prepared for histological examination. The clinical and histological assessments revealed that oral hygiene measures alone 1) reduced the overt signs of inflammation, 2) had a limited effect on the probing depth, and 3) had no effect on the clinical attachment level. When oral hygiene measures were combined with scaling and root planing, however, there was 1) a pronounced reduction in gingival inflammation, 2) a substantial reduction of the probing depth, and 3) a significant gain of clinical attachment.

The authors concluded that scaling and root planing accompanied by oral hygiene measures resulted in greater improvement of the clinical and histopathological parameters describing periodontal disease than oral hygiene measures alone. In fact, oral hygiene measures in this study had no obvious effect on the inflammatory lesion in the deeper parts of the pockets.

Listgarten et al. (1978) studied the effect of subgingival scaling on periodontal disease in 6 patients with advanced lesions. Following an examination of a number of gingival sites for 1) gingival inflammation, 2) probing depth, 3) probing attachment level, 4) supragingival plaque, and 5) composition of the subgingival microbiota, all patients were given detailed instruction and practice in proper tooth-cleaning measures. This oral hygiene instruction was repeated at several consecutive sessions. With the use of a split-mouth design of therapy the teeth in 2 quadrants were carefully scaled, while in 2 quadrants no professional tooth debridement was performed: 8 and 25 weeks after active therapy the patients were reexamined (Table 24-1 and 24-2).

Table 24-1

	Examinations	Nonscaled	Scaled
Plaque Index	0 week	2	2
(median)	8	0	0
	25	0	0
Gingival Index	0	2	2
(median)	8	1	0.5
	25	1.5	0
Probing depth	0	7.0 ± 0.9	7.0 ± 0.6
(mm; $\bar{x}$)	8	6.5 ± 0.9	5.3 ± 1.0
	25	6.5 ± 0.8	4.5 ± 0.9

Table 24-1 presents the results from the clinical examinations. The Plaque Index score representing the nonscaled and scaled sites revealed that the patients' self-performed oral hygiene was effective in eliminating supragingival deposits (Plaque Index score = 0). But, while in the scaled sites gingival health was established following therapy (Gingival Index score = 0) and the probing depths were reduced from 7.0 to 4.5 mm, there was in the nonscaled areas no significant improvement of either gingival conditions or probing depths (Listgarden et al. 1978).

Badersten et al. (1984) studied the effect of improved "self-performed" oral hygiene measures and subgingival scaling and root planing in 16 patients with advanced periodontitis. After an initial examination including assessments of plaque and gingivitis (bleeding on

Table 24-2

	Examinations	Nonscaled	Scaled
Coccoid cells	0 week	41%	42%
+	8	43%	82%
Straight rods	25	39%	75%
Motile rods	0	55%	49%
+	8	48%	13%
Spirochetes	25	51%	8%

Table 24-2 describes the alterations that occurred in the scaled and nonscaled sites regarding some characteristic features of the subgingival microbiota (assessed by dark-field microscopy). Scaling and root planing resulted in a marked increase of the percentage of coccoid cells and straight rods (bacteria which are associated with periodontal health) and a marked decrease in the percentage of motile rods and spirochetes (bacteria associated with periodontal disease). No such alterations of the microbiota occurred in the nonscaled sites. Listgarten et al. (1978) concluded that in patients with advanced periodontal disease and deep periodontal pockets supragingival plaque control without scaling neither eliminates the subgingival infection nor resolves gingival inflammation. Similar findings were reported by Beltrami et al. (1987) in a short-term study (Listgarden et al. 1978).

probing on the base of the pocket) the patients were, on an individual basis, given a series of oral hygiene instructions to improve their self-performed plaque control. After 3 months of repeated oral hygiene instruction all patients were reexamined and subsequently given a series of treatments including supra-and subgingival scaling and root planing. Reexaminations were performed every 3 months during a 2-year period.

Fig. 24-2 (Badersten 1984; Fig. 2) illustrates the result from this study. While the repeated oral hygiene instructions reduced the plaque scores from 60-80% (at the initial examination) to about 5% at 3 months, no corresponding improvement could (at 3 months) be detected with respect to the gingival conditions. After subgingival instrumentation, however, the frequency of sites that bled on probing was dramatically reduced (from 80% to about 10% of sites). The authors concluded that there was no or only a minimal effect of plaque control measures alone at sites with deep periodontal pockets, while subgingival instrumentation produced a marked improvement of the periodontal conditions.

Conclusion

From the clinical studies reported it can be concluded that self-performed oral hygiene measures used alone have a limited, if any, ef-

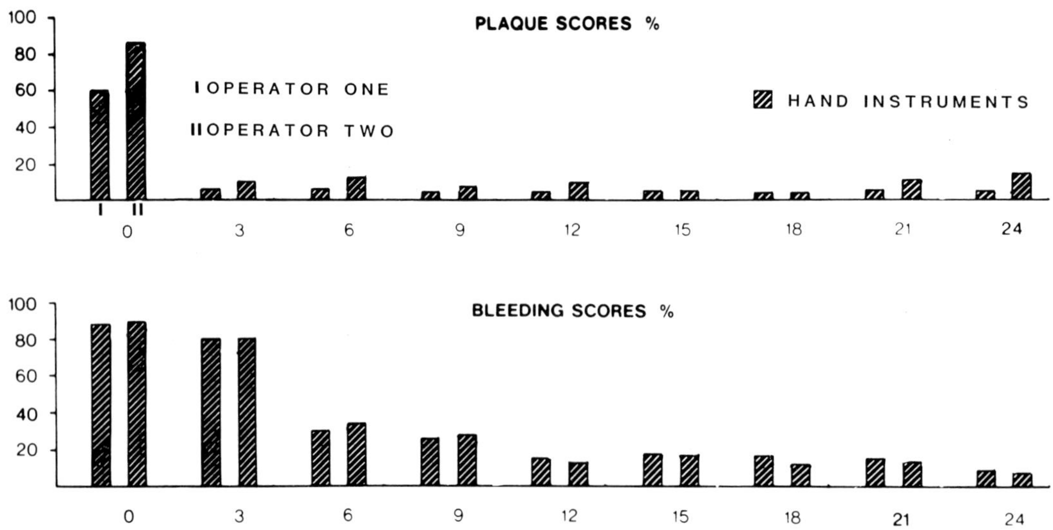

Fig. 24-2.

fect on the subgingival microbiota and the associated signs of inflammation in *deep* periodontal pockets. Oral hygiene measures used alone are therefore not effective in the treatment of periodontal disease at sites with deep pockets.

Scaling and root-planing measures to eliminate inflammation

The potential of scaling and root planing measures to eliminate inflammation and arrest progression of periodontal disease has been studied in a number of clinical trials, e.g. Lövdal et al. (1961), Suomi et al. (1971), Axelsson & Lindhe (1978,1981), Hirschfeld & Wasserman (1978), Morrison et al. (1980), Badersten et al. (1984).

Lövdal et al. (1961) examined around 1,500 individuals in Norway regarding their oral hygiene status, gingival conditions, alveolar bone loss and tooth loss. The patients were subsequently, on an individual basis, given careful oral hygiene instruction, including detailed information in the proper use of toothbrush, toothpick, dental floss, etc. In addition, their teeth were subjected to meticulous supra- and subgingval scaling and root planing. The oral hygiene instruction as well as the scaling and root-planing measures were repeated 2-4 times

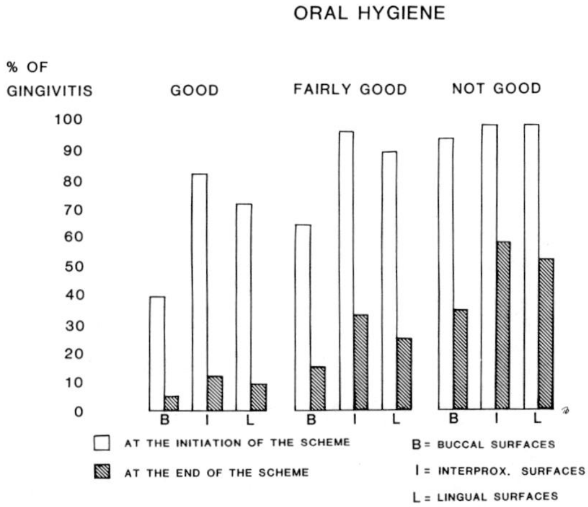

Fig. 24-3. The patients were divided into 3 groups after the initial examination according to their oral hygiene: "good", "fairly good", "not good". During a 5-year period the patients were subjected to scaling and root planing measures 2-4 times per year. The authors noted that in all 3 categories of patients there was a remarkable improvement of gingival conditions after 5 years of repeated plaque control measures. (Data from Lövdal et al. 1961).

per year over a 5-year period at the end of which the patients were reexamined. The authors found (Fig. 24-3; Table 24-3) that "the combined effect of subgingival scaling and controlled oral hygiene definitely reduced the incidence of gingivitis and tooth loss". The improvement was remarkable also in patients whose home-care habits remained improper during the 5 years of trial.

Similar findings were reported by Suomi et al. (1971) from a study comprising 350 individuals in California. A test group of patients received during a 3-year period oral hygiene instruction and scaling 3-4 times per year, while

Table 24-3

Average loss of teeth during the 5-year period and "normal" loss of teeth

	Grade of oral hygiene		
	Good	Fairly good	Not good
"Normal" loss of teeth. Estimate based on the data recorded at the initiation of the period	1.1	1.4	1.8
Actual loss of teeth during the 5-year period	0.4	0.6	0.9

Lövdal et al. 1961

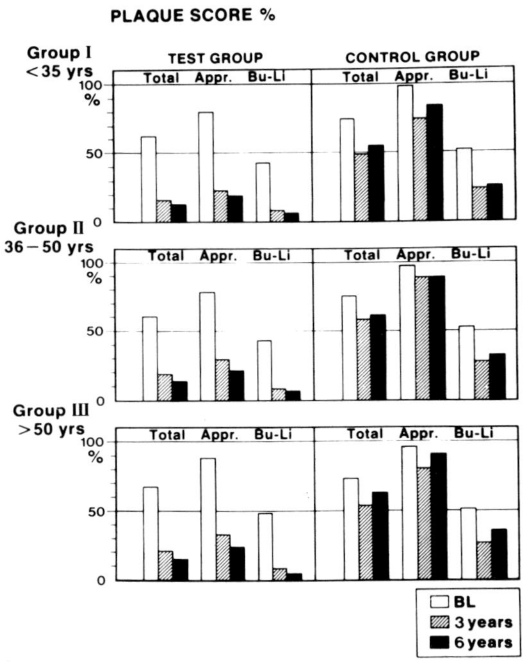

Fig. 24-4. Histogram describing the frequency distribution of tooth surfaces harboring plaque at the baseline examination (BL) (open bars) and at the reexaminations 3 (hatched bars) and 6 (black bars) years later. In the control groups, after 3 and 6 years of trial, there was a tendency towards lower plaque scores on buccal-lingual (Bu-Li) surfaces only. In the test groups the individual mean plaque scores were reduced from 60-70% (BL) to around 10-20% (3 and 6 years). (Data from Axelsson & Lindhe 1981).

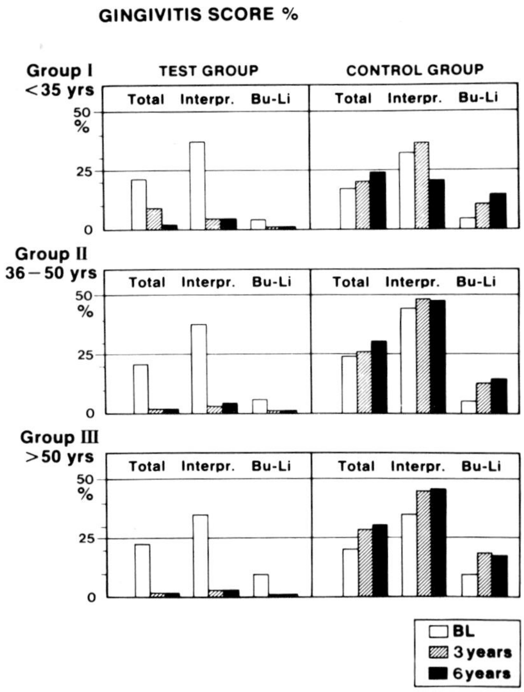

Fig. 24-5. Histogram showing the frequency distribution of inflamed gingival units in the test and control groups at the baseline (open bars) and reexaminations (3 and 6 years; hatched and black bars respectively). The individual mean (total) figures describe unaltered gingival conditions in the control groups but marked improvements in the test groups during the trial. (Data from Axelsson & Lindhe 1981).

a control group during the same period received traditional dental care. At the end of the treatment period the test group patients had significantly less gingivitis and less attachment loss than the controls.

Axelsson & Lindhe (1978, 1981) compared the effect of a prophylactic program including 1) oral hygiene control and 2) scaling and root planing repeated once every 2-3 months over a 6-year period with the effect of traditional dental therapy, i.e. a therapy which was directed towards the symptoms of dental disorders rather than towards the elimination of the etiological factors. Fig. 24-4 depicts alterations regarding oral hygiene that occurred in the test and control groups over the 6 years of observation. In the patients of the control groups there was only a minor improvement in oral hygiene, while in the test groups at the reexaminations after 3 and 6 years, the mean plaque scores were consistently low (< 20%). In the control groups there was no improvement of the gingival conditions (Fig. 24-5), while in the test groups the gingivitis scores had approached 0 values (meaning gingival health) at the reexaminations. Fig. 24-6 gives the attachment level alterations between 1972 and 1978. It can be seen that, while in the patients of the control groups there was a substantial loss of attachment, in the test patients there was no further breakdown of the attachment apparatus.

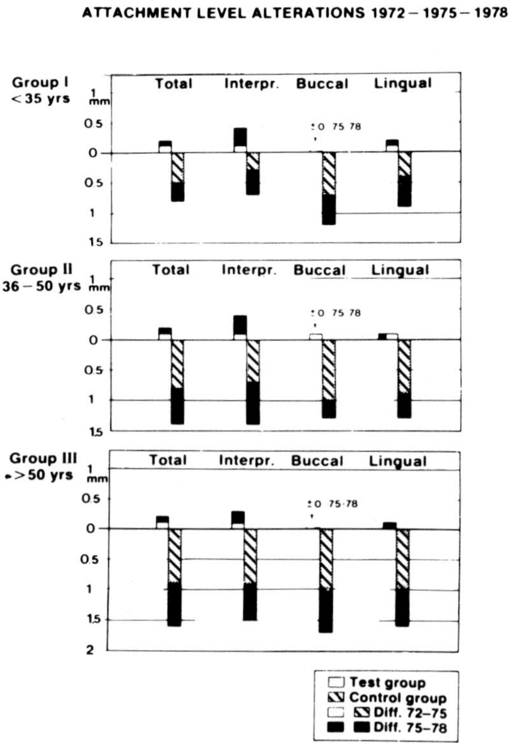

Fig. 24-6. Histogram illustrating alterations of the clinical attachment levels between the baseline (1972) and reexaminations (1975, 1978) in the various test and control groups. The attachment level remained unaltered in the test groups but was reduced in all the control groups (below the O-line). The average attachment loss per year in control groups was: I: 0.13 mm, II: 0.23 mm, III: 0.26 mm. (Data from Axelsson & Lindhe 1981).

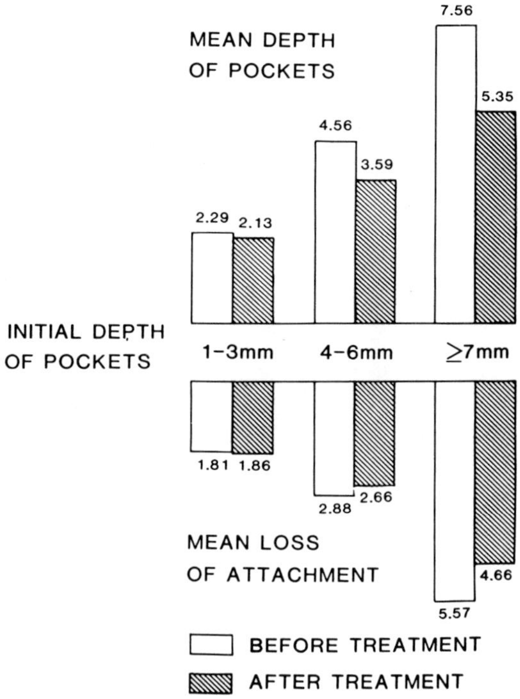

Fig. 24-7. The bars describe reduction of probing depth and some gain of clinical attachment 4 weeks after active therapy comprising subgingival scaling and root planing. (Data from Morrison et al. 1980).

Hirschfeld & Wasserman (1978) presented a long-term-survey of tooth loss in 600 patients treated for periodontal disease. The patients were reexamined at an average of 23 years after the active treatment which included primarily subgingival scaling and root planing followed by careful maintenance therapy. The authors observed that "during the post-treatment period 300 patients had lost no teeth from periodontal disease", and "199 had lost 1-3 teeth...". This means that periodontal therapy directed towards the elimination of the subgingival infection using a nonsurgical approach can be effective in preventing tooth loss in most patients and also in those with advanced periodontal disease.

Morrison et al. (1980) studied the *short-term* effect of nonsurgical treatment in 90 subjects with moderately advanced periodontal disease. Following an initial examination the patients were given oral hygiene instruction and the pockets were treated by subgingival scaling and root planing. Reexamination performed 4 weeks after active therapy revealed that 1) the patients had improved their oral hygiene, 2) the gingivitis scores had decreased, and 3) the initial depth of the periodontal pockets was substantially reduced (Fig. 24-7). The authors concluded that already 1 month following the hygienic phase of periodontal therapy the clinical severity of periodontal disease can be markedly reduced.

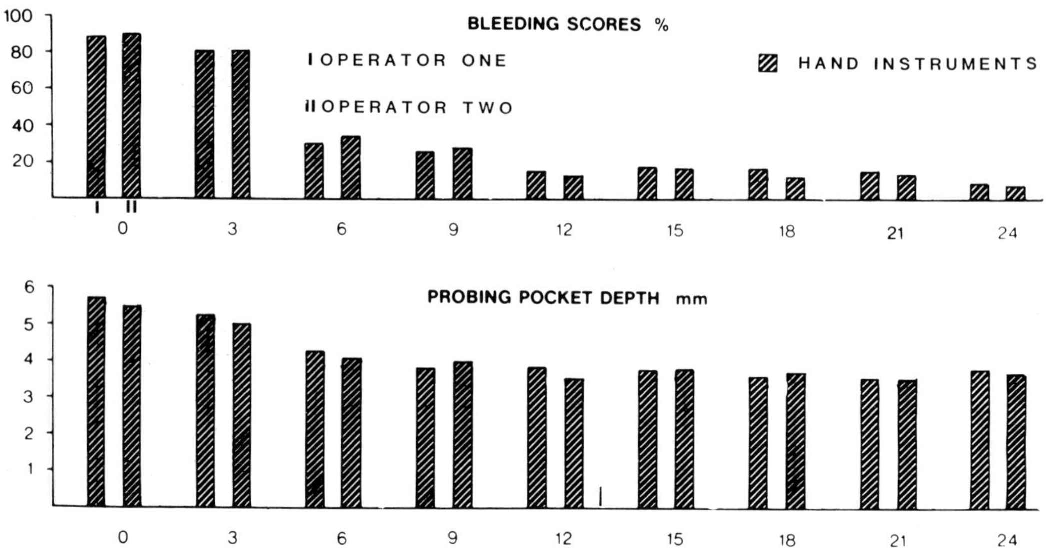

Fig. 24-8.

Badersten et al. (1984) studied, as discussed above, the effect of nonsurgical periodontal therapy in 16 patients with periodontitis. Following an initial examination the patients received oral hygiene instruction and all single-rooted teeth were exposed to meticulous subgingival debridement using either handscalers or an ultrasonic device. Reexamination carried out 2 years after initial therapy showed that this nonsurgical treatment had resulted in the establishment of healthy gingival conditions (only about 10% of the gingival sites examined bled on probing to the base of the pocket) and in a marked reduction in the overall probing depth (Fig. 24-8, Badersten 1984). The authors concluded that careful subgingival scaling and root planing was an effective means to eliminate gingivitis and reduce the probing depth even at sites with initially extremely deep (> 9 mm) periodontal pockets. Similar observations have also been reported by Magnusson et al. (1984)

Conclusion

The above review of some important clinical trials demonstrates that subgingival scaling and root planing are measures which can be effective in 1) eliminating inflammation also in deep periodontal pockets, 2) in reducing probing depths, and 3) in improving clinical attachment levels. This does not mean that scaling and root planing are always the only measures that are required in order to properly eliminate subgingival infection in deep pockets. Thus, studies by e.g. Waerhaug (1978), Rabbani et al. (1981), Magnusson et al. (1984) have revealed that in such pockets residual calculus and plaque may be found even after meticulous subgingival instrumentation. This means that the clinician has to examine carefully all sites in all his patients and monitor the alterations obtained by the nonsurgical therapy. If, following scaling and root planing, signs of "bleeding on probing to the bottom of the pocket" persist, and if the clinical attachment level fails to improve, surgical therapy should be considered since this treatment may facilitate more adequate root debridement (Eaton et al. 1985, Caffesse et al. 1986).

Periodontal surgery-access for proper debridement

Curettage/gingivectomy/flap procedures

The potential of surgical techniques to enable the operator to gain access to the root surfaces for proper debridement and to establish optimal conditions for healing and maintenance therapy has been examined in a number of clinical trials (e.g. Ramfjord et al. 1968, 1973, 1975, Lindhe & Nyman 1975, 1984, Rosling et al. 1976 b, Knowles et al. 1979, Nyman & Lindhe 1979, Isidor 1981, Philstrom et al. 1981, Lindhe et al. 1982a, Westfelt et a1 1985).

Ramfjord and coworkers (Knowles et al. 1979) reported on the effect of periodontal treatment in 43 patients with advanced periodontal disease. The patients received a treatment which included oral hygiene instruction, scaling and root planing followed by either subgingival curettage, modified Widman flap surgery, or the apically positioned flap procedure. Following active therapy the patients were, over an 8-year period, recalled once every 3 months for prophylaxis. The annual examinations revealed that periodontal pockets were reduced in depth and stayed reduced and that the clinical attachment levels were improved over 8 years following either mode of therapy in properly maintained patients (Fig. 24-9).

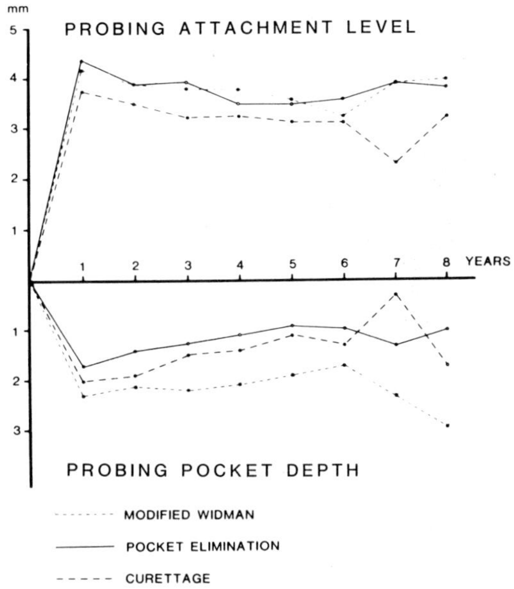

Fig. 24-9. Active therapy including either curettage, modified Widman flap surgery or the apically positioned flap procedure (Pocket elimination) was carried out during year 0. The patients were maintained by prophylaxis every 3 months over an 8-year period. The probing depths were reduced and stayed reduced and the clinical attachment levels were improved and remained improved in all 3 treatment categories. (Data from Knowles et al. 1979).

Lindhe & Nyman (1975,1984) and Nyman & Lindhe (1979) described the long-term effect of treatment in 75 patients who initially suffered from advanced periodontal disease. The patients who were enrolled in the study had lost more than 50% of the supporting apparatus. Following an initial therapy which included instruction in oral hygiene measures and scaling, all patients were treated surgically using an apically positioned flap technique. In some cases bone recontouring was used to eliminate osseous defects. Following active therapy, the patients were, as in the Ramfjord group study described above, for 14 years placed on a maintenance program which included prophylaxis once every 3-6 months. The reexamination performed immediately after healing revealed that the therapeutic measures used had resulted in low Plaque and Gingival Index scores, markedly reduced probing depths and in the maintenance of the height of the alveolar bone around all remaining teeth. Reexaminations 5, 8 and 14 years later disclosed that the maintenance care delivered almost entirely prevented recurrence of symptoms of gingivitis and periodontal disease.

In 1976 Rosling et al. (1976b) described the result of treatment of 50 patients who initially

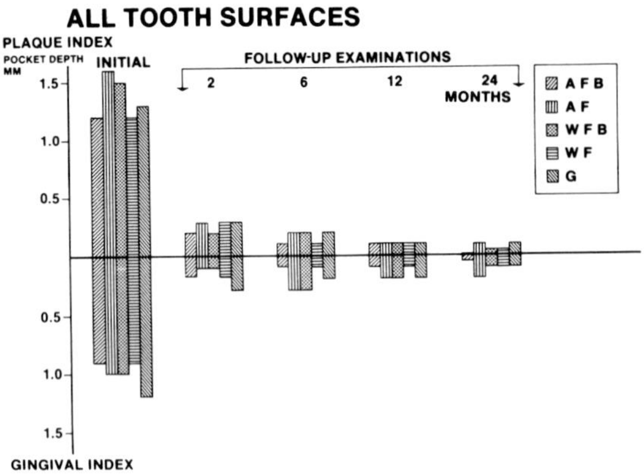

Fig. 24-10. The various treatment modalities (AFB, AF, WFB, WF, and G) are identified in the upper right corner of the diagram. In all 5 categories of patients low Plaque and Gingival Index scores were obtained following active therapy. The low Plaque and Gingival Index scores were maintained during the 24 months of observation. (Data from Rosling et al. 1976).

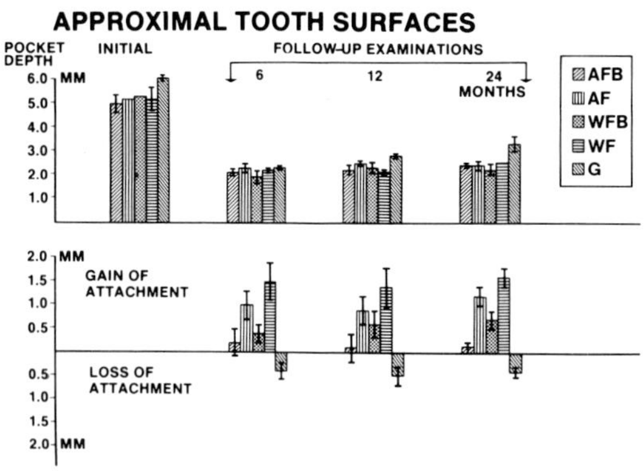

Fig. 24-12. Probing depth and attachment level alterations between the initial examination and the 24-month reexamination are described. During the observation period no loss of clinical attachment occurred in the 5 treatment groups. In patients subjected to flap surgery without additional bone resection there was a substantial gain of clinical attachment. (Data from Rosling et al. 1976; see. Fig 24-10).

suffered from advanced periodontal disease associated with multiple angular bony defects. Following an initial examination the participants in this trial were distributed into 5 different treatment groups. In 2 groups the periodontal lesions were treated with the *apically positioned flap* technique, in 2 other groups the

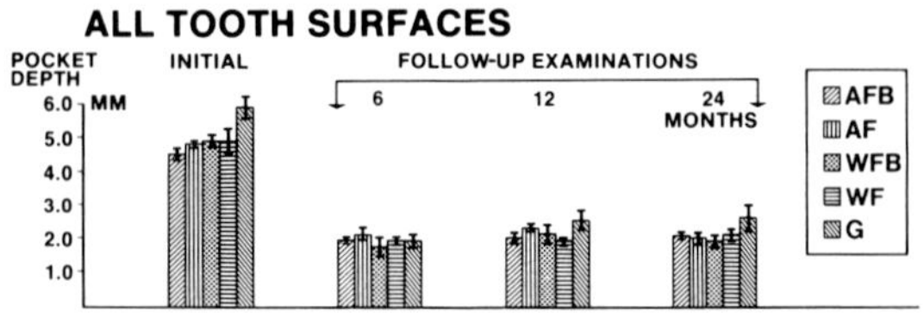

Fig. 24-11. In all 5 groups of patients shallow pockets resulted and remained shallow during the maintenance period. (Data from Rosling et al 1976: see Fig. 24-10).

modified Widman flap technique was used, and in the 5th group the periodontal pockets were eliminated with a *gingivectomy* technique. In 1 of each of the 2 flap treatment groups, bone recontouring was carried out to eliminate angular bony defects, while in the remaining groups the infrabony defects were treated by curettage without osseous surgery. Immediately after treatment the patients were placed on a plaque control regimen which included chlorhexidine mouth rinsing (for 2 months) and professional tooth cleaning once every 2 weeks for 2 years. The reexaminations 2, 6, 12 and 24 months after surgery revealed that all patients had maintained a high standard of oral hygiene (Fig. 24-10). Gingival health was established and maintained for 2 years in most parts of the dentitions. Shallow pockets had resulted (Fig. 24-11) and at interproximal sites at which a flap technique without bone recontouring measures had been utilized there was substantial gain of clinical attachment (Fig. 24-12).

Westfelt and coworkers (1985) treated 16 patients with periodontitis using 6 different techniques: scaling and root planing (S) as a single measure or combined with gingivectomy (G), apically positioned flap without (A) or including bone recontouring (AB), modified Widman flap without (W) or including bone recontouring (WB). During a 6-month period after treatment the patients were recalled once every 2 weeks for professional tooth cleaning. The reexamination performed after 6 months revealed that, irrespective of treatment technique used, low plaque and gingival bleeding scores had

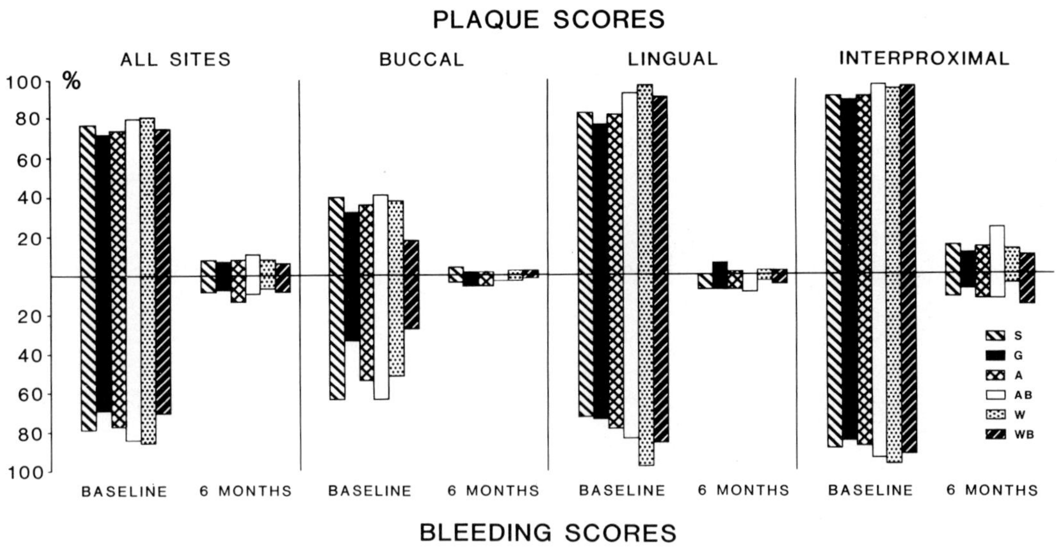

Fig. 24-13.

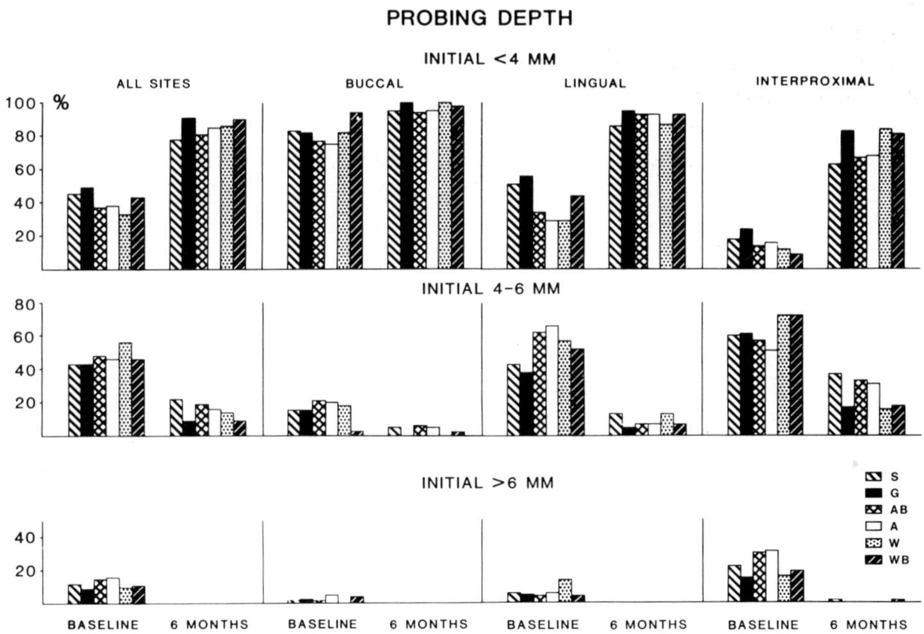

Fig. 24-14a.

resulted (Fig. 24-13; Westfelt Fig. 1). Furthermore, the 6 treatment groups showed similar degree of probing pocket depth improvement (Fig. 24-14; Westfelt Fig. 2), similar change with respect to attachment level changes (Fig. 24-14a) and recession of the gingival margin

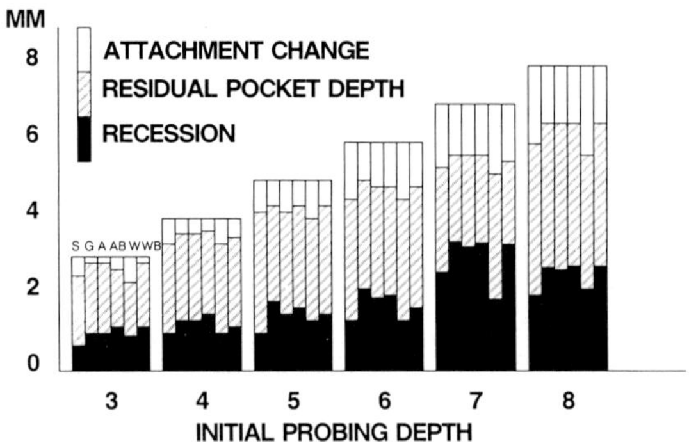

Fig. 24-14b.

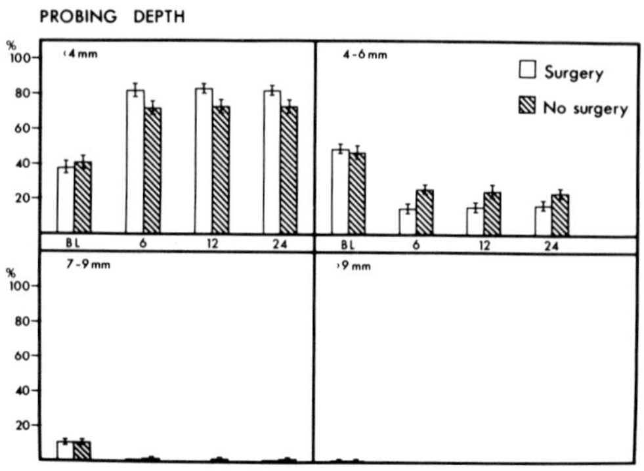

Fig. 24-15. Probing depths. Frequency distribution of probing depths < 4 mm, 4-6 mm, 7-9 mm and > 9 mm calculated from measurements made at the baseline (BL) and reexaminations. At the reexaminations the frequency of probing depths < 4 mm was higher in the Surgery than in the No-Surgery group. (Data from Lindhe et al. 1982).

(Fig. 24-14b). Thus, at sites with initially shallow pockets there was some loss of probing attachment, whereas at sites with initially deep pockets some gain of clinical attachment had occurred. In addition, irrespective of treatment technique used, initially shallow pocket sites had small amounts of gingival recession, while deeper pocket sites showed more pronounced signs of recession of the gingival margin.

Conclusion

The results of the clinical trials described reveal that in patients meeting high requirements of oral hygiene the type of surgical technique used to gain access for proper debridement is of minor importance for the overall result. Since Nyman et al. (1977) demonstrated that, in patients who were *not properly* maintained after surgery, recurrence of periodontal disease developed irrespective of surgical technique used for pocket elimination, the findings reported above point towards the *quality* of the maintenance system as being the discriminating factor for success or failure in surgical treatment of periodontal disease.

Surgical versus nonsurgical approach

Lindhe et al. (1982a) studied healing following one surgical and one nonsurgical approach to treatment of periodontal disease. After a baseline examination patients with moderately advanced disease were subjected to treatment using a split-mouth technique. In the right or left side of the jaw subgingival scaling and root planing were performed in conjunction with the modified Widman flap procedure (surgery group), while in the contralateral jaw quadrants the treatment was restricted to scaling and root planing (nonsurgery group). Following active therapy the patients were recalled for professional tooth cleaning once every 2 weeks (for 6 months) and thereafter for prophylaxis once every 3 months (for 18 months). The results of the study demonstrated that scaling and root planing alone were almost as effective as their use in combination with surgery for establishing clinically healthy gingiva and in preventing further loss of attachment. Both methods of treatment resulted in a high frequency of sites with probing depth of < 4 mm (Fig. 24-15). The reduction of the probing depth was more pronounced in initially deep than in initially shallow pockets and, for initially deep pockets, more marked at sites subjected to surgery than at sites exposed to scaling and root planing alone. The measurements also

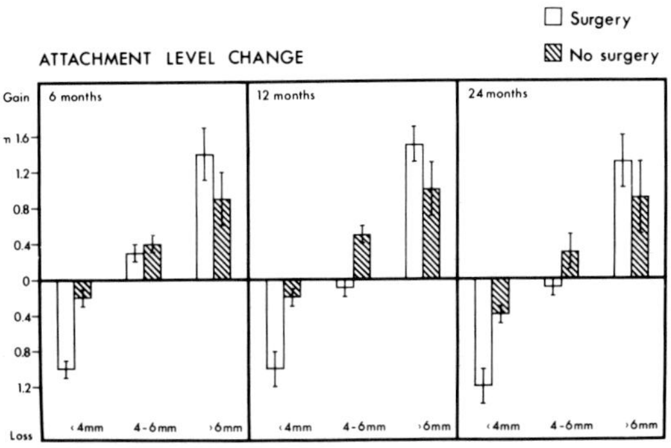

Fig. 24-16. Attachment level change between baseline and the follow-up examinations for probing depths < 4 mm, 4-6 mm and > 6 mm. For sites with probing depths < 4 mm there was loss of attachment while probing depths > 6 mm showed gain of attachment. (Data from Lindhe et al. 1982).

showed that sites with initially deep pockets exhibited more gain of clinical attachment than sites with initially shallower pockets (Fig. 24-16).

Similar findings were reported by Isidor (1981), who studied the effect of surgical and nonsurgical methods of periodontal therapy in 17 patients with moderately advanced periodontal disease. Examinations, performed over a 6-month period following treatment, failed to reveal any marked differences in the effect of therapy between the surgical and nonsurgical approaches. In a 4-year study Pihlstrom et al. (1981) compared the effect of a surgical (modified Widman flap) and a nonsurgical mode of therapy and concluded that both procedures were almost equally effective in reducing signs of periodontal disease, but that the additional flap procedure tended to result in greater pocket reduction and clinical attachment gain in initially deep pockets (Fig. 24-17).

On the other hand Hill et al. (1981), who examined the effect of 4 different types of periodontal treatment in 19 patients reported that none of the surgical modalities of therapy was better than scaling and root planing alone for the maintenance of clinical attachment levels.

When the findings from clinical research are evaluated, it is important to realize that clinical

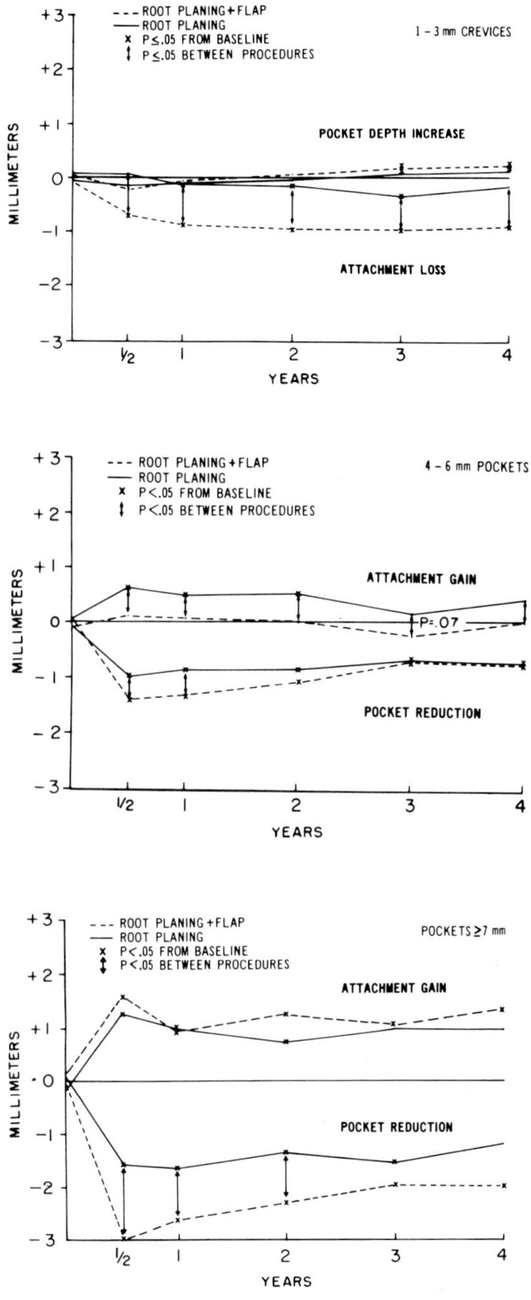

Fig. 24-17. Data from Pihlstrom et al. (1981).

assessments of attachment gain and attachment loss are associated with errors (See Chapter 12). At gingival sites with inflammation and pockets the dentogingival epithelium offers no resistance to the probe. Thus, at probing, the apical base of the inflammatory cell infiltrate

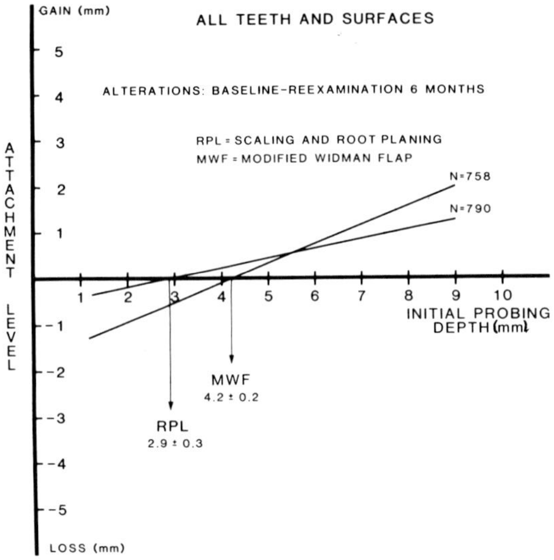

Fig. 24-18. Diagram illustrating alterations in attachment level (gain and loss) between the baseline examination and reexamination after 6 months. The initial probing depth values are described on the X-axis. The regression lines illustrating the effect of scaling and root planing (RPL) and periodontal surgery (MWF) intersect the X-axis at points representing initial probing depths of 2.9 ± 0.3 (RPL) and 4.2 ± 0.2 (MWF). (Data from Lindhe et al. 1982).

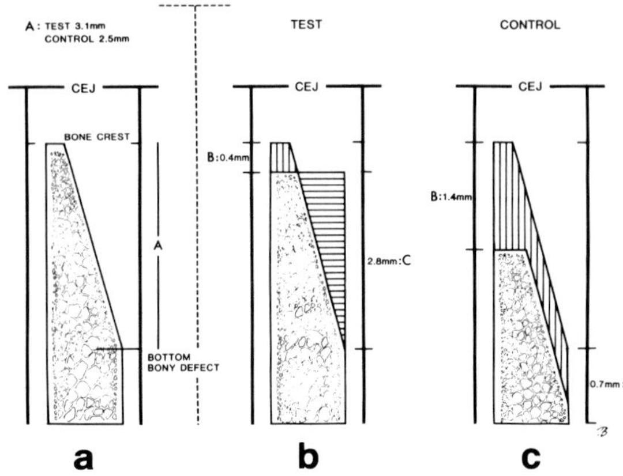

Figs. 24-19 a-c. Schematic drawings illustrating alterations in the level of the marginal alveolar bone crest and the level of the bottom of the bony defects in the test and control groups. Distance A denotes the bony defect (a). In the test group patients this distance was 3.1 mm at the initial examination. The corresponding value in the controls was 2.5 mm. Distance B denotes resorption of the marginal alveolar crest. This distance was 0.4 mm in the test patients and 1.4 mm in the controls (b,c). Distance C denotes gain or loss of bone in the apical portion of the defect. There was a refill of bone in test patients amounting to 2.8 mm, whereas an apical displacement of 0.7 mm of the bottom of the bony defects occurred in the control patients (b,c). (Data from Rosling et al 1976).

rather than the base of the pocket is being identified. After treatment, the elimination of the infiltrate and the replacement of the infiltrate with collagen result in a tighter adaptation of the gingiva to the tooth. The probe, following healing and the ensuing increased tissue tone, can often penetrate only a distance of ≤ 4-5 mm below the gingival margin, i.e. the probe may now fail to reach the apical cells of the dentogingival epithelium. This means that the deeper the inflamed periodontal pocket was at the initial examination, the more gain of clinical attachment is measured following proper healing. Thus, gain of clinical attachment following treatment may rather reflect an error inherent in the measurement technique than a real gain of connective tissue attachment.

The important criterion of periodontitis is "bleeding on probing", and the important criterion of periodontal health is "no bleeding on probing". In the studies referred to above it was demonstrated that "no bleeding on probing" can result from both surgical and nonsurgical approaches to therapy.

"Critical probing depth"

The above reported investigations, describing the effect of surgical and nonsurgical therapy in patients with periodontal disease, have demonstrated that while periodontal sites with initially deep pockets tend to gain clinical attachment, sites with initially shallow pockets tend to lose attachment (Ramfjord et al. 1973, 1975, Knowles et al. 1979, Pihlstrom et al. 1981, Lindhe et al. 1982 a,b, Westfelt et al. 1985). In the study by Lindhe et al. (1982b), regression analysis was used to identify so-called "critical probing depths", i.e. initial probing depth values of sites from different groups of teeth and tooth surfaces below which loss of attachment is likely to occur and above which clinical attachment gain often results following therapy. By means of this method of analysis it was observed that the "critical probing depth" value for scaling and root planing used as the only measure of therapy was significantly smaller than the corresponding value for scaling and root planing used in combination with a modified Widman flap technique of surgery. The slope of the regression lines for the 2 modalities (Fig. 24-18) also indicates, however, that at sites with an initial probing depth above the "critical probing depth" more gain of clinical attachment can be expected to occur following Widman flap surgery than following the nonsurgical modality. On the other hand, the surgical approach may result in more attachment loss than scaling and root planing alone, when used at sites with initially shallow pockets. The findings thus reported may be interpreted to mean that, in patients with a large number of periodontal sites with shallow probing depths, a nonsurgical approach to therapy should be preferred, while in patients with a large number of deep pockets, surgical treatment may result in greater gain of clinical attachment.

Conclusion

Findings from clinical trials reported during the last few years have obviously indicated that nonsurgical approaches to periodontal therapy may be as effective as treatment modalities which also include periodontal surgery. The efficacy of therapy in the studies described has been expressed in terms of 1) resolution of gingivitis, 2) probing pocket depth reduction, 3) gingival recession, and 4) gain of probing attachment.

The student of the above findings must be aware, however, that data describing healing following periodontal therapy have consistently been expressed in terms of *mean values* for individuals or groups of individuals. In other words, the patient (as a whole) has been used as the "experimental unit". There are of course compelling reasons for this choice. Sites (teeth, tooth surfaces) in the same mouth can be viewed as being related samples; they exist in the same host with the same nutritional, endocrinological, immunological etc. status; in designing experiments the subjects can be conveniently randomly assigned to one of several treatment modalities. The concept of using the subject as the "experimental unit" fits rather uncomfortably, however, with the recognition of the site-specific nature of periodontal disease. It is clear that different sites within the same individual show different patterns of disease progression and "lesion morphology" and often respond differently to periodontal therapy. Thus, while the lesion which is associated with a deep angular bony defect often responds to a treatment with considerable probing attachment gain and bone fill, a lesion with a "horizontal" bony defect and suprabony pocket hardly ever responds with regrowth of bone and only occasionally with substantial probing attachment gain. This suggests that there is marked degree of *independence* between the different periodontal sites, a hypothesis which is further validated by the remarkable difference that exists in the composition of the subgingival microbiota from one periodontal site to another in the same patient. The above discussion implies that pooling of treatment data from within the same individual may obscure meaningful differences that may arise at individual sites. Mean values representing individual patients or groups of patients participating in clinical research, therefore, should be used by the clinician as guidelines rather than as recipes when he/she is in the process of planning the treatment for a given patient and a given set of periodontal sites within the patient. The clinician should recognize the fact that both nonsurgical and surgical treatment techniques at many sites may meet her/his objectives. At some sites, however, e.g. at furcation-involved molars, surgical therapy may be the only method that permits proper root debridement. At other sites a nonsurgical approach to therapy may be preferred for esthetical reasons. Irrespective of method of therapy used, the end point of active treatment should ideally be that no periodontal site is present at which bleeding can be provoked by gentle probing to the base of the pocket.

Periodontal surgery used to establish conditions which favor regain of supporting tissue

Under this heading, methods are discussed which are used to obtain a *zone of keratinized and attached gingiva and also methods which favor regrowth of alveolar bone, periodontal ligament and root cementum.*

Keratinized and attached gingiva for the maintenance of gingival health

It has often been claimed that the presence of a zone of keratinized and attached gingiva is necessary for the maintenance of gingival health.

Consequently, a number of surgical procedures have been developed to maintain or establish a zone of such gingiva or to increase its width as part of the overall treatment of periodontal disease. But what is indeed regarded as an adequate zone, in terms of millimeters of keratinized and attached gingiva?

Bowers (1963) stated that it is possible to maintain a clinically healthy gingiva in humans despite a narrow zone of attached gingiva (< 1 mm). However, Bowers also claimed that when there was no attached gingiva present at all, the marginal tissue was usually inflamed.

Lang & Löe (1972) described the results from a clinical trial in humans in which the relationship between the width of keratinized gingiva and gingival health was studied. A group of test subjects without any pathologically deepened pockets first went through a preparatory period of 6 weeks during which their oral hygiene was supervised on a daily basis. Buccal and lingual units were examined at the end of this hygienic phase, for 1) the width of the keratinized gingiva, 2) Gingival Index and Plaque Index scores, and 3) the amount of gingival exudate that could be harvested from plaque-free gingival units with < 2 mm of keratinized gingiva and with > 2 mm of keratinized gingiva. Lang & Löe concluded that gingival health is compatible with a very narrow zone of the gingiva. They also observed, however, that in areas with < 2 mm of keratinized gingiva, clinical signs of inflammation persisted in spite of effective oral hygiene. A subsequent study by Miyasato et al. (1977), on the contrary, indicated that there may be no requirement at all for a minimum width of the attached gingiva for the maintenance of gingival health, provided proper plaque control is established.

Wennström et al. (1981) studied the role of keratinized gingiva for gingival health in an experiment in beagle dogs. Cotton floss ligatures were placed around the teeth on the right side (experimental side) of the jaws in 5 dogs and plaque was allowed to accumulate in order to induce periodontal tissue breakdown. After 150 days the inflamed periodontal tissues around the experimental teeth were removed by surgical means using either a "gingivectomy" or a "flap" procedure. In the "gingivectomy" procedure the entire zone of the keratinized gingiva was excised while with the flap procedure the main part of the keratinized tissue was maintained. During 120 days of healing a high standard of plaque control was maintained by daily professional tooth cleaning. On the left side of the jaw (controls side) proper tooth cleaning was performed daily during the entire observation period of 270 days.

The results of this study demonstrated that, during a 270-day period of careful plaque control, the width of the keratinized gingiva on the control side was maintained unaltered. In comparison, the phase of experimental periodontitis on the test side resulted in a substantial decrease in the width of the keratinized gingiva. Subsequent to the excision ("gingivectomy") of the inflamed periodontal tissue (which in some areas included the entire zone of the keratinized gingiva) a new, although much shorter and thinner, gingival unit developed at most sites. At a few sites, however, no keratinized gingiva reformed. In most respects the structural composition of the regenerated units was similar to that of a normal noninflamed unit. Furthermore, independent of whether keratinized gingiva was present or not and independent of the width of the keratinized zone, in the absence of plaque, the regenerated soft tissue was consistently found to be free from signs of inflammation.

On day 270 in the dog experiment (Wennström et al. 1982) all tooth-cleaning measures were abolished. After 40 days of plaque accumulation, clinical examination was repeated and biopsies were sampled. The biopsy material was subjected to histometric and morphometric analysis. The results demonstrated that the regenerated free gingiva at sites with a wide as well as with a very narrow (< 1 mm) zone of keratinized gingiva responded to mircrobial colonization by an inflammatory reaction, the location and extension of which did not vary with the width of the keratinized zone. It was concluded that, in the presence of plaque, a dentogingival unit with a narrow zone of – or entirely lacking – keratinized gingiva has an equal capacity for inflammatory response against infection as does a unit with a wide zone of keratinized gingiva.

Dorfman & Kennedy (1981) studied the development of gingivitis in 20 patients who at bilateral sites with gingival recession had no attached gingiva present. In one of these bilateral sites an autogenous gingival graft was placed and allowed to heal. The patients were placed on a plaque control program during a subsequent preparatory period until gingival health had been established. At this point in time all patients ceased oral hygiene measures for 21 days. At the end of the plaque accumulation period an examination revealed that there was no difference between grafted and nongrafted sites regarding the number of gingival units that changed from Gingival Index score 0 to scores 1 or 2. Furthermore, there was no difference regarding the net change of gingival fluid flow. Dorfman & Kennedy concluded that recession sites with no attached gingiva are not more susceptible to inflammation than areas with attached gingiva.

Conclusion

The conclusion that can be drawn from the experiments and trials reported above suggests that a certain minimum width of keratinized and attached gingiva is *not necessary* for the maintenance of healthy marginal tissue. Furthermore, nonkeratinized dentogingival tissue has a capacity equal to keratinized gingiva to react with an inflammatory response to plaque accumulation. The inflammatory lesion in nonkeratinized tissue does not spread in apical direction at a more rapid rate than the lesion in keratinized gingival tissue.

Presence of a zone of keratinized and attached gingiva for the prevention of gingival recession

The claim has been made that a zone of keratinized and attached gingiva is necessary to prevent recession of the gingival margin (e.g. Ochsenbein & Maynard 1974, Gartell & Matthews 1976, Boyd 1978). Results from long-term studies by Dorfman et al. (1980), Hangorsky & Bissada (1980), Lindhe & Nyman (1980) and Wennström (1983, 1987) make it reasonable to question this hypothesis.

Dorfman et al. (1980) presented results regarding the effect of the placement of free autogenous gingival grafts in 107 sites with gingival recession and "inadequate" zone of keratinized gingiva. Contralateral sites with corresponding deficiencies served as controls and remained non-operated. The patients were, following active therapy, recalled for scaling and plaque control at 3-month intervals. After an observation period of 2 years, no further loss of attachment had occurred in either grafted or nongrafted sites. In a follow-up study from 1985, Kennedy et al. reported the 6-year data from the same patient sample. They found that the placement of a gingival graft at sites with recession and no attached gingiva may over time provide some gain in clinical attachment ("creeping reattachment"). Hangorsky & Bissada (1980) evaluated the long-term effect of gingival grafts on the condition of the periodontium. A total of 43 gingival grafts were placed in 34 patients with nongrafted contralateral sites serving as controls. One to 8 years after treatment such clinical parameters as width of keratinized gingiva, probing pocket depth, gingival recession, amount of plaque and degree of gingivitis were examined. The authors concluded that "while the free gingival graft is an effective means to widen the zone of the attached and keratinized gingiva, there is no indication that this increase bears direct influence upon periodontal health".

Lindhe & Nyman (1980) in a retrospective study examined alterations of the position of the marginal soft tissue following periodontal surgery. Forty-three subjects with advanced periodontal disease were in 1969 subjected to periodontal therapy, including periodontal surgery using the apically positioned flap technique. After active therapy the patients were placed on a maintenance program which included prophylaxis once every 3-6 months for 10-11 years. They were examined for the distance in mm between the cementoenamel junction and the gingival margin at buccal surfaces of all teeth, with as well as without a zone of keratinized gingiva. The examinations were performed prior to surgery, after 2 months of healing and then after 10-11 years of maintenance care. Lindhe & Nyman reported that gingival recession is a common feature of advanced periodontal disease. As a result of periodontal treatment the position of the gingival margin is often further displaced in apical direction. This displacement, however, is followed by a minor coronal "regrowth" during a 10-11 year period of supervised maintenance. It was further observed that the alterations in the position of the gingival margin followed a similar pattern in areas with and without a zone of keratinized gingiva.

Wennström (1983, 1987) studied the regeneration of the gingiva following surgical excision of the entire gingiva in 6 subjects who had bilateral buccal sites with only a narrow zone of keratinized gingiva present. At the sites to be treated the probing depth and the clinical attachment levels were determined as well as the position of the gingival margin and the width of the keratinized and attached gingiva. Excision of the keratinized gingiva was performed using either a gingivectomy technique or a "flap excision procedure". Following "flap excision procedure" the oral mucosa was coronally positioned to establish the "gingival margin". The patients were subsequently placed on a careful plaque control program and reexamined during a 5-year period after treatment. Wennström reported that following excision of the entire gingiva a zone of keratinized gingiva always reformed but that attached gingiva did not always become established. He also concluded that *independent* of whether a zone of attached gingiva reformed or not the soft-margin tissue could be maintained in a healthy condition and without signs of recession and attachment loss.

In another experiment Wennström et al. (1987) studied gingival tissue reactions in monkeys exposed to orthodontic therapy. They observed that when teeth were moved out through the envelop of the alveolar process there was, at sites with a thin and inflamed gingiva, a risk that recession and loss of connective tissue attachment might occur. These phenomena did not occur at sites with a thick zone of gingiva or oral mucosa. Similar observations were reported by Steiner et al. (1981), who exposed monkey incisors to labial tipping movements. The authors reported that recession, accompanied by attachment loss, could occur under such experimental conditions.

Another situation which may result in gingival recession was described by Ericsson & Lindhe (1984). In an experimental study in the dog the inflammatory response of the gingival tissue was assessed subsequent to the placement of "restorations" with subgingivally located margins. Dogs with advanced periodontitis were first treated using either an "apically placed flap" or a "gingivectomy" procedure. In the flap procedure the main portion of the keratinized gingiva was retained, while in the gingivectomy procedure the *keratinized part of the gingiva was removed in toto*. After healing, gingival sites which had been exposed to "gingivectomy" (test sites) frequently had a thin and "inadequately" wide zone of keratinized gingiva. Flap-treated sites (control sites) consistently had a normal width of keratinized tissue. Restorations (steel bands) were cemented to the test and control teeth so that their apical border was located below the gingival margin. The dogs at this stage were fed a diet which allowed for plaque accumulation and gingivititis development. After 6 months on a plaque-forming diet, it was observed that the placement of a "restoration" in a subgingival position at gingival sites that were also allowed to accumulate plaque established conditions which promoted the development of severe gingivitits. At sites with an "inadequate" width of keratinized gingiva, the inflammatory reaction was consistently accompanied by recession of the gingival margin. Recession did not occur at sites with a normal width of keratinized tissue.

The authors suggested that the placement of restorations in a subgingival position at sites with a narrow zone of – or lacking – keratinized gingiva may in the presence of subgingival plaque favor an inflammatory tissue reaction which results in loss of gingival tissue, i.e. in the apical displacement of the soft-tissue margin.

Conclusion

The results from the human studies described above question the need for zone of keratinized and attached gingiva to prevent recession of the gingival margin in patients enrolled in a properly designed maintenance-care program. Findings from animal research, however, have identified situations which may call for the presence of a zone of keratinized gingiva in order to prevent recession from occurring. Such situations are related to orthodontic or restorative therapy. If during orthodontic treatment a tooth is moved through the envelop of the alveolar process, and if the margin of a restoration is placed subgingivally, there is, at sites with a thin and inflamed gingiva, a risk that gingival recession may occur.

Surgical procedures which favor regrowth of bone, periodontal ligament and root cementum

Regrowth of periodontal tissues has mainly been studied in sites with angular bony defects and infrabony pockets.

Regrowth of periodontal tissues in infrabony pockets treated without grafts

Prichard (1957) and Patur & Glickman (1962) suggested that curettage and root planing of infrabony pockets in conjunction with a flap procedure often resulted in significant gain of periodontal tissue. Ellegaard & Löe (1971) reported the results of a similar modality of treatment of 191 angular bony defects. After a healing period of 2-3 years the patients were reexamined and the authors found that "complete healing" of the angular defects had occurred in 110 out of 191 sites examined. Partial healing had occurred in an additional 28 sites. Rosling et al. (1976a, b) studied the effect of treatment of 124 angular bony defects in 12 patients. All defects were treated with a modified Widman flap procedure, including careful curettage of the bony defect and proper root debridement. Following surgery, the patients were placed on a maintenance program which included professional tooth cleaning (Axelsson & Lindhe 1974) once every 2 weeks. A control group of 12 patients received an identical initial therapy, but was not enrolled in a corresponding maintenance program. Reexaminations carried out 6, 12 and 24 months after therapy demonstrated that the properly maintained patients had experienced a mean gain of clinical attachment in the angular bony defects amounting to around 3 mm. Measurements performed on radiographs or in conjunction with so-called "reentry" procedures revealed that the test sites had lost 0.4 mm of the bone crest, but that the remaining portion of the angular bony defect (2.8 mm) was refilled with bone. In the control patients most of the sites treated showed signs of recurrent periodontal disease, including further loss of clinical attachment and alveolar bone (Fig. 24-19).

Polson & Heijl (1978) described healing in 15 angular bony defects in 9 patients. All defects were treated using a modified Widman flap technique, curettage of the bony defect and proper root planing. Following surgery the patients were, during a 6-month period, placed on a professional tooth-cleaning program. At "re-entry" operations 6-8 months after surgery, Polson & Heijl found that "the behavior of an osseous defect throughout its circumferential extent was characterized by a combination of coronal bone regeneration (77%) and marginal bone resorption (18%)". Infrabony periodontal defects "may predictably remodel after surgical debridement and establishment of optimal plaque control".

Conclusion

The results from the studies referred to demonstrate that significant bone fill can occur in angular bony defects of single-rooted teeth provided postoperative plaque control is of a high standard. It should be observed, however, that clinical measures describing bone fill cannot identify the quality of the attachment between the tooth and the newly formed bone tissue, i.e. whether this attachment is of epithelial or connective tissue nature. It has previously been assumed that bone fill in angular defects was accompanied by the formation of new root cementum and periodontal ligament. However, Caton & Zander (1976) reported from a study in monkeys that "repair of an osseous defect can occur opposite junctional epithelium ...without new attachment of connective tissue". Similar findings were described in a human case report by Moskow et al. (1979). In fact, more recently published animal studies (Caton et al. 1980) have shown that the dentogingival epithelium during healing consistently migrates to a position close to the presurgical level of the pocket epithelium on the root surface irrespective of the occurrence of suprabony or infrabony pockets, and independent of whether bone fill has resulted from the treatment. For details regarding new attachment, see Chapter 19.

Regrowth of periodontal tissues in infrabony pockets treated with grafts

According to the literature the use of grafts in the treatment of angular and infrabony pockets has the following objectives: 1) to restore the lost alveolar bone tissue, 2) to facilitate regeneration of a functional attachment apparatus, i.e. regeneration of root cementum and periodontal ligament, 3) to provide ideal conditions for proper maintenance, and 4) to improve esthetics. The graft materials used to meet these objectives may according to Schallhorn (1977) be divided into:

1. Autografts (a graft which is transferred from one position to another within the same individual)
   A. Cortical bone ("osseous coagulum")
   B. Combination of cortical and cancellous bone ("bone blend")
   C. Cancellous bone and marrow (intraoral donor site/extraoral donor site)

2. Allografts (a graft which is transferred between genetically dissimilar members of the same species)
   A. Freeze dried bone
   B. "Viable" cancellous bone and marrow
   C. "Sterilized" cancellous bone and marrow.

Besides autografts and allografts, synthetic materials have also been used in attempts to improve healing conditions in angular bony defects.

According to Schallhorn (1977) sufficient information exists on the clinical aspects of osseous grafting therapy to justify the inclusion of osseous grafts into the armamentarium of accepted treatment. A major concern, however, in evaluating the proper benefits of the *use of grafts in new attachment procedures* rests in the problem of determining whether new connective tissue attachment indeed formed during healing or if *bone fill* was the sole outcome of treatment. In most of the publications so far presented the conclusions drawn seem to be based on results from measurements such as clinical probing, radiographic examination, re-entry operation, etc. As discussed in Chapter 19 such methods cannot be used to identify the formation of new attachment. They may provide information on bone repair ("bone fill") in angular bony defects but are entirely unreliable in documenting the formation of new attachment.

In some clinical studies, the clinical and radiographic methods of examination were combined with a histological analysis of block sections obtained from the treated areas after healing. Such studies, however, also have a limited value in determining if the connective tissue attachment level has shifted coronally. The reason is the following: in the experiments referred to, the coronal level of the "connective tissue attachment" before treatment was "documented" by clinical probing (a reference groove was prepared in the root surface at this level). But since it is *impossible* to identify the apical extension of the pocket epithelium by probing before therapy (see Chapter 12), the histological analysis of the tissues after healing may not disclose whether new connective tisssue attachment has formed in root-surface areas located coronal to the pre-operative attachment level. The problems inherent in the evaluation of results from "new attachment" procedures are further discussed in Chapter 19.

Conclusion

So far no clinical study presented in the literature has provided conclusive evidence that new connective tissue attachment (i.e. the formation of new root cementum and periodontal ligament) *predictably* may occur following traditional surgical therapy with or without the use of graft materials. In other words, the potential of bone grafts to induce regeneration of the attachment apparatus, including new cementum, alveolar bone and a functionally

Table 24-4

Test sites		
	Distance	
B-A1	B-A2	
x̄ S.D.	x̄ S.D.	
3.02 ± 1.1	3.03 ± 1.1	N.S.
C-B1	C-B2	
x̄ S.D.	x̄ S.D.	
1.41 ± 0.5	1.17 ± 0.5	p < 0.001
Control sites		
	Distance	
b-al	b-a2	
x̄ S.D.	x̄ S.D.	
4.52 ± 1.6	4.36 ± 1.6	N.S.

Table 24-4. The length of distances B-A (base of angular bony defect and apex of test sites), C-B (crest of bone to base of defect at test sites), b-a (crest of bone to apex of control sites) measured in radiographs and expressed as BONE SCORE UNITS. A1, B1, a1 = initial examination. A2, B2, a2 = final examination (5-16 years after treatment).

oriented periodontal ligament, *has not so far been unequivocally established.*

Maintenance of the angular bony defect

The angular bony defect, its formation and treatment has for many years interested and confused the clinician. It has been suggested that an angular bony defect often occurs at periodontally involved teeth that are also exposed to trauma from occlusion (see Chapter 8), or may develop at root surfaces with deficient cementum (Gottlieb 1946, Blomlöf et al. 1987) or may simply form as a consequence of apically migrating subgingival plaque (Lindhe et al. 1975, Waerhaug 1979). It has been claimed that, in the treatment of periodontal disease, angular bony defects must be eliminated since, otherwise, deep pockets and destructive periodontitis invariably recur (see Barrington 1981). Consequently, measures are frequently included in periodontal therapy which, as discussed above, are aimed at actively eliminating the bony defect. Such measures may involve bone resection or recontouring, the placements of grafts in the defects, orthodontic tooth movement etc. It should be realized, however, that no research data have been presented which support the concept that the periodontal site associated with an angular bony defect constitutes a locus minoris resistentiae for recurrent periodontitis. Recently, Pontoriero et al. (1988) reported on a retrospective study performed to evaluate some long-term alteration of the alveolar bone level at periodontal sites with angular and even patterns of bone loss. The study included 48 patients who, following treatment for advanced periodontal disease, had been placed in a maintenance-care program which included recall appointments every 3-6 months for a period of 5 to 16 years. The study included all teeth with angular bony defects that could be detected in a full-mouth series of radiographs obtained at the end of the active treatment phase. Alterations in the position of 1) the *marginal alveolar bone crest* and 2) the *base of the osseous defect* which took place during the maintenance period, were assessed by comparing the post-treatment radiographs with a second set of radiographs obtained at the examination 5-16 years later. In the same 48 patients an equal number of contralateral or neighboring teeth at which bone loss in the radiographs had an even or "horizontal" character were included as controls.

Pontoriero and co-workers observed that periodontal sites which following active therapy displayed either angular or "horizontal" patterns of alveolar bone loss underwent, during a 5-16 year period of maintenance, only minor additional bone level alterations. Additional loss of supporting bone occurred equally frequently at sites with "horizontal" and at sites with angular patterns of bone loss (Table 24-4).

Thus the findings from this study failed to discriminate sites with angular bony defects as being particularly susceptible to recurrent destructive periodontitis. It may thus be concluded that sites which after treatment are associated with an angular bony defect are no more prone to additional bone loss in well-maintained patients than sites with a "horizontal" bone level.

Occlusal adjustment-splinting to maintain/regain stability of teeth

Occlusal adjustment and splinting are measures which may be used in order to reduce increased tooth mobility. In a longitudinal study describing the effect of periodontal therapy in patients with advanced periodontal disease (Lindhe & Nyman 1975, Nyman & Lindhe 1979), 676 teeth were treated which initially exhibited not only advanced loss of supporting tissues but also markedly increased mobility. At the initial examination, 78 of these teeth were found to have established premature contact either in the intercuspal position (IP), or in the movement between the retruded position (RP) and IP, or in lateral or frontal excursive movements of the mandible. In these 78 teeth, occlusal adjustment was performed during the presurgical phase of therapy. This therapy resulted, within a few weeks in most cases, in an obvious reduction in tooth mobility. After a few months it was possible to observe in the radiographs that the angular bony defects that were present around some of these teeth were reduced in size, i.e. a narrowing of the periodontal ligament space had occurred. All patients were subsequently surgically treated by means of the apically positioned flap technique. At the termination of the initial 5-year follow-up period, 113 teeth still exhibited a mobility of Degree 1 or 2. In spite of this persisting hypermobility during a 5- to 8-year period, none of the teeth showed a further breakdown of the attachment apparatus.

Rosling et al. (1976a) studied the effect of periodontal therapy in 12 patients who initially showed signs of advanced periodontal disease combined with multiple angular osseous defects. Of 216 teeth which were subjected to treatment, 37 showed an advanced mobility (Degree 2) at the initial examination. Occlusal adjustment was performed in only 8 of these teeth due to obvious premature contact relationships. Following a presurgical treatment phase, all 216 teeth were subjected to periodontal surgery using the modified Widman flap procedure. In no case was resection of the alveolar bone performed, but treatment was restricted to curettage of the angular bony defects in combination with scaling and root planing. After completion of active therapy, the patients were enrolled in a careful plaque control program which included maintenance therapy once every 2 weeks. An examination performed 2 years after therapy revealed that all the infrabony defects had healed with almost complete bone fill, despite the fact that 12 of the initially hypermobile teeth still exhibited increased mobility (Degree 2).

It may be concluded from the above that periodontal therapy, directed towards the elimination of plaque and calculus, results in proper healing of the periodontal tissues also around hypermobile teeth. This conclusion is supported by observations made in animal experiments (Lindhe & Ericsson 1976) showing that trauma from occlusion and resulting tooth hypermobility does not detrimentally influence healing of the supporting tissues following proper treatment of the plaque-associated lesion.

In order to understand the overall effect of periodontal therapy on tooth mobility, the following fact should be borne in mind: the vast majority of the initially hypermobile teeth described in the studies by Lindhe & Nyman (1975), Rosling et al. (1976a) and Nyman & Lindhe (1979) showed no signs of increased mobility at the termination of the observation period. Thus, elimination of the chronically inflamed periodontal tissues and the establishment of a proper oral hygiene program are in many instances sufficient to normalize the mobility of the teeth.

There are, however, reasons to analyze the occlusion and to eliminate occlusal interferences, if such are present, when teeth, following periodontal treatment, still exhibit permanently increased mobility. This form of occlusal therapy may then result in a narrowing of the periodontal ligament space and a stabilization of the tooth. If such an effort does not diminish the mobility of the tooth (teeth), splinting of the tooth (teeth) may be considered. The mobility of a single tooth is dependent not only on the width and quality of the periodontal ligament but also on the height of the remaining supporting bone. This means that teeth investigated in a reduced, but healthy, periodontium may exhibit increased mobility even if the remaining periodontal ligament space is not widened. In this context, it should be understood that occlusal adjustment and splinting are treatment procedures which are ineffective in the management of plaque-associated periodontal disease (Ericsson & Lindhe 1982), but which are effective in reducing the mobility of hypermobile teeth (Renggli & Mühlemann 1970, Renggli & Schweizer 1974).

References

Axelsson, P. & Lindhe, J. (1974) The effect of preventive programme on dental plaque, gingivitis and caries in schoolchildren. Results after one and two years. *Journal of Clinical Periodontology* **1**, 126-138.

Axelsson, P. & Lindhe, J. (1978) Effect of controlled oral hygiene procedures on caries and periodontal disease in adults. *Journal of Clinical Periodontology* **5**, 133-151.

Axelsson, P. & Lindhe, J. (1981) The significance of maintenance care in the treatment of periodontal disease. *Journal of Clinical Periodontology* **8**, 281-294.

Badersten, A., Nilvens, R. & Egelberg, J. (1984) Effect of nonsurgical periodontal therapy II. Severely advanced periodontitis. *Journal of Clinical Periodontology* **11**, 63-76.

Beltrami, M., Bickel, M. & Baehni, P.C. (1987) The effect of supragingival plaque control on the composition of the subgingival microbiota in human periodontitis. *Journal of Clinical Periodontolgy* **14**, in press

Bowers, G.M. (1963) A study of the width of attached gingiva. *Journal of Periodontology* **34**, 201-209.

Boyd, R.L. (1978) Mucogingival considerations and their relationship to orthodontics. *Journal of Periodontology* **49**, 67-76.

Caffesse, R.G., Sweeney, P.L. & Smith, B.A. (1986) Scaling and root planing with and without periodontal flap surgery. *Journal of Clinical Periodontology* **13**, 205-210.

Caton, J., Nyman, S. & Zander, H. (1980) Histometric evaluation of periodontal surgery, II. Connective tissue attachment levels after four regenerative procedures. *Journal of Clinical Periodontology* **7**, 224-231.

Caton, J. & Zander, H.A. (1976) Osseous repair of an infrabony pocket without new attachment of connective tissue. *Journal of Clinical Periodontology* **3**, 54-58.

Dorfman, H.S. & Kennedy, J. (1981) Gingival parameters associated with varying widths of attached gingiva. *Journal of Dental Research* **60**. Special Issue A, Abstract No. 301.

Dorfman H.S., Kennedy, J.E. & Bird W.C. (1980) Longitudinal evaluation of free autogenous gingival grafts. *Journal of Clinical Periodontology* **7** 216-224.

Eaton, K.A., Kieser, J.B., & Davies, R.M. (1985) The removal of root surface deposits. *Journal of Clinical Periodontology* **12**, 141-112.

Ellegaard, B. & Löe, H. (1971) New attachment of periodontal tissues after treatment of infrabony lesions. *Journal of Periodontology* **42**, 648-652.

Ericsson, I. & Lindhe, J. (1982) The effect of longstanding jiggling on experimental marginal periodontitis in the beagle dog. *Journal of Clinical*

Periodontology **9**, 497-503.

Ericsson, I. & Lindhe, J., (1984) Recession in sites with inadequate width of the keratinized gingiva. *Journal of Clinical Periodontology* **11**, 95-103.

Gartell, J.R. & Matthews, D.P. (1976) Gingival recession, the condition, process and treatment. *Dental Clinics of North America* **20**, 199-213.

Hangorsky, U. & Bissada, N.B. (1980) Clinical assessment of free gingival graft effectiveness on the maintenance of periodontal health. *Journal of Periodontology* **51**, 274-278.

Hill, R.W., Ramfjord, S.P., Morrison, E.C., Appelberry, E.A., Caffesse, R.G., Kerry, G.J., & Nissle, R.R. (1981) Four types of periodontal treatment compared over two years. *Journal of Periodontology* **52**, 655-662.

Hirschfeld, L. & Wasserman, B. (1978) A longterm survey of tooth loss in 600 treated periodontal patients. *Journal of Periodontology* **5**, 225-237.

Isidor, F. (1981) Effekt af parodontalkirurgi. Institut for Parodontologi, Arhus Tandlægeh¢jskole. *Thesis.*

Kennedy, J.E., Bird, W.C., Palcanis, K.G., & Dorfman, H.S. (1985) A longitudinal evaluation of varying widths of attached gingiva. *Journal of Clinical Periodontolgy* **12**, 667-675.

Knowles, J.W., Burgett, F.G., Nissle, R.R., Schick, R.A., Morrison, E.C. & Ramfjord, S.P. (1979) Results of periodontal treatment related to pocket depth and attachment level. Eight years. *Journal of Periodontology* **5**, 225-233.

Lang, N.P. & Löe, H. (1972) The relationship between the width of keratinized gingiva and gingival health. *Journal of Periodontology* **43**, 623-627.

Lindhe, J. & Ericsson, T. (1976) The influence of trauma from occlusion on reduced but healthy periodontal tissues in dogs. *Journal of Clinical Periodontology* **3**, 110-122.

Lindhe, J. & Nyman, S. (1975) The effect of plaque control and surgical pocket elimination on the establishment and maintenance of periodontal health. A longitudinal study of periodontal therapy in cases of advanced disease. *Journal of Clinical Periodontology* **2**, 67-79.

Lindhe, J. & Nyman, S. (1980) Alterations of the position of the marginal soft tissue following periodontal surgery. *Journal of Clinical Periodontology* **7**, 525-530.

Lindhe, J., Socransky, S.S., Nyman, S., Haffajee, A. & Westfelt, E. (1982b) "Critical probing depths" in periodontal therapy. *Journal of Clinical Periodontology* **9**, 323-336.

Lindhe, J., Westfelt, E., Nyman, S., Socransky, S.S., Heijl, L. & Bratthall, G. (1982a) Healing following surgical/non-surgical treatment of periodontal disease. A clinical study. *Journal of Clinical Periodontology* **9**, 115-128.

Listgarten, M.A., Lindhe, J. & Hellden, L. (1978) Effect of tetracycline and/or scaling on human periodontal disease. Clinical, microbiological and histological observations. *Journal of Clinical Periodontology* **5**, 246-271.

Lövdal, A., Arno, A., Schei, 0. & Waerhaug, J. (1961) Combined effect of subgingival scaling and controlled oral hygiene on the incidence of gingivitis. *Acta Odontologica Scandinavica* **19**, 537-555.

Magnusson, I., Lindhe, J., Yoneyama, T. & Liljenberg, B. (1984) Recolonization of a subgingival microbiota following scaling in deep pockets. *Journal of Clinical Periodontology* **11**, 193-207.

Miyasato, M., Crigger, M. & Egelberg, J. (1977) Gingival condition in areas of minimal and appreciable width of keratinized gingiva. *Journal of Clinical Periodontology* **4**, 200-209.

Morrison, E.C., Ramfjord, S.P. & Hill, R.W. (1980) Short-term effects of initial, non-surgical periodontal treatment (hygienic phase). *Journal of Clinical Periodontology* **7**, 199-211.

Moskow, B.S., Karsh, F. & Stein, S.D. (1979) Histological assessment of bone graft.A case report and critical evaluation. *Journal of Periodontology* **50**, 291-304.

Nyman, S. & Lindhe, J. (1979) A longitudinal study of combined periodontal and prosthetic treatment of patients with advanced periodontal disease. *Journal of Periodontology* **4**, 163-169.

Nyman, S., Lindhe, J. & Rosling, B. (1977) Periodontal surgery in plaqueinfected dentitions. *Journal of Clinical Periodontology* **4**, 240-249.

Ochsenbein, C. & Maynard, J. G. (1974) The problem of attached gingiva in children. *Journal of Dentistry for Children* **41**, 263-272.

Patur, B. & Glickman, I. (1962) Clinical and roentgenographic evaluation of the post-treatment healing of infrabony pockets. *Journal of Periodontology* **33**, 164-171.

Pihlstrom, B.L., Ortiz-Campos, C. & McHugh, R.B. (1981) A randomized four-year study of periodontal therapy. *Journal of Periodontology* **52**, 227-242.

Polson, A.M. & Heijl, L.C. (1978) Osseous repair in infrabony periodontal defects. *Journal of Clinical Periodontology* **5**, 13-23.

Pontoriero, R., Nyman, S., Lindhe, J., (1988) The angular bony defect in the maintenance of the periodontal patient. *Journal of Clinical Periodontology* **15**, in press.

Prichard, J.S. (1957) The infrabony technique as a predictable procedure. *Journal of Periodontology* **28**, 202-216.

Rabbani, G.M., Ash, M.M. & Caffesse, R.G. (1981) The effectiveness of subgingival scaling and root planing in calculus removal. *Journal of Periodontology* **52**, 119-123.

Ramfjord, S.P., Knowles, J.W., Nissle, R.R., Burgett, F.G. & Schick, R.A. (1975) Results following three modalities of periodontal therapy. *Journal of Periodontology* **46**, 522-526.

Ramfjord, S.P., Knowles, J.W., Nissle, R.R., Schick, R.A. & Burgett, F.G. (1973) Longitudinal study of periodontal therapy. *Journal of Periodontology* **44**, 66-77.

Ramfjord, S.P., Nissle, R.R., Schick, R.A. & Cooper Jr., H. (1968) Subgingival curettage versus surgical elimination of periodontal pockets. *Journal of Periodontology* **39**, 167-175.

Renggli, H.H. & Mühlemann, H.R. (1970) Zahnbeweglichkeit, marginale Parodontalentzündung und okklusales Trauma. *Parodontologie* **24**, 39-48.

Renggli, H.H. & Schweizer, H. (1974) Splinting of teeth with removable bridges - Biological effects. *Journal of Clinical Periodontology* **1**, 43-46.

Rosling, B., Nyman, S. & Lindhe, J. (1976a) The effect of systematic plaque control on bone regeneration in infrabony pockets. *Journal of Clinical Periodontology* **3**, 38-53.

Rosling B., Nyman, S., Lindhe, J. & Jern, B. (1976b) The healing potential of the periodontal tissues following different techniques of periodontal surgery in plaque-free dentitions. A 2-year clinical study. *Journal of Clinical Periodontology* **3**, 233-255.

Schallhorn, R.G. (1977) Present status of osseous grafting procedures. *Journal of Periodontology* **48**, 570-576.

Suomi, J.D., Greene, J.C., Vermillion, J.R., Doyle, J., Chang, J.J. & Leatherwood, E.C. (1971) The effect of controlled oral hygiene procedures on the progression of periodontal disease in adults: Results after third and final year. *Journal of Periodontology* **42**, 152-160.

Tagge, D.L., O'Leary, T.J. & El-Kafrawy, A. H. (1975) The clinical and histological response of periodontal pockets to root planing and oral hygiene. *Journal of Periodontology* **46**, 527-533.

Waerhaug, J. (1978) Healing of the dento-epithelial junction following subgingival plaque control. II. As observed on extracted teeth. *Journal of Periodontology* **49**, 119-134.

Wennström, J., Lindhe, J. & Nyman, S. (1981) Role of keratinized gingiva for gingival health. Clinical and histologic study of normal and regenerated gingival tissue in dogs. *Journal of Clinical Periodontology* **8**, 311-328.

Wennström, J., Lindhe, J. & Nyman, S. (1982) The role of keratinized gingiva in plaque-associated gingivitis in dogs. *Journal of Clinical Periodontology* **9**, 75-85.

Wennström, J., Lindhe, J., Sinclair, F. & Thilander, B., (1987) Some periodontal tissue reaction to orthodontic tooth movement in monkeys. *Journal of Clinical Periodontology* **14**, in press

Wennström, J. (1987) Lack of association between width of attached gingiva and development of soft-tissue recession. A five-year longitudinal study. *Journal of Clinical Periodontology* **14**, in press

Westfelt, E., Bragd, L., Socransky, S.S., Haffajee, A.D., Nyman, S. & Lindhe, J. (1985) Improved periodontal conditions following therapy. *Journal of Clinical Periodontology* **12**, 283-293.

CHAPTER 25

The Maintenance Phase of Periodontal Therapy

Definition

The primary objectives of periodontal therapy are to establish conditions that are conducive to future optimal plaque control and to prevent subgingival bacterial growth so that inflammation and further loss of periodontal attachment can be prevented or reduced to a minimum. The maintenance of periodontal health often requires considerable effort from the patient in maintaining a careful and thorough program of oral hygiene. It also requires considerable effort on the part of the dental health team. Thus, following the completion of active therapy most patients need professional assistance at regular intervals involving 1) renewed motivation for and instruction in oral hygiene, 2) elimination of calculus and other plaque-retentive factors, and 3) thorough professional cleaning of the teeth. Without such assistance, periodontal therapy will in many cases eventually and inevitably fail. Obviously, it is also necessary to repeatedly examine the patient's periodontal tissues in order to be able to take proper action at an early stage against possible disease recurrence and further destruction of supporting tissues.

Such professional assistance has been termed *maintenance therapy* or *maintenance care*. The treatment given in this context by the dentist and his auxiliary personnel has also been termed *supportive therapy*.

The rationale for maintenance therapy

Prevention and treatment of gingivitis and periodontitis through plaque control have been practiced for many decades. "Clinical experience" indicates that such treatment may be successful. The extent to which the prevention of

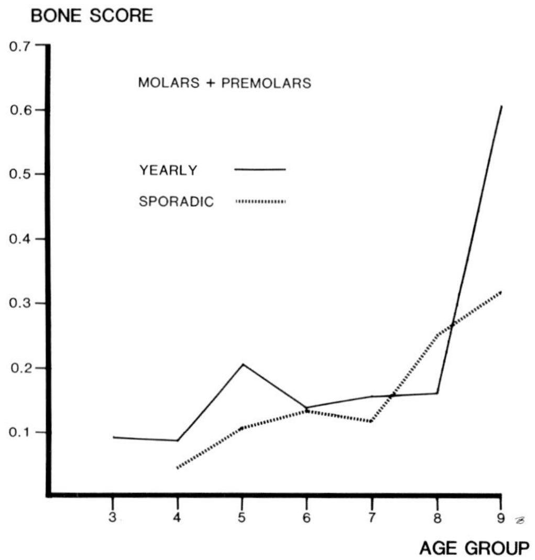

Fig. 25-1. Periodontal bone loss (recorded as increase in "Bone score") over a 6-year period in different age groups in Björn's study (1974). Age group 3 was 25-29 years of age. Age group 9 was 54-59 years of age at the start of the investigation. The loss of bone was more marked in the older age groups, but there was little difference between those who had seen a dentist regularly, at least once per year, and those who only visited sporadically.

supra- and subgingival plaque formation is successful determines the degree of success of the therapy. If the attempts at plaque control are inadequate or unsuccessful in one or more sites of the dentition, inflammatory changes will ensue in these sites and further loss of periodontal attachment often results. This unfortunately occurs too often, since the continuous maintenance of a sufficiently high level of plaque control is demanding both for the dental health personnel and for the patient.

In recent years the "clinical experience" of the beneficial effect of proper plaque control has been supported by results from controlled clinical trials. The causal relationship between the accumulation of bacterial plaque and the development of gingivitis has been experimentally verified in humans (Löe et al. 1965). In animal experiments it has also been shown that accumulation of bacterial plaque over extended periods of time results in the development of periodontitis with pocket formation, loss of attachment and resorption of alveolar bone (Saxe et al. 1967, Lindhe et al. 1973). Conversely, studies in humans have demonstrated that development of gingivitis and periodontitis can be prevented through measures aimed at preventing or reducing plaque formation (Lövdal et al. 1961, Suomi et al. 1971, Axelsson & Lindhe 1978, 1981a). Considerable knowledge has also been gained regarding the mechanisms through which plaque bacteria produce gingival inflammation and destruction of the attachment apparatus.

In general terms, the etiology of gingivitis and periodontitis is therefore fairly well understood. Unfortunately, the causative agents, *i.e.* the microbiota which induce and maintain the inflammatory changes, cannot be eliminated completely from the tooth surfaces for any length of time. Professional treatment can only temporarily reduce the amount of plaque on the tooth surfaces. The microorganisms are still present in the oral cavity and will rapidly recolonize the teeth following professional tooth cleaning. Plaque formation will thus start again and recurrence of the disease will ensue. Controlled, well-documented investigations and experiments over extended periods of time have shown that this development can be prevented only through a maintenance program aiming at regularly repeated removal of plaque. Such investigations have furnished us with clinically applicable knowledge and some of them will be briefly reviewed.

Loss of attachment as a result of inadequate plaque control

Investigations by H. Björn (1971), A.-L. Björn (1974) and Håkansson (1978) indicate that loss of periodontal support in population groups of the same age proceeds at almost the same rate in individuals who receive regular, "traditional dental care" and in individuals who visit the

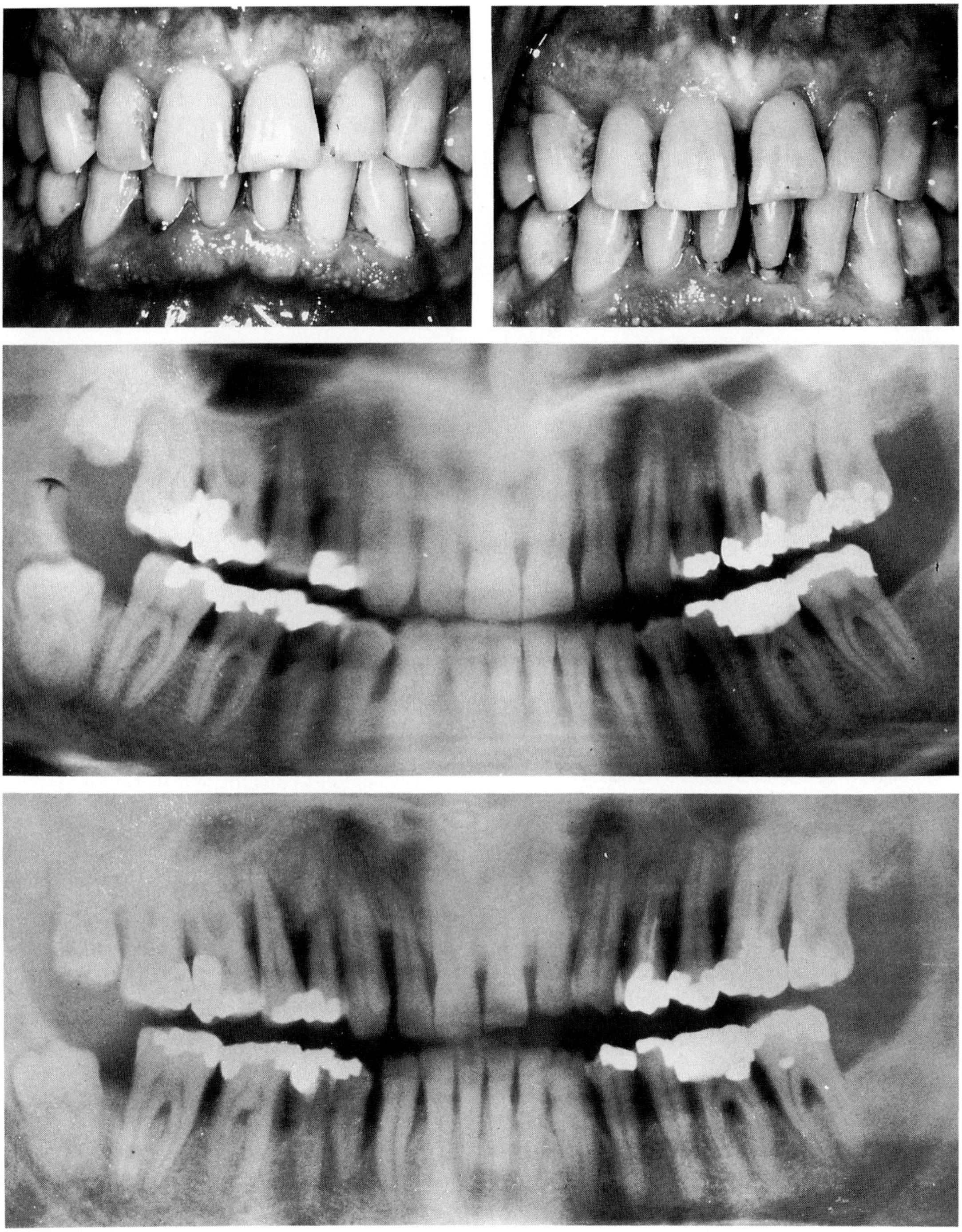

Fig. 25-2a-d. These clinical pictures and radiographs show characteristic changes in one of the subjects included in Björn's investigation (1974). The patient, a 35-year-old man, had visited his dentist at least once per year. (a) is a clinical photo and (c), an orthopantomograph taken at the start of the investigation, (b) and (d) are corresponding pictures taken 6 years later. Considerable gingival recession has occurred, particularly in the lower anterior teeth, and tooth 21 shows evidence of migration. Considerable amounts of restorative and endodontic therapy have been given during the 6-year period. The original orthopantomographs also show the presence of considerable amounts of subgingival calculus. The loss of alveolar bone which was already rather advanced at the initial examination (c) has progressed further around all teeth (d), so that the prognosis for several of them was poor at the 6-year examination.

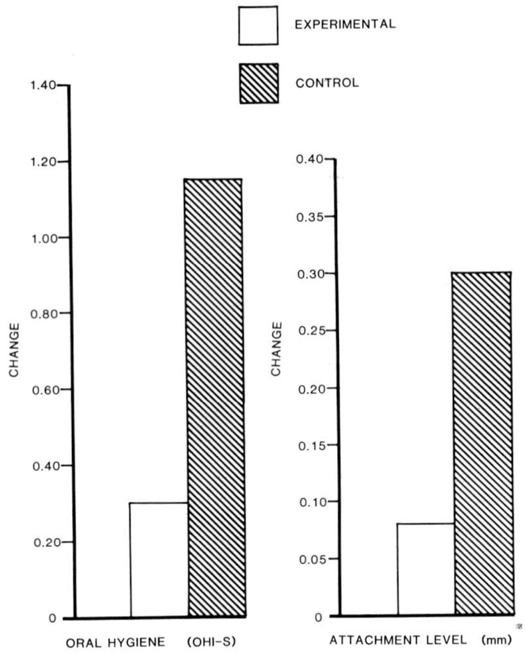

Fig. 25-3. Changes in oral hygiene (plaque scores) and in clinically measured loss of periodontal tissue support over a 3-year period. The experimental group received scaling, polishing and oral hygiene instructions every 3 months. The control group received "traditional dental care", without special measures to improve oral hygiene. The groups were "matched",so that at the start of the experiments they were similar with respect to loss of periodontal support, caries, oral hygiene and in other factors that might be of importance for the comparison. (Adapted from Suomi et al. 1971).

dentist only sporadically (Fig. 25-1). The reason is that "traditional dental care" does not adequately emphasize plaque control, and does not include depuration and periodontal therapy in general (Fig. 25-2).

The rate at which periodontal breakdown and loss of teeth are likely to proceed under such conditions has not been determined exactly and may vary between different individuals. In patients who had received treatment for advanced periodontitis, but who thereafter had only been examined once a year without special efforts to reinforce plaque control, it was shown that the clinically measurable loss of periodontal support may proceed at an average rate as high as 1 mm per tooth surface per year (Nyman et al. 1975). From other, similar investigations in which patients who did not have advanced periodontitis and who received only "traditional" symptomatic dental treatment without adequate emphasis on oral hygiene, Suomi et al. (1971) and Axelsson & Lindhe (1978) reported a somewhat lower annual loss of periodontal support, ranging from 0.1 mm per tooth surface in young adults to 0.3 mm in persons over 50 years of age. Some investigations seem to indicate that with inadequate plaque control and maintenance care, loss of support and bone resorption occur faster with increasing age (Axelsson & Lindhe 1978, Löe et al. 1978). This does not mean, however, that age in itself is a causative factor in the destruction of the periodontal tissues. Plaque-retentive factors, such as calculus and ill-fitting margins of restorations, usually accumulate with age, a process which can be expected to contribute to a more rapid progression of periodontal destruction.

Effect on periodontal conditions of maintenance care including plaque control

The available information indicates that the success or failure of attempts to prevent inflammation and loss of attachment over ex-

Figs. 25-4a-h. The pictures illustrate oral conditions in one of the test group patients in the investigation of Nyman et al (1975) (cf. text, Table 25-1). (a) and (b) illustrate the clinical condition immediately before surgical treatment (a) and after 2 years (b). (c) and (d) show the condition around the teeth of the left side before surgical treatment (c) and 2 years later (d). The radiographs are from corresponding segments before treatment (e, f) and after 2 years (g, h). Tooth 27 was extracted during periodontal surgery. Professional tooth cleaning and oral hygiene instruction were given every 2 weeks. The level of the alveolar bone has been maintained very well over the period of observation or there is possibly some regeneration of alveolar bone. Clinically there was no further loss of periodontal support and in no area did the pocket depth exceed 3 mm.

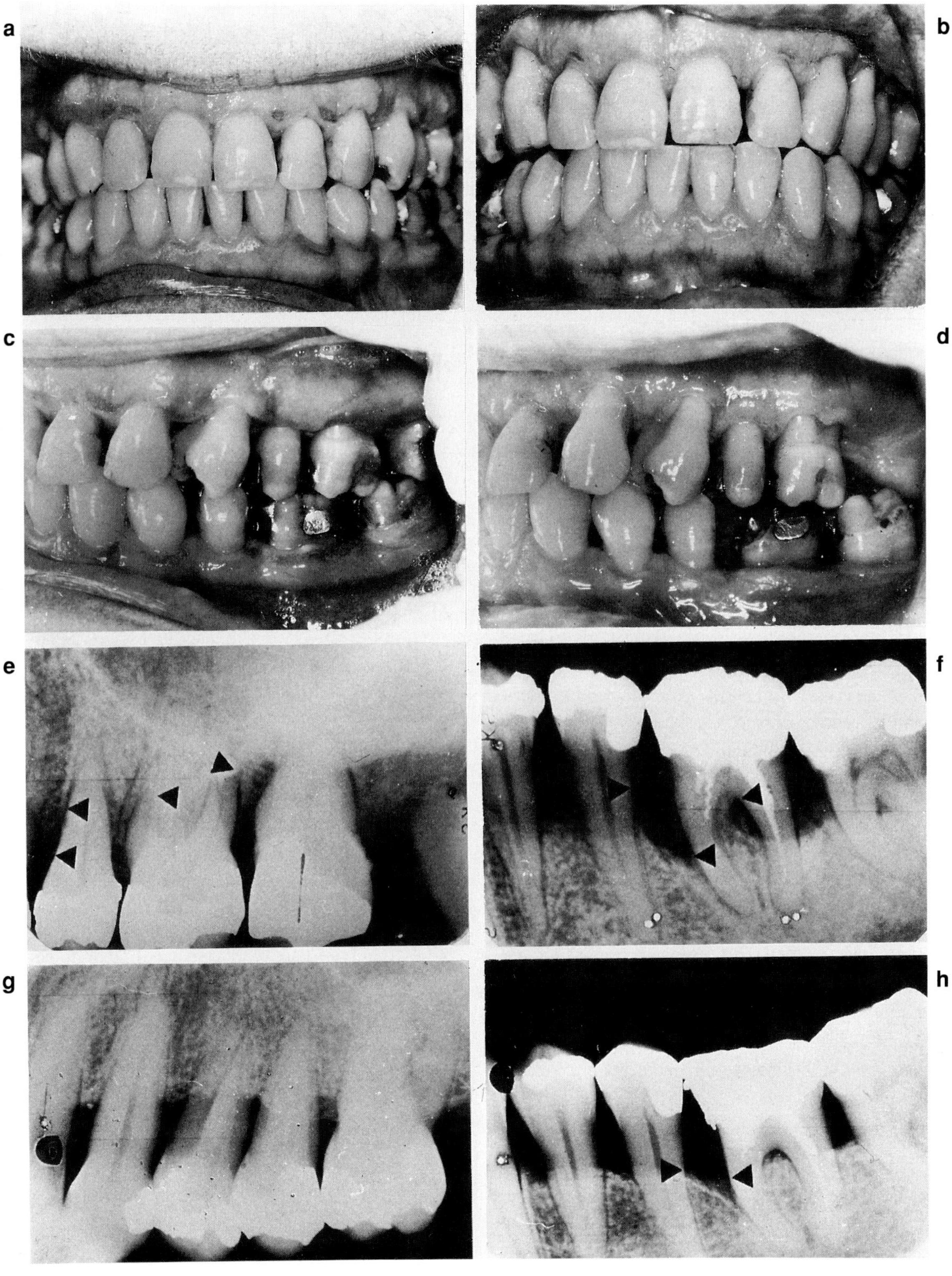

Table 25-1

Mean values for Plaque Index, Gingival Index, pocket depths (mm) and clinical attachment level (mm) registered before treatment and 12 and 24 months after completed periodontal therapy. The test group was given professional cleaning and instructions in oral hygiene every 2 weeks. The control group was only recalled for scaling every 6 months. The average clinically measured loss of periodontal support in the control group over 2 years was 2.2 mm and the pocket depth was almost the same as before treatment. The test group had pockets of less than 3 mm and no further loss of periodontal support (Adapted from Nyman et al. 1975).

Parameter	Examination					
	Initial		12 months		24 months	
	Test	Control	Test	Control	Test	Control
Plaque Index	1.4	1.3	0.3	1.3	0.1	1.5
Gingival Index	1.5	1.6	0.1	1.1	0.1	1.7
Pocket depth (mm)	4.3	4.7	2.7	3.2	2.5	4.0
Attachment gained (+) or lost (-) (mm)			+ 0.3	- 1.2	+ 0.1	- 2.2

tended periods of time depends primarily upon the level of oral hygiene but also upon other measures taken to reduce the accumulation of supra- and subgingival plaque. Whether the patient has received proper treatment for any preexisting periodontal disease also seems to be of importance.

The significance of the patient's oral hygiene and of regular control visits, including debridement for the maintenance of periodontal health over longer periods of time, was studied by Waerhaug and his collaborators (Lövdal et al. 1961). They recorded gingival conditions in 1428 individuals, 20-60 years of age, in an industrial company in Oslo, Norway. Over a period of 5 years, during which the patients were regularly recalled (2-4 times per year) for instruction in oral hygiene and supra- and subgingival scaling, gingival conditions improved by about 60%. Loss of teeth was reduced to about 50% of what would have been expected without these oral hygiene efforts. No surgical treatment of periodontal pockets was performed in this trial, and the investigators found that satisfactory results were very difficult to achieve in areas where pockets were more than 5 mm deep.

Suomi et al. (1971) measured loss of periodontal tissue support in young individuals who only had gingivitis or who had lost only a small amount of the attachment apparatus. An experimental group received scaling and instruction in oral hygiene measures every 3 months over a 3-year period (Fig. 25-3). Plaque accumulation and gingival inflammation were significantly reduced and the mean value for clinically measurable loss of attachment was only 0.08 mm per surface over the observation period as compared to 0.30 mm (= 0.10 mm per year) in a control group in which no special measures were instituted to improve oral hygiene.

In longitudinal studies on the effects of various modalities of periodontal therapy in 104

Figs. 25-5a-d. Clinical pictures and radiographs of one of the patients in the control group (Nyman et al 1975) (cf. text, Table 25-1). The pictures illustrate the conditions before surgical treatment (a, c) and after 2 years (b,d). The patient had been recalled for routine depuration every 6 months but received no oral hygiene instruction. Tooth No. 26 had to be extracted at the start of periodontal therapy. Tooth No. 24 exfoliated spontaneously during the period of observation. The radiographs show that the loss of periodontal support had continued around almost all teeth. Note in particular the rapid loss of alveolar bone around the mandibular teeth.

a b

c

d

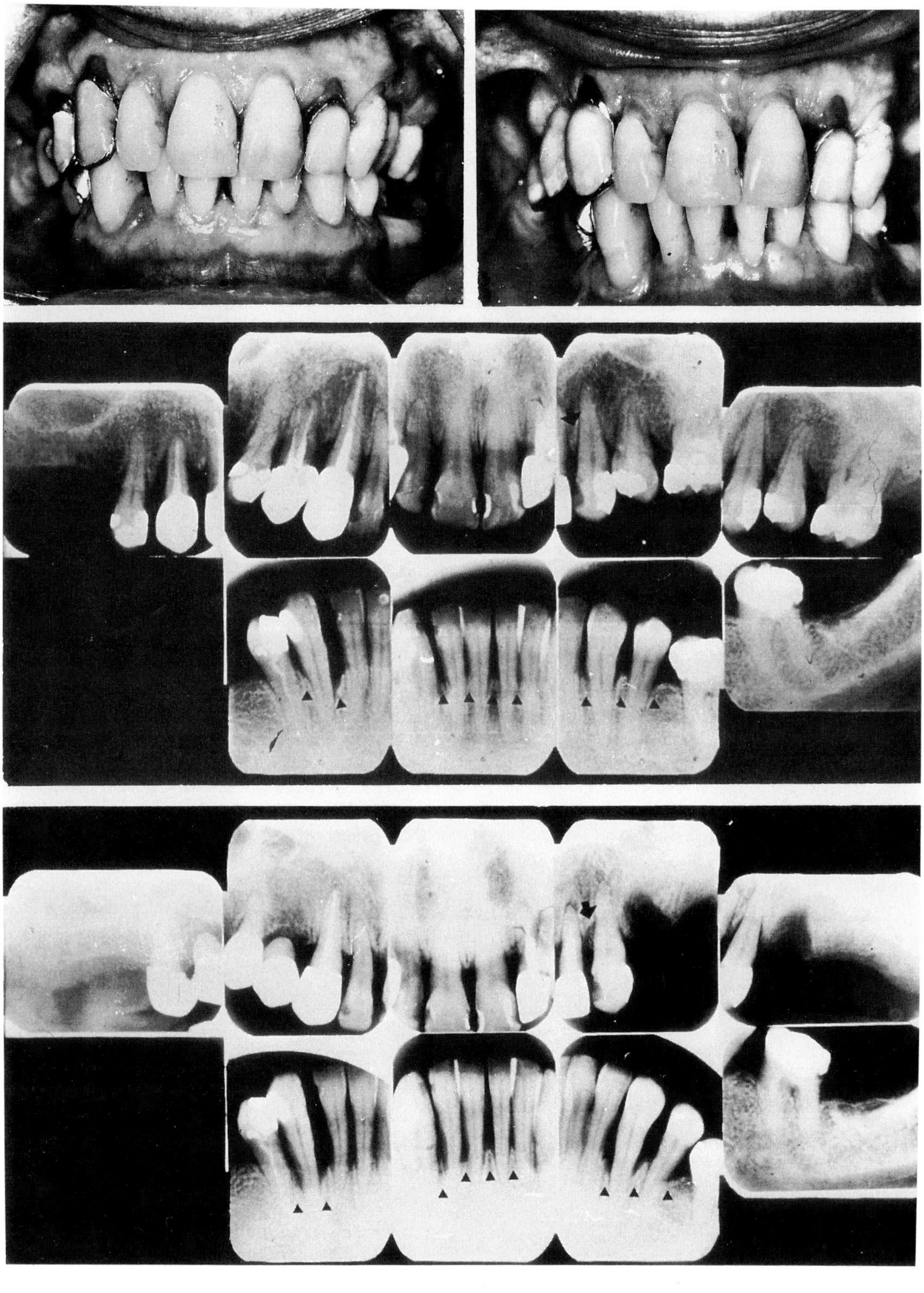

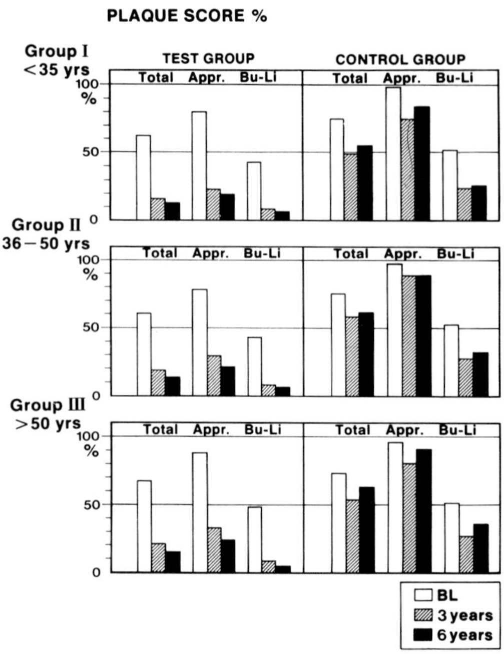

Fig. 25-6a.

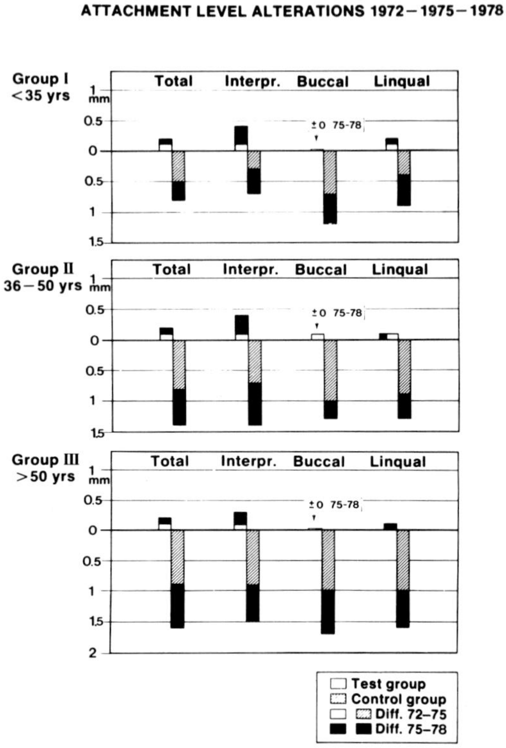

Fig. 25-6b.

Figs. 25-6a, b. Plaque scores (a) (percentage of tooth surfaces harboring visible plaque) and clinical changes in the level of the supporting tissue (b) in test and control groups in Axelsson & Lindhe's investigation (1978) (cf. explanation in the text).The control group which only received "traditional dental care" once per year for 3 years showed little change in plaque scores. The loss of periodontal support was 0.17-0.30 mm per year in the various age groups. In the test group which received professional cleaning and oral hygiene instructions every 2-3 months, plaque scores were low and no further loss of periodontal support could be demonstrated during the 3-year period of observation.

Table 25-2

Change in attachment level	Percentage of surfaces showing change	
	Recall	Non-recall
Attachment level improved	17	1
No change	72	10
Attachment level worse by		
≤ 1 mm	10	34
2 to 5 mm	1	55

Table 25-2. Percentage of sites showing various changes in clinical attachment level between baseline examination 2 months after completion of periodontal surgery and follow-up examination 6 years later. See text for explanation. (Adapted from Axelsson & Lindhe 1981b)

patients, 13-64 years of age, with advanced periodontitis, Ramfjord et al. (1973) recorded an annual mean loss of attachment amounting to 0.04 mm per tooth surface over a 7-year period. All patients received thorough professional tooth cleaning, polishing and oral hygiene instruction every 3 months. Although there were variations in the effectiveness of the patients' self-performed plaque control, this intensive supportive therapy resulted in excellent maintenance of postoperative levels of attachment in all patients. Nevertheless, the results were more favorable in patients with good plaque control than in those with poor oral hygiene (Knowles 1973, Ramfjord et al. 1982).

Table 25-3

Percentage of pockets of various depths in recall and non-recall patients at the initial examination, 2 months after treatment and at 3- and 6-year follow-up visits. See text further explanation. (Adapted from Axelsson & Lindhe 1981b)

Examinations	Percentage of pockets of various depths					
	≤ 3 mm		4-6 mm		≥ 7 mm	
	Recall	Non-recall	Recall	Non-recall	Recall	Non-recall
Initial	35	50	58	38	8	12
Baseline	99	99	1	1	0	0
3 years	99	91	1	9	0	0
6 years	99	80	1	19	0	1

In an investigation by Nyman et al. (1975) in which 20 patients with advanced periodontitis were surgically treated and where the experimental group subsequently received thorough professional cleaning of the teeth and instruction in oral hygiene every 2 weeks (Table 25-1), no further loss of attachment could be demonstrated by clinical examination after 2 years (Fig. 25-4). The patients in the control group, who received the same initial treatment including surgical pocket therapy, were recalled for scaling every 6 months postoperatively, but other measures aiming to maintain plaque control were not instituted. After 2 years, these control patients exhibited an average clinical loss of attachment of around 2 mm. This represents a very rapid progression of periodontal destruction and may indicate that, in the absence of proper maintenance, surgical periodontal treatment can in fact be more harmful than beneficial. The pocket depths 2 years postoperatively were also approximately the same as before surgical therapy in the patients of the control group, whereas in the experimental group, the pocket depths were maintained at the immediately postoperative level (Fig. 25-5). The results from investigations by Axelsson & Lindhe (1978, 1981a) show that even with somewhat less frequent professional tooth cleaning and oral hygiene instruction, sufficiently low values of plaque scores can be maintained to prevent further pocket formation and loss of attachment (Figs. 25-6a, b). Over a 3-year period when an experimental group of 375 adult persons, aged 20-71 years, received thorough professional prophylaxis and oral hygiene instructions every 2 months for the first 2 years and every 3 months during the 3rd year, pocket depths were reduced by approximately 0.5 mm in spite of the fact that they were not originally very deep (on the average 2.0-3.2 mm in the various age groups). Little or no loss of attachment was found in these patients, whereas a control group of patients who were seen annually for "traditional dental care" exhibited a yearly loss of attachment of 0.17-0.30 mm per surface in the various age groups. In the control group pocket depths increased by about 0.5 mm during the experimental period. After 3 more years during which the same regimens were followed, Axelsson & Lindhe (1981a) found that the average annual loss of attachment in the test groups was less than 0.04 mm per tooth surface. In the control groups the loss of support proceeded at approximately the same rate as during the first 3 years.

Axelsson & Lindhe (1981b) also demonstrated the value of a carefully designed maintenance program for patients who had been treated for advanced periodontal disease. They examined 77 patients before treatment, 2

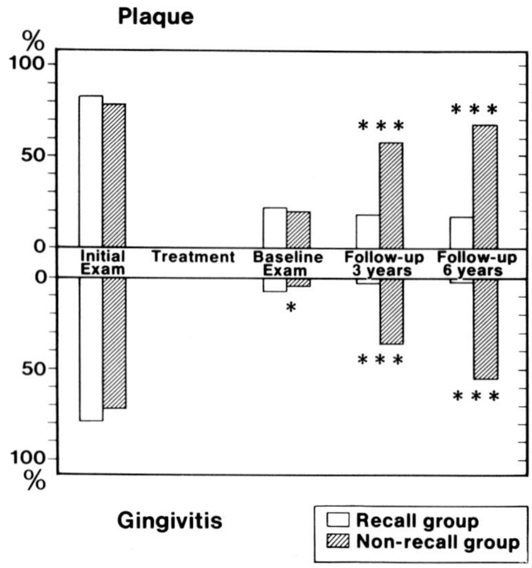

Fig. 25-7a.

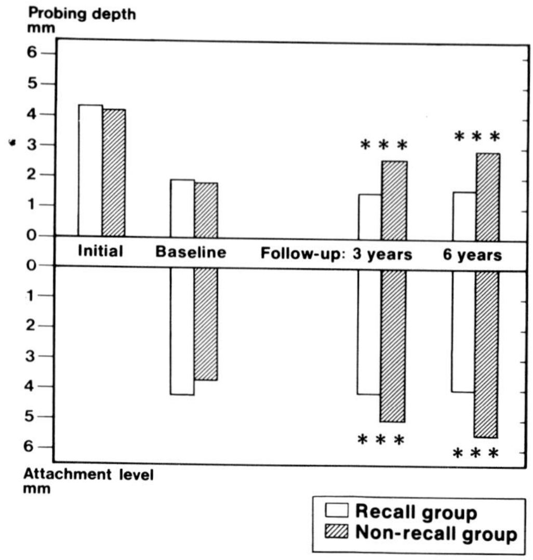

Fig. 25-7b.

Figs. 25-7a, b. Histograms showing (a) average percentages of tooth surfaces harboring visible plaque (above) and inflamed gingival units (bleeding on probing, below), and (b) average pocket depth (above) and clinically measurable attachment levels (below), at initial, baseline and follow-up examinations in Axelsson & Lindhe's study (1981 b). The recall patients were seen every 2-3 months for oral hygiene instructions, meticulous scaling and professional cleaning. See text for further explanation and details.

months after the last surgical procedure, and after 3 and 6 years. Two out of 3 patients (52) were placed on a supervised maintenance program which included oral hygiene instruction, meticulous scaling and professional tooth cleaning every 2 months for the first 2 years and every 3 months for the last 4 years of the observation period (recall group). The remaining patients (25) were sent back to the referring dentist, who was informed of the importance of checking their oral hygiene, calculus formation and gingival and periodontal conditions (non-recall group). The data obtained from the second examination showed that the effect of the initial treatment was good in both groups. Subsequently, the recall patients were able to maintain proper oral hygiene and unaltered attachment levels. In the non-recall group, plaque scores increased markedly from the baseline values, as did the number of inflamed gingival units (Fig. 25-7a). Concomitantly, there were obvious signs of recurrent periodontitis. The mean values for pocket depth and attachment levels at the 3- and 6-year examinations were higher than at baseline (Fig. 25-7b). In the recall group approximately 99% of the tooth surfaces showed either improvement, no change or less than 1 mm loss of attachment, compared to 45% in the non-recall group (Table 25-2). In the latter patients, 55% of the sites showed 2-5 mm further loss of attachment at the 6-year examination, and 20% of the pockets were 4 mm deep or more (Tables 25-2; 25-3).

Söderholm (1979) instituted a program of dental care including 3-monthly professional tooth cleaning and oral hygiene instruction in 443 shipyard employees who had previously been examined by H. Björn (1971) and A.-L. Björn (1974). After 3-4 years, the dental health program had resulted in an improved standard of oral hygiene, and the progressive loss of alveolar bone had been arrested. There was also a decrease in the number of new carious lesions and the need for dental restorations and the rate of tooth mortality had been reduced.

In patients who are well motivated for self-performed oral hygiene, the interval between recall sessions may be prolonged according to the observations by Lindhe & Nyman (1975). In 75 such patients who had been treated for very advanced periodontitis with loss of alveolar bone amounting to half the length of the roots or more, and who were seen for professional tooth cleaning and instruction every 3-6 months, no further loss of alveolar bone could be demonstrated radiologically after 5 years. However, for most patients frequent recalls are of utmost importance. The duration of the effects achieved through motivation and oral hygiene instructions in most patients is rather limited (Elliott et al. 1972, Dennison et al. 1974). Without frequent recalls, including renewed oral hygiene instructions, patients tend to revert to their earlier behavior with respect to oral hygiene habits after a relatively short period of time.

In addition to the favorable effects on the periodontal tissues, a systematic thorough maintenance regimen will apparently also significantly reduce the occurrence of caries (Lindhe & Nyman 1975, Axelsson & Lindhe 1978, 1981a, Söderholm 1979), even in patients in whom large areas of the root surfaces have been exposed after treatment of advanced periodontitis (Lindhe & Nyman 1975).

It should be noted that the above results from clinical investigations, carried out under controlled experimental conditions, are supported by a series of documented reviews of patients, treated and maintained for up to 50 years in various dental practices (Oliver 1969, Ross 1971, Hirschfeld & Wasserman 1978). The patients studied had been referred to specialists for treatment of periodontal disease, and the majority of the cases had advanced disease. In all 3 studies the average annual loss of teeth was drastically reduced so that fewer teeth were lost per patient than in the general population. One of the studies (Hirschfeld & Wasserman 1978) reported loss of teeth in 600 patients who had been maintained for 15-53 years (average 22 years). Over the entire observation period the average loss of teeth was 1.8 per individual. Half the number of patients lost no teeth at all, 199 patients lost 1-3 teeth, whereas 25 patients (i.e. 4.2% of the total sample) lost 13.3 teeth per individual. This study, therefore, not only demonstrates the efficacy of periodontal maintenance therapy but also illustrates the variation in response to such treatment.

When should maintenance start?

After initial therapy in periodontitis cases, adaptive changes in gingival form, bone contour and depth of crevice may take place over several years, but in terms of clinical attachment levels the results are usually fairly stable after 6 months. It was therefore suggested that the first 6 months after completion of therapy for periodontal pockets be considered as a "healing phase" (Westfelt et al. 1983b). Recall visits, which include professional tooth cleaning every 2 weeks during this period, have been recommended, followed by a maintenance program with a prophylaxis every 3 months (Westfelt 1983b). Others have suggested weekly professional cleaning during a 4 weeks' healing period followed by maintenance care every 3 months (Knowles et al. 1979, Ramfjord 1987). Though the efficacy of these two regimens have not been directly compared, the similarities in long-term results indicate that the differences are small, and it has been found that the patients' own plaque control is particularly important during the "healing phase" (Ramfjord et al. 1982).

Objectives of maintenance therapy

Plaque control

Plaque is formed so rapidly and its removal by the patient is so difficult that complete freedom from plaque over extended periods of time is an unrealistic goal. However, although it has been documented that periodontal therapy which is not followed by proper plaque control will inevitably fail (Nyman et al. 1975, Axelsson & Lindhe 1981b), both "clinical experience" and controlled clinical trials have shown that with regular maintenance including professional tooth cleaning, attachment levels can be maintained for several years, even in patients with less than perfect oral hygiene (Axelsson & Lindhe 1978, 1981a,b, Knowles et al. 1979, Ramfjord et al. 1982). For instance, in patients in whom about 5% of the buccal and 25% of the approximal tooth surfaces harbored plaque (average for all surfaces about 16%) there was little or no progression of periodontitis during a 6-year period following active treatment (Axelsson & Lindhe 1981b; cf. Figs. 25-7a,b). One explanation that has been offered (Ramfjord et al. 1982) is that after one episode of proper removal of supra- and subgingival plaque, the complex plaque flora needs some time for reestablishment (Socransky 1977, Listgarten et al. 1978).

It is important, however, to be aware of individual variations, both with respect to the individual patient's ability and motivation to carry out proper oral hygiene procedures and regarding the rate of plaque formation and the response of the tissues to plaque.

Pockets and attachment levels

After pocket elimination, for instance by gingivectomy, Waerhaug (1955) and others have shown that a new dentogingival junction with a clinically measurable pocket of an average depth of 1-3 mm will be established. Under favorable conditions, *i.e.* with good plaque control and minute signs of gingival inflammation, this pocket is not formed at the expense of periodontal tissue support and should therefore be regarded as a reestablishment of normal anatomical relations. Recurrence of pathologically deepened pockets with loss of attachment, on the other hand, will occur, and may occur relatively rapidly following treatment if plaque control is inadequate (Nyman et al. 1975, Axelsson & Lindhe 1981b). It has been clearly demonstrated that with optimal plaque control, recurrence of pockets with loss of attachment can be avoided for at least 5 years (Lindhe & Nyman 1975) and that periodontal health could be maintained in most of 75 patients who originally had "extremely advanced periodontal disease" for at least 14 years (Lindhe & Nyman 1984). In these patients recurrent disease of a significant severity occurred in only a few patients and sites.

In longitudinal clinical studies it has repeatedly been observed that even with good plaque control programs, some sites tend to lose periodontal support slowly over time, with little or no visible inflammation or pocket formation (Knowles et al. 1979, 1980, Badersten et al. 1985a). Such "recession" mostly occurs where the original pocket is shallow, particularly on buccal surfaces. The cause is poorly understood, but inflammation is not a prominent feature in the process. It may go on for some years, and then usually levels off without causing serious problems. It may occur regardless of the type of initial therapy performed and apparently is neither related to plaque formation nor to trauma from tooth brushing.

Practical routines

Maintenance work should be adjusted to the needs of the individual patient both in order to economize with resources and because such an individual approach is more effective. It is important, however, to institute standardized routines for the maintenance work, routines which can be modified to fit the individual case (Robinson 1980). By following standardized routines, omissions can be avoided and standardized routines in themselves allow the operator to work more efficiently. Routines for maintenance care should include:

1. Examination and evaluation :
   Periodontal conditions.
   The patient's standard of plaque control.
2. Supportive treatment (as needed):
   Information and motivation.
   Instruction in methods for plaque control.
   Scaling and polishing.
3. Treatment of recurrence of gingivitis and periodontal disease.

Examination and evaluation

Examination during periodontal maintenance care should include:

A. Periodontal conditions:
   1) Gingival inflammation.
   2) Loss of periodontal tissue support.
   3) Furcation involvements and other special problems.

B. The patient's standard of plaque control:
   1) Registration of residual plaque.
   2) Retentive factors.

Periodontal conditions

Loss of periodontal tissue support can be measured in several ways. Usually this is done simply by *probing for pocket depths*, assuming that increased pocket depth reflects progression of the disease and further destruction of the attachment apparatus. *Measurement of clinical attachment levels, i.e.* measurements of the distance from a fixed point on the tooth, usually the cementoenamel junction, to the bottom of the clinical pocket, is probably a more relevant and precise way to examine alterations in attachment levels. The procedure requires 2 measurements: 1) from the gingival margin to the bottom of the clinical pocket and 2) from the gingival margin to the cementoenamel junction. Many clinicians find this procedure more difficult and time-consuming than pocket measurements. On the other hand, since the pocket depth is recorded simultaneously, a double set of relevant information is obtained through attachment level measurements.

Assessment of changes in tooth mobility may also yield information concerning possible progression of periodontal breakdown, although increased mobility may have other causes than further progression of marginal periodontitis.

Radiographic examination may give important information concerning possible further progression of periodontal disease. Exposure time, tube angulation and procedures for developing radiographs should be standardized as much as possible. Bite-wing exposures may be useful for examination of marginal osseous contours when bone loss is minimal. In patients who have experienced advanced bone loss, however, periapical exposures, preferably using a paralleling long-cone technique, are indispensable.

It is an obvious shortcoming of radiographs that they do not as a rule give information regarding the level and outline of the alveolar bone crest at the labial and lingual/palatal aspects of the teeth. On the other hand, radiographs give valuable supplementary information, *e.g.* of the presence of caries and periapical lesions.

For the registration of *gingival inflammation* one of the indices for scoring of gingivitis may be used. The *Gingival Index system* of Löe & Silness (1963), particularly if combined with the *Plaque Index system* according to Silness &

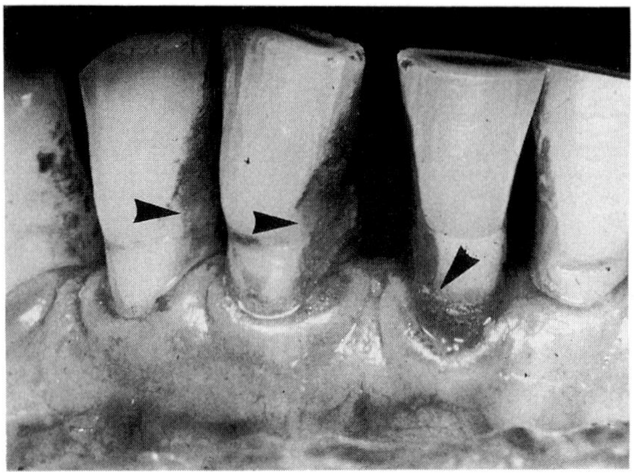

Fig. 25-8a.

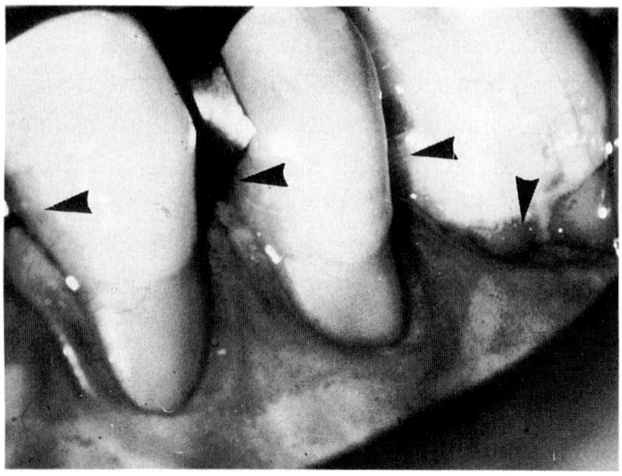

Fig. 25-8b.

Figs. 25-8a, b. Demonstration of plaque by use of disclosing tablets in recall patients. (a) There is plaque on the interproximal tooth surfaces and the patient has also "missed" the facial surfaces on teeth 41 and 31. Bleeding was provoked by probing facially to tooth No. 3. (b) This patient has maintained relatively good oral hygiene during the 4 months since the last maintenance visit. It is characteristic that plaque can be demonstrated particularly in the interproximal areas and in the concavity coronally to the bifurcation area on tooth No. 36 (arrows).

Löe (1964), gives detailed and precise information. Many clinicians, however, find these indices too time-consuming for routine clinical use. An index based on the registration of one single characteristic of gingival inflammation, namely "bleeding on probing", has been presented by Ainamo & Bay (1976): *"The Gingival Bleeding Index"*. Gingival bleeding after gentle probing with a blunt periodontal probe strongly indicates inflammation and suggests the presence of subgingival plaque and possibly calculus or other retentive factors. (For a detailed discussion on examination procedures see Chapter 12).

Tooth brushing trauma or other traumata resulting from faulty oral hygiene practices should be assessed separately.

Furcation involvements are best probed by means of curettes. Radiographs may also give information concerning further progression of periodontal breakdown in furcation areas.

For *scoring and recording of plaque*, a disclosing solution or disclosing tablets should be used, since in this way any remaining plaque is made visible to the operator as well as the patient (Fig. 25-8). This method is helpful both in motivation and instruction in oral hygiene measures. By counting the number of tooth surfaces (mesial, buccal, distal, oral) harboring stained plaque and expressing this number as a percentage of the total number of tooth surfaces present (4 surfaces per tooth); a numerical expression for the situation with respect to plaque control can be obtained. Scoring and recording of plaque is probably the most important part of the examination, from which both operator and patient will obtain useful information and directives.

Retentive factors such as supra- and subgingival calculus and ill-fitting restoration margins may be assessed merely by recording their localization.

Examination of the periodontium and the patient's plaque control should, of course, constitute an integral part of the overall examination of the dental conditions, *i.e.* along with registration of caries and other pathological findings. The findings recorded should give guidelines for the supportive or maintenance therapy. They should also form a basis for evaluation of alterations in the dental and periodontal status of the patient which may occur with time. The findings, therefore, should be recorded on simple and easy-to-follow charts.

The examination performed during routine maintenance visits must be repeated several times over the years. They should therefore be as efficient and simple as possible and at the same time as complete and comprehensive as necessary. In patients who have not developed advanced periodontitis, the routine examination can probably be somewhat simplified. Oliver (1977) found that a "screening examination" which included measurements of pocket depths mesiobuccally and distobuccally, registration of bleeding provoked in the same locations through probing, and assessment of mobility in all teeth would detect 90% of all cases of periodontitis. The cases studied were untreated patients with manifest gingivitis or with established periodontitis. Such simplified examination procedures may be useful for screening of patients on a larger scale, aiming to classify them according to their treatment needs. They can also be used for surveillance after treatment of simple gingivitis without complicating factors such as loss of attachment in furcation areas, etc. But they will probably not be sufficiently exact and thorough when the aim is to monitor alterations in periodontal conditions in individuals who have been treated for advanced forms of periodontitis (see Chapter 2).

Supportive treatment

Information and reinforcement of motivation

Patients expect to be informed about their dental conditions and about the effects of their oral hygiene efforts. If the dentist or the auxiliary personnel does not satisfy the patient's need for information, they may be left with the impression that the dentist is not overly interested in, or even concerned about, their dental health. Both motivation to maintain dental health and confidence in the dentist may suffer. This is particularly true of patients who make great efforts and spend considerable time on oral hygiene procedures, and who may have been subjected to extensive and expensive dental treatment.

Demonstration in the patient's own mouth is usually regarded as being most efficient. Display of bleeding gingival units, deepened pockets and plaque after the use of a disclosing solution is informative and convincing. Many patients need renewal or reinforcement of their motivation for plaque control. To remotivate the patients every time they are seen for control may be tiresome and tedious for the dentist. If such motivating sessions consist primarily of critical remarks they become tiresome and tedious to the patient as well. The effect of this type of motivation is often poor. It is important for both parties that motivation is carried out in a constructive way, so that patients receive the impression that the dentist is genuinely interested in their dental health. Encouragement generally works better than negative criticism (Derbyshire 1980).

During remotivation it is important that the message is varied, so that the patient does not always hear the same "lecture" over again. A program of recalls at regular intervals for control of the periodontal situation in itself probably serves to maintain the patient's motivation, a fact which constitutes one more reason for frequent regular-control visits, particularly for patients with advanced disease.

Instructions for plaque control

Scoring and recording of plaque during recall visits frequently reveals that the patient is in need of renewed instruction in oral hygiene methods. In many instances the patient may not have the manual dexterity necessary to carry out the oral hygiene program that was demonstrated previously, or the patient has not managed to get used to the program and accept it as part of habitual behavior. Undesirable habits which prevent the efficient removal of plaque from certain areas of the dentition may also

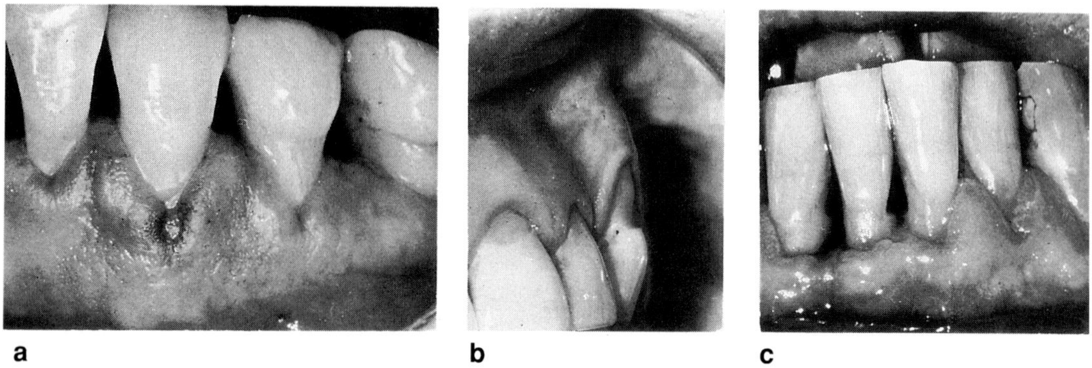

Figs. 25-9a-c. Trauma resulting from faulty oral hygiene habits. (a) Acute tooth brushing trauma on tooth No. 33 and a mild chronic trauma (Y-shaped defect of the "Stillman's cleft" type on tooth 34). Such defects will as a rule heal completely when the method of toothbrushing is corrected. (b) Extensive chronic toothbrushing trauma with defects in hard as well as soft tissues. (c) Hard-tissue defects interproximally in the lower incisors caused by long-term energetic use of wooden toothpicks in a 44-year-old dentist. Note that denuded root surfaces apically to defects will most likely not be cleaned by the toothpick.

have been acquired (Fig. 25-8), or the patient may have discontinued the use of one or more of the means or methods of oral hygiene which were introduced. It may become necessary to reevaluate the initial program on the basis of subsequent experience. In any case, the plaque control program should not be made more complicated than is necessary for the maintenance of a healthy periodontium. Following periodontal surgery, but also as a result of gingival recession or shrinkage, the morphology in the dentogingival region may be changed so that it is necessary to introduce other methods or means of oral hygiene than those recommended during the initial phase. Such changes are frequently seen in interproximal areas, where the space between the teeth becomes somewhat wider. Insertion of new restorations such as fillings, crowns or bridges may also necessitate the introduction of new or additional hygiene methods.

During the maintenance phase, the patient should be examined for possible self-inflicted trauma due to faulty oral hygiene techniques. Such traumatic lesions may be acute and manifest themselves as epithelial abrasion and varying degrees of ulceration of the gingiva. They can be seen both interdentally, labially and even on the lingual/palatal gingival surfaces (Figs. 25-9a-c).

Acute traumata usually heal after a few days when the faulty oral hygiene habits have been corrected. In rare instances, it may be necessary to discontinue mechanical cleaning in the affected area for a few days. Daily mouth rinsing with 0.2% chlorhexidine may be useful during such periods.

A special type of acute trauma may arise when the patient fractures a wooden toothpick so that a part of it becomes firmly lodged in an interproximal area. If such a foreign body becomes wedged into close contact with soft tissues, an acute inflammatory condition or even a periodontal abscess with considerable tissue damage may develop. Patients should be instructed to contact their dentist immediately if they notice symptoms indicative of such a situation.

Chronic traumata are usually seen as gingival retractions and wedge-shaped defects both on vestibular and lingual/palatal surfaces and occasionally on approximal surfaces (Figs. 25-9b,c). Gingival defects of the "Stillman's cleft" type (Fig. 25-9a) generally disappear after some time when the patient is instructed in correct, gentle but thorough oral hygiene methods in the area. Special techniques for tooth cleansing, for instance use of a single-tufted toothbrush, may be indicated. Clinical photographs and casts may be useful adjuncts for monitoring gingival retractions and other chronic defects.

Scaling and professional tooth cleaning

Scaling (depuration) includes removal of supra- and subgingival plaque and calculus, removal of other plaque retentive factors and root planing. Roughness and furrows in the tooth surfaces should be regarded as retentive factors. Plaque may form more rapidly on rough than on smooth surfaces (Waerhaug 1956, Mörmann et al. 1974). In addition, such areas are difficult for the patient to clean. It is therefore justifiable and desirable to smoothen and polish the surfaces of teeth and restorations.

Removal of supragingival plaque and calculus is technically a relatively simple procedure. Subgingival scaling and root planing, on the other hand, are difficult and time-consuming. If the patient has many pockets which are deeper than 3 mm, either because they have not been reduced during surgical therapy or new pockets have formed, several appointments may be required to complete the debridement. In deep pockets the complete removal of all accretions is extremely difficult even for the trained and experienced operator. If subgingival calculus is left behind, inflammation with further loss of attachment may result. The choice of treatment mode during planning of the initial treatment as well as thoroughness and meticulous care in its implementation is therefore of utmost importance for the future maintenance work. The choice of instruments for scaling may also have important consequences. Through improper instrumentation, regular scaling over many years may produce furrows and notches in the root surfaces which are extremely difficult to remove and almost impossible to keep clean. Such furrows and notches are most frequently produced by instruments such as hoes and sickles, in which the working edge ends in a sharp corner or a point (Fig. 25-10). Curettes are probably the best and most versatile instruments for scaling and root planing. Rotating instruments such as diamonds produce rough surfaces and considerable loss of tooth substance (Fig. 25-11a). Scaling with ultrasonic instruments is generally considered to be less efficient and produces somewhat rougher surfaces than scaling by means of curettes (Fig. 25-11b). Improper use of ultrasonic instruments easily

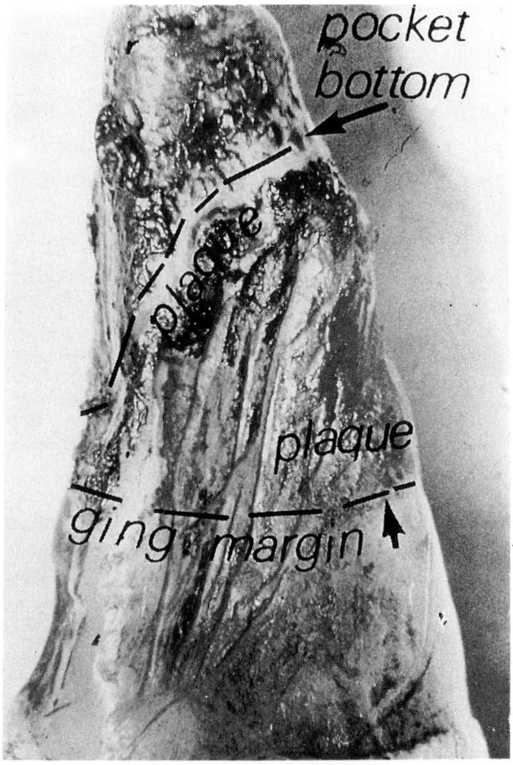

Fig. 25-10. Scratches and furrows after attempts at subgingival scaling in the surface of a tooth which had to be extracted because of recurrent periodontitis. Such scratches frequently result from the use of hand instruments where the working edge ends in a sharp corner (hoes) or a point (sickles). The pocket was deep. Note that in spite of energetic and repeated attempts plaque was still present on the tooth surface. Dental calculus can also be seen, particularly near the bottom of the pocket. (Courtesy of Dr. Waerhaug).

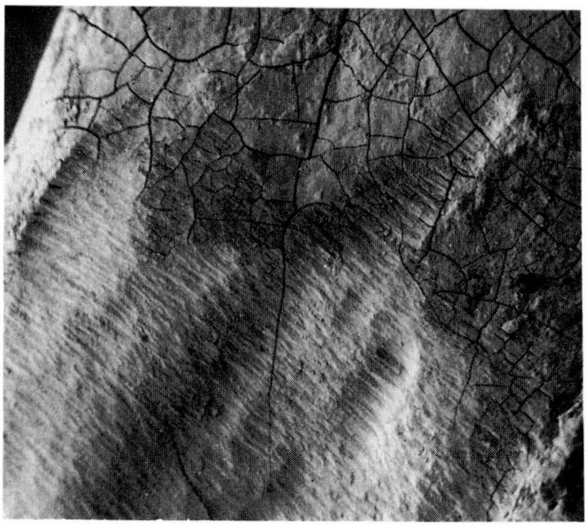

Fig. 25-11a.

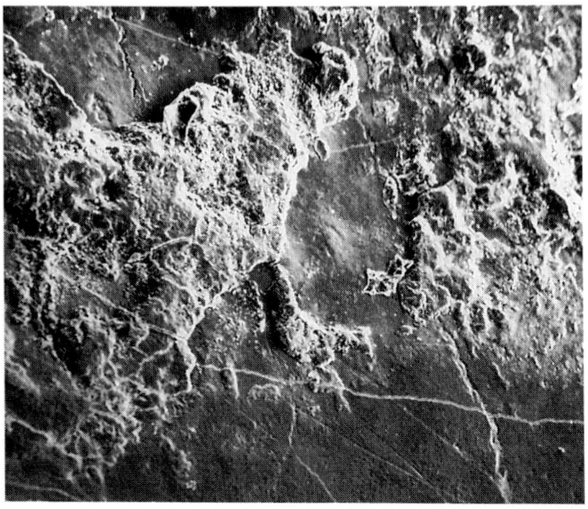

Fig. 25-11b.

Figs. 25-11a, b. Root surfaces after scaling with a fine diamond (a) or an ultrasonic instrument (b). The pictures are taken in a scanning electron microscope and are from investigations by Lie & Meyer (1977) and Meyer & Lie (1977). The surface which has been treated with a fine-grained flame-shaped diamond (a) is uneven and there is considerable loss of tooth substance. (The cracks in the upper part of the picture are due to desiccation during preparation). The surface where attempts were made to scale with an ultrasonic instrument (b) felt entirely smooth upon probing. Nevertheless, remnants of calculus can still be observed.

produces roughness and scratches in metal restorations.

The surface structure and marginal fit of restorations made of amalgam change and deteriorate with time, resulting in increased plaque retention. By careful use of small diamond points or wedge-shaped EVA diamonds, such fillings can often be properly recontoured. For smoothing and polishing, rubber polishers and abrasive paper strips are useful.

Final polishing of all tooth surfaces should be performed with brushes, rubber cups, dental tape and points as carriers for polishing pastes with decreasing grain size and preferably containing fluoride.

Drugs in maintenance care

Drugs for chemical plaque control and other antimicrobial drugs as well as their mode of action and indications for their use in cause-related therapy have been discussed in Chapter 15. The use of drugs in treatment of recurrences will be discussed under "Treatment of recurrent periodontitis" below.

Chemical plaque control. In maintenance care, drugs for chemical plaque control would seem to offer somepromise, particularly chlorhexidine which in 0.2% solution is convenient, easy and reasonably safe to use as a mouthwash. Even in countries where it is readily available the use of chlorhexidine mouthwash has not become as widespread and popular as one would expect. This is probably due to its objectionable side effects (taste, discoloration) and because the drug cannot compensate for inadequate mechanical therapy. Nevertheless, if an ideal oral hygiene is required, chlorhexidine may be a valuable adjunct where mechanical plaque control measures are particularly difficult. As a 1% gel used as a toothpaste it reduced both plaque and gingivitis scores significantly compared to a placebo gel in a group of patients who had been treated for advanced periodontal disease and who had poor oral hygiene (Lie & Enersen 1986). During the "healing phase" after initial therapy 0.2% chlorhexidine mouthrinses may be used, although intensive mechanical tooth cleaning may provide even better results (Westfelt et al. 1983a).

Table 25-4

Conditions which may influence the frequency of maintenance care visits

Related to plaque control	Patient's motivation
	Patient's knowledge and ability to carry out oral hygiene procedures
	Rate of plaque formation
	Retentive factors complicating or preventing effective oral hygiene
	Rate of calculus formation
	Special periodontal risk factors (furcations, furrows, remaining calculus, etc.)
	Toothbrushing and other oral hygiene trauma
Related to tissue destruction	Tendency for development of gingivitis and for tissue destruction
	Host tissue resistance
	Pathogenicity of plaque bacteria
Other	Occlusal relations
	Caries activity

Chlorhexidine mouthrinses may be used during periods of intermaxillary fixation. In the form of a mouthrinse, gel or spray chlorhexidine may also be helpful in physically or mentally handicapped individuals (Joyston-Bechal 1987).

Antibiotics and other antimicrobial drugs. For systemic use over prolonged periods antibiotics should in general be avoided, since results have not been convincing and the risk of development of resistant bacterial strains is considerable (Kornman & Karl 1982, Joyston-Bechal 1987).

Pocket irrigation and slow release devices. Pocket irrigation with antimicrobial drugs has so far failed to show any great value in maintenance care. Results obtained with slow release devices are interesting, but more work is needed before the use of such devices can be recommended (Joyston-Bechal 1987).

Treatment of recurrent periodontal disease

Choice of treatment for possible recurrences of periodontal disease must be based on an analysis of the causes of the recurrence.

Generalized recurrences are most frequently due to deficient maintenance care. Reappearance of signs of gingivitis at regular 3-monthly recall visits do not necessarily mean recurrence of actively destructive periodontitis, but may call for more intensive maintenance care. Pockets which bleed on gentle probing or secrete pus should be noted and the teeth scaled and root planed prior to regular professional cleaning. The patient should then be recalled 2-3 weeks later. At this time retreatment should be decided (see below). Frequent maintenance visits are particularly important in patients who have been treated for advanced periodontitis, particularly during the "healing phase" (Westfelt et al. 1983b, Ramfjord 1987).

Local recurrences are sometimes caused by failure of the plaque control in the local area. The cause of such failure may be faulty or inadequate oral hygiene practices or the presence of retentive factors for which the oral hygiene procedures cannot compensate. More often local recurrences can be traced back to inadequacies in the initial planning or implementation of periodontal therapy. Inspection of the roots of treated teeth which have had to be extracted for periodontal reasons almost always have calculus on them (Ramfjord 1987, cfr.

also Fig. 25-10). Clinical observations have suggested that failure to remove all plaque or calculus is not unusual (Chace 1977). Recent controlled experiments indicate that this occurs much more often than is commonly assumed, even with skilled operators and whether scaling is performed with or without flap surgery (Hunter et al. 1984, Eaton et al. 1985, Caffessee et al. 1986). Furcations, concavities and root furrows may make plaque and calculus difficult to remove, if not entirely inaccessible, and so can subgingival ill-fitting margins of restorations. The possible presence of a root fracture should be considered in endodontically treated teeth, particularly if the tooth carries an artificial crown with a post inserted in the root canal.

Actively progressive periodontal disease can at best only be diagnosed retrospectively, by *e.g.* radiologic or clinical attachment level measurements. There has been some uncertainty regarding criteria on which early retreatment should be undertaken, since neither bleeding on probing, suppuration, pocket depths nor various microbiological parameters have been found to reliably predict progression of periodontal disease (Badersten et al. 1985b, Lang et al. 1986, Listgarten et al. 1986). Bleeding on gentle probing a couple of weeks after a recall visit with professional tooth cleaning and oral hygiene instructions, or bleeding from the same site on several consecutive recall visits, may indicate a need for retreatment (Lang et al. 1986, Ramfjord 1987). Such retreatment can usually be accomplished by thorough scaling and root planing with or without limited flap surgery for access. Such retreatment will usually halt further progression of periodontitis (Ramfjord et al. 1987). If the recurrence is the result of faulty or deficient oral hygiene efforts by the patient, surgical intervention should be postponed until the patient's plaque control has been brought to an acceptable level. At this time surgery may no longer be indicated. It has been suggested that "recalcitrant" as well as recurrent periodontal disease could be caused by infection or reinfection with specific microorganisms, but the evidence can best be described as soft (Listgarten et al. 1986, Moore 1987). Investigations have failed to demonstrate a clear-cut connection between recurrent or refractory periodontitis and any one specific microorganism or combination of organisms (Haffajee et al. 1988). Treatment of recurrent periodontitis with antimicrobial drugs such as tetracycline cannot substitute for proper mechanical retreatment. As supplement to mechanical therapy, systemic antimicrobials may enhance the short-term response to treatment, although a combination of antimicrobial drugs and mechanical therapy has not been shown to have a long-term beneficial effect over mechanical therapy alone. If a systemic antibiotic is to be used, this requires a proper microbiological test and diagnosis which should include tests for antibiotic sensitivity of the suspected organisms. The treatment should preferably be followed up with microbiologic monitoring.

Frequency of maintenance visits

General rules regarding frequency of maintenance visits cannot be given. A number of studies have shown that maintenance based on 3-monthly recalls is sufficient for most patients (Suomi et al. 1971, Ramfjord et al. 1973 1982, Axelsson & Lindhe 1978, 1981a,b, Söderholm 1979). However, some patients may need less frequent visits (Lindhe & Nyman 1975, 1984). It is in the interest of both the patient and the health-care system to avoid "overtreatment" and yet to see the patient as often as the individual case requires.

It is often recommended that the patient be seen relatively frequently during the "healing phase", *i.e.* first 6-month period after completion of the initial periodontal treatment (see under "When should maintenance phase start?", above) and thereafter to adjust the frequency of maintenance-care visits as well as the procedures performed during these visits, as experience is gained with respect to the needs of the individual patient.

The most important factor to consider when deciding the frequency of recall visits is the patient's level of plaque control (Table 25-4). Most often this reflects the patient's motivation to carry out the oral hygiene program. But the degree of understanding and knowledge, as well as manual dexterity, differ from patient to patient (Kenney et al. 1976). The durability of the motivation that the patient has received also varies between patients. In addition, plaque may form at different rates in different individuals. After tooth cleansing, plaque may form less rapidly and probably reaches "mature" composition more slowly if oral hygiene has been proper and the gingiva has been free of inflammation during a period of time preceding the cleansing than if hygiene has been poor and the gingiva has been inflamed (Hillam & Hull 1977, Socransky 1977, Listgarten et al. 1978). This may be an argument in favor of frequent visits for professional tooth cleaning and oral hygiene instruction, particularly in patients with poor oral hygiene or poor resistance to plaque infection.

Even more important are variations in local conditions which increase plaque retention and complicate plaque removal. Along with calculus, restorations constitute the most important retention factors, particularly if the margins of the restorations are located subgingivally or close to the gingival margin (Silness 1978). Patients with many such restorations are more exposed to plaque retention and may require more frequent maintenance visits. The position and anatomy of the teeth may further complicate the patient's plaque control (Ainamo 1972). Furrows and concavities in the exposed root surface, frequently found *e.g.* coronally to furcations, may present obstacles to plaque removal. Some patients appear to have a stronger tendency for calculus formation than others. It may be desirable to see such patients more often for this reason.

Patients also respond differently to plaque infection with variations in the rate of development of inflammation and in the tendency to destruction of the supporting tissues (Hirschfeld & Wasserman 1978). This may be due to variations in host resistance or to variations in the composition of the plaque microbiota. Clinically applicable and reliable methods for evaluating the pathogenicity of the bacterial flora involved in periodontal disease are not as yet available (Moore 1987). Certain bacterial morphological forms are associated with diseased periodontal pockets, whereas few of these forms are found at healthy sites (Listgarten & Helldén 1978), and it has been suggested that differential dark field microscopic bacterial counts could help to identify patients at risk for recurrences of their periodontitis (Listgarten & Levin 1981). Studies were therefore undertaken in treated periodontitis patients, as well as patients with simple gingivitis, to find out if a test based on the relatively simple and rapid method of differential dark-field microscopy could be used to customize recall intervals for individual patients. These studies have yielded interesting results, but so far such microbiological tests are not recommended for general use, particularly because they fail to predict recurrences of disease (Listgarten et al. 1985, 1986).

Only rarely can host tissue resistance to periodontal breakdown be related in practice to well-defined systemic conditions which can be diagnosed. One such condition is diabetes mellitus. For the vast majority of patients, however, host-tissue response can only be evaluated by recording the loss of periodontal support with time and relating this to the patient's plaque control and other measures taken against the plaque bacteria. However, the clinician may be able to form an opinion about the patient's susceptibility to periodontal disease before treatment by considering the degree of periodontal tissue destruction present in relation to the patient's age. Reduced host tissue response is obvious when there is considerable periodontal breakdown in relatively young patients, as in patients with juvenile periodontitis. Advanced loss of periodontal support in older patients, on the other hand, does not necessarily reflect reduced host tissue resistance, even though the amount of plaque bacteria present at the moment is moderate. Tissue breakdown may have progressed over considerable periods of time and under varying conditions with respect to the amount of plaque and types of bacteria present.

Teeth with reduced periodontal support frequently exhibit increased mobility, even after completion of successful periodontal therapy. Such teeth may also develop hypermobility at a later stage if exposed to unfavorable occlusal forces. Even if unfavorable occlusal relations have been corrected in order to avoid such a development, the situation should be supervised since occlusal relations and habits may change with time (Ramfjord & Ash 1983). Only rarely, however, do such conditions necessitate more frequent recall visits than those required for the maintenance of proper plaque control.

Finally, the question of frequency of maintenance visits has certain practical and economical aspects. Most patients who have been subjected to periodontal treatment, including a "healing phase" (Westfelt et al. 1983b), should be recalled after a month. Subsequently, 3-monthly recalls are instituted. If plaque control continues to be proper and other reasons for more frequent visits do not exist after a year or so, the interval between the appointments can be extended to once every 4th or 6th month. Otherwise, visits every 3 months are continued or the frequency of visits can be increased. For patients who maintain excellent oral hygiene and who show good resistance to periodontal breakdown and low caries activity, yearly controls may be sufficient.

All patients who have received comprehensive periodontal therapy should have a thorough examination with respect to loss of gingival inflammation, furcation involvements, etc., at least once a year. Radiographs should be taken at regular intervals.

Responsibilities of the dental team

The responsibility for periodontal maintenance rests primarily with the patient's general dental practitioner. The patient obviously has a responsibility, but it rests with the dentist to supervise the patient's endeavors to meet the requirements of proper tooth cleaning. It is also the responsibility of the general dental practitioner to diagnose and to treat recurrence of the disease, at least as long as the level of severity and difficulty of the particular case do not exceed the dentist's competence. If so, the patient should be referred to a periodontist for retreatment.

If the patient has been referred to a periodontist for the initial periodontal therapy, the specialist will frequently supervise the case during the first months following treatment. When the periodontist subsequently sends the patient back to the referring dentist, the latter again assumes responsibility for the maintenance care. The general practitioner may then expect the specialist to submit a written evaluation of the patient's plaque control, prognosis, particular risk areas and preferably also suggestions concerning the future maintenance care and supportive therapy.

Important parts of the supportive therapy such as reinstruction, scaling and professional tooth cleaning can be performed by a dental hygienist. Other specially trained auxiliaries, *e.g.* "oral hygiene nurses", can also perform such work within the limits of their qualifications and authorization (Söderholm 1979, Hetland et al. 1982). The main responsibility, however, for the treatment that is given by auxiliary personnel still rests with the dentist, who should therefore personally examine the patient at regular intervals and supervise the work he/she has delegated to the auxiliaries. Firm administrative routines are of great value in this context, particularly with regard to communication between the different members of the dental health team.

References

Ainamo, J. (1972) Relationship between malalignment of teeth and periodontal disease. *Scandinavian Journal of Dental Research* **80**, 104-110.

Ainamo, J. & Bay, I. (1976) Problems and proposals for recording gingivitis and plaque. *International Dental Journal* **25**, 229-235.

Axelsson, P. & Lindhe, J. (1978) Effect of controlled oral hygiene procedures on caries and periodontal disease in adults. *Journal of Clinical Periodontology* **5**, 133-151.

Axelsson,P. &Lindhe J.(1981a) The effect of controlled oral hygiene procedures on caries and periodontal disease in adults. Results after 6 years. *Journal of Clinical Periodontology* **8**, 239-248.

Axelsson, P. & Lindhe, J. (1981b) The significance of maintenance care in the treatment of periodontal disease. *Journal of Clinical Periodontology* **8**, 281-294.

Badersten, A., Nilvéus, R. & Egelberg, J. (1985a) Effect of non-surgical periodontal therapy. VI. Localization of sites with probing attachment loss. *Journal of Clinical Periodontology* **12**, 351-359.

Badersten, A., Nilvéus, R. & Egelberg, J. (1985b) Effect of non-surgical periodontal therapy. VII. Bleeding, suppuration and probing depth in sites with probing attachment loss. *Journal of Clinical Periodontology* **12**, 432-440.

Björn, A.-L. (1974)Dental health in relation to age and dental care. *Odontologisk Revy*, Supplement 29.

Björn, H. (1971) Tandhälsotillståndet hos manliga anställda vid en svensk industri. *Tandläkartidningen* **63**, 4-21.

Caffessee, R.G., Sweeney, P.L. & Smith, B.A. (1986) Scaling and root planing with and without periodontal flap surgery. *Journal of Clinical Periodontology* **13**, 205-210.

Chace, R. (1977) Retreatment in periodontal practice. *Journal of Periodontology* **48**, 410-412.

Dennison, D., Lucye, H. & Suomi, J.D. (1974) Effects of dental health instruction on university students. *Journal of the American Dental Association* **89**, 1313-1317.

Derbyshire, J.C. (1980) Patient motivation. In *Periodontal Therapy*, ed. Goldman, H.M. & Cohen, D.W., 6th ed., pp. 516-534. St. Louis: C.V. Mosby Co.

Eaton, K.A., Kieser, J.B. & Davies, R.M. (1985) The removal of root surface deposits. *Journal of Clinical Periodontology* **12**, 141-152.

Elliott, J.R., Bowers, G.M., Clemmer, B.A. & Rovelstad, G.H. (1972) Evaluation of an oral physiotherapy center in the reduction of bacterial plaque and periodontal disease. *Journal of Periodontology* **43**, 221-224.

Haffajee, A.D., Socransky, S.S., Dzink, J.L. & Taubman, M.A. (1988) Clinical, microbiological and immunological features of subjects with refractory periodontal diseases. *Journal of Clinical Periodontology.*

Hetland, L., Midtun, N. & Kristoffersen, T. (1982) Effect of oral hygiene instruction given by paraprofessional personnel. *Community Dentistry and Oral Epidemiology* **10**, 8-14.

Hillam, D.G. & Hull, P.S. (1977) The influence of experimental gingivitis on plaque formation. *Journal of Clinical Periodontology* **4**, 56-61.

Hirschfeld, L. & Wasserman, B. (1978) A long-term survey of tooth loss in 600 treated periodontal patients. *Journal of Periodontology* **49**, 225-237.

Hunter, R.K., O'Leary, T.J. & Kafrawy, A.H. (1984) The effectiveness of hand versus ultrasonic instrumentation in open flap root planing. *Journal of Periodontology* **55**, 697-703.

Håkansson, J. (1978) Dental care habits, attitudes towards dental health and dental status among 20-to-60-year-old individuals in Sweden. Thesis. University of Lund. Lund, Sweden: Bokförlaget Dialog.

Joyston-Bechal, S. (1987) Topical and systemic antimicrobial agents in the treatment of chronic gingivitis and periodontitis. F.D.I. Technical Report No. 26. *International Dental Journal* **37**, 52-62.

Kenney, E.B., Saxe, S.R., Lenox, J.A. et al (1976) The relation or manual dexterity and knowledge to performance of oral hygiene. *Journal of Periodontal Research* **11**, 67-73.

Knowles, J.W. (1973) Oral hygiene related to long-term effects of periodontal therapy. *Journal of the Michigan State Dental Association* **55**, 147-150.

Knowles, J.W., Burgett, F., Nissle, R.R. et al (1979) Results of periodontal treatment related to pocket depth and attachment level. Eight years. *Journal of Periodontology* **50**, 225-233.

Knowles J., Burgett, P., Morrison, R. et al (1980) Comparison of results following three modalities of periodontal therapy related to tooth type and initial pocket depth. *Journal of Clinical Periodontology* **7**, 32-47.

Kornman, K.S. & Karl, E.H. (1982) The effect of long- term low-dose tetracycline therapy on the subgingival microflora in refractory adult periodontitis. *Journal of Periodontology* **53**, 604-610.

Lang, N. Joss, Orsanic, T. et al (1986) Bleeding on probing. A predictor for the progression of periodontal disease? *Journal of Clinical Periodontology* **13**, 590-596.

Lie, T. & Enersen, M. (1986) Effects of chlorhexidine gel in a group of maintenance-care patients with poor oral hygiene. *Journal of Periodontology* **57**, 364-369.

Lie, T. & Meyer, K.(1977)Calculus removal and loss of tooth substance in response to different periodontal instruments. *Journal of Clinical Periodontology* **4**, 250-262.

Lindhe, J., Hamp, S.-E. & Löe, H. (1973) Experimental periodontitis in the Beagle dog. *Journal of Periodontal Research* **8**, 1-10.

Lindhe, J. & Nyman, S. (1975) The effect of plaque control and surgical pocket elimination on the establishment and maintenance of periodontal health. A longitudinal study of periodontal therapy in cases of advanced disease. *Journal of Clinical Periodontology* **2**, 67-79.

Lindhe, J. & Nyman, S. (1984) Long-term maintenance of patients treated for advanced periodontal disease. *Journal of Clinical Periodontology* **11**, 504-514.

Listgarten, M.A. & Helldén, L. (1978) Relative distribution of bacteria at clinically healthy and periodontally diseased sites in humans. *Journal of Clinical Periodontology* **5**, 115-132.

Listgarten, M.A. & Levin, S. (1981) Positive correlation between the proportions of subgingival spirochetes and motile bacteria and susceptibility of human subjects to periodontal deterioration. *Journal of Clinical Periodontology* **8**, 122-138.

Listgarten, M.A., Lindhe, J. & Helldén, L. (1978) Effect of tetracycline and/or scaling on human periodontal disease. Clinical, microbiological and histological observations. *Journal of Clinical Periodontology* **5**, 246-271.

Listgarten, M.A., Schifter, C.C. & Laster, L. (1985) 3-year longitudinal study of the periodontal status of an adult population with gingivitis. *Journal of Clinical Periodontology* **12**, 225-238.

Listgarten, M.A., Schifter, C.C., Sullivan, P. et al (1986) Failure of a microbial assay to reliably predict disease recurrence in a treated periodontitis population receiving regularly scheduled prophylaxes. *Journal of Clinical Periodontology* **13**, 768-773.

Löe, H. & Silness, J. (1963) Periodontal disease in pregnancy. I. Prevalence and severity. *Acta Odontologica Scandinavica* **21**, 533-551.

Löe, H., Theilade, E. & Jensen, S.B. (1965) Experimental gingivitis in man. *Journal of Periodontology* **36**, 177-187.

Löe, H., Ånerud, Å., Boysen, H. & Smith, M. (1978) The natural history of periodontal disease in man. The rate of periodontal destruction before 40 years of age. *Journal of Periodontology* **49**, 607-620.

Lövdal, A., Arnö, A., Schei, 0. & Waerhaug, J. (1961) Combined effect of subgingival scaling and controlled oral hygiene on the incidence of gingivitis. *Acta Odontologica Scandinavica* **19**, 537-553.

Meyer, K. & Lie, T. (1977) Root surface roughness in response to periodontal instrumentation studied by combined use of microroughness measurements and scanning electron microscopy. *Journal of Clinical Periodontology* **4**, 77-91.

Moore, W.E.C. (1987) Microbiology of periodontal disease. *Journal of Periodontal Research* **22**, 335-341.

Mörmann, W., Regolati, B. & Renggli, H.H. (1974) Gingival reaction to well-fitted subgingival proximal gold inlays. *Journal of Clinical Periodontology* **1**, 120-125.

Nyman, S., Rosling, B. & Lindhe, J. (1975) Effect of professional tooth cleaning on healing after periodontal surgery. *Journal of Clinical Periodontology* **2**, 80-86.

Oliver, R.C. (1969) Tooth loss with and without periodontal therapy. *Periodontal Abstracts* **17**, 8-9.

Oliver, R.C. (1977) Patient evaluation. *International Dental Journal* **27**, 103-106.

Ramfjord,S.P.(1987) Maintenance care for treated periodontitis patients. *Journal of Clinical Periodontology* **14**, 433-437.

Ramfjord, S.P. & Ash, M.M. (1983) *Occlusion.* 3rd ed. Philadelphia, London, Toronto: W.B. Saunders Co.

Ramfjord, S.P., Knowles, J.W., Nissle, R.R. et al (1973) Longitudinal study of periodontal therapy. *Journal of Periodontology* **44**, 66-77.

Ramfjord, S.P., Morrison, E.C., Burgett, F.G. et al (1982) Oral hygiene and maintenance of periodontal support. *Journal of Periodontology* **53**, 26-30.

Ramfjord, S.P., Caffessee, R.G., Morrison, E.C. et al (1987) 4 modalities of periodontal treatment compared over 5 years. *Journal of Clinical Periodontology* **14**, 445-452.

Robinson, R.E. (1980) Maintenance of the periodontally treated patient. In *Periodontal Therapy*, ed. Goldman, H.M. & Cohen, D.W. 6th ed., pp. 1155-1178. St. Louis: C.V. Mosby Co.

Ross, I. F. (1971) The results of treatment. A long-term study of one hundred and eighty patients. *Parodontologie* **25**, 125-134.

Saxe, S.R., Greene, J.C., Bohannan, H.M. & Vermillion, J.R. (1967) Oral debris, calculus and periodontal disease in the Beagle dog. *Periodontics* **5**, 217-225.

Silness, J. (1978) Placement of margins. *In Prosthodontic treatment for partially edentulous patients.* ed. Zarb, G.A., Berman, B., Clayton, J.A. & MacKay, H. F. St. Louis: C.V. Mosby Co.

Silness, J. & Löe, H. (1964)Periodontal disease in pregnancy. II. Correlation between oral hygiene and periodontal condition. *Acta Odontologica Scandinavica* **22**, 121-135.

Socransky, S.S. (1977) Microbiology of periodontal disease. Present status and future considerations. *Journal of Periodontology* **48**, 497-504.

Söderholm, G. (1979) Effect of a dentalcare program on al health conditions. A study of employees of a Swedish shipyard. Thesis. University of Lund.

Suomi, J.D., Greene, J.C., Vermillion, J.R., Doyle, Chang, J.J. & Leatherwood, E.C. (1971) The effect of controlled oral hygiene procedures on the progression of periodontal disease in adults: Results after third and final year. *Journal of Periodontology* **42**, 152-160.

Waerhaug, J. (1955) Depth of incision in gingivectomy. *Oral Surgery, Oral Medicine and Oral Patholoqy* **8**, 707-718.

Waerhaug, J. (1956) Effect of rough surfaces upon gingival tissue. *Journal of Dental Research* **35**, 323-325.

Westfelt, E., Nyman, S., Lindhe, J. & Socransky, S. S. (1983a) Use of chlorhexidine as a plaque control measure following surgical treatment of periodontal disease. *Journal of Clinical Periodontology* **10**, 22-36.

Westfelt, E., Nyman, S., Socransky, S.S. & Lindhe, J. (1983b) Significance of frequency of professional tooth cleaning for healing following periodontal surgery. *Journal of Clinical Periodontology* **10**, 148-156.

Index